CHILDBEARING:
a nursing perspective

Childbearing: A Nursing Perspective

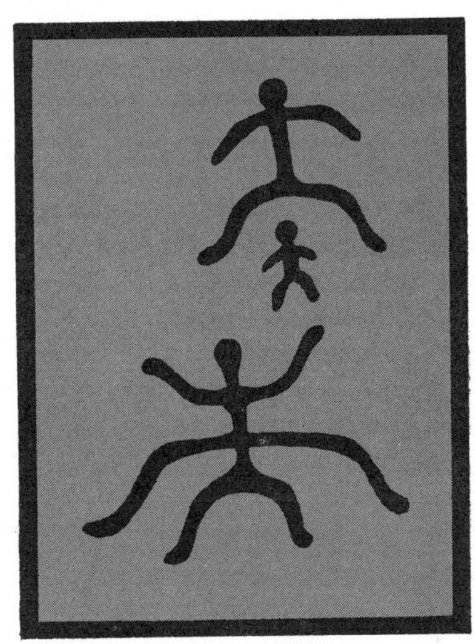

Ann L Clark

Formerly, Professor and Chairman
Department of Maternal and Child Nursing
Rutgers University College of Nursing
Newark, New Jersey

Dyanne D Affonso

Assistant Professor
University of Arizona
College of Nursing
Tucson, Arizona

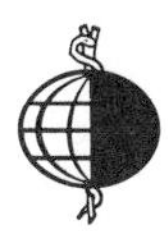

F. A. DAVIS COMPANY, Philadelphia

Second printing 1976
Third printing 1977
Fourth printing 1978

Printed in the United States of America

Library of Congress Cataloging in Publication Data
Main entry under title:

Childbearing: a nursing perspective.

Includes bibliographical references and index.
1. Obstetrical nursing. 2. Childbirth. I. Clark, Ann L. II. Affonso, Dyanne D.
[DNLM: 1. Obstetrical nursing. 2. Pregnancy—Nursing texts. 3. Psychology, Social—Nursing texts. WY157 C536]
RG951.C45 610.73'678 75-40100
ISBN 0-8036-1830-1

This book is dedicated to

William, Kevin, and Javey Affonso
and to Marshall Clark.

Me Ke Aloha Pumehana.

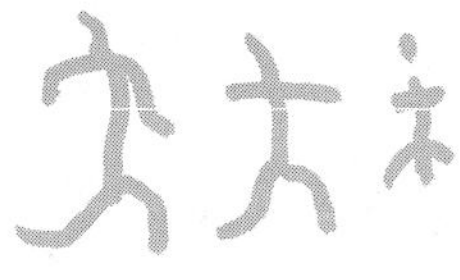

Family

To Our Readers

Family

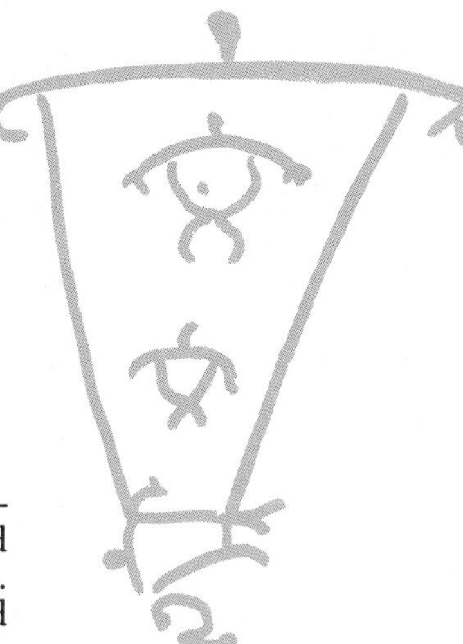

Pregnancy and Birth

The designs around this page are petroglyphs. Petroglyphs can be found in almost all parts of the world and are man's permanent record of his ancient culture. These are Hawaiian petroglyphs. Hawaiians produced many such figures. Indeed of all the Polynesians, they were the most prolific in this manner.

These petroglyphs are included in this publication which focuses on maternal and child nursing for two reasons. The first reason is that the meanings of an overwhelming majority of Hawaiian petroglyphs revolve around an ardent desire for fertility and procreation. Many petroglyphs depict pregnancy, birth scenes, and families. The second reason is that the authors are daughters of Hawaii, one a natural-born daughter and the other a daughter by adoption. We wanted to share with you some of the ancient heritage of the Polynesians. We hope you enjoy it.

Data from Cox, J. H. and Stasok, E.: *Hawaiian Petroglyphs*. Bishop Museum Press, Honolulu, Hawaii, 1970.

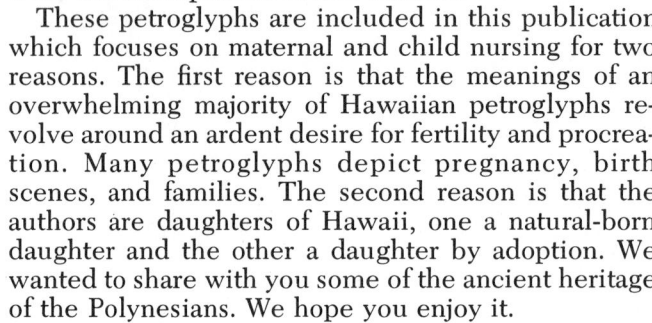

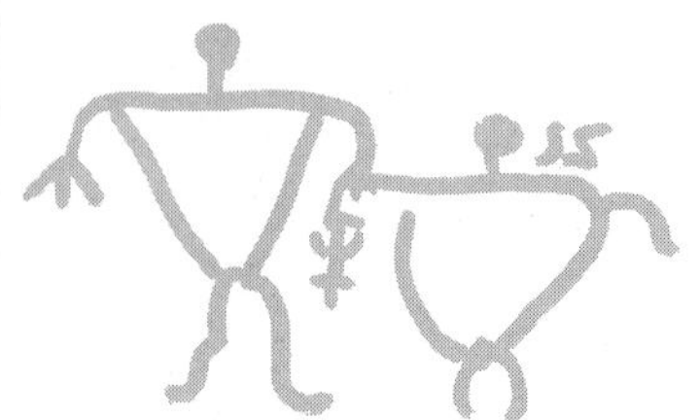

Birth Scene

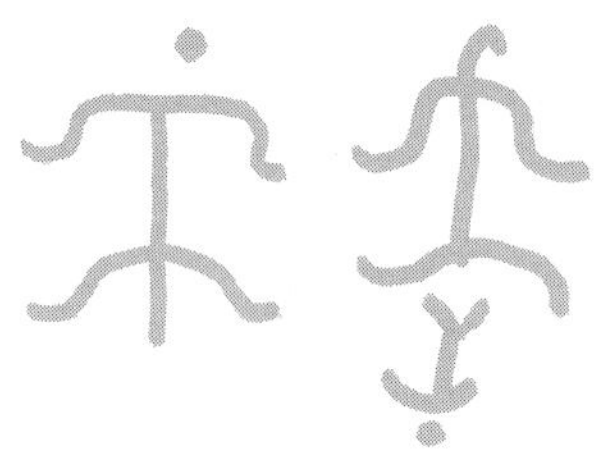

Birth Scene

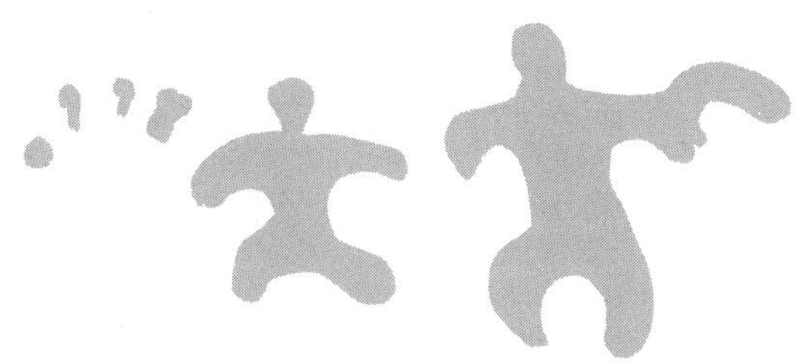

Family

Foreword

The context of patient care in maternity nursing is four-dimensional: 1) the physical or bodily changes in accommodation to childbearing and the puerperium, 2) the complete social involvement in the act of childbearing, including the nurturance of the child, 3) the psychologic sphere that bridges the physical and social worlds, and 4) the continuities and discontinuities of the physical, social, and psychologic experiences over a considerable period.

Childbearing: A Nursing Perspective is a basic obstetrical nursing text which introduces the nurse to these broader dimensions of maternity nursing.

The careerist in maternity nursing soon realizes that there is a complex social context in which nursing care is given. The maternity patient is not socially dysfunctional because of a physical condition. On the contrary. The maternity patient is, in a very intimately physical and totally involved way, performing society's most essential task. At every social level —the family, the neighborhood, the city, the state, the nation—the intensely personal experience of childbearing contributes to the viability, immortality, and renewal of the social group and the transmission of its valued cultural attainments, giving meaning and purpose to these attainments and providing hope for the pursuit of attainments not yet achieved.

A nation, a religion, a community and a family are dependent on the feminine capacity and ability for childbearing for their survival and for the quality of that survival. The dependency is intense. The impact of society's wishes and hopes on the childbearing woman comes in the form of moral and ethical persuasions, in help and understanding of her feminine tasks, and in honor and respect to her when she successfully becomes a mother.

Nursing help and care in this complex, four-dimensional field of maternity nursing requires a vast store of knowledge and a large repertoire of skills upon which to draw eclectically and appropriately to meet the unique needs of the patient in her particular situation. No two patients are in the same situation, no two childbearing situations are the same for the same woman, and no two situations within the childbearing trimesters or in childbearing, childbirth, and childrearing are the same for any one woman.

Reva Rubin
Professor and Director
Graduate Programs
in Maternity Nursing
University of Pittsburgh
School of Nursing

Preface

A conceptual frame of reference is one way to organize knowledge and to apply it appropriately for nursing intervention. The concepts in this book were selected to best exemplify the biologic, psychosocial, and cultural forces influencing childbearing. Conceptual overviews were written especially for this book by experts in the fields of nursing, medicine, psychology, and sociology. They provide the basis for nursing intervention.

Nursing intervention, as discussed in this book, encompasses common themes described below:

1. The impact of the childbearing experience on the individual and the family is explored in relation to relevant psychosocial and cultural concepts. For example, self concept and role transition during pregnancy, labor, delivery, and the puerperium are highlighted.
2. Nursing assessment is viewed as a critical aspect of the nursing process. Assessment allows nursing care to be relevant to the unique needs of the individual childbearing family. Therefore, a major portion of each unit directs itself to a discussion of the biologic, psychosocial, and cultural factors the nurse should incorporate into the assessment process.
3. The plans for nursing intervention in this book are based on scientific rationale which emerges from the application of biologic, psychosocial, and cultural concepts. The authors sought creative approaches to identifying nursing actions. One approach was to utilize a theme of protection, nurturance, and stimulation of the childbearing family.
4. The role of the nurse as presented in the various phases of the childbearing experience is viewed as one which allows the practitioner to utilize the potential for extension of the nursing role.

This book was written for the student learning the profession of nursing. Content is based on the assumption that the reader has had formal basic preparation in the natural and behavioral sciences. Nurses in clinical practice will find the book useful for reviewing contemporary maternal-neonatal nursing. The reader is encouraged to search for new solutions to clinical nursing problems. It is hoped that this book will be a stimulus for creative approaches to maternal-neonatal nursing practice.

ANN L. CLARK
DYANNE D. AFFONSO

Acknowledgments

This book does not propose to be the exclusive beliefs and values of the two coauthors. Our parents, our teachers, our professional colleagues in nursing and in the broad field of health science, our students, and hundreds of childbearing families are all a part of what we have come to value in nursing practice. We wish to express our gratitude and appreciation to all of them.

We are particularly indebted to many who have offered constructive criticism, valuable suggestions and who have shared illustrations and other materials for the book. We want to particularly acknowledge the assistance of Nancy Okamoto, R.N., Eleanor Smith, R.N., Thomas R. Harris, M.D., Paul McCallin, M.D., Marjorie Abel, Emilie Henning, R.N., Mary Fowler, R.N., Mimi Bronner, R.N., Louise Childs, M.D., Beverly McCord, R.N., Kathy Puls, R.N., Marshall Klaus, M.D., T. Barry Brazelton, M.D., Katherine Barnard, R.N., Diane M. Nunnally, R.N., Jeanette Junti, R.N.

To the contributing authors go our very special thanks. They have provided the basic framework for the structure of this nursing text.

We are especially grateful to Dr. Thomas R. Harris, who not only became a contributor, but also reviewed most of the neonatal content in this book. His suggestions were invaluable in assuring that the content on the well and sick neonate reflects the most current and in-depth knowledge.

We also thank the nursing staff at Tucson Medical Center Neonatal Intensive Care Nursery for so generously sharing their clinical expertise with us.

We thank Caroline Affonso, Barbara Herman, Dave Fisher and the audiovisual staff at the University of Arizona for preparation of many original drawings and photographs for this book. We also thank Teresa Marsico, Judy Funches, and Margaret Bean, of the Division of Nurse Midwifery, Martland Hospital, Newark, New Jersey, for their help in providing material for original photographs.

The literature search was facilitated by the excellent assistance of several librarians. We would particularly like to thank Peggy Place and Esther Nekomoto at Tripler Army Medical Center; Ann Kota, Madeline Fisher, and other members of the staff at Hawaii Medical Library; Clyde Winters of Health Information Network of the Pacific; and Marian Chavez, Fred Heidenreich, and the staff at the University of Arizona Medical Library. Their assistance, interest, and concern went far beyond the call of duty.

We thank those who carefully typed and proofread the manuscript: Judy Goo, Marjorie Middlebrook, Penelope Burton, and Dorothy Galvez.

We are especially appreciative of the encouragement and assistance of Judith M. Kim, Nursing Editor, and Mary Helen Jacob, Copy Editor, F. A. Davis Company.

Finally, we say mahalo nui loa to our long-suffering families who encouraged and sustained us during the book's preparation.

ANN L. CLARK
DYANNE D. AFFONSO

Contributors

ABEL, MARJORIE, M.S.
Public Health Consultant, Maternal and Child Health Branch, and Chief, Nutrition Branch, Hawaii Department of Health, Honolulu, Hawaii.

AKAMATSU, TOSHIO J., M.D.
Associate Professor and Chief, Division of Obstetrical Anesthesia, Department of Anesthesiology and Anesthesia Research Center, University of Washington School of Medicine, Seattle, Washington.

AGUILERA, DONNA C., Ph.D., F.A.A.N.
Associate Professor, Department of Nursing, California State University, Los Angeles, California

BEDNAR, JOHN, M.D.
Major, Army Medical Corps, formerly of the Department of Obstetrics and Gynecology, Tripler Army Medical Center, Honolulu, Hawaii

BENOLIEL, JEANNE Q., R.N., D.NSc.
Professor and Chairman, Department of Comparative Nursing Care Systems, School of Nursing, University of Washington, Seattle, Washington

BINTLIFF, SHARON, M.D.
Associate Professor of Pediatrics and Genetics, University of Hawaii, School of Medicine, and Pediatric Staff, Kauikeolani Children's Hospital, Honolulu, Hawaii

BONICA, JOHN J., M.D.
Professor and Chairman, Department of Anesthesiology and Anesthesia Research Center, University of Washington School of Medicine, Seattle, Washington

BRAZELTON, T. BARRY, M.D.
Associate Professor of Pediatrics, Harvard Medical School, Children's Hospital Medical Center, Boston, Massachusetts

DANFORTH, DAVID D., M.D.
Walkins Professor and Chairman, Department of Obstetrics and Gynecology, Northwestern University School of Medicine, Chicago, Illinois

DEFEO, VINCENT J., Ph.D.
Professor of Anatomy and Reproductive Biology, University of Hawaii School of Medicine, Honolulu, Hawaii

FINNEY, RUTH, Ph.D.
Assistant Professor, Department of Human Development, University of Hawaii, Honolulu, Hawaii

GILES, HARLAN R., M.D.
Assistant Professor and Director, Genetic Information and Perinatal Reference Unit, University of Arizona College of Medicine, Tucson, Arizona

HALE, RALPH W., M.D.
Associate Professor and Chairman, Department of Obstetrics and Gynecology, University of Hawaii School of Medicine, Honolulu, Hawaii

HARRIS, THOMAS R., M.D.
Neonatology Division Head, and Associate Professor, Department of Pediatrics, University of Arizona College of Medicine, Tucson, Arizona

HEINE, M. WAYNE, M.D.
Professor, Department of Obstetrics and Gynecology, University of Arizona College of Medicine, Tucson, Arizona

Henning, Emilie D., R.N., Ed.D.
Associate Professor of Nursing and Director, Graduate Program in Maternal-Child Nursing, Rutgers University College of Nursing, Newark, New Jersey

Hommel, Flora, R.N., B.S.
Executive Director, Childbirth Without Pain Education Association, Detroit, Michigan

Hong, Suk Ki, M.D., Ph.D.
Professor of Physiology, Schools of Medicine and Dentistry, State University of New York at Buffalo, Buffalo, New York

Lego, Suzanne, R.N., Ph.D.
Adjunct Associate Professor, Graduate Program in Advanced Psychiatric Nursing, Rutgers University College of Nursing, New Brunswick, New Jersey

Lum, Jean, L. J., R.N., Ph.D.
Associate Professor, Department of Professional Nursing, University of Hawaii School of Nursing, Honolulu, Hawaii

Messick, Janice M., R.N., M.S.
Clinical Program Evaluation Specialist, Program Evaluation Service, Veterans Administration Hospital, Brentwood, Los Angeles, California

Morgan, Marie Grannan, R.N., M.S.
Supervisor, Nursing Quality Control, Queen's Medical Center, Honolulu, Hawaii

Newton, Niles, Ph.D.
Professor, Division of Psychology, Department of Psychiatry, Northwestern University Medical School, Chicago, Illinois

Peplau, Hildegard E., R.N., Ed.D.
Professor Emeritus, Department of Psychiatric Nursing, Rutgers University College of Nursing, New Brunswick, New Jersey

Puls, Kathy, R.N., C.N.M.
Supervisor of Nurse-Midwifery Services, Chicago Department of Health, Chicago, Illinois

Contents

UNIT 10—Crises during Childbearing

UNIT 11—Current Issues

APPENDICES

UNIT 1

INTRODUCTION

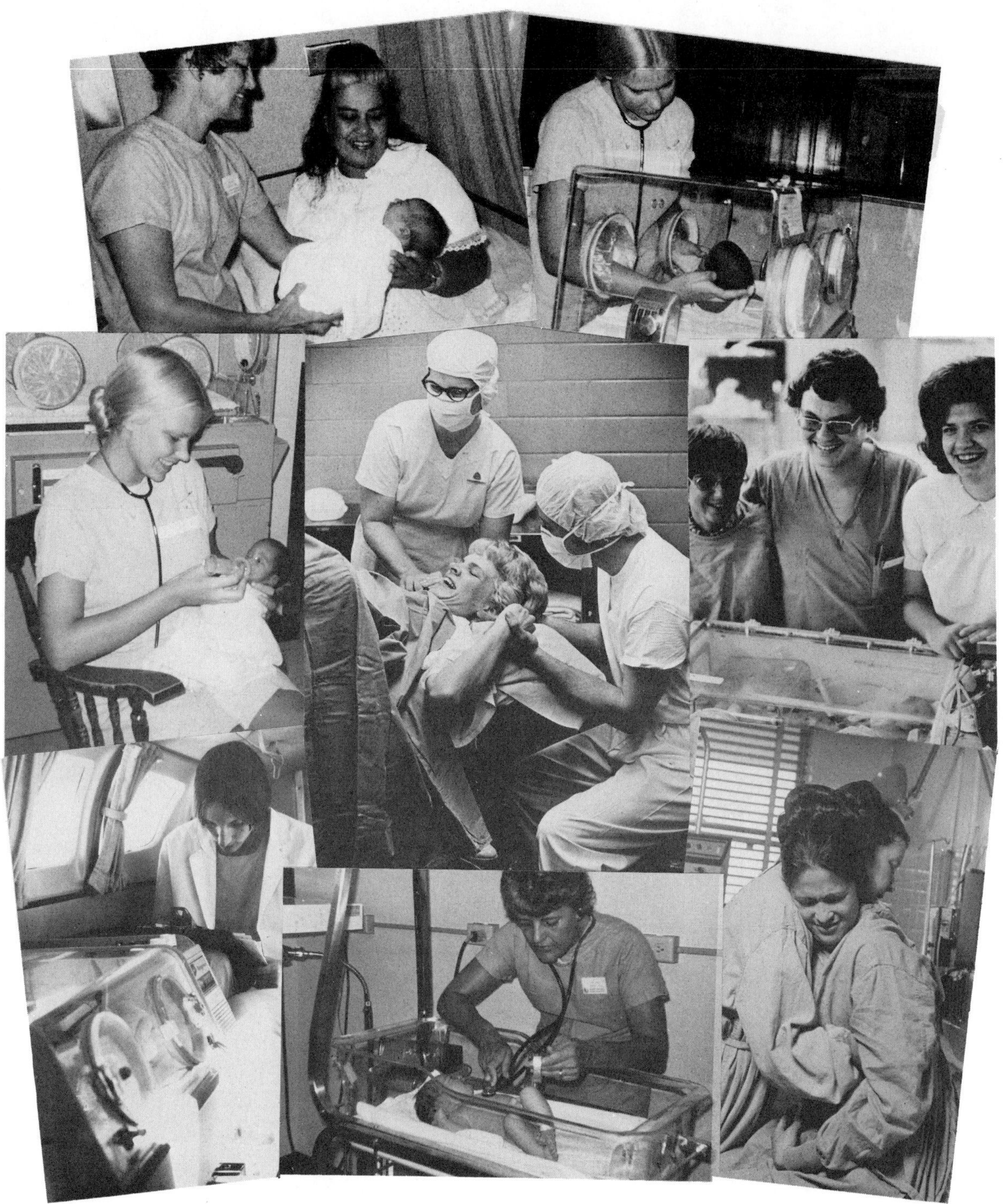

1 Maternal and Child Health Nursing

DYANNE D. AFFONSO, R.N., M.N.
ANN L. CLARK, R.N., M.A.

Some health care needs are manifested at specific developmental phases of the life cycle, with nursing care focusing on primary prevention, promotion, and maintenance of optimal health. This describes *maternal and child health nursing*. Nursing during the childbearing and childrearing phases of life assumes the responsibility for assisting families to achieve their own goals within the concept of high-level wellness. Maternal and child health nursing provides those essential services to promote and maintain well-being for the childbearing family as a unit and for each individual within the family. It includes such activities as:

Assisting the expectant family to determine and meet their own health goals.

Assisting the expectant family to understand and cope with the impact of pregnancy and parenthood.

Assessing the health status of the expectant mother and of the family as a unit.

Intervening to create an atmosphere in which the individual and family can make appropriate adjustments to their current life situation and prepare for the next phase of the life cycle.

Helping the individual and family to understand their personal reactions to events of childbearing and to utilize their strengths in coping with normal life situations.

Creating a supportive environment in the clinic, hospital, and home which will promote as positive an experience as possible, both biophysically and psychosocially, for expectant and new parents.

Appropriately intervening in crisis situations to support the family.

Assisting individuals and family to prepare for healthy and wanted pregnancies through family planning.

Helping through educational means to prepare females of all ages to become healthy women.

Teaching or assuring the teaching of family life education which includes human sexuality, taught in a manner which is acceptable, understandable, and appropriate to the age group for which it is intended.

Placing special emphasis through education on adequate nutrition during all phases of the life cycle.

Preparing the expectant family to achieve a satisfying labor.

Teaching and promoting appropriate parenting skills.

Performing selective diagnostic and therapeutic procedures.

Remaining alert to deviations from normal and caring for them or referring them to colleagues on the health team as appropriate.

Coordinating health care needs of the individual and family. Acting as patient advocate as appropriate. Collaborating with other health team members to assure quality health care.

Making referrals to appropriate agencies for specialized care and/or continuity of care.

Identifying aspects of the community which are or may be detrimental to the health of families and assuming responsibility by collaborating with appropriate agencies to remove these deterrents to health.

Promoting legislation in the interest of mothers, children, and families.*

The American Nurses' Association, through its Division on Maternal and Child Health Nursing Practice has stated the premises on which maternal and child health nursing practice is based, and the aims of that practice in the following manner:

Maternal and child health nursing practice is based on the following premises:

1. Survival and the level of health of a society is inextricably bound to maternal and child health nursing practice.
2. Maternal and child health nursing practice respects the human dignity and rights of individuals.
3. Maternal and child health nursing practice is family-centered.
4. Maternal and child health nursing practice focuses on the childbearing, childrearing phases of the life cycle which include the development of sexuality, family planning, interconceptual care and child health from conception through adolescence.
5. Maternal and child health nursing makes a significant difference to society in achieving its health goals.
6. Man is a total human being. His psychosocial and biophysical self are interrelated.
7. Human behavior shapes and is shaped by environmental forces and as such sets into motion a multitude of reciprocal responses.
8. Through his own process of self-regulation the human being attempts to maintain equilibrium amidst constant change.
9. All behavior has meaning and is influenced by past experiences, the individual's perception of those experiences, and forces impinging upon the present.
10. Growth and development is ordered and evolves in sequential stages.
11. Substantive knowledge of the principles of human growth and development, including normative data, is essential to effective maternal and child health nursing practice.
12. Periods of developmental and traumatic crises during the life cycle pose internal and external stresses and may have a positive or negative effect.
13. Maternal and child health nursing practice provides for continuity of care and is not bound by artificial barriers and exclusive categories which tend to restrict and delimit practice.
14. *All* people have a right to receive the benefit of the delivery of optimal health services.

Maternal and child health nursing practice is aimed at:

1. Promoting and maintaining optimal health of each individual and the family unit.
2. Improving and/or supporting family solidarity.
3. Early identification and treatment of vulnerable families.
4. Preventing environmental conditions

*These activities are derived, in part, from *Statement about Maternal and Child Health Nursing*, American Nurses' Association Division on Maternal and Child Health Nursing Practice.

which block attainment of optimal health.
5. Prevention and early detection of deviations from health.
6. Reducing stresses which interfere with optimal functioning.
7. Assisting the family to understand and/or cope with the developmental and traumatic situations which occur during childbearing and childrearing.
8. Facilitating survival, recovery and growth when the individual is ill or needs health care.
9. Reducing reproductive wastage occurring at any point on the continuum.
10. Continuously improving the quality of care in maternal and child health nursing practice.
11. Reducing inequalities in the delivery of health care services.

Maternal and child nursing differs from the practice of clinical nursing in other specialties in that:

1. The focus of the practice is on a process (childbearing) which is considered a normal, healthy experience in the life cycle. Thus the nursing goals are primarily to promote and maintain health. When the process deviates from normal, nursing action then more nearly resembles the nursing practice of other clinical specialties.
2. Nursing focuses on both the promotion of physical health and the potential for optimal emotional development. The latter is an important component of maternal and child nursing because growth and development of the child are influenced by his prenatal environment and the quality of the parenting he receives. Ultimately, these early life experiences influence his adaptation to society.
3. The transmission of culture is provided by the family unit, and therefore is inextricably bound to maternal and child health. Nursing activities during childbearing have multiple outcomes in terms of the immediate and future health of both the individual and the society.
4. Unlike many other health conditions, childbearing should be, and very often is, a joyous experience. Nursing intervention can help assure that the event is a joyous one.

THE UNIQUE ROLE OF THE NURSE

Ideally, meeting the health needs of the expectant and new family takes a team of professional health workers. The nurse learns to collaborate and coordinate her role with physicians, medical social workers, dieticians, and an increasing number of technicians. What then is the nurse's unique role?

Nursing is unique in its interaction with people in the delivery of health care primarily because it is in a *position of closeness* in relation to the individual, the family, and the community. This closeness develops because the nurse is able to witness health-illness life experiences due to proximity in terms of time, person, and place.

Proximity in Time. Nursing care is provided and made available to individuals almost continuously. In hospitals, it is provided 24 hours daily. In community health services, nursing care and consultation are available every day. Moreover, childbearing encompasses a relatively long period of time—nine months of pregnancy during which the family usually seeks care at frequent intervals, a period of labor when the parturient receives intensive nursing care, two or three days of hospital stay when the mother and infant are given 24-hour nursing care, and a postpartal period, generally regarded as six weeks, when less intensive care is provided for the expanded family. This results in a period of life during which nurses and families have frequent contacts. The nurse can, therefore, make unique contributions toward satisfying the health needs of families through initial assessment, by shaping the environment so that it is supportive to the developmental and situational crises that arise, by fashioning a satisfying health care system, and by building a trusting relationship with individuals within that system.

Proximity in Person. Nursing care requires the physical presence of the nurse. Since it focuses on helping individuals maintain their daily life patterns, nursing care is delivered primarily through the use of self, by the giving and teaching of health care. The nurse does use technologic devices to extend her delivery of care, but is physically present when they are used. The nurse's use of self occurs through her sensory modalities. For example, visual capacities allow observations during the assessment process. Auditory capacities are used in determining needs and goals of the individual. Tactile capacities are employed in providing physical care and stimulating behavioral development.

Proximity in Place. In every geographic locale where expanding families are found nursing care can be provided. In homes, hospitals, schools, clinics, and industry, nurses are available to individuals whenever health care needs are manifested.

No other member of the health care team has the same opportunity to meet the health care needs of childbearing families. Nursing is unique in its proximity of time, person, and place to expanding and new families. Patient advocacy and coordination of health care needs of individuals are natural results of this special relationship.

THE NURSING PROCESS

Now that the components of maternal and child nursing have been identified, it is imperative to examine how nurses can implement a philosophy reflecting their unique purposes and goals. The activities of nursing involve a process: a deliberate, systematic, intelligent way of thinking, learning, and working with individuals and communities. The process is referred to as *the nursing process.* It involves the manner in which nurses select, pattern, and blend knowledges from the natural and behavioral sciences (as well as from accumulated knowledge from nursing research), utilizing cognitive and psychomotor skills to:

Identify existing and potential problems.

Make inferences as to what factors are causing or contributing to the problems.

Set nursing goals to solve or manage the problems.

Formulate a plan of action to achieve nursing goals.

Implement the plan, either by self or in collaboration with others.

Evaluate the results and make any necessary modifications to ensure that problems, goals, and actions remain relevant to the unique needs of the individual.

Nursing literature contains many different interpretations of the components of the nursing process. In general, the components are:

1. Assessment. This is the orderly investigation of data and knowledges to determine the nature of a problem. The following steps help the nurse complete the assessment phase:
   a. *Data collection.* This consists of gathering information on factors influencing the individual's state of health and his ability to cope with his health situation. In this book such influences are referred to as the biologic, psychologic, and sociocultural factors which affect a person's health status.
   b. *Interpretation or analysis of the data with theoretic knowledge.* The nurse considers the data in light of theoretic norms to help identify deviations as well as the possible causes for devia-

tions which are creating a health problem. Collection of additional data may be necessary to validate or reject tentative problems.

c. *Nursing diagnosis.* Analysis leads to the identification of the problem, also known as the *nursing diagnosis.* This results from recognition of a pattern derived from a nursing investigation of the patient. The nursing diagnosis states that aspect of the person's health to which the nurse will address herself. These aspects are described by Hall[1] as:

    (1) Nurturing aspect: a close interpersonal relationship concerned with the intimate bodily care of the person.
    (2) Medical aspect: shared with the medical profession, the nurse is concerned with assisting the person with the medical deviations which are affecting his health.
    (3) Helping aspect: shared with all professional persons, the nurse is concerned with assisting the person in "self-actualization." Travelbee[2] refers to this aspect of nursing as helping the individual find meaning in the experience which has changed his health status.

2. Goal Setting. Nursing goals should be related to the problem, realistic and attainable, mutually set by the patient and nurse, and expressed in ways which allow measurement and evaluation of attainment.
3. Nursing Actions. Actions should be based on scientific rationale and be logically related to the goal. They should be stated explicitly so that there will be consistency in implementation among members of the health care team.
4. Evaluation and Reassessment. Evaluation describes the effects of nursing actions on the patient. It involves a description of the individual's responses and reactions to a nursing care regimen at a specified point in time.[3] A reassessment of the problem-solving approaches used is also done to determine the necessity of modifying the plan of nursing care. Modification may be necessary when a particular plan of care has failed to achieve the nursing goal, or when the health needs of the patient have changed.

SCIENTIFIC RATIONALE FOR NURSING ACTION

The knowledge base is a vital aspect of maternal and child nursing. The biologic, psychologic, and sociocultural concepts and principles form the basis for nursing action. It is for this reason that this book presents overviews and provides bibliographies for indepth study of relevant concepts and principles. The following statement by the American Nurses' Association expands this rationale:

> Maternal and child health nursing practice is based on nursing knowledge, principles and concepts drawn from the biological, physical and social sciences and from the humanities. These principles and concepts are selected and synthesized into the theoretical basis for maternal and child health nursing practice. Regardless of the setting in which nursing is practiced (hospital, home, school, community, etc.), basic concepts and principles are used to describe, explain, and predict human development and behavior potential. A thorough understanding of the interrelatedness of the cultural, psychosocial, spiritual, and physiological influence on the individual and the family is essential to effective practice.[4]

CREATIVITY IN NURSING ACTION

Hopefully, greater creativity in nursing action will be forthcoming, both by identifying nursing activities in effective and novel ways, and by stimulating nursing students to develop creative approaches to nursing. One such novel approach is to classify nursing care as being *protective, nurturing* and/or *stimulating* to individuals involved in the childbearing experience. Parts of this book discuss nursing care in this manner.

Nursing Actions Which Protect. The nature of this action is to protect the individual from potentially hazardous conditions or stimuli. The goal is to block stimuli which may threaten the person's health status and/or behavioral stability. For example, the nurse who suctions the trachea of a neonate to prevent obstruction of the airway, or who moistens the lips of a woman in active labor to prevent them from drying and cracking, is implementing protective nursing actions.

Nursing Actions Which Nurture. These assist an individual to maintain a degree of stability in his health status and his activities of daily living. The nurse is offering nurturance when her actions focus on activities such as ingestion, elimination, rest, sleep, and comfort. Nurturing actions also focus on providing emotional support so that the individual and his family can cope optimally with the health-illness event. For example, nurturance is being provided when the nurse remains physically present with a grieving family.

Nursing Actions Which Stimulate. These involve some action which becomes a stimulus intended to help the individual maximize his potential for physical and behavioral growth and development. Implicit in these actions is a behavioral change toward a more positive health status. Two of the processes the nurse may use in these actions are teaching-learning and motivation. For example, the nurse may teach the family how to use environmental resources to improve their health, or motivate families to use nutrition to promote optimal growth and development for the fetus, the expectant mother, and the entire family. Stimuli, in the interest of the behavioral development of the neonate, can be used by the nurse and taught to the parents.

Nursing actions which protect, nurture, and stimulate are not terminal in themselves. Rather, there exists a cyclic relationship among them. Let us examine the nursing activities in helping a newborn with his first feeding. First, providing nutrients in the form of breast milk or formula *protects* the neonate from hypoglycemia. Second, the feeding marks the beginning of a patterned activity which will maintain the neonate's nutritional needs (*nurture*). Third, in the process of feeding the baby, the nurse or mother can *stimulate* his behavioral development by providing sensory input using her face, voice, and touch. This cyclic relationship clearly indicates that nursing activities have multiple consequences.

EMERGING ROLES IN NURSING PRACTICE

We live in a dynamic society with ever-changing societal conditions and needs which affect the health care system. The consumer is now becoming an active participant in this system. He is better informed and is demanding that health care is a *right* of all Americans. In order that health care needs may be met, the health team is reviewing the functions and roles of each member. Decisions are being made that will better utilize the expertise of each discipline. Today's nursing student is entering the field of maternal and child health care at an exciting time when nursing is expanding its role beyond traditional functions and beyond the traditional health care settings. For example:

> Nurses are now providing primary care to expectant mothers assessed to be normal healthy women.

Nurses are assuming greater responsibility for the conduct of normal labors.

Nurses are assessing the neonate both physically and behaviorally.

Nurses are assuming greater responsibility for the new mother, e.g., assessing her physical readiness to return home and helping with parenting skills.

Nurses are assuming responsibility in their communities and in the nation to ensure protection of the health of our country's mothers and children through provision of health care facilities and through legislation to protect and provide resources for improved health care delivery.

STANDARDS FOR MATERNAL AND CHILD HEALTH NURSING

Nursing is the largest of all health professions. With over 800,000 members,[5] it can play a major role in improving the quality of health care for the mothers and children of this nation. One way in which the professional organization of nurses is moving toward guaranteeing quality of service is through the development of *Standards.* The Standards are stated according to the systematic approach to nursing practice as related earlier in this chapter (assessment, nursing goals, nursing actions, evaluation, and reassessment). These standards provide a means of determining the quality of care which our clients and patients receive.

These Standards will unquestionably undergo revision as the scope of nursing practice continues to enlarge and the theoretic basis upon which the practice rests becomes more sharply delineated. In the meantime, every practitioner of nursing and every student of nursing has a responsibility to make her unique contribution toward fulfilling these Standards. The remainder of this chapter contains the *Standards of Maternal and Child Health Nursing Practice,** along with brief examples of the obstacles to achieving these Standards and a look at the challenges still facing the nursing profession. *Attaining these Standards is the challenge of today.*

STANDARD I

Maternal and child health nursing practice is characterized by the continual questioning of the assumptions upon which practice is based, retaining those which are valid and searching for and using new knowledge.

Rationale: Since knowledge is not static, all assumptions are derived from knowledge or findings of research which are subject to additional testing and revision. They are carefully selected and tested and reflect utilization of present and new knowledge. Effective utilization of these knowledges stimulates more astute observations and provides new insights into the effects of nursing upon the individual and family. To question assumptions implies that nursing practice is not based on stereotyped or ritualistic procedures or methods of intervention; rather, practice exemplifies an objective, systematic and logical investigation of a phenomenon or problem.

Assessment Factors: Therefore in practice, the maternal and child health nurse:

1. Critically examines and questions accepted modes of practice rather than relying on ritualistic or routinized modes of practice.
2. Utilizes current and new knowledge in identifying and questioning the validity of the assumptions which form the bases of nursing practice.

**Standards of Maternal and Child Health Nursing Practice,* American Nurses Association, 1973, with permission.

3. Continuously expands and improves nursing practice by utilizing theories and research findings in search of alternative solutions.
4. Actively shares new knowledge and approaches with colleagues and others in the community.

Maternal and child nursing has often been described as routine, unchallenging, and uninteresting. It is true that many aspects of maternity care have remained static for several decades. What is most tragic is that there is useful research in the behavioral sciences which has not reached the patient and brought about needed changes in maternal and child care. All of this is beginning to change, and, what is more exciting, nurses themselves are undertaking clinical studies to improve the quality of nursing care.

The challenge to nursing in this area is to continually question all practice that is based on empirical observations, to become involved in data collection that will lead to accepting or rejecting traditional practice, and to develop improved methods of communicating ongoing research so that every nurse will have the opportunity to improve her present practice.

The biophysical and psychosocial aspects of reproduction are complex. Although the woman alone is physically pregnant, the entire family is affected by the pregnancy in a psychosocial manner. The basic needs of each family member change and these changes are reflected in the responses of other members of the family to the coming event. A deep and thorough understanding of the following standard is essential.

STANDARD II

Maternal and child health nursing practice is based upon knowledge of the biophysical and psychosocial development of individuals from conception through the childrearing phase of development and upon knowledge of the basic needs for optimum development.

Rationale: A knowledge and understanding of the principles and normal ranges in human growth, development, and behavior are essential to maternal and child health nursing practice. Concomitant with this knowledge is the recognition and consideration of the psychosocial, environmental, nutritional, spiritual, and cognitive factors that enhance or deter the biophysical and psychological maturation of the individual and his family.

Assessment Factors: Therefore in practice, the maternal and child health nurse:

1. Observes, assesses, and describes the developmental level and/or needs of the individual within the family before performing any actions.
2. Involves the individual and family in the assessment and planning of care.
3. Works with individuals and groups utilizing knowledge of the psychosocial, environmental, nutritional, spiritual, and cognitive factors inherent in the family or group environment.

The challenge to nurses is to eradicate every vestige of nursing that focuses on the physical to the exclusion of the psychosocial. For too many years the pregnant woman was viewed as a "shell" to house her gravid uterus. The impact of pregnancy and parenthood on the individual and family has more recently been recognized. Even today, the care offered is too frequently not family-centered. There is a wealth of knowledge now available to nurses that will give useful direction in planning family-centered care.

Data collection is an all-important aspect of assessment and problem solving in nursing.

The assessment factors are well enumerated in the following Standard.

STANDARD III

The collection of data about the health status of the client/patient is systematic and continuous. The data are accessible, communicated, and recorded.

Rational: Comprehensive care requires complete and ongoing collection of data about the client/patient to determine the nursing care needs and other health care needs of the client/patient. All health status data about the client/patient must be available for all members of the health care team.

Assessment Factors:

1. Health status data include
   a. growth and development
   b. biophysical status
   c. emotional status
   d. cultural, religious, socioeconomic background
   e. performance of activities of daily living
   f. patterns of coping
   g. interaction patterns
   h. client's/patient's perception and satisfaction with his health status
   i. client/patient health goals
   j. environment (physical, social, emotional, ecological)
   k. available and accessible human and material resources
2. Data are collected from
   a. client/patient, family, significant others
   b. health care personnel
   c. individuals within the immediate environment and/or the community
3. Data are obtained by
   a. interview
   b. examination
   c. observation
   d. reading records, reports, etc.
4. Format for the collection of data
   a. provides for a systematic collection of data
   b. facilitates the completeness of data collection
5. Continuous collection of data is evident by
   a. frequent updating
   b. recording of changes in health status
6. The data are
   a. accessible on the client/patient records
   b. retrievable form record-keeping systems
   c. confidential when appropriate

New tools and instruments are being developed to facilitate data collection. One challenge to maternal and child nursing is to remain aware of these instruments and develop ways of using them for assessment purposes. Traditional methods must be reviewed in the anticipation that better methods can be found. History taking must move away from the "routine" in which questions are asked and answers laboriously recorded with little meaningful interaction between the nurse and client. Therefore, interviewing skills for all nurses must be improved. Teaching must move away from the didactic to a dialogue in which feelings are explored, solutions to problems are searched for, realistic expectations are shared, and anticipitory guidance is provided. Data collection must be cumulative and shared with all members of the health team. Assessment data relating to the expectant family is also relevant to the labor experience and parenting.

Nurses need sufficient data concerning the health status of the mother or infant to reach a substantive decision about the nursing needs of the patient. In maternal and child nursing, unlike many other types of nursing, physical normalcy is the expected health status. Accurate and complete assessment will determine if there are deviations from this base. In such cases the woman or infant is considered to be *at risk*.

STANDARD IV

Nursing diagnoses are derived from data about the health status of the client/patient.

Rationale: The health status of the client/patient is the basis for determining the nursing care needs. The data are analyzed and compared to norms.

Assessment Factors:

1. The client's/patient's health status is compared to the norm to determine if there is a deviation, the degree and direction of deviation.
2. The client's/patient's capabilities and limitations are identified.
3. The nursing diagnoses are related to and comparable to the totality of the client's/patient's health care.

As an example, let us apply this standard to a young adolescent unwed mother. The health status of this individual includes her physical, emotional, and mental growth and development. Her pelvis may not yet have developed sufficiently to allow vaginal delivery. Her emotional growth may not have progressed to such an extent that her developmental tasks of adolescence have been completed. In such a case, one of the goals of nursing care would be to help the family or a community agency provide the necessary parenting to the infant until the mother is able to do so.

Pregnancy is generally accepted as a normal life experience; however, deviations can and do occur. Such deviations may be physical or emotional, affecting the individual and the entire family.

STANDARD V

Maternal and child health nursing practice recognizes deviations from expected patterns of physiologic activity and anatomic and psychosocial development.

Rationale: Early detection of deviations and therapeutic intervention are essential to the prevention of illness, to facilitating growth and developmental potential, and to the promotion of optimal health for the individual and the family.

Early detection requires that minute deviations be recognized, often before the individual or his family is aware that such deviations exist. The nurse has a unique opportunity to observe and assess the patient and his family, particularly in the community setting.

Assessment Factors: Therefore in practice, the maternal and child health nurse:

1. Demonstrates a thorough understanding of the range of normal body structure and function by detecting signs and symptoms which are not within normal limits.
2. Identifies the variety of coping mechanisms which may serve an adaptive function or represent maladaptive patterns of response.
3. Searches for improved means of detecting impairment of physical and emotional function.
4. Searches for improved means of detecting physical, psychological or environmental situations which may lead to impaired functioning.
5. Instructs the individual and family in recognizing and understanding deviations.

In the last decade, crisis theory has been applied more and more to the nursing care of individuals. The challenge lies in recognizing individuals and families vulnerable to crisis during the childbearing experience and assuring that therapeutic intervention is available as needed.

Another challenge is assessment to identify individuals at risk, both physically and emotionally. Such assessment should include detection of behavioral responses not within normal limits and environmental conditions which may lead to impaired functioning.

Nursing goals must be congruent with the goals of the expanding family. Although the expanding family's main goal is that of adding a new member to the family, there are also many lesser goals. The nurse must be aware of all these goals in order to formulate realistic and relevant nursing goals for maximizing functional capacities during pregnancy and parenthood.

STANDARD VI

The plan of nursing care includes goals derived from the nursing diagnoses.

Rationale: The determination of the desired results from nursing actions is an essential part of planning care.

Assessment Factors:

1. Goals are mutually set with the client/patient and significant others
   a. they are congruent with other planned therapies.
   b. they are stated in realistic and measurable terms.
   c. they are assigned a time schedule for achievement.
2. Goals are established to maximize functional capabilities and are congruent with
   a. growth and development
   b. biophysical status
   c. behavioral patterns
   d. human and material resources

In nursing practice, priorities must be set since all nursing needs cannot be met at the same time. The promotion, maintenance, and restoration of health includes a number of physical, emotional and informational needs. The assessment process gives direction as to which ones must be given priority. A knowledge base facilitates this process and aids in setting goals and planning and timing nursing intervention. It is possible that more than one goal can be accomplished at the same time or by the same act.

STANDARD VII

The plan of nursing care includes priorities and the prescribed nursing approaches or measures to achieve the goals derived from the nursing diagnoses.

Rationale: Nursing actions are planned to promote, maintain and restore the client's/patient's well-being.

Assessment Factors:

1. Physical measures are planned to manage (prevent or control) specific client/patient problems and clearly relate to the nursing diagnoses and goals of care, e.g., ADL, use of self-help devices, etc.
2. Psychosocial measures are specific to the client's/patient's nursing care needs and to the nursing care goals, e.g., techniques to control aggression.
3. Teaching-learning principles are incorporated into the plan of care and the objectives for learning stated in behavioral terms, e.g., specification of content for learner's level, reinforcement, readiness, etc.

4. Approaches are planned to provide for a therapeutic environment
   a. physical environmental factors are used to influence the therapeutic environment, e.g., control of noise, control of temperature, etc.
   b. psychosocial measures are used to structure the environment for therapeutic ends, e.g., paternal participation in all phases of the maternity experience.
   c. group behaviors are used to structure interaction and influence the therapeutic environment, e.g., conformity, territorial rights, locomotion, etc.
5. Approaches are specified for orientation of the client/patient to
   a. new roles and relationships
   b. relevant health (human and material) resources
   c. modifications in the plan of nursing care
   d. relationship of the modifications in the nursing care plan to the total care plan
6. The plan includes the utilization of available and appropriate resources
   a. human resources—other health professionals
   b. material resources
   c. community
7. The plan is an ordered sequence of proposed nursing actions.
8. Nursing approaches are planned on the basis of current knowledge.

For example, immediately following birth there are goals to be reached for both the mother and her infant. Vital signs are monitored to assure health *maintenance.* The mother must be protected from undue blood loss, infection, and sensory overload. *Promotion* of mother-infant relationships is also a goal. These two goals can be achieved simultaneously under usual conditions. The nurse's knowledge and assessment of factors are used to determine how and when this is done. *Restoration* for the mother is another goal. However, rest, an important part of restoration, is usually possible only after her vital signs are stabilized, she is assured her child is well, and she receives positive reinforcement from her mate.

Participation by the individual or family in maintaining, promoting, or restoring health is especially relevant in maternal and child nursing. A good example is when a premature infant is born. The health problems of the infant may be so acute, at first, that the health professionals alone must assume responsibility for the promotion and maintenance of the infant's health. The maternal-infant attachment process would also be a nursing goal, and maternal care of the infant would be the ultimate goal. While the infant is ill, the mother would begin to see and touch her infant. She would learn about the life-supporting measures used in the interest of her child, but see them as temporary. Gradually she would begin to provide care for her child. This Standard recognizes that such parent participation is valued and fosters growth for both the mother and the child.

STANDARD VIII

Nursing actions provide for client/patient participation in health promotion, maintenance and restoration.

Rationale: The client/patient and family are provided the opportunity to participate in the nursing care. Such provision is made based upon theoretical and experiential evidence that participation of client/patient and family may foster growth.

Assessment Factors:

1. The client/patient and family are kept informed about
   a. current health status
   b. changes in health status
   c. total health care plan
   d. nursing care plan
   e. roles of health care personnel
   f. health care resources
2. The client/patient and family are provided with the information needed to make decisions and choices about
   a. promoting, maintaining and restoring health
   b. seeking and utilizing appropriate health care personnel
   c. maintaining and using health care resources

The challenge to maternal and child nursing is to utilize all available knowledge and resources in the interest of fostering growth.

STANDARD IX

Maternal and child health nursing practice provides for the use and coordination of all services that assist individuals to prepare for responsible sexual roles.

Rationale: People are prepared for sexual roles through a process of socialization that takes place from birth to adulthood. This process of socialization, to a large extent, is carried out within the family structure. Social control over child care increases in importance as humans become increasingly dependent on the culture rather than upon the family unit. The culture of any society is maintained by the transmission of its specific values, attitudes and behaviors from generation to generation. Attitudes and values concerning male and female roles develop as part of the socialization process. Attitudes toward self, the opposite sex, and parents will influence the roles each individual assumes in adulthood and the responsibilities accepted.

Assessment Factors: Therefore in practice, the maternal and child health nurse:

1. Utilizes resources available in the social and behavioral sciences to help her understand the attitudes and values of individuals and families with whom she is working.
2. Utilizes opportunities available to her to promote those attitudes and values conducive to emotional and physical health and family solidarity, without imposing her own value system.
3. Encourages society to provide the resources needed to help people prepare for responsible sexual roles.
4. Interprets to other health personnel the needs of individuals and families as she sees them and attempts to understand the needs as seen by other health personnel.
5. Works with other health personnel to develop services which promote optimal health and family solidarity.

Helping individuals prepare for responsible sex roles has great relevance for maternal and child nursing. Nurses teach expectant parent classes and have been responsible for instituting family life courses in secondary schools. These activities of nursing are movements toward achieving the above Standard. Today, the challenges to nursing are at least three in number. First, nursing must motivate the public to value expectant parent education so that all expectant parents are prepared for the transition into their new roles of mother or father. There must be dynamic programs in sufficient numbers and in appropriate places to meet needs. Second, nurses must take the leadership in encouraging schools to provide all adolescents with appropriate family life courses which will help prepare them for responsible sexual roles. Third, the nurse herself must provide positive reinforcement of responsible parenting behavior, thereby encouraging a sense of worth and prestige in the role of parent.

Our society manifests the belief that every individual should be given the opportunity to achieve his optimal potential for health. Although this has not been accomplished for all, there is movement toward this goal.

STANDARD X

Nursing actions assist the client/patient to maximize his health capabilities.

Rationale: Nursing actions are designed to promote, maintain, and restore health. A knowledge and understanding of the principles and normal ranges in human growth, development, and behavior are essential to maternal and child health nursing practice.

Assessment Factors:

1. Nursing actions
   a. are consistent with the plan of care
   b. are based on scientific principles
   c. are individualized to the specific situation
   c. are used to provide a safe and therapeutic environment
   e. employ teaching-learning opportunities for the client/patient
   f. include utilization of appropriate resources
2. Nursing actions are directed to the physical, psychological, and social behavior associated with
   a. ingestion of food, fluid, and nutrients
   b. elimination of body wastes
   c. locomotion, exercise
   d. temperature and other regulatory mechanisms
   e. self-fulfillment
   f. relating to others

Opportunity to achieve optimum health should be provided from the very beginning of life. When an individual is born he is totally dependent on others to assist him in maximizing his capabilities. The nurse is an important part of that early environment. The challenge to nursing is to ensure that every newborn is provided with optimal care that will assure optimal physical growth and behavioral development. This includes more than the physical components of care, and encompasses psychologic and social components as well.

Clearly, no one has greater interest in the outcome of nursing care than the patient herself. By sharing nursing goals and their evaluation with the expectant and new mother, the nurse can better determine their relevance to her. The mother can provide the best data to evaluate whether nursing goals are being met and what effects nursing action has had on her health care.

STANDARD XI

The client's/patient's progress or lack of progress toward goal achievement is determined by the client/patient and the nurse.

Rationale: The quality of nursing care depends upon comprehensive and intelligent determination of the impact of nursing upon the health status of the client/patient. The client/patient is an essential part of this determination.

Assessment Factors:

1. Current data about the client/patient

are used to measure his progress toward goal achievement.
2. Nursing actions are analyzed for their effectiveness in goal achievement of the client/patient.
3. The client/patient evaluates nursing actions and goal achievement.
4. Provision is made for nursing follow-up of particular clients/patients to determine the long-term effects of nursing care.

Not all goals are achieved. It may be necessary to reassess, reorder priorities, and set new goals. A new plan of nursing care then evolves.

STANDARD XII

The client's/patient's progress or lack of progress toward goal achievement directs reassessment, reordering of priorities, new goal setting and revision of the plan of nursing care.

Rationale: The nursing process remains the same, but the input of new information may dictate new or revised approaches.

Assessment Factors:
1. Reassessment is directed by goal achievement or lack of goal achievement.
2. New priorities and goals are determined and additional nursing approaches are prescribed appropriately.
3. New nursing actions are accurately and appropriately initiated.

A good example of the application of this Standard is found in labor. Psychophysical preparation for labor has as its goal a normal, controlled labor. Progress toward this goal may be blocked by conditions not under the control of the individual or nurse, e.g., abnormal position of the fetus or ineffective labor contractions. In some cases, a cesarean section may be necessary. The nurse and patient must then effect a change in goals. One goal would be to keep the anxiety level of the patient at a minimum. The new plan for nursing care would use knowledge of the concept of anxiety to facilitate learning on the part of the patient rather than permitting her to panic.

Statistical evidence shows the disparity of health care services offered expectant parents and their families and the differential care given to various socioeconomic and racial groups. Moreover, there is a real challenge to America to lower its mortality and morbidity rates of infants. Despite America's material wealth our status of infant health, although greatly improved, is not as satisfactory as that of certain other nations. Progress is currently being made toward better utilization of personnel delivering health care services to mothers and infants. Gaps in health care services are being filled by nurses in expanded roles. Such expansion of roles is a response to the application of this Standard.

STANDARD XIII

Maternal and child health nursing practice evidences active participation with others in evaluating the availability, accessibility and acceptability of services for parents and children and cooperating and/or taking leadership in extending and developing needed services in the community.

Rationale: Knowledge of services presently offered parents and children is the first step in determining the effectiveness of health care to all in the community. When it is recognized that needed services are not available, accessible or acceptable, the nurse takes leadership in working with consumers, other health disciplines, the community and governmental agencies in extending and/or developing these services. Services must be continually evaluated, expanded, and changed if they are to improve the health and well-being of all parents and children within our society.

Assessment Factors: Therefore in practice, the maternal and child health nurse:

1. Applies and shares the cultural and socioeconomic concepts which help her understand the differences in the unique needs of individuals and families.
2. Recognizes the need for available health services for all parents and children in the community.
3. Utilizes the services and resources presently available.
4. Works with consumers, nurse colleagues, other health disciplines, the community and governmental agencies in evaluating the availability, accessibility, and acceptability of services to all parents and children in the community.
5. Participates actively with significant others in initiating changes in the delivery of health services and/or developing new services to enable each individual in the family to function at his optimum capacity and to enhance family unity.

REFERENCES

1. Hall, L.: *Nursing—What Is It?* (revised, mimeograph) Loeb Center, April 26, 1963, pp. 1–5.
2. Travelbee, J.: *Interpersonal Aspects of Nursing,* ed. 2. F. A. Davis, Philadelphia, 1972, p. 157.
3. Mayers, M.: *A Systematic Approach to the Nursing Care Plan.* Appleton-Century-Crofts, New York, 1972, p. 139.
4. *Standards of Maternal and Child Health Nursing Practice.* American Nurses' Association, Kansas City, 1973, p. 3.
5. Munger, M. D.: *ANA program to promote collective bargaining.* Hospital Topics 52:23, 1974.

2 Historical Perspectives

ANN L. CLARK, R.N., M.A.

Understanding contemporary maternal and child care must be based on a knowledge of its historical past. In this way, the nurse can better understand the system that has developed to provide family care during the childbearing phase of life. This includes the health care structure, federal support for care, education, and research, as well as national and worldwide organizations. The nurse must also recognize the strengths of the system and barriers that still block provisions for better maternal and child care in this country.

EARLY INFLUENCES

Prior to the twentieth century the expectant mother was not a visable part of the health care system. She generally received no prenatal care. The family physician was engaged, but did not usually see his patient until he was called to deliver the mother in her own home. Many women were never seen by a physician at all. A midwife, who had usually learned her skills from another "granny midwife," was engaged to care for the woman during the "birthing" process and often to care for the woman and her household after the delivery. The family was present during the birth and the extended family was available to help the mother care for her infant and other members of the immediate family.

This system had the advantage of making the transition to parenthood less of a crisis. Young people had numerous opportunities to observe others during pregnancy and since the birth occurred at home they sometimes even witnessed it. Also, large families gave the adolescent adequate opportunity to practice infant and child care. However, there were great disadvantages in terms of maternal and infant morbidity and mortality. Many women died giving birth and a large number of infants did not survive or were left with handicapping neurosensory defects.

The latter part of the nineteenth century brought the Industrial Revolution with its social and economic changes, many of which had great impact on maternal and infant care. Many Americans moved from farms into the cities to work in factories. This caused crowding and the creation of slums which in turn brought about menacing health problems. Proceduralized work routines and task distribution resulted in greater productivity but also caused depersonalization of the individual worker. At this time, fundamental patterns of family relationships changed. The center of productivity shifted from the home to the factory. Women took jobs outside the home and the roles of male and female, long stable, now began to be modified. Very young children were pressed into the labor market and infants often received a minimum of care.

Scientific knowledge of disease was still relatively limited. Death from puerperal sepsis was common. Large numbers of infants and young children died from infant diarrhea largely due to lack of knowledge of safe pasteurization of milk.[1] However, the Industrial Revolution was inseparably connected with parallel progress in the physical sciences. Through advancements in the field of immunology the way was paved by the opening of the twentieth century for a sharp reversal in morbidity and mortality.[2] Safe water, refrigeration, improved sewage disposal, and control of some of the infectious and communicable diseases were some of the advancements which benefited maternal and child health. Other improvements included higher standards of living and increased availability of public education.

MODERN MATERNAL CARE

Prenatal care was initiated by nurses and made available in 1901 through the Instructive Nursing Association of Boston Lying-In Hospital. It was instituted to safeguard the lives of expectant mothers and their infants.

Today, physicians are generally responsible for providing prenatal care for the American mother, but it must be recognized that many women, even though delivered by a physician, receive little or no prenatal care. As there has never been a national survey to determine how many women receive prenatal care, it is not possible to give a representative picture of the United States, but it is known that due to socioeconomic factors a number of women receive little or no care. As related later in this chapter, Federal legislation is extending and improving maternity care on a comprehensive basis, especially to women of high risk who cannot afford prenatal care.[3]

Women who are not delivered by physicians are usually delivered by nurse-midwives, or "other midwives." Nurse-midwives are registered professional nurses who are certified as such by the American College of Nurse-Midwifery upon graduation from a nurse-midwifery school. These schools' programs may be six to eight months in length or may be placed in a university setting and are an integral part of the master's degree program. A few states license professional nurse-midwives to practice under medical supervision and many states are attempting to modify laws to include their registration. The number of certified nurse-midwives is increasing.

There are no schools for "other midwives" but short programs are developed by health departments in some states where "granny midwives" practice. States which recognize these midwives require licensure with annual renewal. The number of these midwives is decreasing.

Over the years an increasing number of births have taken place in hospitals rather than in the home. This has been largely responsible for the reduction in maternal and neonatal mortality. At the same time, however, the family-centered approach to family expansion has been lost. Mothers labor in strange environments, often with a minimum of support. Hospital delivery means that childbirth is treated much like a dysfunctional process. The mother, father, infant, and other children are separated resulting in increased anxiety. The central nursery, once necessary to protect the infant, now separates him from his well and would-be comforting mother and is also viewed as a possible source of cross-contamination. The individual needs of the infant could often be better met by its own mother.

Indeed, as the hospital began substituting for the home in caring for mothers and infants in the early twentieth century, hospital care paralleled the mechinization occurring in industry. Bottle feeding was largely substituted for breast feeding. Care was dispensed as though the hospital were a kind of a production system—a machine turning out its product by the application of a controlled technical device with "routine" the accepted method. The declining death rate was taken as the index for a measurable performance.[4]

Presently, approximately 97 per cent of all births occur in hospitals (99 per cent of white patients and 85 per cent of non-white patients). These hospitals are licensed by the state and may seek accreditation by the Joint Commission on Accreditation of Hospitals. The hospital stay, originally two to three weeks, has slowly been reduced. The average stay for a mother is now three to four days, with many women leaving the hospital after a stay of only 24 hours. The mother's and infant's care while in the hospital is supervised by physicians and nurses, but little follow-up care is usually provided until the mother receives her six week's checkup.

Today, if a woman decides to deliver at home she will have difficulty finding a physician to attend her. In some areas a certified nurse-midwife, working in close association with a physician, may be available. A few women are choosing to deliver at home using lay assistance.

The infant's care is usually supervised by the family physician, a pediatrician, pediatric nurse practitioner, pediatric clinic, or government-supported Child Health Conference. Public health nurses make visits to selected new mothers and infants, but these encompass a very small percentage of those who could be benefited by such continuous care.

BIRTH RATE

The United States registered its lowest annual birth rate in 1972 according to the National Center for Health Statistics. Total births were estimated at 3,256,000. Figure 2-1 shows the census clock at the U. S. Department of Commerce, Bureau of the Census, in Washington, D. C., which registers all additions and reductions in our national population. Note that when this photograph was taken (1975) there was a birth somewhere in the United States every 10 seconds. Our population is increasing, but this is due to an *excess of births over deaths* and not an increased birth rate.

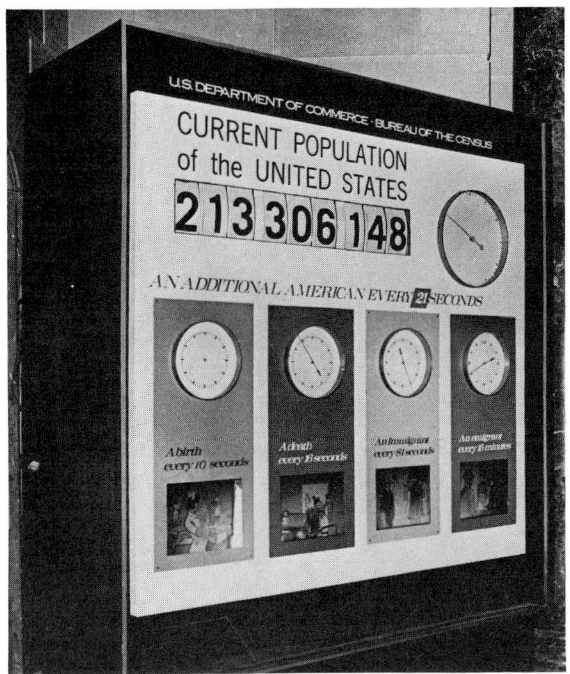
U.S. DEPARTMENT OF COMMERCE · BUREAU OF THE CENSUS
CURRENT POPULATION
of the UNITED STATES
213 306 148
AN ADDITIONAL AMERICAN EVERY 21 SECONDS
A birth
every 10 seconds

FIGURE 2-1. Census clock at the U.S. Department of Commerce, Bureau of the Census, Washington, D.C.

In the last decade we have seen changes in the birth rate. In 1975 there were 25 million women between the ages of 20 and 35. These are the usual childbearing years, and the potential for additional changes in the birth rate must be recognized and considered in planning for maternal and child health care.

MATERNAL MORTALITY

In 1915 the maternal mortality rate was 60.8 per 10,000 births. Since then, it has been reduced by 94 per cent until now it is considered to be an almost irreducible minimum. In 1972 the deaths of an estimated 780 women were attributed to complications of pregnancy, childbirth, and the puerperium. As seen in Table 2-1, except after 1971 when the rate was unusually low, the maternal mortality rate has declined each year. Factors which have contributed to this improvement include research in pregnancy and its complications, increased prenatal care, increased hospital deliveries, readily available blood transfusions, and widespread use of antibiotics.[5]

TABLE 2-1. Maternal Mortality Rate

Year	*Maternal Mortality Rate*
1972	24.0 (est.)
1971	20.5 (est.)
1970	24.7 (est.)
1969	27.4 (est.)
1968	24.5
1967	28.0
1966	29.1
1965	31.6
1964	33.3
1963	35.8
1962	35.2
1961	36.9
1960	37.1
1950	83.3

(From *Vital Statistics Report, Annual Summary for the United States, 1972.* U. S. Department of Health, Education and Welfare.)

INFANT MORTALITY

The infant mortality rate in 1900, from those states then reporting these statistics, was 200 per 1,000 births. Since then, it has been reduced by more than 80 per cent, with a drastic reduction occurring in the 1930s when antibiotics were discovered. The reduction, as shown in Figure 2-2, has continued into the present decade. Although these figures are impressive, a great deal remains to be done. The United States rated sixteenth in infant mortality rates among 25 selected countries in both 1971 and 1972 (Table 2-2). These comparisons persist even though the United States reached a new low level of infant deaths in 1972. There were 60,200 estimated deaths, which represents a rate of 18.5 per cent per 1,000 live births.

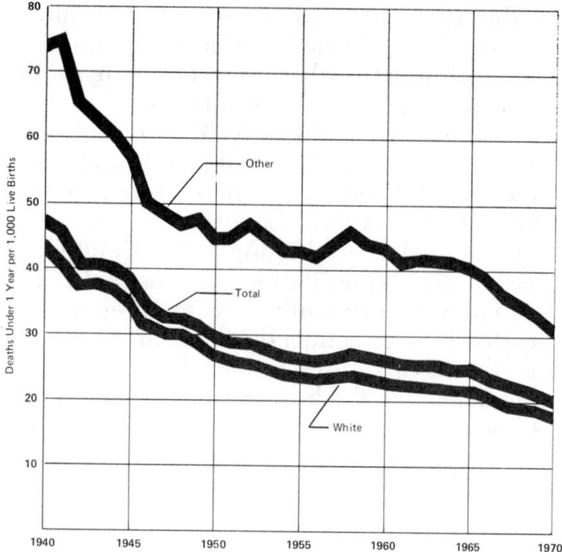

FIGURE 2-2. Infant mortality trends, 1940 to 1970. (Source of data: Maternal and Child Health Project, George Washington University.)

As shown in Table 2-3, infant mortality rates by race strongly indicate a great need to focus on improving care to the non-white population. The total infant mortality rate for "all other" races continues to be roughly 80 per cent higher than for the "white" race. Since 1950 the latter has declined almost 40 per cent, while the former has declined 35 per cent. It is likely that these rates of decline would converge if social and health measures were equally applied to both groups.[6]

TABLE 2-2. Infant Mortality Rates for Selected Countries

Country	*Infant Mortality Rate* 1971	1972
Sweden	11.1	10.8
Netherlands	11.1	11.4
Finland	11.8	11.3
Japan	12.4	11.7
Norway	12.8	11.3
Denmark	13.5	
France	14.4	13.3
Switzerland	14.4	13.0
New Zealand	16.6	
Australia	17.3	16.7
Canada	17.6	17.1
United Kingdom	17.9	
German Democratic Republic	18.0	17.7
Ireland	18.0	17.7
Hong Kong	18.4	17.5
United States	19.2	18.5
Belgium	19.8	20.5
Israel	21.3	
Czechoslovakia	21.6	
U.S.S.R.	22.6	24.3
German Federal Republic	23.1	22.5
Bulgaria	24.9	25.8
Spain	25.2	18.5
Austria	26.1	25.1
Greece	26.9	26.9

Data are provisional. Infant mortality rate per 1,000 live births. (From Puffee, R. R. and Serrano, C. V.: *Patterns of Mortality in Childhood.* Scientific Publications No. 262. Pan American Health Organization, Washington, D. C., 1973.)

The infant mortality rate also varies from state to state as shown in Table 2-4. There is a marked reduction in many states and twice as many show declines as show increases. The state with the highest rate for 1972, Mississippi, has a declining rate when compared with 1971. However, it is still one-third higher than the national average. Utah has the lowest rate in the nation, 14.4.

GOVERNMENT ACTIONS

Federal and state governments have assumed a significant role in the improvement of maternal and child care.

WHITE HOUSE CONFERENCES

President Theodore Roosevelt, in 1909, called the first White House Conference to identify problems of maternal and child health services. These White House Conferences have been called each decade since, to review current needs of mothers, children, and youth. The 1930 Conference developed *The Children's Charter,* which served as a model for the United Nations Declaration of the Rights of the Child. The theme of the 1960 Conference was Opportunities for Children and Youth to Realize Their Full Potential for Creative Life in Freedom and Dignity. The 1970 Conference was established:

> To enhance and cherish the individuality and identity of each child through the recognition and encouragement of his or her own development, regardless of environmental conditions or circumstances of birth.
>
> Goals
>
> To discover what will best promote the development of the American child through the remaining years of the Twentieth Century.
>
> To establish priorities among those issues and problems known to affect the child in the United States.
>
> To predict problems or issues which may emerge to threaten the life, health, or well-being of the total child during the next decade, and create plans and policies to deal with them.
>
> To act as a vehicle for the recognition of

TABLE 2-3. Infant Mortality Rates by Age and Color: United States, 1950 and 1960 to 1972

	Total			*White*			*All Other*		
Year	*under 1 year*	*under 28 days*	*28 days to 11 months*	*under 1 year*	*under 28 days*	*28 days to 11 months*	*under 1 year*	*under 28 days*	*28 days to 11 months*
1972 (est.)	18.5	13.7	4.8	16.3	12.3	4.0	29.0	20.6	8.5
1971 (est.)	19.2	14.3	4.9	16.8	12.9	3.9	30.2	20.8	9.4
1970 (est.)	19.8	14.9	4.9	17.4	13.5	3.9	31.4	21.6	9.8
1969 (est.)	20.7	15.4	5.4	18.4	14.1	4.4	31.6	21.6	10.0
1968	21.8	16.1	5.7	19.2	14.7	4.5	34.5	23.0	11.6
1967	22.4	16.5	5.9	19.7	15.0	4.7	35.9	23.8	12.1
1966	23.7	17.2	6.5	20.6	15.6	5.0	38.8	24.8	13.9
1965	24.7	17.7	7.0	21.5	16.1	5.4	40.3	25.4	14.9
1964	24.8	17.9	6.9	21.6	16.2	5.4	41.1	26.5	14.6
1963	25.2	18.2	7.0	22.2	16.7	5.5	41.5	26.1	15.4
1962	25.3	18.3	7.0	22.3	16.9	5.5	41.4	26.1	15.3
1961	25.3	18.4	6.9	22.4	16.9	5.5	40.7	26.2	14.5
1960	26.0	18.7	7.3	22.9	17.2	5.7	43.2	26.9	16.4
1950	29.2	20.5	8.7	26.8	19.4	7.4	44.5	27.5	16.9

For 1969 to 1972, based on a 10 per cent sample of deaths; for all other years, based on final data. Rates per 1,000 live births. (From National Center for Health Statistics, Monthly Vital Statistics Report, Vol. 21, No. 13, June 27, 1973.)

the child as a valuable and precious resource to be cherished and protected.

To identify and encourage resources which would be committed toward solving the issues and problems confronting the American child.

To establish orderly and effective procedures for a national effort, having as its goal the enhanced development of the American child through the remaining years of the Twentieth Century.[7]

These Conferences have been responsible for the development of standards to improve services to mothers and children, and the promotion of such programs as The Children's Bureau and maternal and child health care under the Social Security Act.

THE CHILDREN'S BUREAU

Established in 1912, The Children's Bureau was originally organized to protect children in the labor market. Today its overall objective is to promote the health of mothers and children. The Bureau initiated early studies of maternal and infant mortality and has been responsible for improved prenatal care and reduced infant mortality. It is mainly through this agency that funds are made available, studies are conducted, projects are developed, and information is published in the area of child welfare.

THE SOCIAL SECURITY ACT

In 1963, Federal legislation amended the Social Security Act (Public Law 88-156). This legislation is known as *Mental Retardation and Maternal and Child Health.* Funds, through The Children's Bureau, are provided on a project basis to local and state health departments to develop *maternal and infant care projects* "in order to help reduce the incidence of mental retardation caused by complications associated with childbearing," and to provide "necessary health care to pro-

TABLE 2-4. Live Births, Birth Rates, and Infant Mortality Rates, by Place of Occurrence

Area	*Live Births*		*Infant Mortality Rate*	
	1972 number	*1972 rate*	*1972*	*1971*
New England	166,513	13.8	17.0	16.6
Maine	15,892	15.4	16.7	16.3
New Hampshire	11,294	14.6	14.8	15.6
Vermont	7,180	15.5	15.9	15.0
Massachusetts	79,522	13.7	17.4	17.1
Rhode Island	13,495	13.9	19.0	18.9
Connecticut	39,130	12.7	16.3	15.5
Middle Atlantic	516,702	13.7	17.8	18.4
New York	254,431	13.9	18.1	18.6
New Jersey	97,529	13.2	17.1	18.0
Pennsylvania	164,742	13.8	17.7	18.1
East North Central	644,471	15.7	18.4	18.8
Ohio	170,347	15.8	17.6	18.2
Indiana	87,191	16.5	19.2	18.0
Illinois	175,604	15.6	20.0	20.7
Michigan	147,187	16.2	18.4	19.2
Wisconsin	64,142	14.2	15.3	15.7
West North Central	249,435	15.0	17.6	18.1
Minnesota	56,629	14.5	17.4	17.8
Iowa	41,383	14.4	17.4	17.0
Missouri	74,981	15.8	18.2	19.0
North Dakota	10,577	16.7	15.7	15.3
South Dakota	10,728	15.8	21.3	17.1
Nebraska	23,500	15.4	17.7	17.2
Kansas	31,637	14.0	16.4	19.8
South Atlantic	514,943	16.2	20.8	21.3
Delaware	8,867	15.7	18.9	14.4
Maryland	51,059	12.6	15.8	18.0
District of Columbia	21,579	28.8	25.5	28.5
Virginia	71,939	15.1	20.6	20.8
West Virginia	26,679	16.7	20.8	21.9
North Carolina	89,491	17.2	23.0	22.2
South Carolina	49,007	18.4	21.8	22.5
Georgia	84,337	17.9	21.2	21.3
Florida	108,985	15.0	19.9	20.7
East South Central	232,489	17.7	22.0	22.8
Kentucky	55,419	16.8	19.3	20.4
Tennessee	69,752	17.3	22.2	21.6
Alabama	61,869	17.6	22.2	23.6
Mississippi	45,449	20.1	24.7	26.6
West South Central	362,664	18.2	19.1	19.9
Arkansas	32,985	16.7	16.8	19.9
Louisiana	68,611	18.4	19.8	22.1
Oklahoma	41,246	15.7	18.6	18.4
Texas	219,882	18.9	19.4	19.5

TABLE 2-4—*Continued*

Area	*Live Births*		*Infant Mortality Rate*	
	1972 number	*1972 rate*	*1972*	*1971*
Mountain	165,446	18.7	17.1	18.3
Montana	11,361	15.8	18.3	20.7
Idaho	13,828	18.3	15.5	16.6
Wyoming	5,814	16.9	20.1	21.1
Colorado	39,869	16.9	17.6	18.0
New Mexico	20,589	19.3	19.9	20.9
Arizona	37,258	19.2	16.4	18.3
Utah	27,934	24.8	14.4	14.1
Nevada	8,793	16.7	18.1	22.9
Pacific	405,114	14.9	16.0	17.1
Washington	47,148	13.7	15.9	18.6
Oregon	32,303	14.8	16.6	18.1
California	303,542	14.8	15.8	16.8
Alaska	6,797	20.9	16.5	18.3
Hawaii	15,324	18.9	17.5	16.2
Puerto Rico	—	—	—	24.5
Virgin Islands (U.S.)	—	—	—	25.6

Data are provisional. Birth rate per 1,000 total population. Infant mortality rate per 1,000 live births. (From National Center for Health Statistics, Report 21, No. 13, June 27, 1973.)

spective mothers who have or are likely to have conditions associated with childbearing which will increase the hazards to the health of the mothers or their infants and whom the state and local health agency determines will not receive the necessary health care because they are from low income families or for other reasons beyond their control."[8] The medical and hospital costs are borne by the project, supplemented by state and local funds on a 1:3 basis. Clinics are reporting improvements in prenatal care rates, neonatal death rates, and premature birth rates.[9, 10]

A program of *formulae grants* to states for maternal and child health and crippled children's services was authorized under Title V when the Social Security Act was passed in 1935. Since then, Title V has been extended to include a program of *special projects* to promote the health of mothers and children through maternity and infant care covering the period of pregnancy and the first year of the baby's life, intensive care for the high-risk newborn, and comprehensive health services and dental care for children. In 1975 this program of special projects was combined with the formulae grants and each state is required to have such a program as a condition for receiving Federal funds.

Title V provides funds for 20 university-affiliated programs which train health personnel from many disciplines to work with handicapped and retarded children. It also supports research on maternal and child health and crippled children.

By 1974 the maternal and child health programs included 56 maternity and infant care projects, 8 infant intensive care projects, 59 projects for comprehensive health care of children, and 18 dental health projects. It is supporting 77 research projects and sponsoring both training and research abroad.

Also authorized under Title V are *family planning projects.* These are designed to help families plan for the number of children they want, and to space their children to protect the health of both the mother and child. In 1975 the capacity of these services was 1.9 million individuals. Family planning is an integral part of maternal and child health programs, neighborhood health centers, and migrant health services.

RESEARCH

An enormous study was initiated in 1958 under a grant from the National Institutes of Health known as *The Collaborative Prenatal Study.*[11] During the years 1959 to 1965, 55,000 pregnant women were registered for prenatal care and study in 14 collaborating medical centers. This was a prospective as well as retrospective study to accumulate data for analysis regarding pregnancy, labor and delivery, and the child's development. The broad objectives of the study were to:

1. Determine the relationship between factors in the prenatal environment and the continuum of human reproductive failure, with particular reference to the central nervous system for
   a. early manifestations of deficits (infancy and early childhood)
   b. later manifestations of deficits (5 to 15 years).
2. Study the effect of the extra-uterine environment on fetal development (e.g., family situation, socioeconomic factors).
3. Determine the relationship of prematurity to factors in the perinatal environment and to the continuum of human reproductive failure, with particular reference to the central nervous system.
4. Determine the relationship between factors in the postnatal environment, up to 15 years, and the development of neurologic and sensory disorders.
5. Determine the relationship between genetic factors and the continuum of human reproductive failure, with particular reference to the central nervous system.
6. Study clinico-pathological correlations in the continuum of human reproductive failure, with particular reference to the central nervous system.
7. Improve the classification, treatment and prevention of cerebral palsy.

Data in this study are still being accumulated on the children as they develop and analysis of the data continues. Table 2-5 shows the characteristics and conditions of pregnancy of the women in this study. The perinatal death rate of white infants is shown to be 35.1, while that for black infants is 41.9. Likewise, the birth-weight rate below 2,501 grams is 71.4 for white patients and 134.2 for black patients.

Table 2-6 shows the total figures of the study

TABLE 2-5. Characteristics and Conditions of Pregnancy

	White with Condition			*Black with Condition*		
Condition	*%*	*perinatal death rate*	*birthweight rate <2,501 g.*	*%*	*perinatal death rate*	*birthweight rate <2,501 g.*
Organic heart disease	1.44	55.2	176.5	1.76	71.4	189.0
Pneumonia during pregnancy	.57	27.8	103.8	.44	56.8	139.5
Bronchial asthma	.93	28.4	105.3	1.42	70.4	159.3
Diabetes	.66	144.0	95.7	.65	139.5	149.1
Convulsions, not eclamptic	.35	30.3	46.9	.21	119.1	194.4
Psychosis or neurosis	4.71	36.0	89.7	1.69	29.6	186.8
Hyperemesis gravidarum	1.64	35.7	66.7	.71	35.5	117.7
Incompetent cervix	.34	323.1	614.0	.36	478.9	679.3
Hydramnios	1.54	137.9	86.5	1.26	99.2	87.9
Placenta previa	.77	176.1	328.2	.56	190.9	529.4
Abruptio placentae	2.39	195.5	263.0	1.90	360.7	476.9
Prolapse of cord	1.10	168.3	118.6	.78	298.0	235.3
All cases	—	35.1	71.4	—	41.9	134.2

(From Niswander and Gordon.[11])

TABLE 2-6. Outcomes by Race

	White			*Black*		
Outcomes	*all cases*	*number*	*rate*	*all cases*	*number*	*rate*
Births	19,048			20,167		
Perinatal deaths		668	35.07		845	41.90
Stillbirths		415	21.79		457	22.66
Fresh stillbirths		200	10.50		246	12.20
Livebirths	18,633			19,710		
Neonatal deaths		253	13.58		388	19.69
Livebirths with known birthweight	18,481			19,504		
Birthweight <2,501 g.		1,319	71.37		2,617	134.18
Mean birthweight, g.	3,272			3,039		
One year exams	14,662			17,123		
Neurologically abnormal at 1 yr.		253	17.26		274	16.00

(From Niswander and Gordon.[11])

in relation to the above figures. Note that, except for neurologic abnormalities at the end of the first year of life, the rate of fetal wastage and number of high-risk infants born are higher for blacks in every instance.

BIRTH REGISTRATION

In 1915 the Federal Government began birth registration, but it was not until 1930 that every state was reporting this information. The birth is first registered by a local or state registrar and then reported to the National Office of Vital Statistics in Washington, D. C. Data related to births, deaths, and other population figures are all compiled by the National Office of Vital Statistics.

The *birth certificate* (Figs. 2-3 and 2-4) is a valuable legal document. It is the official record of a person's full name, parentage, and the date, place, and time of birth. Proof of the facts of birth are needed for entrance to school, work permit, license to drive, entrance into Armed Forces, marriage license, passport, welfare benefits, retirement pensions, Social Security benefits, and others.

ORGANIZATIONS

World Health Organization (WHO). In 1948 the United Nations founded this specialized agency as an international cooperative for health. Its goal is "the attainment by all people of the highest possible level of health," with health defined as "a state of complete physical, mental, and social well-being and not merely the absence of infirmity."[12]

WHO activities are divided into several categories:

1. Directing and coordinating authority on international health work.
2. Providing demonstration teams for teaching disease control.
3. Compiling world health statistics.
4. Promoting medical research and distributing technical publications.
5. Providing international standardization of drugs, vaccines and other medical supplies for the administration of international sanitary regulations.

WHO has made dramatic contributions to world health through large scale campaigns against preventable disease. There are also various WHO committees which specialize in maternal and child care, e.g., WHO Expert Committee on Maternity Care and WHO Expert Committee on Nutrition in Pregnancy and Lactation.

United Nations International Children's Emergency Fund (UNICEF). This agency was established in 1946 to meet the needs of children of World War II. It is now known as the *United Nations Children's Fund* and concerns itself with maternal and child health services, control of disease, nutrition projects, and family and child welfare clinics. UNICEF is supported by voluntary contributions rather than the regular United Nations budget. The *Declaration of the Rights of the Child* (Appendix 4) was developed by this agency and adopted by the United Nations General Assembly in 1959.

La Leche League. This organization was established in 1956 in the United States but has now become an international organization. Its objectives are to foster breast feeding and to support women who are breast feeding their infants. It conducts meetings, offers individual counseling and support, and distributes publications. In many cities, hospitals and public health nursing agencies work in a cooperative manner with the La Leche League by making referrals to help assure continuity of care for the lactating woman.

Planned Parenthood Federation of America. This organization offers services in family planning through publications and clinics throughout the United States. Through the

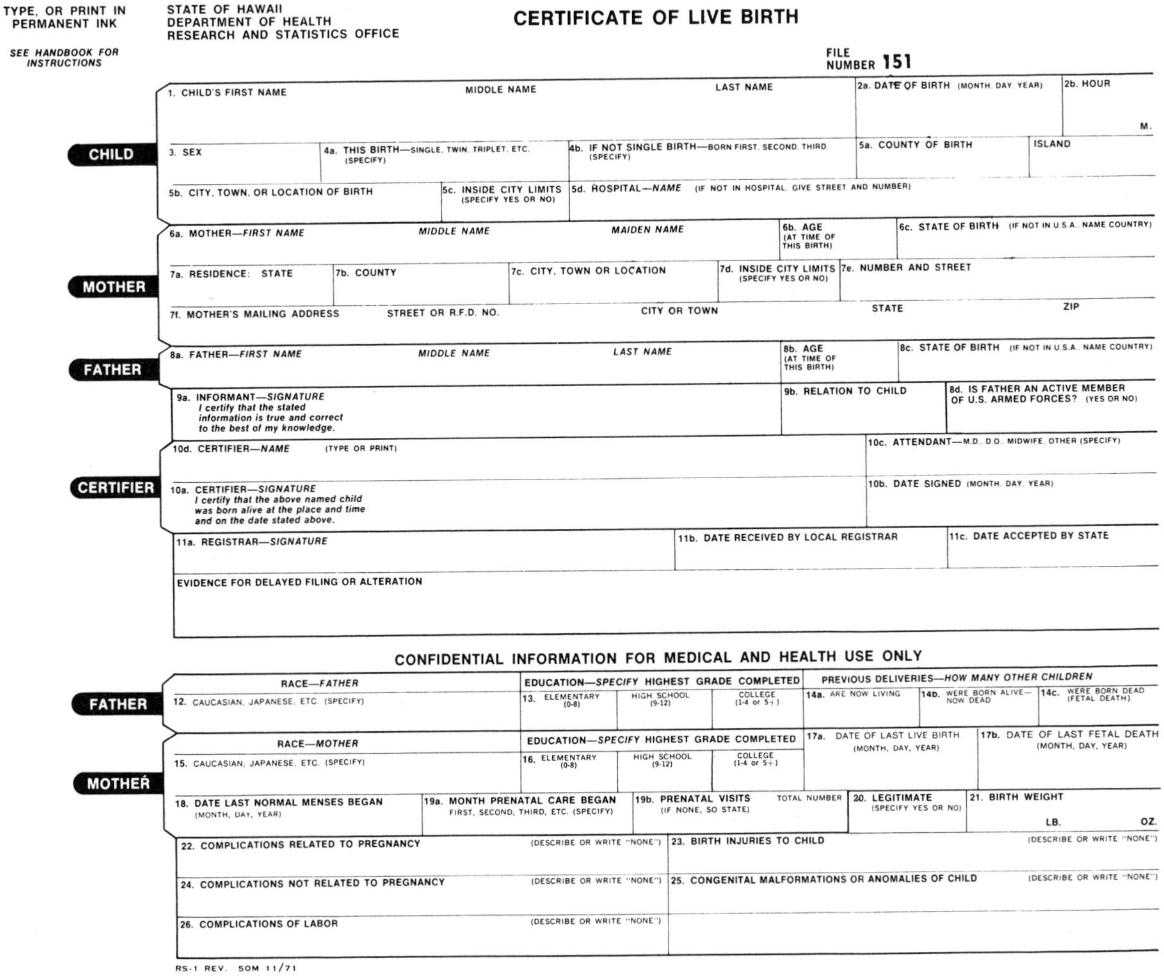

TYPE, OR PRINT IN PERMANENT INK

SEE HANDBOOK FOR INSTRUCTIONS

STATE OF HAWAII
DEPARTMENT OF HEALTH
RESEARCH AND STATISTICS OFFICE

CERTIFICATE OF LIVE BIRTH

FILE NUMBER **151**

CHILD

1. CHILD'S FIRST NAME | MIDDLE NAME | LAST NAME | 2a. DATE OF BIRTH (MONTH, DAY, YEAR) | 2b. HOUR M.

3. SEX | 4a. THIS BIRTH—SINGLE, TWIN, TRIPLET, ETC. (SPECIFY) | 4b. IF NOT SINGLE BIRTH—BORN FIRST, SECOND, THIRD (SPECIFY) | 5a. COUNTY OF BIRTH | ISLAND

5b. CITY, TOWN, OR LOCATION OF BIRTH | 5c. INSIDE CITY LIMITS (SPECIFY YES OR NO) | 5d. HOSPITAL—*NAME* (IF NOT IN HOSPITAL, GIVE STREET AND NUMBER)

MOTHER

6a. MOTHER—*FIRST NAME* | *MIDDLE NAME* | *MAIDEN NAME* | 6b. AGE (AT TIME OF THIS BIRTH) | 6c. STATE OF BIRTH (IF NOT IN U.S.A., NAME COUNTRY)

7a. RESIDENCE: STATE | 7b. COUNTY | 7c. CITY, TOWN OR LOCATION | 7d. INSIDE CITY LIMITS (SPECIFY YES OR NO) | 7e. NUMBER AND STREET

7f. MOTHER'S MAILING ADDRESS | STREET OR R.F.D. NO. | CITY OR TOWN | STATE | ZIP

FATHER

8a. FATHER—*FIRST NAME* | *MIDDLE NAME* | *LAST NAME* | 8b. AGE (AT TIME OF THIS BIRTH) | 8c. STATE OF BIRTH (IF NOT IN U.S.A., NAME COUNTRY)

9a. INFORMANT—*SIGNATURE* *I certify that the stated information is true and correct to the best of my knowledge.* | 9b. RELATION TO CHILD | 8d. IS FATHER AN ACTIVE MEMBER OF U.S. ARMED FORCES? (YES OR NO)

CERTIFIER

10d. CERTIFIER—*NAME* (TYPE OR PRINT) | 10c. ATTENDANT—M.D., D.O., MIDWIFE, OTHER (SPECIFY)

10a. CERTIFIER—*SIGNATURE* *I certify that the above named child was born alive at the place and time and on the date stated above.* | 10b. DATE SIGNED (MONTH, DAY, YEAR)

11a. REGISTRAR—*SIGNATURE* | 11b. DATE RECEIVED BY LOCAL REGISTRAR | 11c. DATE ACCEPTED BY STATE

EVIDENCE FOR DELAYED FILING OR ALTERATION

CONFIDENTIAL INFORMATION FOR MEDICAL AND HEALTH USE ONLY

FATHER

RACE—*FATHER* 12. CAUCASIAN, JAPANESE, ETC. (SPECIFY) | EDUCATION—*SPECIFY* HIGHEST GRADE COMPLETED 13. ELEMENTARY (0-8) | HIGH SCHOOL (9-12) | COLLEGE (1-4 or 5+) | PREVIOUS DELIVERIES—*HOW MANY OTHER CHILDREN* 14a. ARE NOW LIVING | 14b. WERE BORN ALIVE—NOW DEAD | 14c. WERE BORN DEAD (FETAL DEATH)

MOTHER

RACE—*MOTHER* 15. CAUCASIAN, JAPANESE, ETC. (SPECIFY) | EDUCATION—*SPECIFY* HIGHEST GRADE COMPLETED 16. ELEMENTARY (0-8) | HIGH SCHOOL (9-12) | COLLEGE (1-4 or 5+) | 17a. DATE OF LAST LIVE BIRTH (MONTH, DAY, YEAR) | 17b. DATE OF LAST FETAL DEATH (MONTH, DAY, YEAR)

18. DATE LAST NORMAL MENSES BEGAN (MONTH, DAY, YEAR) | 19a. MONTH PRENATAL CARE BEGAN FIRST, SECOND, THIRD, ETC. (SPECIFY) | 19b. PRENATAL VISITS (IF NONE, SO STATE) TOTAL NUMBER | 20. LEGITIMATE (SPECIFY YES OR NO) | 21. BIRTH WEIGHT LB. OZ.

22. COMPLICATIONS RELATED TO PREGNANCY (DESCRIBE OR WRITE "NONE") | 23. BIRTH INJURIES TO CHILD (DESCRIBE OR WRITE "NONE")

24. COMPLICATIONS NOT RELATED TO PREGNANCY (DESCRIBE OR WRITE "NONE") | 25. CONGENITAL MALFORMATIONS OR ANOMALIES OF CHILD (DESCRIBE OR WRITE "NONE")

26. COMPLICATIONS OF LABOR (DESCRIBE OR WRITE "NONE")

RS-1 REV. 50M 11/71

FIGURE 2-3. Certificate of live birth, State of Hawaii.

Margaret Sanger Research Bureau, research on infertility and contraception is conducted and marriage counseling services are offered.

International Childbirth Education Association (ICEA). Federations of this organization are made up of lay individuals, nurses, and physicians in every state and in a number of foreign countries. This organization fosters family-centered maternal and infant care and education for childbirth through conferences, workshops, and publications. In some communities it has become a strong voice of the public to communicate health needs and concerns to health care providers.

CURRENT CHALLENGES AND GOALS

Improving the health of families during childbearing and childrearing involves com-

H105. 142 REV. 3-72
500M 3-72

Local Registrar's No. COPY.
Primary Dist. No.

COMMONWEALTH OF PENNSYLVANIA
DEPARTMENT OF HEALTH
VITAL STATISTICS
CERTIFICATE OF LIVE BIRTH

COPY.

1. PLACE OF BIRTH a. County | 2. MOTHER'S MAILING ADDRESS a. Street address, R.D. or box number
b. City, borough, or township | b. Post office, state, and zip code
c. Name of hospital or institution | 3. INFORMANT

A__________
B__________
C__________
D__________
E__________
F__________
G__________
H__________
I__________

CHILD
4. THIS CHILD'S NAME a. (First) b. (Middle) c. (Last)
5. THIS CHILD'S SEX | 6 a. THIS BIRTH WAS Single ☐ Twin ☐ Triplet ☐ | 6 b. If TWIN or TRIPLET. This child was born: 1st ☐ 2nd ☐ 3rd ☐ | 7. DATE OF BIRTH (Month) (Day) (Year)

FATHER
8. FATHER'S FULL NAME a. (First) b. (Middle) c. (Last) | 9. HIS AGE Years
10. HIS BIRTHPLACE (State or foreign country) | 11. a. HIS USUAL OCCUPATION | 11. b. KIND OF BUSINESS OR INDUSTRY

MOTHER
12. MOTHER'S FULL MAIDEN NAME a. (First) b. (Middle) c. (Last) | 13. HER AGE Years
14. HER BIRTHPLACE (State or foreign country) | 15. WHERE DOES MOTHER ACTUALLY LIVE? a. State b. County
16. CHILDREN Previously Born to This Mother (DO NOT include this child) a. How many are NOW living? b. How many were born alive but are NOW DEAD? c. How many were delivered dead after sixteen weeks pregnancy? | c. Does Mother Live in a Township? (NOT within the limit of a city or borough) ☐ YES, she lives in__________ Township. ☐ NO, she lives within the actual limits of__________ City or Borough.

17. I hereby certify that this child was born alive on the date stated above at __________ m., E. T.
Signed __________ ☐ M.D. ☐ D.O. ☐ Other (Specify) Certifier's Address __________
Date Signed __________

18. DATE RECEIVED FOR FILING | 19. LOCAL REGISTRAR'S SIGNATURE S.S. No.

NOTICE

Make certain that the appropriate Letter "D" or "S" is inserted in the Time Element in Item 17.

CONFIDENTIAL medical report below MUST be completed for MEDICAL and HEALTH use

20. FATHER'S RACE | 21. MOTHER'S RACE | 22 a. LENGTH of PREGNANCY in _____ COMPLETED WEEKS | 22 b. WEIGHT OF CHILD AT BIRTH _____ grams or _____ lbs. _____ oz. | 23. LEGITIMATE? Yes ☐ No ☐
24. IN WHAT TRIMESTER WAS FIRST VISIT PRENATAL CARE? 1st ☐ 2nd ☐ 3rd ☐ No visit ☐ Unknown ☐ | 25. SEROLOGIC TEST for SYPHILIS Yes ☐ No ☐ Date | 26. METHOD OF DELIVERY
27. DESCRIBE ANY CONGENITAL MALFORMATION | 28. DESCRIBE ANY COMPLICATION OF LABOR
29. DESCRIBE ANY BIRTH INJURY | 30. DESCRIBE ANY COMPLICATION OF PREGNANCY

FIGURE 2-4. Certificate of live birth, Commonwealth of Pennsylvania.

plex problems relating to the economic and social conditions in our nation. About 20 per cent of American families have incomes below the demarcated poverty line.[13] During the last two decades many of these people have moved into cities while large segments of the middle-income group have moved to the suburbs.[14] *Standards of living* for those persons at the bottom of the socioeconomic scale must be improved. Health care, in the broadest sense of the word, must be recognized as a right of citizenship. It is forecast that within the next decade prepaid comprehensive health care on a per capita basis will be enacted. While we are trying to achieve this goal, there are other problems requiring studies and solutions for improved health care. These are considered briefly here and are discussed in more detail throughout the remainder of the book. The problems are:

Making family planning and birth control safe, effective, available, and acceptable.

Reducing maternal morbidity and mortality to a minimum.

Assuring that all expectant and new parents obtain preparation for parenthood.

Making high quality prenatal care acceptable and available to all expectant mothers.

Humanizing all aspects of maternal and child health.

Reducing perinatal morbidity and mortality to a minimum.

Utilizing all health care professionals appropriately.

Making available comprehensive services to adolescent parents.

Assuring continuity of care from one conception to the next (interconception care).

Birth control methods, although relatively safe and effective, are not 100 per cent so, and are not yet available to all at a price they can afford. However, ongoing research and provision of more comprehensive health care services are expected to improve this situation. Also, many women are not motivated to control conception, but to control births. As a result, abortion is being utilized for population control. Motivation studies are needed in this area. Some couples find all present forms of conception control unacceptable. Research to find more acceptable methods is needed. Public education on the need for population control must be continued and expanded.

Causes of *maternal mortality*, especially toxemia, hemorrhage, and infection, require continued research on their causes and treatments. Morbidity, both physiologic and psychologic, occurs during pregnancy to an unacceptable degree. Causes must be discovered and high quality health care made available to all women.

Preparation for pregnancy, labor, the puerperium, and parenting must be made available to all. Family life education should be offered beginning in secondary schools. The quality of expectant parent classes must be upgraded to meet the needs of widely diverse cultural groups. Classes must include parent-infant adaptation and parental guidance.

Prenatal care must be of the highest quality and made available and acceptable to all expectant mothers. There are many deterrents to prenatal care which need to be rectified.[15–19] Impersonal and even rude routine care, long waiting periods on uncomfortable benches, transportation, and preschool child care are some of the problems which require attention. Financial and motivational problems need the attention of legislators as well as health professionals. Satellite clinics with evening and weekend hours are needed to meet expectant mothers' needs. Special emphasis must be placed on high quality nutritional intake for expectant mothers.

All routines should be scrutinized to assure that *humanized care* is provided. Within the environment of the traditional hospital maternity unit, primary emphasis is too often placed on rigidity of controls and the immediacy of patient care needs. This tends to fragment the care process, disregarding the principle of individual differences and ignoring both the social and cultural past of the patient as well as the impact of ongoing hospital experiences upon the mother's and infant's future psychologic well-being.[20] A warm, secure, family-centered birth experience should not be too much to expect. The new parents should not have difficulty in being together and having free access to their infant. We need to experiment with simpler facilities for the safe care of mothers and infants.

Perinatal morbidity and mortality, particularly deaths during the first week of life, are too high. Prematurity, asphyxia, atelectasis, congenital malformation, and birth trauma are the main causes of infant mortality and require further research. Safe access to intensive care nurseries should be provided in addition to centralization for judicious use of health personnel.

Judicious use of health personnel to improve delivery of maternal and child health care is exemplified by the extended role of the professional nurse, e.g., maternal health nurse practitioners and pediatric nurse practitioners, as well as maternal and child clinical nurse specialists, perinatal clinical nurse specialists, and certified nurse-midwives. In this way, professional nurses can more fully utilize their knowledge and skills. Physicians have too long used their expert knowledge and skills with expectant and new mothers who could be given safe and acceptable care by nurses.

All *adolescent parents* need comprehensive services for health care. To make these services accesible will take the coordinated efforts of many disciplines. Educational programs for all adolescents should include courses in human sexuality and family living. Educational programs for pregnant schoolgirls need to be provided, not only to meet the special needs that result from the pregnancy, but to permit these young women to continue their education.

Continuity of care should include the entire childbearing and childrearing period. During pregnancy, care must be provided in a less fragmented manner. The psychosocial well-being of the entire family unit must be considered. One serious gap in the total care of the family occurs in the immediate postpartal period. Many women experience anxiety, fatigue, and depression in the early weeks following hospital discharge. Ways must be developed to assist them.

Realization of the above goals involves more than a commitment to saving lives. It must also include a commitment to improve the quality of life. Nursing must help individuals and families achieve a life worth living.

REFERENCES

1. Wooden, H. E.: *Impact of the Industrial Revolution on hospital maternity care.* Nurs. Forum 1:91, 1961.
2. Ibid.
3. *Maternity Care in the World.* Pergamon Press, London, 1966, p. 173.
4. Wooden: op. cit., p. 96.
5. Hardy, W.: *A ten year review of maternal mortality.* Obstet. Gynecol. 43:65, 1971.
6. Wegman, M. E.: *Vital statistics, 1972, with observations on China.* Pediatrics 52:873, 1973.
7. Publication OL-400-908. U. S. Government Printing Office, Washington, D.C.
8. Anderson, E. H. and Lesser, A. J.: *Maternity care in the United States: gains and gaps.* Am. J. Nurs. 66:1539, 1966.
9. Slatin, M.: *Extra protection for high risk mothers and babies.* Am. J. Nurs. 67:1241, 1967.
10. Pearse, W. H.: *The maternity and infant care program.* Obstet. Gynecol. 35:114, 1970.
11. Niswander, K. and Gordon, M.: *The Collaborative Perinatal Study: The Women and Their Pregnancies.* W. B. Saunders, Philadelphia, 1972.
12. *World Health Organization Technical Report Series, No. 51.* World Health Organization, Geneva, Switzerland, 1952.
13. U. S. Children's Bureau: *Some Facts—Figures about Children and Youth.* U. S. Government Printing Office, Washington, D. C., 1963.
14. Gold, E. M.: *A broad view of maternity care.* Children 9:52, 1962.
15. *Prelude to Action.* Maternity Center Association, New York, 1968, pp. 29–51.
16. Monahan, H. and Spenser, E.: *Deterrents to prenatal care.* Children 9:114, 1962.
17. Hilliard, M. E.: *New horizons in maternity care.* Nurs. Outlook 15:33, 1967.
18. Slatin, M.: *Why mothers bypass prenatal care.* Am. J. Nurs. 71:1388, 1971.
19. Ely, C., et al.: *Are maternity clinic dropouts necessary?* Am. J. Nurs. 67:41, 1967.
20. Wooden, H. E.: *The family-centered approach to maternity care.* Nurs. Forum 1:63, 1962.

UNIT 2

PSYCHOSOCIAL CONCEPTS

3 *Identity and the Self System*

RUTH FINNEY, Ph.D.

So great is our concern in the United States of the 70s with "identity"—its nature, pursuit, and possible loss—that ours has been described as the Identity Society.[1] The ability to contemplate self has long been considered uniquely human. Although recent work by Gallup[2] suggests that chimpanzees can become self-aware, apparently only humans become *preoccupied* with trying to answer the question "Who am I?" This chapter first defines the issues basic to a discussion of the concept of the self system. Some of the processes involved in the formation of self and identity are highlighted, with Erikson's theory presented as an example of one theory on the concept of identity. Finally, sex identity is explored, partly because we are so actively re-examining sex roles today but also because childbearing and childrearing are so obviously enmeshed in sex identity.

BASIC ISSUES

Gordon[3] asks people to answer the question "Who am I?" in order to measure self-concept. By asking this question of oneself and attending to the additional questions that come to mind while seeking the answer, one can anticipate the issues that are most important in determining definitions of self and identity.

Should one answer only about the way one is now? What about the past? Does that count? Perhaps one is trying to become something different in the future. Is that anticipated self, or even the effort toward it, part of who one is? There may also be a particular way one does not want to be and tries to avoid. Does one include that? Does one describe the way one is (or is not) in a single situation, or in many? If one thinks of many different situations or times, does one describe the way one *usually* is? What about the various ways, but perhaps only fleetingly displayed or experienced, in which one does different things in different places with different people? What about the things that other people think about one? Is that who one is? Perhaps one has a sense of a private person behind what others see and react to, and that is *really* who one is.

Now, if one goes on to wonder whether or not questions like these should be answered in terms of the way one is described in the answers, or in terms of the part of oneself that is doing the answering, or the part somehow observing the creating and answering of questions, one has covered the important issues that scholars consider when they both ask and seek to answer "What is identity?" "What is self?" "How are they different?"

Gergen[4] suggests five issues as the most important in discussions on self:

1. Fact or fiction?
2. The knower or the known?

3. A structure or a process?
4. One or many?
5. Consistent or inconsistent?

In addition, he feels that any definition should permit measurements to be made and predictions tested, that in some way "self" should be scientifically useful. Concerning his own definition, he states:

> In the search for a viable definition of self, we have had to face up to issues that have long provoked argument in the field. Perhaps we can crystallize the biases we have developed this far into a definition. The notion of self can be defined first as process and then as structure. On the former level we shall be concerned with that process by which the person conceptualizes (or categorizes) his behavior—both his external conduct and his internal states. On a structural level, our concern is with the system of concepts available to the person in attempting to define himself.[5]

THE ROLE OF OTHERS

The influence of other individuals plays an extremely important part in the development and maintenance of one's self and identity. Cooley[6] proposed the idea of the *looking glass self* which arises from social interaction and what one imagines are the results of others' appraisals of oneself. G. H. Mead[7] developed the idea further. One comes to see the way one is, he said, reflected in the ways others actually behave toward one, and then goes on to copy their behaviors and attitudes toward the self and to shape it accordingly. In the sixties, Kluckhohn[8] described a version of this line of thought when she suggested that families inadvertently influence their children's development with *implicit role models,* e.g., a parent might call one child "the little professor," and another "the dumbie." Thereby both the way others think of and act toward the children and the children's way of experiencing themselves could be affected. The verbal models would imply that different behaviors were to be rewarded in the children as well as rewarding to them. The work of Spiegel,[9] Kluckhohn's colleague, prompted De Levita[10] to stress the care that adults should take when they address or discuss the young in the latter's presence. Anyone on whom another is dependent should be cautioned similarly.

Gergen[11] points out that a parallel between what others think of one and what one thinks of oneself could result from one's influence on others rather than the reverse. Work by Videbeck[12] demonstrated that there was a direct effect on one's concept of self that resulted from the appraisals of others. Weinstein[13] offers the term altercasting for the process, which we all engage in, of expecting others to behave in particular ways according to the roles in which we cast them.

According to Gergen,[14] five processes contribute to the development of self-concept:

1. Labeling of dominant behavior patterns
2. Reflected appraisal
3. Social comparison
4. Biased scanning
5. Role-playing.

Biased scanning refers to the selective attention one can pay to the environment and memory in order to gather evidence that will reinforce an identity one favors. Role-playing can be limited to an "appropriate" time and place (when the complementary status is most clearly relevant), or extend into other situations if one identifies with the role even when "off stage," so to speak. Regarding reflected appraisal, he suggests that its effect on self-concept is greatest when the other 1) is believable as well as personalistic, 2) is for great change in self-conception and suggests this often, 3) is not contradicted, and 4) offers a positive appraisal.[15] To illustrate social comparison, he cites an experiment that he and Morse[16] conducted which showed that comparison of self with others could lead one to raise or lower self-esteem, depending on whether one appeared to be more or less of something socially desirable (or undesirable). He states:

> Such findings have broad implications. We have already discussed the significance that high self-esteem may have for one's mental well-being. These results suggest that one's level of self-regard may be vitally affected by the social surroundings in which he happened to find himself.[17]

Thus others affect self-concept to different degrees depending on the circumstances, including how important they are to us, in what way, how they present their attitudes or expectations, and whether these conflict with or complement those of others and ourselves. How and why we process, register, and respond varies and is a matter of ongoing research. However, minimum prerequisites for the development of self and identity are:

1. An individual
2. Significant others (as defined by family, peer or work group, ethnicity, history, or culture)
3. Recognition by others who can and do satisfy basic needs
4. Experience in separation from others
5. Ability to discriminate between others and self
6. Ability to copy others
7. Linguistic skills for communication
8. Ability to integrate and organize disparate experiences.

We tend to associate the development of self and identity with childhood, but when they are defined as processes there is no clear-cut time for their beginning and no necessary cut-off point during the life cycle. Horrocks and Jackson suggest that "a complete examination of the genesis of self should certainly give some consideration to the possibility of embryological origins."[18] They call attention to the work of Sontag and Wallace[19] on the reactions of the developing human organism in utero and state ". . . in the months before birth rudimentary aspects of a preself-awareness may be posited."[20] They refer to this as a "somatic self . . . probably the result of uterine circumstances, including stress experienced by the mother. . . ."[21] They feel that this is the foundation for more refined perceptions of the self which will be developed in interactions with others after birth.

BODY SCHEMA AND BODY IMAGE

In his review of body schema and body image, Nash[22] writes that these are sometimes incorrectly used as though they are interchangeable with self-concept. Head[23] introduced "body schema" and Schilder[24] provided the best known discussion of "body image." Nash distinguishes *body schema* as a " 'diagram' of the body . . . built up in the brain . . . by which coordinated, purposeful movements are carried out and by which the body parts and the body itself are oriented in space."[25] This schema may be influenced genetically, in utero, and by later learning. When the infant becomes aware of his or her body one then speaks of *body image*. The parents' cuddling and handling of their child helps achieve this awareness. Body image involves evaluations of the body:

> The child's concept of himself as a physical person is difficult to separate from the concept that he builds up of himself as a total person. There are periods in development when emphasis on the physical qualities of the individual become particularly marked, and at these times his physical attractions or deficiencies (whether actual or imagined)

may have a considerable influence on the development of his concept of himself as a person.[26]

Body image is but one part of self-concept, and is not equivalent to it, despite its importance and very basic contribution to it.

A survey by Berscheid and associates[27] reveals that Americans in general are more satisfied with their bodies than might be predicted, given the emphasis in our culture on attractive physical appearance. Nonetheless, "almost half of the women and about one third of the men said they are unhappy about their weight and twice as many women as men are *very* dissatisfied (21 per cent to 10 per cent)."[28] It was also found that the more attractive a woman is in her twenties the less happy and well adjusted she may be in her forties, a relationship perhaps influenced by the more dramatic changes likely in her physical appearance. As Americans grow older they may tend to gain weight and become dissatisfied with their appearance. This can generalize to include aspects of self or identity other than body image. During pregnancy, the effects of weight gain and other physical changes on the mother's body image must be considered when planning and providing nursing care. The nurse who gratuitously speculates about the likelihood of permanent changes in the body (size of parts, stria, etc.) may not be helping the pregnant woman cope with her changing body image. Also, there is some threat to the ego during pregnancy and this may affect body image.[29] Understanding the different ways in which women experience changes in their bodies during and after pregnancy is extremely relevant for nursing and requires further research.

ERIKSON, THE GARDENER OF IDENTITY

Since Erikson's work during the forties and fifties, psychologists have shown greater interest than ever in both self and identity. De Levita observes that growing interest within psychology in related areas of behavior, role, and function "made 'identity' shoot up like a miraculous tree with Erikson as its brilliant gardener, and its use has now become so common that writers no longer feel obliged to define the term."[30] Erikson himself comments, "The more one writes about this subject, the more the word becomes a term for something as unfathomable as it is all-pervasive."[31] After more than two hundred pages of his book *Identity, Youth and Crises,* Erikson looks back and remarks:

> So far I have tried out the term identity almost deliberately—I like to think—in many different connotations. At one time it seemed to refer to a conscious sense of individual uniqueness, at another to an unconscious striving for a continuity of experience and at a third as a solidarity with a group's ideal. . . .[32]

In his many-faceted explorations of identity, Erikson employs terms that may be new and confusing to the reader. For this reason, a discussion of some of these concepts is included here.

EGO IDENTITY AND IDENTITY CRISIS

For Erikson, the goals of identity might be said to include:

1. A consistent style of integrating past, present, and future choices and actions.
2. Self-awareness of a continuity of style.
3. Integration of disparate roles.
4. Acceptance by a group in a firm position that does not conflict with one's self-perceived style.
5. Self-esteem.

Erikson uses the term ego to refer to the

psychoanalytic concept for that part of a person that tests reality, organizes experiences with and within it, and in general is involved in the understanding and enjoyment of it to provide self-esteem and mutuality with others. Ego identity is not usually achieved before the end of childhood and is influenced by outcomes of previous developmental crises. Erikson believes that in adolescence there is a trial period immediately preceding the establishment of ego identity. During this time there is identity crisis, when different roles and styles may be tried out. This is a normal part of development and should not be confused with crises in later life when a person who has achieved ego identity loses it, perhaps never to regain it again depending on how the problem is viewed and treated.

NEGATIVE IDENTITY

Erikson's discussion of negative identity is particularly relevant for all concerned with youth. He describes psychiatric patients who are unable to achieve a positive ego identity and who, rather than remain confused, prefer—perhaps consciously—to commit themselves to being all the things "presented to them as most undesirable or dangerous and yet as most real."[33] In this way they are at least something. Adults in positions of authority who deal with young people should ask themselves if they respond in terms of what they don't (so they say) want the young to be rather than in terms of the positive things the young show capacities to become, but which may not be so real to the adults. Adults may want things for the young that were impossible for themselves and which may also be impossible for the next generation, which then sees how unrealistic their elders are and seeks a reality of sorts by becoming the opposite. We all know stories of perfection-demanding fathers whose sons became alcoholics, of would-be ladies whose daughters are devotedly not so. To Erikson these cases may be temporary and desperate efforts by the young to regain mastery of choice. However, by responding as though it is permanent, adults can lock the young into the negative identity.

Based on his work with psychiatric patients, Erikson sees a common pattern in the family backgrounds of young people with negative identities. The mothers are concerned with status and appearances rather than with real feelings. They love, but in an intrusive way that shows their own insatiable hunger for approval. They are apt to be jealous of the father as an object of the child's affections. Because of the impossibility of satisfying such a mother's needs, her child may gain a basic sense of failure. The father is apt to be successful or even outstanding in his work, but dependent on his wife and jealous of his child. With so little gratification forthcoming from parents, the children are likely to show especially strong attachments to any siblings, and/or early autism, and perhaps to have suffered some trauma involving separation from home.

Erikson believes that negative identity can be avoided if identity confusion is not treated as a permanent illness but as a route to possible wholeness:

> Teachers, judges, and psychiatrists [and nurses?] who deal with youth came to be significant representatives of that strategic act of "recognition," the act through which society "identifies" and "confirms" its young members and thus contributes to their developing identity. . . . If, for simplicity's sake or in order to accommodate ingrown habits of law or psychiatry, they diagnose and treat as a criminal, a constitutional misfit, as a derelict doomed by his upbringing, or indeed as a deranged patient, a young person who, for reasons of parental or social marginality, is close to choosing a negative identity, that young person may well put his energy into becoming exactly what the care-

> less and fearful community expects him to be—and make a total job of it.[34]

THE EPIGENETIC PRINCIPLE

This forms the basis for understanding the importance of history, culture, and ethnicity in identity formation. The epigenetic principle is derived from knowledge of how organisms systematically develop in a set way. Erikson says:

> Somewhat generalized, this principle states that anything that grows has a ground plan, and that out of this ground plan the parts arise, each part having its time of special ascendancy until all parts have arisen to form a functioning whole.[35]

If one could see a human sperm and ovum immediately after the sperm had penetrated, one would scarcely guess that a complex organism would result, one which we would recognize as a human baby. But that is what will happen, and in the same sequence for every fertilized egg of the same species. Once born, the organism continues to develop in a set way. Both before and after birth, the time of ascendancy for each part is also the critical period, the time when it is most vulnerable to danger and defect. The form to emerge exists before we see it and is influenced by the environment in which it develops. For Erikson, the rules derived from the epigenetic principle are true for psychosocial as well as physiologic development.

Application of the epigenetic principle to the formation of identity proposes that for all human beings in all periods of history the same developmental tasks appear in the same order and at the same rate. Interestingly, this view actually enhances the importance of culture. The *way* in which tasks are presented and the solutions emphasized as more or less likely and desirable depend on historical period, culture, and ethnicity.

GROUP IDENTITY

Erikson is suggesting, then, that the individual's life cycle and the history of his society are intrinsically bound. It is the family which first translates the values of a culture as seen in its institutions into what is "good" or "bad"—an opportunity for growth or crises—for the child. Erikson defines child training and group identity as:

> Child training . . . is the method by which a group's basic ways of organizing experience, or what we may call group identity, is transmitted to the infant's early bodily experiences, and, through them, to the beginnings of his ego.[36]

It was during his time spent with American Indians that the mutual complementation of ego identity and group identity became so clear to Erikson. Among them, he saw that individual acts, ceremonies, and rituals could become important symbols of their common methods for solving tasks at the critical periods of psychosocial development. One's developmental crises had been shared by others in the same group and solved in similar ways with similar lasting effects and styles of integrating experiences. Thus later, at the group level, symbols could both elicit and contribute shared meanings and energies.

WHOLENESS VERSUS TOTALITY

These are the two kinds of choices one makes throughout the life cycle. Erikson uses wholeness to refer to an assembly of very different parts into a whole which is productive and yet open to possible rearrangement of its parts or even the addition of new ones. By totality he means an entity with its parts set in one arrangement without any consideration of alternative ones and to which no other part may be added. The important distinction is that in wholeness, choice, organization, and integration are ongoing, but in a totality, there is no choice after the initial organization is made. Erikson believes that people's psyches can be organized by these principles. Wholeness in humans is healthy. Totality is not, except perhaps in an emergency.

Erikson speaks of wholeness in two ways. One refers to the continuity of self over time and space. The other refers to the complementary link between individual and group identity. So far as the latter is concerned, its achievement is the product of a series of crises of wholeness that develop following the epigenetic principle. Thus wholeness can only be achieved over time. It integrates the different times, events, and persons involved in one's life yet leaves one open to new growth through new experiences. This is done through the ego which not only offers a consistent style linking person and group but an ongoing one that blends self with ideal self throughout the life cycle.

CHOICES DURING THE EIGHT AGES OF MAN

Erikson proposes a series of developmental crises during the life cycle which offer choices between a positive (wholeness) and a negative (totality) outcome. What is chosen at an early crisis determines whether or not there is any real choice later. Only an early wholeness choice can leave one open to something new instead of the closed system of totality.

There are eight major choices accompanying different developmental periods (Fig. 3-1). As would be predicted by the epigenetic principle, each comes in the same order, at the same rate, for every human being. The first term of each pair is the wholeness choice; choosing it makes a later wholeness choice possible. The second term is the totality choice; choosing it prevents a later wholeness choice. At stake are the things that make life meaningful and satisfying to oneself and those with whom one lives. At the time of each choice crisis there is an opportunity for new growth, a refocusing of energy and relationship to one's group and its institutions. However, there is also a new, specific area of vulnerability.

The first choice, between a sense of basic trust or mistrust, comes during infancy. The second, which usually occurs in the second year, is between a sense of autonomy or shame. The third, which comes towards the end of the third year, is between a sense of initiative or guilt. The fourth choice is characteristic of the school years and involves a sense of industry or inferiority. The fifth choice, typical of adolescence, is crucial: a sense of identity or identity confusion. The task at this time is to bind into one all the part identifications of the past, along with the ideal identification, others' opinions, and new roles. When this fails, one has a negative (totality) outcome: one is not being what one really is. If one is to be able to make positive (wholeness) choices throughout the rest of life, one must first have a sense of identity. The sixth choice, between a sense of intimacy or isolation, comes in early adulthood. The seventh choice is between a sense of generativity or stagnation in adulthood. The eighth choice, that of the aging person, is between integrity or despair.

Erikson uses the following statements to characterize the parts of the sense of identity involved in these choices. These are the positive (wholeness) outcomes of each stage in turn:

1. I am what I hope to have and give.
2. I am what I can will freely.
3. I am what I imagine I can be.
4. I am what I can learn to make work.
5. I am what I might become; followed by: I am what I am.
6. I am what I love.
7. I am what I care for.
8. I am what survives of me.[37]

The seriousness of all that is involved is best conveyed by Erikson himself:

From the stages of life, then, such disposi-

VIII MATURITY								EGO INTEGRITY VS. DESPAIR
VII ADULTHOOD							GENERATIVITY VS. STAGNATION	
VI YOUNG ADULTHOOD						INTIMACY VS. ISOLATION		
V PUBERTY AND ADOLESCENCE					IDENTITY VS. ROLE CONFUSION			
IV LATENCY				INDUSTRY VS. INFERIORITY				
III LOCOMOTOR-GENITAL			INITIATIVE VS. GUILT					
II MUSCULAR-ANAL		AUTONOMY VS. SHAME, DOUBT						
I ORAL SENSORY	BASIC TRUST VS. MISTRUST							
	1	2	3	4	5	6	7	8

FIGURE 3-1. The eight ages of man. (From Erikson, E. H.: *Childhood and Society*, ed. 2, revised. W. W. Norton, New York, 1963, with permission.)

tions as faith, will power, purposefulness, competence, fidelity, love, care, wisdom—all criteria of vital individual strength—also flow into the life of institutions. Without them, institutions wilt; but without the spirit of institutions pervading the patterns of care and love, instruction and training, no strength could emerge from the sequence of generations.[38]

SEX IDENTITY AND CHANGING SEX ROLES

Kagan observes that "of the many attributes that go into concept of self one of the most important is sex-role identity."[39] Children learn sex-role standards as they do other categories and the content varies according to time and place. After all, how does one judge "masculinity" or "femininity" if not with regard to "what most men do" and "what most women do." When a person's subjective judgment of self matches the standards of the ideal for a person of the same sex in the same community, Kagan says there is a firm sex-role identity; when it does not, a weak one. In our own society, sex-role standards are being actively re-examined and ideals may be shifting. Yet "traditional" standards still wield considerable influence on individual sex-role identities and on the way we experience others.

The work of Broverman and associates[40] suggests that in our culture members of the mental health professions—both male and female—equate characteristics of "healthy adult" with those of "healthy male," but not "healthy female." Independence, objectivity, aggression, dominance, adventurousness, and self-confidence are not considered healthy so often for women as for men. Instead,

> . . . clinicians are more likely to suggest that healthy women differ from healthy men by being more submissive, less independent, less adventurous, more easily influenced, less aggressive, less competitive, more excitable in minor crises, having their feelings more easily hurt, being more emotional, more conceited about their appearance, less objective, and disliking math and science. This constellation seems a most unusual way of describing any mature, healthy individual.[41]

Chesler[42] has conducted extensive interviews which further substantiate the view that clinicians are prejudiced against women as being much less than healthy adults.

Whether or not nurses and obstetricians share these views would be an interesting research question. For instance, might the woman patient who knows exactly what kind of delivery she wants and who seeks information about her progress in technical terms be viewed as "unhealthy" because she is not "submissive" and thus not "feminine"? This could also make her threatening to female nurses and doctors who pride themselves on being more traditional. It is interesting to note that in Tanzer's[43] report a sample of women who chose natural rather than "traditional" childbirth methods were *not* significantly different physiologically or psychologically from those who chose the latter. She observes, "Contrary to a common assumption, it is not a certain 'type' of woman who chooses natural childbirth."[44] Instead, she argues, it is exposure to a course in natural childbirth methods that makes the difference.

Bardwick's[45] review helps clarify Freud's theories related to the development of sex identity which are an important source of bias against women. According to Freud, the young boy may resolve his conflict with his father over the mother as a sex object by identifying with the father. To do this successfully requires the development of a strong super-ego which can transform into identification the son's hostile feelings toward the father and his fears that the father will retaliate and castrate him. For the young girl there is penis envy which Freud says gives her "natural" feelings of inferiority. She blames her mother "for cheating her of a penis and turns to her father for a penis or a child."[46] Instead of being competitive with boys (said to reflect a state of penis envy) the healthy girl, according to Freud,[47] will seek a penis as an organ to give her a child, preferably one with a penis to compensate for her own lack. Both passivity and masochism are regarded by Freudians as truly feminine, as are greater anxiety and dependence, all the result, in the Freudian view, of the young female not needing to resolve an Oedipus complex in the same dramatic way as is required of a boy. The result is that a woman's super-ego is "naturally" weaker.

Although Bardwick does not agree with Freud's reasons for it, she does observe that females demonstrate less often than males the traits which Broverman's subjects cite as healthy in adults. Her own view is that this results from strong biologic influences. In support of this, she cites examples of sex differences among 3-year-olds, and claims they are evidence that cultural influences cannot be paramount. However, recent work by Goldberg and Lewis[48] has shown that mothers do handle boys and girls in markedly different ways even before the children are 6 months old. The differences can be systematically related to contrasting behaviors displayed at 13 months of age by the two sexes toward their mothers. Cultural influences, then, can hardly be excluded when considering sex-role differences.

Money and Ehrhandt's[49] studies of hermaphrodites also attest to the influence upbringing has on sex-identity. When sex assignment for hermaphrodites varied but gonadal sex was constant, their subjective gender identity tended to be that of assignment. Whiting's[50] discussion of sex-identity indicates that there may be different conscious and unconscious components. One's primary identity is said to be the same as that of the parent who controlled resources important to one as an infant and who was then "copied" in an effort to gain that control for oneself. The sex of the secondary identity is thought to be influenced by one's peers during adolescence. Thus, there may be conflict between the two. For example, a male with a primary female sex identity may engage in super-masculine "protest" behavior as an adolescent in an effort to prove to peers and himself that he is really male.

One of the classics on culture and sex-role differences is M. Mead's *Sex and Temperment in Three Primitive Societies*[51] which offers an example of one culture wherein the healthy female is dominant and aggressive while the male is nurturant. In a second culture, both male and female resemble the "healthy male" of the Broverman study, and in a third culture, both are more like her "healthy female." Rosenberg and Sutton-Smith regard the assumption of inevitable sex-role differences between the sexes as perhaps "archaic and a typological error."[52] They point out that in the past individuals have been assumed to be divisable into types that are no longer considered applicable. They note that perhaps the most important areas of change relevant to sex-role alternatives are childbirth and childrearing "which no longer seem to be the irrevocable barrier they once were to the removal of sex role stereotypes."[53] Not only are women taking a more independent role in these areas, but men are taking a more nurturant one.

Young boys, too, are being exposed to new alternatives for sex roles that sanction participation in child care as an appropriate part of masculinity. *Free to be You and Me*[54] and *William's Doll*[55] are examples of changing sex roles being presented in today's children's literature.

Brazelton[56] has observed that he knows of no society which depends on the strength of the male for its economic production and which also permits males to participate in the birth process, because males would be "hooked" through ethologically based "signals" from the newborn infant which would release nurturant behavior in the new fathers and thus distract them from their vital role in the economy. Jobs in our own industrial, mechanized economy are not so intrinsically "sexist" as those in, say, a hunting culture, so far as the economic survival of a society is concerned. Thus, males may participate more freely during delivery. This participation has many potential benefits. In addition to leading to a possible peak for the mother in natural childbirth, it can lay the basis for stronger family relations and a more nurturant role for fathers.

Nurses must become aware of any prejudices which they or their coworkers may have toward women or toward the expectant father's participation in the childbirth process. In these days of shifting sex roles it is more appropriate to think of *parent* and child rather than mother and child as the appropriate unit for health care. Psychology and the helping sciences related to it have too long neglected the role of the father.[57] Bailyn[58] emphasizes the perhaps surprising extent to which men may already derive primary satisfaction from their families rather than their work alone. She points out that identifying the conditions under which men find it possible to give primary emphasis to their families while at the same time functioning satisfactorily in their own careers may be particularly important for understanding and supporting new alternatives for sex-role standards.

Hopefully, open-minded professionals in all health fields can and will provide health care environments that both recognize and sanction new alternatives for both sexes' participation in the anticipation, delivery, and care of children, without threat to the sex identities of those concerned.

REFERENCES

1. Glasser, W.: *The Identity Society.* Harper and Row, New York, 1972.
2. Gallup, Jr., G.: *It's Done with Mirrors—Chimps and Self-Concept.* Psychology Today 4:58, 1971.
3. Gordon, C.: *Self-conceptions: configurations of content.* In Gordon, C. and Gergen, K. J. (eds.): *Self in Social Interaction.* Wiley, New York, 1968.
4. Gergen, K. J.: *The Concept of Self.* Holt, Rinehart and Winston, New York, 1971, p. 13.
5. Ibid., pp. 22, 23.
6. Cooley, C. H.: *Human Nature and the Social Order.* Scribner, New York, 1922.
7. Mead, G. H.: *Mind, Self and Society.* University of Chicago Press, Chicago, 1934.
8. Kluckhohn, F.: Unpublished lecture. Prosemenar in social relations, Harvard University, Cambridge, Massachusetts, 1962.
9. Spiegel, L.: *The self, the sense of self and perception.* Psychoanal. Study Child, XIV:81, 1959.
10. De Levita, D. J.: *The Concept of Identity.* Mouton & Co., Paris, 1965.
11. Gergen: op. cit., p. 41.
12. Videbeck, R.: *Self-Conception and the Reaction of Others.* Sociometry 23:351, 1960.
13. Weinstein, A.: *Altercasting and interpersonal relations.* In Secord, P. and Bachman, C. (eds.): *Readings in Social Psychology.* Prentice-Hall, Englewood Cliffs, 1967.
14. Gergen: loc. cit.
15. Ibid., p. 49.
16. Gergen, K. J. and Morse, S. J.: *Self-consistency: measurement and validation.* Proceedings of the American Psychological Association, 1967, pp. 207, 208.
17. Ibid., p. 52.
18. Horrocks, J. E. and Jackson, D. W.: *Self and Role: A Theory of Self Process and Role Behavior.* Houghton Mifflin, Boston, 1972, pp. 11, 12.
19. Sontag, L. W. and Wallace, R. F.: *The movement response of the human fetus to sound stimuli.* Child Dev. 6:253, 1935.
20. Hurrocks and Jackson: op. cit., p. 10.
21. Ibid.
22. Nash, J.: *Developmental Psychology, A Psychobiological Approach.* Prentice-Hall, Englewood Cliffs, 1970.
23. Head, H.: *Studies and Neurology, vol. II.* Hodder and Stoughton and Oxford University Press, London, 1920.
24. Schilder, P.: *The Image and Appearance of the Human Body.* International University Press, New York, 1950.
25. Nash: op. cit., p. 461.
26. Ibid., p. 464.
27. Berscheid, E., Walster, E. and Bohrnstedt, G.: *Body image, the happy American body: A Survey Report.* Psychology Today 7:119, 1974.
28. Ibid., p. 121.
29. McConnell, O. L. and Daston, P. G.: *Body image changes in pregnancy.* J. Project. Techn. 25:451, 1962.
30. De Levita: op. cit., p. 65.
31. Erikson, E. H.: *Identity, Youth and Crises.* Norton, New York, 1958, p. 9.
32. Ibid., p. 208.
33. Ibid., p. 174.
34. Ibid., p. 196.
35. Ibid., p. 92.
36. Ibid., pp. 47, 48.
37. Ibid., pp. 107, 114, 122, 127, 138, 141.
38. Ibid., p. 141.
39. Kagan, J.: *Check one: □ male □ female.* In *The Female Experience.* C.R.M., Inc., Del Mar, 1974, p. 51.
40. Broverman, I., et al.: *Sex-role stereotypes and clinical judgments of mental health.* In Bardwick, J. (ed.): *Readings in the Psychology of Women.* Harper and Row, New York, 1972.
41. Ibid., p. 322.
42. Chesler, P.: *Women and Madness.* Avon Books. New York, 1973, p. 23.
43. Tanzer, D.: *Natural childbirth: pain or peak experience.* In *The Female Experience.* C.R.M., Inc., Del Mar, 1974.
44. Ibid., p. 28.

45. Bardwick, J. *The Psychology of Women: A Study of Biocultural Conflicts.* Harper and Row, New York, 1971.
46. Ibid., p. 6.
47. Freud, S.: *The psychology of women.* In *New Introductory Lectures on Psychoanalysis,* trans. W. J. H. Sprott. Norton, New York, 1933.
48. Goldberg, S. and Lewis, M.: *Play behavior in the year-old infant: early sex differences.* In Bardwick, J. (ed.): *Readings on the Psychology of Women.* Harper and Row, New York, 1972.
49. Money, J. and Ehrhardt, A.: *Man & Woman, Boy & Girl.* Johns Hopkins University Press, Baltimore, 1972.
50. Whiting, J. W. M.: *Comment.* Am. J. Sociol., 67:391, 1962.
51. Mead, M.: *Sex and Temperment in Three Primitive Societies.* William Morrow, New York, 1932.
52. Rosenberg, B. G. and Sutton-Smith, B.: *Sex and Identity.* Holt, Rinehart and Winston, New York, 1972.
53. Ibid., pp. 88, 89.
54. Thomas, M.: *Free to be You and Me,* McGraw-Hill, New York, 1974.
55. Zolotow, C.: *William's Doll.* Harper and Row, New York, 1972.
56. Brazelton, B.: Unpublished lecture. School of Public Health, University of Hawaii, December, 1973.
57. Benson, J.: *Fatherhood, a Sociological Perspective.* Random House, New York, 1968.
58. Bailyn, L.: *Career and family orientations of husbands and wives in relation to marital happiness.* In Bardwick, J. (ed.): *Readings in the Psychology of Women.* Harper and Row, New York, 1972.

BIBLIOGRAPHY

Bardwick, J.: *The Psychology of Woman, A Study of Biocultural Conflicts.* Harper and Row, New York, 1971.

Benson, J.: *Fatherhood, a Sociological Perspective.* Random House, New York, 1968.

De Levita, D. J.: *The Concept of Identity.* Mouton & Co., Paris, 1965.

Erikson, E. H.: *Identity, Youth and Crises.* Norton, New York, 1958.

Gergen, K. J.: *The Concept of Self.* Holt, Rinehart and Winston, New York, 1971.

Glasser, W.: *The Identity Society.* Harper and Row, New York, 1972.

Gordon, C. and Gergen, K. J. (eds.): *Self in Social Interaction.* Wiley, New York, 1968.

Horrocks, J. E. and Jackson, D. W.: *Self and Role: A Theory of Self Process and Role Behavior.* Houghton Mifflin, Boston, 1972.

Mead, G. H.: *Mind, Self and Society.* University of Chicago Press, Chicago, 1934.

Mead, M.: *Sex and Temperment in Three Primitive Societies.* William Morrow, New York, 1932.

Money, J. and Ehrhardt, A.: *Man & Woman, Boy & Girl.* Johns Hopkins University Press, Baltimore, 1972.

Rosenberg, B. G. and Sutton-Smith, B.: *Sex and Identity.* Holt, Rinehart and Winston, New York, 1972.

4 *Role Theory*

JEAN L. J. LUM, R.N., Ph.D.

Individuals occupy numerous positions in society. In the course of interacting with one another, stable, recognizable patterns of behavior emerge. How and why does this phenomenon occur? Role theory provides a conceptual orientation for understanding how individuals function and affect one another within a social context.

The term *role* refers to "the functions a person performs when occupying a particular characterization (position) within a particular social context."[1] It thus includes both the position itself as well as its associated expectations. Various roles are interrelated since one person's role is partially dependent upon the roles of related others in the social context. The term *theory* refers to a set of interrelated hypotheses or propositions concerning a phenomenon or set of phenomena. Theory provides a convenient way of organizing data. In addition, it helps us to move beyond empirical data and recognize implications and relationships not evident from any single datum. It guides research and leads to predictions about events not yet observed. Theory seeks to explain, predict, and control phenomenon.

While the field of role has many of the components which comprise a theory (e.g., a body of knowledge, a characteristic research endeavor, a domain of study, many hypotheses and theories concerning particular aspects of its domain, a particular perspective, and a rich language system), it has yet to be integrated into a single monolithic theory that the term role theory implies.[2] Therefore, in this chapter role theory is viewed as a conceptual framework or orientation presenting a set of concepts, rather than as a deductive system yielding highly integrated propositions.

BASIC ROLE CONCEPTS

The concepts of role theory provide an excellent approach for analyzing and understanding social behavior. A *concept* is a word that expresses an abstraction based on observed events or their inferences. Concepts and their definitions make up the language of role theory and provide the means for communication about the objects of study. There are scores of words in the role vocabulary, and elaboration and refinement of its language continue. Thus, the following discussion presents only the most important and relevant concepts of role theory.

POSITION

A *position* is a collectively recognized category of persons occupying a specified place in a social structure. Persons in a particular category are thus recognized because they possess certain common attributes, exhibit similar behaviors, or evoke common reactions from others toward themselves.

Age, sex, and ethnic background are examples of common attributes which distinguish people of different categories. The positions of children, teenager, and adult are age-graded; male and female denote sex differences; and Scandinavian, Hawaiian, and Oriental designate ethnic derivations. Persons occupying positions such as teacher, student, and nurse behave similarly in selected ways. Categories of persons designated as minorities, scapegoats, and outcasts are differentiated mainly by the similar ways in which other people treat them. Thus a person may simultaneously occupy numerous positions, e.g., a young female, wife, mother, daughter, aunt, nurse, Hawaiian, college-educated person, club member, and many others.

Some positions are ascribed on the basis of what a person is in terms of age, sex, or family connections (e.g., a 25-year-old wife). Others are achieved based on what the person can do (e.g., nurse and teacher). A position may involve life-long tenure (e.g., female and daughter), or may only be briefly held (e.g., club member). They also vary in the degree of ease with which the individual moves from one position to another and in the degree to which the position is collectively recognized. Positions are necessarily a relational concept and thus denote complementary positions. For example, the complementary position for teacher is student; for daughter, parents; for wife, husband; for nurse, patient; and so forth.

To function appropriately, the individual must be able to accurately locate himself in relation to others in the social structure. He must consider the position of others on the basis of observed cues, appearances, and behaviors. Identifying symbols include names for the position (e.g., physician, policeman), clothing and artifacts (e.g., uniforms, badges of office, jewelry), speech, gestures, and facial expressions (e.g., salutes, bows), and physical location (e.g., home, school, office). The accuracy which which a person recognizes such cues and draws conclusions about the position of the other is directly related to the accuracy with which he locates his position. Recognition of these cues about others and location of self in the social structure lead to predictable role behaviors in interactional situations. These behaviors are largely determined by the role expectations associated with respective positions.

ROLE EXPECTATIONS

The concept of role expectations is central to role theory. A wide range of interchangeable terms is used for this concept including norms, prescriptions, rule, and role demands. *Role expectations* refer to "the rights and privileges, the duties and obligations, of any occupant of a social position in relation to persons occupying other positions in the social structure."[3] Role expectations serve as significant guides and standards for appropriate conduct and behavior.

Secord and Backman[4] discuss role expectations in terms of their anticipatory and normative qualities of interaction. Anticipatory expectations are used by a person to predict the manner in which another will respond to him or to a particular situation. These anticipations and predictions are usually made on the basis of past experiences. The normative nature of role expectations refers to the obligatory qualities of a given position. Normative expectations represent what a person "should" or "ought" to do in a given position and situation. Biddle and Thomas[5] refer to the "shoulds" and "oughts" that are internalized as norms while those that are overtly expressed are referred to as role demands. In the course of socialization, many role demands are internalized by the person and become covertly held norms.

Role expectations differ in content and structure as a function of the viewpoint perceived by the person assessing the role expectations. Smooth social interaction occurs when persons hold reciprocal knowledge of one another's role expectations and take into account the role behavior of their partner in the interaction. For example, in the categories of husband and wife, the role obligations of the husband specify certain rights and privileges for the wife, and the role obligations of the wife specify certain rights and privileges for the husband. This relationship consists of expectations applicable to the occupant of a position in relation to occupant of a single complementary position. Generally, however, the occupant of a particular position interacts with occupants of numerous complementary positions. For example, a college president is involved in a set of expectations with such role partners as faculty member, student, dean, and regent. In all of these situations, the person remains in the position of college president but behaves differently during interaction with each of the occupants of the complementary roles as specified by appropriate role expectations. Role expectations generally facilitate social interaction by providing a means of reciprocal prediction of behavior for the interactants.

A qualitative note is also incorporated into role expectations in that the occupant of a position is not only expected to perform certain acts and not others, but is also expected to perform actions in specified ways. Thus, a mother is expected not only to feed and clothe her child but also to demonstrate qualities of love, affection, warmth, and tenderness while performing her acts of nurturance.

Role expectations are influenced by many other important factors. They vary in terms of their generality or specificity. In highly structured bureaucracies, precise behaviors are outlined while in other situations, role expectations provide only broad guidelines, leaving the occupant of the position a wide range of acceptable behaviors from which to choose. There are also differences in the area of extensiveness. Some role expectations have relevance only to a narrowly circumscribed portion of a person's position. Others, particularly those related to age and sex roles, apply to a larger proportion of a person's role repertoire. Role expectations vary in relation to formal or informal positions. Those for many formal positions are well known to most people while those for informal roles are less clear. They also differ in their degree of clarity. Thus expectations vary in permissiveness, completeness, complexity, and in the degree to which they are understood and accepted. Diversity among the dimensions of role expectations can lead to discrepancies in predictions of behaviors and thus affect social interaction.

ROLE PERFORMANCE

Role performance refers to behaviors displayed by a person which are relevant to the role he is enacting. Role expectations and role performance should be distinguished from each other. In contrast to normative role expectations which specify how a person is supposed to behave, role performance refers to the actual behaviors displayed in a particular interactional situation. These behaviors may or may not conform to expectations. The actual behavior of particular individuals may deviate markedly from normative expectations if they do not fit their roles very well.

In addition, considerable variation may be observed in the manner in which different persons behave while enacting the same role or in which the same person behaves while enacting the same role on different occasions. This is possible because role expectations provide a relatively wide range of acceptable behaviors. Many different behaviors may fulfill the expectations for a given role. For example, if disciplining children is perceived to be an expectation of the father role, particular fathers may discipline their children in different ways (e.g., by physical punishment, psychologic deprivation, tongue lashing, and so forth). Role theory thus allows for the enactment of alternative acceptable modes of role behaviors while classifying persons into categories and attributing relatively uniform expectations to a given category.

The number of roles which a person enacts also influences his role performance ability. A person with a repertoire of a variety of well practiced, realistic social roles is better able to meet new and critical situations and to deal effectively with others than the person with a meager, relatively unpracticed, and socially unrealistic repertoire.

The intensity with which a person enacts various roles is another area in which variations in role performance are observed. Sarbin[6] proposes seven levels of organismic involvement in the degree to which the self is involved during role enactment. His levels range from noninvolvement at the lowest level of enactment, to a ritualistic, mechanical performance where the self and role are clearly differentiated, to a level of complete integration of self and role at the highest level of enactment. In this highest level, the performance is so intensified that self and role become undifferentiated.

Along another dimension, Goffman[7] discusses the particular impressions an individual attempts to make on others during his presentation of performance. He was particularly interested in the expressive characteristics of role performance and in the individual's attempts to convey to others, either covertly or overtly, those aspects of himself that he wished to be known. The concept of front was used to refer to that part of an individual's performance which he constructed to define the situation for those who observed the performance in order to impress them with the fact that he was living up to the idealized aspects of a given role. For example, a college professor might display numerous scholarly journals on his bookshelves to convey to others that he is living up to expectations of himself as a scholar while concealing his interest in detective stories by keeping these out of sight. He thus constructs a role-consistent front which impresses others with his fulfillment of role expectations by selectively exposing limited facets of himself.

Role performance is also influenced by the amount of time a person spends in one role relative to the amount he spends in other roles. Generally, greater variability in time spent in a given role is associated with roles of an achieved rather than an ascribed nature. For example, ascribed positions such as female, adult, and mother involve being in the role all the time. However, a person can move in and out of an achieved position such as nurse, teacher, or musician.

SELF-ROLE CONGRUENCE

Social roles are perceived and enacted against the background of the self and the individual personality. In the process of interacting with the social environment, a person begins to experience a sense of self and assumes characteristics as a consequence of the roles he enacts. He recognizes that others react to him, and he in turn begins to react to his own actions as he expects others to react. In taking the viewpoint of others and seeing oneself as an object, a person begins to develop a *self-concept* with corresponding beliefs and attitudes about himself.[8] He then attempts to behave, and tries to get others to behave toward him, in ways that are consistent with his self-concept. Other things being equal, role enactment is more effective, proper, appropriate, and convincing when self-characteristics are congruent with role expectations and requirements. In addition, the presence or absence of particular attributes may facilitate or interfere with successful role enactment on the basis of the individual's physical characteristics, abilities, skills, personality traits, academic degree or other evidence of certification. In situations in which a person is assigned a role within his capabilities, incompatibilities in role performance may still result if the role does not allow him to make use of his skills and abilities, is not suited to his personality and temperament, or otherwise does not meet his needs. Conditions and circumstances which make it difficult for a person to perform in accordance with role expectation result in role strain. Congruence of self and role along the dimensions of similarity in traits, values, beliefs, and skills, leads to more effective social interaction and a more enjoyable, involved, and committed role performance.

MULTIPLE ROLES

A person usually occupies many positions and enacts numerous roles during the course of a typical day. Some roles are enacted successively while in other situations multiple role obligations occur simultaneously. In some instances successive role enactment is cyclic in nature. For example, the succession from occupational role during working hours to father role at home is repeated daily. In other instances successive enactment of many different roles over a period of time is nonrepetitive. An example is the successive enactment of age roles as an individual moves through the life cycle. Ceremonies and other rites of passage facilitate transitions into successive roles by specifying the abandonment of old roles and the acquisition of new ones (e.g., graduation, marriage and the honeymoon, retirement).

In the simultaneous enactment of two or more roles a person may activate one role while keeping the others latent, may alternate roles within a given period of time, or may integrate several roles in his performance. Multiple role demands may pose serious difficulties to a person's ability to fulfill role obligations unless the allocation of time and resources among the various roles is handled in a satisfactory manner. Important factors influencing this allocation are the individual's norm commitment and the reaction by role partners in terms of anticipated rewards or punishments. Some roles are more important to the person than others and therefore take precedence. In addition, there is a socially accepted hierarchy of role evaluation in which crisis determines priority.

Enactment of a large number of roles has advantages in better preparing individuals to meet life experiences. However, a lack of effective coordination among multiple roles can result in conflicting expectations and other difficulties.

ROLE CONSENSUS AND CONFLICT

As mentioned previously, role behavior does not always conform to the expectations associated with a role category. The degree of consensus for various aspects of a role varies from complete agreement (*consensus*), through polarization (*conflict*), to complete disagreement (*dissensus*). The concepts of role consensus and role conflict are explored here in greater detail in terms of their importance in meeting role expectations.

Clarity and Consensus

The degree of clarity and consensus regarding role expectations for various role categories differs among people in a society. Generally, when role expectations are explicit it is easier to conform to them. However, when they are unclear, different interpretations arise and an individual is uncertain as to what is expected of him. Newly emerging roles, in particular, often lack clarity. Also, successive or rapid changes in a role result in unclear expectations. For example, the women's liberation movement has resulted in changes in the expectations of the role of women in society. Men and women are thus in the process of redefining expectations for themselves and redefining their relations to each other.

Various types of disagreement concerning role expectations are recognized as a consequence of lack of clarity and consensus. These include disagreement on 1) what expectations are included for a given position, 2) the range of permitted or prohibited behavior, 3) the situations to which the role expectations apply, 4) whether the expected behavior is mandatory or preferred, 5) which expectations should take precedence when there are conflicts, and 6) what constitutes an equitable exchange in role rights and obligations.[9]

Mechanisms to increase clarity and consensus involve various communication strategies to reconcile and accommodate differences. Such attempts may range from informal "heart to heart" talks to formal written statements of expectations. Compatibility of norms affects reciprocal expectations in role performance. Role fulfillment is enhanced when there is clarity and consensus and is inhibited when they are lacking.

Conflict and Competition

Simultaneous occupancy of two or more positions having incompatible role expectations results in inter-role conflict. Contradictory expectations held by two or more persons or groups regarding the same role results in intrarole conflict. Competition among expectations occurs when time limitations affect a person's ability to fulfill two or more expectations. An example of conflict between role expectations is that of the military chaplain performing the incompatible roles of religious leader and military officer. Competition due to time allocation is exemplified by a university professor who must allocate time to fulfill his responsibilities in teaching, research, and community service.

Various measures can be employed to reduce conflicts in role expectations. Arranging role obligations in a hierarchy of priorities aids in determining which take precedence over others. Structural features for reducing conflict include the differences in the power of the various role partners to exert sanctions, restrictions on multiple position occupancy, temporal and spatial separation of situations involving conflicting expectations, and insulation from observations of complementary position occupants. Compromising conflicting roles by merging them into a single role also helps reduce strain. Other techniques involve changing beliefs regarding incompatible roles by providing meanings and interpretations which make them compatible. A past history of success in using a particular technique, social reinforcement from significant others, and availability of particular measures influence the selection of strategies to resolve strain arising from incompatible role expectations.

ROLE LEARNING

Most role behavior is learned behavior. It is through the process of socialization that role learning takes place. *Socialization* is the interactional process whereby a person's behavior is modified to conform to the expectations of the group or groups to which he belongs. It includes not only a child's acquisition of adult behaviors but also an adult's acquisition of behaviors appropriate to the expectations associated with new positions in the larger society. Thus, socialization continues throughout the life cycle.

Role learning includes learning role expectations associated with the individual's own role as well as the specifications for other complementary roles. Therefore, adequately learning a role requires the learning of the entire role set. In many instances, the role aspirant acquires the attitudes, beliefs, values, and skills associated with a new role from the more experienced occupants of the position. Strauss[10] refers to this integral part of teaching the inexperienced as coaching. The coach, using his own special skills and prior training, can guide and advise the novice and thus help him to master his new role. The coach also serves as a model for the learner. In such relationships, learning results from identification with and imitation of the role model. In addition, the coach or teacher serves an important function by providing social reinforcement to the learner through positive and negative sanctions. Praise and criticism not only provide incentives for the learner, but also furnish feedback on the progress he is making in his performance.

In other cases, the individual may utilize anticipatory socialization to acquire new behaviors characteristic of a position which he is about to occupy but of which he is not currently a member.[11] By anticipating what these new behaviors are, an individual prepares himself and eases his entry into the new role. Role-taking and role-playing are other terms used to describe the interrelated processes of acquisition, training, practice, and preparation for a new role. In role-taking the person constructs the other's role in his imagination, while in role-playing he enacts what he conceives to be his appropriate role in a given situation. In this manner both complementary and self-roles can be rehearsed. Through evaluation and validation by self and others, the individual acquires appropriate role expectations and behaviors for given positions in a particular social context according to some adopted standard. Such a standard for normative and comparative measures is provided by an individual's reference group or groups. The reference group thus sets and enforces standards of conduct and belief against which the person compares himself and others. A reference group may be a membership or a nonmembership group. While groups to which a person belongs serve as a frame of reference for self-evaluation and attitude formation, a person may not need to be an actual member of a group to use it as a reference group. These significant others provide additional social support in helping a person function appropriately in his social roles.

REFERENCES

1. Shaw, M. E. and Costanzo, P. R.: *Theories of Social Psychology.* McGraw-Hill, New York, 1970, p. 326.
2. Thomas, E. J. and Biddle, B. J.: *The nature and history of role theory.* In Biddle, B. J. and Thomas E. J. (eds.): *Role Theory: Concepts and Research.* John Wiley & Sons, New York, 1966, pp. 3–19.
3. Sarbin, T. R. and Allen, V. L.: *Role theory.* In Lindzey, G. and Aronson, E. (eds.): *The Handbook of Social Psychology, vol. 1.* Addison-Wesley, Reading, 1968, p. 497.
4. Secord, P. F. and Backman, C. W.: *Social Psychology.* McGraw-Hill, New York, 1964, pp. 453–467.
5. Biddle, B. J. and Thomas, E. J. (eds.): *Role Theory: Concepts and Research.* John Wiley & Sons, New York, 1966.
6. Sarbin and Allen: op. cit., pp. 492–497.
7. Goffman, E.: *The Presentation of Self in Everday Life.* Doubleday, New York, 1959.
8. Mead, G. H.: *Mind, Self, and Society.* University of Chicago Press, Chicago, 1934.
9. Secord and Backman: op. cit., pp. 468–493.
10. Strauss, A. L.: *Mirrors and Masks.* The Free Press, Glencoe, 1959.
11. Morton, R. K.: *Social Theory and Social Structure.* The Free Press, New York, 1957, pp. 265–271.

BIBLIOGRAPHY

Biddle, B. J. and Thomas, E. J.: *Role Theory: Concepts and Research.* John Wiley & Sons, New York, 1966.

Clausen, J. A. (ed.): *Socialization and Society.* Little, Brown and Company, Boston, 1968.

Deutsch, M. and Krauss, R. M.: *Theories in Social Psychology.* Basic Books, New York, 1965.

Goffman, E.: *The Presentation of Self in Everyday Life.* Doubleday, New York, 1959.

Gordon, C. and Gergen, K. J. (eds.): *The Self in Social Interaction.* John Wiley & Sons, New York, 1968.

Goslin, D. A. (ed.): *Handbook of Socialization Theory and Research.* Rand McNally, Chicago, 1969.

Homans, G. C.: *Contemporary theory in sociology.* In Faris, R. E. (ed.): *Handbook of Modern Sociology.* Rand McNally, Chicago, 1964.

Mead, G. H.: *Mind, Self, and Society.* University of Chicago Press, Chicago, 1934.

Morton, R. K.: *Social Theory and Social Structure.* The Free Press, New York, 1957.

Sarbin, T. R. and Allen, V. L.: *Role theory.* In Lindzey, G. and Aronson, E. (eds.): *The Handbook of Social Psychology, vol. 1.* Addison-Wesley, Reading, 1968.

Secord, P. F. and Backman, C. W.: *Social Psychology.* McGraw-Hill, New York, 1964.

Shaw, M. E. and Costanzo, P. R.: *Theories of Social Psychology.* McGraw-Hill, New York, 1970.

Strauss, A. L.: *Mirrors and Masks.* The Free Press, Glencoe, 1959.

5 *Joy*

EMILIE D. HENNING, R.N., Ed.D.

Understanding the concept of joy and its influence on human behavior is essential to the practice of maternal and child care nursing. What is joy? What are the sources of joy? How can one attain joy? In answering these questions, descriptions and theories related to joy are discussed with emphasis on its implications for the family during childbearing and childrearing.

DEFINITIONS

Joy has been defined in many ways. Basically, it is an emotion. An emotion is defined sharply as a cerebral state. As such, it affects both the mental and motor systems of the person experiencing a specific emotion. Recall the behavior of a joyous person. Such a person is usually depicted with a smile on the face, a twinkle in the eyes, and with self-assurance and excitement conveyed by body movements and verbal communications. All of these reactions are by-products of the internal feeling being experienced. These visible responses support the fact that behavior is an expression of the inner state of the organism.

Joy, along with sadness, anger, and fear, is included by many persons in their classification of the four basic emotions. But note that joy is the only positive emotion in this list. Izard classifies joy as "one of the earliest fundamental emotions to be clearly expressed by a well-recognized facial pattern, the smile."[1] The smile plays an important role in the early development of affectional patterns between the infant and his parents. Because of its early appearance and significance in infancy, Izard considers joy not only one of the basic emotions but also one of the simplest.

McDougall,[2] however, classifies joy as one of the complex, secondary emotions. According to him, it is complex because it is a sentiment, composed of the primary emotions of aesthetic pleasure, sympathetic pleasure, tender emotion (love), and positive self-feeling. It is secondary because it evolves from these more basic or fundamental feelings. Sorrow is another complex secondary emotion, a composite of tender emotion (love) and negative self-feeling (loss).

Philosophers have also added to our understanding of joy. Heidigger states that "the original essence of joy is the process of becoming at home in proximity to the source."[3] By *source*, he means the *actuality of being*, and by *joy*, the *feeling of self-fulfillment in the presence of being*. Schutz defines joy as "the feeling that comes from the fulfillment of one's potential."[4] Tillich considers joy to be "nothing else than the awareness of our being fulfilled in our true being, in our personal center."[5] Existentialists, especially existentialist psychologists such as May, argue that "it

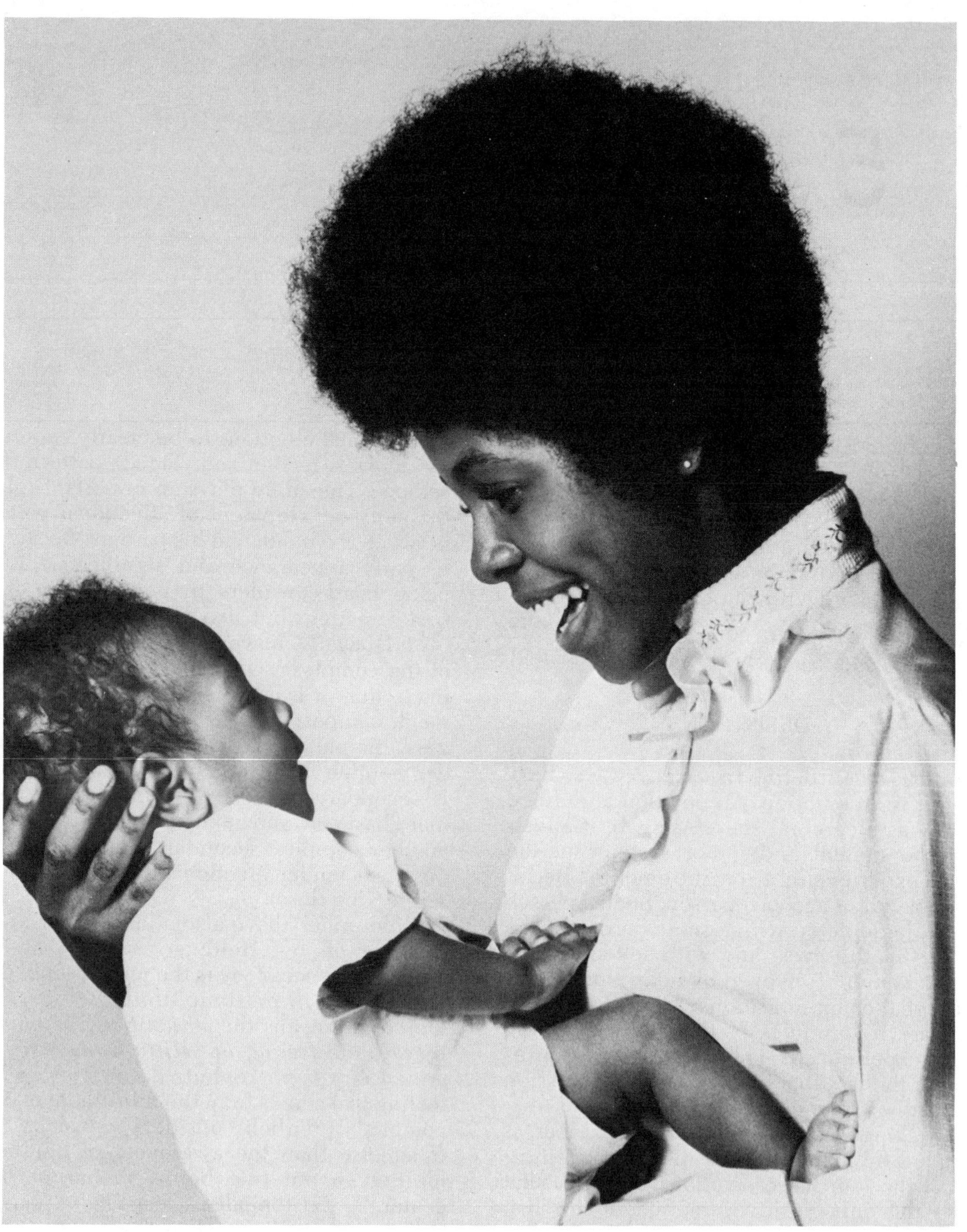

is more than awareness, it is consciousness."[6] Consciousness is considered a higher level in that one not only sees the self is threatened but one has the insight to do something about it. This concept is used by sensitivity and encounter groups which are discussed later.

SOURCES

It is possible to identify experiences which make a person joyous as he progresses through the developmental stages of life. Maslow's hierarchy of basic human needs is used as the framework. Beginning with the most basic, Maslow identifies the five kinds of needs as 1) physiologic, 2) safety and security, 3) belongingness and affection, 4) respect for self and others, and 5) self-actualization.[7] According to his theory, a new and higher human need emerges when a lower need is fulfilled by being sufficiently gratified. If there is a deficiency in the gratification of any of these needs, the person will develop some type of personality dysfunction. These dysfunctions vary in degree, and range from simple dependency on others to actual neuroses. If persons strive for gratification of these basic needs in the proper sequence, they will be growth-motivated; that is, they will aspire to attain self-achievement through goal setting and thus gain increased satisfaction and enjoyment from life—the signs of a healthy personality.

The pleasure one derives from meeting these basic needs also gives joy. Buhler,[8] in a study of 69 infants over a period of months, investigated the relationship of internal states, as evidenced by pleasure and displeasure, to positively and negatively expressed movements. She found that during the first few months of life, signs of displeasure occurred far more often than signs of pleasure. Positively directed expressive movements, e.g., lifting of the corners of the mouth, flowing eyes, and firming of the facial muscles, occurred after the baby was made warm and comfortable and were correlated with a pleasurable internal state. This study supports Maslow's theory about gratification of basic needs. Thus, the pleasure derived from the fulfillment of physiologic needs is a source of joy.

Gratification of the need for safety and security is another source of joy. This is exemplified by the toddler who is free of anxiety when exploring his environment in the presence of his mother. However, if his mother leaves the room, he looses the feeling of safety and security, becomes anxious, and shows his displeasure by crying.

The need for love, referred to by Maslow as the need for belongingness and affection, must be met in order for a person to be joyous. Maslow states, "if this deficiency love (D-love) in infants is satiated, it results in love for Being (B-Love) in adults."[9] Persons with B-love are more able to offer and accept love. The fulfillment of the love needs of children is essential for the development of adults with B-love. Such persons are joyous, independent individuals capable of giving love to others and possessing a minimum of anxiety and hostility. In this way, love becomes a source of joy.

As children master various psychomotor and intellectual tasks, they learn to respect themselves as a result of praise and rewards by significant others, such as parents, relatives, and teachers. As they continue to grow and their world enlarges, they interact with others and jointly master tasks. Through these experiences, they gain respect for others. Thus, respect for self and others resulting from the accomplishment of tasks, either individually or cooperatively, is a source of joy.

The constant striving for and periodic attainment of another basic need, self-actualization, also provides joy. Self-actualization occurs when one attains a highly desired goal. This gives one a great feeling of inner satisfaction and fulfillment. Examples are the attainment of a high grade in an examination or the receipt of one's baccalaureate degree. A less tangible example is the intense love and involvement a mother and father feel for their newborn child. Self-actualization has as its purpose the accomplishment of a growth-motivating goal, a goal that has great significance to the individual. However, it should be remembered that attainment of such a goal is not the end of this process. It is merely the achievement of one goal in a continuous series of goals for each individual. It is possible that the need for self-actualization may never be totally gratified since it depends upon the specific goals and the number of them that an individual sets for himself.

Schutz[10] identifies other sources of joy which apply to both the child, as a developing person, and to the mature individual. The first is a healthy body or smoothly functioning physical structure. The second is personal functioning which refers to full development of the body. This includes optimal neuromuscular control, sensory acuteness, physical stamina, cognitive ability, and emotional control. The outcome is complete development and integrated functioning of the body. Because man is also a social animal, the third source is the development of interpersonal relations which are rewarding to all concerned. This means that the needs of inclusion, control, and affection are adequately balanced among interactants, resulting in interpersonal joy. Since man lives in a society composed of a variety of social institutions, organizational relations are another potential source of joy. A society and culture that support and enhance the individual are essential for self-actualization, a prerequisite and a source of joy. Schutz summarizes by stating:

> Joy is the feeling that comes from the fulfillment of one's potential. Fulfillment brings to an individual the feeling that he can cope with his environment; the sense of confidence in himself as a significant, competent, lovable person who is capable of handling situations as they arise, able to use fully his own capacities, and free to express his feelings. Joy requires a vital, alive body, self-contentment, productive and satisfying relations with others, and a successful relation to society.[11]

ATTAINMENT

You are probably thinking that this discussion sounds very idealistic. How can all of these sources of joy be successfully recognized and utilized by each person? It is possible, but unfortunately much of the effort must be devoted to undoing. Our society has placed greater emphasis on guilt, shame, embarrassment, failure, and retribution—all negative self-feelings which must be overcome in order for joy to become dominant. Training in the ability to overcome these negative feelings is provided by consciousness-raising groups which are becoming increasingly popular. These groups, through the guidance of a trained leader, help persons to understand their feeling states and to develop directness and honesty within themselves and their interpersonal relations in order to gain an internalized feeling of satisfaction which ultimately leads to joy. Their goal is to help persons develop to their fullest potential. Thus, they attempt to help persons attain peak experiences.

What are peak experiences? They are those experiences which cause one to feel a deep sense of inner satisfaction and joy. During peak experiences, an individual perceives his potential to be far greater than he ever thought. As a result, he sees himself as a new person who is able to cope with his feelings more effectively and to reach a point of accepting, respecting, and loving himself more. Peak experiences have a wide range of sources. They can result from simply having a physiologic need met, or from having reached a certain highly desired goal or objective in one's life. They can be experienced by an individual, a couple, or even a crowd if a common goal is achieved.

Maslow believes that "peak experiences have aftereffects upon the person which may validate the experiences."[12] His proposed affirmations about these aftereffects include the following: Peak experiences have therapeutic effects in the sense of removing symptoms, especially those of a neurotic nature. They can change a person's view of himself, his relations with others and the world. They foster creativity and expressiveness within the individual. The individual remembers the peak experience as a very important and desirable happening and strives to repeat it. The person is "recharged" by feeling that life is worth living, regardless of how drab and ungratifying it may be.

Peak experiences, then, produce an altered state of consciousness within the individual experiencing them. He feels more integrated (whole); more egoless; more fully and easily functioning; more responsible and active in his activities; free of blocks, fears, and inhibitions; more creative, spontaneous, expressive, and uncontrolled; and lucky, fortunate, and grateful. Peak experiences are possible during all stages of development during the life cycle.

Pregnancy and childbirth are examples of potential sources of peak experiences. Pregnancy is literally a representation of the physiologic union of the two partners into one. The creation of another human being, a mystic symbol of their love, can result in joy to such a degree that it becomes a peak experience. Pregnancy may also be the first occasion in a marriage when the partners realize the extent to which they are psychologically, socially, and economically interdependent.

The birth of the child indicates to the mother the fulfillment of her function as a woman and the beginning of her mothering role in assuming the care of her child. To the father, supporting his wife during labor and delivery can be a source of great inner satisfaction. His presence during the birth makes it an experience in which they can share in each other's joy at their accomplishment. Thus, as Howells states, "pregnancy and childbirth may nurture and enhance the gay and joyful functioning of a family group."[13]

REFERENCES

1. Izard, C. E.: *The Face of Emotion.* Appleton-Century-Crofts, New York, 1971, p. 46.
2. McDougall, W.: *An Introduction to Social Psychology.* Methuen, London, 1923.
3. Heidegger, M.: *Existence in Being.* Henry Regenry Company, Chicago, 1949, p. 260.
4. Schutz, W. C.: *Joy.* Grove Press, New York, 1967, p. 17.
5. Tillich, P.: *The New Being.* Charles Scribner's Sons, New York, 1955, p. 146.
6. May, R.: *Existential Psychology.* Random House, New York, 1961, p. 14.
7. Maslow, A. H.: *Toward a Psychology of Being,* ed. 2. Van Nostrand Reinhold Company, New York, 1968.
8. Buhler, C.: *The First Years of Life.* John Day, New York, 1930.
9. Maslow: op. cit., p. 34.
10. Schutz: op. cit.
11. Ibid., p. 17.
12. Maslow: op. cit., p. 101.
13. Howells, J. G.: *Childbirth is a family experience.* In Howells, J. G. (ed.): *Modern Perspectives in Psycho-Obstetrics.* Brunner/Mazel, New York, 1972, p. 130.

BIBLIOGRAPHY

Benedek, T.: *The family as a psychologic field.* In Anthony, E. J. and Benedek. T. (eds.): *Parenthood: Its Psychology and Psychopathology.* Little, Brown and Company, Boston, 1970.

Clark, A. L.: *The adaptation problems and patterns of an expanding family: The neonatal period.* Nurs. Forum V:92, 1966.

Clark, A. L., Bunnell, M. and Henning, E. D. (eds.): *Parent-Child Relationships: Role of the Nurse.* Rutgers University, The State University of New Jersey, New Brunswick, New Jersey, 1968.

Colman, A. D.: *Psychological state during first pregnancy.* Am. J. Orthopsychiatry 39:792, 1969.

Colman, L. L. and Colman, A. D.: *Pregnancy as an altered state of consciousness.* Birth and the Family 1:7, 1973.

Duvall, E.: *Family Development.* J. B. Lippincott, Philadelphia, 1971.

Fraiberg, S.: *The Magic Years.* Charles Scribner's Sons, New York, 1959.

Gibert, H.: *Love in Marriage.* Hawthorne Books, New York, 1964.

Hines, J.: *Father: The forgotten man.* Nurs. Forum X:176, 1971.

Leibman, S.: *Emotional Forces in the Family.* J. B. Lippincott, Philadelphia, 1950.

Lidz, T.: *The Person: His Development throughout the Life Cycle.* Basic Books, New York, 1968.

Metzler, D. (ed.): *Birth.* Ballantine Books, New York, 1973.

Richardson, S. and Guttmacher, A.: *Childbearing: Its Social and Psychological Aspects.* Williams & Wilkins, Baltimore, 1965.

Rubin, R.: *Cognitive style in pregnancy.* Am. J. Nurs. 70:502, 1970.

Rubin, R.: *The family-child relationship and nursing care.* Nurs. Outlook 12:36, 1964.

Schaefer, G. and Zisowitz, M.: *The Expectant Father.* Simon & Schuster, New York, 1964.

Shainess, N.: *The psychologic experience of labor.* Child and Family V:12, 1966.

Ulin, P. R.: *The exhilarating moment of birth.* Am. J. Nurs. 6:60, 1963.

Wessman, A. E. and Ricks, D. F.: *Mood and Personality.* Holt, Rinehart & Winston, New York, 1966.

Wonnell, E. B.: *The education of the expectant father for childbirth.* Nurs. Cin. North Am. 6:591, 1971.

6 *Touch and Sensuality*

VINCENT J. DeFEO, Ph.D.

Pause for a moment . . . and from your experience recall—a pleasant sound—a pleasant sight—a pleasant smell—a pleasant taste—a pleasant motion—a pleasant touch. What kind of touch? Was it light, firm, deep, holding, caressing, tickling, warm, moist, or some other? The pleasant sensations which you have just identified are evidence of your own sensuality. We are all born with a great capacity for such awareness. It is part of our biology and hence must be important in order for it to have been retained through the long span of human evolution.

EARLY SENSUAL DEVELOPMENT

As a parasitic embryo and fetus whose organ systems were dedicated to survival, the strange environment into which we were suddenly extruded at birth became a continuous threat to our existence. Unlike our intrauterine home, we were now confronted with uncertainties. Every so often, we needed to be reassured that we were "going to make it." The reassurance came to us mainly through our senses of physical *contact* and *motion*, but in nonthreatening ways. We learned through repeated touch, caresses, fondling, snuggling, warmth, physical comfort, holding, and gentle movement that we were in a safe place. We felt that we were secure and could trust this setting to continue to provide for our needs. When other sensory systems (auditory, gustatory, olfactory, and visual) were incorporated into this association, they reinforced and expanded this trust. As we gained in comfortableness, we increased this awareness of pleasant sensations. Thus our sensuality developed with our needs and we experienced a freedom—to flow with the stimuli, to experiment without being self-conscious, and we learned to give as well as to receive. At various stages of our infancy and childhood, however, depending upon the attitudes and the degree of uncomfortableness of our parents or their equivalents, attempts were made to bring these feelings (sensations) under control and admonitions were often placed on certain aspects of our sensuality, e.g., our wanting to look, listen, touch, or be touched. The reason for the controls, particularly of touch, were likely based on parental concerns arising from future sexual implications and its potential threat to parental self-image, especially if pregnancy were involved. Because of its power, touch was both appreciated and feared.

Touching is a unique part of our sensuality and perhaps derives its power and importance because, unlike the other senses, it provides a simultaneous communication between individuals. One cannot, under normal circumstances, touch someone without the awareness of being touched. In other words, it

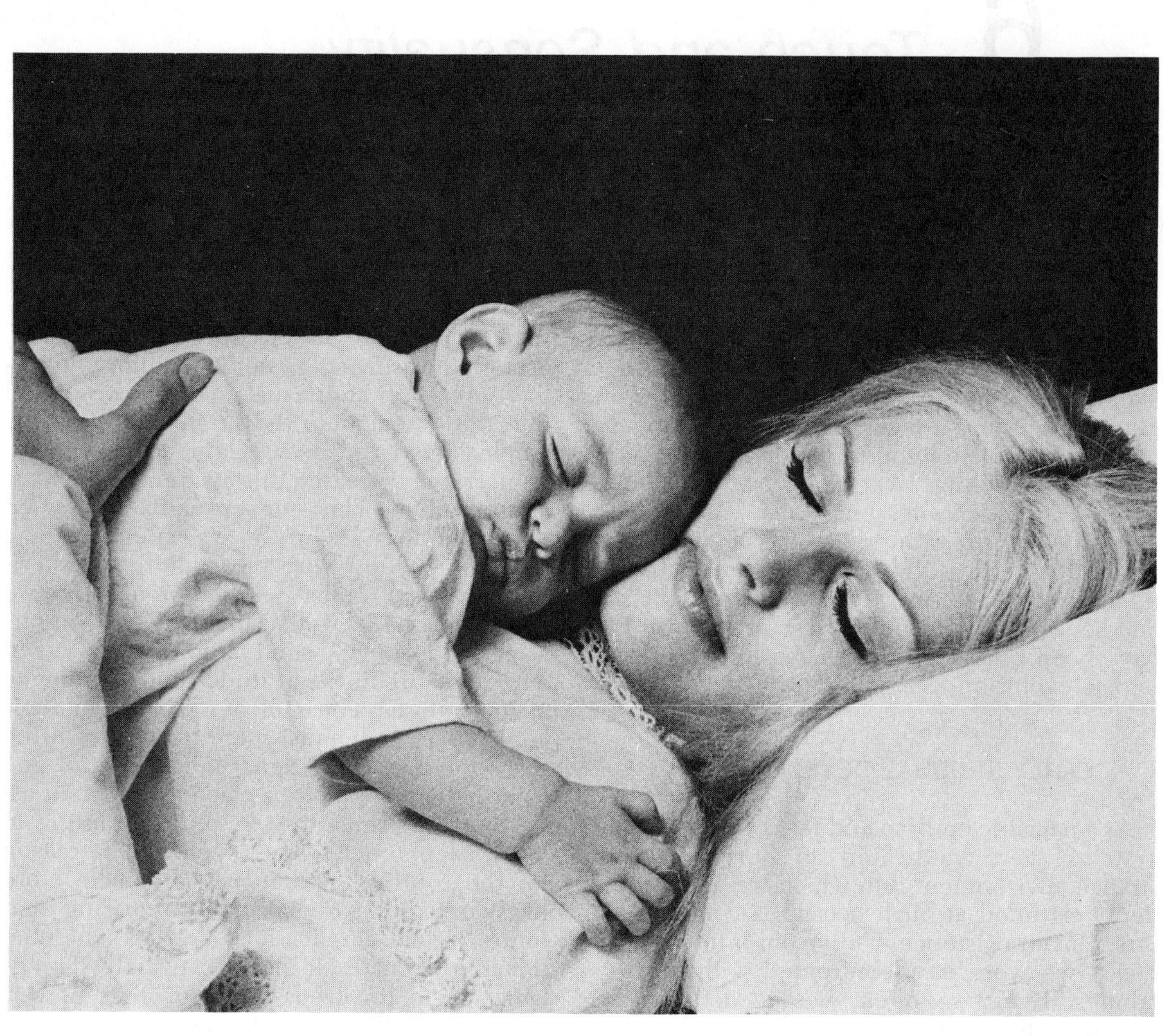

is impossible to be a giver without also being a receiver. Touching is therefore an effective way of demonstrating interest in someone. We can use touch to let someone know that we care, and also to find out if they care. They show this by the manner in which they accept our touch.

SKIN HUNGER

The term skin hunger refers to the desire for physical contact associated with acceptance and lovingness—a desire shared by both females and males as neonates. In preparation for their feminine role as future nurturers, girls are allowed to continue to seek the satisfaction of their skin hunger and can easily associate touch with affection among girlfriends as well as parents. Boys, however, in the establishment of their role identity, have unfortunately been encouraged to regard touching as "sissy" or non-masculine. Because of the possibility of rejection, touching can produce anxiety in a male, no matter to which sex the touch is directed. The opportunity for satisfaction of his skin hunger may therefore become limited. Uncomfortableness with touch causes some males to transfer the entire responsibility for this satisfaction to the skin of their penis—an acceptable touch organ because it is an unmistakable symbol of masculinity. Women are occasionally aware of their own skin hunger and their need to be held which is often independent of sex.[1] However, sex may sometimes be the price a woman is willing to pay for the attempt to satisfy her skin hunger. In some relationships, the occasion for sexual involvement provides the only opportunity for physical closeness and the temporary manifestation of acceptance and caring. It is also not surprising that prolonged sex play can develop into an important prerequisite for sexual intercourse.

The need for satisfaction of skin hunger in adolescent girls may create problems for some fathers who, instead of simply recognizing his daughter's sensual (not sexual) desire for physical contact, may become appalled and frightened as he becomes aware of his arousal and feelings which *he* construes as sexual (not sensual). Instead of accepting the naturalness of such sensual feelings, including the arousal, some fathers become filled with feelings of guilt or a fear that they may lose control and thus might act on those sensual feelings. These intense feelings of guilt or fear may emerge as anger directed toward the girl who becomes confused by this parental rejection and learns an unforgettable lesson about her developing womanhood as she is pushed away.[2] There is a need for better communication to avoid misunderstanding in this area. However, this need also extends to most of us in the health professions to whom the consumer looks for leadership, guidance, and permission. Effectiveness in helping a patient deal with her/his sensual-sexual concerns (e.g., arousal and orgasm during breast feeding) varies according to the nurse's or doctor's sexual comfort. Whenever professionals show discomfort or bias, they rapidly lose the opportunity to help dispel fear, confusion, and anxiety. The hospital setting itself also encourages physical and psychologic distance between an adult patient and a loved one. The fear of potential embarrassment and disapproval from hospital staff interferes with the demonstration of real warmth, affection, and caring, all of which may be desperately needed by the patient. Although at present it may be a fantasy, it would be very humane if hospitals included some form of nurturing based on touch (e.g., a sensuous, nongenital, regional or total massage) as a component of nursing care and as a contrast to procedures which are often uncomfortable if not actually painful.

Sometimes people feel lonely when they do not have someone who accepts their touch and who touches them in return. Such is often the case among the aged. Perhaps the affinity between children and their grandparents derives in part from their mutual need for touch. If the aged in institutions had similar, approved, touch opportunities through sensuous, nongenital massage which they could learn to give each other, there might be an improvement in their well-being and they might feel less rejection. We must become more comfortable about our own gift of touch in order to be able to give permission and approval to those whose lives we influence and control.

SENSUALITY AND SEXUALITY

Some of our uncomfortableness about touch comes from our society's apprehension about the overlap of that which is sensual and that which is sexual. A certain touch may be experienced as disgusting, neutral, sensual, or sexual in each of us, depending entirely upon the situation as it reflects on our ego state. The touch itself is only a sensation, no matter what organ is involved. Hence, the capacity for our sexual responsiveness resides within our brain rather than our sex organ, and *we* are responsible for the turn on or the turn off. It is we who choose to convert a sensual feeling into a sexual one—no one can do that to us, or for us. The escalation of sexual tension and its culmination in orgasm (release of that tension) is the result of our willingness to focus increasing amounts of awareness on our genitals and then letting go of our ego control. Some writers[3] limit the term sexuality to the orgasm and resolution phase of the sexual response cycle described by Masters and Johnson[4] and refer to the cycle's excitement and tension build-up phase (plateau) as still part of sensuality. While it is true for most individuals that the touching of sex organs is essential for the build-up of sex tension and orgasm, it is not absolutely necessary in all cases, e.g., in males during nocturnal emission, and in some females as a result of kissing. The implications of this ability are important in helping patients with spinal cord injuries to develop their sexual feelings even though there may be an absence of genital sensations. The point is: All that is sexual is not genital, and all that is genital is not sexual. The stroking of a penis and the caressing of a vulva can be as sensual and as similar as the stroking of an arm or the caress of a face. It is we who chose to make it different.

Parents sometimes become alarmed over a child's interest in touching her/his own genitals. The child's motivation is quite likely to be sensual rather than sexual. The prohibition of infant and childhood exploration of the genitals is among the earliest taboos we experience as human beings. These negative attitudes discourage an important form of self-discovery and cause problems, especially for girls whose parents are most concerned about the later consequences (social stigma) which they fear may be an outgrowth of such early experience. For the girl, the attitudes which accompany parental desires to control such experience may be difficult to shed later. Unlike the male, who from childhood has been given permission, indeed required, to hold his penis for the purpose of accurately directing his urine stream, women have been discouraged from touching their genitals. Nevertheless, taking that responsibility is an important step, even though uncomfortable for some. More and more, one now finds sex counselors, psychotherapists, clergy, and groups concerned with women's liberation giving women strong endorsement to practice genital caressing.* Regarding this topic, Kinsey stated that for women, "it is doubtful if any type of therapy has ever been as effective as early experience in orgasm, in reducing the incidences of unresponsiveness in marital coitus, and in increasing the frequencies of response to orgasm in that coitus."[5]

---

* The term genital caressing is more than a euphemism for masturbation. It also connotes a state of affection and lovingness—and what is wrong in applying this to ourselves as we do to others?

The capabilities for sexual responsiveness certainly exist before puberty. In an excellently presented study of the sexual experiences and reactions of 30 women, Shaffer[6] found that 13 recalled being involved in their own genital caressing or stimulation before the age of 12 and of these, 7 reached orgasms. The earliest experience of orgasm reported for the group was that of a woman who at the age of 4 discovered the pleasure associated with the exposure of her genitals to the forceful stream of water in the bathtub. She still recalls the experience of being caught by her mother and the anger displayed in her frozen face and stern eyes, in addition to the reprimand she received. With such early experiences, it is no wonder that many adults still feel anxiety and guilt when they engage in their own genital caressing. It is also not surprising to learn that there are women who have never seen their own genitals in a mirror. Other women, however, express curiosity about what their vagina and cervix look like but lack the courage to ask the physician or nurse to help her visualize these organs in conjunction with a pelvic examination. Recently, the proliferation of women's self-help groups has enabled women to teach one another. The book *Our Bodies, Ourselves*,[7] written by women, for women, is a basic text providing excellent attitudes and information. However, no book exists in the area of sensuality and sexuality which can tell us about our feelings as an individual. Each of us is the only expert and it is up to us to discover those pleasant sensations and to communicate that information openly and unashamedly to our love partner. The devaluation of pleasure has been a part of our Western heritage and has taken the form of a work ethic which Masters and Johnson[8] discuss in terms of its cost in marital disharmony and sexual dysfunction. Marital disharmony often responds to improvement in verbal communications while sexual dysfunction often responds to improvement in both verbal and nonverbal communications. The latter involves training in sensual (not sexual) activity utilizing touching and caressing without any demands or performance expectations. Through the reestablishment of this close, nongenital touching, the person experiences the partner as a caring, nurturing, loving person and the most frequent sexual dysfunctions (anorgasmia, impotence, and premature ejaculation) are more readily responsive to treatment.[9,10] This approach to sexual therapy underscores the importance of our sensuality.

It is a serious mistake, however, to believe that that is what sensuality is all about, i.e., to enable us to become sexually functional. Although it contributes to sexuality, sensuality is important in its own right, long before we were ever aware of sex.

SENSORY DEPRIVATION

Considerable attention has been devoted to research in the area of sensory deprivation. The early work of the Harlows[11–13] on rhesus monkeys reared in isolation with stationary, wire or cloth covered surrogate mothers convincingly demonstrated the serious consequences of sensual deprivation. The excellent film "Rock-A-Bye Baby"[14] shows two monkeys' violent and aggressive behavior toward each other during their first touch-contact after many years of isolation rearing beginning at birth. Such monkeys have difficulty with social interactions, including their mating behavior. If mating does occur, such females become poor mothers and are known to attack their infant offspring. A similar parallel exists for humans in which it is noted that parents who abuse their children were themselves the victims of insufficient mothering.[15]

Prescott[16] prefers the term *somatosensory* deprivation, especially in relation to the newborn. He includes in this term not only those afferents which are cutaneous and visceral, but also those which are muscle-joint related and vestibular. Of these four, he regards the vestibular component which provides a cerebellar input as being especially important during neonatal and postnatal development. (He postulates that afferent stimulation of this circuit may be occurring even during fetal development as a result of maternal activities.) Whereas sensory stimulation during development contributes to increased growth of the particular system which is being enriched, sensory deprivation is like malnutrition and adversely affects the brain.[17,18] Such deprivation is similar to a functional deafferentation, and in experimental animals produces stimulus-seeking behaviors as if to maximize the sensory stimulation of which they were deprived during development.[19] For example, cats born and maintained in a visually deprived environment (darkness) for 1 year and then deprived of food for 24 hours, would choose to stimulate (bar press) for light rather than food.[20] The animals would work to obtain light until they were fatigued. Isolation-reared monkeys show stimulus-seeking behavior in the form of self-clutching, rocking behavior, and thumb, toe, and penis sucking.[21] But when isolated infant monkeys are reared with a *moving* surrogate mother, the rocking behavior does not appear[22] nor does it appear in visually deprived monkeys,[23] cats,[24] or congenitally blind children,[25] provided that somatosensory stimulation is adequate. Although neonatal movement is synchronous with the structure of adult speech as early as the first day of life,[26] it nevertheless appears that even severe sound deprivation has no significant influence in a number of measurements relating to emotional and social adjustment.[27] Distance receptors (sight and hearing) are thus apparently not as important as near receptors (touch and, especially, motion) for infant motor-mental and emotional-social development.[28,29] Institutionalized children, like isolation-reared monkeys, also develop perseverative rocking behavior attributed to reduced body contact and movement. Furthermore, immobilization of infants and children in plaster casts or other restraining devices is associated with depression, hyperactivity, and outbursts of violence.[30]

Prescott[31] views the cerebellum as the regulator of sensory-emotional-motor processes in the phenomenon of maternal-social deprivation. This is based on: the processing of sensory information by the cerebellum; its influence upon autonomic functions; its interaction with the limbic system; its relationship to cerebral mechanisms; its regulation of motor functions; and its developmental immaturity, including its postnatal growth which thus makes it susceptible to insults, e.g., insufficient sensory stimulation, neonatal anoxia, malnutrition, and viral infections. Maternal-social deprivation can be interpreted as a special case of partial, functional, somatosensory denervation resulting later in cerebellar supersensitivity and hyperexcitability according to Cannon's law of denervation sensitivity.[32] The denervation supersensitivity may be a precursor to transneuronal agenesis and/or degeneration. Through its connections with the frontal cortex and the limbic and reticular systems, a neuronal model is suggested which involves the cerebellum and accounts for the withdrawn autistic behaviors as well as the violent, aggressive behaviors that accompany isolation rearing. Attachment and dependency behaviors can also be related to the somatosensory system in which the former is associated with somatosensory stimulation and the latter with somatosensory deprivation.[33] Appropriate, enriched, sensory stimulation can be beneficial in emotionally disturbed and hyperactive children.[34] One can thus begin to understand the paradoxical effect of drug stimulants which are capable of quieting the hyperactive child. Prescott[35] hypothesizes that the need for drugs (abuse) may be linked with early somatosensory deprivation and his suggestion that drug stimulation is a substitute for somatosensory stimulation merits further study. Cannon's law of denervation supersensitivity applies to the drug dependency phenomenon and has been used to account for the seizures of barbituate withdrawal as well as the depression from amphetamine withdrawal.[36] A recently discovered treatment for the symptoms of heroin and opium withdrawal involving use of acupuncture stimulation of the ears is certain to generate further research and may provide additional support for the somatosensory deprivation hypothesis.[37,38]

A cross-cultural study by Prescott and McCay[39,40] based on the somatosensory hypothesis statistically linked the deprivation of physical affection and physical pleasure (somatosensory deprivation) to the expression of physical violence. The investigators used Textor's[41] publication of coded, cross-cultural data for 400 cultures around the world. The variables that were searched related to the presence or absence of physical, affectional, or other pleasurable somatosensory-related processes, including sex. The cultures possessing these variables were then re-examined with regard to activity characterized by physical violence and crime. Correlations were calculated and some of the conclusions were as follows:

> Societies characterized by high infant physical affection (overall infant indulgence, prolonged breast feeding, low commitment to religious and supernatural belief systems, low child anxiety over performance in obedience and responsibility) were also characterized by low theft, and negligible or absent killing, torture, or mutilation of the enemy (N = 49, P = .004*).
>
> Societies that used physical punishment of infants and children for disciplinary purposes were characterized by infant and child neglect (N = 66, P = .00001).
>
> Most (83%) of the 11 societies with repressive premarital sexual behaviors offset the advantage of high infant physical affection and showed high adult physical violence.
>
> All societies with permissive premarital sexual behaviors compensated for the detrimental effects of infant physical affectional deprivation and showed low adult physical violence.
>
> Societies characterized by both high infant physical affection and permissive premarital sexual behavior showed a *rare probability* (8 times in a million) of being physically violent (N = 25).
>
> Societies characterized by both high infant physical affection and permissive extramarital behavior showed a *low probability* (9 times in a thousand) of becoming violent (N = 18).

Based on the above findings, they feel that "serious questions should be raised concerning the values of virginity, chastity and monogamous sexual relationships in human societies because the cost of such a value system is extremely high, namely high personal crime, chronic warfare and interpersonal physical violence."[42] In many animals, there is a reciprocal relationship between those brain areas associated with physical pleasure and those areas associated with physical violence so that activation of one causes an inhibition of the other.[43–45] The same may also be true for humans. Prescott[46] contends that somatosensory deprivation and the consequent lack of experiencing body pleasure during formative periods influences the development, organization, and function of the brain so that violence centers are later predisposed to a dominant activity over the brain's pleasure centers. If so, then those value systems which ignore, condemn, or deprive humans of their basic sensual nature will predispose them toward physical violence rather than a state of peace and joy.

There is the need in our country to encourage the development and growth of sensuality so that it will someday be unthinkable to do

---

* N = number of cultures; P = probability level (significant).

violence to anyone else's body or to anyone else's mind.

REFERENCES

1. Hollender, M. H.: *Women's wish to be held: Sexual and nonsexual aspects.* Medical Aspects of Human Sexuality 10:12, 1971.
2. Schaefer, L. C.: *Women and Sex.* Random House, New York, 1973.
3. Rosenberg, J. L.: *Total Orgasm.* Random House, New York, 1973.
4. Masters, W. H. and Johnson, V. E.: *Human Sexual Response.* Little, Brown and Company, Boston, 1966.
5. Kinsey, A. C., et al.: *Sexual Behavior in the Human Female.* W. B. Saunders, Philadelphia, 1953, p. 385.
6. Schaefer: op. cit.
7. Boston Women's Health Book Collective: *Our Bodies, Ourselves.* Simon and Schuster, New York, 1973.
8. Masters, W. H. and Johnson, V. E.: *Contemporary influences on sexual response. 1. The work ethic.* Presented at the Second Annual Siecus Citation Dinner, New York, October, 1972.
9. Ibid.: *Human Sexual Inadequacy.* Little, Brown and Company, Boston, 1970.
10. Hartman, W. E. and Fithian, M. A.: *Treatment of Sexual Dysfunction.* Center for Marital and Sexual Studies, Long Beach, 1972.
11. Harlow, H. F.: *The nature of love.* Am. Psychol., 13:673, 1958.
12. Harlow, H. F. and Harlow, M. K.: *The affectional systems.* In Schrier, A. M., Harlow, H. F. and Stollnitz, F. (eds.): *Behavior of Nonhuman Primates, vol. II.* Academic Press, New York, 1965.
13. Harlow, H. F., *Learning to Love.* Albion, San Francisco, 1971.
14. Dokecki, P. R.: *When the bough breaks . . . what will happen to baby?* Film review of *Rock-A-Bye Baby* (Time-Life Films, New York). Contemporary Psychology 18:64, 1973.
15. Steele, B. F. and Pollack, C. B.: *A psychiatric study of parents who abuse infants and small children.* In Helfer, R. E. and Kempe, C. H. (eds.): The Battered Child. University of Chicago Press, Chicago, 1968.
16. Prescott, J. W.: *Early somatosensory deprivation as an ontogenetic process in the abnormal development of the brain and behavior.* In Goldsmith, I. E. and Moor-Jankowski, J. (eds.): *Medical Primatology, 1970.* Karger, Basel, 1971, p. 356.
17. Rosenzweig, M. R., et al.: *Modifying brain chemistry and anatomy by enrichment or impoverishment of experience.* In Newton, G. and Levine, S. (eds.): *Early Experience and Behavior.* Charles C Thomas, Springfield, 1968.
18. Prescott, J. W.: *Developmental neuro-psychophysics.* In Prescott, J. W., Read, M. S. and Coursin, D. B. (eds.): *Malnutrition and Brain Function: Neuropsychological Methods of Assessment.* In press.
19. Ibid.: *Cannon's Law of denervation supersensitivity: Implications for psychophysiological assessment* (abstract). Psychophysiology 9:279, 1972.
20. Ibid.: *Invited commentary: Central nervous system functioning in altered sensory environments* (C. I. Cohen). In Appley, M. H. and Trumbull, R. (eds.): *Psychological Stress.* Appleton-Century-Crofts, New York, 1967, p. 113.
21. Harlow, H. F.: *Learning to Love.* op. cit.
22. Mason, W. A.: *Early social deprivation in the nonhuman primates: Implications for human behavior.* In Glass, D. E. (ed.): *Environmental Influences.* The Rockefeller University Press and Russell Sage Foundation, New York, 1968.
23. Berkson, G.: *Social responses of animals to infants with defects.* In Lewis, M. and Rosenblum, L. (eds.): *The Origins of Behavior.* New York, John Wiley, 1973.
24. Riesen, A. H.: *Effects of visual deprivation on perceptual function and the neural substrate.* In *D'Ajuriaguerra Deafferentation Experimentale et Clinique* (symposium). Bel Air, 1964.
25. Fraiberg, S.: *Parallel and divergent patterns in blind and sighted infants.* Psychoanal. Study Child XXIII:264, 1968.
26. Condon, W. S. and Sander, L. W.: *Neonate movement is synchronized with adult speech: Interactional participation and language acquisition.* Science 183:99, 1974.
27. Bowyer, L. R. and Gillies, J.: *The social and emotional adjustment of deaf and partially deaf children.* Br. J. Educ. Psychol. 43:305, 1972.
28. Prescott, J. W.: *Somatosensory deprivation and its relationship to the blind.* Presented at Research Conference on the Effects of Blindness and Other Impairments on Early Development, American Foundation for the Blind, Inc., New York, April, 1972.
29. Klaus, M. H., et al.: *Maternal attachment: Importance of the first post-partum days.* N. Engl. J. Med. 286:460, 1972.
30. Friedman, C. J., et al.: *Sensory restriction and isolation experiences in children with phenylketonuria,* J. Abnorm. Psychol. 73(4):294, 1968.
31. Prescott, J. W.: *A developmental neural-behavior theory of socialization.* In *Maternal-Social Deprivation as Functional Somatosensory Deafferentation in the Abnormal Development of the Brain and Behavior* (symposium). 78th Annual Convention, American Psychological Association, Miami, September, 1970.
32. Cannon, W. B. and Rosenblueth, A.: *The Supersensitivity of Denervated Structures.* Macmillan, New York, 1949.

33. Ainsworth, M. D.: *Attachment and dependency: A comparison.* In Gerwitz, J. L. (ed.): *Attachment and Dependency.* V. H. Winston and Sons, 1972.
34. Nyhan, W. L.: *Behavioral phenotypes in organic genetic disease.* Pediatr. Res. 6:1, 1972.
35. Prescott, J. W.: *Before ethics and morality.* The Humanist 32:19, 1972.
36. Sharpless, S. K.: *Isolated and deafferented neurons: Disuse supersensitivity.* In Jasper, H., Ward, A. and Pope, A. (eds.): *Basic Mechanisms of the Epilepsies.* Little, Brown and Company, New York, 1969.
37. Wen, H. L. and Cheung, S. Y. C.: *Treatment of drug addiction by acupuncture and electric stimulation.* Asian J. Med. 9:138, 1973.
38. Ibid.: *How Acupuncture Can Help Addicts.* Drugs and Society 2(8):18, 1973.
39. Prescott, J. W. and McKay, C.: *Somatosensory deprivation and the pleasure principle: Neurobiological and cross-cultural perspectives of sexual, sadistic and affectional behaviors.* Presented at Society of Biological Psychiatry 27th Annual Convention, Dallas, April, 1972.
40. Ibid.: *Child abuse and child care: some cross-cultural and anthropological perspectives.* Presented at Research Workshop National Conference on Child Abuse, Washington, June, 1973.
41. Textor, R. B.: *A Cross-Cultural Summary.* HRAF Press, New Haven, 1967.
42. Prescott and McKay: *Child abuse and child care.* op. cit.
43. Heath, R. G.: *Pleasure and brain activity in man.* J. Nerv. Ment. Dis. 154:3, 1972.
44. Delgado, J. M.: *Brain research and behavioral activity.* Endeavour XXVI:149, 1967.
45. Mark, V. H. and Ervin, F. R.: *Violence and the Brain.* Harper and Row, New York, 1970.
46. Prescott and McKay: *Child abuse and child care.* op. cit.

BIBLIOGRAPHY

Comfort, A.: *The Joy of Sex: A Gourmet Guide to Love Making.* Crown Publishers, New York, 1972.

LeBoyer, F.: *Birth Without Violence.* Alfred Knopf, New York, 1975.

Libby, R. W. and Whitehurst, R. N.: *Renovating Marriage toward New Sexual Life-Styles.* Consensus Publishers, 1973.

Lidz, T.: *The Person: His Development throughout the Life Cycle.* Basic Books, 1968.

Montagu, A.: *Touching: The Human Significance of the Skin.* Columbia University Press, 1971.

Whitehurst, R. N.: *Violence and the family: Violence potential in extramarital responses.* Journal of Marriage and the Family 33:683, 1971.

7 Sensory Alteration

MARIE GRANNAN MORGAN, R.N., M.S.

The environment of today's efficient and highly mechanized hospital differs greatly from the surroundings of most people's everyday lives. Patients in health care settings may experience unusual effects when in situations of altered sensory input. In addition, the entire childbearing experience exposes the pregnant woman, her family, and the new infant to changes in their normal patterns of sensory input. Nurses must have an understanding of the sensory alteration that occurs during the childbearing process, especially during the period of hospitalization. Only through an awareness of such changes and their effects can modifications of health care settings and nursing interventions be used to improve patient care.

DEFINITIONS

Many terms are used more or less interchangeably to identify the phenomena caused by alterations in sensory input. A few of the most frequently used terms are discussed here.

SENSORY DEPRIVATION

This state occurs when the amount or intensity of stimulation received by the sensory modalities (vision, hearing, taste, smell, touch, and kinesthesia) is greatly reduced. This may result from lack of stimuli, presence of low grade monotonous stimuli, or impaired functioning or loss of sense organs. For example, during pregnancy a woman may experience sensory deprivation resulting from restrictions on her usual work and recreation activities, and changes in her eating and sleeping patterns. In the hospital, restrictions concerning position, visitors, usual patterns of intake and output, and the attitude and behavior of the staff may cause sensory deprivation.

PERCEPTUAL DEPRIVATION

In this situation the patterning or meaningfulness of stimuli received through the senses is reduced or changed. This may result from the presence of new or strange stimuli, masking or distortion of familiar stimuli, or inability of the brain to interpret the significance of the sensations received. Frequently, the definitions of sensory deprivation and perceptual deprivation are combined, using the term sensory deprivation to include both situations.

SENSORY OVERLOAD

This state results from an increase in the amount, intensity, and/or complexity of stimuli impinging simultaneously on two or more sensory modalities. For example, sensory overload may result from the procedures, equipment, sights, sounds, and strange faces in the hospital. Infant care tasks may cause the parents to feel overwhelmed by routines for feeding, bathing, diapering, and washing clothes. Ironically, with such sensory overload, a feeling of deprivation may also occur. Parents may feel deprived by not being able to perform their usual routines for deriving pleasure and relaxation.

SENSORY ALTERATION

Since sensory deprivation, perceptual deprivation, and sensory overload may be experienced singly or in various combinations, a comprehensive term, sensory alteration, is suggested by Jackson and Ellis[1] to indicate that sensory input or the interpretation of it is altered from the usual. Therefore, sensory alteration refers to any situation in which there is a decrease or increase in the amount, intensity, patterning, or meaningfulness of sensory stimulation.

BEHAVIORAL EFFECTS

It must be remembered that the experiences reported and observed while subjects are undergoing sensory alteration are not psychotic reactions, but are the results of altered sensory input.

One of the first responses to sensory deprivation is to spend an increased amount of time asleep. An individual needs stimulation that is varied and meaningful, and will do anything to change a situation lacking it. Sleeping is one of the easiest ways to do this. It is after a maximum amount of sleep is obtained that other experiences occur. These vary in range and intensity and include perceptual, somatic, emotional, and intellectual disturbances as well as noncompliance behavior.

Perceptual disturbances include those frequently labeled hallucinations and may be visual, auditory, gustatory, or olfactory. The person may see textured surfaces, colors, geometric designs, people, objects, and even whole landscapes or scenes. Sounds of wind, water, ticking clocks, or music may be heard. Time distortion, usually experienced as underestimation of time intervals, may occur making it difficult to note relationships of past, present, and future, and to relate the sequence of events.

Somatic disturbances include such objectively measured physiologic aspects as changes in the electrical patterns of the brain, the electrical conductivity of the skin, and secretions of gastric juices. There may be increased sensitivity to touch, pain, sound, smell, and taste, as well as various bodily discomforts.

Various degrees of emotional impairment are possible with great individual differences. They may include fear, mild to severe anxiety, and rapid, marked mood swings.

Intellectual disturbances include an inability to concentrate and a lack of clarity and organization of thought. This may be mild to severe and the latter may include bizarre or paranoid ideas.

Noncompliance behavior is unintentional interference with goal-directed behavior. The individual displaying this would probably be labeled as "uncooperative" since he would be acting against the specific directions he had been given. His behavior, however, is not intentional and he may report that "it just happened."

It must be remembered that there may be a wide range of individual responses to altered sensory input. The differences occur not only from study to study but also among subjects participating in the same experiment. Some people experience very vivid reactions. Others have moderate to mild responses, while still others have none at all. The experiences themselves are frightening to some people, while others are not in the least disturbed and even find them rather interesting.

FACTORS INFLUENCING BEHAVIOR

The following factors can influence the type and degree of reaction in a person experiencing sensory alteration.

1. Restriction of movement, with or without various attachments to the body and regardless of normal or altered sensory environment, produces intellectual and perceptual disturbances. Immobilization reduces tactile and kinesthetic stimulation thus decreasing sensory input. However, placing a person in a recumbent position without imposing restriction of movement does not cause these effects.
2. Perceptual deprivation seems to produce greater intellectual and behavioral impairment then sensory deprivation.
3. Exercise may decrease many of the disturbances caused by perceptual deprivation. Movement provided by exercise may cause enough kinesthetic and proprioceptive stimulation to offset the lack of stimulation in other sensory modalities.
4. Most gross perceptual and thought disorganization occurs during periods of low level arousal, such as in hypnagogic and hypnopompic states (the intervals between wakefulness and sleep, and sleep and wakefulness, respectively).
5. Stress responses are increased by putting subjects in a deprivation environment with an indefinite time limit to the situation and telling them of the passage of time. This fosters a feeling of lack of control over the situation and its termination.
6. Repeated exposures to sensory deprivation do not indicate an adaptive mechanism for many of the reactions; however, there is a drastic decrease in verbal stress response. In other words, a person may experience similar effects every time he is in a deprivation situation, but simply not talk as much about it.
7. Quantity and intensity of experiences are minimized by telling a person that unusual effects "sometimes" occur. Some frequent and extreme impairments may be generated by a panic state following milder disturbances which caused the individual to question his sanity. Reassurance allays his fears and prevents panic.
8. Although it is very difficult to make predictions based on personalities, the following types seem to experience more stress: impulsive, independent, introverted, and those with low pain tolerance.

Again, these factors cannot be applied to all persons in these circumstances, but they are relevant to the experiences manifested by many individuals.

THE RECTICULAR FORMATION THEORY

The large number of studies done in the field of sensory alteration have yielded vast amounts of data. Several different theories have been offered, but none has been accepted as explaining the many different facets of the phenomena. Many theorists have used an approach with a neurophysiologic basis. Lindsley[2] has been one of the leading proponents of a theory centered around the recticular formation.

The reticular formation is a core of intertwining small neurons located in the midventral portion of the primitive brainstem. It extends from the medulla to the thalamus and consists of two components, the descending reticular activating system (DRAS) and the ascending reticular activating system (ARAS). The DRAS exerts influence on spinal motor reflexes and voluntary control of muscles. The ARAS conducts impulses received from all sensory modalities to the cortex where effective cognition or perception takes place. It can also exert a facilitating or inhibiting effect on these impulses by providing a mechanism which maintains general arousal and focuses attention.

Another system, the corticofugal system, feeds into the reticular formation. It is a pathway from the cortex into the ARAS through which cognition or ideation can also initiate arousal. In addition, there is a mechanism in the sensory pathways called centrifugal control which monitors the levels of stimulation coming from the sense organs and the levels of cortical and reticular activity. In a feedback system, the control automatically regulates the amount of sensory input entering the cortex.

Thus, the reticular formation acts as a regulator for input-output levels and is able to adapt to varied levels of activity within certain limits. The adaptation level is then projected to the cortex. When stimulation reaching the ARAS exceeds either the upper or lower end of these limits, as in sensory overload or deprivation, there appears to be an overwhelming inhibition or facilitation of the impulses and behavior becomes disorganized.

Although this theory does not answer all of the numerous questions raised by the phenomenon of altered sensory input, it can be used as a foundation for beginning to understand what may occur in an individual under certain circumstances. It can provide a basis for formulating possible nursing interventions for patient care.

EVALUATION OF POTENTIAL FOR SENSORY ALTERATION

Nursing deals with helping the patient cope with stresses of the environment until he is able to cope on his own. It is necessary, then, to realize the impact of sensory alteration on patients and be aware of implications for modifying the environment and for employing nursing interventions to assist the individual in coping with such changes. The checklist below is provided as a guide for evaluating the environment and patient to obtain an estimate of the amount of sensory alteration possibly occurring. Each condition stated in the list increases the likelihood of the patient experiencing effects of sensory alteration. The use of such a checklist helps make the nurse aware of gross changes in sensory input for a patient, and enables her to focus on specific conditions contributing to the alteration which need special consideration when planning nursing care.

It is important to remember that the conditions in the checklist have not been proven as causative factors for sensory alteration. It is not a foolproof way to determine which patients will experience effects of sensory alteration, or the degree to which those affected will be disturbed by the experiences. It will, however, give the nurse a starting point from which to develop awareness and provide patient care relative to these phenomena.

SENSORY ALTERATION CHECKLIST*

Evaluation of the Environment

1. Alteration in the amount or intensity of stimulation for each sensory modality.
2. Alteration in the patterning or meaningfulness of stimulation for each sensory modality.
3. Restrictions imposed on movement or body position.
4. Use of medications for sedation or analgesia.
5. Lack of time-orienting factors (day/night light cycles, meal times, clock, calendar)
6. Lack of adequate sleep periods.
7. Increased degree of social isolation.
8. Increased duration of altered stimulation.

---

* Modified from Jackson and Ellis.[1]

9. Presence of realistic dangers in the situation.

Evaluation of the Patient

1. Impairment or loss of any sensory modality.
2. Decreased amount of control over the situation.
3. Decreased amount of control over termination of the situation.
4. Decreased knowledge about duration of the situation.
5. Increased severity of illness.
6. Presence of severe or unalleviated pain.
7. Child or elderly person.
8. Foreign ethnic background.
9. Presence of abnormal personality characteristics.

REFERENCES

1. Jackson, C. W., Jr. and Ellis, R.: *Sensory deprivation as a field of study.* Nurs. Res. 20:46, 1971.
2. Lindsley, D. B.: *Common factors in sensory deprivation, sensory distortion, and sensory overload.* In Solomon, P., et al. (eds.): *Sensory Deprivation.* Harvard University Press, Cambridge, 1961, pp. 174–194.

BIBLIOGRAPHY

Cameron, C. F., et al.: *When sensory deprivation occurs. . . .* The Canadian Nurse 68:32, 1972.

Chodil, J. and Williams, B.: *The concept of sensory deprivation.* Nurs. Clin. North Am. 5:453, 1970.

DeMeyer, J.: *The environment of the intensive care unit.* Nurs. Forum 6:262, 1967.

Ellis, R.: *Unusual sensory and thought disturbances after cardiac surgery.* Am. J. Nurs. 72:2021, 1972.

Jackson, C. W., Jr. and Ellis, R.: *Sensory deprivation as a field of study.* Nurs. Res. 20:46, 1971.

Ohno, M.: *The eye-patched patient.* Am. J. Nurs. 71:271, 1971

Schultz, D. P.: *Sensory Restriction: Effects on Behavior.* Academic Press, New York, 1965.

Solomon, P., et al. (eds.): *Sensory Deprivation.* Harvard University Press, Cambridge, 1961.

Thomson, L.: *Sensory deprivation: A personal experience.* Am. J. Nurs. 73:266, 1973.

Vernon, J. A.: *Inside the Black Room.* Clarkson N. Potter, Inc., New York, 1963.

Zubek, J. P. (ed.): *Sensory Deprivation: Fifteen Years of Research.* Appleton-Century-Crofts, New York, 1969.

8 *Frustration and Conflict*

SUZANNE LEGO, R.N., Ph.D.

Although frustration and conflict are two separate concepts, they are so closely related that they are usually discussed together. Some authors believe that frustration leads to conflict; others that conflict leads to frustration; and still others that conflict and frustration are synonomous terms.[1] In this discussion, each concept is examined separately so that its operations or process may be carefully understood.

FRUSTRATION

Most people experience frustration frequently in the normal course of daily living. It occurs when obstacles prevent achievement of a goal. When this happens, people have characteristic ways of responding. For this reason, frustration is sometimes viewed as an event and sometimes as a state. A frustrating *event* is one in which goal-directed activity is blocked in some way, while a frustrating *state* is one in which the person whose goals has been blocked feels the consequences of this blocking. These effects vary among individuals and include anger, aggression, withdrawal, rigidity, fantasy, regression, fixation, repression and learning.

Let us use as an example a woman who has been married for several years and wants very much to have a child. Though she and her husband have visited doctors who found no physiologic reason why they should be unable to conceive, they cannot. Thus, the inability to conceive is a frustrating event, and the woman is in a frustrated state. She may respond in any of the ways described above. Anger may lead her to exclaim, "This is unfair!" Her anger may expand to *aggression* and she may lash out at her husband, "You are to blame!" If she has experienced frustration repeatedly, the woman may *withdraw* from the frustrating event by stopping sexual relations altogether. *Rigidity* may show itself in this situation by an inflexibility in attempting to deal with the obstacle. If her doctor suggests intercourse at various times and ways during her menstrual cycle, she may react by rigidly sticking to one method and time, e.g., only when she thinks she is ovulating. Paradoxically, instead of fighting the obstacle this may perpetuate her frustration. The woman's frustration over her inability to bear children may lead to *fantasy* on her part that she is pregnant, when in reality she is not. *Regression,* a retreat to early forms of behavior, may also occur. Thus, the woman may resort to frequent crying or retreat to bed with "colds" or "fatigue." At times, *repression* is also a result of frustration. In this case, the woman may repress her feelings by consciously failing to pay attention to the frustrating situation. Finally, *learning* may take place under conditions of frustration. The woman who is unable to conceive may try new methods, times of the month, or even ways of relaxing which may ultimately help remove the obstacle to her goal.

CONFLICT

Conflict results from the simultaneous presence of opposing goals of equal strength. The person in a state of conflict feels pulled in different directions at the same time. Conflict has been categorized as:

1. Approach-approach conflict, involving equally attractive but mutually exclusive goals.
2. Avoidance-avoidance conflict, involving equally unattractive goals.
3. Approach-avoidance conflict, involving an equally attractive and repulsive goal.

We can now see how conflict is tied to frustration. For the attainment of a goal is here blocked by the pull to another goal. Thus, it is not surprising that the effects of conflict are identical or similar to those of frustration. They include withdrawal, hesitation, vacillation, tension, and blocking.

Approach-approach conflict often is experienced when pregnancy is diagnosed. To continue a desirable career and be gainfully employed (goal) may be a direct barrier to being pregnant and becoming a mother (goal). During early pregnancy you may observe considerable vascillation as the pregnant woman considers both goals and moves back and forth between them, depleting vital energy.

Avoidance-avoidance conflict may also arise during pregnancy. For example, the new parents may need assistance in meeting the costs of medical care, furnishings (crib, bottles, highchair, and so forth), and clothing (maternity clothes for the mother and diapers and baby clothes for the infant). They are faced with two possibilities. They could ask their parents for the money. This is unattractive, because they wish to remain independent. On the other hand, they could borrow money from the bank. In this case, they must pay interest. In either case a goal is thwarted, and both choices are unattractive.

In considering *approach-avoidance conflict* it is necessary and most interesting to examine the classic work of Miller.[2] Based on experimental studies, he determined four principles of approach-avoidance conflict.

1. The tendency to approach an "approach goal" is stronger the nearer the subject is to it.
2. The tendency to avoid an "avoid goal" is stronger the nearer the subject is to it.
3. The strength of avoidance increases more rapidly with nearness than does that of approach.
4. The strength of the tendencies to approach and avoid varies with the strength of the drive upon which they are based.

Let us return to the example of the woman who is unable to conceive, and examine these principles. For the sake of understanding, let us assume that the woman is experiencing unconscious conflict in that she simultaneously wants a child and does not want a child. The woman decides, based on her "approach goals," to visit a family planning agency. As she nears the agency her tendency to talk with them increases (Principle 1). However, her tendency to avoid the "avoid goal" also increases (Principle 2). The tendency to avoid overpowers the tendency to approach (Principle 3). Thus, she "retreats" by avoiding the agency or "forgetting" what the family counselor tells her. This avoidance behavior causes her avoidance tendency to grow weaker. Thus, her approach tendency grows stronger and she again desires to have the baby, visit the agency, and hear the counselor (Principle 4). This example illustrates the effects of conflict cited above, i.e., withdrawal, hesitation, vacillation, tension, and blocking.

BEHAVIORAL CONSIDERATIONS

Nurses are often bewildered by patients who exhibit frustration and conflict. In order to help these individuals she must understand the underlying processes responsible for their behavior. In this way she can then work with the person to minimize frustrations and solve conflicts. Let us consider the example of a patient who is told she must follow a dietary regime. If she likes food which is not included in the diet, she is immediately faced with frustration. This may be viewed in two ways. First, the patient wants a particular food but it is forbidden. In this case, her goal of eating the food she likes is blocked by the diet. The second way is to view maintenance of her diet as the goal. In this case, eating the forbidden food is a block to her goal. In either situation the nurse observes that the patient exhibits anger, aggression, withdrawal and/or the other behaviors characteristic of the frustrated individual. In addition, this patient is experiencing approach-avoidance conflict. She wants to approach the forbidden food, but her diet states that she must avoid it. At times, the tendencies to approach and avoid will be of approximately equal strength. The nurse will then observe the patient hesitate, vacillate, block, and display other signs of conflict. Understanding the reasons for these behaviors helps the nurse trace the important process in operation and then intervene appropriately.

The nurse will also observe frustration and conflict in the realm of human relations. For example, the patient states that she wants nothing more than to be close to other individuals and to have permanent relationships. This is her goal and she expresses aloud her frustration that this does not happen. The nurse observes, however, that the woman herself puts up the blocks to this goal. In her behavior with members of the health team she is abrupt and arrogant, preventing any possibility of close feelings toward her. In addition, she repeatedly chooses friends who are unable or unwilling to commit themselves to another person. Again her goal of closeness is frustrated, but she has provided the block by her choice of friends. This person is also in conflict. She both wants closeness (is attracted to it) but is frightened by it (avoids it). Her conflict may be clearly observed by her otherwise unexplainable changes in mood. Just as she seems to be getting along well with people, she does something which drives them away. It must be remembered that part of this conflict is unconscious. Only the desire to approach the goal is conscious. The desire to avoid the goal is unconscious. An awareness of this aspect of conflict is necessary in order to understand the process involved and initiate appropriate intervention to help this patient resolve her frustrations and conflicts.

REFERENCES

1. Yates, A.: *Frustration and Conflict.* John Wiley and Sons, New York, 1962, pp. 174, 175.
2. Miller, N.: *Experimental studies of conflict.* In Hunt, J. (ed.): *Personality and the Behavior Disorders.* Ronald Press, New York, 1944, pp. 433, 434.

BIBLIOGRAPHY

Hilgard, E.: *Introduction to Psychology.* Harcourt, Brace and Company, New York, 1953.

Lewin, K.: *Behavior and development as a function of the total situation.* In Cartwright, D. (ed.): *Field Theory in Social Science.* Harper Torch Books, New York, 1951.

Manaser, J. and Werner, A.: *Instruments for the Study of Nurse-Patient Interaction.* Macmillan, New York, 1964.

Miller, N.: *Experimental studies of conflict.* In Hunt, J. (ed.): *Personality and the Behavior Disorders.* Ronald Press, New York, 1944.

Morgan, C. *Introduction to Psychology.* McGraw-Hill, New York, 1961.

Munn, N.: *Psychology: The Fundamentals of Human Adjustment,* ed. 4. Houghton Mifflin, Boston, 1961.

Peplau, H.: *Interpersonal Relations in Nursing.* G. P. Putnam's Sons, New York, 1952.

Rosenzweig, S.: *An outline of frustration theory.* In Hunt, J. (ed.): *Personality and the Behavior Disorders.* Ronald Press, New York, 1944.

Rouslin, S.: *Conflict and frustration.* In Clark, A., Bunnell, M. and Henning, E. (eds.): *Parent-Child Relationships: Role of the Nurse.* Rutgers, The State University of New Jersey, New Brunswick, 1968, pp. 63–66.

Yates, A.: *Frustration and Conflict.* John Wiley and Sons, New York, 1962.

9 *Anxiety*

HILDEGARD E. PEPLAU, R.N., Ed.D.

In order to understand and apply the concept of anxiety in nursing practice it is necessary to distinguish between tension and anxiety. Both are internally experienced forms of discomfort that provide energy which is transformed into tension-reducing or anxiety-reducing behaviors. Tension, however, pertains to inborn biologic needs while anxiety pertains to acquired sociocultural needs.[1] In newborn infants this distinction is easily observable since all of their needs are biologically determined. The need for food evokes bodily tensions in the infant, which, when transformed into sucking behavior as a food resource is presented, lead to satiation of the need. Adults usually experience mixtures of biologic (inborn) and sociocultural (acquired) needs. For example, food that would relieve hunger might not, at the same time, satisfy acquired status needs.

SOURCES

Anxiety arises from two sources: *interpersonal transmission* and *unmet expectations* related to acquired needs.[2] Before an infant develops any acquired sociocultural needs, the only possible source through which the infant experiences anxiety is through a mother or mother-surrogate who is anxious. This interpersonal transmission occurs through empathic observation; the infant feels within himself the anxiety that is being experienced by the mothering-one. This ability to feel within oneself the feelings being experienced by another person who is in the same situation is called empathic observation.

Nurses can easily observe empathic transmission of anxiety from mother to infant in the feeding situation. The behavior of the infant may be the only clue to anxiety in the mother if she is unaware of her own anxiety-related behavior. A non-anxious infant usually takes the mother's nipple readily, sucks steadily, and as the need for food is satiated becomes drowsy, disinterested in obtaining more food, and then falls asleep. Infants who empathize the mother's anxiety use one of the two principal patterns of behavior: 1) the infant will suck–stop–cry–suck again–stop–cry– and eventually vomit, or 2) the infant will suck–stop–cry–refuse to suck–continue to cry– and finally use somnolent detachment. In both instances need–satisfaction has been replaced by the extreme discomfort of anxiety, and new behaviors have been evolved to relieve, reduce, or prevent more anxiety. In both instances, if a non-anxious nurse takes the infant and bottle-feeds it, the infant will revert to the earlier pattern of need–satisfaction.

The anxiety of the mother (or mother-surrogate), whether recognized or not, which is communicated empathically and known by the infant as a "felt relation" can be a major factor in the feeding situation that disrupts the expectation of mutual satisfaction, i.e., satiation of the infant's need for food and satisfaction of the mother's acquired sociocultural need to successfully feed her infant.

The second source of anxiety in the infant is the same as that which gives rise to the mother's anxiety—acquired sociocultural needs. These needs can more simply be referred to as expectations; some synonyms are wishes, wants, anticipations, desires, and goals. Acquired needs include needs for prestige, status, esteem, and the need to confirm prevailing self-views. In the infant, in contrast to the mother, such expectations or acquired needs are in a very early stage of development. They are simple, connected with daily experiences in meeting biologic needs, and are not intellectually known as they would be for a child or an adult. They are known as "felt relations," i.e., the perception of connections among a series of events that is apprehended at an emotional rather than an intellectual level.

At birth, an infant has no expectations of himself or of others. He has biologic needs which produce tensions in bodily organs and muscles and which evoke tension-reducing behaviors such as sucking, defecating, or urinating. Expectations begin to develop through his social experiences, his interactions with others. Again, the feeding situation serves as a primary learning event through which the infant gradually acquires expectations. The infant begins to foresee what will happen on the basis of what has happened. He comes to expect that which has occurred with regularity in his experience. If, for example, the following sequence occurs regularly, the infant will begin to expect the sequence once he gives the signal: 1) the infant cries to signal his need, 2) the mothering-one hears the cry, comes promptly, attends to and feeds the infant, 3) the infant feels need–satisfaction and sleep intervenes. Nurses can observe that within a few weeks infants will cry and then wait for the sequence to follow. This observation suggests that momentary delay of need–satisfaction is initiated by the infant in anticipation of a sequence that has been experienced regularly, in which an expectation of need–satisfaction has unfailingly been met.

Anxiety arises when expectations that are held, and are active and operative at a particular time, are not met for some reason. It is then that acute discomfort is experienced, followed almost immediately by anxiety-relieving behaviors, and then usually by justification or rationalization for those behaviors.

Not all expectations that are held can be met. Some are unreasonable, e.g., a person who recurringly expects love from a nonloving mother or spouse has a built-in perpetuation of anxiety. Some expectations are too specific when they should be more general, e.g., a mother who wants to give birth to a boy but delivers a girl would have been fortified against anxiety by expecting to accept whatever she delivers because it is hers. Some expectations must be made known and be acceptable to others in order to be met. Some expectations of others are beyond their intellectual or interpersonal competencies or their economic means. Not all expectations are clearly within the awareness of a particular individual, e.g., acquired needs for prestige, status, and esteem are not always fully recognized. Self-views also operate as expectations in the sense that the views an individual has of himself will impel him toward actions to confirm those views. An individual whose self-views are primarily derogatory will tend to expect belittling from others and feel anxious if it is not forthcoming. Working with an anxious person to help him understand what he expected and what happened instead is more often than not a difficult professional service.

Not all unmet expectations evoke anxiety. The strength of the acquired need, the degree of awareness of it, the competence of an individual to observe and accommodate to discrepancies between what is wanted and what occurs, and the extent of automatic responding to everyday experiences are all involved.

APPLICATION OF CONCEPT

The application of the concept of anxiety shown in Table 9-1 provides both an explanation of the development of anxiety and a framework for nursing interventions when the concept is applied during a professional interaction with a client. It presents the essence of observations and interventions related to the development and resolution of this phenomenon. However, there is more to be known in a general way. An understanding of the considerations discussed below is necessary for the useful application of the concept.

RELIEF BEHAVIORS

Anxiety is energy. It is not directly observable. What can be noticed are its antecedents and the transformations of the energy into behavior. In working with mothers and newborn infants the nurse will probably first observe one of the two patterns of infant response to empathized mother-anxiety noted previously. In adults, the behavior used to relieve anxiety may run the gamut from helplessness to violent rage. The most common relief behaviors include restlessness, irritability, and anger, although apathy, fantasy, and somnolent detachment are also frequently seen.

Most textbooks suggest two overall patterns of response: fight and flight. Another categorization of general response tendencies includes four major patterns: 1) *Somatization*—using a bodily organ to express the problem symbolically, using the energy of anxiety through organ behaviors. Vomiting by the infant may exemplify this mode of anxiety-relieving behavior. Similarly, ulcers in adults are generally considered to be psychosomatic responses to anxiety. 2) *Acting out*—using externally-directed behaviors such as pacing, fighting, violence, and drug abuse. 3) *Introspection*—using autistic invention as a highly private mode of thought in order to attempt in a solitary way to solve the problem. 4) *Investigation*—talking with others to describe, analyze, formulate, and validate the meaning of various aspects of an anxiety-producing experience and thus deduce a learning product from it that will provide foresight to prevent anxiety in

TABLE 9-1. Application of the Concept of Anxiety

Development of Anxiety	*Resolution of Anxiety*
1. Expectations are held, and are active and operative (wishes, wants, goals, needs for status, prestige, esteem, etc.)	3. Work with the person to recognize, formulate, and state the expectations that were operative just before anxiety was felt.
2. Those expectations are not met.	4. Work with the person to recognize, formulate, state, and consider the reasonableness of how and why the operative expectations were not met.
3. An acute, extreme bodily discomfort is experienced.	1. Work with the person to recognize and name and the anxiety.
4. Behaviors that relieve, reduce, or prevent more anxiety are evolved or such automatic behaviors that worked similarly in the past are evoked.	2. Work with the person to connect the named anxiety and the behavior presently used to relieve it.
5. The relief behaviors are justified or rationalized.	

similar situations in the future. Only this fourth pattern has growth-provoking usefulness; but it requires sustaining the discomfort in order to use the energy of anxiety while learning something new, rather than seeking immediate relief from anxiety.

Relief behaviors tend to become automatic. They are evoked to reduce, relieve, or prevent more anxiety and, if successful, tend to be used recurringly, instantly, without thought, and without the person being aware of the anxiety-relieving function. "Nonstop talkers" are usually persons who relieve anxiety by out-talking others who are present in a situation with them. At the other extreme, withdrawal and use of private fantasy is another behavioral pattern used to relieve anxiety. It is only through sensitive observation, interviewing, and the use of judgment that fairly accurate inferences can be made concerning whether a particular person is or is not using certain behaviors merely to restore comfort when an unmet expectation evokes anxiety.

The problem with automatic relief behaviors is that they do not lead to an understanding of anxiety-producing antecedents, i.e., expectations held and how they were unmet, and thus foresight for the prevention of additional anxiety does not develop. Consequently, relief behaviors must again be evolved in later situations and in relation to increases in the amount of anxiety experienced. In situations of extreme anxiety, when it is absolutely necessary to have and to be able to use competence is in analyzing complex events while experiencing extreme discomfort, there is a very good possibility that automatic relief behaviors will fail to work. In that event, a psychotic breakdown, a psychosomatic illness, or acting out of "blind rage" usually occurs. The prevention of postpartum psychosis is in part related to the ability of the mother to recognize and discuss freely data related to the first four steps in the development of anxiety (see Table 9-1).

DEGREES OF ANXIETY

Anxiety also occurs in different degrees: mild, moderate, severe, and panic. Mild and moderate anxiety are experienced by everyone and need not interfere with functioning in a productive manner, providing there is awareness of the anxiety, ability to name it, and willingness to work toward determining the antecedent factors. However, severe anxiety and panic usually require reduction to mild or moderate levels before productive functioning can proceed. The basic difference in the various degrees of anxiety is reflected in their effects on the perceptual field of the anxious individual. What can be seen, heard, and comprehended during severe anxiety or panic is greatly limited by constriction of the perceptual field. Therefore, when talking to patients in panic, it is necessary to restrict input to short sentences that can be heard and acted upon.[3]

Another important problem is the rapid escalation of anxiety from moderate to severe or panic degrees. Measures for preventing such increases include recognition of lesser degrees, naming the anxiety, and talking about the situation in which it arose.

The energy provided by anxiety can be used for problem solving, i.e., talking about the event in which anxiety was evoked so that its problematic aspects can be identified, analyzed, and understood. This is the main point in nursing practice.[4]

REFERENCES

1. Peplau, H.: *Therapeutic concepts.* In *Aspects of Psychiatric Nursing.* The League Exchange, 26B, 1957.
2. Ibid.: *Anxiety in the mother-infant relationship.* Nursing World 134:11, 1960.
3. Ibid.: "Anxiety." Videotape by Video Nursing Inc., 1968. Available through the American Journal of Nursing.
4. Ibid.: "Psychiatric Nursing." Audiotape series 100-200. PSF Corporation, San Antonio.

BIBLIOGRAPHY

Brody, S. and Axelrad, S.: *Anxiety and Ego Formation in Infancy.* International University Press, New York, 1970.

Hoch, P. H. and Zubin, J.: *Anxiety.* Grune and Stratton, New York, 1950.

Janis, I. L.: *Psychological Stress.* John Wiley & Sons, New York, 1958.

Levitt, E. E.: *The Psychology of Anxiety.* Bobbs-Merrill, Indianapolis, 1967.

May, R.: *The Meaning of Anxiety.* Ronald Press, New York, 1950.

Roche Laboratories: *Aspects of Anxiety,* ed. 2. J. B. Lippincott, New York, 1968.

Spielberger, C. D.: *Anxiety: Current Trends in Theory and Research, vol. II.* Academic Press, New York, 1972.

Sullivan, H. S.: *The Interpersonal Theory of Psychiatry.* W. W. Norton, New York, 1953.

10 *Loss*

JEANNE Q. BENOLIEL, R.N., D.N.Sc.

Helping patients and families experiencing loss and grief to adapt to the personal and social changes that follow requires health care personnel who are knowledgeable about the origins and manifestations of these states and who appreciate the variability in human responses resulting from culturally learned patterns of expression. Ultimately the value of knowledge about loss and grief lies in its usefulness as a resource from which to develop a repertoire of approaches and methods for assisting people to cope with the consequences of serious loss.

EARLY INFLUENCES

If loss is defined as a state of being deprived of something that once was available, then loss is clearly a normal part of human experience. Birth itself can be viewed as a loss in the sense that the infant moves from a warm and protective intrauterine environment into the harsh realities of a world where he must learn to fend for himself. Heavily dependent on those who take care of his fundamental needs for food, warmth, and physical comfort, the newborn learns through experience that gratification of his needs depends on the availability and good graces of other people. He learns to associate separation from or withdrawal by others (his mother in particular) as a threat to his own survival.

At the same time that the infant is being introduced to the experience of separation, he is also beginning the process of development of an autonomous self. Through contacts with people and inanimate objects, he develops various emotional attachments to them—some bring pleasure and others bring pain. How he learns to think and feel about these different relationships, as he develops cognitively and socially, depends largely on the characteristics and meanings of his primary relationships—with mother, father, siblings, peers, and others in positions of authority. According to Peretz,[1] how the child learns to think and feel about himself is closely related to his identification with the thoughts, feelings, traits, and behaviors of the significant adults who are his parents. (In some societies, the significant adults in a child's world include members of the extended family and other adults in addition to or in place of his natural parents.)

The child's capacity to cope with loss begins during these early years when his sense of self and feelings of personal worth are being formed. As developmental changes alter him or his social environment, the child faces many losses, each of which makes demands on his capacity to cope. Some of these changes are trivial, but others involve the severance of important relationships. For example, at some point in time a young child who has been breast-fed from birth learns that his mother's breast is no longer available to him on demand. Similarly, when a second child is born into a family, the first child loses his primary position of central importance and now must learn to share parental attention with someone else—someone whose demands usually take precedence over his. Losses of valued relationships such as these put a heavy strain on the child's capacities to adapt.

COPING MECHANISMS

Since loss is such a central part of human experience, it is not surprising that coping mechanisms develop at each level of existence. At the most primitive level are the physiologic protective responses of aggressive activity and loud protest—external manifestations of internal "fight or flight" reactions. At the psychologic level, protection occurs through the development of mechanisms of psychologic defense, such as repression, projection, guilt, displacement of feelings, substitution of attachment, rationalization of behavior, denial of feelings, denial of reality, and regression to earlier patterns of behavior. Social norms and rules governing proper behavior provide mechanisms for coping with the effects of loss in the interactional sphere of human relationships. At the broadest level of existence are the institutionalized cultural patterns of coping that derive from the primary values and beliefs of a society (or subcultural group) and determine the bereavement behaviors expected of members of that society in response to serious loss.[2]

TYPES OF LOSS

Throughout life, each individual experiences losses that require him to adapt in minimal or major ways depending on the type of loss and the circumstances under which it takes place. The normal process of growth and maturation introduces the child to many kinds of losses, and through these experiences he develops techniques of adaptation which eventually become part of his fundamental personality.

Loss of a Significant Relationship. This type of loss refers to the loss of any human relationship to which an individual has strong attachments and from which he gains emotional gratification. It is by far the most critical loss experience and may even be of a life-threatening nature. According to Bowley,[3] loss of the maternal relationship in early infancy has been found to interfere with normal psychologic development.

Loss of External Objects or Possessions. Objects to which individuals form attachments are many and varied. They include money, jewels, home, country, books, cars, and many other tangible items on which people depend for personal gratification and reward.

Loss of Some Aspect of the Self. This type of loss involves a change in self-perception due to the removal or disappearance of a personally valued attribute, physical ability, or social role. Loss of this nature can be precipitated by any change which dramatically alters in negative ways an individual's mental image of himself. Chronic illness, for example, can contribute to such a change by interfering with a person's ability to engage in activities which he formerly took for granted. So, too, can the birth of a baby cause a mother to experience loss of freedom to pursue her own interests, but loss of this sort is often hidden because of the cultural expectation that babies bring joy.

Partial Loss. This term is sometimes used to refer to physical and social changes that seriously impinge on an individual's sense of personal identity and self-esteem, and necessitate major changes in styles of living. Partial loss includes such critical changes as sexual impotence, amputation of a part of the body, development of sensory deficiencies, surgical removal of an internal organ, disfigurement caused by accident or surgery, and decreases in physical prowess due to the aging process.

REACTIONS TO LOSS

Reactions to loss depend on a combination of circumstances and not simply on loss per se. These reactions are determined by several interacting elements: the special meaning of a relationship that is gone, the degree to which the relationship is replaceable, the level of personal and social disruption produced by a loss, the time in the life cycle when loss occurs, and the availability of adaptive capacities and coping resources for responding to the effects of the change.

Severe and intense reactions to loss occur whenever a key relationship disappears, but even severe reactions can be attenuated if a new relationship replaces that which is gone. Thus, widowhood among elderly persons is usually a more serious loss than it is among young adults, primarily because the latter group has access to many more replacement relationships than does the former. Severe reactions are also likely to occur when a person's coping capacity is limited or undeveloped, and in this regard, the very young and the very old are high-risk groups through their vulnerabiity to the effects of loss.

In psychiatric theory, as Peretz[4] has pointed out, a person's reaction to loss is determined by the depth of his psychologic dependency on the lost relationship. Utilizing a sociologic framework, Weiss[5] identifies five categories of human-to-human relationship that are necessary for the well-being of the person and for satisfaction in living. In his view, people need relationships that provide opportunity for intimacy, social integration, nurturance, reassurance of worth, and assistance; and loss of any relationship that serves a singular function in human existence leads to social and personal disorganization. He also believes that the psychologic impact of a lost relationship comes from the significance of the relationship to the person and not from the type of relationship per se. Benoliel[6] has noted that reactions to lost relationships are intensified in a context of multiple losses and multiple problems.

GROUP LOSS

Groups, as well as individuals, experience loss. The death of any member of a family results in a reorganization of family relationships, with disruption more likely when the person lost is a child or young adult. The family expresses grief in a variety of ways depending on religious, cultural, and social factors. Bereavement is also affected by whether or not death is expected. Families are usually not well equipped to cope with the complexities of unexpected and sudden loss through death.

A family may also have the problem of adapting to incomplete or partial loss produced by chronic illness, disability, or fatal illness in one of its members. For example, the impact of juvenile-onset diabetes on patients and their families may be both traumatic and never-ending in its influence, and some family systems are better able than others to adapt to the change in constructive ways. In fatal diseases, anticipatory mourning is often part of a family's preparation for the death that eventually must come. According to Futterman and associates,[7] the process of anticipatory mourning in parents of leukemic children is a functionally essential component of successful adaptation to the difficult and serious loss they must face.

Groups other than families may also be affected by the loss of significant members, and even societies as totalities may engage in bereavement, as happened in the United States when President Kennedy was killed. Within the hospital, death on a ward may be extremely disruptive to both personnel and patients, e.g., when a favorite patient dies or there are several deaths at one time. In fact, wards where death is frequent can be considered high-risk work settings because of the high grief potential they carry for personnel who work there.

PROCESS OF GRIEVING

Loss produces a state of sorrow and deprivation, but not all losses result in the experience of grief. According to Parkes[8] and to Switzer,[9] *grief* is a total organismic response to the loss of a significant relationship, and *grieving* is the psychobiologic process of assimilating the change and its meaning into a new definition of reality.

Initially, acute loss produces a feeling of separation anxiety and a sense of deprivation, and response to these reactions is both physiologic and emotional. In a study of human reactions following acute loss, Lindemann[10] identified five characteristics that he considered to be pathognomonic for grief: somatic distress and tension; preoccupation with an image of the lost person or relationship; feelings of guilt; hostility and anger; and changes in ordinary patterns of conduct or behavior. The process of grieving consists of responses that usually occur in the following pattern: a period of numbness and shock; feelings of anger and fear; a sense of helplessness and a wish to be helped; feelings of despair and emptiness, sometimes coupled with guilt and shame; and finally, a renewal of hope and a reorganization of behavior directed toward a new relationship or reconstruction of the old one.

Psychologic recovery from the pain of significant loss is a process that requires time. In a general sense, the more significant the relationship, the more time will be needed to grieve until resolution is reached. Time alone is not sufficient, however, and resolution of loss can only come about through the psychologic process of "giving up" the relationship that is gone. Grief work is a term frequently used to describe the emotional experience of finding emancipation from a lost relationship, but not all people are successful in reaching this point.

BEREAVEMENT AND MOURNING

Cultural conditions and socializing influences determine to a great extent how individuals learn to experience and express grief. Bereavement behavior is a socially-learned pattern of conduct in response to loss, especially loss through death. There are many variations in the types of bereavement behavior expected and encouraged in different cultural and subcultural groups. Mourning practices are rooted in the fundamental values and beliefs of a society and are often bound by its religious traditions and customs. For example, Racy[11] states that in the traditional Arab culture expression of grief is not permitted in the presence of a dying person, but after the death everyone expresses his pain and sorrow openly and loudly and is expected to do so. These practices have their origins in the kinship patterns of Arab communities and the meaning of death as proclaimed by Islam.

The dominant cultural emphasis in the United States fosters a social role of bereaved persons preoccupied with grief expression but often without socially sanctioned outlets for other strong emotions. Even though the dominant Anglo influence stresses control of public display of feelings, there clearly are differences among people from various ethnic backgrounds. Persons of Italian and Jewish background, for example, are frequently more open in grief expression than are people whose ancestors came from northern Europe.

The conduct of bereavement for any person emerges from a complex interplay involving his inner personal experience and the outer social world with its explicit and implicit rules for proper behavior. His conduct is also influenced by the meaning of the lost relationship, his past experience with loss, and his present capacity to adapt to the stresses of change. In a study of grief and mourning behavior in the United Kingdom, Gorer[12] identified eight different styles of mourning based on time used by the mourning person: denial of mourning, absence of mourning, hiding grief, time-limited mourning, mourning before death, unlimited mourning—the "never get over" group, unlimited mourning—mummification, and unlimited mourning—despair. Some of these behavioral patterns clearly fall into the category of maladaptive reactions.

MALADAPTIVE REACTIONS

The normal process of grieving is an effective and necessary means of resolving the consequences of serious loss. There are, however, other types of grief reaction described as maladaptive, which are characterized by a failure to cut the ties with the lost relationship. Parkes[13] describes two features characteristic of atypical grief: an intense separation anxiety, and a strong but only partially successful effort to avoid grieving. Inability to resolve the loss means that the individual carries the loss within him in a form that interferes with his capacity to function as a social being in a maximally effective way. Maladaptive grief reactions in individuals include depression, hypochondriasis, alcoholism, psychosomatic illness, acting-out behaviors, and neurotic and psychotic states.

In a similar manner, families and other groups can manifest grief in ways that are destructive to the group rather than enabling movement toward resolution of the lost relationship. Thus, whether significant loss involves an individual or a group of individuals, the outcomes of bereavement are determined by a complex meshing of antecedent, concurrent, and subsequent events that together influence the meaning of loss, grief, and change. Vollman and associates[14] studied families to identify those capable of coping with sudden death and those prone to develop maladaptive patterns of response. They found that families with few social ties or connections with other families or groups in the society were more likely to develop maladaptive grief reactions than were families with established ties or memberships in well-defined cultural subgroups.

ASSISTANCE SERVICES

The development of mechanisms for offering assessment and assistance services to those facing significant losses has to date been essentially ad hoc in nature and often dependent on the special interests of one committed person. An example of such commitment is the hospice for terminal cancer patients developed in England under the leadership of Cicely Saunders.[15] In the United States many health care institutions provide generalized services to a broad spectrum of people rather than to a single group with specialized problems. The development of effective helping services requires consideration of several different types of grief-producing situations. In general, helping services in organized health care systems need to provide assistance for at least two major types of problems: acute grief reactions resulting from sudden and unexpected deaths or other significant personal losses, and chronic and prolonged transitions involving individuals and/or groups in the problems of adapting to partial losses.

CRISIS INTERVENTION

The concept of crisis intervention derived from the work of Caplan[16] provides the basis for active treatment of persons and groups involved in acute psychosocial crises that overstress their available coping resources. The goal of crisis intervention is to prevent maladaptive grief reactions by offering psychologic assistance during periods of high vulnerability. On a pragmatic basis, crisis intervention services require a team of well-trained people available at all times. The appearance of crisis clinics in many communities over the past few years is an indication of the rising demand for services of this nature. However, similar types of crisis intervention services are needed in hospitals and other health care institutions to help personnel as well as patients and their families cope with the stresses of loss and grief.

TRANSITION SERVICES

The development of services for persons and groups who are trying to cope with chronic grief and the interminable transitions produced by partial losses is a difficult problem. Assistance in these situations may require the availability of replacement or substitution services for aspects of living formerly viewed as familial rather than health care concerns. Also, manifestations of grief may appear in disguised form, e.g., as hypochondriasis or alcoholism, and not be recognized as related to the significant loss. In another instance, the problem may concern a group of people engaged in chronic grief, e.g., in custodial institutions where the elderly, infirm, or mentally retarded are housed indefinitely.

Recognition of the need for special services to help people in these prolonged and psychologically depleting situations has come slowly, but recent years have seen the appearance of new forms of transition assistance. For example, hospital chaplaincy programs in many general hospitals have expanded to provide ongoing counseling services for those involved with the problems of long term and fatal illnesses. Self-help groups such as Parents without Partners, Lamplighters, diabetic summer camps, and many others have been created to offer support and guidance within the context of shared experience. Hoffman and Futterman[17] introduced play therapy in the waiting room of an oncology clinic to create a milieu which would encourage leukemic children and their parents to participate actively in the coping tasks of anticipatory mourning and maintenance of mastery in the face of helplessness and hopelessness.

Although mechanisms are clearly needed for building psychologic services into the health care system, the effectiveness of these services ultimately depends on health care personnel who are sensitive to the nuances of grief and able to contend with its intricacies and uncertainties. Nurses are often in a position to assist people in coping productively with the different stages of the grieving process. To do so, however, they must learn to cope with their own feelings of loss and grief, and find flexible ways of helping other people deal with theirs. Writing about the disruptive effects of untimely deaths, Weisman[18] proposes that the goal of psychologic intervention is twofold: to foster an appropriate and timely bereavement process similar to that considered appropriate for an individual patient dying of long term disease, and to transform highly calamitous deaths into forms that permit resolution of loss in appropriate and timely ways. This goal offers a perspective applicable to any and all grief-producing situations, and provides direction to assist in making decisions under different sets of social and cultural conditions.

REFERENCES

1. Peretz, D.: *Development, object-relationships, and loss.* In Schoenberg, B., et al. (eds.): *Loss and Grief: Psychological Management in Medical Practice.* Columbia University Press, New York, 1970.
2. Volkart, E. H.: *Bereavement and mental health.* In Leighton, A. H., Clausen, J. A. and Wilson, R. E. (eds.): *Explorations in Social Psychiatry.* Basic Books, New York, 1957.

3. Bowlby, J.: *Pathological mourning and childhood mourning.* J. Am. Psychoanal. Assoc. 11:500, 1963.
4. Peretz: op. cit.
5. Weiss, R. S.: *The fund of sociability.* Trans-action 6:39, 1969.
6. Benoliel, J. Q.: *Assessments of loss and grief.* Journal of Thanatology 1:182, 1971.
7. Futterman, E. H., Hoffman, I. and Sabshin, M.: *Parental anticipatory mourning.* In Schoenberg, B. et al. (eds.): *Psychosocial Aspects of Terminal Care.* Columbia University Press, New York, 1972.
8. Parkes, C. M.: *Bereavement.* International Universities Press, New York, 1972.
9. Switzer, D. K.: *The Dynamics of Grief.* Abingdon Press, New York, 1970.
10. Lindemann, E.: *Symptomatology and management of acute grief.* Am. J. Psychiatry 101:144, 1944.
11. Racy, J.: *Death in an Arab culture.* Ann. N. Y. Acad. Sci. 164:874, 1969.
12. Gorer, G.: *Death, Grief, and Mourning.* Anchor Books, Garden City, 1967.
13. Parkes: op. cit.
14. Vollman, R. R., et al.: *The reactions of family systems to sudden and unexpected death.* Omega 2:105, 1971.
15. Saunders, C.: *The last stages of life.* Am. J. Nurs. 65:70, 1965.
16. Caplan, G.: *Principles of Preventive Psychiatry.* Grune and Stratton, New York, 1964.
17. Hoffman, I. and Futterman, E. H.: *Coping with waiting: Psychiatric intervention and study in the waiting room of a pediatric oncology clinic.* Compr. Psychiatry 12:79, 1971.
18. Weisman, A. D.: *Coping with untimely death.* Psychiatry 36:374, 1973.

BIBLIOGRAPHY

Bowlby, J.: *Process of Mourning.* Int. J. Psychoanal. 42:317, 1961.

David, R. H. and Neiswender, M. (eds.): *Dealing with Death.* University of Southern California, Los Angeles, 1973.

Engel, G. L.: *Grief and Grieving.* Am. J. Nurs. 64:97, 1964.

Fulton, R. (ed.): *Death and Identity.* John Wiley & Sons, New York, 1965.

Gorer, G.: *Death, Grief, and Mourning.* Anchor Books, Garden City, 1967.

Kubler-Ross, E.: *On Death and Dying.* Macmillan, New York, 1969.

Moriarty, D. M. (ed.): *The Loss of Loved Ones.* Charles C Thomas, Springfield, 1967.

Parkes, C. M.: *Bereavement.* International Universities Press, New York, 1972.

Schmale, A. H.: *Normal grief is not a disease.* Journal of Thanatology 2:807, 1972.

Schoenberg, B., et al. (eds.): *Loss and Grief: Psychological Management in Medical Practice.* Columbia University Press, New York, 1970.

11 *Crisis*

JANICE M. MESSICK, R.N., M.S.
DONNA C. AGUILERA, Ph.D., F.A.A.N.

A person in crisis is at a turning point. He faces a problem that he cannot readily solve using the coping mechanisms that have worked for him before. As a result, his tension and anxiety increase, and he becomes less able to find a solution. A person in this situation feels helpless—he is caught in a state of great emotional upset and feels unable to take action on his own to solve his problem. The two cardinal symptoms of crisis are increased anxiety and increased depression.

Crisis intervention can offer the immediate help that a person in crisis needs in order to re-establish equilibrium. It is short-term therapy that focuses on solving the immediate problem. An understanding of crisis theory is necessary in order to assess, anticipate, formulate plans, and appropriately intervene when the equilibrium of patients and their families is threatened.

CRISIS THEORY

Caplan[1] views the individual as living in a state of emotional equilibrium with his goal always to return to or maintain that state. When customary problem-solving techniques cannot be used to meet a particular problem, the balance of equilibrium is upset. The individual must either problem-solve or adapt to nonsolution. In either case a new state of equilibrium will ensue, sometimes better and sometimes worse insofar as positive mental health is concerned. When the individual faces a problem that he cannot solve there is a rise in frustration, signs of anxiety, and disorganization of function, resulting in a period of protracted emotional upset. This state is referred to as *crisis*.

Caplan emphasizes that crisis is characteristically self-limiting and lasts from four to six weeks. This constitutes a transitional period, representing both the danger of increased psychologic vulnerability and an opportunity for personality growth. The outcome of a crisis is determined by the kind of interaction which takes place during this period between the individual and the key figures in his emotional milieu.

TYPES OF CRISES

An individual is continually exposed to change, and thus potential crisis, by the ongoing processes of maturational development, shifting situations within his environment, or a combination of both. Potential crisis areas occur during the period of great social, physical, and psychologic change experienced by all human beings in the normal growth process. These changes may occur during concomitant biologic and social role transitions, e.g., puberty, young adulthood, marriage, and parenthood.

MATURATIONAL CRISES

Maturational crises have been described as normal processes of growth and development. These usually evolve over an extended period of time, such as during the transition into adulthood, and frequently require that the individual make many characterologic changes. There may be an awareness of increased feelings of disequilibrium, and intellectual understanding of any correlation with normal developmental change may be inadequate. Erikson[2] feels that each transitional stage must be successfully negotiated, or it will create problems in later life. These stages are: preschool, school age, preadolescence, adolescence, young adulthood, adulthood, late adulthood, and finally, old age.

SITUATIONAL CRISES

Situational crises are those events which occur in the environment and may be stressful to the individual and thus may evoke a crisis. One such event could be the birth of a baby: this requires a change in living patterns. There may be feelings of inadequacy in caring for the child or resentment because of a loss of freedom, either of which may be compounded by fatigue. Even more stressful could be the birth of a premature or handicapped infant. This may involve feelings of guilt, shame, and resentment.

There are many other situations that may be stressful, such as loss of job, divorce, death of a loved one—anything that involves loss or change. This is why it is frequently difficult to determine if a crisis is due to situational events or maturational events. Often there is an overlap, with one compounding the other.

BALANCING FACTORS

Why is it that some people experience crisis and others do not? Let us use the example of two mothers: Sue and Mary. Both have just given birth to premature infants. Sue is upset, naturally, but doesn't go into crisis; however, Mary does go into crisis. Why? Why does Sue react in one way and Mary in a different way to the same stress? What factors decide whether a person will regain a state of equilibrium, or enter a state of crisis? Three factors have been isolated and identified that seem to make the difference: perception of the event, situational support, and coping mechanisms. Figure 11-1 demonstrates a paradigm of the effects of a stressful event on the human organism. The upper portion illustrates the "normal" initial reaction of an individual to a stressful event. In column A, the balancing factors are operating and crisis is avoided. In column B, the absence of one or more of these balancing factors may block resolution of the problem, thus increasing disequilibrium and precipitating a crisis.

PERCEPTION OF THE EVENT

In other words, What does it mean to the person? How does he think it will affect his future? Can he look at the event realistically, or does he distort its meaning? For example, Sue views the birth of a premature infant as upsetting and realizes that some changes will have to be made in her plans, but she feels fulfilled as a mother and accepts and loves her premature child because it is hers. However, Mary views her premature infant as evidence that she is a failure as a mother. The infant threatens her self-esteem and she feels guilty, ashamed, and resentful.

SITUATIONAL SUPPORT

This refers to those persons in the environment upon whom an individual can depend for

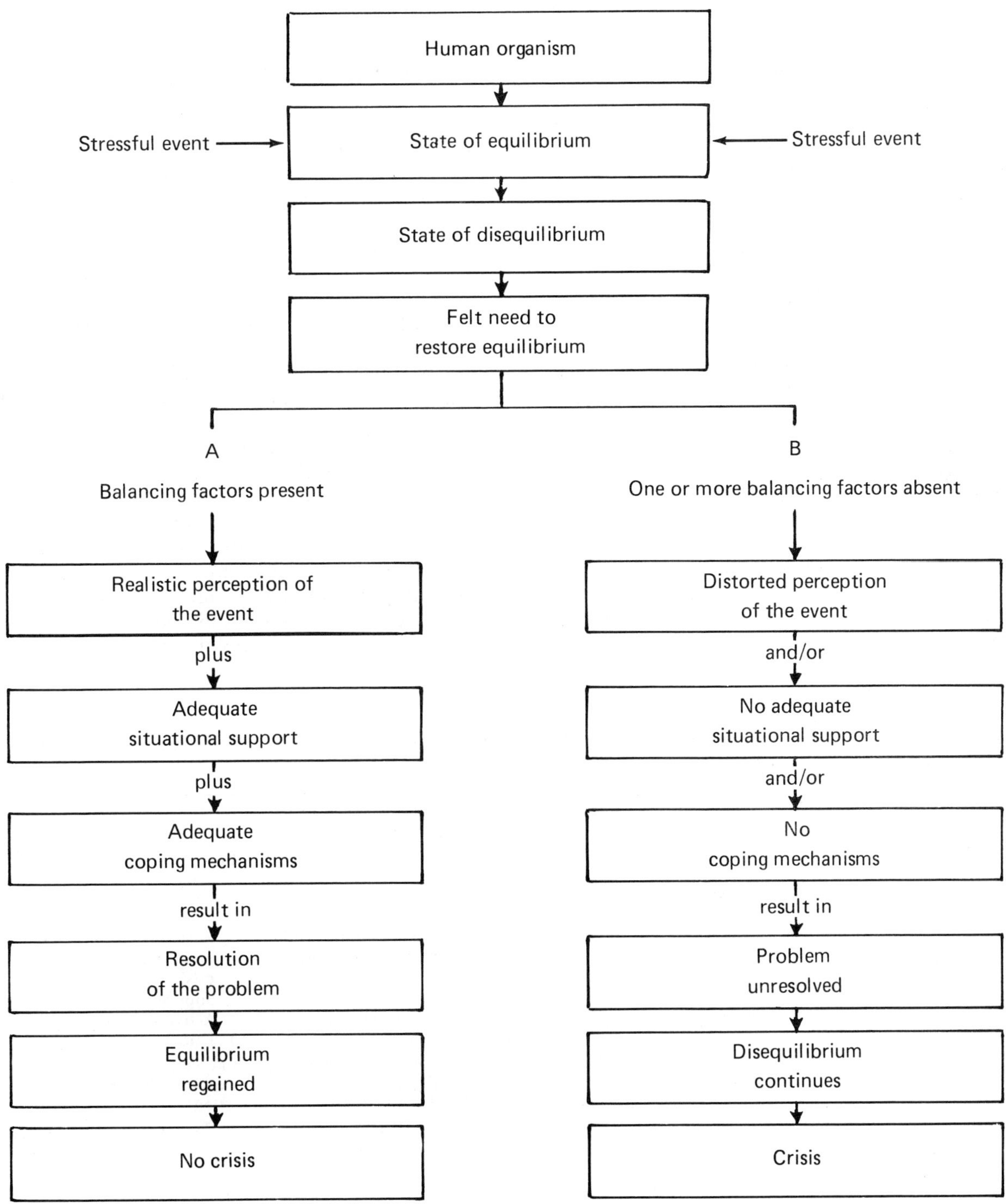

FIGURE 11-1. Effects of balancing factors in a stressful event. (From Aguilera and Messick, [3] with permission.)

help. To whom can the person turn? Who is available to talk with them about the stressful event? Spouse? Family? Friends? For example, Sue seeks and receives support from her husband and family. Mary, however, refuses to turn to anyone for assistance, and refuses any help that is offered.

COPING MECHANISMS

These are the activities which help a person resolve problems. What does he usually do? Sit down and try to think it out? Have a good cry? Get angry and shout? Talk with someone about the problem? Sue's coping mechanism is to discuss the situation. She is able to problem-solve and plan for the changes made necessary by the event. Her anxiety and depression are reduced, equilibrium is restored, and crisis is avoided. Mary withdraws from the situation. She is unable to problem-solve. Her anxiety and depression increase, and crisis is evoked.

CRISIS INTERVENTION

The goal of crisis intervention is the resolution of an immediate crisis. Its focus is on the genetic present with the restoration of the individual to his pre-crisis level of functioning or possibly to a higher level of functioning. The therapist's role is direct, suppressive, supportive, and that of an active participant. Techniques are varied, and limited only by the flexibility and creativity of the therapist. These may include helping the individual gain an intellectual understanding of his crisis, assisting the individual in bringing his feelings out into the open, exploring past and present coping mechanisms, finding and using situational supports, and anticipatory planning with the individual to reduce the possibility of future crises. Indication for this type of therapy would be an individual's (or family's) sudden loss of ability to cope with a life situation. The average length of treatment is from one to six sessions. Some of the major differences among psychoanalysis, brief

TABLE 11-1. Major Differences between Psychoanalysis, Brief Psychotherapy, and Crisis Intervention Methodology*

	Psychoanalysis	*Brief Psychotherapy*	*Crisis Intervention*
Goals of therapy	Restructuring the personality	Removal of specific symptoms	Resolution of immediate crisis
Focus of treatment	1. Genetic past	1. Genetic past as it relates to present situation	1. Genetic present
	2. Freeing the unconscious	2. Repression of unconscious and restraining of drives	2. Restortion to level of functioning prior to crisis
Usual activity of therapist	1. Exploratory 2. Passive observer 3. Nondirective	1. Suppressive 2. Participant observer 3. Indirect	1. Suppressive 2. Active participant 3. Direct
Indications	Neurotic personality patterns	Acutely disruptive emotional pain and severely disruptive circumstances	Sudden loss of ability to cope with a life situation
Average length of treatment	Indefinite	From 1 to 20 sessions	From 1 to 6 sessions

* From Aguilera and Messick,[3] with permission.

psychotherapy, and crisis intervention methodology are presented in Table 11-1.

Because a crisis state is short, usually lasting no more than a few weeks, intervention must begin as soon as possible. The outcome of a crisis is governed by the interaction, the help received, during this period. If no help is sought or given the crisis may be resolved, but the level of functioning, the state of equilibrium, will usually be at a lower level than it was before the crisis. If, on the other hand, help with a crisis situation is sought and given, the level of functioning and state of equilibrium can return to the pre-crisis level and there may be an increase in problem-solving abilities and more effective coping skills may be learned.

REFERENCES

1. Caplan, G.: *Concepts of Mental Health and Consultation.* U. S. Department of Health, Education and Welfare, Washington, D. C., pp. 183–206.
2. Erikson, E.: *Identity: Youth and Crisis.* Norton, New York, 1968.
3. Aguilera, D. C. and Messick, J. M.: *Crisis Intervention: Theory and Methodology.* C. V. Mosby, St. Louis, 1974.

BIBLIOGRAPHY

Aguilera, D. C.: *Sociocultural factors: Barriers to therapeutic intervention.* J. Psychiatr. Nurs. 8:14, 1970.

Aguilera, D. C., and Messick, J. M.: *Crisis: The psychiatric nurse intervenes.* J. Psychiatr. Nurs. 5:233, 1967.

Ibid.: *Crisis Intervention: Theory and Methodology,* ed. 2. C. V. Mosby, St. Louis, 1974.

Berliner, B.: *Nursing the patient in crisis.* Am. J. Nurs. 70:2154, 1970.

Brandon, S.: *Crisis theory and possibilities of therapeutic intervention.* Br. J. Psychiatry 117:541, 1970.

Chandler, H. M.: *Family Crisis Intervention.* J. Natl. Med. Assoc. 64:211, 1972.

Donner, G. J.: *Parenthood as a crisis.* Perspect. Psychiatr. Care X:84, 1972.

Flomenhaft, K. and Langsley, D. G.: *After the crisis.* Mental Hygiene 55:473, 1971.

Lindemann, E.: *The meaning of crisis in individual and family.* Teachers Coll. Rec. 57:310, 1956.

Maloney, E. M.: *The subjective and objective definition of crisis.* Perspect. Psychiatr. Care IX:257, 1971.

McClellan, M. S.: *Crisis groups in special care areas.* Nurs. Clin. North Am. 7:2, 1972.

Messick, J. M.: *Crisis intervention concepts: Implications for nursing practices.* J. Psychiatr. Nurs. 10:3, 1972.

Morley, W. E., Messick, J. M. and Aguilera, D. C.: *Crisis: Paradigms of intervention.* J. Psychiatr. Nurs. 5:31, 1967.

Ovesy, L. and Jameson, J.: *Adaptational techniques of psychodynamic therapy.* In Rado, S. and Daniels, G. (eds.): *Changing Concepts of Psychoanalytic Medicine.* Grune & Stratton, New York, 1956.

Rapaport, L.: *The State of Crisis: Some Theoretical Considerations.* University of Chicago Press, Chicago, 1972.

Raphael, B.: *Crisis intervention: Theoretical and methodological considerations.* Aust. N. Z. J. Psychiatry 5:183, 1971.

Williams, F.: *Intervention in maturational crisis.* Perspect. Psychiatr. Care IX:240, 1971.

UNIT 3

THE CONCEPT OF CULTURE

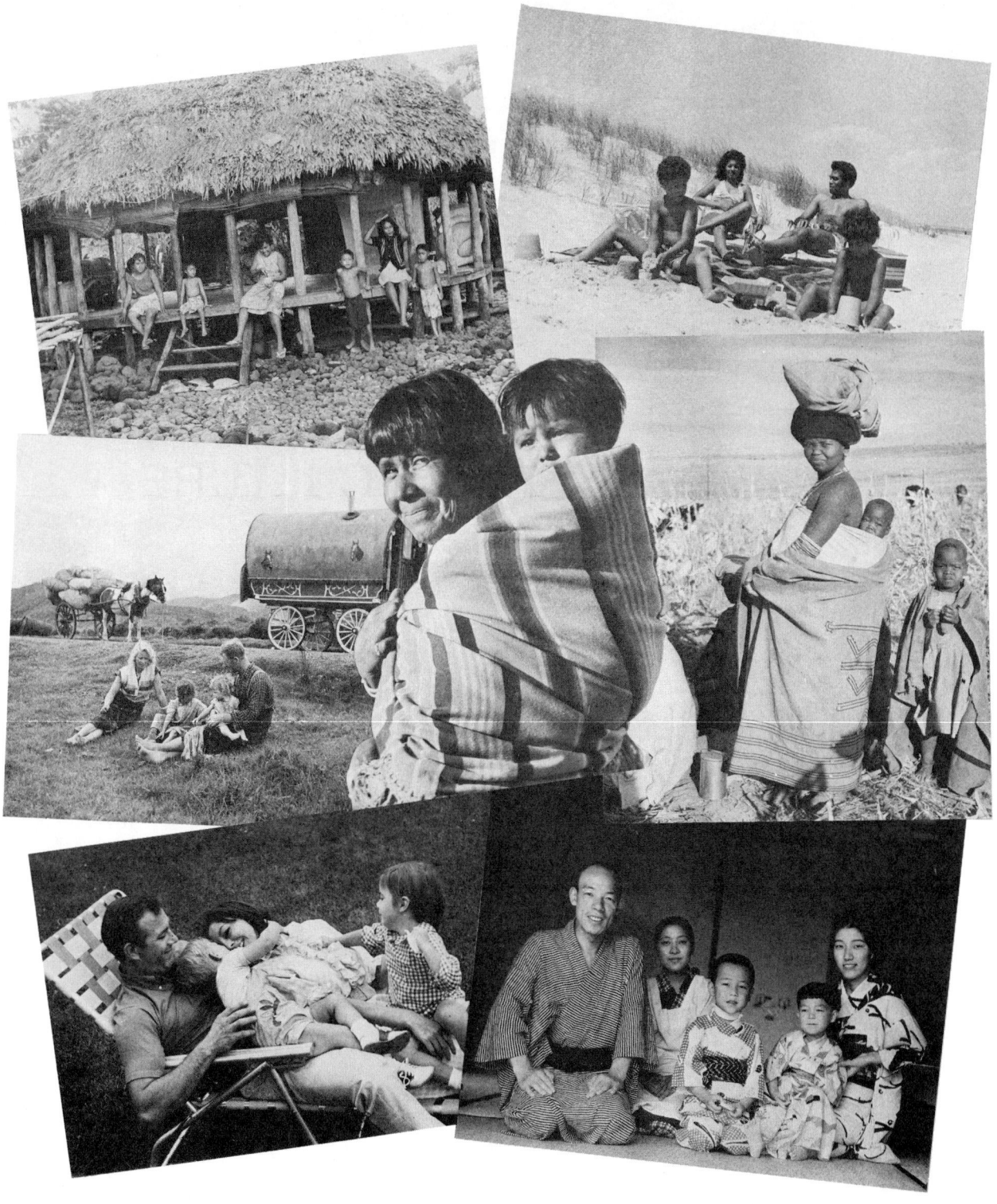

12 *Cross-Cultural Perspectives*

NILES NEWTON, Ph.D.

In order to provide humanized, family-centered nursing care during childbearing and childrearing it is necessary to understand variations in attitude and behavior which result from cultural influences. The nurse, frequently in contact with people from many social groups, is in an especially good position to make use of this knowledge. This chapter discusses the importance of the concept of cultural patterning using illustrations of nurturant care during childbirth and the postpartum period.

ADVANTAGES OF CROSS-CULTURAL STUDIES

What do the various customs of other people have to do with an understanding of modern obstetric nursing care? Why bother to discuss what is done in other parts of the world or at other times in history? The main value to be gained from studying the behavior of ancient, traditional, and far-off peoples is that they demonstrate a wide range of potential behavior and can help us to see more clearly the effects of our own society on our own behavior. This knowledge helps us to be more understanding of other ways of doing things. For example, a woman breast feeding her frightened two-year-old in the emergency room might receive more sympathetic treatment from a nurse who is aware that long-term nursing was an accepted custom in this country several generations ago and is still practiced in many parts of the world.

Cross-cultural studies can also give us insights into different views of health care by distinguishing practices based on biologic necessity from those based on social customs. For example, in our society there is a tendency to feel that it is a physical necessity to keep a woman lying down during labor and delivery, possibly because we tend to think of birth in terms of sickness and surgical techniques. Actually, many mothers find other positions comfortable. A survey of birth positions in 76 non-European societies found that 62 of them use upright positions, usually kneeling, sitting, or squatting.[1] Once we understand that various birth positions are possible, we can examine more meaningfully the social and psychologic reasons why our society favors the position it does.

LIMITATIONS OF CROSS-CULTURAL STUDIES

Although we can get ideas from other people in other places, it must be remembered that it is impossible to "transplant" customs. Each society translates customs and their meanings into its own terms. For example, the Espanos, a Peruvian village people, when confronted with the idea of vitamins, concluded that vitamin-rich foods were too strong for infants, too fattening during pregnancy, and thus should be avoided.[2]

Any single social practice is intimately connected with many other customs and attitudes. For example, obstetric care in the Netherlands demonstrates that home delivery can be physically safe and offers certain psychologic and psychosomatic advantages. In fact, the Dutch, who still depend very heavily on home deliveries, have much more favorable maternal and child health statistics than those of the United States. However, such a home delivery system could not be transplanted to this country without major changes in attitudes toward birth and the role of health professionals. It seems natural in Holland to keep laboring women at home since childbearing is seen as a normal physiologic phenomenon. Pregnant and laboring women are called "mothers" not "patients" unless pathology has become apparent. The Dutch have many highly trained midwives whose obstetric training lasts three years, and also midwives' assistants who give less technical home nursing care. Thus, health care practices are interrelated to other practices and attitudes within the society. They are part of a whole that must be considered and dealt with as a whole.

THE MOTHER DURING LABOR

This discussion examines how nurturant care is patterned during labor, noting variations from one culture to another. Feeding and medicating are important parts of nurturant care during labor. Some societies emphasize nutrition while others emphasize medication and still others give both. It should be noted that customs often change radically within a short period of time under the impact of contact with Western industrial culture. The customs described existed at the time of observation and recording but may have disappeared since then.

FOOD AND DRINK

Various nutritional approaches have been found in primitive labor. The African Hottentots fed soups to laboring women to strengthen them. The Yumans and the Pawnee, both of North America, developed a strong prohibition against drinking water during labor; it must cease with the first labor pain. Maternal death was ascribed to breaking this taboo. The Bahaya of Africa permitted drinking during labor but prohibited eating.

Current patterns in the United States are similar to these restrictive preliterate groups except that *both* food and drink are taboo in most institutions. Although it is currently believed that these restrictions are to prevent aspiration of vomitus during inhalation anesthesia, safe labors are being managed in many parts of the world giving food and drink as part of their nurturing pattern.

Current European medicine often does not place restrictions on food during labor to the same extent. For example, British customs in this regard allow both food and drink. In normal cases, three meals a day during labor are recommended. Breakfast is to consist of tea, thinly cut and lightly buttered toast, "jelly" marmalade, and an egg if the patient wishes. Lunch includes strained chicken broth, sieved meat or fish with no fat, and sieved fruits (except citrus fruits). Supper is similar to breakfast. When general anesthesia is anticipated, the women in early labor are still permitted strained chicken soup, sieved fruit, tea, toast, a lightly boiled egg, and fruit juice.[3]

American traditions of nurturant care in the past included giving nourishment during labor. An early nineteenth century obstetric text states: "She should be supplied from time to time with mild bland nourishment in moderate quantities. Tea, coffee, gruel, barley water, milk and water, broths, etc. may safely be allowed."[4]

MEDICATION

Within the last 150 years biochemical support of women in labor in the United States has changed from food to drugs. In fact, anesthesia and analgesia are perhaps the chief forms of their nurturant care at the present time.

Medication during labor is not a new or modern nurturant technique. The first act of the Ukrainian midwife was to give the mother a generous dose of whisky to ease her pains. The Amhara of Ethiopia gave a drink of mashed linseed to relax the birth tract and lessen the pain. On the other side of the world in North America, Indian midwives used plant preparations to ease pain during birth. Drugs for stimulating labor are also not limited to modern industrial society. The Bahaya who live near Lake Victoria in Africa used such a potent oxytocic drug that many cases of ruptured uteri were reported. The Sierra Tarascans of Mexico had a drug sufficiently strong that it was used not only to accelerate labor but also to induce abortion.

AUDITORY STIMULATION

In many societies, nurturant care during labor involves sensory stimulation. Some methods emphasize an auditory approach while others use cutaneous stimulation.

Laotians in Indochina, the Navajo of North America and the Cuna of Panama used music during labor. Stimulating conversation was used by some primitive groups who patterned labor as a social event where people gathered around the laboring woman. For example, among the Navajo the hogan was open when a baby was being born. Anyone who came to lend moral support was invited to stay and eat. In America music is now frequently used and soothing conversation with the laboring woman is advocated by natural childbirth and Lamaze proponents.

CUTANEOUS STIMULATION

A common form of sensory stimulation is abdominal stimulation. This technique was employed during labor among the Kurtatchi of the Solomon Islands. A woman attendant chewed special roots and vegetation. She spat the resulting red saliva on her hands and rubbed the laboring woman's abdomen, using a circular motion, all round the edge of the belly. Occasionally the attendant knelt behind the laboring woman and moved clasped hands from the top of the protuberant abdomen to the bottom shaking it violently. This pattern of abdominal stimulation appeared among other widely separated primitive people, indicating independent invention of the techniques. The Yahgan midwife of Tierra del Fuego, at the southern tip of South America, made circular strokes on the abdomen with the flat of her hand to stimulate birth. The Punjab midwife rubbed melted butter on the abdomen.

An American version of abdominal stimulation is the technique of abdomen rubbing taught to women in the Lamaze program. Bing recommends it, stating "soothe the pain by massaging your abdomen gently in time with your breathing."[5] Notice that in America it is recommended that the woman give herself this nurturant care, whereas in the cultures cited previously, the midwives did it.

The natural childbirth technique of having the husband rub the woman's back has its counterpart in a number of preliterate cultures. Among the Pukapuka of New Zealand, a medicine man specializing in obstetrics helped a woman in delivery by pushing with the heel or palm of the hand on the small of her back. The Kurtatchi and the Kazakhs of Asia used knee pressure of the attendant holding the woman from behind.

In times of stress it is comforting to be held by another person. This is a frequent method of showing cherishing nurturance. Such physical contact helps give emotional as well as physical support. Ford's[6] survey of preliterate cultures indicated that 25 such societies supported women from behind as they labored. In Sweden and the Netherlands the husband supports the woman's back during the second stage of labor. In the United States the woman usually receives almost no body contact during the second stage of labor. Her legs are held by mechanical devices and if she is having a Lamaze or natural childbirth delivery her back is sometimes supported by inanimate objects, a back rest or triangular pillow.

THE LEISURELY APPROACH

Another basic difference in the patterning of nurturant behavior during labor is whether attempts are made to speed labor or whether a leisurely approach is used.

The following account by Holmberg of one such leisurely approach describes the Siriono, an extremely primitive group that lived in Bolivia. The mother receives little nurturant care except psychologic support.

> Of the eight births which I had the good fortune to witness among the Siriono, four took place during the day and four at night. In the former cases the mothers received no help whatever, either during the preparations for the births or during the births themselves. In the other four cases the husbands assisted to the extent of setting fire to a few dried leaves of motacu palm in order to light up the immediate environs of the hammock, but beyond this they gave no help.
>
> At all of the births a crowd of women were present, standing by or sitting in adjoining hammocks, gossiping about what it was like when they had their last child or speculating as to whether the prospective child would be a boy or girl. Not a move was made by these onlookers to assist the parturient woman, except in one case when twins were born. . . . To exert force during labor a woman grasps the rope strung above her hammock which the mother herself has hung.
>
> In all of the births which I witnessed, except that of the twins, the mothers had no difficulty in delivery. The time of labor varied from 1 to 3 hours, but never extended beyond that limit. In all instances the babies were born head first.
>
> The infant, in being born, slides off the outside strings of the hammock on to the soft earth below. Since hammocks are not hung more than a few inches above the floor, the shock to the infant of falling to the ground is not great, yet it is probably sufficient to start it breathing and induce it to show other signs of life. In no case did I see an infant slapped to give life. All of them started breathing immediately after the shock of birth.
>
> Immediately after the birth the mother gets out of her hammock and kneels on the floor to one side of the infant until the afterbirth is expelled. . . . If the father is present the umbilical cord is cut at once; if not, the mother must await his arrival. The cord is cut by the father with a bamboo knife.[7]

THE LABOR-SPEEDING APPROACH

In contrast to the Siriono, other primitive peoples managed labor on the "maximum assistance" principle. Feelings of impatience were often quite openly expressed. A prolonged labor among the Pukapuka of New Zealand was described this way: "At times there were at least ten persons all pushing parts of her body and calling to her to push the child out."[8] The mother was accused of being afraid to press down and was constantly scolded for not telling her attendants when the pains were starting. In Jordan, the village women dropped in to see how things were going. In the case of a slow labor they would comment, "Hurry up. We wish to see thy son before we go to bed!"

Vigorous physical measures were used in many parts of the world to speed labor. The Hottentots of South Africa pulled the baby out, grasping it by the chin once the head emerged. If the baby was delayed in spite of strong labor contractions, attempts were made to stretch the vagina, and sometimes the area was deliberately torn to make room. The Chagga of Tanganyika also developed a kind of episiotomy. In extremely difficult labors, primigravidas would be cut to facilitate delivery.

Pressure on the abdomen is the most commonly reported mechanical labor-speeding device. This can be applied as a violent manipulation, as firm pushing during contraction, or as constant pressure maintained by means of a tight belt or binder. An extreme example of this was the practice of the Karen midwives of Burma who, according to Marshall, "believed in aiding nature rather than letting nature take its own course, even in normal cases. . . . They resorted to massage to hasten the birth and in stubborn cases they tread on the abdomen to expel the fetus."[9]

HISTORIC VIEW OF LABOR SPEEDING

Contrasting patterns of nurturant care can also be found within Western traditions. At certain times active speeding was considered to be most helpful to the woman and at other times reliance on supporting natural physiologic processes was advocated.

Hippocrates advised leaving the placenta alone even if it remained unexpelled for three or four days. while Celsus, a Roman medical authority, advocated inserting the hand into the uterus as soon as the baby was born and removing the placenta. Some physicians advocated cutting the perineum in order to hasten delivery while others felt that preserving the perineum was of positive value. Ould,[10] in 1742, believed in cutting the vulvar outlet when it offered too great resistance and Michaelis,[11] in 1810, felt that the perineum should be incised to avoid a dangerous tear. However, a popular textbook[12] of 1831 emphasized the importance of preserving the perineum and discussed in detail labor-slowing techniques whereby this could be accomplished.

The "laissez faire" school of obstetrics was once popular in the United States. In 1816 Merriman stated: "Natural labour requires but little assistance on the part of the accoucheur. He must recollect that the dilation of the soft parts will be effected by the natural pains, assisted by the bag of waters gradually insinuating itself through the uterus and vagina, much more easily and more safely, than by any artificial means that he can employ."[13] Almost a century later, in 1913, DeLee wrote: "The treatment of the first stage is one of watchful expectancy. The duty of the accoucheur is to observe the efforts of nature, not to aid, until she has proven herself unequal to the task. Only when nature fails, is art to enter. Nothing is so reprehensible as meddlesome midwifery."[14]

Current patterns of obstetric care in the United States tend to reflect the belief that the shorter the labor the better. First stage labor is frequently speeded with surgical rupture of the membranes, administration of oxytocin, or both. The laboring woman is urged to push hard and bear down during the second stage of labor in order to exert maximum force during contractions, thus speeding labor. "Prophylactic forceps" and "prophylactic episiotomies," which hasten the second stage of labor, are routinely used on many patients. The rapid delivery of the placenta, accomplished by manual manipulation of the fundus, is a widely practiced obstetric technique.

THE POSTPARTUM MOTHER

REST AFTER BIRTH

A few preliterate groups stress resumed activity. Among the most extreme are the Yahgan near the South Pole. The community gives help to the mother of a newborn baby, but the rest period after delivery lasts one day or less. Yahgan women were seen "almost directly after birth" or "one quarter hour after delivery" going about their work of gathering shellfish, lifting loads, and rowing as if nothing had happened.[15]

Although this description fits many American notions of primitive childbearing, actually the majority of preliterate societies give a great deal of nurturant care to women after delivery, permitting them to rest in seclusion. A survey by Ford of 64 preliterate societies states: "The majority of societies require the mother to remain in seclusion for three to seven days, either isolating her in a special shelter or confining her to her dwelling. During the period of strict confinement, the woman remains indoors with her baby. Only a few specified visitors are permitted to enter the hut. During this time it is only the mother or her special nurse who tends the infant. In a few tribes the period of seclusion extends to two weeks or a month—rarely longer. Some tribes, though requiring strict isolation for a few days only, continue to restrict the woman's activities for a month or so after birth."[16]

These patterns correspond with the type of advice given to American women a hundred years ago by Chavasse: "The horizontal—or level—position for either ten days or a fortnight after labor is important. A lady frequently fancies that if she supports her legs, it is all that is necessary. Now this is absurd—it is the womb, not the legs that require rest, and the only way to obtain it is by lying flat either on a bed or sofa."[17]

Several decades ago a hospital stay of ten days after a normal delivery was not unusual in the United States. Currently, mothers are being discharged three or four days after birth, or even sooner, and the help they get at home is minimal. I recently helped to organize a study of 200 postpartum mothers who delivered in the Chicago area. The large majority reported they did receive some help with the housework the first week, but little after that. With grandmothers working and relatives far away, the American mother is getting to be more like the Yahgan woman rather than her own great grandmother who often received considerable nurturant care from a larger family group after delivery.

THE CARE GIVER

There is one aspect of childbearing in which cultural patterning is so uniform that it strongly suggests a biologic base. This is with regard to *who* gives nurturant care to childbearing women. All over the world, in all societies, it is women who overwhelmingly give the most nurturant care to other women.

Jelliffe and Bennett[18] have discussed the childbearing practices of traditional cultures, noting that the work of caring for a large family and producing food during the last months of pregnancy may have been eased by relocation of the family members—toddlers may be sent to relatives or the woman herself may return to her own mother. Another solution is to "import" into the family an older child of a relative. The Chagga appointed a young girl to cook for the mother and baby during her confinement. For four days after delivery the Tewa mother lay supine while friends and relatives did the housework. Not until the eighth day did they leave, when the mother herself began to assume household work.

Often in traditional cultures birth took place in the home of the mother's or the father's mother. Thus, care of the parturient woman was provided by the grandmother and her younger daughters. The Punjab girl leaves her husband and mother-in-law, with whom she still feels shy, and travels to the home of her birth to be with her own mother and the village midwife, whom she has known for years. This same return to the mother's home for the first baby has been reported among peoples in Africa, North America, South America, the Middle East, and in the Pacific Islands. The importance of this custom is highlighted by the fact that it is practiced by many people living thousands of miles apart.

In some cultures, co-wives may also be a source of childbearing assistance. Jelliffe and Bennett[19] state, "Polygamy was an obvious advantage during pregnancy as there were other adult and responsible women present to care for everything—provided the polygamous marriage was harmonious." Hamer,[20] in a study of 29 African societies, found that lower infant mortality rates were associated with a high incidence of polygamous marriages.

In preliterate cultures all over the world, the elderly woman, rather than the skilled man, was the predominant attendant at normal labor. Ford[21] noted that in 58 of such cultures elderly women were reported to assist at birth and their absence was noted in only two.

We tend to feel that today in the United States male physicians are the prime givers of care in childbearing—but think a moment—is this really so? Think of the time that nurses and other female helpers spend with the patient during office and clinic visits. Consider who actually provides nurturant care for the woman in the labor suite and postpartum. Although the era of the famous midwives is over and males now get the majority of credit for obstetrics, *in terms of hours spent* giving care to childbearing women, women still overwhelmingly do the most work. The change pertains to *which* women give the care. It used to be relatives and friends who helped before, during, and after delivery. Now, during the perinatal period, strange women have been substituted for familiar ones.

NURTURANT CARE OF THE INFANT

MOTHER-BABY CLOSENESS

Many traditional and preliterate cultures emphasize physical closeness between mother and child and immediate attention to crying. Mother-baby closeness among the Aymara of Bolivia was described in this way by Tichauer: "Wherever the mother went, even to a dance, the baby would go, with her little head close to hers and easily slung forward in front of her in case of need. . . . No modesty was attached to nursing even in public places. . . . At night the child slept next to his mother. This continued until he was about two years old or until the next child was born. Nursing had precedence over any other activity in which the mother might have been engaged, such as selling her vegetables in the market, for instance, although she may have been extremely anxious to make the sale."[22]

In the Jordan village of the Middle East, a totally different social setting, the same degree of closeness was reported by Granqvist: "Even after birth the mother and child were closely connected for a long period. To be fed the baby required its mother all the time for it must not be hungry. Both in everyday life and at festivals one can observe how, as soon as the little child cried or showed the least sign of restlessness, it was at once laid to the mother's breast. Very often a woman who was nursing a child had an opening in her dress over each breast and thus she could feed it at once. And she did it unhesitatingly in any place, at any time and very often."[23] The breast was considered the symbol of compassion in Jordan. A woman who had something special to ask God would bare her breast and then make her appeal.

Frick described the closeness of mother and baby in China: "The mother puts her child to her breasts as often as he becomes restless or cries, and this day or night. Nobody can tell how often the infant is nursed and for how long. It is never limited to a few months, but lasts for years (five years is no rarity). Usually the nursing period lasts until the birth of another child. It is looked at as very natural when the mother nurses her child and she therefore carries him always with her."[24]

Inner Mongolian farmers' wives indicated their acceptance of breast feeding in their mode of dress. Grandmothers and unmarried girls wore jackets but Cammann states: "The nursing mothers, which means all women with young children, did not wear jackets. Instead, they had a remarkable upper garment. . . . It was a very narrow bib which extended from neck to trousers, between the breasts, leaving the latter exposed. They nursed the children until they were two or three; and sometimes the older children, youngsters of six or seven, would also 'step up for a drink,' "[25]

Half way around the world, a similar closeness exists. Beals writes about the Sierra Tarascans in Mexico: "Children are nursed freely whenever they desire the breast. . . . Nursing takes place in a variety of public circumstances on the street or on the roads and even while riding on the burro. Through the first year or so the child sleeps with the nipple of the mother's breast in its mouth at night."[26]

Societies without industrial economies usually nurse children a long time. A study of 46 preliterate cultures disclosed that 31 of them weaned infants beginning at 2 or 3 years of age, 13 began weaning at 18 months, and one weaned at 6 months.[27] Another example is the traditional culture of Pakistan where a study of 127 children between 18 months and 2 years revealed that every one of them was still getting some breast milk.[28]

SEPARATION OF MOTHER AND BABY

It would, however, be a mistake to think that all traditional cultures have close mother-child relations. The Tewa of the southwestern United States put considerable distance between mother and child. Whitman[29] reports that pottery making supplied the families not only with the livelihood but with a surplus over and above the necessities of life. Because pottery making was primarily woman's work, it gave women an economic and social importance they had never had before. Babies were kept in beds (or less frequently in cribs) until they were a year old. They were left alone in the bedroom and not taken up except for feeding and bathing. Weaning was begun when the baby was a year old. The mother was pleased if the baby stopped nursing because then she could get more work done.

The women of Alor, an island in Indonesia, provided the chief economic support of the family by cultivating crops. They returned to the fields ten days to two weeks after childbirth, leaving the infant in the care of a relative. However, when the mother came home from the fields in the late afternoon, she usually immediately nursed and fondled the infant and carried it until bedtime, offering the breast whenever the child was restless. At night, mother and infant slept together on the same mat.

The United States leads the world in this more separated pattern of mothering. Most children are not breast fed and even when breast feeding occurs it is usually "token" breast feeding, a pattern which still permits considerable distance between mother and baby. I have summarized it this way:

> Token breast feeding is characterized by severe limitations of sucking by social custom from the day of birth to the day of eventual total weaning, which usually occurs within a few weeks. There are rules restricting the number of feedings, the duration of feedings, the amount of time between feedings, and the amount of mother-baby contact that stimulates the urge to suck. Infants and mothers are frequently housed

in different rooms. Sleeping in bed with the mother is considered dangerous. The strength of the infant's breast sucking is limited by teaching it bottle sucking techniques, by dulling the appetite with glucose water, formula and semisolid foods. The practice of feeding the baby by the clock may result in a baby too worn out with crying to suck well, or a baby too sleepy to show persistent strong sucking.

Even during this brief time of breast feeding the infant is likely to have had much other substance besides breast milk. A survey of 49 physicians found that 44 of them believed breast feeding should be supplemented. The custom of feeding cereal at a very early age regardless of feeding method may be very common. Of the infants studied in one recent survey, 79.4% received cereal by one month of age.

Token breast feeding is the most common pattern of breast feeding in some fully industrialized countries, and is closely related to total artificial feeding. For instance, a recent sample of all women—1,476—delivered at a university teaching county hospital in a Midwest low income city neighborhood indicated that 11% of the mothers tried to breast feed. Of those who tried to nurse, 69% gave up breast feeding within 4 to 6 weeks after delivery.

The occasional mother who does nurse longer still usually appears to practice only partial breast feeding. Of a sample of Boston mothers who nursed their babies for three months or longer, 70% gave bottles to their babies, and 71% introduced solid foods before the baby was 3 months old.[30]

The change in American customs has been rapid. Between 1911 and 1916, studies on over 22,000 city babies indicated 58 per cent were breast fed in the twelfth month of life. A textbook of pediatrics in 1906 recommended night feedings through the first month.[31] Four nursings were advocated on the first postpartum day and six on the second. Ten nursings per day were considered correct for the rest of the first month, eight per day for the second and third months, seven per day for the fourth and fifth months, and six per day from the sixth to eleventh months.

Toleration of a considerable amount of crying has also become part of the modern American pattern of nurturant care of babies. Spock[32] indicates the amount of crying acceptable in current American patterns: "If a baby has been crying hard for 15 minutes or more and if it's more than two hours after the last feeding—or even if it is less than 2 hours after a *very small* feeding—give him another feeding. If it's less than 2 hours after a *full* feeding, it's unlikely that he's hungry. Let him fuss or cry for 15 or 20 minutes more, if you can stand it. . . ." With regard to crying when put down to sleep, he advises: "Let him cry for 15 or 30 minutes if he has to. Some babies fall asleep faster if left in the crib, and this is the method to strive for in the long run."

A study[33] in an American hospital nursery which recorded infants' behavior 24 hours a day, found that the infants cried an average of 113.2 minutes daily. An inverse relationship was found between crying and nursing care—crying decreased when the amount of nursing care increased.

HISTORIC AND ECONOMIC PERSPECTIVES

It is important to recognize that the changes in nurturant care of infants during this century are a culmination of trends started in the seventeenth and eighteenth centuries.

Ryerson[34] has written a remarkable review of childcare customs. She based her data on medical texts published between 1550 and 1900, written or translated in English. After 1800, she used only medical texts published in America. Between 1550 and 1750 medical texts were unanimous in recommending that a newborn baby be given a purge or laxative as a matter of course. This custom disappeared within the next 50 years so that by 1800 no texts recommended purging. Swaddling the baby so that he could not freely move his hands and feet was favored by all medical writers until 1675. However, none of the writers advocated swaddling after 1800.

Feeding schedules for infants were not mentioned in texts published between 1550 and 1725. Thereafter, some sort of scheduling was advocated by a few texts. Between 1825 and 1850 the majority mentioned scheduling. By 1875 all books advocated some sort of scheduled restriction.

The most remarkable changes were in the recommended dates of weaning from the breast. From 1550 to 1650 all texts agreed that two years was the correct age of weaning. By 1850 this had been lowered to one year. In 1875 nursing a child for two years was considered reprehensible and the recommended weaning age was less than one year.

Mother-baby closeness began to erode quickly at the time of the Industrial Revolution. This was reflected not only in weaning age, but also with regard to sleeping habits. Before 1750, children slept in bed with their mothers until weaning at about age two. After the child left his parents' bed, he usually had someone else to sleep with—a brother, sister, or servant.

One of the greatest puzzles in the field of cultural patterning of childbearing is determining the underlying cause of such changes. Why did we gradually lower the recommended weaning age and invent schedules? Why did DeLee's horror at "meddlesome midwifery" change to the custom of speeding labor as much as possible?

My belief is that the answer can be found in economics. Before the Industrial Revolution children represented badly needed hands to help with the work and also security in old age. Now children are an economic handicap, with the potential to greatly reduce their parents' standard of living. Whereas childbearing women were once an asset since their product was needed and useful, they are now often viewed as contributors to pollution and overpopulation. Such economically-determined attitudes toward children and childbearing women are reflected in the amount and type of nurturant care they receive.

REFERENCES

References originating from the Human Relations Area Files are marked with an asterisk (*). In cases where foreign language texts from Human Relations Area Files are quoted, the translations into English are those of the Human Relations Area Files.

1. Naroll, F., Naroll, R. and Howard, F. H.: *Position of women in childbirth.* Am. J. Obstet. Gynecol. 32:943, 1961.
2. Wellin, F.: *Maternal and infant feeding practices in a Peruvian village.* J. Am. Diet. Assoc. 31:889, 1955.
3. Baird, D.: *Combined Textbook of Obstetrics and Gynecology,* ed. 8. E. S. Livingston, Edinburgh, 1968.
4. Merriman, S. (with notes and additions by James, T. C.): *A Synopsis of the Various Kinds of Difficult Parturition, with Practical Remarks on the Management of Labours.* Stone House, Philadelphia, 1816, pp. 20–22.
5. Bing, E.: *Six Practical Lessons for Easier Childbirth.* Bantam, New York, 1969.
6. Ford. C. S.: *A Comparative Study of Human Reproduction.* Yale University Publications in Anthropology, No. 32, 1945.
7. *Holmberg, A. R.: *Nomads of the Long Bow: The Siriono of Eastern Bolivia.* Publication No. 10, Smithsonian Institute, Institute of Social Anthropology, Washington, 1950, pp. 67, 68.
8. *Beaglehole, E. and Beaglehole, P.: *Ethnology of Pukapuka.* Bernice P. Bishop Museum Bulletin 150, Honolulu, 1938.
9. *Marshall, H. I.: *The Karen People of Burma: A Study in Anthropology and Ethnology.* Ohio State University Bulletin, 26, No. 13, 1922.
10. DeLee, J. B.: *The Principles and Practice of Obstetrics.* W. B. Saunders, Philadelphia, 1913, p. 291.
11. Ibid.: p. 296.
12. Burns, J. (with improvements and notes by James, T. C.): *The Principles of Midwifery: Including the Diseases of Women and Children.* Clafton and Van Norden Printers, New York, 1831.
13. Merriman: op. cit.
14. DeLee: op. cit.

15. *Gusinde, M.: *Die Yamana: vom Leben und Denken der Wassernomaden am Kap Hoorn, vol. II.* Mudling bei Wien, Anthrpos-Bibliothek, 1937.
16. Ford: op. cit., p. 66.
17. Chavasse, P.H.: *Woman as a Wife and Mother.* Evans, Philadelphia, 1870, p. 246.
18. Jelliffe, D. B. and Bennett, F. J.: *World-wide care of the mother and newborn child.* Clin. Obstet. Gynecol. 5:64, 1962, p. 66.
19. Ibid.
20. Hamer, J. H.: *The Cultural Aspects of Infant Mortality in Subsaharan Africa.* Doctoral dissertation (anthropology), Northwestern University, Ann Arbor, University Microfilms, 1962.
21. Ford: op. cit.
22. Tichauer, R.: *The Aymara children of Bolivia.* J. Pediatr. 62:399, 1963, pp. 405, 406.
23. *Grangvist, H.: *Birth and Childhood among the Arabs: Studies in a Muhammadan Village in Palestine.* Söderström, Helsingiors, 1947.
24. Frick, J.: *Mutter und Kind bei den Chineson in Tsinghai: III. das Neugeborene.* Anthropos 51:513, 1956.
25. Cammann, S.: *The Land of the Camel: Tents and Temples of Inner Mongolia.* Ronald Press, New York, 1951, p. 39.
26. *Beals, R. L.: *Cheran: A Sierra Tarascan Village.* Publication No. 2, Smithsonian Institute of Social Anthropology, Washington, 1946, p. 170a.
27. Ford: op. cit.
28. Jelliffe, D. B.: *Infant Nutrition in the Subtropics and Tropics.* World Health Organization, Geneva, 1955.
29. *Whitman, W.: *The Pueblo Indians of San Ildefonso.* Columbia University Press, New York, 1947.
30. Newton, N.: *Psychologic differences between breast and bottle feeding.* Am. J. Clin. Nutr. 24:993, 1971.
31. Southworth, T. S.: *Maternal feeding.* In Carr, W. L. (ed.): *Practice of Pediatrics.* Lea Brothers, Philadelphia, 1906.
32. Spock, B.: *Baby and Child Care,* revised ed. Pocket Books, New York, 1968, pp. 184, 186.
33. Aldrich, C. A., Sung, C. and Knop, C.: *The crying of newly born babies.* J. Pediatr. 26:313, 1945.
34. Reyerson, A. J.: *Medical Advice on Child Rearing, 1550-1900.* Harvard Ed. Review 31:302, 1961.

BIBLIOGRAPHY

Brown, E.: *New Dimensions of Patient Care—Patients as People.* Russel Sage Foundation, New York, 1964.

Bullough, B. and Bullough, V. I.: Poverty, Ethnic Identity and Health Care. *Appleton, Century, Crofts,* New York, 1972.

Ford, C. S.: *A Comparative Study of Human Reproduction.* Yale University, Publications in Autopology, No. 32, 1945.

Ford, C. S. and Beach, F. A.: *Patterns of Sexual Behavior.* Harper, New York, 1951.

Haire, D.: *The Cultural Warping of Childbirth.* International Childbirth Education Supplies Center, Seattle, 1972.

Howells, J. G.: *Modern Perspectives in Psycho-obstetrics.* Oliver & Boyd, Edinburgh, 1972, and Brunner/mazel, New York, 1973.

Leininger, M.: *Nursing and Anthropology: Two Worlds to Blend.* Wiley, New York, 1970.

Marshall, D. S. and Suggs, R. C. (eds.): *Human Sexual Behavior: Variations in Ethnographic Spectrum.* Basic Books, New York, 1971.

Mead, M. and Newton, N.: *Cultural patterning of perinatal behavior.* In Richardson, S. A. and Guttmacher, A. F. (eds.): *Childbearing: Its Social and Psychological Aspects.* Williams & Wilkins, Baltimore, 1967.

Morris, N. (ed.): *Psychosomatic Medicine in Obstetrics and Gynecology.* S. Karger, Basel, 1972.

Newton, N. and Newton, M.: *Psychologic aspects of lactation.* N. Engl. J. Med. 277:1179, 1967.

Newton, N.: *Population limitation in cross cultural perspective: 1. Patterns of contraception.* J. Reprod. Med. 1:343, 1968.

Ibid.: *Ease of childbirth: Combined cross cultural and experimental approach.* Journal of Cross-Cultural Psychology 1:85, 1970.

Ibid.: *Psychological differences between breast and bottle feeding.* Am. J. Clin. Nutr. 24:993, 1971.

Ibid.: *Childbearing in broad perspectives: Some key issues.* In *New Horizon in Midwifery.* Proceedings of the 16th Triennial Congress of the International Confederation of Midwives, International Confederation of Midwives, London, 1973.

Ibid.: *Inter-relationships between sexual responsiveness, birth and breast feeding behavior.* In Zubin, J. and Money, J. (eds.): *Critical Issues in Contemporary Sexual Behavior.* Johns Hopkins Press, Baltimore, 1973.

Ibid.: *Birth Rituals in Cross-Cultural Perspective: Some Practical Applications.* Proceedings of the 9th International Congress of Anthropological and Ethnological Sciences, Section on Status of Female: Reproduction. In *World Anthropology.* Co-libri, The Hague, Netherlands (in press).

Ryerson, A. J.: *Medical advice on child rearing, 1550-1900.* Harvard Educational Review 31(3):302, 1961.

Saunders, L.: *Cultural Differences and Medical Care–The Case of the Spanish-speaking People of the Southwest.* Russel Sage Foundation, New York, 1954.

Toms, Herbert: *Our Obstetric Heritage.* Shoe String Press, Hamden, 1960.

Whiting, B. B.: *Six Cultures, Studies of Child Rearing.* John Wiley & Sons, New York, 1963.

William, C. D. and Jelliffee, D. B.: *Mother and Child Health: Delivering the Services.* Oxford University Press, London, 1972.

13 Framework for Cultural Assessment

DYANNE D. AFFONSO, R.N., M.N.

Theoretical knowledge of cultural patterns in and of itself is useless to the nurse. Facts, principles, and generalizations of the culture concept become meaningful when this knowledge is applied to formulate nursing goals and identify how such goals can be attained. A family's perception of health and illness is culturally derived, and delivery of health care must be congruent with cultural life styles. Culture is especially significant to the childbearing process because it defines the meaning of the experience and designates appropriate behaviors for reacting to and coping with events. All behavior is meaningful and should not be ridiculed, judged negatively, or ignored. At times, an individual's behavior may perplex the nurse because it seems inappropriate or in conflict with good health care. Macgregor illustrates how noncompliant behaviors may be related to ethnocentricity:

> The behavior of noncompliant patients, however deviant or seemingly inappropriate, is not a matter of mere capriciousness. There are reasons why they respond as they do, and apart from reasons that are solely physiologic or organic, explanations may be found on other levels: psychologic, sociologic, and/or cultural.
>
> One cannot underestimate the tenacity of cultural patterns and the hold they have on patients even when health is at stake.[1]

Nurses are in a unique position to observe and assess the behavior of individuals and families during the childbearing experience. The following discussion is a guide to the type of information the nurse should assess to gain a better understanding of a family's responses during childbearing, and to plan nursing approaches which will be culturally acceptable.

PREGNANCY

Newton states, "In no known culture is pregnancy ignored or treated with total indifference; instead it elicits a gamut of emotions and feelings."[2] In her extensive exploration of cross-cultural patternings during pregnancy, she suggests the following for assessment:

What Is the Meaning and Value of Reproduction to the Culture?

In some cultures "reproduction may be the best road to social status."[3] Children definitely increase the status of the parents and a woman is viewed as being more attractive, receiving more attention, and bringing honor upon the entire extended family when she produces a new family member. In contrast, some cultures feel that childbearing makes a woman less attractive, weaker, and may contribute to endangering the entire society. This type of assessment data is important because it influences whether a woman and her family will be supported through the experience or whether childbearing will become a stressful life event. When parenthood is valued, the woman's ego will be enhanced. When the culture does not value parenthood, the woman may be plagued by feelings of guilt, shame, and possibly ridicule. The greatest danger is a conflict between the cultural value of the person and that of the health professionals. For example, a family with their eighth pregnancy may not understand why the health team appears perturbed by this, and the health team may not appreciate why the family allows another pregnancy to occur. One of the challenges in modern health care is to work with families whose health is jeopardized by increased pregnancies and help them value family planning without destroying their cultural value on the importance of reproduction.

What Feelings of Responsibility Are Imposed on the Parents as a Result of Pregnancy?

Newton states that the "most prominent feeling about pregnancy is a sense of responsibility for the development of the fetus."[4] This sense of responsibility is usually exhibited through prescriptions or prohibitions on the behaviors of both the mother and father. The belief is that the life style (values and practices) of the parents directly affects the welfare of the fetus and neonate, and also determines whether birth will be normal or difficult. Should the pregnancy or its outcome deviate from normal, the nurse must be prepared to deal with feelings of guilt and blame on the part of the parents. She must be able to communicate to them that certain aspects of gestation are beyond their voluntary control.

Assess the Ways a Culture Expresses Its Beliefs about Prenatal Influences.

According to Ferreira,[5] attitudes and beliefs about prenatal influences fall into three classifications: taboos, external influences, and internal influences.

Taboos. These are prohibitions on certain behaviors, e.g., engaging in sexual intercourse, or eating particular foods. Indulgence in the forbidden behaviors is believed to jeopardize the pregnancy, as well as the mother and baby. For example, in some cultures, hot, spicy foods are forbidden in order to protect the mother and fetus from the effects of heat such as burning, scarring (birthmarks), and dryness of the skin.

Taboos are one of the richest aspects of folklore during pregnancy, and the most prominent taboos are those on dietary restrictions to ensure a healthy baby. The assessment on food taboos not only involves identifying the specific foods a pregnant woman is forbidden to eat but also collecting information concerning how many meals should be eaten, when and with whom meals are to be eaten, any special rituals or prohibitions in the preparation of the meals, and what foods are deemed necessary for a healthy gestational outcome. This information helps the nurse present teachings about prenatal nutrition by working within the dietary patterns of the family, and modify (as feasible) meals during hospitalization to better approximate the woman's cultural eating patterns.

Data on sexual taboos during pregnancy help provide meaning to behaviors which may otherwise perplex the nurse. For example, a woman may be physically separated in another room from her husband to enforce the taboo. The nurse should not always expect a taboo on sex since some cultures advocate increased coitus as a protective measure during pregnancy (the giving of strength to the fetus by the father).

External Influences. These are believed to be sources of evil which are detrimental to the outcome of childbearing. The nurse needs to appreciate cultural norms for protecting the mother and baby from "evil sources." One of the most prominent cultural patterns is avoidance of the "evil eye" on a pregnant mother or a neonate. The evil eye is defined in various ways, e.g., being looked upon by a stranger or a condemned member of the society. Some examples of cultural measures to protect the mother and fetus or baby from evil sources are:

Special cleaning rituals to rid the home of evil spirits.

Use of special objects inside and/or outside the home to ward off evil spirits.

Family or community members (especially the prospective father) may be called upon to perform rituals or stand guard around the dwelling of the pregnant mother.

Substances believed to have protective qualities may be applied or placed on various parts of the mother's and/or neonate's body.

An extreme cultural patterning is total isolation of the mother to prevent her from having contact with any external source with the potential for evil.

The nurse should not interfere with any cultural ritual. Ridicule or creating obstacles to the performance of such tasks can generate unnecessary anxiety in the prospective parents and their family. The nurse must also understand that a family may be forced to modify their cultural protective measures when childbearing occurs in a new environment, such as a woman of a foreign ethnic heritage in an American health care system. If the woman or her family feels unable to perform all the behaviors in the prescribed manner, there may be increased anxiety because protection is incomplete. Cultural protective behaviors may seem bizarre to the American health professional. Hopefully, it is the nurse who becomes an advocate for the family by conveying the meaningfulness of the behaviors to other members of the health team.

Internal Influences. These are believed to originate from the mother's own feelings, attitudes, and behaviors which can adversely affect the fetus. Some examples of such cultural beliefs include:

A pregnant woman (and her husband) should not ridicule or criticize the appearance of other babies or their child may bear the features that are being judged negatively.

The family (especially the pregnant mother and/or husband) should not engage in any cutting or killing activities or the child is likely to be malformed or even die.

Many Polynesian cultures believe that jewelry around the neck should not be worn, and activities involving tying or knotting ropes or strings should be avoided to prevent knotting of the umbilical cord or its wrapping around the baby's neck.

Birthmarks on an infant are frequently attributed to maternal behaviors during pregnancy such as being frightened, sustaining injuries such as falls, or not satisfying maternal food cravings.

The nurse must appreciate that a pregnant woman, in addition to experiencing the physiologic aspects of the pregnancy, may also feel that it is necessary to closely monitor her feelings and behaviors to avoid becoming a source of danger to the fetus. Thus, a woman's perception of priorities to ensure a healthy gestation may differ considerably from those of the health team. For example, the physician or nurse may emphasize the value of adequate nutrition, while the woman may feel that good prenatal care is not so much what she eats but what she avoids doing (such as not looking at or dreaming of dead things, or the child will be born dead).

How Is Pregnancy Viewed by the Society?

Some examples of the different feelings pregnancy can evoke in a social group include:

Pregnancy can be a time of increased stress, vulnerability, and debility, thus creating a potentially dangerous period for mother and baby.

Pregnancy can be a time of shame and reticence during which patterns of shyness and secrecy are manifested.

Pregnancy can be a time of pride and joy during which heightened solicitude is expressed for the pregnant woman. (Thus a woman may receive increased attention during this period of her life.)

Pregnancy may be a reflection of sexual adequacy or triumph.

This type of assessment data serves two important nursing purposes: 1) it gives meaning to the behaviors manifested and 2) it helps the nurse to respond appropriately. For example, when pregnancy is viewed as a time of vulnerability, the woman's behaviors may approximate those of a sick role. Rather than being judgmental or perturbed by such behaviors, the nurse should focus on helping the woman to identify specifically what she is fearful of so that appropriate actions to minimize or eliminate perceived dangers can be taken.

INTRAPARTAL PERIOD

Cultural determinants relating to the process of labor and delivery greatly influence a woman's attitudes and behaviors during this time. Suggested areas for nursing assessment include:

Is Birth Seen as a Normal Physiologic Process or Is It Related to Pathology or Illness?

This is a significant area to explore because it influences a woman's reactions to pregnancy and how she will be treated by others (including the type of health care delivered by physicians and nurses). This type of assessment data can help the nurse predict the degree to which labor and birth are perceived as threatening to a woman's life. For example, one woman may believe that labor is not very different from her other bodily functions and approach labor ready to accept whatever events occur and the sensations to be felt. Another woman may approach labor with fear and dread because she has been conditioned by stories describing labor as dangerous and comparable to being sick. Attitudes as to whether labor is a normal or pathologic process also influence the health team members' perception of their roles. For example, the need for and amount of medications used throughout pregnancy, labor, and delivery is determined by the physician's perception of how much medicinal help is necessary to enhance the process. In America there is often the attitude that delivery necessitates medical intervention. Thus, a woman may undergo various procedures which in themselves may become a greater source of stress than the childbirth process itself. Therefore, it is very important that the nurse take the initiative to assess the impact of medical intervention on the woman and answer questions or provide information when necessary. This will minimize the woman's (or husband's) need to resort to fantasies and will prevent increased anxiety which might otherwise result from the perplexing and seemingly inappropriate behavior of the medical staff.

Is Birth Considered a Private or Social Event?

Some cultures exhibit a need for birth to be a secretive and private event. In such cultures there usually is a lack of adequate knowledge about the physiologic processes involved and there are restrictions as to who may witness and participate in the birth process. Many Americans are examples of this type of cultural patterning as reflected in the fact that the topic of exactly how birth occurs is largely avoided and stories about the stork or other fantasies are invented about childbirth. However, in the Navaho culture birth is regarded as a social event which everyone is invited to witness.

This type of assessment data has several implications for the nurse:

It influences whether family members are permitted to be present during the event. Often in the American health care system there is a conflict between the staff's norms and those of the family. This conflict may be manifested not only by prohibiting the husband's presence in the delivery room, but also when he is allowed, by medical routines that greatly interfere with his ability to view the event and support or to be near his wife.

It indicates the degree of modesty or privacy desired by the woman and her husband. This influences the importance of such simple actions as use of curtains, draping the legs during vaginal exams, and ensuring privacy when procedures are done. In some societies it is considered "shameful" for a woman to be attended by men, and these women will prefer that their husbands not be present during delivery.

It guides the nurse in predicting the amount and type of information a woman and her husband will have about events during childbirth. It must be remembered that many cultural life styles do not advocate information about birth. Therefore, health professionals are acting unrealistically when they expect that all women with previous pregnancies will have accurate knowledge of the childbearing process. Nurses should provide such information, considering appropriate cultural influences, during each contact with the woman and her family.

Does Birth Represent a Sense of Personal Achievement or Is It an Event Dictating Payment by the Mother and/or Others?

Some cultures view birth as an act of achievement for the mother and thus praises and gifts are showered on the woman. In contrast, other cultures believe that a woman or her family must render payment in the form of praise, gifts, or fees to the attendants of the birth process. In American society both types of cultural patterning can be found. For example, the new mother is usually praised and given gifts by family members and friends in recognition of her achievement. However, the new parents give monetary rewards and praise to the obstetrician and hospital. This has important implications for nursing. Nurses must remember that the primary focus during childbirth should be on the woman and her family, and thus direct praise and comments accordingly.

POSTPARTAL MATERNAL CARE

After delivery, a woman and her family may exhibit behaviors that appear to conflict with the nurse's or physician's concept of good postpartal care. Therefore, it is necessary to explore cultural patternings regarding protection to the mother after childbirth. Examples of areas for nursing assessment are:

What Norms Are Prescribed Regarding Dietary Intake, Restrictions, and Preparation of Food?

Many cultures have prescribed eating patterns to assure that the womb and vagina heal, and that the breasts will be adequately filled with milk. The nurse needs to assess whether the postpartal dietary intake is adequately supporting physiologic recovery. For example, maternal anemia in the postpartal period may be related to the taboo of foods high in iron and/or protein, and does not necessarily mean that the family is irresponsible about the mother's welfare.

What Norms Are Prescribed Regarding Types of Maternal Activities Allowed and Amount of Maternal Responsibility for Household Duties and Infant Care?

Knowledge about these factors will guide the nurse as to whether such measures as postpartal exercises are appropriate content for teaching. It also helps the nurse to understand dependent or independent behaviors exhibited by the mother after childbirth.

What Precautions Are Prescribed to Protect the Mother from Dangers and to Enhance Postpartal Recovery?

In some cultures it is believed that the use of abdominal binders will aid the involution of the uterus. Other rituals may relate to cleanliness or disposal of wastes such as the lochia to ensure good maternal health. No matter how strange cultural patterns may appear, the nurse should not force the woman to abandon them. This would cause the woman to feel vulnerable to danger or even death.

What Type of Help Is Acceptable and Who Is to Provide This Support?

This assessment question has important implications concerning those persons with whom the nurse must work in order to deliver efficient and effective health care. Frequently a husband, relative, or important member of the society is called upon to help the new mother meet her daily needs. The nurse needs to utilize the prescribed "support system" when delivering health care. Otherwise, the mother may ignore the nurse's information and suggestions because they are not sanctioned by her cultural group. Likewise, when the nurse wants to reinforce good health care behaviors, praise must be given not only to the mother, but also to members in the support system.

ROLE OF THE FATHER DURING CHILDBEARING

The role of the father during childbearing is very important in many cultures. *Couvade* is the practice of childbearing rituals, taboos, and duties by the father, and is sometimes viewed as the male version of childbirth. Couvade is so widespread that its significance cannot be ignored. In various societies couvade:

Establishes biological paternity and legitimacy of the birth. This is important because in some cultures illegitimacy can jeopardize the right of a mother and child to live.

Provides economic and social support toward women and children. This emphasizes the responsibility of the man for the welfare of his family.

Ensures protection for the health and development of the fetus because it is a common belief that the father's behaviors and attitudes can affect the fetus.

Couvade emphasizes the father's role and responsibilities for the birth of each child. The beneficial effects can be manifested in his identification and appreciation of what childbearing entails since he can easily identify with his wife. Such active participation in rituals and duties also helps the father to establish a relationship with his new child. It is interesting to note that while most cultures greatly emphasize male participation during childbearing, the American culture has largely ignored the father's role. Simmons comments, "We moderns are about the only people on earth who prescribe for the father an idle, nervous, inconsequential role in this critical period."[6]

Nurses must assess the cultural norms dictating the father's role during childbearing. Behaviors reflecting taboos and rituals mimicking childbirth should be supported and acknowledged as being a significant contribution, rather than ridiculed. Nurses also need to make more deliberate efforts to involve the father in ways which emphasize his ability to make significant contributions to the experience. Thus, health professionals may find that fathers do not necessarily "get in the way," and the long-term effects on father-child and father-mother relationships may also be positively affected.

PARENT-INFANT INTERACTIONS

It is important to remember that parental behaviors which may seem harsh, cruel, or negligent may merely reflect cultural patterning for childrearing. Suggested areas for nursing assessment are:

What Is the Meaning of Children to the Culture?

The ascribed meaning or value of children to the culture greatly influences the physical and emotional care given to the child, as well as who delivers such care. The degree to which a child is seen as making an important contribution to the social group determines how the child is treated. The nurse should also explore the parent's commitment toward meeting the child's daily needs. Sometimes a grandparent, relative, or sibling is the primary provider of infant care. At times the value of a child carries a degree of sexual discrimination. The nurse may observe different responses to a child of the preferred sex.

Are There Cultural Patterns Related to Infant Care?

Nurses should investigate how a family is expected by its society to feed, groom, discipline, and meet the infant's daily needs. This data helps in understanding behaviors related to infant care which may appear contradictory to good health habits. Also, what is valued by the American health system may not be valued by a different cultural group. For example, it is advocated that the newborn be exposed to various stimuli to arouse his senses and enhance behavioral development. However, a person from another culture may be appalled by a nurse's action to stimulate a newborn because of beliefs that the baby must be protected from evil sources such as the evil eye.

Are There Cultural Norms Regarding Parental Responses to the Behaviors or Appearance of the Infant?

There is a tendency to label parental behaviors as good or bad. However, the nurse must appreciate that a parent's reactions may have cultural significance. For example, a particular culture may dictate that a mother immediately put a crying, fussy baby to her breast. Another culture may believe that crying is good for the lungs and thus a mother may ignore crying behaviors for a length of time. A culture may also have prescribed behaviors for reacting to a child who deviates from normal. An example of this is the killing of badly deformed babies. The nurse needs to understand that parental responses are reflective of their life style and that if parents respond in ways not sanctioned by their culture, serious repercussions may occur to the family. Therefore, the nurse should avoid hasty criticism of parental responses but should be prepared to become an advocate of the child when his safety and well-being are truly threatened.

OTHER CULTURAL DETERMINANTS

In addition to assessing various aspects of the childbearing process, the nurse must also obtain information about the meaning and acceptable responses during such life experiences as pain, anxiety, and crisis. Examples of areas for assessment when exploring these experiences are:

When are such experiences viewed as valid and acceptable during the childbearing process? For example, is the pain experience recognized as an integral part of childbirth?

What are acceptable behaviors for reacting to and coping with such experiences? For example, what responses are expected during a situational crisis such as the death of an infant?

Is there an accountability factor associated with the experience, and if so, who is accountable? For example, are there feelings of guilt or blame during pain or loss and if so, whom are these feelings directed toward (mother, father, relatives)?

What are acceptable means for receiving help and support during such experiences?

CHALLENGES OF CROSS-CULTURAL ENCOUNTERS

When working with individuals of another culture, the nurse is challenged to achieve the following objectives:

Understand how the individuals perceive their health situation in terms of what they identify as health care needs and services desired.

Appreciate cultural norms which influence communication patterns between the nurse and the individual or family.

Implement nursing approaches to effect desired changes in health practices in a manner congruent with the cultural life style.

Meaningful communication is the means by which these goals may be achieved. In order to do this, the nurse must assess the cultural influences on communication behaviors—her own as well as the client's. Hall states, "Culture is the link between human beings and the means they have of interacting with others."[7] Unfortunately, our health care system overemphasizes verbal communication. Patients are *told* facts about their health conditions and encouraged to *ask* questions. Thus, health professionals frequently fail to appreciate that a patient and his family may be actively communicating even if no words are spoken. The way a person uses his body, has eye contact or not, and his distance or closeness to another person are all part of a communicative process. This aspect of communication is highy significant because it reflects patterned behaviors relative to daily living (culture). Davis emphasizes this:

> And so it might be, if words were all. But they are only the beginning, for beyond words lies the bedrock on which human relationships are built—non-verbal communication. Words are beautiful, exciting, important, but we have overestimated them badly—since they are not all or even half the message. In fact, as one scientist suggested, "Words may be what men use when all else fails."[8]

Therefore, the nurse should become aware of cultural dictates which guide communication patterns on the following levels:

Paralinguistic behaviors refer to the tone of voice and the pitch and speed of vocalizations. For example, speaking loudly may be objectionable in one culture and valued in another.

Kinesic behaviors refer to the expressive behaviors of the body in terms of facial expressions, eye contact, body posture, and use of hands or other parts of the body as signals or messages (gestures). Some cultures may be suspicious of a nurse who does not use kinesic behaviors while others may be perplexed or distracted by such behaviors.

Proxemic behaviors refer to the spatial relationships during the interaction. Influential factors are the size of the room, arrangement of furniture, proximity of the individuals, and seating arrangements. A good example concerns the position of the nurse during an interaction with a patient. Behaviors of the nurse, such as standing at the door, the foot of the bed, or near the head of the bed, may communicate a reluctance or a desire for interaction. Thus proxemic behaviors can promote or hinder the development of a successful nurse-patient relationship.

Tactile behaviors refer to the use or prohibition of touching acts during an interaction. Some cultures view touch as a way of obtaining information about the other party and thus have prolonged tactile contacts, such as a long handshake. Other cultures may be deeply offended if a stranger attempts to touch them.

In addition to assessing the other person's cultural patterns the nurse must realize that she brings her own cultural heritage to an interaction and thus may unconsciously transmit messages on the paralinguistic, kinesic, proxemic, and tactile levels. Hall states, "Not only almost totally ignorant of what is expected in other countries, we are equally ignorant of what we are communicating to other people by our own natural behaviors."[9] Thus it is essential that nurses recognize and assess their own cultural biases. The cultural impact on communication patterns cannot be treated lightly. It is the foundation upon which the nursing process develops from assessment, through implementing actions, to evaluation of the care delivered.

When a nurse is able to understand and appreciate a family's cultural life style through successful communication, the next step is to deliver nursing care. One of the most difficult tasks confronting the health care system is how to deliver care which necessitates a change in the present health patterns in order to move the family toward a higher level of wellness. The following is a very important concept the nurse must value if success is to be achieved when change in cultural patterning is mandatory:

> It is doubtful that anyone ever really changes culture in the sense that this term is generally used. What happens is that small informal adaptations are continually being made in the day to day process of living.
>
> If a person really wants to help introduce cultural change, he should find out what is happening on the informal level and pinpoint which informal adaptations seem to be most successful in daily operations, bringing these to the level of awareness.[10]

What does this mean to the nurse? First, the nurse needs to understand that a cultural group will do what they feel works best or brings them pleasure and success in daily living. For example, members of a particular culture may bind a newborn's umbilical cord and place oils or other substances on the area in the belief that this will promote healing.

They will continue this practice until the nurse can prove to them that another alternative can also be successful. Proof is demanded in the form of a living example of a healthy infant whose umbilical area was exposed to air instead of being bound and treated with oils. All the nurse's explanations and pictures of infections will have no impact on the culture because these words and pictures are not an integral part of their process of daily living. Effecting change of a cultural pattern is a process that demands patience and perseverance. The desired changes may be manifested much later, e.g., in another generation's childbearing practices. The process is also time consuming because nursing actions must always reinforce cultural values rather than ridicule or label them as wrong. Remember, culture is intended to safeguard one's physical, emotional, and social health. It is unrealistic to expect a person or a society to discard a cultural pattern until it can be replaced with a better one.

REFERENCES

1. Macgregor, F.: *Uncooperative patients: Some cultural interpretations.* Am. J. Nurs. 67:88, 1967.
2. Newton, N.: *Pregnancy, childbirth, and outcome: A review of patterns of culture and future needs.* In Richardson, S. and Guttmacher, A. (eds.): *Childbearing—Its Social and Psychological Aspects.* Williams & Wilkins, Baltimore, 1964, p. 164.
3. Ibid., p. 158.
4. Ibid., p. 164.
5. Ferreira, A.: *Prenatal Environment.* Charles C Thomas, Springfield, 1969, p. 14.
6. Simmons, L.: *Effects of Changing Culture on Childbearing and Family Life,* Report of a Work Conference, Maternity Center Association, New York, 1962, p. 34.
7. Hall, E.: *The Hidden Dimension.* Doubleday, New York, 1966, p. 213.
8. Davis, F.: *Inside Intuition: What We Know about Nonverbal Communication.* McGraw-Hill, New York, 1973, p. 5.
9. Hall, E.: *The Silent Language.* Fawcett World Library, New York, 1969, p. 9.
10. Ibid., pp. 90, 91.

BIBLIOGRAPHY

Bardwich, J. M.: *Psychology of Women: A Study of Bio-Cultural Conflicts.* Harper and Row, New York, 1971.

Biesanz, J. and Biesanz, M.: *Modern Society.* Prentice-Hall, Englewood Cliffs, 1954.

Blaylock, J.: *The psychological and cultural influences on the reaction to pain: A review of the literature.* Nurs. Forum 7:262, 1968.

Brown, M. I.: *Implications of cultural change for maternal and child health nursing.* American Nurses Association, Clinical Sessions, Monograph 18, 1962.

Caudill, W. A.: *Tiny dramas: vocal communication between mother and infant in Japanese and American families.* In Lebra, W. P. (ed.): *Transcultural Research in Mental Health, Vol. II of Mental Health Research in Asia and the Pacific.* University Press of Hawaii, Honolulu, 1972.

Caudill, W. A. and Schooler, C.: *Child behavior and childbearing in Japan and in the United States: An interim report.* J. Nerv. Ment. Dis. 157:323, 1973.

Elonen, A. S.: *The effect of childrearing on behavior in different cultures.* Am. J. Orthopsychiatry 31:505, 1961.

Goodman, M. E.: *The Culture of Childhood.* Teachers College Press, Columbia University, New York, 1967.

Handy, E. S., Graighill, P. and Kawena, M.: *The Polynesian Family System in Ka'u, Hawaii.* Tuttle, Rutland, 1958.

Horton, P. B.: *Sociology and the Health Science.* McGraw-Hill, New York, 1965.

Jekel, J. F., et al.: *Factors associated with rapid subsequent pregnancies among school age mothers.* Am. J. Public Health 63:769, 1973.

Josselyn, I. M.: *Cultural forces, motherliness and fatherliness.* Am. J. Orthopsychiatry 26:264, 1956.

Linder, E. M.: *Childbirth practices in two primitive cultures—Implications for modern maternity care.* Bulletin of American College of Nurse-Midwifery 11:126, 1966.

Lloyd-Jones, E.: *Cultural influences on interpersonal dynamics.* Nurs. World 132:15, 1958.

Lubic, R.: *Socio-cultural aspects of maternity care.* Briefs 33:131, 1969.

MacBride, A.: *Maternal and infant care customs among Hawaiians today.* Public Health Nursing 44:439, 1952.

Mead, M.: *Understanding cultural patterns.* Nurs. Outlook 4:260, 1956.

Minturn, L., et al.: *Mothers of Six Cultures: Antecedents to Childrearing.* John Wiley, New York, 1964.

Moss, F. T. and Meyer, B.: *The effects of nursing interaction upon pain relief in patients.* Nurs. Res. 15:303, 1966.

Newton, N.: *Childbirth and culture.* Psychology Today 4:74, 1970.

Opler, M. K.: *Cultural values and attitudes in child care.* Children 2:45, 1955.

Queen, S. A. and Habenstein, R.: *The Family in Various Cultures,* ed. 3. Lippincott, Philadelphia, 1967.

Reichert, C.: *Cultural bases of sex attitudes.* In Taylor, D. L. (ed.): *Human Sexual Development.* F. A. Davis, Philadelphia, 1970.

Simmons, L. W.: *Cultural patterns in childbirth.* Am. J. Nurs. 52:989, 1952.

Smoyak, S.: *Cultural incongruence: the effect on nurses perception.* Nurs. Forum 7:234, 1968.

Sottong, P.: *The dilemma of the parent as culture bearer.* Social Casework 36:302, 1955.

Tulkin, S. R., Leiderman, P. H.: *Infancy in a cultural convent.* J. Nerv. Ment. Dis. 157:320, 1973.

Walker, F.: *Bridging a cultural gap for better patient care.* Milit. Med. 139:26, 1974.

Whiting, B. E.: *Six Cultures: Studies of Childrearing.* John Wiley, New York, 1973.

Zborowski, M.: *Cultural components in response to pain.* In Apple, D. (ed.): *Sociological Studies of Health and Sickness.* McGraw-Hill, New York, 1960.

UNIT 4

PHYSIOLOGIC PERSPECTIVES

14 Maternal-Fetal Growth

RALPH W. HALE, M.D.

Knowledge of the maternal-fetal growth process during childbearing is essential in order to plan and implement the best possible care during this period. The nurse must understand the origins and significance of the various physiologic and psychologic changes which occur during this unique interaction.

DETERMINATION OF PREGNANCY

Positive determination of pregnancy is difficult during the very early stages of gestation. Unfortunately, this is also the time when the woman and physician are most interested in establishing whether or not conception has occurred. Therefore, it is necessary that the early signs and symptoms of pregnancy are understood as well as the relative importance of each.

The clinical diagnosis of pregnancy is based upon those physical changes which occur in the gravid patient and her subjective sensations in association with these changes. These manifestations are divided into:

Presumptive signs of pregnancy—these lead one to suggest pregnancy.

Probable signs of pregnancy—pregnancy is most likely present.

Positive signs of pregnancy—definitive evidence of pregnancy.

PRESUMPTIVE SIGNS

Many of the presumptive signs of pregnancy are subjective symptoms recognized by the patient herself. The signs include amenorrhea, nausea with or without vomiting, changes in the breast (increased size, vascularity, tingling, tenderness), weight gain, urinary frequency, sensations of fetal movement (quickening), pigmentation of the skin, abdominal striae, fatigue, and lassitude.

Amenorrhea. This is the most important presumptive sign. Whenever it is present in a woman during the childbearing years, pregnancy must be considered. In a woman who menstruates regularly it is a valuable clue, but is not infallible. Absence of menstruation may result from a number of other conditions, such as emotional stress, chronic disease, and environmental changes. The nurse must also be aware of additional considerations pertaining to menstruation and pregnancy. For example, gestation can begin without prior menstruation in young girls. Occasionally, uterine bleeding which simulates menstruation occurs during early pregnancy. Nursing mothers, who rarely menstruate during lactation, may conceive. Even women who believe they have passed the period of menopause may become pregnant.

Nausea and Vomiting. During pregnancy this condition often occurs. It is referred to as "morning sickness" since it is usually noted in the morning upon arising. However, it may persist throughout the day, and in some women it is worse in the evening. Women are often affected by odors of cooking and by smoking. This symptom, particularly if it persists, is a presumptive sign of pregnancy. It is not a positive sign since nausea and vomiting also occur with many other conditions.

Changes in the Breasts. During the early weeks of pregnancy, the woman may complain of tingling and tenderness in the breasts. By the second month, the breasts begin to increase in size due to development of the alveolar system. As the pregnancy progresses, the areolae become increasingly pigmented. Late in pregnancy the veins become prominent and striae may appear.

Urinary Frequency. Frequency of urination may occur in the early weeks of pregnancy due to pelvic congestion from the increased vascularity of the pelvic organs. Pressure on the bladder by the enlarging uterus can also cause frequent micturition. However, other conditions may be responsible, and the possibility of urinary tract infection must be considered.

Quickening. Sensations of fetal movements may be perceived by the woman as early as the sixteenth week of pregnancy. However, they are often confused with intestinal peristalsis and are significant only in collaboration with other signs.

Pigmentation of the Skin. Discoloration in the midline of the abdomen (linea nigra) and of the face (mask of pregnancy) may be noted as the pregnancy progresses. These phenomena occur earlier in a multigravida than in a primigravida. The mask of pregnancy disappears after pregnancy, but the linea nigra usually remains as a faint line.

Abdominal Changes. Cutaneous manifestations of the abdomen, such as enlargement and striae, are commonly associated with pregnancy but are not positive signs. Enlargement, for example, may result from tumors or ascites. Striae are caused by separation of the collagenous fibers of the skin.

Fatigue. Fatigue and somnolence frequently accompany the first trimester of pregnancy, but are too nonspecific to be considered evidence of pregnancy.

Chadwick's Sign. This is a bluish discoloration of the vaginal mucosa due to intense congestion of the pelvic organs. It is not conclusive evidence of pregnancy since other conditions may also cause pelvic congestion.

PROBABLE SIGNS

The probable signs of pregnancy include many of the presumptive signs. It is the changes in their physical manifestations which indicate that pregnancy is probable, rather than merely presumptive. These include an increase in uterine size, the uterine souffle, changes in the cervix, uterine contractions, ballottement, and results of laboratory tests.

Uterine Size and Shape. Measured over a period of time, the gravid uterus shows an increase in size. During the first few weeks this is limited almost entirely to the anterioposterior diameter, but at a later period the body of the uterus becomes almost globular. The uterus changes from a small, firm, pear-shaped organ to a large, soft, spherical one.[1]

Hegar's Sign. More characteristic than the change in shape of the uterus is the change in consistency. The uterine body feels doughy or elastic. The lower segment of the uterus becomes so soft that on bimanual examination there may seem to be nothing between the cervix and the body of the uterus. This marked softening is known as Hegar's sign. However, this is not a positive sign of pregnancy since the walls of a nonpregnant uterus may also become excessively soft.

Goodell's Sign. The cervix, which is normally firm, becomes soft by the second month of pregnancy. This is known as Goodell's sign. Since other conditions may also cause softening of the cervix, this is a probable sign of pregnancy but not definite proof.

Uterine Souffle. This is a soft blowing sound heard on auscultation of the uterus. It indicates an increase in the maternal blood flow to the uterus and is therefore considered a probable sign of pregnancy.

Braxton Hicks Contractions. The pregnant uterus produces these painless, palpable contractions at irregular intervals beginning very early in pregnancy. They may occasionally be felt in early pregnancy during bimanual examination and in later pregnancy by abdominal examination. Since they may also occasionally occur in a nonpregnant uterus, they are only a probable sign of pregnancy.

Ballottement. The amount of amniotic fluid is large in comparison with the fetus during the fourth and fifth months of pregnancy. By percussing the uterus, the part of the fetus nearest the pressure seems to float away and then return to its original position. This rebounding of the fetal parts is known as ballottement. However, both the abdominal and vaginal methods of detecting the fetus in this way are subject to error since tumors in the abdomen or ascites may give the same sign.

Laboratory Tests. Human chorionic gonadotrophin (HCG) is produced by the trophoblasts in the placenta. Its presence in maternal plasma and its excretion in the urine of the pregnant woman provide the basis for the endocrine tests for pregnancy. HCG may be identified by any one of a variety of immunoassays or bioassays. Unfortunately, such laboratory tests do not absolutely identify the presence or absence of pregnancy.[2] The basic problem in most assay procedures arises from the immunologic and biologic similarities between HCG formed by the trophoblast and the luteinizing hormone secreted by the pituitary. In most tests, the luteinizing hormone cross-reacts with the antibody to HCG.

Among the most frequently used immunoassays are latex inhibition slide tests, hemagglutination inhibition tube tests, and direct latex agglutination slide tests. Inhibition of agglutination indicates that HCG was present in the fluid tested. The results of immunoassays are usually available in a few hours.

Bioassays, long in use, are still occasionally employed to aid in determining pregnancy. They depend on the reaction of an animal's sex organ to HCG present in injected urine. Bioassays may give false results unless the urine specimen is collected with care. In addition, these tests usually require several days to obtain results and the care of the test animals constitutes an added expense.

Recently, the technique of radioimmunoassay has been developed as a test of pregnancy.[3] This test is based on the antigen-antibody reaction in animals and HCG is measured by sensitive radioisotope techniques (Fig. 14-1).

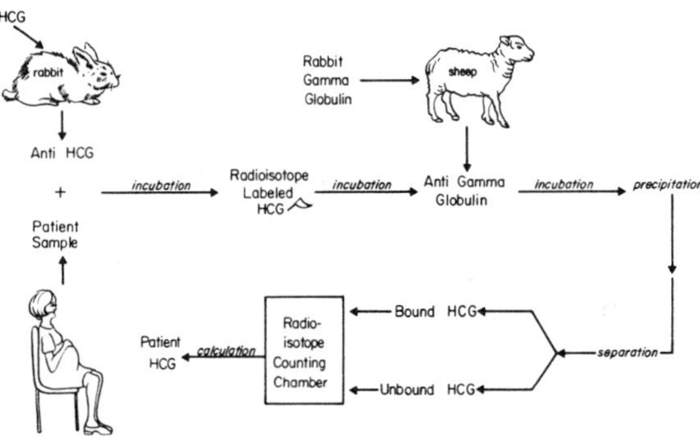

FIGURE 14-1. Radioimmunoassay test for pregnancy.

An even more sensitive technique for use in the research laboratory has been developed to test for the β subunit of HCG.[4] By use of this method, pregnancy can be confirmed before the woman misses a menstrual period.

POSITIVE SIGNS

The positive signs of pregnancy are rarely present before the fourth month of gestation.

They include auscultation of fetal heart tones, palpation of fetal parts, roentgenograms of the fetal skeleton, and ultrasound scanning of the fetus. These constitute legal as well as medical proof of pregnancy.

Auscultation of Fetal Heart Tones. Hearing and counting the fetal heart pulsations provides definitive evidence of pregnancy. The fetal heart can usually be heard using a head stethoscope after the twenty-second week of gestation, although this varies with the thickness of the abdominal wall. It sounds similar to the tick of a watch under a pillow and is distinct from the maternal heartbeat. More sophisticated instruments, such as those using ultrasound, may also be used to ascertain fetal heart rate.

Palpation of Fetal Parts. After the first trimester, fetal parts can usually be differentiated by palpation.

Roentgenograms of Fetal Skeleton. Although these provide proof of pregnancy after the fourth lunar month of gestation, the procedure is not usually employed due to the possibility of harmful effects on fetal development.

Ultrasound Scanning of Fetus. In this procedure, ultrasonic waves are used to measure the size and shape of the fetus. In most cases pregnancy can be confirmed before the end of the first trimester.

In the determination of pregnancy it must be remembered that many other conditions may present similar physiologic and psychologic manifestations. For example, endocrine disturbances or emotional stress may cause amenorrhea. Tumors or ascites may be responsible for an increase in the size of the abdomen. In addition, one must always be aware of the possibility of pseudocyesis (imaginary pregnancy). In this condition a woman develops the classic signs of pregnancy, such as amenorrhea, morning sickness, changes in the breasts, weight gain, abdominal enlargement, quickening, and even labor, but she is not physically pregnant. This usually occurs in women with an intense emotional desire to become pregnant.

DURATION OF PREGNANCY

Once pregnancy has been confirmed, one of the next major concerns is to assess the duration of pregnancy and estimate the time of delivery. The usual time is 10 lunar months (nine calendar months) after the last menstrual period. The actual length of gestation is 266 days, but due to many possible biologic variations a woman usually gives birth somewhere within two weeks of this estimated date. There is, therefore, no precise way to predict the length of a particular pregnancy. The usual method of estimating the expected date of delivery is calculation by *Nägeles Rule.* This method involves taking the first day of the last normal menstrual period, adding seven days and then subtracting three months from this date. The year will also change in most calculations. The resulting date is referred to as the estimated date of delivery. Since this rule is based on the ideal 28 day cycle with ovulation occurring on approximately the fourteenth day, its reliability depends upon how closely a particular woman's menstrual cycle coincides with this pattern. However, it does give an accurate estimate of the time for delivery.

If the woman is unsure of her last normal menstrual period other techniques may be used, as gestation progresses, to establish the duration of pregnancy. The date of first movement felt by the mother and the first time fetal heart tones are ausculated are important dates for evaluation, although again these times may vary. The method most commonly used is *McDonald's Rule.* By use of this technique the growth of the uterus is measured from the pubic symphysis to the highest point in the abdomen in centimeters. When this figure is multiplied by two and then divided by seven, the duration of pregnancy in lunar months is obtained. If it is multiplied by eight and di-

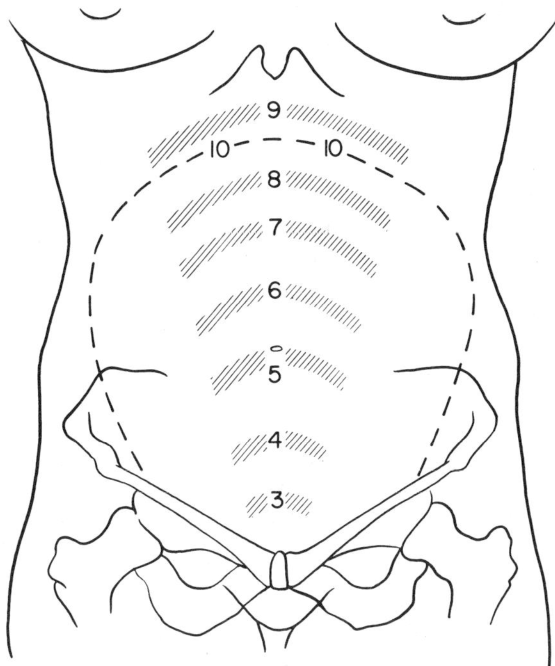

FIGURE 14-2. Height of the fundus at various lunar months of pregnancy.

vided by seven, the duration of pregnancy in weeks is obtained. Although this is a useful estimate of fetal development, it cannot be considered accurate in obese women, women with ascites, multiple pregnancy, or even women with large or small babies.

It is also possible to estimate the stage of gestation by virtue of the relative position of the uterus in the abdominal cavity (Fig. 14-2). *Bartholomew's Rule* is a helpful technique. The distance between the pubic symphysis and the umbilicus is divided into four equal parts. At two months of gestation, the uterus is one fourth of the distance, at three months it is three fourths the distance, and at five months it reaches the umbilicus. A similar procedure is carried out between the umbilicus and the lower sternal border. When the uterus reaches each of the plateaus, one month is added. In addition, as the uterus reaches the fifth or sixth month of gestation it may gradually rotate to the right. This is called dextrorotation and occurs in approximately 80 per cent of pregnancies.

If it is necessary to obtain a more accurate estimate of the length of gestation, e.g., in cases of diabetes mellitus in the mother or Rh sensitization in the infant, more sophisticated methods of evaluation, such as amniocentesis and evaluation of the amniotic fluid for creatinine or the lecithin-sphingomyelin ratio, may be used to ascertain fetal maturity.[5] In the later stages of pregnancy, roentgenograms may also be of help in establishing fetal maturity, since the distal femoral epiphysis begins to ossify at 36 week of gestation. However, this is not 100 per cent accurate and must be viewed from that aspect.

TERM PREGNANCY

When the fetus reaches the stage of intrauterine development in which it has maximum chance for extrauterine survival, the pregnancy is referred to as a term pregnancy. This usually applies after the thirty-sixth week of gestation. Determination is based on the estimated date of delivery and other evaluations of fetal growth. As with all measurements, however, additional factors must be considered. These include, for example, a small or large baby, any intrauterine disease, and previous obstetric and menstrual histories.

When evaluating for term pregnancy there are several clinical findings which may be of assistance. In the woman having her first pregnancy, engagement may be helpful. *Engagement* is frequently referred to as *lightening*, and is the process by which the fetal head suddenly descends into the pelvic cavity. In the primigravida this usually occurs approximately two weeks prior to the time of delivery. In addition, cervical changes in the primigravida may be helpful in determining whether the pregnancy has reached term. As the cervix effaces and begins to dilate and soften, it is relatively certain that term is fast approaching. The multigravida, however, does not have the same signs as the primigravida and one must rely on clinical judgment based on all of the factors utilized in determining the duration of pregnancy.

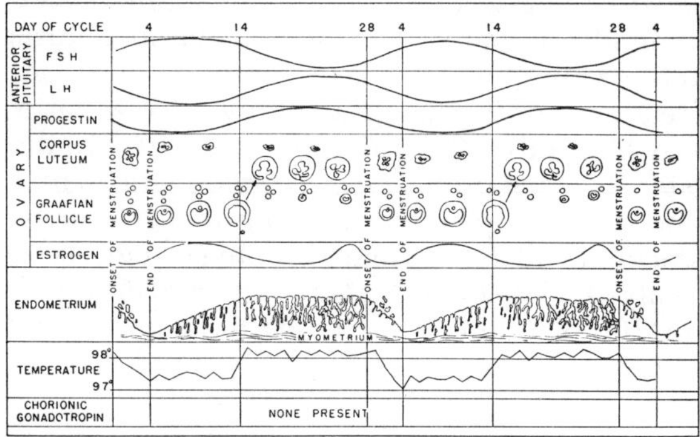

FIGURE 14-3. Schematic diagram of the variations in hormone secretion, anatomic changes in the ovary and endometrium, and oral temperature during two successive normal menstrual cycles. (From Bryant R. D. and overland, A. E.: *Woodward and Gardner's Obstetric Management and Nursing*. F. A. Davis, Philadelphia, 1966, with permission.)

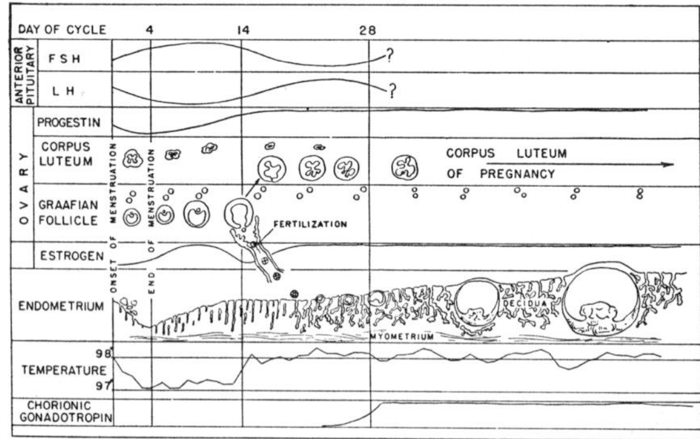

FIGURE 14-4. Schematic diagram of the hormonal, anatomic, and temperature variations preceding and following conception. (From Bryant, R. D. and Overland, A. E.: *Woodward and Garner's Obstetric Management and Nursing*. F. A. Davis, Philadelphia, 1966, with permission.)

PRETERM PREGNANCY

Some women give birth before reaching the stage of pregnancy in which they are at term. Premature infants are those born before they have had sufficient time to achieve optimal intrauterine development. Evaluation of maturity is based on gestational age and birth weight. Prematurity usually presents problems associated with inadequate development of body organs and systems due to the shortened period of gestation.

POST-TERM PREGNANCY

Occasionally a woman reaches the stage of pregnancy in which she is at term, and yet labor does not ensue. When this continues for two weeks or longer beyond the estimated date of delivery, fetal postmaturity must be suspected. This is a difficult decision to make and currently there is dispute as to whether such a condition actually does exist. However, it is generally accepted that there is such a condition and that it will present increased problems due to placental insufficiency and the predisposition of the infant to feto-pelvic disproportion.

MATERNAL ADAPTATION

REPRODUCTIVE SYSTEM

The changes in the reproductive organs of the female during pregnancy are those most specifically related to the increase in vascularity, elevation of the level of reproductive hormones, and increase in size of the uterus (Figs. 14-3 and 14-4).

During pregnancy, the *vulva* and *vagina* gradually become more vascular and edematous. This increase in vascularity leads to the bluish discoloration of Chadwick's Sign. In addition, the patient may notice occasional development of varices and gradual loosening and relaxing of the supportive tissues of the vagina and vulvar area. These conditions reduce rapidly after pregnancy and have very few associated side effects.

In the *uterus*, both the corpus and cervix undergo many changes during pregnancy. The *cervix* begins to develop cyanosis and softening due to increased vascularity. In addition, it begins to shorten and develop a tenacious mucous plug which seals the cervical canal. As pregnancy progresses, the cervix continues to become shorter and thinner, a process called *effacement*, and in the muligravida may show slight dilatation starting in the thirty-second week of pregnancy. The mucous plug usually remains intact until at least 48 hours before delivery.

The changes in the *corpus* of the uterus are those associated with hyperplasia and hypertrophy of the uterine muscular fibers. The nonpregnant uterus which weighs between 50 and 80 g. will grow to a term size of approximately 700 to 800 g. Although this increase is due mainly to proliferation of new myometrial tissue, hyperplasia of the muscle cells and mitosis also contribute. Uterine growth results from the hormonal effects of the pregnancy as well as the distention and stretching caused by the developing embryo.

Other changes are related to the hormone production of the corpus luteum and placenta. In the *ovary*, cells may develop a deciduous reaction due to an increase in circulating hormones. However, it is not normal to develop large ovarian cysts, and if these occur, a careful evaluation is necessary.

The *breasts* are also affected by the elevated levels of hormones. They gradually enlarge and may occasionally become quite large. They may also become painful, a condition referred to as mastalgia. The vascularity of the breasts increases during pregnancy. This is first noted as a pink discoloration which gradually darkens. As the pregnancy continues, the veins may become prominent. There is an increase in the size and pigmentation of the areolae. Small glands in the periareolar area, called Montgomery's glands, are also noted to enlarge.

URINARY SYSTEM

The urinary system also undergoes marked changes during pregnancy. The renal plasma flow increases approximately 20 to 25 per cent with a resulting 50 per cent increase in glomerular filtration rate. Hydroureter occurs and is considered normal during pregnancy. This is especially noticeable in the right kidney and is possibly related to the pressure of the uterus which is dextrorotated on the pelvic brim, and elevated progesterone levels which cause general dilatation of smooth muscles. Occasionally, there may be stasis of urine in the ureters, pelvis, kidney, and bladder which may predispose to urinary tract infection. Asymptomatic bacteriuria occurs in approximately 6 per cent of pregnancies.

GASTROINTESTINAL SYSTEM

Most of the changes in the gastrointestinal system during pregnancy are related to the change in smooth muscle tone due to elevated levels of circulating progesterone. Occasionally a woman develops an appetite for unusual foods or even substances which are not fit to be consumed, e.g., clay or plaster. This latter condition is called pica. Hypertrophy of the gums occurs during pregnancy and may occasionally produce bleeding. Constipation is a very common complaint, especially in the later stages of pregnancy when relaxation of smooth muscles and the physical bulk of the large uterus tend to decrease intestinal motility. Another condition which may occur in the pregnant woman is relaxation at the cardiac sphincter of the esophagus with subsequent reflux of gastric acids. This causes chronic esophagitis and the complaint of heartburn. Although annoying, these gastrointestinal changes rarely cause any significant harm to the pregnant woman.

METABOLIC SYSTEM

Many metabolic changes are due to the effect of the various steroid and protein hormones of pregnancy. Others are due to the altered utilization of food substances, vitamins, minerals, and so forth. Although these changes are frequently evaluated only in research laboratories or in the presence of illness, it is important to realize that such changes do take place. However, it must be remembered that all changes in a pregnant woman are closely interrelated and cannot easily be discriminated from other physiologic changes which are taking place. These changes must be viewed in relationship to the primary organ system responsible for their control.

The blood level of total lipids rises during pregnancy with a compensatory rise in serum cholesterol levels. Although the exact reason for this is unknown, it is speculated that the increased estrogen levels of pregnancy may cause this alteration. Fat storage is also a common finding during pregnancy. This is related to the total weight gain and food intake of the individual patient.

Most of the endocrine glands continue to produce at normal levels throughout pregnancy. However, there is evidence that plasma insulin levels may increase. Women who are latent diabetics will frequently become actual diabetics during pregnancy. There is also an increase in the amount of mineral storage. This is especially noticeable in sodium, potassium, and calcium levels. The largest amount of storage occurs in the fetus, but there are also elevated levels in the amniotic fluid, and accumulation in the placenta and uterus. These are but a few of the general metabolic changes which occur during pregnancy. This subject is discussed in more detail in Chapter 15. Although these changes rarely cause problems, in certain state of stress or disease they may become grossly altered. Individuals with pre-existing diseases, e.g., hyperthyroidism, hypothyroidism, or diabetes mellitus, must be carefully monitored to assure correct functioning of their metabolic systems.

PRENATAL DEVELOPMENT

The three stages of prenatal development are:

Ovum—from fertilization until establishment of primitive villi at approximately 12 to 14 days of gestation.

Embryo—following ovum stage until a crown-rump length of approximately 32 mm. is reached, usually 54 to 56 days of gestation.

Fetus—following embryo stage until the end of pregnancy.

FERTILIZATION

When sperm is ejaculated into the vagina of the female, it immediately invades the cervical mucus. If the cervical mucus is in the proper stage of receptiveness, as occurs during the luteal phase of the menstrual cycle, the sperm migrates through the uterine cavity into the

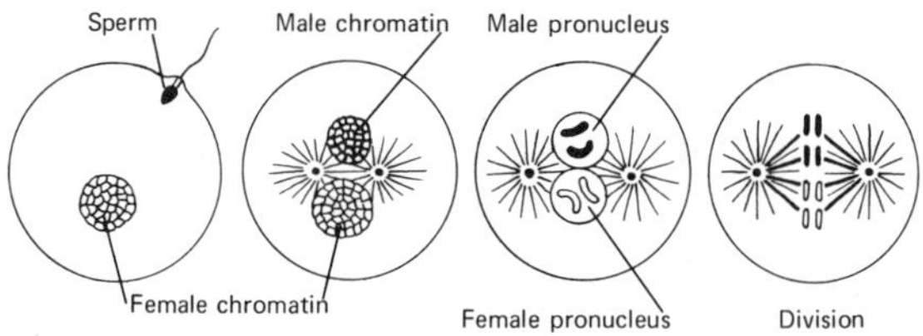

FIGURE 14-5. The fertilization process. (From *Taber's Cyclopedic Medical Dictionary*, ed. 12. F. A. Davis, Philadelphia, 1973, with permission.)

cornual end of the fallopian tube to meet the ovum in the distal third where fertilization will occur. The sperm penetrates the ovum, their pronuclei join, and pregnancy is initiated (Fig. 14-5).

IMPLANTATION

After fertilization, the ovum migrates through the fallopian tube by peristalsis and ciliary activity. It takes two to three days for the ovum to reach the uterine cavity. During this time, mitotic cell division has been occurring and the ovum is now in its morula stage. It remains in the uterine cavity for three to four days and continues its development to a blastocyst form. On approximately the sixth day after fertilization, implantation occurs. In this process, the ovum attaches itself to the wall of the uterus. Throughout this time, the corpus luteum of the ovary has been secreting progesterone in large quantities to prepare the endometrium for implantation. Once the process of implantation begins, it takes approximately 24 hours for the blastocyst to embed in the endometrium with subsequent proliferation of the endometrium over the implanting blastocyst. Once this occurs, the advancing trophoblast, which is entirely syncytiotrophoblast, begins to invade the endometrium. This invading syncytiotrophoblast begins to provide an exchange between the developing embryo and the maternal circulation. This forms the early primitive placenta. Almost immediately after implantation, the trophoblast begins to produce the hormone human chorionic gonadotrophin.

THE PLACENTA

The physiologic function of the placenta is to deliver all necessary food substances and

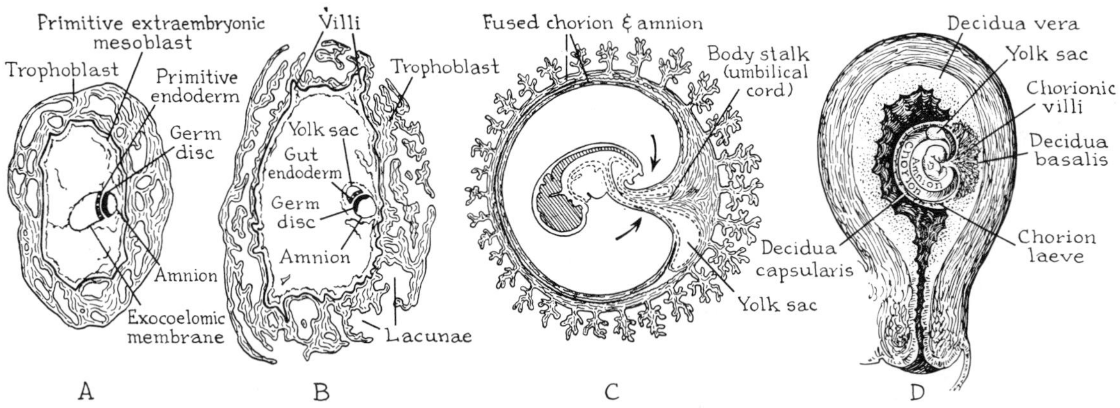

FIGURE 14-6. Development of placenta and fetal membranes. *A*, At 12 days the lacunae are present and contain blood, the blastocyst cavity has already become distended and lined with mesoblast to form the exocoelomic cavity. *B*, At 13 days the primitive unbranched villi appear consisting of mesodermal cores in cytotrophoblastic protrusions covered by syncytiotrophoblast that lines the intervillous space (lacunae). *C*, Development of amniotic cavity, yolk sac, allantois and umbilical cord. The amniotic sac which at first overlies the embryonic rudiment, comes to surround it in the manner indicated by the arrows. These two growing margins finally merge into the body stalk. The amniotic cavity accumulates fluid in which the embryo floats. The villi have undergone significant branching, those near the body stalk much more than the others. *D*, At 6 weeks the villi have largely disappeared from the side bulging into the uterine cavity (decidua capsularis). The chorion laeve is atrophic and the chorionic villi are proliferating into the decidua basalis. (From Bonica, J.: *Obstetric Analgesia and Anesthesia*. F. A. Davis, Philadelphia, 1972, with permission.)

materials to the developing embryo, and to remove from the embryo its excretory products. After implantation, the growth process of the placenta continues in an orderly fashion (Fig. 14-6). In development of the early placenta, the cytotrophoblast spreads out through the columns in asociation with the syncytiotrophoblast to develop primary villi. In association with these primary villi, *lacunae* appear and develop into a network, and the circulation of the early placenta is established. By this time, the endometrium has undergone marked hypertrophy and is now referred to as the *decidua*. The part underlying the developing embryo is called the *decidua basalis*. The part covering the embryo is called the *decidua capsularis*. The part lining the remainder of the uterine cavity is called the *decidua parietalis*.

The outer layer of the fetal membranes is called the *chorion*. As the developing placenta begins to grow more into the endometrial tissue and develops an extensive villous network, that part of the chorion closest to the maternal blood supply is called the *chorion frondosum*. This is the site of the development of the placenta. The remainder of the chorion which covers the developing embryo is called the *chorion laeve*, but this will soon atrophy and remain the chorionic part of the fetal membranes. Within the chorion, the embryo is developing in the amnionic cavity. As this fluid-filled cavity enlarges, it pushes the outer layer of cells against the chorion laeve, forming the inner layer of the fetal membranes, called the *amnion*. As the placenta continues to develop, its maternal surface divides into *cotyledons* which become subdivisions of the placenta. Communication within these cotyledons is by vascular supply into the developing embryo. The placenta continues its growth process until approximately the fourth or fifth month of gestation, at which time the syncytiotrophoblast begins to disappear and the cytotrophoblast remains. The mature placenta at term is a rounded, flattened organ approximately one sixth the weight of the newborn infant.

The *umbilical cord* forms the attachment between the developing embryo and the placenta. It is derived from the primitive germ disk which differentiates so that the cord is directed into the chorion frondosum with its vascular supply. At term, the umbilical cord is approximately 50 cm. in length, 1 to 2 cm. in diameter, and contains a mucous substance, called *Wharton's jelly*, within a loose connective tissue framework. The umbilical cord usually has two arteries and one vein.

FETAL GROWTH

The nine calendar months of pregnancy may be divided into three groups of three months each, referred to as the first, second, and third trimesters of pregnancy.

The First Trimester. This is a period of remarkable growth. By the end of the second week of gestation, the embryo contains three distinct germ layers from which body organs and systems develop:

Ectoderm—epidermis, including hair and nails; epithelium of internal and external ear, nasal cavity, mouth, and anus; nervous tissue; and glands.

Mesoderm—connective tissue; blood vessels; lymphatic tissue; kidneys; pleura; peritoneum; pericardium; muscles; and skeleton.

Entoderm—respiratory tract (except nose); digestive tract (except mouth and anus); bladder (except trigone); liver; and pancreas.

At 24 days of gestation the heart consists of one large chamber, the lung buds first appear, and a rudimentary kidney and gut exist. However, by the end of the first trimester, the heart has compartmentalized, limbs are differentiated, and the lung buds have branched into bronchi.

The gut is fairly well developed, as are the liver, pancreas, gallbladder, and spleen. Sex can now be distinguished, and the fetus has unmistakable human features. At this time the fetus weighs approximately 1 oz. and is about 3 in. long.

The Second Trimester. During this period organogenesis continues and the fetus undergoes further maturation. Facial features become defined. Fine body hair called *lanugo* appears. *Vernix caseosa*, a white, cheeselike, fatty substance, is produced to protect the fetal skin which lacks subcutaneous fat deposits. *Meconium,* the mucous substance which constitutes the first stools, begins to appear in the intestines. Body organs and systems of the fetus become functional, but are still immature. At the end of the second trimester, the fetus weighs approximately 1½ lb. and is about 12 in. long.

The Third Trimester. The third trimester is characterized by rapid weight gain and final maturation of the fetus. Subcutaneous fat deposits appear, making the skin less red and wrinkled. Lanugo is shed, and weight increases give the fetus a more rounded body shape. At the end of the third timester, body organs and systems attain optimal intrauterine development and the fetus begins to prepare for the birth process. At this time the fetus weighs approximately 7 lb. and is about 20 in. long.

REFERENCES

1. Beazley, J. M. and Underhill, R. A.: *Fallacy of fundal height.* Br. Med. J. 4:404, 1970.
2. Kerber, K. J., et al.: *Immunologic test for pregnancy, a comparison.* Obstet. Gynecol. 36:37, 1970.
3. Midgley, A. R.: *Radioimmunoassay: A method for human chorionic gonadotropin and human luteinizing hormone,* Endocrinology 79:10, 1966.
4. Kosasa, T. S., et al.: *Evaluation of radioimmunoassay kits for the beta subunit of HCG, FSH and HLH.* Obstet. Gynecol. 43:481, 1974.
5. Gluck, L., et al.: *Diagnosis of respiratory distress syndrome by amniocentesis.* Am. J. Obstet. Gynecol. 109:440, 1971.

BIBLIOGRAPHY

Davis, M. E. and Rubin, R.: *DeLee's Obstetrics for Nurses,* ed. 18. W. B. Saunders, Philadelphia, 1966.

Eastman, N.: *Expectant Motherhood,* ed. 5. Little, Brown and Company, Boston, 1970.

Hellman, L. and Pritchard, J.: *Williams Obstetrics,* ed. 14. Appleton-Century-Crofts, New York, 1971.

Patten, B. M.: *Human Embryology.* McGraw-Hill, New York, 1968.

Pitkin, R. M.: *Prenatal estimation of fetal maturity.* Int. J. Gynecol. Obstet. 7:199, 1969.

15 *Hormones*

M. WAYNE HEINE, M.D.

In the ever-expanding role of the nurse in the primary care of women, an understanding of the role of hormones throughout the menstrual cycle and pregnancy is essential. This chapter discusses hormonal changes and their effects during the childbearing years of a woman's life.

THE MENSTRUAL CYCLE

The interaction of the central nervous system with other endocrine glands is the controlling factor of the female reproductive cycle. The central nervous system exercises this control by means of complex interactions of special neurohumoral cells of the hypothalamus, hypophyseal portal system, and anterior pituitary. The hypothalamus exerts its effect by means of neurotransmitters called releasing factors or inhibiting factors. Control of the reproductive cycle depends on the interrelationship of releasing factors, other neurohumors, pituitary gonadotrophins, and gonadal steroids. The rising levels of estrogens cause the anterior hypothalamic area to react with a cyclic surge of luteinizing hormone (LH). Ovulation occurs within a few hours after the LH surge. The cycle may be affected by feedback effects of gonadal steroids, signals from the external environment, as well as feedback from the pituitary to the hypothalamus itself.

Prior to puberty, the ovary is fully capable of responding to follicle stimulating hormone (FSH) and LH, but gonadotrophin levels remain low during the prepubertal age. The onset of puberty is variable and is influenced by general health as well as genetics. The exact mechanism by which the central nervous system exerts its inhibitory effect on the hypothalamic pituitary axis is not known.

The sequence of development begins with a gradual rise of gonadotrophins followed by a gradual rise of estrogens. The estrogens stimulate breast budding and development called *thelarche*. This is followed by increased adrenal and ovarian androgens associated with sexual hair growth which is called *pubarche*. When sufficient estrogenic stimulation of the endometrium has taken place, menstrual bleeding occurs with fluctuation of estrogen levels. Initial cycles are often anovulatory.

Puberty usually occurs between the eighth and fourteenth years of life. Development of secondary sexual characteristics prior to age eight is considered precocious and requires investigation. Occasionally there is only precocious thelarche or pubarche. This is associated with increased end organ sensitivity to physiologic levels of hormones. The majority of cases of precocious puberty are idiopathic and due to premature release of the inhibitory effects of the central nervous system on the hypothalamic pituitary axis. However, it is always necessary to consider the possibility of central nervous system, adrenal, and gonadal tumors.

By age 16, 95 per cent of females who are going to have ovulatory cycles will have done so. If spontaneous menstruation does not occur by age 18, the condition known as *primary amenorrhea* exists.

The menstrual cycle of the reproductive-age female requires precise and dynamic interrelationship between the hypothalamic pituitary axis, gonadal steroids, and the end organ response of the uterus. The occurrence of ovulation divides the cycle into two phases. The *follicular phase* precedes ovulation and the *luteal phase* follows ovulation.

FOLLICULAR PHASE

During the follicular phase, a number of primordial follicles in the ovary undergo devel-under the influence of FSH. Ovulation, however, is not stimulated by FSH alone. One follicle develops exactly to the point where ovulation can occur should the correct stimulation be applied. Why only one follicle reaches this point of development is not known. A rise in serum estrogen occurs about seven to eight days prior to ovulation, reaching a peak shortly before the LH surge. LH increases gradually throughout the follicular phase with a dramatic surge just after the peak of estrogen.

During ovulation, LH is released in a pulsatile fashion at high levels for approximately 24 hours. The follicle at the appropriate stage of maturity is released near the fallopian tube within a few hours after the LH surge. Thus, ovulation is completed and the luteal phase begins.

LUTEAL PHASE

After ovulation, the ovum undergoes *luteinization,* the process by which the corpus luteum is developed. At this time there is also an increase in the production of progesterone and estrogen. The peak level of progesterone occurs seven to nine days after ovulation. If fertilization does not take place, regression of the corpus luteum with a gradual decline in progesterone production occurs approximately eleven to twelve days after ovulation. The exact mechanism controlling the life span of the corpus luteum and the progesterone production is unknown. The endometrium changes in response to progesterone and estrogen production. Endometrial glands become secretory and more tortuous. If fertilization and implantation do not occur, there is a loss of height of the endometrium and a decrease in blood flow due to constriction and retraction of the spiral arteries. This is followed by progressive endometrial ischemia and finally hemorrhage and menstruation.

If fertilization does take place, the ovum is unattached for approximately five to seven days, allowing the endometrial glands to fill with nutrient secretions. By this time, the ovum has become a blastocyst and is ready for implantation if the endometrium has sufficient depth, vascularity, and secretory activity. After implantation, the blastocyst begins to secrete human chorionic gonadotrophin and the hormonal changes of pregnancy begin.

ENDOCRINE ALTERATIONS DURING PREGNANCY

During pregnancy, dramatic endocrine alterations produce a close metabolic relationship between the mother and fetus. Early in pregnancy, the synthesis of human chorionic gonadotrophin helps stimulate the corpus luteum to produce estrogen and progesterone which help maintain the nutritional environment of the early embryo. These steroids also alter uterine growth and tone, and aid in preparation of the breasts for lactation. Later in pregnancy, the placenta supplies most of the estrogen and progesterone. The placenta also produces human placental lactogen which is important for lactation and aids fetal anabolism. Many of the humoral agents and adjustments of pregnancy are only now being recognized and are as yet poorly understood. It is hoped that in the near future, with improved assay techniques, a better understanding of the physiologic function of these various humoral agents will be achieved. This will make possible the earlier detection of any abnormalities, more accurate estimates of their significance, and improved plans of care.

HUMAN CHORIONIC GONADOTROPHIN

Human chorionic gonadotrophin (HCG) is one of the earliest known hormones secreted by trophoblastic tissue. It has some FSH-like activity but mainly LH-like activity. Immunologically, it is also similar to LH. Factors which control production and secretion rates are as yet unknown. HCG production reaches its highest level in the third month of pregnancy and then levels off (Fig. 15-1). Its clearance rate is approximately 1 ml. per unit with 6 to 8 per cent of the HCG in the active form. Approximately 90 per cent of HCG in the urine is inactive. Biosynthesis and metabolic breakdown of HCG are not known. Biologic and immunologic assays are available for measurement of HCG and are used to aid in the determination of pregnancy.

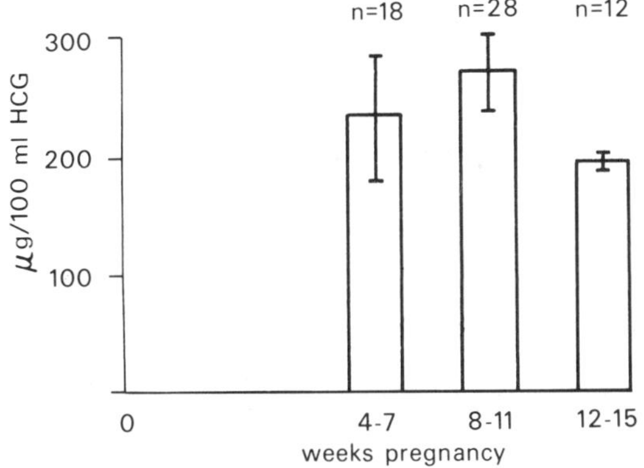

FIGURE 15-1. Chroionic gonadotrophin levels during pregnancy.

The role of HCG in pregnancy is not fully established. It may help maintain the corpus luteum by production of various steroids and therefore aid in the continued growth and increased blood supply to the embryo. It is also postulated that it affects the maternal immune mechanism, thus preventing the rejection of the fetus.

HUMAN PLACENTAL LACTOGEN

Human placental lactogen (HPL) is another of the protein hormones produced by the placenta. It has growth-like activity and is associated with the mobilization of fatty acid and nitrogen retention in the mother and fetus. It also appears to have lactogenic and luteotropic activity. HPL is a polypeptide with a molecular weight between 19,000 and 30,000. Immunologically, it is similar to human pituitary growth hormone. Placental growth is very closely related to the production of HPL with the majority being secreted into the maternal blood stream. Only 0.3 per cent of the maternal values are found in the fetus.

By being glucose-sparing in the mother, HPL allows increasing amounts of glucose to the fetus. HPL measurements are useful in determining growth of the placenta, but are not useful in predicting fetal distress since it may continue to be secreted after fetal death as long as the placental circulation is intact.

PROGESTERONE

Progesterone, a C-21 steroid, is supplied mainly by the corpus luteum during the first 12 weeks of pregnancy. The trophoblastic production of progesterone begins during the second or third weeks after ovulation. The highest levels of progesterone are found in umbilical and uterine venous blood. Thus, it appears to be produced in the placenta with the precursors coming from the maternal circulation. The three biologically active progestogens in the human, progesterone, 20α-dihydroprogesterone, and 20β-dihydroprogesterone are not excreted in the urine. They are, however, metabolized and broken down into pregnanediol which is excreted in the maternal urine. Urinary pregnanediol and blood serum progesterone levels show a gradual rise throughout the course of pregnancy. The increase in serum progesterone is closely related to the increase in placental weight. It will, however, be produced even after fetal death, as has been shown in patients receiving intra-amniotic hypertonic saline solution for therapeutic abortions. In these cases, urinary pregnanediol and serum progesterone levels fell only 20 per cent while estrogen levels fell approximately 80 per cent.

The function of progesterone is not fully understood. It appears to serve as a precursor to the fetal adrenal gland in the production of corticoids. It also appears to cause a decrease in myometrial activity. However, progesterone levels do not fall before labor, and its exact role during labor is not known.

CORTISOL

Maternal plasma levels of cortisol increase throughout pregnancy, but the circadian rhythm is unaffected. This increase is probably due to increased transcortin levels with free cortisol levels remaining essentially unchanged, since 24-hour urinary cortisol levels remain the same or are only slightly increased.

Although the fetus is capable of synthesizing cortisol and may utilize placental progesterone as a precusor, the majority of cortisone comes from the mother. When the fetal adrenal matures and is able to synthesize more cortisone, fetal cortisone may then play a part in initiating labor.

ALDOSTERONE

Aldosterone is the most biologically active mineralocorticoid. During pregnancy, aldosterone levels gradually increase beginning about the fifteenth week. The reason for this increase is not known, but progesterone, a known aldosterone antagonist, increases throughout pregnancy and may cause a compensatory rise in aldosterone.

ANDROGENS

Production of androgens (C-19 steroids) by the fetus has been noted as early as six weeks of gestation. The genital ridge begins production of androgens, and levels gradually increase until approximately the twentieth week of gestation. The fetal adrenal, however, produces dehydroepiandrosterone which is circulated through the fetal liver to form 15α and 16α hydroxylated steroids. These compounds are then transferred to the placenta where they can be converted to estriol.

ESTROGEN

Although it has been known for some time that there is a dramatic rise in estrogen levels during pregnancy (Fig. 15-2), it has only been during the past 15 years that the complex interrelationship between the placenta and fetus and the active role of the fetus in production of estrogens have been elucidated. Steroid precursors are transferred to the fetus from the mother and the placenta. The fetal adrenal produces a precursor which is circulated through the fetal liver and then transferred to the placenta where estriol is formed. Estriol is then transferred to the maternal

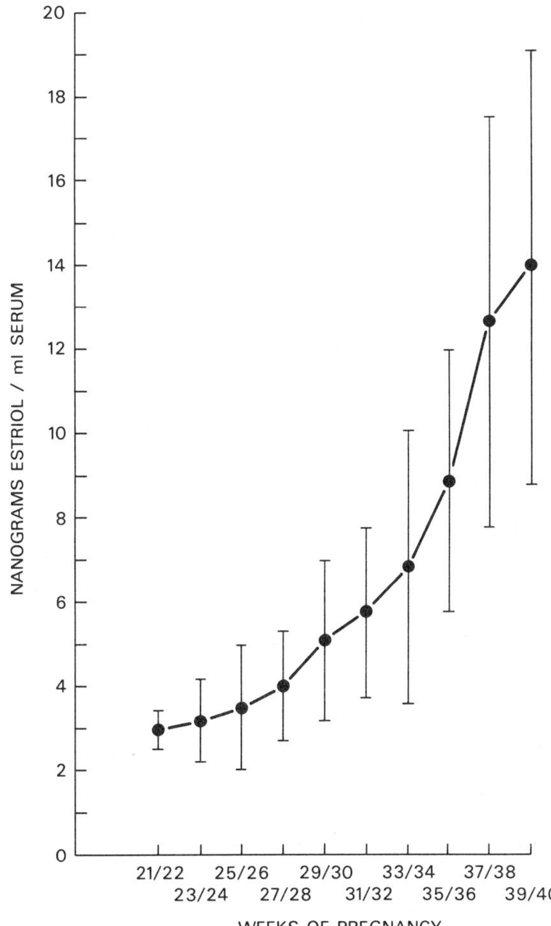

FIGURE 15-2. Estriol levels during pregnancy.

circulation and is excreted in maternal urine.

The functional role of high estrogen levels is not known but they are probably involved in maintaining fetal nutrition and regulating uterine and fetal growth and development.

Since normal production of estrogen requires a functional relationship between the fetal-placental unit and the mother, serial estrogen determinations may be used to monitor certain high-risk pregnancies, such as those involving hypertension, preeclampsia, prior stillborns, and diabetes. Since there may be a marked fall of estriol within 24 to 48 hours of fetal-placental difficulty, it is important that determinations be run frequently. With the newer automated urinary methods and serum radioimmunoassay methods, the time and cost involved have decreased sufficiently to make this feasible. It should be remembered that a drop in estriol values is the result, not the cause, of fetal-placental difficulty.

LACTATION

Growth and development of the breasts depends on many hormones. During puberty, growth is stimulated by increased levels of estrogen. Progesterone is associated with lobular alveolar maturation. Other hormones, especially prolactin, are needed for final differentiation into mature alveolar epithelia. During pregnancy, there is a dramatic increase in estrogen, progesterone, and prolactin. In addition, the placenta secretes increasing amounts of HPL which stimulate even further growth and maturation of the breasts. At the time of labor, the levels of these hormones fall. During puerperal suckling, however, there is a transient spike in prolactin levels. These transient peaks plus the increased cortisol associated with the stress of labor may be the initiator of milk production. The prolactin peaks enhance milk production while oxytocin from the posterior pituitary stimulates milk ejection. Suckling maintains prolactin and oxytocin release. Mothers not wishing to nurse are often given androgen and/or estrogens which appear to depress milk production at the alveolar level.

Most medications and drugs cross the plasma-milk barrier. Therefore, careful consideration must be given to the potential effect on the infant of any drug the mother may receive.

MENSTRUAL IRREGULARITY

The female reproductive cycle involves a very delicate balance between the central nervous system, various other endocrine glands, and the reproductive tract. Almost any disturbance of this system of checks and balances will result in menstrual irregularity. Therefore, it is important to remember that all these checks and balances must be evaluated in the patient with menstrual irregularity if it persists beyond what would be three normal cycles.

Amenorrhea is the complete cessation of menses. Anovulation may be associated with either amenorrhea or irregular menstrual bleeding. Since some causes are common to both anovulation and amenorrhea, these conditions are discussed together.

It must be remembered that a lack of menstrual regularity is a symptom and not a disease in itself. It is extremely important that the cause of the irregularity be investigated and not merely masked by exogenous hormone therapy.

One of the common causes of irregular menstrual bleeding associated with ovulation is pregnancy, either intrauterine or extrauterine. The possibility of pregnancy must always be kept in mind. Occasionally, leukemia results in excessive or intermenstrual vaginal bleeding. Submucous myomas which press on the endometrium are often associated with excessive menstrual flow. In any patient with a cyclic pattern of abnormal bleeding, be it excessive or intermenstrual, it is important to investigate for a bleeding disorder.

A patient may have normal secondary sexual characteristics and be ovulating regularly, but experience amenorrhea due to a mullerian duct defect such as an imperforate hymen, transverse septum across the vagina, or even vaginal, uterine, or endometrial agenesis. Amenorrhea may also be caused by insufficient ovarian development or a lack of gonadotrophic hormone production. Ovarian agenesis or dysgenesis may or may not be associated with a sex chromosomal abnormality. The patient who has never had a menstrual period but has high levels of gonadotrophic hormones is likely to have an ovarian developmental defect.

Cessation of ovarian function associated with high levels of gonadotrophins prior to age 40 is termed premature menopause. This usually includes the signs and symptoms of menopause with high levels of gonadotrophic hormones.

Another cause of irregular or anovulatory cycles, with or without obesity and hirsutism, may be polycystic ovaries. In this syndrome there is a steady level of FSH associated with a slight increase in LH. This results in multiple follicular development but lack of ovulation with an associated increase in production of ovarian androgens and a constant level of estrogen. It is not known whether this is an ovarian defect or a result of abnormal hypothalamic-pituitary stimulation. Due to the constant level of unopposed estrogen, these patients may develop endometrial hyperplasia and, occasionally, endometrial carcinoma.

The treatment of polycystic ovarian syndrome depends on the patient's priorities. If she is desirous of pregnancy, clomiphene citrate therapy or a wedge resection of the ovary may be beneficial if all other fertility factors are normal. If excessive hair growth is a concern, suppression of ovarian androgens by exogenous estrogen and progestins found in the combination birth control pill is often helpful. If profuse and irregular bleeding is the only complaint, cyclic progestins will regulate the periods and counteract endometrial hyperplasia.

Ovarian tumors producing estrogen and/or androgen may cause similar symptoms. These patients usually have low FSH and LH levels and will not improve with cyclic hormonal therapy. If the tumors are not palpable, endoscopic examinations, such as laparoscopy or culdoscopy, are indicated.

Dysfunction of almost any endocrine gland in the reproductive-age female is usually associated with menstrual irregularity. Hypothyroidism may result in excessive, prolonged menses and hyperthyroidism often results in scant, irregular menses. Tumors or hyperplasticity of the adrenal gland may cause excessive secretion of androgens and/or cortisone. These patients usually exhibit hirsutism and virilization in addition to menstrual irregularity.

Occasionally, a juvenille diabetic will have delayed onset of menses. However, since the advent of insulin, if the patient is under reasonable diabetic control, she will usually have fairly normal cycles unless there is some other cause for irregularity.

The central nervous system exerts dramatic control over the menstrual cycle in the female. It is not unusual for a woman to miss a period when under severe psychologic or physiologic stress. A dramatic example of this is the patient who has anorexia nervosa, a compulsion against food. This patient will usually have amenorrhea from the time that her weight loss begins. Tumors of the central nervous system, especially in the hypothalamic or pituitary area, often result in amenorrhea and/or galactorrhea. If a woman experiences lactation not associated with pregnancy, she may have up to a 40 per cent chance of eventually developing a hypothalamic or pituitary tumor. For this reason, skull films with visual field examinations should be performed on all patients with amenorrhea.

INFERTILITY

Approximately 15 per cent of married couples experience involuntary infertility. Infertility is defined as the condition in which pregnancy does not occur within one year of unprotected intercourse. Most investigators, however, will evaluate patients if conception does not occur after six months of unprotected intercourse.

When evaluating the infertile couple, it is extremely important to establish good rapport in view of the great emotional impact this condition may have. It is vital that the couple understand that time and patience are needed, and that the probability of successful resolution is approximately 50 per cent depending on the factors involved (Table 15-1).

TABLE 15-1. Etiologic Factors in Infertility

Factors	*Occurrence (%)*
Female	
Anovulation	20
Tubal factors	35
Cervical factors	5
Endometriosis	10
Male	
Low sperm count	20
Unknown	10
Two or More Factors	40

The initial evaluation should reveal a thorough medical history of both the husband and wife, including prior fertility of either partner, reproductive tract or abdominal infection or surgery, chronic or hereditary diseases, and exposure to chemicals, x-rays, or extreme temperature changes.

The physical examination should include careful evaluation of organs and parts of the body with special attention given to fat and hair distribution. Pelvic examination of the female should reveal the state of hair distribution, clitoral size, evidence of vaginal infection, normality of the cervix, size and configuration of the uterus, and any adnexal or pelvic masses. The husband's genital exam should reveal the size of the penis, placement of the urethra, testicular size and consistency, and any abnormality of the epididymis or prostate. Although the physical examination is extremely important, it will reveal the cause of infertility in only five per cent of cases.

Since a low sperm count is the primary cause of infertility in 20 per cent of cases and a contributing cause in an additional 20 per cent, a sperm count is one of the first tests to be obtained in the evaluation of an infertile couple. A normal sperm count is usually over 60 million per cc. with a volume of 2.5 to 5 cc. per ejaculation.

A thorough menstrual history of the wife must be obtained. If the periods suggest anovulation, an endocrine evaluation should be done. If the periods are regular, the patency of the tubes should be evaluated. This may be done in the office with the passage of carbon dioxide through the uterus and tubes. Hysterosalpingography requires special x-ray equipment, but may be more revealing since it allows evaluation of the endometrial cavity, size and configuration of the tubes, and may occasionally be therapeutic if there is minor obstruction. Tubal patency tests are usually done during the follicular phase of the cycle.

During the ovulatory shift of the menstrual cycle, there is a change in the character of the cervical mucus. Normally, the cervical mucus is very viscid, but during this time it becomes thin with few white cells and is easily penetrated by sperm. An evaluation of the cervical mucus within 24 hours after intercourse showing five or more motile sperm per high-power field indicates that cervical penetrability is normal.

It has been postulated that sperm allergies in the female are one of the unexplained causes of infertility. This may be due to an antibody in the female reacting to the sperm or to bacteria which is carried on the surface of the sperm or in the seminal fluid. If the allergy is secondary to infection, it may be treated with antibiotics with up to a 50 per cent probability of success. When it is due to an allergy to sperm, the success rate may be as low as 10 per cent even after using a condum for as long as one year.

The properties of the cervical mucus may be improved by low-dose estrogens, or if infection is present, topical or systemic antibiotics. If neither treatment results in improvement in the presence of erosion, cervical cryosurgery or cauterization may be necessary.

MENOPAUSE

Menopause denotes the physiologic cessation of menses usually occurring between age 40 and 55. A more accurate term may be climacteric since there is usually a gradual transition from fully-ovulatory, normal cycles to the complete cessation of menses with estrogen deficiency. Between age 35 and 45, many patients notice premenstrual spotting. Evaluation of progesterone levels and basal body temperatures suggest that there is some corpus luteal inadequacy. This may be followed by menstrual irregularity with anovulatory cycles. During this period of time, estrogen levels gradually decrease. Eventually, the follicles become refractory to gonadotrophic hormones and ovulation ceases with a continued fall in estrogen production. As the estrogen levels fall, symptoms of estrogen deficiencies, such as the vasomotor symptoms of hot flushes and sweats, increase. Other signs of estrogen deficiency include atrophy of the vaginal and bladder epithelium, some loss of skin tone, and occasionally osteopetrosis.

Menopause may also be associated with variable psychologic symptoms such as irritability, mood fluctuations, and depression. It is difficult to predict which symptoms a patient will develop, and which women will require symptomatic treatment for estrogen deficiency. Approximately 25 to 30 per cent of patients experience the climacteric so gradually and with so few symptoms that they may not require estrogen replacement. However, most women present symptoms of estrogen deficiency and require estrogen replacement therapy. It is important to remember that this is the time of life when endometrial carcinoma often develops, and any irregular bleeding while on hormone replacement therapy requires careful investigation.

BIBLIOGRAPHY

Fuchs, F. and Klopper, A.: *Endocrinology of Pregnancy.* Harper and Row, New York, 1971.

Lox, C. D., et al.: *Estriol—The hormone of pregnancy.* Arizona Medicine, 30:623, 1973.

Joel, C. A. (ed.): *Fertility Disturbances in Men and Women.* S. Karger, Basel, 1971.

Speroff, L., et al.: *Clinical Gynecologic Endocrinology and Infertility.* Williams & Wilkins, Baltimore, 1973.

16 *Transport of Essential Elements in Maternal System*

SUK KI HONG, M.D., Ph.D.

Profound local and systemic changes in maternal physiology are initiated by conception and continued throughout pregnancy. After expulsion of the placenta many of these changes are rapidly reversed. Although many of these changes occur in the interests of the growing embryo or fetus, the maternal body also reacts with a series of adjustments required for her own interests.

The complex and multiple endocrinologic alterations during pregnancy are responsible for many changes observed in pregnant women. However, the presence of the growing embryo or fetus imposes a considerable additional physiologic load on the mother. In this chapter, the functions of various maternal physiologic systems involved in transport of essential elements are discussed.

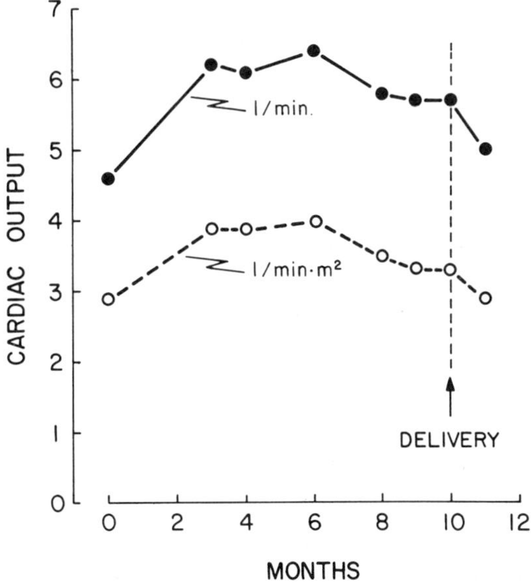

FIGURE 16-1. Changes in the cardiac output (l./min.) and cardiac index (l./min./m.²) during pregnancy. (Based on data of Palmer, A. J. and Walker, A. H. C.: *The maternal circulation in normal pregnancy.* J. Obstet. Gynecol. Brit Emp. 56:537, 1949.)

CARDIOVASCULAR CHANGES

From a clinical viewpoint, the cardiovascular changes of pregnancy are of paramount importance, particularly in patients with any form of heart disease.

CARDIAC OUTPUT AND HEART RATE

In nonpregnant women, the resting cardiac output is approximately 4.5 l. per min. (or 3 l. per min. per m.² body surface). As shown in Figure 16-1, the cardiac output increases approximately 35 per cent by the end of the first trimester, and this increase seems to persist until term. Although there is a slight tendency for reduction near term, the validity of this reduction has been challenged.[1] In contrast to this marked increase in the cardiac output, the resting heart rate increases only 5 to 10 beats per min., an increase of approximately 6 to 12 per cent. This means that the observed increase in cardiac output is due largely to an increase in the stroke volume. The cause of this early increase in cardiac output is unknown, but it may be related to the hormonal changes. Although the blood volume also increases during pregnancy, it is not evident during the first trimester, and thus cannot account for the early increase in cardiac output. Oxygen consumption also increases during pregnancy but the magnitude of the increase is significantly less than that observed in cardiac output.

During labor, cardiac output increases 15 to 20 per cent with each uterine contraction. This does not seem to be due to pain, for the increase cannot be abolished by regional anesthesia. In addition, there is an overall increase in cardiac output of approximately 40 per cent by the end of the second stage of labor which is largely abolished by caudal analgesia.

HEMODYNAMICS

Mean arterial blood pressure remains essentially normal during the first trimester, shows a slight reduction by 3 to 6 mm. Hg during the second trimester, and returns to the normal range during the third trimester. Since cardiac output is already considerably increased during the second trimester, the reduction in mean arterial pressure must mean that total peripheral resistance (pressure/flow or cardiac output) is significantly lowered during this period. Bader and associates[2] estimated that there is approximately a 25 per cent reduction in total peripheral resistance after five months of pregnancy. A major part of the reduced peripheral resistance is apparently in the uteroplacental circulation, which constitutes a low resistance shunt. During labor, mean arterial blood pressure increases with each uterine contraction. Simultaneously, cardiac output also increases, and thus the work of the heart must increase significantly. The administration of ergometrine for its oxytocic effect concomitantly increases the mean blood pressure in many women (especially hypertensives), further increasing the work of the heart.

Venous pressure measured in the anticubital region remains normal. However, the femoral venous pressure rises 10 to 15 cm. H_2O above normal as a result of the pressure exerted by the enlarging uterus on the pelvic veins. This factor contributes to the development of ankle edema and varicose veins.

In the last trimester of pregnancy, approximately 8 per cent of women who lie on their backs complain of faintness. This is accompanied by a large reduction (30 per cent or more) in systolic blood pressure and by bradycardia, a decrease in the heart rate. This combination of hypotension and bradycardia is termed *supine hypotensive syndrome* and reduces the cardiac output approximately 50 per cent. If position is changed, the above symptoms disappear almost immediately. Since this phenomenon is due to compression of the inferior vena cava by the heavy uterus, it is also known as *vena cava syndrome*. Such a compression of the vena cava would impede the venous return to the heart and cause a precipitous fall in arterial pressure.

Capillary pressure remains relatively unchanged, except in the lower extremities where it is considerably elevated.

REGIONAL BLOOD FLOWS

Neither hepatic nor cerebral blood flow shows any changes during pregnancy. However, renal blood flow increases markedly during the first trimester. A detailed discussion of renal blood flow appears later in this chapter. The forearm blood flow (primarily flow to the muscle) shows an almost fourfold increase during the third trimester, accompanied by a 90 per cent reduction in peripheral resistance within the forearm. The most important organ in pregnancy is, of course, the uterus (and its placenta) which must support the fetus. It is estimated that blood flow through the maternal circulation of the placenta reaches as high as 750 ml. per min. during the later phases of gestation. It is further estimated that about 500 ml. of blood are squeezed into the central blood volume very early in the uterine contraction phase of delivery. At the height of the uterine contraction, the uteroplacental circulation, which represents an area of low resistance, is temporarily excluded, thereby raising the mean blood pressure and decreasing the cardiac output. Immediately following delivery, the uterus contracts firmly, and again there is an autotransfusion effect. However, this is largely balanced by external blood loss, which averages 300 ml. before and after delivery of the placenta.[3]

HEMATOLOGICAL CHANGES

BLOOD VOLUME

The average total blood volume in nonpregnant women is approximately 4 l. In pregnancy, the blood volume does not change appreciably during the first trimester. Thereafter, it increases almost linearly until nine months. The blood volume at nine months of pregnancy is approximately 30 to 50 per cent (1.5 l.) greater than the normal level (Fig. 16-2). This increase in blood volume is due to increases in both plasma volume and blood cell mass. However, the expansion of plasma volume (approximately 1.25 l) is far greater than that of the red cell mass (approximately 0.25 l.), and thus results in a reduced erythrocyte count, hematocrit ratio, and hemoglobin concentration.

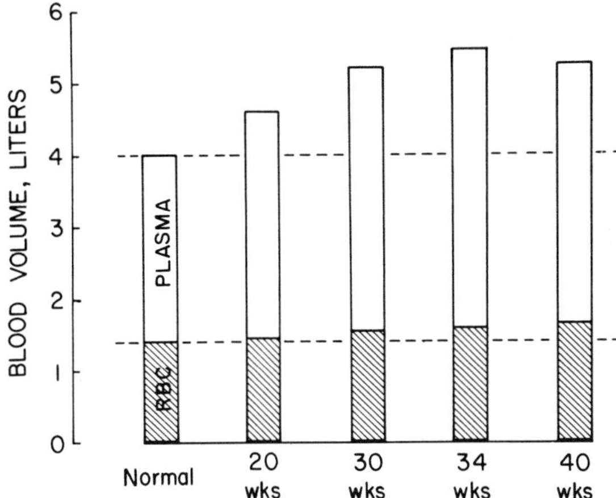

FIGURE 16-2. Changes in total blood volume during pregnancy. The shaded and open bars represent the red blood cell mass and plasma volume, respectively. (Based on data of Hytten and Leitch.[7])

The increase in plasma volume may be explained as follows: 1) a retention of body fluid resulting from increased secretion of adrenocortical hormones, estrogen and progesterone, and 2) a decrease in the capillary pressure due to shunting of blood through the uteroplacental circulation. The increase in red cell mass is associated with hyperplasia of bone marrow which is demonstrable throughout pregnancy and for approximately two months postpartum. Gemzell and associates[4] suggested that the increased hematopoiesis may be related to the rise in adrenal steroids which occurs in the first half of pregnancy.

ERYTHROCYTES, HEMATOCRIT, AND HEMOGLOBIN

As stated previously, the plasma volume expands more than the red cell mass. Consequently, the erythrocyte (RBC) count, hematocrit ratio (RBC mass/blood volume) and hemoglobin concentration decrease almost 10 per cent during the last two trimesters (Fig. 16-3). This is sometimes referred to as *the*

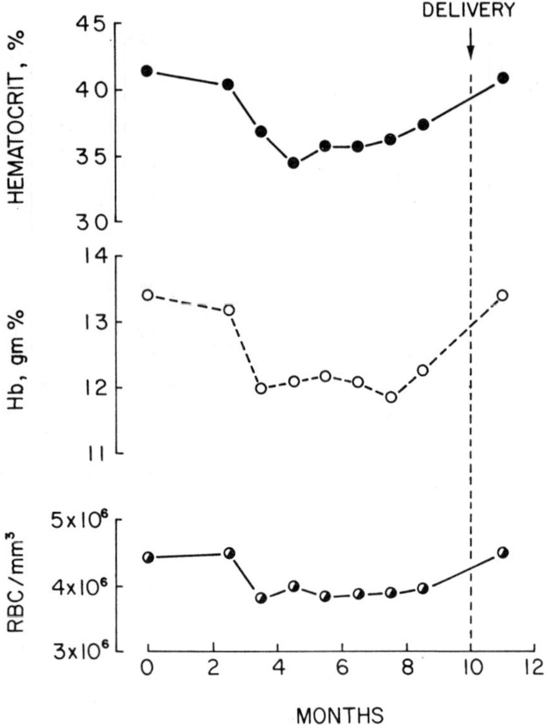

FIGURE 16-3. Changes in the erythrocyte count, hematocrit ratio, and hemoglobin concentration during pregnancy. (Based on data of Holby, R. G.: *The iron and iron-binding capacity of serum and the erythrocyte protoporphyrin in pregnancy.* Obstet. Gynecol. 2:119, 1953.)

physiologic anemia of pregnancy. However, in the majority of instances when adequate amounts of iron are supplied, the drop in hemoglobin concentration is quite modest, approximately 1 g.%. Hemoglobin values below 11.5 g.% suggest iron deficiency. Within one month after delivery, these reduced values return to the normal range.

LEUKOCYTES

In contrast to a reduction in erythrocyte counts, there is a consistent increase in leukocyte counts throughout pregnancy. A leukocytosis in the range of 10,000 to 12,000 per mm.[3] is reported. This increase is largely due to an increase in polymorphonuclear cells. In fact, both eosinophils and lymphocytes decrease somewhat during pregnancy. During labor and the first week postpartum, these changes in leukocytes are even more exaggerated. Leukocyte counts do not return to the normal range until approximately six weeks postpartum. The meaning of these changes in leukocytes during pregnancy is not clear.

IRON METABOLISM

The iron requirement increases greatly during pregnancy. In addition to increased erythropoiesis in the mother, she must also supply sufficient amounts of iron to the fetus. It is estimated that the mother needs about 600 mg. of iron to form her own extra blood while the fetus needs about 375 mg. to form its blood. Therefore, the total iron requirements is about 1,000 mg. The normal iron store (nonhemoglobin) in average women is only about 100 mg. Thus, about 900 mg. of iron must be supplied to a pregnant woman or she will develop a significant anemia due to iron deficiency. Since the average American diet does not contain sufficient amounts of iron to meet this need, routine iron supplements are indicated, especially in the second half of pregnancy. The concentration of iron in the blood usually decreases from the normal level of about 150 μg.% to 80 to 90 μg.% during the second half of pregnancy.

BLOOD COAGULATION

During pregnancy, fibrinogen levels increase by about 50 per cent (300 mg.% in nonpregnant women and 450 mg.% at term). Certain other factors of the coagulation system, e.g., proconvertin and Stuart factor, are also appreciably increased. In addition, there is a modest increase in the platelet count. It is believed that these changes are brought about by the influence of estrogen and progesterone. Due to these changes, the overall coagulability of blood (reaction time plus fibrin formation time) decreases from 12 to 8 minutes, and in addition, there is a significant reduction in the fibrinolysis time. However, there is no evidence to indicate that normal pregnancy is complicated by an increased incidence of spontaneous thromboses before the time of delivery.

RESPIRATORY CHANGES

LUNG VOLUMES

Due to the ease of measurement, vital capacity has received repeated attention. Findings indicate that there is no significant change in vital capacity during pregnancy. Any decrease in vital capacity is important. In pregnant women with pulmonary or cardiac disease, particularly mitral stenosis, reduced vital capacity is one of the earliest signs of impending failure.[5]

Various subdivisions of lung volumes show more definite changes during pregnancy (Table 16-1). Inspiratory capacity (tidal volume plus inspiratory reserve volume) increases by 120 ml. (5 per cent of normal value) in late pregnancy. This means that the expiratory reserve volume (vital capacity minus inspiratory capacity) must be reduced by about 120 ml. (15 per cent of normal value). The residual volume also decreases by 200 ml. (20 per cent of normal value) and hence, both the total lung capacity (vital capacity plus residual volume) and the functional residual capacity (expiratory reserve volume plus residual volume) are decreased. In other words, all the changes in various lung volumes during pregnancy are primarily due to reductions in the residual volume and the expiratory reserve volume, which can be attributed to the mechanical effect of the enlarging uterus. Later in gestation, when intra-abdominal pressure is increased, the thoracic cage is pushed upward and the lower half widens. The diaphragm is accordingly elevated, especially at the periphery. The central portion may appear flattened and its excursion reduced. In addition to these anatomic considerations, there is a possibility that the reduced residual volume could be partly due to an increase in pulmonary blood volume. As discussed earlier, pregnancy is associated with significant increases in cardiac output and total blood volume. Despite these increases, the pressure in the right ventricle and the pulmonary vessels appears normal. This indicates a reduced resistance to flow, most probably the result of a dilatation of the pulmonary vascular bed.

TABLE 16-1. Changes in Lung Volumes (ml.) during Pregnancy

Lung Volumes	*Nonpregnant*	*Pregnant**	*Difference*
Residual volume	965	770	−195
Expiratory reserve volume	655	555	−100
Inspiratory capacity	2625	2745	+120
Vital capacity	3280	3300	+ 20
Total lung capacity	4245	4070	−175
Functional residual capacity	1620	1325	−295

*Last trimester.
(Based on data of Cugell et al.[6])

VENTILATION

During pregnancy, oxygen consumption increases considerably to support the fetus. This is achieved primarily by increasing the pulmonary ventilation (Table 16-2). On the average, the tidal volume increases nearly 40 per cent at term. In general, there is a linear increase in the tidal volume from three months of pregnancy until term. The respiratory rate rises relatively little, if at all, and is maintained

TABLE 16-2. Changes in Pulmonary Ventilation and Gas Exchange During Pregnancy

	Nonpregnant	*Pregnant*†	*Difference*
Tidal volume, ml.	487.0	678.0	+191.0 (40%)
Respiratory rate/min.	15.0	15.0	0.0
Minute volume, l./min.	7.3	10.3	+3.0 (42%)
Dead space ventilation,* l./min.	2.1	2.1	0.0
Alveolar ventilation, l./min.	5.2	8.2	+3.0 (58%)
Oxygen consumption, ml./min.	196.0	238.0	+42.0 (22%)
Ventilatory equivalent (min.vol./O_2 consump.) l./100 ml.	3.7	4.3	+0.6 (16%)

*Based on an assumed dead space of 140 ml. in both groups. (Based on data of Cugell et al.[6])

†Last trimester.

at about 15 to 16 per min. Thus, the pregnant woman breathes more deeply, but not more frequently. Although the reasons for this interesting breathing pattern are not clear, it is important in that it increases the efficiency of ventilation. Whenever the respiratory rate increases, the dead space ventilation also increases, and therefore, the alveolar ventilation (minute volume minus dead space ventilation) increases relatively less.

The minute volume (tidal volume × respiratory rate) averages 7 l. per min. in nonpregnant women and increases to about 10 l. per min. during pregnancy (approximately a 40 per cent increase). Assuming a constant dead space of 140 ml., alveolar ventilation increases from the normal level of 5.2 l. per min. to 8.6 l. per min. at term. This represents a 65 per cent increase and is considerably greater than the 40 per cent increase in minute volume.

As discussed previously, there is a 20 per cent reduction in the functional residual capacity in late pregnancy. This means that the increased volume of tidal air mixes with a smaller volume of residual air in the lungs, thus expanding the margin of safety for the fetus.

GAS EXCHANGE

Oxygen consumption increases substantially during pregnancy due to the additional oxygen consumed by the fetus. In late pregnancy, the consumption is about 20 per cent higher than normal (see Table 16-2). It is estimated that two thirds of this increment is consumed by the fetus and the rest is consumed by the mother to support increased cardiac and respiratory work, and additional breast tissue and uterine muscle.

The first step in meeting this increased demand for oxygen is to increase the pulmonary ventilation so that more oxygen molecules reach the alveoli. As discussed above, minute volume and alveolar ventilation increase greatly during pregnancy. However, there is a significant difference in the magnitude of increase in ventilation and that in oxygen consumption. As compared in Table 16-2, the percentage of increase of the minute volume in late pregnancy is nearly twice that of the oxygen consumption. In nonpregnant women, 7.3 l. per min. of ventilation are needed to supply about 200 ml. of oxygen per min. Thus, the ventilatory equivalent for oxygen is 3.7 l. per 100 ml. of oxygen consumption, in contrast to 4.3 l. in late pregnancy. Since the relative increase in alveolar ventilation during pregnancy is even greater than the minute volume, the above difference in ventilatory equivalent is even more impressive if alveolar ventilation is used in place of minute volume. It is clear that there is considerable hyperventilation, or overbreathing, in pregnancy.

While overbreathing in pregnancy may assure a supply of needed oxygen to the lungs, it also causes carbon dioxide to be washed out of the lungs. As a result, the alveolar concentration of CO_2 is lower than in the nonpregnant women. The partial pressure of CO_2 (P_{CO_2}) in the alveolus is rather precisely controlled at approximately 38 to 40 mm. Hg. It decreases to a mean value of approximately 30 mm. Hg by the end of the second trimester and remains at this level until delivery.

CHANGES IN RENAL FUNCTIONS AND BODY FLUID

Clinically, the various changes in renal functions associated with alterations of body fluid volume and composition are extremely important.

RENAL HEMODYNAMICS

Certain weak organic acids are powerfully secreted by the renal tubule and under appropriate conditions their plasma clearance [(urine flow × urinary concentration)/plasma concentration] can be used as a measure of the renal plasma flow, i.e., the volume of plasma flowing through the kidneys every minute. The most widely used organic acid for this purpose is para-aminohippuric acid (PAH). Once the renal plasma flow is measured by determining the plasma clearance of PAH (C_{PAH}), the renal blood flow can be calculated using the following formula:

Renal blood flow (ml/min.)

$$= \frac{100 \times C_{PAH}\ (\text{ml./min.})}{100 - \text{hematocrit}\ (\%)}$$

The renal plasma flow in nonpregnant women is about 600 ml. per min. per 1.73 m.^{2} body surface. In pregnancy, this increases to 900 ml. at 3 months, declines somewhat during the remainder of pregnancy, and returns to normal at term (Fig. 16-4). Strangely enough, the renal plasma flow falls during the postpartum period. The renal blood flow has a pattern similar to the plasma flow, but due to the decreasing hematocrit level, it tends to fall slightly throughout pregnancy and then more rapidly near term.

The early increase in renal plasma and blood flow is due to the corresponding increase in cardiac output. The continuous decline in renal blood flow toward the end of pregnancy may be related to body position. Most studies have been carried out with the

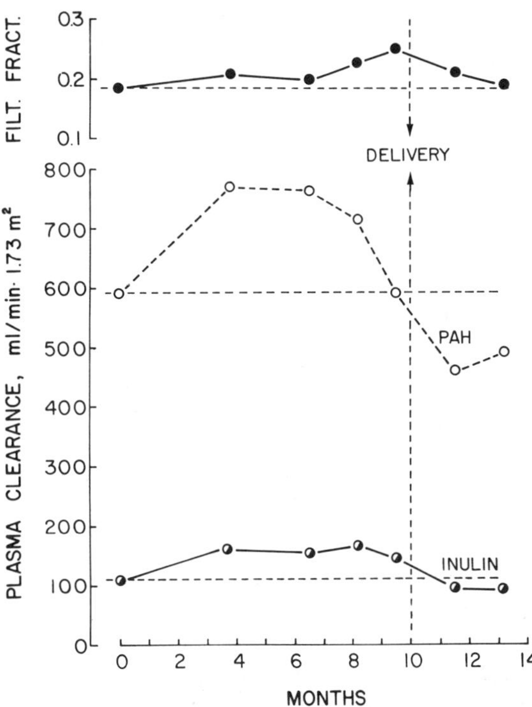

FIGURE 16-4. Changes in renal hemodynamics during pregnancy. (Based on data of Sims, E. A. H. and Krantz, K. E.: *Serial studies of renal function during pregnancy and the pureperium in normal women.* J. Clin. Invest. 37:1763, 1958.)

patient supine. As discussed earlier in connection with the supine hypotensive syndrome, when a woman in the later stages of pregnancy lies on her back, cardiac output decreases due to compression of the vena cava and bradycardia. Such a reduction in cardiac output could reduce renal blood flow.

The glomerular filtration rate (GFR) is usually determined by the plasma clearance of inulin (C_{IN}), an agent which is filtered but is neither reabsorbed nor secreted by the renal tubule. In nonpregnant women, it is about 110 ml. per min. per 1.73 $m.^2$ body surface. This value increases to 150 to 160 ml. by the end of the first trimester and, unlike renal plasma flow, is more or less maintained at this elevated level throughout pregnancy. Following delivery, it returns to the normal range.

Since the GFR increases more during pregnancy than the renal plasma flow, the proportion of the plasma flow which is filtered (filtration fraction: C_{IN}/C_{PAH}) is raised above the nonpregnant level (0.18). On the average, it increases to 0.20 during most of pregnancy and to 0.25 during the last two months.

This increase in filtration fraction is probably due to the reduction in plasma protein concentration found during pregnancy (Fig. 16-5). Such a reduction in plasma protein concentration decreases the colloid osmotic pressure of plasma, which in turn increases the effective filtration pressure (capillary hydrostatic pressure minus colloid osmotic pressure) in the absence of any blood pressure change.

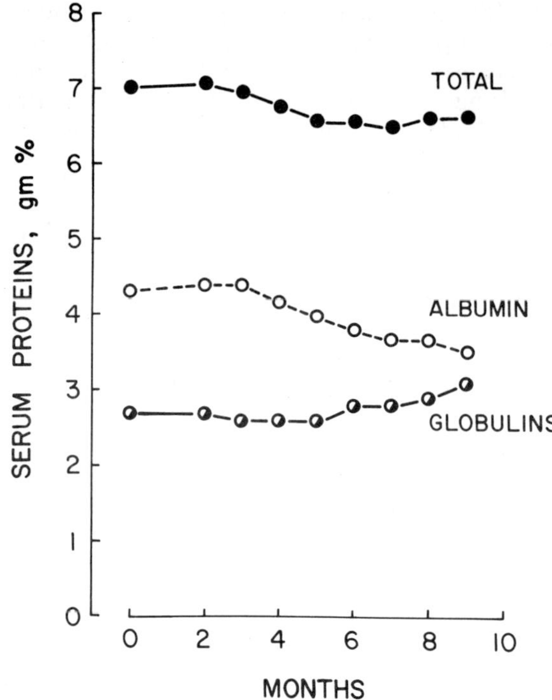

FIGURE 16-5. Changes in the serum concentration of total protein, albumin, and globulins during pregnancy. (Based on data of Von Studnitz, W.: *Studies on serum lipids and lipoproteins in pregnancy.* Scand. J. Clin. Lab. Invest. 7:329, 1955.)

URINARY EXCRETION OF VARIOUS SUBSTANCES

The increase in GFR considerably increases the load of substances presented to the renal tubules for reabsorption. As a result, the overall rate of excretion of filtered substances (especially those which are passively reabsorbed, e.g., urea) should increase until a new steady state is established. However, the mechanism of reabsorption is different for individual substances and therefore each substance is discussed separately.

Water. Although much has been written about body water during pregnancy, surprisingly few investigations have been made concerning the way the kidney handles water during pregnancy. Moreover, it has never been clearly established whether or not the urine flow is indeed increased. There is, however, evidence to indicate that the rate of elimination of a given water load is considerably greater during the second trimester, but is dramatically reduced during the third trimester.[7] In early pregnancy, thirst is one of the most common symptoms, perhaps suggesting that there is dehydration due to increased water excretion. The marked decline in ability to eliminate a given water load during the last trimester may be related to certain hormonal changes which tend to cause retention of sodium and water.

Sugar. Benign glycosuria is common during pregnancy with an incidence of 35 per cent. In normal nonpregnant women, all the filtered glucose is reabsorbed in the proximal tubule by an active transport system. This system is characterized by the presence of a clearly defined maximal rate of reabsorption (TM_G). The TM_G for normal women is about 300 mg. per min. per 1.73 m.^{2} body surface and does not seem to change during pregnancy. However, it must be remembered that there are about two million nephrons in two kidneys and also that there is a certain degree of imbalance, or heterogeneity, between the glomerular filtration rate and the TM_G among different nephrons. When the amount of filtered glucose increases from the normal level of about 110 mg. per min. to 160 mg. per min. in pregnancy due to the increased GFR, the amount of glucose filtered is still below the TM_G. However, some glucose may appear in urine if the amount of glucose filtered in particular nephrons becomes larger than the TM_G due to the heterogeneity of nephron functions.

Amino Acids. Pregnancy is also associated with considerable amino aciduria, again largely due to the increased GFR. However, there is considerable variation in the rates of excretion of individual amino acids. In the case of histidine which is excreted in urine in large quantities (more than a threefold increase during pregnancy), there appears to be an inhibition of the reabsorption mechanism.

Urea, Uric Acid, Creatinine, and Iodide. The clearance of these substances also increases along with the GFR during pregnancy. As a result, the plasma concentration of these substances is reduced. Such a reduction in the plasma level of inorganic iodine is almost certainly responsible for the goiter of pregnancy.

Sodium. Maintenance of sodium balance is vital in preserving constancy of the body fluid volume and osmolarity. Although intake of sodium may be regulated, sodium balance is maintained mainly by controlling the urinary excretion of this ion. Since the first process of urine formation is filtration at the glomerulus, the GFR is important in determining how much sodium should be excreted. In general, the rate of sodium excretion is proportional to the amount of sodium filtered, and the GFR is called the *first factor* in sodium regulation. A more subtle adjustment of sodium excretion is carried out at the tubular level by aldosterone and is called the *second factor.* Until recently, these two factors were considered to be entirely responsible for the regulation of sodium excretion under all conditions. However, a critical evaluation of the increased sodium excretion following either the extracellular fluid volume expansion with saline or the blood volume expansion with blood led to the discovery of a yet unidentified *third factor(s)* which induces a natriuresis. Regarding the nature of the third factor(s), there are two schools of thought, one physical and the other humoral.

During normal pregnancy, the GFR is raised and there is a marked increase in the secretion of aldosterone. Therefore, the rate of sodium excretion is determined by the balance of two opposing forces: the increase in GFR increasing the sodium excretion, and the increase in aldosterone secretion decreasing the sodium excretion. In addition, there is a considerable increase in blood volume which is expected to activate the third factor(s) and induce an increase in sodium excretion. Thus, the regulation of sodium excretion during pregnancy is a very complicated process, and it is still not known exactly how the kidneys regulate this excretion. As far as it is known, the concentration of sodium in body fluids is maintained during normal pregnancy at normal nonpregnant levels. Moreover, the ability of the kidneys to eliminate a given salt load is unaltered. In other words, the enhanced filtration of sodium in pregnancy is matched by an equally enhanced ability to reclaim sodium from the filtrate. However, there is a widespread belief that edema is associated with excessive retention of sodium, particularly in preeclamptic toxemia, and dietary restriction of sodium is commonly advised in antenatal clinics. It should also be noted that in the presence of preeclampsia there is a reduction in renal blood flow and glomerular filtration rate.

It is difficult to see the biologic sense in many of the changes described above. While it might seem reasonable for a woman to increase her excretory powers (by increasing both renal blood flow and GFR) to ensure adequate waste disposal for the fetus, it seems unreasonable to make the maximum adjustment early in pregnancy and then reduce it when one would expect the load to be greatest. The basic renal function during pregnancy is still largely unknown and much work needs to be done in this area.

BODY FLUID VOLUME

Due to technical difficulties involved in the measurement of total body fluid volume, there are considerable quantitative differences in the values reported by various investigators. However, it is generally true that the major increase in body water occurs during weeks 12 to 38 of pregnancy. In pregnant women without any detectable sign of edema, the average increases in total body fluid are 3.44 l. during weeks 12 to 30 and 2.28 l. during weeks 30 to 38. The total increase in body water during 40 weeks reaches 6.49 l. (Table 16-3). As expected, the degree of increase in body water during pregnancy is much greater in edematous women. According to Hytten and Leitch,[8] approximately 35 per cent of this increase can be accounted for by fetal body water, 20 per cent by placental water and amniotic fluid, and 15 per cent by water in the uterus and mammary glands. Approximately 30 per cent of the increase is due to expansion of blood volume and of extra- and intra-cellular fluid volumes in organs other than the uterus and the mammary glands.

TABLE 16-3. Mean Increase in Total Body Fluid (l.) during Pregnancy

Period (wks.)	*No Edema*	*Ankle Edema*	*Generalized Edema*
0–12 (estimated)	0.20	0.20	0.20
12–30	3.44	3.65	4.46
30–38	2.28	2.78	5.24
38–40 (extrapolated)	0.57	0.70	1.31
Total (0–40)	6.49	7.33	11.21

(Based on data of Hytten and Thomson in Hytten and Leitch.[7])

Measurement of the extracellular fluid (plasma plus interstitial fluid) volume is also subject to certain variations depending upon the method used. Therefore, any quantitative evaluation of data has to be made with considerable care. It is estimated that the extracellular fluid volume increases by approximately 5 l. during pregnancy. Of this increase, approximately 60 per cent can be accounted for by the fetus, placenta, amniotic fluid, uterus, and mammary glands. The rest is attributed to increases in plasma volume (0.9 l.) and interstitial fluid volume (1.2 l.). Thus, the extracellular fluid volume is not uniformly expanded. Normally, interstitial fluid volume (approximately 15 per cent of body weight) is approximately three times larger than the plasma volume (approximately 5 per cent of body weight). Despite this difference in size between the two fluid compartments, the magnitude of increase in volume during pregnancy is approximately the same in both cases, indicating that expansion of plasma volume is far greater than that of interstitial fluid volume. The reasons for this great expansion of plasma volume have already been discussed.

TABLE 16-4. Changes in Plasma Electrolyte Concentrations (mEq./l.) during Pregnancy.

Electrolyte	*Nonpregnant*	*First Trimester*	*Second Trimester*	*Third Trimester*
Na^+	143.0	139.0	139.0	140.0
K^+	4.3	4.1	4.0	4.0
Ca^{++}	4.9	4.9	4.8	4.7
Mg^{++}	1.7	1.6	1.5	1.5
HCO_3^-	26.0	25.0	24.0	23.0
Cl^-	105.0	103.0	104.0	104.0
HPO_4^{--}	2.0	2.0	1.8	1.8
$Protein^-$	16.5	16.4	15.4	15.1
Total cations	154.0		149.0	
Total anions	149.0		145.0	

(Based on data of Newman in Hytten and Leitch.[7])

Although there is no direct method for measuring intracellular fluid volume, it can be calculated from the difference between total body fluid volume and extracellular fluid volume. Since the average increases in total body fluid and extracellular fluid volumes are 7 and 5 l., respectively, the average increase in intracellular fluid volume should be 2 l. Most of this can be accounted for by the fetus, placenta, uterus, and mammary glands, indicating that there is no significant increase in the intracellular fluid volume of the maternal organs other than the uterus and mammary glands. The only increase noted is in the blood volume, as discussed previously.

As noted above, the increase in interstitial fluid volume is not remarkable compared to that of plasma volume. However, the magnitude of increase in interstitial fluid volume could reach 5 l. in pregnancy associated with generalized edema. Such an increase is associated with the retention of sodium, brought about by hormonal imbalances. Unlike ankle or leg edema which are due to an increase in capillary filtration pressure and are not related to the renal tubular handling of sodium and water, generalized edema involves the upper half of the body. Since generalized edema may be associated with preeclampsia, efforts are made to prevent its occurrence by routine restriction of sodium chloride or treatment of the edema with diuretic drugs.

BODY FLUID COMPOSITION

Changes in plasma electrolytes during pregnancy are minimal, with the exception of protein concentration. As shown in Table 16-4, there is a fall of about 5 mEq. in both cations and anions. It is by no means clear whether such a small decrease is real. If it is real, the osmotic pressure of plasma will be reduced by about 10 mOsm., and this should somewhat increase the cell volume. A reduction in bicarbonate (HCO_3^-) concentration is expected due to the reduction in P_{CO_2} of arterial blood during pregnancy. Pregnant women consistently hyperventilate, and P_{CO_2} decreases to about 30 mm. Hg. The plasma pH is determined using the Hendersen-Hasselbalch equation.

$$pH = 6.1 + \log \frac{(HCO_3^-)}{0.0301 \times P_{CO_2}}$$

Thus, one can calculate the bicarbonate concentration for P_{CO_2} of 30 mm. Hg and pH of 7.4. The value of (HCO_3^-) so calculated is 18 mEq. per l. However, the value would be higher if P_{CO_2} is greater than 30 mm. Hg. There is no evidence to indicate that plasma pH changes during pregnancy.

Although there is complete agreement that serum protein concentration falls during pregnancy, there are considerable differences of opinion as to the extent and pattern of the fall. Total protein concentration decreases most during the second trimester, after which it is maintained. The magnitude of decrease is about 0.5 to 1.0 g.%. This reduction is largely due to the corresponding changes in serum albumin concentration. Actually, the albumin concentration shows a greater and more sustained decrease compared with total protein. On the other hand, the globulin concentration remains stable during the first half of pregnancy, after which it actually increases significantly. Among various fractions (α_1, α_2, β, and γ) of globulin, the β-fraction is primarily responsible for this rise. Although these changes in serum protein concentration have a significant impact on the regulation of blood volume, it is not known how they are produced. The most attractive possibility is to attribute them to "dilution." There is significant expansion of the plasma volume during pregnancy and this could decrease the protein concentration of plasma. However, a careful analysis of the time course of changes in protein concentration and plasma volume indicates that protein concentration falls rather abruptly at a time in pregnancy when plasma volume is just beginning to rise. This suggests that the fall in concentration of plasma proteins is not due to dilution as the plasma volume expands. It is more likely that the fall of plasma protein concentration contributes to the expansion of plasma volume.

The changes in blood concentrations of certain nitrogen compounds and glucose during pregnancy are summarized in Table 16-5. Due to the high GFR during pregnancy, the plasma clearance of substances which are passively reabsorbed in the renal tubule is increased. Urea is in this category. Although the tubular handling of creatinine and uric acid is much more complicated than that of urea, their clearance is also known to increase during pregnancy. As a result, the blood concentration of these substances decreases 30 to 50 per cent. In contrast, the glucose concentration does not seem to decrease significantly although glycosuria is often present in pregnant women. This is probably due to the presence of the extrarenal regulatory mechanism which maintains the blood glucose concentration at a certain level.

TABLE 16-5. Changes in Concentration of Organic Substances (mg. %) in Whole Blood during Pregnancy

Substances	*Nonpregnant*	*Pregnant**
Urea-N	13.10	8.70
Creatinine	0.67	0.46
Uric acid	6.00	3.00
Glucose	80.00	80–90

*Last trimester.
(Based on data of Altman and Dittmer.[9])

The composition of intracellular fluid during pregnancy is entirely unknown. It is likely that the electrolyte concentration is maintained at normal levels while the concentrations of creatinine and urea may be reduced.

REFERENCES

1. Page, E. W., Villee, C. A. and Villee, D. B.: *Human Reproduction—The Core Content of Obstetrics, Gynecology and Perinatal Medicine.* W. B. Saunders, Philadelphia, 1972.
2. Bader, R. A., et al.: *Hemodynamics at rest and during exercise in normal pregnancy as studied by cardiac catheterization.* J. Clin. Invest. 34:1524, 1955.
3. Page, Villee and Villee: op. cit.
4. Gemzelle, C. A., Robbe, H. and Sjostrand, T.: *Blood volume and total amount of hemoglobin in normal pregnancy and the puerperium.* Acta Obstet. Gynecol. Scand. 33:289, 1954.
5. Wilson, J. R., Beecham, C. T. and Carrington, E. R.: *Obstetrics and Gynecology,* ed 3, C. V. Mosby, St. Louis, 1966.
6. Cugell, D. W., et al.: *Pulmonary function in pregnancy.*

I. Serial observations in normal women. Am. Rev. Tuberc 67:568, 1953.

7. Hytten, F. E. and Leitch, I.: *The Physiology of Human Pregnancy.* Blackwell Scientific Publications, Oxford, 1964.
8. Ibid.
9. Altman, P. L. and Dittmer, D. S. (eds.): *Biological Handbook–Blood and Other Body Fluids.* Federation of American Societies for Experimental Biology, Washington,D. C., 1961.

BIBLIOGRAPHY

Cugell, D. W., et al.: *Pulmonary function in pregnancy. I. Serial observations in normal women.* Am. Rev. Tuberc. 67:568, 1953.

Gemzelle, C. A., Robbe, H. and Sjöstrand, T.: *Blood volume and total amount of hemoglobin in normal pregnancy and the puerperium.* Acta Obstet. Gynecol. Scand. 33:289, 1954.

Holby, R. G.: *The iron and iron-binding capacity of serum and the erythrocyte protoporphyrin in pregnancy.* Obstet. Gynecol., 2:119, 1953.

Palmer, A. J. and Walker, A. H. C.: *The maternal circulation in normal pregnancy.* J. Obstet. Gynecol. Brit. Emp. 56:537, 1949.

Sims, E. A. H. and Krantz, K. E.: *Serial studies of renal function during pregnancy and the puerperium in normal women.* J. Clin. Invest. 37:1764, 1958.

Von Studnitz, W.: *Studies on serum lipids and lipoproteins in pregnancy.* Scand. J. Clin. Lab. Invest. 7:329, 1955.

17 *Nutrition*

Part 1—Implications for Maternal, Fetal, and Neonatal Systems

Marjorie Abel, M.S.

> One of the greatest mysteries of life is the power of growth, that harmonious development of composite organs and tissues from protoplasmic cells with the ultimate formation of a complex organism with its orderly adjustment of structure and function—development, growth and vital capacity all depend upon the availability of food in proper amounts and proper qualities.[1]

This statement was quoted by Hunscher to open a symposium on "The Life Cycle and Its Diet."[2] Although it was written in 1907, it is just as true today and provides the appropriate perspective for a discussion of nutrition during pregnancy, lactation, and the first year of life. Throughout history, much attention has been paid to the diets of pregnant women. Although there was some positive advice, the majority seems to have consisted of many restrictions and prohibitions. The special committee on Maternal Nutrition and the Course of Pregnancy appointed by the National Academy of Sciences states, "Even today, some of the views concerning maternal nutrition have little more scientific basis than did the views of the ancients."[3] In addition, much nutritional research is done on animals, and extrapolation of such data to the human situation must be done with extreme caution.

REVIEW OF LITERATURE

In 1936, Garry and Stiven[4] reviewed over 300 studies of pregnancy in animals and humans and concluded that "a mixed diet of natural food stuffs gave the best results." Ten years later, Garry and Wood[5] reviewed 400 contributions to the literature since the review in 1936 and concluded that a more critical attitude was developing among researchers but that there was also an increasing volume of uncritical popular literature. When the propaganda of manufacturers of supplements and vitamins were added, it was difficult to make a objective appraisal.

Keys and associates[6] studied evidence of the effects of extreme starvation on pregnant women in World Wars I and II. They concluded that the size of the newborn is affected by substantial restrictions in the maternal diet and that the effects of maternal undernutrition on prenatal growth are greatest in the third trimester.

Burke and coworkers[7-9] conducted one of the few linear studies on humans. They followed a group of mothers through more than one pregnancy and followed the children into adolescence. Their results demonstrated that adequate prenatal nutrition resulted in a reduction of congenital anomalies and improvement in condition of the infants. Of 216 pregnancies studied, 28 cases of toxemia occurred: 44 per cent were among patients with "poor" or "very poor" diets and 8 per cent were among those whose diets were "fair." Not a single case occurred in the women whose diets were rated "good" or "excellent."

A report on Maternal Nutrition and Child Health was published by the National Research Council in 1950.[10] It pointed out that from Pearl Harbor to V. J. Day there were 281,000 Americans killed in action. In the same period, December 7, 1941 to August 12, 1945, 430,000 babies in the United States died during the first year of life. Factors involved in this failure of reproduction also produce an army of handicapped and mentally defective children and weakened mothers. These tragedies are largely preventable. Knowledge gained in this century indicates that a better understanding of the role of nutrition in reproduction would result in greatly decreased mortality and morbidity among both mothers and infants.

In 1955, the Milbank Memorial Fund published papers presented at a conference on the Promotion of Maternal and Newborn Health.[11] The forword states that "in the past, infant mortality was chiefly a problem of infant care and control of external environment, but today the picture has changed and the major problems of infancy are in the newborn and are closely linked to the reproductive process and its management." Tompkins and associates reported on maternal nutrition studies at the Philadelphia Lying-in Hospital. Approximately 60 per cent of infant deaths were occurring in the first week of life. This study pointed out that mothers who were underweight had a higher incidence of infants with birth weights of less than five pounds, while obese mothers had a much lower incidence of low-birth-weight infants.

In 1965, the World Health Organization published a report on Nutrition in Pregnancy and Lactation.[12] This widely distributed report also helped to advance the growing idea that it was time to pay more attention to nutrtion as it relates to the childbearing experience.

NUTRITION BEFORE PREGNANCY

Pitkin[13] states that there is a considerable body of evidence suggesting that a woman's total nutritional background, extending even to the time of her own intrauterine experience, is of particular importance in determining her reproductive efficiency. He feels that a woman's nutrition during childhood and earlier may be of greater significance than that during pregnancy, especially if medical care is not available early in pregnancy.

Nutrition has profound effects on fertility. Severe malnutrition is associated with infertility. The mechanism involves alterations in hypothalmic-pituitary functions with resultant interference in production or release of gonadotrophic hormones.

Although the maternal mortality rate in the United States has steadily declined, there is little evidence that nutritional care has improved. Some of this is due to poverty, but more is due to lack of nutrition education and poor information on the needs of pregnancy.

When maternal mortality rates are low, fetal and infant mortality becomes a more sensitive indicator of reproductive efficiency. Other measures of maternal inefficiency are the proportion of low-birth-weight infants, the prevalence of perinatal handicaps, injuries, and failure of the newborn to adapt. There is a growing volume of evidence to include failure of normal brain development among these hazards. Factors affecting these poor outcomes of pregnancy include biologic immaturity of the mother (under 17 years of age), high parity, short stature, low prepregnancy weight for height, low weight gain during pregnancy, poor nutritional status, smoking, certain infectious agents, chronic disease, complications of pregnancy, and a history of unsuccessful pregnancies.

Socioeconomic factors also contribute. Women at highest risk are likely to have been born and brought up in poor homes and large families having little access to good medical care, food, and eduction. Poor quality crowded housing favors the spread of infectious diseases. Children grow up with poor health habits and poor food habits. Girls tend to bear children early and must rear them in the same surroundings. The girls may not have developed to their full genetic potential and enter pregnancy in suboptional health and nutritional status, adding the requirements of pregnancy to those of adolescence.

Poverty is ordinarily believed to be central to these factors, but there are also women with adequate incomes who put themselves at equal risk by constantly dieting for slimness, who smoke excessively, and who arrive at childbearing age in a poor state of nutrition and with poor food habits and poor health habits.

Thus, as Stearns[14] states, the best insurance for a healthy infant is a mother who is healthy and well nourished throughout her entire life as well as during the pregnancy itself.

WEIGHT GAIN

Available statistics on the amount gained during pregnancy in the United States reflect the fact that many obstetricians advise patients to eat less than their appetites dictate. However, during pregnancy a weight gain of at least 24 pounds is desirable and should be encouraged. Such weight gains are associated with the lowest incidence of preeclampsia, low birth weight, and perinatal mortality.

The products of conception include the fetus, placenta, and amniotic fluid. These account for approximately half of the total weight gained. The weight of the expanded maternal blood is known fairly accurately and estimates for enlargement of the uterus and the breasts can be made. The total of these leaves approximately 5 kg. unexplained. There is some disagreement as to the composition of this extra weight. Early investigations indicated that this weight might be protein. However, more recent research indicates that it is largely fat which represents an energy store to sustain fetal growth in the last half of pregnancy or to support the energy drain of lactation. The mechanism for fat storage appears to return to normal after delivery.

There is a wide variability of weight gain even when the pregnant woman is allowed to eat according to her appetite. Some women gain very little, others gain more than twice the averge of 12.5 kg. Young women tend to gain slightly more weight than older women, primigravidas slightly more than multigravidas, and thin women slightly more than fat women. There is evidence that healthy, well nourished women with a high weight for height may gain large amounts of water. Women who are underweight for height gain more fat. The energy needed to gain and maintain added tissues and storage is influenced by the size of the woman and her activity. Women in less developed countries use more energy than those in developed countries. The National Research Council's Recommended Dietary Allowances[15] provide an additional 300 calories daily during pregnancy. Unless activity is very restricted this additional intake will rarely result in excessive weight gain and the possible stored fat seems to disappear spontaneously in most cases.

A particular pattern of weight gain has been found to be associated with a better than average course of pregnancy and healthier babies. This involves a gain of 1.5 to 3.0 lb. during the first trimester, increasing steadily to approximately 14 lb. at the end of the second trimester, and approximately 24 lb. at the end of the third trimester. The gain in the second trimester represents storage in the mother's body. In the third trimester the fetus increases in size and storage of nutrients. There seems to be no scientific justification for routine limitations of weight gain to lesser amounts, although individual differences must be considered in all biologic measurements. The pattern of weight gain may be of greater importance than the total amount. A sudden sharp increase near the twentieth week of pregnancy may indicte water retention and possible beginning of preeclampsia.

The Committee on Maternal Nutrition[16] notes that one of the drawbacks in the use of body weight is that total body weight includes water, muscle mass, bone, and adipose tissue. Increased weight may be an increase in any of these parameters. The same principle applies to birth weight if this is the only measurement used. For example, it has been found that starvation as a means of weight reduction in obese persons resulted in the loss of more water and protein than of fat. The Committee concluded that although healthy women on well balanced diets who eat to appetite will have a wide range of weight gain, a gain of 20 to 25 lb. is a reasonable average. Current obstetric practices that restrict weight gain by limiting caloric intake may contribute to the large number of low-birth-weight infants and the high perinatal and infant mortality rates.

PROTEIN

All living matter so far discovered contains protein. Proteins are structural elements. They also participate in every biologic process at every level. They are enzymes or essential components of enzymes. They function in intracellular and extracellular structures of the body. Antibodies and some hormones are proteins. In combination with nucleic acid they carry inheritance factors. Proteins provide nitrogen and amino acids to form body proteins and other nitrogen-containing substances.

Proteins are complex molecules constructed with amino acids as building blocks. The human body cannot synthesize all 20 of the amino acids. Those that cannot be synthesized by the cells are called *essential* since these must be supplied in the food. The human adult must be provided with eight essential amino acids: isoleucine, leucine, lysine, methionine, phenylalanine, threonine, tryptophan, and valine. In addition, infants also need histidine. The other amino acids, which can be synthesized by the body, are termed *nonessential.* Knowledge of the human requirement for amino acids at various developmental stages is not complete, nor is knowledge of the amino acid content of many food proteins. By chemical analysis and feeding tests, proteins can be given a biologic value. Meat, fish, milk, and egg proteins have complete amino acid compositions and high digestibility. They are said to have a high biologic value. Most of the vegetable and grain proteins are low in some of the essential amino acids and some are low in digestibility. Used by themselves, such proteins have low biologic values. However, when supplemented with some of the animal proteins, the total supply of amino acids will be adequate. If the various amino acid contents of grains, fruits, and vegetables are known, these may be combined to supply protein of a satisfactory biologic value. However, it is safer to use a combination of animal and vegetable proteins at all times.

During pregnancy and other periods of rapid growth when the total protein rquirement is increased, it is best to use additional animal protein. Both mother and infant need protein for growth and maintenance. It is estimated that approximately 950 g. of protein are deposited during the last six months of pregnancy. This represents an increase in maternal tissues and blood and in fetal tissues. The recommended daily allowance of protein for women 19 to 50 years old is 46 g. An additional 30 g. per day is recommended during pregnancy, with a further addition of 20 g. per day during lactation. The Committee on Maternal Nutrition[17] reports that research has indicated that as the protein intake of pregnant women is increased the efficiency of utilization of protein declines. They arrived at an intake figure of 92

g. daily as the point of maximum use. This is in agreement with Burke's findings.[18] Burke reported that with up to 90 g. of protein daily there was steady improvement in the condition of both mother and baby, but that beyond that point there was no additional improvement.

DIETARY RESTRICTIONS

The idea of restriction of calories to prevent weight gain during pregnancy as a protection against toxemias can be traced to World War I experiences. Because of food scarcities, women gained less weight. It was also found that there were fewer toxemias and other complications. Although there was no scientific testing of any relationship, this idea found its way into obstetric texts and became widely used. Experiences in Russia and Holland during World War II seemed to confirm this idea, although in Great Britain, where maternal diets were fortified, the number of premature births dropped 25 per cent.

In the United States, some authorities suspect that the decrease in the incidence of toxemias might be caused by the increase in the amount and quality of proteins used. The proportion of calories furnished by protein has remained at 11 to 12 per cent of the total intake for 55 years. The amount of animal protein of high biologic value has increased with the shift away from cereals and other vegetable proteins of lower biological value.

Animal experiments have shown conclusively that restriction of either calories or protein causes inferior results of pregnancy, including deficiencies in intellectual function. However, such animal research is not always applicable to humans and results should be viewed cautiously. The amount of evidence in humans is growing. Caloric and protein restriction to limit maternal gain has profound results on fetal growth and development. Larger maternal weight gain is generally associated with a larger birth weight, and mechanical difficulties during delivery are not increased. Thus, the hazards of the low-birth-weight infant could often be avoided.

Two main factors are involved in dietary restrictions: 1) common obstetric practice almost routinely limits calories to restrict weight gain during pregnancy, and 2) many women take the opportunity of pregnancy to lose unwanted pounds. Pitkin and associates[19] warn that excess weight gained in pregnancy and not lost between pregnancies may contribute to obesity in the mother. For this reason, they recommend that it is both reasonable and defensible to limit weight gain to some extent. The pattern and amount of gain should be considered. If the patient gains the full amount of 10 to 12 kg. during the first half or two thirds of pregnancy, they suggest that further weight gain be limited to 0.3 kg. per week rather than the standard 0.8 kg. Any drastic treatment for obesity should be done between pregnancies rather than during a pregnancy.

Various recommended daily allowances for women are shown in Table 17-1 with additional recommendations for pregnancy and lactation. Appropriate caloric restriction requires considerable understanding of the nutritive value of foods. When weight control is mentioned, there is a tendency on the part of patients to think in terms of the popular publications on the subject. For several years, the main emphasis in these fad diets has been on limiting carbohydrate intake to 50 g. per day or less. Protein and fat are allowed in almost unlimited amounts. These diets ignore two important facts about carbohydrates, especially starches: 1) in the absence of adequate caloric supply in the form of carbohydrates and fats, dietary amino acids cannot be utilized efficiently, and 2) fat burns in the flame of carbohydrates. The energy requirement of the organism must be satisfied first. Unless 50 to 60 per cent of the caloric requirement is supplied by fat and carbohydrates, amino acids cannot be used for protein synthesis or

TABLE 17-1. Recommended Daily Allowances for Women

	Age (yrs.)					
	*11–14**	*15–18†*	*19–22‡*	*23–50§*	*Pregnancy*	*Lactation*
Calories (kcal.)	2,400	2,100	2,100	2,000	+300	+500
Protein (g.)	44	48	46	46	+30	+20
Vitamin A (I.U.)	4,000	4,000	4,000	4,000	5,000	6,000
Vitamin D (I.U.)	400	400	400	400	400	400
Vitamin E (I.U.)	10	11	12	12	15	15
Ascorbic Acid (mg.)	45	45	45	45	60	60
Folacin (μg.)	400	400	400	400	800**	600
Niacin (mg. equiv.)	16	14	14	13	+2	+4
Riboflavin (mg.)	1.3	1.4	1.4	1.2	+0.3	+0.5
Thiamin (mg.)	1.2	1.1	1.1	1.0	+0.3	+0.3
Vitamin B_6 (mg.)	1.6	2.0	2.0	2.0	2.5	2.5
Vitamin B_{12} (μg.)	3.0	3.0	3.0	3.0	4.0	4.0
Calcium (g.)	1.2	1.2	0.8	0.8	1.2	1.2
Phosphorus (g.)	1.2	1.2	0.8	0.8	1.2	1.2
Iodine (μg.)	115	115	100	100	125	125
Iron (mg.)	18	18	18	18	18+††	18
Magnesium (mg.)	300	300	300	300	450	450
Zinc (mg.)	15	15	15	15	20	25

* Body size 44 kg.; height 155 cm.
† Body size 54 kg.; height 162 cm.
‡ Body size 58 kg.; height 162 cm.
§ Body size 58 kg.; height 162 cm.
** The diet may be supplemented with 0.2–0.4 of folacin daily.
†† It is recommended that the diet be supplemented with 30–60 mg. of iron daily.
(From *Recommended Dietary Allowances.*[15])

other specific purposes. Protein, unlike fat, cannot be stored in any amount. Consequently, amino acids in excess of the requirement are further broken down and enter the energy pathways. This is uneconomical use of expensive high protein foods.

A high protein, high fat, and low carbohydrate diet may result in the formation of ketone bodies. Both saturated fatty acids and some amino acids may be involved in this process. Ketone bodies may cause maternal acetonuria which has been reported to result in neuropsychologic defects in the offspring. The effects are most pronounced in the third trimester. When dietary restriction reaches a point where the mother's reserves are depleted and nutrients supplied by the mother to the fetus are insufficient, breakdown of fats occurs and the danger of ketosis increases. If a reducing diet is used during pregnancy, these possibilities should be considered.

Caloric restriction inevitably results in restriction of other nutrients since nutrients supplying calories are also carriers of essential minerals and vitamins. Without carefully balanced supplements, it is impossible to meet the recommended daily allowances for pregnancy at any caloric level below 1,600. Yet many women are using diets of 1,000 calories or less during pregnancy.

ANEMIAS

Normal hematopoiesis requires a nutritionally adequate diet. Hemoglobin is a complex molecule of protein and iron. Its production requires an ample supply of protein to provide the essential amino acids. There must be sufficient calories from sources other than protein in order to protect the protein from being used as a source of energy. There must be sufficient additional iron to balance the increase in volume of maternal blood and to provide a fetal store of about 300 mg. of iron. Other minerals are required, including copper and zinc, as well as vitamins such as folic acid, vitamin B_{12}, and several others, to serve as cofactors in the synthesis of heme and globin.

The two most common types of anemia in pregnancy are iron deficiency anemia and megaloblastic anemia due to a deficiency of folic acid. Of these, iron deficiency anemia occurs more often.

The recommended daily allowance of iron is 18 mg. for all females from 11 to 55 years of age, supplemented with 30 to 60 mg. per day during pregnancy. Absorption of iron is a complex process influenced by the intestinal mucosa and the amount of available iron in the food ingested. Absorption is selective and the amount absorbed will be enough to maintain a body store of about 300 mg. Not all forms of iron are equally available for absorption. In general, animal sources appear superior to vegetable sources.

During normal pregnancy, there is an increase in blood volume which is only partially balanced by an increase in circulating blood cells and hemoglobin. If iron is available to the bone marrow, approximately 500 mg. will be used for the increase in maternal blood, and approximately 250 to 300 mg. will go to the fetus and the placenta. Thus, the iron used during pregnancy amounts to about 800 mg. with a single fetus and more with multiple births. Iron needed during pregnancy comes from the following sources:

Maternal Iron Stores. Iron stores in many women of childbearing age are deficient and may become even more depleted during pregnancy.

Diet. The average diet of young women seldom provides more than 6 to 10 mg. of iron daily. Since absorption is no more than 10 to 20 per cent of the food iron, many women enter prgnancy with inadequate iron stores. Iron occurs in small amounts in many foods but not enough to add up to 18 mg. daily from the current diets eaten by women of childbearing years who are trying to stay slim. All animal livers are high in iron, ranging from 6.5 to 19.0 mg. of iron per 100 g. Oysters, dark green leafy vegetables, dried beans and peas, some dried fruits, eggs and some seaweeds are other good sources of iron. Few of these foods are eaten regularly by young women.

Supplementation with Ferrous Iron. Iron supplementation in the form of ferrous salts by mouth is recommended if the pregnant woman will take it regularly. It is recommended that all women receive 30 to 60 mg. of iron as a daily supplement during the second and third trimesters. Women who have been given this iron supplementation average 12 g. of hemoglobin per 100 ml. of blood regardless of socioeconomic status.

Megaloblastic anemia due to a deficiency of folic acid has been mentioned as a possible occurrence during pregnancy. The vitamin in this deficiency is variously known as folic acid, folacin, or folate. It exists in many chemical forms and occurs in a wide variety of foods of animal and vegetable origin, particularly glandular meats, yeasts, and green leafy vegetables. Vitamin B_{12} appears to be involved in some of the reactions in which folate serves as a coenzyme. A folate deficiency may arise from four main causes: inadequate dietary intake, impaired absorption, excessive demands by tissues of the body, and metabolic derangements. Megaloblastic anemia due to maternal folate deficiency is not common in the United States but it does occur. Supplementation with folate is recommended since requirements may be higher during pregnancy and vitamin preparations including more than 0.1 mg. of folate require a prescription. This restriction resulted from the observation that more than 0.1 mg. per day prevents the appearance of pernicious anemia in some patients although the neurologic manifestations of this disease may progress.

WATER AND ELECTROLYTES

Water and electrolytes provide essential building materials for the protoplasm, just as proteins do. Water represents from 45 to 65 per cent of the total body weight, depending on the amount of fat. Most of the water is divided into the intracellular compartment and the extracellular compartment. *Sodium* is the principal cation (positive ion) of the extracellular fluid, and *potassium* is the principal cation of the intracellular fluid. Sodium functions in the maintenance of osmotic equilibrium and body fluid volume; potassium functions in cellular enzyme activity. The differential concentration of sodium and potassium across the cell wall determines the electric potential of the cell membrane and thus cellular excitability and nerve-impulse conduction. Deficiences of either cation retard growth in animals.

The body content of sodium is under homeostatic control. Moderately high intakes are promptly excreted in the urine, and the level quickly drops when intake is reduced. The usual intake of sodium as sodium chloride is from 6 to 18 g. daily. With the increase of processed foods in the United States this intake may be increasing. Occasionally, control mechanisms may break down and abnormal intakes or losses of sodium exceed the body's ability to cope. Abnormal losses may result from diarrhea, vomiting, chronic renal disease, prolonged use of diuretics, or excessive perspiration. When water intake exceeds 4 liters, extra salt may be indicated.

Diets restricted in sodium are used in the treatment of a number of conditions. During pregnancy, they are often used if there is excessive weight gain or edema with or without hypertension.

Potassium is widely distributed in foods. Potassium deficiency is a well defined syndrome that complicates many pathologic states. Potassium deficiency may occur during prolonged intravenous feeding, after severe diarrhea or diabetic acidosis, and when diuretics are given with a low sodium diet. High levels of serum potassium lead to toxicity in cardiac failure and renal failure.

Chloride is the most important negative ion in maintenance of fluid and electrolyte balance.

TOXEMIAS

The causes and mechanisms of the toxemias of pregnancy have always been a subject of controversy. The relationship of weight gain to toxemias has been discussed under topics of Weight Gain and Dietary Restrictions.

Preeclampsia is more common in women who are markedly underweight at conception and who do not gain normally during the pregnancy. The pattern of gain is also important. Sharp increases beginning near the twentieth week are a danger sign.

The centers of controversy regarding caloric and protein intake and have already been discussed. Caloric and protein restriction have been used widely without scientific evidence, despite work suggesting that hypoproteinemia and the resulting edema may be a primary factor in the etiology of toxemia.[20] Proteinuria is one of the principal signs of toxemia, yet very little research has been done on this relationship.

Vitamin B_6 is involved in at least 30 enzyme systems functioning in carbohydrate, fat, and protein metabolism. Evidence has accumulated that vitamin B_6 will prevent early nausea and vomiting and possible toxemias of pregnancy.

The relationship between sodium retention and extracellular edema is well established.

Preeclamptic patients hold large amounts of sodium. Measurements of exchangeable sodium show excessive amounts both in absolute terms and in relation to body water. Increased intake of salt has been known to trigger preclampsia. Thus, it is not surprising that restriction of salt during pregnancy is widespread and that diuretics are commonly used in connection with salt restriction.

The kidney normally returns all the nutrients in the filtrate to the plasma. The quantity varies with both the nutrient and the plasma level. Pike and associates[21] have done extensive research on the effect of sodium restriction in rats. Damage to the adrenals and kidneys of the rats may be cause to look more carefully at the use of salt restriction and diuretics in pregnant women. The amount of sodium restriction in the rats was comparable to that in a human diet using no salt in cooking or at the table. When diuretics are used in combination with that limitation of sodium, the damage to kidneys and adrenals must be seriously considered. Pitkin states that there is no reason for routine restriction of dietary sodium in normal patients.[22]

The recommended daily allowance for adults is 2.3 g. of sodium or 5.8 g. of sodium chloride.

MINERALS

CALCIUM AND PHOSPHORUS

Calcium is a major structural component of the body composing 1.5 to 2.0 per cent of the body weight of the mature human. More than 99 per cent of this calcium is in bones and teeth. Bone formation is an active process, constantly removing calcium from body fluids or returning it to them. The small remaining amount of calcium in body fluids is important. It contributes to blood coagulation, neuromuscular irritability, muscle contractility, and myocardial function. Unlike sodium and potassium, calcium is not completely absorbed. The amount absorbed is increased by intestinal secretions. Vitamin D is needed for efficient absorption. Phytate, oxalate, and fatty acids of the diet form poorly soluble calcium complexes interfering with absorption. If a person has been using high level of calcium intake, the intestine rejects a large portion of the calcium intake. A decrease of dietary calcium leads to a negative balance, but if the low level continues, absorption is increased and a positive balance may return. A reverse adaptation takes place when a low calcium supply is increased. Children in growth periods and pregnant or lactating women increase their intestinal uptake of calcium. The recommended daily allowance for girls from 11 years to 18 years of age is 1.2 g. For women 19 years of age and over, it drops to 0.8 g. per day. It is recommended that during pregnancy the allowance be raised 0.4 g. daily despite improved efficiency of intestinal absorption.

Calcium and phosphorus are major mineral constituents of bones and teeth. The ratio of calcium to phosphorus is 2:1. In addition, phosphorus is present in blood and cells as soluble phosphate ions as well as in lipids, proteins, carbohydrates, and energy transfer enzymes.

TRACE ELEMENTS

In many cases, research in inorganic elements began with the idea that the substance was toxic. In comparatively large amounts most of them are toxic, but in very small amounts they have been established as dietary essentials for humans.

Iron has already been discussed under the topic of Anemias.

Copper is an essential nutrient for all mammals. Copper deficiency is rare in man but it has been found in patients with iron deficiency anemia and as a result of increased loss in sprue. Copper is widely distributed in foods. The richest sources are liver, kidney, shellfish, nuts, raisins, and dried legumes. Milk is poor in both iron and copper. Recommended daily allowances for copper have not been set.

Fluorine is present in small but widely varying amounts in practically all soils, water supplies, plants, and animals. It is a normal constituent of all diets. The highest amounts in man and animals are found in bones and teeth. In teeth, fluoride seems to be localized in the enamel and makes the teeth more resistant to acid-producing bacteria. There is some evidence that fluoride protects bones against osteoporosis.

Iodine is an integral part of the thyroid hormones which have important metabolic roles. Iodine is an essential nutrient for man. Sources are food and water. Where the soils are low in iodine and seafoods are not available, iodized salt should be used.

Magnesium is an essential nutrient for plants and animals. It is an important constituent of all soft tissue and bone, and is an activator of many enzymes. Low serum magnesium levels have been observed in alcoholism, diabetes, malabsorption syndromes, kwashiorkor, neuromuscular disorders, surgical patients receiving fluids parenterally or on very restricted dietary regimens, and persons receiving diuretics. This may have application to pregnant women. There is evidence that magnesium, calcium, and phosphorus may be related in the human. The average American diet has been estimated to contain 120 mg. of magnesium per 1,000 calories.

Chromium may be a required nutrient with a possible role in carbohydrate metabolism in the human.

Cobalt is an integral part of vitamin B_{12} which is involved in a number of body processes, including utilization of iron.

Manganese is an essential element needed for normal bone structure. It has been shown to be part of enzyme systems in man.

Zinc is an essential element for animals and man, but no uncomplicated zinc deficiency has been shown.

Potassium has been discussed in the section on Water and Electrolytes.

A mixed diet containing green leafy vegetables, fruit, whole grains, organ meats and lean meats will usually supply adequate amounts of these elements.

VITAMINS

There is a tendency to believe that all is well nutritionally provided an adequate supply of vitamins is available. In addition, some seem to believe that if a little is good, more is better. Vitamins are essential. They are chemically unrelated substances which are grouped together because they are essential in minute amounts for specific metabolic reactions within the cell. A particular vitamin may be essential for one species but not for another. For example, ascorbic acid (vitamin C) is essential for man, monkey and the guinea pig because these species lack a metabolic pathway to synthesize adequate amounts of this vitamin. Vitamins are classified as water-soluble or fat-soluble since this property determines the patterns of transport, excretion, and storage. There are many forms of some of the vitamins. Usually one form is most active in humans, although other forms may be altered for use in the body. All vitamins act as catalysts for specific metabolic reactions. In this function they are similar to hormones. Without other nutrients, vitamins cannot build or maintain the body. With the single exception of folic acid there is no scientific justification for prescribing vitamin supplements to healthy pregnant women on adequate diets. The indiscriminate use of high concentration vitamin preparations is potentially dangerous and may give a false sense of security to women with poor food habits.

FAT-SOLUBLE VITAMINS

Vitamin A is a fat-soluble substance which is found in two similar isomers in mammals and saltwater fish. Much of the vitamin A activity in our diets is in the form of provitamin A carotenoids. The greatest amount of vitamin A is provided by conversion of β-carotene in the intestinal walls. Vitamin A is essential for the integrity of epithelial cells and as a stimulus for new cell growth. It aids in maintaining resistance to infections. These functions are particularly applicable to pregnancy.

Excessive carotene may produce carotenemia due to the inability of the body to convert large amounts of carotene into vitamin A. This may result in a yellow discoloration of the skin. Hypervitaminosis A can produce excessive bone fragility, enlargement of the liver and spleen, and drying and peeling of the skin.

The recommended daily allowance for vitamin A is 4,000 I.U. The body does store vitamin A in the liver.

There is an increased need for vitamin A during infancy, pregnancy, and lactation. An additional 1,000 I.U. of vitamin A are needed during the second and third trimesters since the nutritional well-being of the rapidly growing fetus is dependent on the mother's intake. To assure that the infant receives adequate vitamin A, an additional increase of 1,000 I.U. is recommended during lactation.

Vitamin A deficiency may result from poor absorption of vitamin A or conditions that interfere with digestion or absorption of fat. In underdeveloped countries, deficiencies in the supply of fat often lead to vitamin A deficiency. Use of mineral oil in salad dressings or other uses in the diet may cause poor absorption of vitamin A.

Vitamin D is essential at all ages for maintenance of calcium homeostasis and skeletal integrity. As with a number of other vitamins, vitamin D occurs in several forms. Vitamin D_3 is made in the human body by action of ultraviolet rays. Inadequate supplies of vitamin D will cause rickets in infants and young children. Occasional cases of rickets in adolescents suggest that it is required throughout the growing years. As little as 100 I.U. daily has prevented rickets in normal infants and 300 I.U. has cured rickets. The requirement of vitamin D in adult life is not known but 400 I.U. daily is recommended during pregnancy and lactation.

It has long been known that excessive amounts of vitamin D (1,000 to 3,000 I.U. per kg. per day) are potentially dangerous to children and adults. Excessive doses mobilize phosphorus and calcium from the tissues, thus reversing the effect of normal doses. Vitamin D hypervitaminosis may cause nausea, anorexia, diuresis, and headaches. Food intake decreases and calcium and phosphorus retentions are lowered. Fortification of various foods with vitamin D may lead to overdoses in infants and young children. Vitamin preparations often contain 400 I.U. of vitamin D or more. Milk is fortified with vitamins A and D. Vitamin D is added to cereals and other inappropriate foods. Thus, it is possible for an infant to receive 1,000 I.U. or more.

Vitamin E is an essential nutrient in more than 20 vertebrate species, including man. The forms of vitamin E are tocopherols. α-Tocopherol has the highest biologic activity and δ-tocopherol is the most active antioxident. Tocopherols, as antioxidents, preserve easily oxidizable vitamin A and unsaturated fatty acids in foods or in the body. The earliest investigations of vitamin E deficiency were done in rats. Females became pregnant, but all the fetuses were resorbed. A great deal of research has since been done in rats, cattle, sheep, rabbits, dogs, chickens, and other species. Damage was considerable but different in each species. It was not possible to give human diets lacking in vitamin E, but controlled studies of the treatment of similar symptoms could be made. Vitamin E was given to women with a history of spontaneous abortions but results were negative. Horwitt[23] studied the long-term results of low vitamin E diets in humans. Thirty-eight men were carefully monitored during the eight years of the study. There was no apparent physical or mental impairment caused by the restricted intake of vitamin E. The men were in satisfactory health when their blood levels were lowered by 80 per cent. However, red blood cells had shorter survival times and for this reason the study was discontinued. The conclusions was that humans need some vitamin E, but can be satisfied by everyday diets which include leafy vegetables, whole grain products, and fats, especially vegetable oils. The recommended daily allowance of vitamin E for women 19 to 50 years old is 12 I.U. An additional 3 I.U. per day is recommended during pregnancy and lactation. Very low levels of vitamin E have been found in patients with diseases that impair the absorption of fat. Vitamin E does not cause the disease; the disease prevents the absorption of vitamin E. The human need for vitamin E was confirmed when premature infants suffering from hemolytic anemia were studied. These infants were being fed a synthetic commercial milk substitute which was low in vitamin E. When given a supplement of vitamin E, the anemia improved. The normal resistance of red blood cells to rupture by oxidizing agents in markedly reduced in vitamin E deficiency. The amount necessary to prevent hemolysis is between 2 and 10 I.U.

Vitamin K occurs widely throughout nature. Again, the term vitamin K covers a family of related substances. Vitamin K is required in microgram amounts by man and certain animals to maintain prothrombin and other clotting factors. It acts in the synthesis of clotting-proteins in the liver. Green leafy vegetables are high in vitamin K, and it is also synthesized by bacteria in the human intestine. Infants do not have the necessary bacterial flora during the first few days of life and this may lead to "hemorrhagic disease of the newborn." Fomon[24] recommends a combination of prenatal administration of 5 mg. of vitamin K for two weeks before the estimated date of delivery and a single does of 1 mg. to the infant soon after birth. Except for this specialized need and others connected with specific diseases, the average individual has no known need for vitamin K supplementation.

WATER-SOLUBLE VITAMINS

Ascorbic Acid (Vitamin C). Most animals have a metabolic pathway by which they are able to synthesize adequate amounts of ascorbic acid. However, man, monkey, and guinea pig lack this pathway. In these species a lack of ascorbic acid leads to the development of a deficiency disease called *scurvy.*

Ascorbic acid has multiple functions in the animal body. It is the least stable of the vitamins, sensitive to alkalies and to oxidation especially in the presence of iron or copper ions, but it is fairly stable in acid solution. It is involved in the synthesis of intercellular substances (reticulum and collagen). It is also involved with dentine, cartilage, and the protein matrix of bone. Therefore, it plays an important role in tooth formation, bone formation and repair, and wound healing. It functions in the metabolism of phenylalanine and tyrosine, and is probably also related to capillary integrity. Ascorbic acid may be involved in the synthesis of certain steroids in the adrenal glands. There is a high concentration of ascorbic acid in the adrenal glands as well as in the corpus luteum and the pituitary gland.

Evidence indicates that 10 mg. of ascorbic acid will prevent scurvy. The recommended daily allowance of ascorbic acid is 20 mg. in the United Kingdom, and 30 mg. in Canada, Australia, and Norway. In the United States, 45 mg. per day is recommended for nonpregnant women of all ages. For many years, it was thought that ascorbic acid was not stored by humans. However, research with healthy men using radioactive isotopes to study body pools indicates that tissues store 4 to 5 g. of ascorbic acid. These same studies indicate a mean utilization of 21.5 mg. with a standard deviation of 8.1 mg. Thus the recommended daily allowance provides generous amounts of ascorbic acid under normal conditions. During pregnancy and lactation, 60 mg. per day is recommended. This amount allows for higher tissue levels in order to give added protection to health. Smoking interferes with the absorption of ascorbic acid and some authorities suggest that those who smoke need to double the recommended amount.

Recently the suggestion has been made that large doses of ascorbic acid (1 to 5 g. daily) are useful in the prevention and treatment of the common cold. There is little responsible research to support this contention, and many reputable researchers have pointed out results that should lead to caution in using more than the recommended daily allowance. Goldsmith[25] points out that 1 g. daily may cause diarrhea and that amounts of 4 to 12 g. daily can lead to formation of urate and cystine stones in the gallbladder. It is also reported that infants born to mothers who took excessive doses of ascorbic acid during pregnancy were conditioned to this intake and needed additional ascorbic acid to prevent scurvy. Schrauzer[26] notes that an individual adapted to large doses of ascorbic acid develops stress symptoms when the dosage is stopped. Also, subjects using daily doses of 200 to 550 mg. retained no more than 91 mg., regardless of level of intake.

Biotin. Biotin is essential for the activity of many enzyme systems in bacteria, animals, and probably man. Biotin combines with avidin in raw egg white to from a stable complex which cannot be broken down by proteolytic digestion. It can be broken down only by heat. Biotin combined in this way is nutritionally unavailable. Avidin was the first known example of an antivitamin. Deficiency states have been recognized in man only when diets have included large amounts of raw egg white. Minimum daily requirements have not been established, but diets providing a daily intake of 150 to 300 μg. of biotin are considered adequate. Pregnancy and lactation require an increased amount. Biotin is found in many foods. Some of the richest sources are liver, kidney, milk, eggs, nuts (especially peanuts), cauliflower, mushrooms, dried beans and peas, chocolate, and yeast.

Folacin (Folic Acid, Folate, Pteroylmonoglutamic Acid). Folacin has been discussed in detail in the section on Anemias. Approximately 20 per cent of megaloblastic anemas involve folacin deficiency. This may occur in persons over the age of 65, in infants on unsupplemented proprietary formulas or goat's milk, and in patients suffering from malabsorption syndromes.

The recommended daily allowance of folacin is 400 μg. This should be increased to 800 μg. during pregnancy, and 600 μg. during lactation.

Niacin. The term niacin is used to denote both nicotinic acid and nicotinamide. Nicotinic acid is a vasodilator and side effects of its use include increased skin temperature, disturbances of pulse rate and intensity of heart beat, and increased peristalsis. Nicotinic acid is used as medication when these effects are desired. However, nicotinamide, which does not cause these side effects, is used more frequently.

Pellagra was endemic in many parts of the world for several centuries. It was endemic in the southern part of the United States early in this century. In 1914, a U. S. Public Health team headed by Dr. Joseph Goldberger was sent to determine the cause of the disease. Early symptoms are lassitude, weakness, and diarrhea. It was called the disease of the four Ds—dermititis, diarrhea, dementia, and death. In 1926, Goldberger found that the typical diet of pellagrins also caused black tongue disease in dogs. In 1937, Elvehjem discovered that niacin would cure black tongue disease in dogs. As work proceeded on pellagra, it became clear that it was not a simple deficiency of niacin. One of the amino acids, tryptophan, acts as a precursor of niacin. Corn diets, low in protein and niacin, were also low in other vitamins in the B group. In cereals, niacin is in a bound form that must be hydrolyzed in order to become nutritionally available. Thus, the daily requirement of niacin is influenced by the amount and kind of protein available. Animal proteins (milk, eggs, meats) contain about 1.4 per cent tyrptophan. Proteins of vegetable origin (cereals and legumes) usually contain about 1 per cent tryptophan. Corn is low in tryptophan. An average of 60 mg. of dietary tryptophan is equivalent to 1 mg. of niacin. The minimum amount of niacin equivalents is also related to caloric intake. The recommended daily allowance is expressed as 6.6 equivalents per 1,000 calories, with no fewer than 13 equivalents when intake is less than 2,000 calories. During pregnancy there is an increased conversion of tryptophan to niacin. An increase of 2.0 equivalents of niacin per day based on the increased caloric intake is recommended.

Pantothenic Acid. Pantothenic acid is one of the group of B vitamins. It is widely distributed. Especially good sources are animal tissues, whole grain cereals, and legumes. Lesser amounts are found in milk, vegetables, and fruits. A diet adequate in the B-complex vitamins will also be adequate in pantothenic acid. Perhaps for this reason, deficiency occurs as part of restriction of many nutrients. This is important since pantothenic acid is incorporated into coenzyme A which is involved in the release of energy from carbohydrates, degradation and metabolism of fatty acids, and synthesis of sterols, steroid hormones, prophyrins, and acetylcholine. Biochemical defects may exist undetected for some time, but ultimately, symptoms of tissue failure appear. In man, deficiencies are slow to develop even on a diet essentially free of pantothenic acid for six to nine months. If an antivitamin is given with a deficient diet, within a few months an illness develops similar to that which develops in animals. The most important feature of pantothenic acid deficiency in both animals and man is loss of antibody production. The recommended daily allowance is 5 to 10 mg. There is no evidence either for or against an increase during pregnancy and lactation.

Riboflavin. This vitamin is slightly solvent in water where it shows a yellow-green fluorescence. It is very soluble in alkali and is insoluble in fat or fat solvents except alcohol. It is sensitive to light, especially in the presence of alkali. Riboflavin functions as a coenzyme or as an active prosthetic group of flavoproteins concerned with the oxidative processes. The human requirement for riboflavin is related to body size, metabolic rate, and rate of growth.

Riboflavin is involved in the conversion of tryptophan to niacin. It is present in the retinal pigment of the eye and plays a part in light adaptation. When there is a deficiency of riboflavin, the eye suffers a number of symptoms, including burning, itching, and impairment of visual acuity. Some of the skin reactions to deficiency are inflammation of the tip and sides of the tongue, and lesions on the lips and corners of the mouth. There are also symptoms of damage to the nervous system and to the blood.

The recommended daily allowance during pregnancy is 1.5 mg. which considers the increased metabolic rate and body size due to growth of the fetus and accessory tissues.

Thiamin. Thiamin functions in carbohydrate metabolism and it has been assumed that the thiamin need depends on the amount of carbohydrate in the diet. Thimain deficiency may be caused by a diet low or lacking in thiamin or by antivitamins that are antagonistic to it. Thiamin deficiency results in the disease called *beriberi* which is characterized by nervous and cardiovascular symptoms, mental confusion, muscular weakness, loss of ankle and knee jerks, cramps in the muscles of the calf, edema (wet beriberi), and muscle wasting (dry beriberi). Early symptoms are loss of appetite and growth failure. Thiamin is not stored and the total amount in the body is only enough to last a few days. The recommended 1.0 mg. per day is adequate for normal adults. During pregnancy, an additional allowance of 0.3 mg. per day is recommended.

Principal food sources of thiamine are pork, dried beans and peas, liver, lamb, veal, nuts, and whole grain cereals. Destruction of thiamin is retarded in acid media and accelerated in alkaline media.

Vitamin B_6. Vitamin B_6, like many vitamins, is a term used to denote a group of naturally occurring pyridines that are metabolically and functionally interrelated. This nutrient has been found to be essential in over 30 enzymatic reactions. It functions in carbohydrate, fat, and protein metabolism, though its major functions seem to be related to protein and amino acids. Adults fed diets low in vitamin B_6 developed biochemical signs of deficiency within a period of one to six weeks. The recommended daily allowance, to allow a margin of safety, provides 2.0 mg. with 100 gm. or more of protein. During pregnancy, abnormalities have appeared in women on apparently normal diets. The placenta actively transports vitamin B_6 to attain an increase in fetal blood of five times the level of mother's blood. The recommended 2.5 mg. per day during pregnancy should meet this need.

Vitamin B_{12}. Vitamin B_{12} occurs predominantly in animal foods bound to protein. This vitamin is often the limiting factor in the most carefully planned vegetarian diets. When liver was found to be effective in treating prenicious anemia, the search for the active ingredient began. Finally, crystalline vitamin B_{12} was isolated and found to be identical to an animal protein factor which was involved with growth. Although this vitamin appears in sevral forms, the principal form is a large molecule with a cyanide group attached to the central cobalt. Vitamin B_{12} is involved in at least five different coenzymes. The absorption of the large, complex molecule of vitamin B_{12} is not yet fully understood. An even larger gastric molecule called the intrinsic factor is required to assist in the process. An inadequate amount of intrinsic factor leads to inadequate absorption of vitamin B_{12}. Calcium is also involved in this absorption mechanism.

Vitamin B_{12} is essential for normal functioning of all cells, particularly cells of the bone marrow, nervous system, and gastrointestinal tract. It is probably involved in the metabolism of protein, fat, and carbohydrate, but its most important function seems to be in the metabolism of nucleic and folic acids. Megaloblastic anemias resulting from vitamin B_{12} deficiency appear to be the result of damage to the ability of cells to form deoxyribonucleic acid and involve a disturbance in folic acid metabolism.

The recommended daily allowance is 3.0 μg. to replace normal losses. If body stores are depleted, 15 μg. per day will gradually replenish these stores. During pregnancy and lactation, 4.0 μg. per day is recommended.

CHOLINE

Choline is not a vitamin. It is an essential metaboilite which, at one time, was generally classified as a vitamin. It may be synthesized in the cell if the amino acids serine and methionine are present. Dietary choline protects against poor growth, fatty liver development, and renal damage in many experimental animals. However, choline deficiency has never been demonstrated in man. The average mixed diet consumed in the United States has been estimated to contain 500 to 900 mg. per day including its natural precursor, betaine. Fresh egg yolk, liver, soy beans, and peas are good sources of choline. There are lesser amounts in other vegetables and milk.

PREGNANCY DURING ADOLESCENCE

The occurrence of pregnancy during adolescence presents both physical and psychologic risks. Girls under age 17 are at greater risk if pregnancy occurs before their own growth is completed. After age 17, hazards are the same as those for the age group of 20 to 24 years old. There is a sharp increase in infant mortality for each year that the mother's age is under 17 years. In developed countries there has been a decline in the age of menarche to a mean of approximately 13 years.

Sexual maturation occurs in an orderly sequence and is closely related to growth and skeletal maturation, although there are individual differences. When maturation is early, the menarche may be coincidental with the peak of adolescent growth and the girl may be capable of conceiving before her skeletal growth, including pelvic capacity, is complete.

In many situations, the pregnant girl is subjected to punitive practices by society and prenatal care is often inadequate. In the United States, live births to mothers 17 years of age or younger have been increasing both in actual numbers and as percentage of live births. In 1965, 29,000 girls under 15 years of age gave birth to live infants out of a total of 197,372 born to girls 17 years and under.

Young teenage mothers have more babies weighing less than 2,500 g. at birth than do older mothers. The overall percentage of such low-birth-weight infants born alive to mothers under 15 years of age in the United States was 18.7 per cent. As maternal age increases, the proportion of low-birth-weight infants decreases up to age 40. Neonatal, postneonatal, and infant mortality rates are all much higher for infants born to young mothers. Multiparity in the young mothers increases the risks.

Before age 17, nutrient requirements reflect the special demands of growth and maturation. Individual differences are great so each girl must be treated differently. Caloric requirements follow the growth curve.

Nutritional status at conception is the result of a girl's lifetime nutritional experience and is an important determinant of reproductive efficiency. As has been pointed out, a well-balanced diet during pregnancy is important to both mother and baby. Since there are great differences in rate of growth and development, and since food habits of the adolescent girl tend to vary widely, a detailed study should be made of each adolescent patient. A team from the University of California at Berkeley conducted a survey and concluded that the diets of pregnant teenagers were less than adequate.[27] They met the recommended daily allowance for protein but lacked sufficient calories. The girls were constantly admonished to watch their weight gain, and thus tended to minimize their total food intake. Many had instructions in low sodium and low calorie diets and the histories show that they tried to follow instructions. Infant birth weights tended to follow the mothers weight gain and the mean birth weight was 3.0 kg. This and other studies emphasize the need for investigation of the current and past food habits of the pregnant adolescent. The social pressure for a slim figure and the wide distribution of unbalanced diets for weight loss must be considered. Many of these diets are low calorie, high protein, low fat and recommend 50 g. of carbohydrate or less. The adolescent with her need for protein for anabolic purposes is placed in the position of catabolizing the protein to supply the needed calories.

CALORIES

Adequate caloric intake is critical to support growth during adolescence. The daily caloric intake for girls under age 17 is often as much as 400 carlories below the recommended daily allowance.[28] In addition, the widespread practice of routinely placing pregnant women on restricted diets is often extended to include pregnant adolescents. The majority of pregnant girls are classified as being poor in vitamin A and ascorbic acid, and borderline in calories, protein, calcium, and iron. Caloric restriction results in significantly lower intakes of protein, iron, and other nutrients, as well as calories.

PROTEIN

During the period of accelerated growth there is increased need for protein and an enhanced ability to retain nitrogen. Teenage growth during pregnancy requires more protein than the amount considered desirable for pregnant women. In addition, teenagers with poor nutritional histories have exceptional protein needs during pregnancy. An intake of 92 g. of protein per day is recommended.

CALCIUM

There is evidence that calcium absorption and retention increase during the growth spurt and the premenarchal period. A mean retention of 400 mg. of calcium per day for several years appears necessary for adequate mineralization of the skeleton. This requires intakes of 1.0 to 1.6 g. per day of calcium and 400 I.U. per day of vitamin D.

IRON

As indicated previously, it is difficult to meet the recommended iron requirements on a normal diet. Despite the greater efficiency of the body's ability to absorb iron during periods of low intake, increased growth rate, and during pregnancy, there is evidence that adolescent girls do not receive enough iron. During pregnancy, additional iron requirements increase this deficiency. Iron supplements of 30 to 60 mg. daily are recommended.

LACTATION

At one time, most infants were breast fed and there currently seems to be a movement back to breast feeding. Psychologic rewards to both mother and infant are likely when the mother desires the experience. Breast feeding may transmit antibacterial and antiviral antibodies that will provide protection to the infant.

The ability of a woman to breast feed her child depends on her general health and nutritional status. The development of the mammary gland is part of the general adjustment of the woman to the whole process of reproduction. When pregnancy is initiated, there is a sudden development of ducts, lobules, and alveoli due to ovarian hormonal influences. During the second half of pregnancy, secretory activity becomes more pronounced. During lactation, the mammary gland is very active. Radioactive sodium given orally was found in human milk 20 minutes later.

With the increasing safety and convenience of formula feeding, the decision to feed by breast or bottle has been left largely to the mother. The frequency of breast feeding during the newborn period decreased from 65 per cent in the 1940s to 26 per cent in 1965. Since 1958, the frequency of breast feeding at one month as been stable at 20 percent, but drops to 8 to 10 per cent at age four months.

The recommended daily allowances during lactation are higher for many nutrients than they are during pregnancy (see Table 17-1). Most of the increases are easily explained. The mean daily excretion of milk over an average lactation period of six months is 850 ml. Actually, the amount varies widely. The basic diet should be supplemented with a variety of foods to supply extra calories as well as other nutrients required. The caloric recommendation during lactation is an additional 500 calories per day, or that amount which will maintain the mother's weight at the desired level. The average protein in human milk is 1.2 g. per 100 ml. The range is wide—from 0.95 to 1.47 g. per ml. To allow for varying biologic values of protein in the diet, an additional 20 g. of protein per day is recommended. Vitamin A should be increased by 1,000 I.U. per day to assure the infant an adequate supply. Increases in niacin and riboflavin are also recommended.

The volume of breast milk is difficult to measure and varies from time to time. An insufficiency of liquids, protein, or calories may reduce the amount of milk, but will not usually affect the composition.

In this age of widespread use of various drugs, it must be remembered that most drugs received by the lactating woman are excreted in her milk. The amount is usually insignificant. However, sometimes the drug concentration is higher in the milk than in the mother's plasma. Unfortunately, very little is known on this subject. Both nicotine and marijuana appear to have adverse effects on the infant.

FETAL NUTRITION

The placenta plays a fundamental role in fetal nutrition, yet little is known about how this function is performed. Very early in gestation, the placenta is responsible for ensuring that all substances needed for growth and development reach the fetus in adequate amounts. It also returns surpluses and waste products to the mother's circulation. The placenta is metabolically active. Transfer of substances may be by diffusion or by active transport. Some substances may be converted to others or actually synthesized in the placenta.

It is known that most nitrogen reaches the placenta as amino acids. The concentrations of amino acids, calcium, and phosphorus are higher in the placenta than in the mother's blood. Carbohydrate reaches the placenta as glucose and is converted to glycogen. There is some evidence that blood glucose of the mother affects fetal growth.

A small placenta does not necessarily limit the size of the fetus, provided the placenta is functioning properly. Malnutrition of the mother and fetus may exist independently if the placenta is defective or if the mother has poor circulation or other conditions that affect the transfer of nutrients. Measurements of wet weight, cell number and size, protein, and trace elements indicate that malnourished mothers have fewer cells in the placenta but that these cells are larger. Birth weight correlates with the number of cells in the placenta. Habitual cigarette smoking and drug usage tend to produce lower birth weights in infants as well as anomalies caused by substances that pass through the placenta and interfere with normal development of the fetus. Various infectious agents are also known to affect the fetus.

NEONATAL NUTRITION

Nutritionally, the newborn infant is the result of a long series of metabolic processes within the mother which, in turn, are the result of metabolic processes in the maternal and paternal body prior to pregnancy. Toverud states, "If mothers were in a nutritionally adequate condition prior to conception and received an adequate diet during pregnancy and lactation, supported by sound medical guidance throughout, maternity would be less hazardous and children would be more apt to receive their rightful nutritional heritage."[29]

Traditionally, birth weight is one index of fetal development and welfare of the newborn. The Committee on Maternal Nutrition considers three categories of small infants: those that are conceived small, those that are born before their time, and those that are small for dates.

The third group gives the best indication of failure in utero. Maternal size is a powerful factor in determining the size of the infant, but nutrition is also important. In Japan birth weights in 1963 were markedly greater than they were in 1945 or even pre-World War II. Many factors were undoubtedly influential, but during those 20 years the quantity and quality of food improved greatly and a nation-wide nutrition education program was implemented.

A major concern is whether retardation of overall physical growth in utero is paralleled by a retardation in mental development which cannot be corrected postnatally. Experiments in rats have shown that restriction of calories and protein in the maternal diet resulted in smaller litters, smaller size of the young, and lower survival rates. In addition, there were deficiencies in intellectual function and metabolic activities.

Recent studies of the cellular aspects of growth may explain these phenomena. DNA exists in the nucleus of the cell and is the index of cell number and protein. RNA is developed by DNA and escapes from the nucleus to form new protein in the cytoplasm. RNA is the index of cell size. Pitkin[30] suggests that the development of an organ or tissue involves sequential phases of hyperplasia (cell division), hyperplasia and hypertrophy (cell growth), and finally hypertrophy alone. It seems logical that restricting essential nutrients during cell division might have permanent effects while the effects of restriction during cell growth might be reversed by adequate nutrition.

What information we have on the human brain is made by autopsy studies and confirms the animal studies. The human brain begins development by the fourth week of gestation. The most rapid growth of the brain is from three months before birth to six months after birth. Approximately 90 per cent of postnatal brain growth is completed before the fourth year. Once growth is completed, the brain does not increase in cell number. The brain is particularly important since specific areas have definite functions which are not duplicated anywhere else and are incapable of pattern regeneration. Even after the structure of the central nervous system is complete, the system is very susceptible to specific types of dietary deficiences, regardless of age. These include thiamin, niacin, vitamin B_{12}, iodine, and iron deficiencies.[31] The effect of malnutrition on development and the functioning of the central nervous system depends on when the deprivation occurs, how long it lasts, and how severe it is. One example of inborn errors of metabolism is phenylketonuria in which the infant is born without a specific enzyme which is needed in the metabolic pathway of phenylalanine. If not treated immediately after birth, the child will have irreversible mental deficiency of varying degrees. Other nutrients involved in such errors include the vitamins B_6 and folic acid, the carbohydrate galactose, and the amino acids methionine and leucine.

Modern mothers cling to the idea that bigger babies are better babies. Purveyors of vitamin supplements and commercial infant formulas are constantly reminding mothers of their duty to the baby. It has been remarked that one virtue of breast feeding is that the mother does not know how much the infant was getting. With formula feeding, she is constantly trying to have the infant finish the recommended amount of foods despite individual differences in appetite and requirement. The result is a continuing increase in the size of infants. The old maxim that a baby doubles his birth weight in five months does not apply to bottle fed babies. Many babies on modern feeding regimens double their weight in three to four months. Height at one year has also increased by seven per cent over the height in the nineteenth century. Overfeeding may not be the only cause. Racial mixtures, disease control, and socioeconomic factors also contribute.

Infant feeding has changed drastically since the introduction of commercial infant foods. When breast feeding first went out of style, it was replaced by evaporated milk formulas with or without added carbohydrate but supplemented by cod liver oil for vitamin D and fruit juice for ascorbic acid since these were the only vitamin deficiences incidental to bottle feeding. The increased production of commercial infant foods, including formulas, cereals, and a large variety of pureed solid foods, has changed the pattern of infant feeding. Forbes[32] points out that the abundant and varied food supply, adequate purchasing power in a large part of the population, promotional advertising, and the value ascribed to "bigness" all contribute to excessive food intake. Formulas of commercial premodified milks are made with water, nonfat milk solids, lactose with or without other sugars, and vegetable oils, usually coconut oil. They are heavily fortified with minerals and vitamins, and usually with large amounts of iron. They have a definitely sweet flavor which introduces infants to sweets without delay. Most other foods are also sweetened and children grow up expecting foods to taste sweet. Formula is often supplemented with cereals and fruit within the first month. Some mothers begin supplementing the formula as early as the first week.

Jacobziner and associates[33] examined 23,000 infants and preschool children and found as many suffering from overfeeding as from undernutrition. Rueda-Williams and Rose[34] found caloric intake in excess of recommendations in a study of infants from 2 to 15 months of age. There is evidence that these excess calories are stored as fat. This excess, during a period of cell division, increases the number of cells in the body to accommodate fat storage. Once the number of fat storage cells is increased, reduction of weight will decrease cell size but not cell numbers. Thus, the overweight infant is predisposed to obesity for the rest of his life.

The following recommended daily allowances provide guidelines, but it must be remembered that children differ greatly.

Energy needs are two to three times as great as the adult in terms of body weight. They are calculated as calories per kg. of body weight. Up to two months of age, the requirement it is 120 calories per kg.; from two to six months, 110 calories per kg.; and from six months to one year it is 100 calories per kg. Practical measures for increasing calories as the infant grows include use of formula more concentrated than 67 calories per 100 ml. and use of cereals and strained foods. Strained foods may be poorer in calories than formula, so the strained foods chosen should be those rich in calories.

Protein allowances are related to age and weight. From birth to two months the recommendation is 2.2 g. per kg.; from two to six months, 2.0 g. per kg.; and from six months to one year, 1.8 g. per kg. This protein should be high in biologic value. The average protein content of human milk is 1.2 g. per 100 ml. Malnutrition has little effect on the quality of milk, but reduces the quantity. Mature cow's milk provides 3.3 g. per 100 ml. Experience has shown that the lower amount of protein from human milk is adequate for growth. Human milk places a smaller load on the kidneys than cow's milk, but an increase in water intake will solve this problem. There seems little difference between human and cow's milk in efficiency for infant development. Infant diets should supply approximately 9 per cent of their calories from protein.

Fats are the most concentrated source of calories, but they also have other metabolic functions. For this reason, skim milk is not desirable in infant feeding unless some form of fat is provided to supply small amounts of linoleic acid and arachidonic acid which are required for normal growth and integrity of the skin. It is recommended that at least 20 per cent of the calories in the diet come from fat.

Carbohydrates provide the rest of the calories needed by the infant. Both human and cow's milk are low in carbohydrate, and lactose is the principal form. Infants may be fed any form of carbohydrate that is included in the adult diet. As the infant becomes ready for solid foods, starches replace or supplement sugars to bring the caloric intake up to that required. It has been suggested that starches produce less fat storage than sugars.

Mineral requirements, with the exception of iron, appear to be adequately met in the breast-fed infant. Formulas and other foods also provide adequate amounts of minerals except iron, unless the formula is fortified with iron. Fomon[35] estimates that the electrolytes—sodium, chloride, and potassium—are needed in amounts larger than have previously been considered adequate. The amounts he suggests for infants up to four months are: sodium, 8 μg. per day; chloride, 8 μg. per day; and potassium, 8 μg. per day. Calcium is needed for growth. Absorption is influenced by the amount of calcium in the formula, its chemical form, the amount of vitamin D, and the type of fat. The advisable intake during the first year is 500 mg. per day which is the amount available in one pint of milk. Phosphorus is absorbed more efficiently than calcium and the advisable intake is 220 mg. per day. Magnesium is also required for tissue synthesis and 21 mg. per day is advised. Other trace elements are also essential for infants but the exact amount is not known.

Iron deserves a discussion of its own. The infant is born with a body store of iron adequate for two to three months, providing the maternal diet was adequate. Anemia in infancy is defined as a condition in which the hemoglobin is less than 10 g. per ml. When the hemoglobin is less than 7 g. per ml., vigorous therapy should be implemented. The requirement for dietary iron is related to: 1) the amount of iron accumulated in the fetus during gestation, 2) the perinatal and subsequent loss of blood, and 3) the rate of growth. The accumulated iron may last two to three months. The bone marrow is relatively inactive for the first month or two and during this period the hemoglobin decreases slowly. At approximately two months the hemoglobin begins to increase. In modern practice, iron supplements are used very early with the aim of providing a net increment of 200 mg. during the first year. Both human and cow's milk are low in iron. However, with the use of formulas providing 8 to 12 mg. of iron per liter and infant cereals fortified with iron, adequate iron absorption is assured. Natural sources of iron should be added as soon as possible to develop the habit of using those foods.

Vitamins are essential at all ages. However, human and cow's milk provide sufficient vitamin A, thiamin, riboflavin, and niacin to protect the infant. In addition, commercial formulas are fortified with these vitamins. Excess in the form of vitamin complexes is not needed. The recommended daily allowances from birth to one year are: vitamin A, 1,500 I.U.; vitamin D, 400 I.U.; and vitamin E, 5 I.U. Excessive intake may result in toxicity. Fomon[36] quotes Caffey, "Hazards of vitamin A poisoning from routine prophylactic feeding of vitamin concentrates A and D to healthy infants and children on good diets are considerably greater than the hazards of vitamin A deficiency without concentrates." The recommended daily allowance for vitamin D is already higher than the actual need. When a concentrate is given in addition to vitamin D fortified milk (400 I.U.), there is a chance of overdosage. The addition of vitamin E to that already present in cow's milk is not considered necessary. Ascorbic acid is low in cow's milk, although adequate amounts are found in human milk. It is advisable to give some form of ascorbic acid to the newborn. Commercial fruit juices for infants are fortified with ascorbic acid in varying amounts ranging from the recommended daily allowance of 35 mg. to as high as 65 mg. When the infant is changed to other forms of fruit or fruit juice, care should be taken to use those that are naturally high in ascorbic acid or are fortified with the vitamin.

Recommended daily allowances for the B vitamins are: birth to two months, thiamin, 2 mg.; riboflavin, 0.4 mg.; niacin, 5 mg. equiv.; vitamin B_6, 0.2 mg.; vitamin B_{12}, 1.0 μg.; folacin, 0.05 mg.; from two to six months, thiamin, 0.4 mg.; riboflavin, 0.5 mg.; niacin, 7 mg. equiv.; vitamin B_6, 0.3 mg.; vitamin B_{12}, 1.5 μg.; folacin, 0.05 mg.

Thiamin plays a key role in carbohydrate metabolism. Unless the infant is on a high carbohydrate diet or one of the soy formulas, the normal milk will supply adequate amounts. Riboflavin is very high in milk and other foods normally fed to infants. The requirement is easily met from meats, milk, eggs, green leavy vegetables, and whole grains. The niacin requirement is met if adequate B_6 and the amino acid tryptophan are present. Both human and cow's milk apparently provide adequate vitamin B_6. Folate from cow's milk, meats, and green leafy vegetables seems adequate for the normal infant. However, the low-birth-weight infant may need supplements to prevent megaloblastic anemia.

SUMMARY

1. It is important to make an assessment of the nutritional status of the pregnant woman as soon as possible after conception. Her dietary history before conception should be taken into consideration. Her diet should be planned and nutrition education continued throughout pregnancy.

2. A weight gain of 24 pounds or more should be encouraged. Caloric intake should not be curbed. There is a strong positive relationship between maternal weight gain and the birth weight of the infant, and between prepregnancy weight and birth weight. Restricting weight gain is particularly harmful for underweight women and pregnant adolescents.

3. There is no evidence that caloric restriction during pregnancy has any effect on the incidence of toxemia and no evidence that women who gain in fatty tissue are more likely to develop toxemia than women who do not. There is no advantage to caloric restriction for the purpose of weight reduction during pregnancy, even for obese women. The possible danger of inducing ketosis with hazard to the neurologic development of the fetus must be considered. Weight reduction should be undertaken after delivery.

4. Severe caloric restriction with adequate protein may result in use of protein for basic energy requirements, thus causing a protein deficiency.

5. The rate of gain is important. After the twentieth week, a sudden gain in weight is cause for suspecting that water is being retained.

6. The widespread practice of routinely limiting sodium during pregnancy and at the same time prescribing diuretics is potentially dangerous.

7. The routine supplementation of the diet during pregnancy with vitamin and mineral preparations is of uncertain value. Except for possible supplements of iron, folacin, and iodine, any addition of vitamin and minerals should be given only until the diet can be improved by addition of required foods. If supplements are used, the concentration should approximate the recommended daily allowance. Vitamin and mineral preparations should not be considered as substitutes for proper food habits.

8. Overnutrition is a serious problem with many infants. The mother's idea that a bigger baby is healthier leads to overfeeding. The use of commercial infant foods, each fortified with many nutrients, leads to duplication of adequate intakes and consequent overnutrition.

9. Too many foods are sweetened, which conditions the infant to prefer a sweet taste and leads to dental caries and overweight.

10. Provided the family diet is adequate,

infants can become accustomed early to the family food pattern through the use of blended or strained family foods rather than commercial infant foods.

REFERENCES

1. Chittenden, R H.: *The Nutrition of Man.* Frederick A. Stokes Company, New York, 1907.
2. Hunscher, H. A.: *Starting the cycle.* From a symposium on The Life Cycle and Its Diet. Journal of Home Economics 29:101, 1957.
3. Committee on Maternal Nutrition, Food and Nutrition Board, National Research Council: *Maternal Nutrition and the Course of Pregnancy.* National Academy of Sciences, Washington, 1970.
4. Garry, R. C. and Stiven, D.: *A review of recent work on dietary requirements in pregnancy and lactation with an attempt to assess human requirements.* Nut. Abstr. Rev. 5:855, 1936.
5. Garry, R. C. and Wood, H. O.: *Dietary requirements in human pregnancy and lactation–A review of recent work.* Nut. Abstr. Rev. 15:591, 1946.
6. Keys, A., et al.: *Growth and development. The Biology of Human Starvation, vol. 2.* University of Minneapolis Press, Minneapolis, 1950.
7. Burke, B. S.: *Nutrition during pregnancy–A review.* J. Am. Diet. Assoc. 20:735, 1944.
8. Burke, B. S., et al.: *Nutrition studies during pregnancy.* Am. J. Obstet. Gynecol. 46:38, 1943.
9. Ibid.: *The influence of nutrition during pregnancy upon the condition of the infant at birth.* J. Nutr. 26:569, 1943.
10. *Maternal Nutrition and Child Health.* Bull. 123. National Research Council, National Academy of Sciences, Washington, 1950.
11. *The Promotion of Maternal and New Born Health.* Papers presented at the 1954 Annual Conference of the Milbank Memorial Fund, New York, 1955.
12. World Health Organization: *Nutrition in Pregnancy and Lactation.* WHO Tech. Rep. Serv. No. 302, Geneva, 1965.
13. Pitkin, R. M.: Nutrition and Reproduction. Unpublished working paper, Workshop on Nutrition and Maternal Health Services, Harvard School of Public Health, 1973.
14. Stearns, G: *Nutritional state of mother prior to conception.* J.A.M.A. 168:1655, 1958.
15. *Recommended Dietary Allowances*, ed. 8. Food and Nutrition Board, National Research Council, National Academy of Sciences, Washington, 1974.
16. *Nutritional Supplementation and the Outcome of Pregnancy.* Proceedings of a Workshop held at Sagamore Beach, Massachusetts. Committee on Maternal Nutrition, National Academy of Science, Washington, 1973.
17. Ibid.
18. Burke: *Nutrition studies*, op. cit.
19. Pitkin, R. M., et al.: *Maternal nutrition, a selective review of clinical topics.* Ostet. Gynecol. 40:773, 1972.
20. Strauss, M. B.: *Observations on the etiology of the toxemias of pregnancy, the relationship of nutritional deficiency, hypoproteinemia and elevated venous pressure to water retention in pregnancy.* Am. J. Med. Sci. 190:811, 1935.
21. Pike, R. L., Miles, J. E. and Wardlaw, J. M.: *Juxtaglomerular degranulation and zona glomerulosa exhaustion in pregnant rats induced by low sodium intakes and reversed by sodium load.* Am. J. Obstet. Gynecol. 95:604, 1966.
22. Pitkin, Roy M.: Nutrition and Reproduction. Unpublished working paper, Workshop on Nutrition and Maternal Health Services, Boston, April 1973.
23. Horwitt, M. K.: *Vitamin E and lipid metabolism in man.* Am. J. Clin. Nutr. 8:451, 1960.
24. Fomon, S. I.: *Infant Nutrition.* W. B. Saunders, Philadelphia, 1967.
25. Goldsmith, G.: *Common cold, prevention and treatment with ascorbic acid not effective.* J.A.M.A. 216:337, 1971.
26. Schrauzer, G.: personal communication.
27. *Nutritional Supplementation and the Outcome of Pregnancy*, op. cit.
28. U. S. Department of Agriculture, Agriculture Research Service: *Food Intake and Nutritive Value of Diets of Men, Women and Children in the United States, Spring 1965. A Preliminary Report.* ARS 62-18. U. S. Government Printing Office, Washington, 1969.
29. *Maternal Nutrition and Child Health*, op. cit.
30. Pitkin et al.: op. cit.
31. Leverton, R. M.: *Facts and fallacies about nutrition and learning.* J. Nutr. Ed.: 1:7, 1959.
32. Forbes, G. B.: *Introductory remarks presented at the Ninth International Congress of Pediatrics.* Am. J. Clin. Nutr. 9:527, 1961.
33. Jacobziner, H., et al.: *How well are well children?* Am. J. Pub. Health 53:1937, 1963.
34. Rueda-Williams, R. and Rose, H. E.: *Growth and nutrition in infants–The influence of diet and other factors on growth.* Pediatrics 30:639, 1962.
35. Fomon: op. cit., p. 141.
36. Ibid, p. 117.

BIBLIOGRAPHY

Committee on Maternal Nutrition, Food and Nutrition Board, National Research Council: *Maternal Nutrition and the Course of Pregnancy.* National Academy of Sciences, Washington, 1970.

Flowers, C. E.: *Nutrition in pregnancy.* J. Reprod. Med. 7:201, 1971.

Fomon, S. I.: *Infant Nutrition.* W. B. Saunders, Philadelphia, 1967.

Hytten, F. E. and Leitch, I.: *The Physiology of Human Pregnancy.* Blackwell, Oxford, 1966.

Naeye, R. L., Blanc, W. and Paul, C.: *Effects of maternal nutrition on the human fetus.* Pediatrics 52:494, 1973.

Pike, R. L. and Smicklas H. A.: *A reappraisal of sodium restriction during pregnancy.* Int. J. Gynaecol Obstet. 10:1, 1972.

Wohl, M. G. and Goodhard, R. S.: *Modern Nutrition in Health and Disease.* Lea and Febiger, Philadelphia, 1968.

Part 2—Framework for Nutritional Assessment and Planning

Ann L. Clark, R.N., M.A.

The importance of nutrition to the pregnant woman, the developing fetus, the entire family, and mankind cannot be overemphasized. Some important considerations are:

1. The woman's prepregnant and prenatal nutrition affects the way she feels during the pregnancy and the outcome of the pregnancy. For example, low iron stores leave the woman feeling fatigued. Malnutrition plays a basic etiologic role in toxemia of pregnancy. Premature separation of the placenta occurs in the absence of folic acid.[1] The lack of vitamins A and E may produce teratogenic effects.[2] Maternal nutrition plays a role in the premature birth of the infant.

2. The placenta does *not* act as a parasite extracting the necessary nutrients for fetal growth and development. This is a myth that should have been discarded long ago. What feeds the expectant mother feeds the embryo and fetus.[3] Poor nutrition leads to poor maternal, fetal, and newborn health. Dietary deficiencies of essential nutrients cannot be made up by supplementation.

3. Nutrition plays a paramount role in labor. Effectiveness of uterine musculature depends upon protein stores, hemoglobin levels, and physical health.

4. Good nutrition during pregnancy sets the stage for successful breast feeding. It is of utmost importance during the period of lactation.

5. Good nutrition during pregnancy speeds recovery during the puerperium. Moreover, good nutrition during the postpartal period results in the mother being better able to cope with experience of mothering.

6. The infant's weight, length, development of the osseous system (including teeth, although not yet erupted), and his brain development all depend on the expectant mother's nutrition.[4] The long-range effects continue to influence the child's entire physical and mental growth and development.

7. The antepartal, postpartal, and lactation periods present unique opportunities for establishing patterns of wise food selection for the entire family. Good nutrition results in improved health and in the control of weight, thereby reducing costs for health maintenance.

It is not an exaggeration to say that *the future health of mankind depends, to a large degree, on the nutritional foundation laid down during prenatal life.*

UNIVERSITY OF OREGON MEDICAL SCHOOL
HOSPITALS AND CLINICS

DIET HISTORY

Date Bldg. Fl. Rm.

Unit No.
Name
Birthdate

Name

Address

Birthdate	Age	G	P	AB	Phone Number

Religion | Allergies to food

Have you ever been on a diet before?

How is your appetite?	Height	Weight before pregnancy	Weight now

What did you eat yesterday for:

Breakfast	Lunch	Dinner	Snacks

INSTRUCTIONS:

Please circle "D" if you eat the following foods **daily**, "W" if you eat them **weekly**, "M" for **monthly**, "S" for **seldom**, and "N" for **never**. Under kinds list specific type if appropriate such as milk, whole milk, 2% milk, skim milk or powdered skim milk. Amounts would be whether it is approximately a cup, a slice or teaspoon, etc.

FOOD	KIND	FREQUENCY	AVERAGE AMOUNT
Milk		D W M S N	
Cheese		D W M S N	
Ice Cream		D W M S N	
Milk in cooking		D W M S N	
Meat:			
Luncheon meat		D W M S N	
Sausage		D W M S N	
Pork, ham, beef		D W M S N	
lamb or venison		D W M S N	
Meat in mixtures as stew, casseroles, taco, tamale, gravy		D W M S N	
Liver		D W M S N	
Poultry		D W M S N	
Fish		D W M S N	
Eggs		D W M S N	
Peanut butter		D W M S N	
Nuts		D W M S N	
Seeds		D W M S N	
Dried peas or beans		D W M S N	
Fruit, raw		D W M S N	
Fruit, canned		D W M S N	
Fruit juice		D W M S N	
Powdered fruit drinks		D W M S N	
Vegetable, cooked		D W M S N	
Vegetable, raw		D W M S N	
Vegetable, salad		D W M S N	
Potato		D W M S N	

FOOD	KIND	FREQUENCY	AMOUNT
Bread or rolls		D W M S N	
Biscuits or cornbread		D W M S N	
Rice, macaroni, etc.		D W M S N	
Tortillas		D W M S N	
Cereal, dry		D W M S N	
Cereal, cooked		D W M S N	
Pancakes or Waffles		D W M S N	
Sweetrolls or doughnuts		D W M S N	
Crackers		D W M S N	
Cake		D W M S N	
Pie		D W M S N	
Potato chips or other chips		D W M S N	
Koolaid or soft drinks		D W M S N	
Candy		D W M S N	
Sugar, syrup or honey		D W M S N	
Jam or jelly		D W M S N	
Popsicles		D W M S N	
Butter or margarine		D W M S N	
Other fats or oils		D W M S N	
Mayonnaise or salad dressing		D W M S N	
Pizza		D W M S N	
Soup		D W M S N	

1. Do you eat at regular times each day?
2. How many days a week do you eat: Breakfast—

   Lunch—

   Dinner—

   During the evening—
3. How many days a week do you snack: Midmorning—

   Afternoon—

   Evening—
4. What foods do you dislike?
5. Do you eat anything or have a craving for anything not normally considered food—e.g., laundry starch, clay?
6. Are you a heavy salter—in cooking? —at the table?
7. Do you do the cooking? the shopping?
8. Do you take a vitamin and/or mineral supplement?

DIET EVALUATION AND RECOMMENDATIONS:

FIGURE 17-1. Diet history. (Courtesy of the University of Oregon Medical School.)

NUTRITIONAL ASSESSMENT

Each expectant mother is an individual whose attitudes toward food, emotional response to food, cultural meaning of food, and knowledge of nutrition are unique by combination.[5] Coupled with this are the woman's attitudes toward health, and toward being pregnant and having a child. Creating a positive attitude toward nutrition during pregnancy requires patience, understanding, and respect for a woman's individual pattern of behavior.

In assessing the woman's nutritional intake it is also necessary to learn:

What are the purchasing practices in the woman's family? Does the expectant mother make the decisions concerning what is to be purchased or does someone else in the family have that prerogative?

What are the cultural values and beliefs related to food and particularly to appropriate food for an expectant mother? Learning the woman's place of birth and early childhood home will help the nurse recognize food patterns that are culturally valued.

What value does food hold for nutrition, status, appetite, customs, and so forth?

What budget is available for food purchases and how adequate is it? How many persons are there in the home for whom food must be purchased and prepared? Are any of these people on special diets?

What facilities are available in the home to store, refrigerate, and prepare food?

Who prepares the food for the family? How much control does the expectant mother have over the preparation of food?

What is the expectant mother's education and what occupation does she pursue?

DIET HISTORY

In order to help an expectant mother meet dietary needs for herself and her developing fetus, a diet history, such as the one shown in Figure 17-1, needs to be completed. During the process of taking diet history, useful information is obtained concerning the woman's level of nutrition knowledge and clues to methods of counseling.

In addition to the kinds of foods eaten, the amounts should also be recorded. Such terms as cup, teaspoon, size, portion eaten, types of bread, and kind of milk become important in arriving at an assessment. The method of food preparation should also be considered in the assessment.

The diet history is one of the important clinical tools for evaluation of the patient's nutritional state. Evaluation is also based on the physical examination. Particular note should be made of the prepregnant weight. Laboratory studies are also an important part of the nutritional assessment. Particularly significant are the hemoglobin levels and the total protein concentration of the blood. Nutritional counseling should utilize all available data.

As in any other teaching and counseling session, provisions must be made for the nutritional assessment. Time must be provided for the woman to discuss her concerns about food and the diet. Good nutrition for the expectant mother can be taught in a class or on an individual basis. The husband should be included whenever possible, for it is essential that he understands the importance of the diet. He can also offer valuable moral support to his wife. The costs of the extra nutrients can be better managed when both husband and wife understand the importance of good nutrition.

Working from the dietary history, the evaluation can be a joint endeavor of the nurse and the expectant mother, or it can become a class project. Using a food value chart,* the expec-

* Such as the one obtainable from the Superintendent of Documents, U.S. Government Printing Office, Washington, D. C. 20402, for 30¢.

tant mother can analyze the diet for calories, protein, calcium, iron, and vitamins A, C, and D. This intake, matched against the recommended daily allowances, gives the counselor an opportunity to emphasize the positive aspects of the diet and, based on individual preferences, to plan for correcting any deficiencies. Fortunately, with our more recent knowledge of maternal nutrition, it is no longer necessary for the expectant mother to feel deprived. The emphasis should be on what she may have and the quality of the increases she may now include in her diet.

BLOCKS TO NUTRITIONAL ADEQUACY

1. Nutrition may not have a top priority for the expectant mother. Considering all the problems with which she may be trying to cope, adequate nutrition may not be of prime importance to her. Indeed, the problems may cause changes that are nutritionally harmful. Some individuals react to stress by overeating; others experience anorexia and do not eat adequately.
2. Individuals may lack knowledge of the importance of nutrition to health and particularly to pregnancy.
3. Cultural factors may be obstructions to proper nutrition during pregnancy.
4. The individual may have no control over the food she is served, thus leaving her to feel helpless in the situation. This often occurs when two generations live together and the older generation makes the final decision about nutritional practices.
5. The individual may be unable to cope with changes brought about by the pregnancy. The woman may be unwilling or unable to accept motherhood. She may be unable to manage the family budget so that adequate nutrition is assured. She may feel a sense of futility. With little to look forward to, her focus may be on satisfactions here and now.

It is not always possible to achieve all desired changes in nutrition. However, any changes are better than none at all. After sufficient data collection, the nurse must decide what is possible and work toward helping the expectant mother reach those goals.

NUTRITIONAL COUNSELING

All the knowledge we have about nutrition and its impact on the mother's health and the health of her fetus is of little value unless it is applied to the pregnant woman. The majority of women are ready, willing, and motivated to make whatever adjustments are needed in their diets. Other women are not able or willing to do so to the fullest extent. For the first group, relating the necessary information to them and showing continued interest in their progress is often all that is needed. The second group requires much more attention. However, the principles of learning are applicable to all.

Learning is more effective when the expectant parents are ready to learn, i.e., they are motivated to learn and have experiential readiness for learning. Moderate anxiety is beneficial to learning, whereas severe anxiety or very low anxiety detracts from learning. The goals to be attained must be clearly identified. They must be realistic (not too high) so that they are attainable, but not so low as to be boring. The nutritional information related to the expectant mother must be meaningful and must not beyond her ability to comprehend and remember. Parallel teaching, i.e., teaching at the individual level, is important. New material must build on what is already known so that it can be readily associated.

Using many senses in learning increases the likelihood that the individual will understand and remember. Nutrition should be taught using visual aids and expectant parents should be given material to take home with them for continued references.

PRINCIPALS OF MOTIVATION

The two principles of health behavior motivation as delineated by Rosenstock[6] are helpful in understanding the nutritional behavior of the expectant mother.

Note that these actions depend on the way the individual *feels* or *believes*. They are not necessarily based on facts. Information the woman has heard may be erroneous or may be accurate, but what is important is how she *believes* it applies to her.

These principles, in addition to helping better understand the expectant mother, also help us to recognize that it is more important to assess her *beliefs* than it is to recognize her *knowledge*. Teaching of facts can then deal with beliefs. Knowledge will be useful in filling in the gaps of information and in correcting misinformation. Our success in changing nutritional behavior will be in direct proportion to our understanding of the woman to whom we are relating. We must adapt nutrition teaching to fit the person, not expect her to fit our program.

We should also ask ourselves the question, how is health through nutrition taught? How are individuals motivated to eat for health? Schools, from the earliest grades, have a role to play. If the school in our community is not filling that role, we have a community responsibility as a health professional to explore our concern.

Principal I

Health behavior is a function of a health motive or threat and the individual's belief about various courses of action open to him.

A. The degree to which a woman *feels* threatened she may become ill or give birth to a damaged child.

B. The degree to which the woman *feels* this occurrence will have serious consequences to her.

C. The degree to which the woman *feels* there is a probability this will occur to *her*.

D. The degree to which the woman *believes* she has one or more courses of action which will reduce the chances of this occurrence.

Principle II

Individuals' motives and beliefs about various courses of action are often in conflict with each other and behavior emerges as the resolution of these conflicts.

A. Two motives may compete with each other for dominance. The woman may want health but also want other things which the family income can buy.

B. An available course of action to satisfy a motive may be intrinsically frustrating. If the prescribed diet is unpleasant, upsetting or causes discomfort, it may be abandoned.

C. The individual may not see any other course of action to satisfy an existing motive. This may increase fear and anxiety so that the woman is no longer able to think objectively. She may lack control of her nutritional intake because others have the prerogative in food selection and food preparation. Cultural or social pressure may be too great.

MENU PLANNING

The U.S. Department of Agriculture has prepared a practical guide for well balanced human nutrition. It is a *base* on which nutrition counseling of the expectant mother is built. It consists of:

1. Milk group
   A quart of milk daily is basic. Cheese and ice cream are also good sources of nutrition.
2. Meat group
   Two or more servings of meat are mandatory. This includes beef, veal, pork, lamb, poultry, fish, and eggs. Dry beans, peas, and nuts are alternates. One serving of liver weekly should be included. One serving equals two to three ounces of boneless cooked meat, poultry, or fish; two eggs; or one cup of cooked dry beans or peas.)
3. Vegetable and fruit group
   Four or more servings which should include a dark green leafy vegetable and a deep yellow vegetable at least every other day, a citrous fruit or other vegetable high in vitamin C, other fruits and vegetables including potato. (One serving equals one-half cup of vegetable or fruit.)
4. Bread and cereal group
   Four or more servings which include whole grain, enriched and restored products. (One serving equals one slice of bread or one-half to three-quarters cup of cooked cereal.)

This will supply one half to two thirds of the caloric requirements during pregnancy and most of the known vitamin requirements. Table 17-1 in the previous section, containing the dietary requirements of women with additions needed for pregnancy and lactation, should be used as a guide for menu planning.

SUMMARY OF MAJOR FUNCTIONS AND SOURCES OF NUTRIENTS*

Protein

Growth of fetus and accessory tissues.

Production of breast milk.

Animal Protein	Vegetable Protein
meat	dried beans
fish	dried peas
poultry	lentils
eggs	nuts
milk	peanut butter
cheese	

Iron

Maintain hemoglobin level of mother.

Maintain mother's stores of iron.

Furnish iron for fetal development.

Furnish infant with iron stores needed for blood formation during neonatal period before food sources of iron and added to diet.

Good Sources	Fair Sources
pork liver	enriched pastas
kidney	spinach
beef liver	canned mackerel
oysters	enriched white bread
clams	kale
canned dried beans	mustard greens
prune juice	whole wheat bread
liverwurst	eggs
heart	brussels sprouts
lean pork	broccoli
lean beef	
raisins	
cooked dried beans	
cooked dried peaches	
cooked dried apricots	
cooked dried prunes	
canned green peas	

* From *The Journal of Reproductive Medicine*, 7:272, 1971, with permission.

Ascorbic Acid

Production of intercellular substances necessary for the development and maintenance of normal connective tissue in bones, cartilage and muscles.

Improves health of bones and teeth.

Increases absorption of iron.

Good Sources	Fair Sources
citrus fruits or juice	asparagus
broccoli	cabbage, raw
brussels sprouts	cauliflower
cantaloupe	chile, fresh or canned
greens—collards, mustard, turnip	kale
peppers	liver
	other melons
	potatoes or sweet potatoes in jackets
	spinach
	tomatoes or prunes

Vitamin D

Promotes absorption and retention of calcium and phosphorous necessary for growth and formation of bones and teeth.

Good Sources
- butter
- egg yolk
- fish oils
- liver
- milk fortified with vitamin D
- other foods may contain added vitamin D—check labels.

Niacin

Helps translate sources of energy into useable form.

Good Sources	Fair Sources
fish	milk
heart	potatoes
lean meat	whole grain and enriched bread
liver	whole grain and enriched cereal
peanuts	
peanut butter	
poultry	

Vitamin A

Tooth formation.

Normal bone growth.

Healthy skin.

Vision—light/dark adaptation.

Vitamin A	Carotenes
butter	dark green and deep yellow vegetables and a few fruits
egg yolk	apricots
fortified margarine	broccoli
kidney	cantaloupe
liver	carrots
whole milk	chard
cream	collards
	kale
	mustard greens
	persimmons
	spinach
	pumpkin
	sweet potatoes
	turnip greens
	winter squash

Thiamin

Appetite and digestion normal.

Nervous system health.

Completion of carbohydrates.

Good Sources	Fair Sources
whole grain and enriched bread	eggs
whole grain and enriched cereals	fish
dried peas	meat
dried beans	poultry
oranges	milk
liver	many vegetables
heart	
kidney	
lean pork	
nuts	
potatoes	
peas	
wheat germ	

Calcium

Skeletal structures of the fetus.

Production of breast milk.

Blood coagulation, neuromuscular irritability and muscle contractility.

Good Sources	Fair Sources
skim milk	dark green leafy vegetables
buttermilk	dried beans
whole milk	broccoli
nonfat dry milk	cottage cheese
cheese	canned fish, including bones
ice milk	oranges
ice cream	

Riboflavin

Functions in number of enzyme systems in tissue respiration.

Metabolism of amino acids and carbohydrates.

Good Sources	Fair Sources
heart	broccoli
kidney	cheese
liver	dark green leafy vegetables
milk	eggs
ice milk	ice cream
	lean meat
	poultry

CONVERTING THE DIETARY REQUIREMENTS

The nurse will often need to help the expectant family convert the recommended dietary allowances into specific foods and in specific amounts. Below, protein, iron, calcium, vitamin A, and ascorbic acid are handled in such a fashion.* These are not the only nutrients needed, but assuring their inclusion will meet the major goals of adequate nutrition during pregnancy and lactation.

* Nutritional values were obtained from Bowles, C. F. and Church, H. N.: *Food Values of Portions Commonly Used*, ed. 11. Lippincott, Philadelphia, 1970.

Protein	
Pregnant adolescent	65–90 g.
Pregnant adult	65–90 g.
Nursing mother	75–105 g.

Foods rich in protein		
meat and poultry	1 oz.	7.0 g.
fish	1 oz.	7.0 g.
eggs	1	6.0 g.
cheese	1 oz.	7.0 g.
cheddar		
processed American	1 oz.	6.5 g.
cottage cheese	¼ cup	7.0 g.
peanut butter	2 tbsp.	7.0 g.
frankfurter	1	7.0 g.
milk (liquid)	8 oz.	9.0 g.
nonfat dry milk	1 oz. (4 tbsp.)	10.0 g.
liquid	8 oz.	8.8 g.
red kidney beans	⅔ cup	7.8 g.
lima beans, dry cooked	⅝ cup	9.4 g.

Certain grains, legumes, nuts, and vegetables can be combined with animal proteins and with each other to produce the daily needs. This is discussed in detail under the topic Vegetarian Diets, appearing later in this chapter.

Example of adequate protein intake	
2 servings (3 oz. of meat, fish or poultry)	42 g.
2 eggs	14 g.
½ cup cottage cheese	14 g.
Total	70 g.

Iron	
Pregnant adolescent	18+ mg.
Pregnant adult	18+ mg.
Nursing mother	18+ mg.

Foods rich in iron		
meat, fish, and poultry	4 oz	3.60 mg.
Liver	1 oz.	2.40 mg.
eggs	1	1.10 mg.
dark green leafy vegetables	½ cup	1.00 mg
bread and cereal	1 serving	0.85 mg.
dried beans and peas	1 oz.	2.30 mg.
some dried fruit	4 halves	0.80 mg.

Superior vegetables include peas,watercrest, mustard greens, beet greens, brussel sprouts, collards, dandelion greens, and escarole. Superior dried fruits include apricots, prunes, and raisins.

Example of an adequate iron intake	
1 serving (3 oz.) of meat, fish or poultry	3.0 mg.
1 serving (3. oz.) of liver	7.2 mg.
2 eggs	2.2 mg.
2 vegetables	2.0 mg.
4 servings of bread or cereal	3.4 mg.
Total	17.8 mg. (near adequate)

Calcium	
Pregnant adolescent	1700 mg.
Pregnant adult	1200 mg.
Nursing mother	1300 mg.

Foods rich in calcium		
milk		
fluid	1 cup	285 mg.
dry milk	1 oz.	367 mg.
cheese	1 oz.	221 mg.
custard, pudding, and ice cream	½ cup	135 mg.
canned salmon	3 oz.	159 mg.
sardines	3 oz.	367 mg.
oysters	1 cup	269 mg.
oranges	1	50 mg.
spinach	½ cup	112 mg.
broccoli	⅔ cup	126 mg.

Example of adequate calcium intake	
2 cups of milk	570 mg.
2 ounces of cheese	441 mg.
one serving of ice cream	135 mg.
one serving of spinach	112 mg.
Total	1258 mg.

Dried milk used in cooking is an excellent source of calcium. If the patient will not or cannot use milk in her diet, the calcium needs will be very difficult to meet.

Vitamin A	
Pregnant adolescent	5000 I.U.
Pregnant adult	5000 I.U.
Nursing mother	6000 I.U.

Foods rich in vitamin A		
spinach	½ cup	6000 I.U.
carrots	⅓ cup	5000 I.U.
sweet potatoes	⅓ cup	6000 I.U.
broccoli	⅓ cup	1700 I.U.
tomato juice	1 cup	2540 I.U.
cooked prunes	⅓ cup	1780 I.U.
green leafy vegetable	⅓ cup	1450 I.U.
cantaloupe	½ cup diced	4100 I.U.
watermelon	1 wedge (4″ × 8″)	2530 I.U.
apricots	3	2890 I.U.
papaya	⅓	1750 I.U.
peach fresh	1	1320 I.U.
canned	½ cup sliced	2230 I.U.
liver	1 oz.	6000 I.U.
eggs	1	590 I.U.

Example of adequate vitamin A intake	
2 eggs	1180 I.U.

4 apricots	3853 I.U.
1 serving of a green leafy vegetable	1450 I.U.
Total	6483 I.U.
or	
1 serving (½ cup) of spinach, carrots, or sweet potatoes	6000 I.U.

Ascorbic Acid	
Pregnant adolescent	60 mg.
Pregnant adult	60 mg.
Nursing mother	60 mg.

Foods rich in ascorbic acid

oranges	1 whole or 4 oz. juice	66 mg.
papayas	⅓	56 mg.
tangerines	1 small	26 mg.
grapefruit	½	50 mg.
cabbage (raw)	½ cup	24 mg.
turnip and other dark greens	⅔ cup	69 mg.
strawberries	1 cup	89 mg.
broccoli	½ cup	55 mg.
tomato juice	8 oz.	38 mg.
cabbage (raw)	1 cup	50 mg.
tomatoes	1 small	35 mg.
sweet potatoes	1 medium	24 mg.
spinach	½ cup	27 mg.
cauliflower	½ cup	17 mg.
pepper	½ medium	40 mg.
watercress	10 sprigs	79 mg.

Example of adequate ascorbic acid intake

8 ounces of tomato juice	38 mg.
1 serving (½ cup) of spinach	27 mg.
1 serving (½ cup) of cauliflower	17 mg.
Total	82 mg.
or	
4 ounces of orange juice	66 mg.

Table 17-2 presents examples of nutritionally adequate prenatal menus for various cultures.

Since vitamins and minerals are so readily available in natural foods, there is no scientific justification for prescribing most vitamin supplements during pregnancy. The use of vitamin and mineral supplements as a substitute for adequate intake of nutrients is an unsound practice, since these supplements do not supply proteins or other nutrient factors found in natural foods. In addition, the cost of supplements may limit the purchase of needed foods.

However, in view of the widespread incidence of iron deficiency anemia and the increased iron requirement of pregnancy, iron supplementation is needed during the second and third trimester of pregnancy in amounts of 30 to 60 mg. daily. A daily supplement of 0.2 to 0.4 mg. of folate during pregnancy is also recommended to prevent folic acid deficiency.

NUTRITIONAL HIGH RISK

The previous application of nutrition to the expectant and lactating mother may need to be modified for some individuals. Many women enter pregnancy with less than optimal health. A number of these women come from homes where they have not had access to good medical care, food, and education, resulting in suboptimal health and nutritional status. There are also women with quite adequate incomes who, for various cultural and personal reasons, arrive at the childbearing age with poor nutrition. Women with poor nutritional habits present a challenge to health professionals—for once tissue is depleted, considerable increase in the essential nutritive factors is necessary, often more than it is possible to obtain from an optimal diet. Nutritional products of modern chemistry are highly useful in this endeavor, but at our present state of technology they can only supplement, they do not replace our natural sources of nutrients. Pregnancy presents a natural opportunity to help women evaluate their health status and

TABLE 17-2. Sample Menus*

The menus below show the cultural variations possible when planning a nutritionally adequate prenatal diet. All meet the Recommended Dietary Allowances for calories, provide a minimum of 90 grams of protein, and exceed the Recommended Dietary Allowances for vitamin A and C and calcium. Only the Black and Mexican dietary pattern meets the Recommended Dietary Allowances for iron, providing 21.9 mg and 23.1 mg. The Regular, American-Indian, and the Oriental pattern provide 15.3 mg, 15.8, and 15.3 respectively. The Lacto-Ovo plan provides only 12.0 mg.

	Regular	*Mexican*	*Black*	*Oriental*	*American Indian*	*Lacto-Ovo*
BREAKFAST:						
2 energy foods	1 cup Cream of Wheat	2 corn tortillas	1 cup grits	1 cup rice	1 cup corn mush	1 cup brown rice
	1 tbsp. sugar	2 tbsp. jelly	1 tbsp. sugar	1 tsp. sugar (in tea)	1 tbsp. sugar	1 tbsp. honey
1 calcium protein food	1 cup milk	½ cup evaporated milk in coffee	1 cup milk	1 cup milk	1 cup milk	1 cup milk
1 vitamin C food	1 cup orange juice	1 cup orange juice	1 cup orange juice	1 cup orange juice	1 cup orange juice	1 cup orange juice
LUNCH:						
1 energy food	1 slice bread	1 tortilla	1 2″ square corn bread	½ cup rice	1 slice Indian fried bread	1 slice whole wheat bread
2 protein foods	2-1 oz. slice cheese	1 cup beans	1 cup pork and beans	3 ½ oz. tofu 1 egg	1 cup pinto beans	1 cup lentils
1 calcium protein food	1 cup milk	½ cup evaporated milk and chocolate	1 cup milk	1 cup milk	1 cup milk	1 cup milk
1 vitamin A food	½ cup spinach	½ cup spinach 1 green pepper	½ cup collard greens	3/5 bok choy	½ cup spinach	½ cup spinach
1 vitamin/mineral food	1 banana	1 banana	1 banana	1 banana	1 apple	1 banana
DINNER:						
1 energy food	1 small baked potato	½ cup Spanish rice	2 halves candied yams	½ cup rice	½ cup fried potatoes	1 small baked potato
3 protein foods	3 oz. beef roast	1 cup beans 1 cup caldo	3 ½ oz. fried pork chops	okazu (stewing beef 3 oz. and ½ cup broccoli and 2 oz. tofu)	3½ oz. fish	3½ oz. cheese (Cheddar)
1 calcium/protein food	1 cup milk	½ cup evaporated milk and coffee	1 cup milk	1 cup milk	1 cup milk 1 stalk broccoli	1 cup milk 1 stalk broccoli
2 vitamin/mineral foods	1 stalk broccoli 1 cup fruited Jello	1 cup fruited Jello	1 cup peas 1 cup fruited Jello	1 cup fruited Jello	1 cup fruited Jello	½ cup fruited Jello
SNACKS:						
1 calcium/protein food	1 cup custard	1 cup flan	1 cup custard	1 cup custard	1 cup custard	1 cup custard
1 vitamin/mineral food	1 pear	1 pear	1 pear	1 pear	1 pear	1 pear
1 energy food	2 oatmeal-raisin cookies	2 oatmeal-raisin cookies	2 oatmeal-raisin cookies	2 oatmeal-raisin cookies	2 oatmeal-raisin cookies	2 oatmeal-raisin cookies

* From Cross, A. T. and Walsh, H. E.: *Prenatal Diet Counseling*. J. Reprod. Med. 7:265, 1971, with permission.

develop good nutritional habits for optimum health.

Women who need to have particular attention paid to their nutrient intake during pregnancy include:

1. Biologically immature expectant mothers, particularly those under 17 years of age in whom the stresses of pregnancy are added to the nutrient needs for growth and development. Poor existing nutritional status may further contribute to a poor pregnancy outcome.
2. Women who have had rapid succession of pregnancies, often depleting the maternal nutrient stores.
3. Women with low prepregnant weight for height.
4. Women with limited weight gain during pregnancy.
5. Overweight expectant mothers. Despite obesity, they may not be well nourished or have adequate intake of essential vitamins and minerals.
6. Women in low socioeconomic situations. Low income makes it very difficult to be well nourished.
7. Women who, for religious or other reasons, limit their food intake to certain groups of foods.
8. Women with health problems resulting from poor nutrition.
9. Healthy women besieged with confusing, conflicting, and misleading information on nutrition.

ANEMIA

Anemia may be due to a number of factors, both acquired and hereditary. Iron stores of women are seldom large enough to meet the iron requirements of pregnancy. Since usual diets in America are not likely to provide sufficient quantities of iron, the Committee on Maternal Nutrition recommends that "all women receive 30 to 60 mg. of iron as a daily supplement during the second and third trimester," and that "supplementation with folic acid is also warranted, especially in instances where folate requirements are high, such as in chronic hemolytic anemia and multiple pregnancy. A daily supplement of 200 to 400 mg. of folic acid should prevent deficiencies in pregnant women."[7]

ADOLESCENCE

Young teenage mothers produce a disproportionate number of low-birth-weight infants. Conception and parenthood, while the body is still in the formative stages, creates physiologic stress to the maternal body. Thus, there is increased need for food to satisfy energy requirements for rapidly enlarging organs and tissues as well as for fetal growth. These demands are further complicated when the adolescent is malnourished. Dietary habits of adolescents are often bizarre. The intake of iron, calcium, vitamin A, and ascorbic acid are often less than optimal. Clinical and nutritional surveys indicate that 19 per cent of American teenagers are underweight and 30 to 35 per cent are overweight.[8] A very careful assessment of the adolescent's nutritional intake is necessary with special focus on calories, protein, and calcium since these elements are critical for the girl's normal growth and development.

TOXEMIA OF PREGNANCY

Two issues involving nutrition during pregnancy are sodium chloride intake and weight gain.

During normal pregnancy, the body goes to considerable lengths to promote sodium retention for maternal and fetal needs. However, there is no supportive data to date that correlates this physiologic process with the development of toxemia. The restriction of sodium during normal pregnancy is therefore not supported, even though this practice is widespread. When toxemia occurs during pregnancy, the restriction of sodium, to reduce the edema, is still frequently prescribed. The evidence as to the value of this practice is conflicting. However, there seems to be general agreement among authorities that the regulation of sodium intake in patients with a definite diagnosis of preeclampsia is not a major part of the treatment.[9] The time for reappraisal of the role of sodium intake during pregnancy is long overdue, and nurses are advised to keep up with the literature as new studies are reported. Nevertheless, if a patient is told to limit her sodium intake, the nurse must be prepared to help her with this dietary restriction.

Three degrees of sodium restriction are generally applied: mild, moderate, and strict, or the diet may be ordered in mEq. or in mg. of sodium (1 mEq. = approx. 23 mg.). Mild restriction allows 100 to 200 mEq. (approx. 2,400 to 4,500 mg.). Moderate restriction allows 43 mEq. (approx. 1,000 mg.). Strict restriction limits to 23 mEq. (approx. 500 mg.).[10]

Fruits and vegetables have relatively low sodium content with the exception of[11]

artichokes	mustard greens
beets	white turnip
beet greens	kale
swiss chard	sauerkraut
celery	spinach
dandelion greens	carrots

Animal proteins, such as meat, poultry, fish, milk, cheese, and eggs are relatively high in sodium. However, these foods are nutrionally essential. There are also other products, used to preserve or enhance the flavor of foods, which contain sodium in other forms. Such items include baking soda, sodium saccharin, sodium benzoate, and monosodium glutomate.

If *mild restriction* is recommended, the patient may eat most food omitting obviously salty foods such as bacon, potato chips, salad dressing, saltwater fish, pickled vegetables, salted nuts, salted pork, luncheon meat, frankfurters, and soy sauce. Other foods may be *lightly* salted during preparation, but *no* salt may be added at the table.

In *moderate restriction*, no salt is used during preparation or at the table, with the exception of *either* ¼ teaspoon of salt used as preferred during the day *or* the eating of regular bakery bread and regular salted butter. (1 slice of bread = 150 mg. sodium. 2 tsp. butter = 100 mg. sodium.) If the patient prefers to use the ¼ teaspoon of salt, she should place it in a separate salt shaker daily and should purchase salt-free bread and sweet butter. She should also avoid the salty foods mentioned above.

If the patient is to *strictly limit* her sodium intake, she should be referred to a dietitian for counseling. When it is not possible to make such a referral, the nurse will need to use a food value chart to select the foods the patient prefers that are in keeping with dietary restrictions.

The lack of salt makes food unpalatable for most people. The patient can be helped to enhance the natural flavor of foods through compatable seasonings, such as:

Beef: bay leaf, thyme, marjoram, onion, dry mustard, parsley, dill, or herb butter.
Pork: garlic, marjoram, or sage.
Lamb: garlic, onion, thyme, parsley, marjoram, mint, or rosemary.
Liver: parsley, onion, chives, or herb butter.
Veal: summer savory, chervil, basil, marjoram, bay leaf, cumin, or oregano.
Poultry: fresh or dried celery leaves, basil, marjoram, parsley, rosemary, summer savory, sage, thyme, or paprika.
Fish: lemon, garlic, dill butter, chopped dill, basil, tarragon leaves, or sweet butter.
Eggs: chives, parsley, basil, marjoram, rosemary, tarragon, thyme, onion, or mushrooms.

Asparagus: chives, lemon, caraway, herb butter, or sweet butter.
Carrots: chives, parsley, mint, or chervil.
Corn: chives, parsley, green pepper, onion, tomato, or chili powder.
Green beans: dill, thyme, marjoram, nutmeg, onion, chives, scallions, rosemary, lemon, or unsalted French dressing.
Peas: chives, mint, parsley, chervil, onion, mushrooms, or lettuce.
Potatoes: parsley, chives, onion, rosemary, mace, or scallions.
Squash: lemon, ginger, mace, basil, cloves, nutmeg, onion, green pepper, or chives.
Tomatoes: garlic, onion, parsley, basil, sage, chervil, or tarragon.*

The patient may use salt substitutes in most instances. These are usually preparations of potassium chloride with the addition of some spices. Since potassium is often deficient in low sodium diets, this may be additionally useful. The patient should be warned not to substitute vegetized salts for table salt, since these also consist of sodium chloride.

The nurse should remember that the signs and symptoms of sodium depletion are similar to those of toxemia (apathy, anorexia, nausea, vomiting, decreased urine volume, and increased serum uric acid). Kidney damage resulting from sodium depletion may also be responsible for albuminurea.[12]

The other issue that arises during pregnancy when toxemia occurs is weight control. Pitkin and colleagues,[13] as well as many others, state that there is no convincing evidence that excessive weight gain, due to tissue deposition, is related to toxemia and that there is no scientific justification for routine weight restriction of less than 22 to 27 pounds. This topic has been discussed in detail in the previous section. It is advised that nurses keep up with the literature as new research is done in this area.

* From Snively, W. D., Beeshear, D. R. and Roberts, K. T.,[11] with permission.

VEGETARIAN DIETS

The nurse, during her professional career, may care for expectant mothers who, for socioeconomic, cultural, religious, or personal reasons, eat a vegetarian diet. Often these individuals exclude meat, fish, and poultry, but include eggs and milk in their diet (lacto-ovo-vegetarian diet). Others exclude eggs and milk as well as meat, fish, and poultry (pure vegetarian diet). Planning a scientifically nutritious vegetarian diet to protect the health of the mother and her developing fetus is indeed a challenge. Without sound nutritional knowledge, following a vegetarian diet can be hazardous. However, it is possible to construct a vegetarian diet which provides all of the essential nutrients.[14] The intake of all essential amino acids presents the greatest problem. Proteins from vegetable sources are not complete proteins. They do not include all of the eight essential amino acids. Therefore, the selection of foods must be carefully made so that the combination results in adequate amounts of all the amino acids eaten simultaneously. Such combinations are:

wheat and peanuts
bread and gelatin
cereal and milk
dried beans and corn

In addition to the proper combinations, the quantity is also important if the diet is to be adequate.

Total proteins and combinations of proteins necessary to give essential amino acids from incomplete protein sources are shown in Table 17-3.

In order to insure an adequate diet, the use of milk, milk products, and eggs should be encouraged. Without these products containing animal protein, it is difficult to get enough protein of high biologic value. In addition, eggs are a good source of iron, and milk is our best source of calcium. Both of

TABLE 17-3. Appropriate Protein Combinations for Vegetarian Diets*

Food	Suggested Serving	Total Protein (g)		Food	Suggested Serving	Total Protein (g)
(choose 1 from this group)			PLUS	(choose 1 from this group)		
LEGUMES				GRAINS†		
canned baked beans	¾ cup cooked	11		barley	1 cup cooked	16
				bulgar	1 cup cooked	8
dried lima beans	¾ cup cooked	12		oatmeal	1 cup cooked	5
kidney beans	¾ cup cooked	11		rice	1 cup cooked	4
lentils	¾ cup cooked	10		rye bread	2 slices	4
navy beans	¾ cup cooked	11		wheat bread	2 slices	6
soybeans	¾ cup cooked	15		white bread	2 slices	4
tofu	2″ × 2″ × 2½″ block	20				
(choose 1 from this group)			PLUS	(choose 1 from this group)		
LEGUMES				NUTS AND SEEDS‡		
canned baked beans	¾ cup	11		Brazil nuts	8 medium	4
				cashew nuts	½ cup	12
dried lima beans	¾ cup cooked	12		pistachio nuts	3 teaspoons	7
kidney beans	¾ cup cooked	11				
lentils	¾ cup cooked	10		sesame kernels	3 teaspoons	6
navy beans	¾ cup cooked	11				
soybeans	¾ cup cooked	15		sunflower seeds	3 teaspoons	8
tofu	2″ × 2″ × 2½ block	20				
(choose 1 from this group)			PLUS	(choose 1 from this group)		
YEAST				GRAINS		
yeast (Brewer's) powder	1 level tsp.	4		barley	1 cup cooked	16
				bulgar	1 cup cooked	8
				oatmeal	1 cup cooked	5
				rice	1 cup cooked	4
				rye bread	2 slices	4
				wheat bread	2 slices	6
				white bread	2 slices	4

* From the Nutrition Branch, Hawaii State Department of Health, with permission.

† Raw cereal products are high in starch which is not readily utilized by the body. Unless they are cooked, the cereal products may have little energy value.

‡ Nuts are high in fat and calories.

TABLE 17-3. *Continued*

(choose 1 from this group)			PLUS (choose 1 from this group)			PLUS (choose 1 from this group)		
			LEGUMES			NUTS AND SEEDS		
peanuts (roasted)	2 tsp.	8	canned baked beans	¾ cup	11	Brazil nuts	8 medium	4
pumpkin kernels	2 tsp.	10	dried lima beans	¾ cup cooked	12	cashew nuts	½ cup	12
squash kernels	2 tsp.	10	kidney beans	¾ cup cooked	11	pistachio nuts	3 tsp.	7
wheat germ	2 tsp.	3	lentils	¾ cup cooked	10	sesame kernels	3 tsp.	6
			navy beans	¾ cup cooked	11	sunflower seeds	3 tsp.	8
			soybeans	¾ cup cooked	15			
			tofu	2″ × 2″ × 2½″ block	20			

these elements are important during rapid growth periods such as pregnancy.

The main difference between *lacto-ovo-vegetarian diets* and an average American diet is the replacement of meat with a variety of legumes, meat analogs, cereals, nuts, and a more generous intake of milk, milk products, and eggs. In planning such a diet, the four basic food groups are still followed:

1. In the *meat (protein) group*, meat will be replaced by the generous intake of a variety of legumes, nuts, and meat analogs made from wheat and/or soy proteins and other formulated plant proteins. A number of markets now produce frozen, dehydrated, and canned analogs. There are also vegetarian recipe books which help the homemaker prepare a number of foods which combine legumes, cereals, and nuts with milk and eggs.
2. The *milk group* will change only in that greater amounts of low-fat milk and milk products such as cheese and cottage cheese will be used. These contribute to the protein intake and provide the necessary vitamin B_{12}.
3. In the *cereal and bread group*, intake will increase somewhat, particularly in the whole grain form.
4. In the *fruit and vegetable group*, selection and amount are important to make up the needed caloric intake.

Planning a *pure vegetarian diet* is more difficult since it is devoid of all animal foods, including milk and eggs. Since many plant foods are low in calories, a large intake of plant foods is necessary to meet caloric needs. Since there is no vitamin B_{12} in plant foods, supplementation is necessary.

Sufficient calcium intake is another problem. Two glasses of fortified soybean milk daily are necessary to meet requirements, plus green leafy vegetables such as collards, turnip greens, kale, mustard greens. One cup of these vegetables provides calcium equal to that in eight ounces of milk. Cabbage, broccoli, and cauliflower also provide lesser quantities of calcium, as do dried fruits, nuts (particularly almonds), and legumes.

A careful assessment of both the lacto-ovo-vegetarian diet and the pure vegetarian diet is essential to insure that the mother and fetus are receiving adequate nutrients. Table

TABLE 17-4. Foods Used by Vegetarians*

Food	Weight (g.)	Serving	Energy	Protein	Calcium (mg.)	Iron (mg.)	Vitamin A (I.U.)	Thiamine (mg.)	Riboflavin (mg.)	Vitamin C (mg.)
Wheat Germ	68	1 cup	245	18.0	49.0	6.4	—	1.360	0.460	—
Coconut										
Water	100	½ cup	11	0.21	12.5	0.07	—	—	0.010	1.4
Flesh, mature nut	100	½ cup	421	3.60	17.1	1.95	—	0.058	0.013	3.8
Milk, with water	100	½ cup	252	3.21	16.3	1.64	—	0.026	0.003	2.8
Brewers Yeast, dry	8	1 tbsp.	25	3.00	17.0	1.40	—	1.250	0.340	—
Nuts										
Almonds, shelled	142	1 cup	850	26.00	332.0	6.70	—	0.340	1.310	—
Brazil nuts	140	1 cup	915	20.00	260.0	4.80	—	1.340	0.170	—
Cashew nuts, roasted	135	1 cup	760	23.00	51.0	5.10	140	0.580	0.330	—
Peanuts, halves	144	1 cup	840	37.00	107.0	3.00	—	0.460	0.190	—
Peanut butter	9	1 tbsp.	55	2.00	7.0	0.20	—	0.030	0.010	—
Pecans, halves	108	1 tbsp.	740	10.00	79.0	2.60	140	0.930	0.140	2.0
Walnuts, black	126	1 cup	790	26.00	—	7.60	380	0.280	0.140	—
Walnuts, English	100	1 cup	650	15.00	99.0	3.10	30	0.330	0.130	3.0
Bean										
Green, raw	100	½ cup	32	1.90	56.0	0.80	600	0.080	0.110	19.0
Green, cooked	100	½ cup	25	1.60	50.0	0.60	540	0.070	0.090	12.0
Soy, raw, immature, shelled	100	⅔ cup	134	10.90	67.0	2.80	690	0.440	0.160	29.0
Soy, cooked, immature, shelled	100	⅔ cup	118	9.80	60.0	2.50	660	0.310	0.130	17.0
Soy bean sprouts, raw	100	1 cup	56	7.90	30.0	1.30	28	0.170	0.140	7.0
Soy, mature seeds, raw	100	1 cup	403	34.10	226.0	2.80	340	0.060	—	2.0
Fruit										
Banana, 6″ × 1½″	150	1	85	1.00	8.0	0.70	190	0.050	0.060	10.0
Avocado, summer	100	⅓ lge.	103	1.40	8.0	0.60	838	0.040	0.117	6.0
Avocado, winter	100	¼ lge.	211	0.20	4.0	0.50	1890	0.050	0.108	4.0
Raisins	160	1 cup	200	1.00	99.0	5.60	30	0.180	0.130	2.0
Papaya, small	97	½	45	0.38	29.0	0.18	1060	0.026	0.042	89.0
Mango	100	1	66	0.50	5.0	0.30	1639	0.037	0.059	70–142
Guava, whole	112	1 med.	73	0.84	10.6	1.67	—	0.041	0.059	78–300
Guava, seeds removed	90	1 med.	50	0.25	13.1	0.26	98	0.050	0.054	90.0

* From the Nutrition Branch, Hawaii State Department of Health, with permission.

17-4 shows the food values of various foods used in vegetarian diets.

NEONATAL NUTRITION

The newborn infant's nutritional requirements must be carefully balanced to include sufficient nutrients, water, and electrolytes to provide for energy and growth, to keep the infant hydrated, and yet not overload his system. The margin for error in infants is rather narrow. Moreover, all infants do not have the same nutritional needs. The size (weight) of the infant and his activity are measures usually used to provide the caloric needs and total fluid requirements. The infant who is breast fed has most of his nutritional requirements met if the mother's nutrition is adequate and her milk supply meets the infant's needs. The addition of iron may be prescribed if the infant was born before his iron stores were fulfilled (prematures, low-birth-weight infants, and twins), and vitamin D, 400 I.U. daily, may be begun at two weeks of age.

When the newborn infant is fed artificially, an attempt is made to modify cow's milk to approximate the composition of human milk. Basically there are three nutritional differences in the composition of cow's and human milk:

	Human milk (%)	*Whole cow's milk* (%)
Protein	1.0–1.5	3.2–4.1
Sugar (lactose)	6.5–7.5	4.5–5.0
Calcium	0.034–0.045	0.122–0.179

The calories per fluid ounce are very similar: 22 calories for human milk, 20 to 21 calories for whole cow's milk. Proprietary milk feedings imitate the composition of breast milk by one or more of the following:

Lowering the protein content

Lowering the mineral content, particularly with regard to calcium

Substituting a vegetable-fat mixture containing more unsaturated fat for the milk fat

Adding carbohydrate, usually lactose, to make up for reduced calories in protein.

NUTRIENTS

Calories. The neonate requires 42 to 50 calories/lb./day (80 to 92 calories/kg./day). Table 17-5 shows ways in which calories are used by the neonate.

TABLE 17-5. Caloric Requirements of the Newborn Period*

Basal metabolic need	48 calories/kg./day
+30% for bodily activity	15 calories/kg./day
+10% for fecal loss	5 calories/kg./day
+12% for specific dynamic action	6 calories/kg./day
+Growth allowance	18 calories/kg./day
Total food requirement	92 calories/kg./day (42 calories/lb./day)

* From Smith, C. A.: *The Physiology of the Newborn Infant,* ed. 3. Charles C Thomas, Springfield, Ill., 1959, with permission.

Protein. 1.5 to 2 g./lb./day (3.5 g./kg./day) are needed. 1 ounce of cow's milk = 1 g. protein. Protein should constitute 10 to 15 per cent of the total calories.

Carbohydrates should constitute 40 to 45 per cent of the total calories. 1 ounce (2 tbsp.) of sugar = 120 calories.

Fat should constitute 30 to 35 per cent of the caloric intake.

Water. The neonate requires 2 to 3 oz./lb./day (8 to 100 ml./kg. on days 1 to 10).

Vitamins. Requirements are: *Vitamin A*, 600 I.U. daily. Human milk, cow's milk, and commercial formulas have sufficient quantities. *Vitamin C*, 25 to 50 mg./day. Breast fed infants need no supplement. Formula fed infants need this supplement as ascorbic acid or orange juice, beginning the second week of life. *Vitamin D*, 400 I.U. daily. Supplementation needed beginning the second week of life.

COMPUTATION OF A FORMULA

The following example shows how these needs can be met through a prepared formula:

Weight of infant: 7 lbs. 8 oz. (7.5 lb.)
Protein
needs: 7.5 lb. × 1.5 g. = 11 g.
Fluid
needs: 7.5 lb. × 2.5 oz. = 19 oz.
Calories
needed: 7.5 lb. × 45.0 Cal. = 337 Cal.
Meeting the protein needs:
11 oz. whole milk
protein (1 oz. = 1 g.) = 11 g.
calories (1 oz. = 20 Cal.) = 220
Meeting fluid needs:
11 oz. milk (listed above) + 8 oz. water = 19 oz.
Meeting caloric needs:
1 oz. (2 tbsp.) sugar = 120 calories
11 oz. milk (listed above) = 220 calories
Total 340 calories

PROPRIETARY FORMULAS

Many liquids and powders are now available which need only the addition of water to make them nutritionally adequate infant feedings. Several of them are reinforced with vitamins and iron. Some examples are Similac, S.M.A., Enfamil, and Bremil. Some are prepared and sold in throwaway nursing bottles, with or without nipples attached.

SPECIAL FORMULAS

Infants who are found to be allergic to cow's milk are ordered formulas made from soybean milk. These are produced commercially under the names of Sobee, Mullsoy, and Soyalac. Goat's milk is also sometimes ordered for these children.

Special formulas are ordered for infants who cannot handle phenylalanine, an amino acid. This condition is known as phenylketonuria (PKU) and such infants are fed a formula known as Lofenalac.

Infants unable to metabolize lactose and galactose because they lack the enzyme galactose-1-phosphate urindyl transferase have a condition known as galactosemia. They are fed Nutramigen or soybean formulas.

REFERENCES

1. Streiff, R. R. and Lutte, A.: *Folic acid deficiency in pregnancy.* N. Engl. J. Med. 276:776, 1967.
2. Reid, D. E., Ryan, K. J. and Benirschke, K.: *Principles and Management of Human Reproduction.* W. B. Saunders, Philadelphia, 1972.
3. Brewer, T. H.: *Human maternal-fetal nutrition.* Obstet. Gynecol. 40:868, 1972.
4. Reid: op. cit.
5. Cross, A. T. and Walsh, H. E.: *Prenatal diet counseling.* J. Reprod. Med. 7:265, 1971.
6. Rosenstock, I. M.: *What research in motivation suggests for public health.* Am. J. Public Health 50:295, 1960.
7. Committee on Maternal Nutrition, Food and Nutrition Board of the National Research Council: *Maternal Nutrition and the Course of Pregnancy.* National Academy of Sciences, Washington, 1970. p. 7.
8. Heald, F. P. and Peckos, P. *Nutrition of adolescents.* Children 11:27, 1964.
9. Pitkin, R. M., et al.: *Maternal nutrition—A selective review of clinical topics.* Obstet. Gynecol. 40:773, 1972.
10. Krause, M. and Hunscher, M.: *Food, Nutrition and Diet Therapy,* ed. 5. W. B. Saunders, Philadelphia, 1972.
11. Snively, W. D., Beshear, D. R. and Roberts, K. T.: *Sodium-restricted diet: review and current status.* Nurs. Forum 13:59, 1974.
12. Pike, R. L. and Smicklas, H. A.: *A reappraisal of sodium restriction during pregnancy.* Int. J. Gynaecol. Obstet. 10:1, 1972.
13. Pitkin: op cit.
14. Register, U. D. and Sonnenberg, L. M.: *The vegetarian diet.* J. Am. Diet Assoc. 62:253, 1973.

BIBLIOGRAPHY

Bowes, C. F. and Church, H. N.: *Food Values of Portions Commonly Used*, ed. 11. J. B. Lippincott, Philadelphia, 1970.

Brazelton, T. Berry: *Assessment of the infant at risk*. Clin. Obstet. Gynecol. 16:361, 1973.

Chesley, L. C.: *Sodium retention and fetal eclampsia*. Am. J. Obstet. Gynecol. 95:127, 1966.

Dahl, L.: *Salt and hypertention*. Am. J. Clin. Nutr. 25:231, 1972.

Ebbs, J. H., Tisdall, F. F. and Scott, W. A.: *The influence of prenatal diet on the mother and child*. J. Nutr. 22:515, 1941.

Flowers, Charles E.: *Nutrition in pregnancy*. J. Reprod. Med. 7:201, 1971.

Food—The Yearbook of Agriculture 1959. The United States Department of Agriculture, Washington, D.C.

Human pregnancy nutrition: a clinical view. Obstet. Gynecol. 30:605, 1967.

Hungerford, M. J.: *Childbirth Education*. Charles C Thomas, Springfield, Ill., 1972.

Jelliffe, D.: *Mothers' milk and other home foods*. The Clinician 37:166, 1973.

Kallen, D. J. (ed.): *Nutrition, Development & Social Behavior*. U. S. Department of Health, Education and Welfare, Washington, D.C., 1973.

Lappe, F. M. *Diet of a Small Planet*. Ballantine Books, New York, 1971.

Miller, H. C. and Hassanein, K.: *Fetal malnutrition in white newborn infants: maternal factors*. Pediatrics 52:504, 1973.

Naeye, R. L., Blanc, W. and Paul, C. *Effects of maternal nutrition on the human fetus*. Pediatrics 52:494, 1973.

Redman, B. K.: *The Process of Patient Teaching in Nursing*. ed. 2. C. V. Mosby, St. Louis, 1972.

Winick, M.: *Malnutrition and brain development*. J. Pediatr. 74:667, 1969.

Winick, M. and Rosso P.: *Head circumference and cellular growth of the brain in normal and marasmic children*. J. Pediatr. 74:774, 1969.

Zamenhof, S., van Marthens, E. and Grauel, L.: *Studies on some factors influencing prenatal brain development*. In R. J. Goss (ed.): *Regulation of Organ and Tissue Growth*. Academic Press, New York, 1972.

Zamenhof, S. and Holzman, G. F.: *Study of correlations between neonatal head circumferences, placental parameters and neonatal body weights*. Obstet. Gynecol. 41:855, 1973.

18 *Genetics*

SHARON J. BINTLIFF, M.D.

The understanding of growth unique to the fetus must begin with an understanding of the interacting influences of genetic factors and environmental experiences. Genetic factors are present at conception and are largely unaltered throughout life (although somatic mutation may occur); environmental experiences are constantly changing. The first and most critical environment for every human being is intrauterine. The general principles of human biologic growth must begin with a discussion of chromosomes, concepts of gene action, control of cell differentiation, and control of growth.

CHROMOSOMES AND CHROMOSOME MUTATION

Man has 23 paired chromosomes in every living cell. These are most clearly seen, with the light microscope, in dividing cells at the metaphase stage. The most accessible and easily studied cell is the blood leukocyte. The study of human chromosomes involves taking a photomicrograph of the chromosome spread from a dividing cell, cutting out the individual chromosomes, and arranging them in pairs. The members of a pair are homologous, complementary in function, and similar in appearance, with the exception of the X and Y chromosomes which are the sex-determining pair in males. According to shape and size, chromosomes are classified into seven groups, A to G, and also numbered from 1 to 22 as shown in Figure 18-1, the twenty-third pair

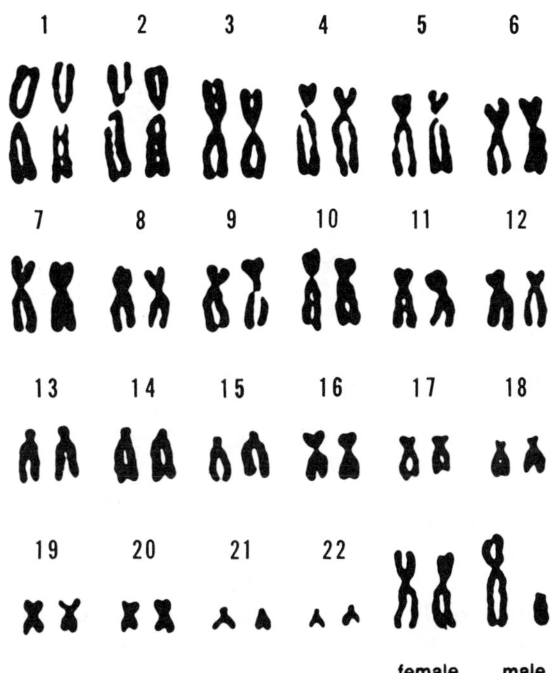

FIGURE 18-1. Paired human chromosomes. (From *Taber's Cyclopedic Medical Dictionary*, ed. 12. F. A. Davis, Philadelphia, 1973, with permission.)

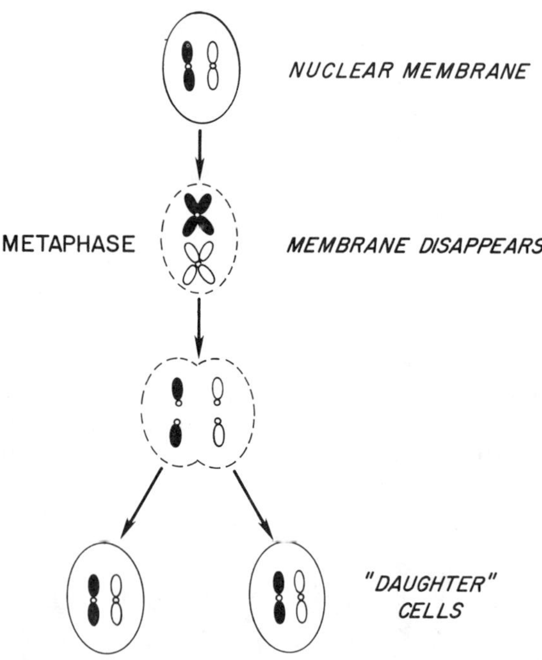

FIGURE 18-2. Cellular division of mitosis.

being the sex chromosomes—XX in women, XY in men.[1] Newer methods of staining now allow us to separate each individual pair within each group.

In somatic cell division (mitosis) the longitudinal separation of each internally replicated chromosome into two chromatids is followed by cell division (Fig. 18-2). As the cell and nucleus divide, the paired chromatids separate and one chromatid passes into each daughter cell and reconstitutes a chromosome. Each daughter cell then has a complete (diploid) set of 23 pairs of chromosomes as did the mother cell. In gamete (germ cell) formation, there are two cell divisions for one division of the chromosome. In the first, the reduction division of the primary spermatocyte (young sperm) or oocyte (young ovum), the chromatids although formed do not separate. Instead, homologous chromosomes pair together and then one member of each chromosome pair enters the daughter cell. The secondary spermatocyte or oocyte thus contains 23 unpaired chromosomes (a haploid set), each split into two chromatids. Then, with the second division, the chromatids separate so that the gametes again contain a haploid set of unpaired chromosomes (Fig. 18-3). In ovum formation, one of the daughter cells produced in both first and second meiotic divisions forms a polar body so that the final product is one and not four ova. With fertilization of the ovum by sperm and the fusion of the two nuclei, the zygote once again has a diploid set of 23 pairs. During pairing, two adjacent chromatids, derived from the homologous chromosomes of a pair, usually exchange genetic material at several points, the other two remaining intact. This process, called crossing over, allows the genes to be recombined in

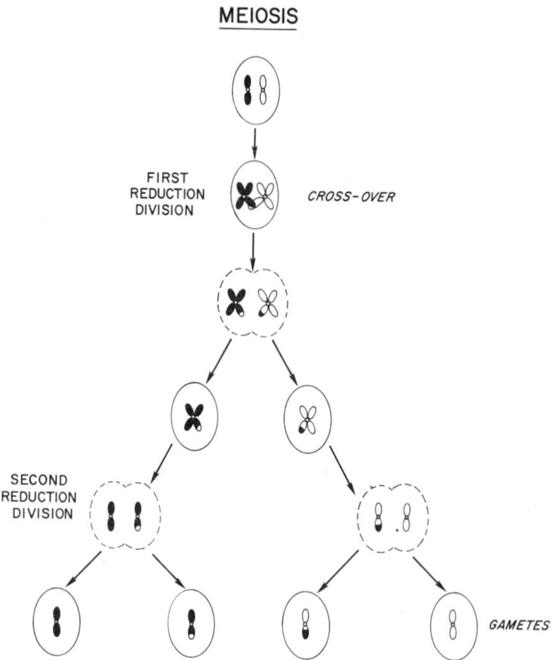

FIGURE 18-3. Cellular division of meiosis.

different ways and thus helps to maintain genetic variability in the offspring.

SEX DETERMINATION

The genetic sex of an individual is determined by the segregation of the father's X and Y chromosomes at the first division of meiosis in sperm formation. At conception, a Y-bearing sperm produces an XY (male) zygote, and an X-bearing sperm produces an XX (female) zygote. The number of X chromosomes present is simply established.

GENES

CHEMICAL STRUCTURE

The genetic information in the chromosomes is now known to be carried in molecules of deoxyribonucleic acid (DNA).[2] These are linked into two strands loosely attached at their bases and twisted round each other in the form of a double-stranded helix, which forms the backbone of the chromosome.

DEFINITION

A gene may be defined in several different ways—as the unit of function (cistron), as the unit of recombination (recon) or as the unit of mutation (muton). The most useful definition is perhaps that of function. In this sense, a gene consists of a length of DNA whose function is to produce a specific protein, polypeptide, which may combine with other polypeptides (produced by other genes) to produce biologically active proteins such as enzymes. There are *structural genes* whose function is to produce messenger ribonucleic acid (RNA) and hence polypeptides or proteins. There are *operator genes*, probably at one end of a series of structural genes, whose function is to activate this production. Another gene, the *regulator gene*, is possibly situated on another chromosome and functions to repress the activity of the operator gene.

NATURE OF MUTATIONS

There is probably more than one type of gene mutation. The most common, however, are true gene mutations and depend on single base substitutions in just one triplet of bases in a structural gene. This mistake in the DNA coding causes the RNA made from this DNA to be incorrect also. Because this messenger RNA is incorrect, the amino acid it is supposed to produce is not made and the subsequent enzyme does not function properly. When an enzyme is made abnormally or not produced at all, the orderly steps in the process of metabolism are disrupted.

MENDELIAN-TYPE INHERITANCE OF MUTANT GENES

Because man is a diploid organism (paired chromosomes), each gene locus has a comparable gene determinant. These pairs of genes are referred to as alleles, or partners, which normally work together. A mutant gene indicates a changed gene. A major mutant gene is defined as a genetic determinant which has been changed in such a way that it can give rise to an abnormal characteristic. If a mutant gene in single dosage gives rise to an abnormal characteristic despite the presence of a normal allele (partner), it is referred to as *dominant* because it causes abnormality even when counterbalanced by a normal gene partner (Fig. 18-4). A mutant gene which only causes an abnormal characteristic when present in double dosage (or single dosage without a normal partner, as for an X-sex linked mutant gene in the male) is referred to as *recessive* (Fig. 18-5). There are gradations of mutant

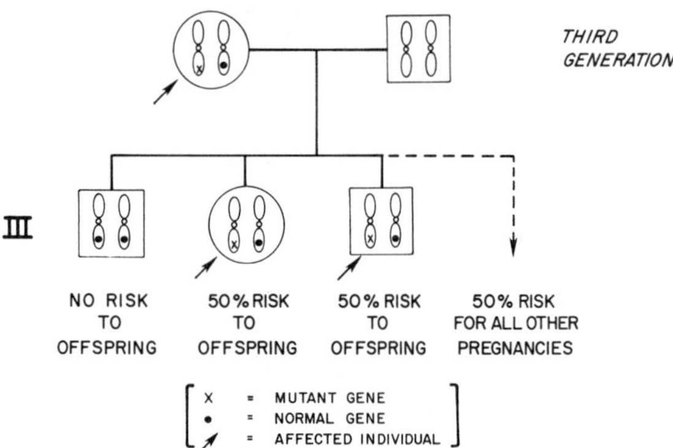

FIGURE 18-4. Dominant inheritance.

genes ranging from those that always cause an abnormal characteristic in single dosage (dominant), to those that occasionally cause some abnormality in single dosage (semi-dominant), to those that never cause an evident alteration except when present in double dosage (recessive).

Expression is a term used to indicate the extent of abnormality that is due to a genetic aberration. The expression may be stated as severe, usual, mild, or no expression, the latter being synonymous with lack of penetrance in an individual who has the genetic aberration.

The basic process of morphogenesis (human development) is genetically controlled, being dependent on the environment for full expression of the genetic potential (for normalcy or disease). This genetic information that guides the morphogenesis and function of an individual is *all* contained within the zygote. After the first few cell divisions, differentiation begins to take place, presumably through activation or inactivation of particular genes, allowing cells to assume diverse roles. The entire process is programmed in a timely and sequential order with little allowance for error, especially in very early development. Despite the almost miraculous breakthrough of genetic coding, relatively little is actually known about the fundamental process that controls morphogenesis. However, the following descriptions and examples of certain normal phenomena known to occur should be helpful.

Cell Migration. This refers to the proper migration of cells to a predestined location critical in the development of many structures. For example, the germ cells move from the

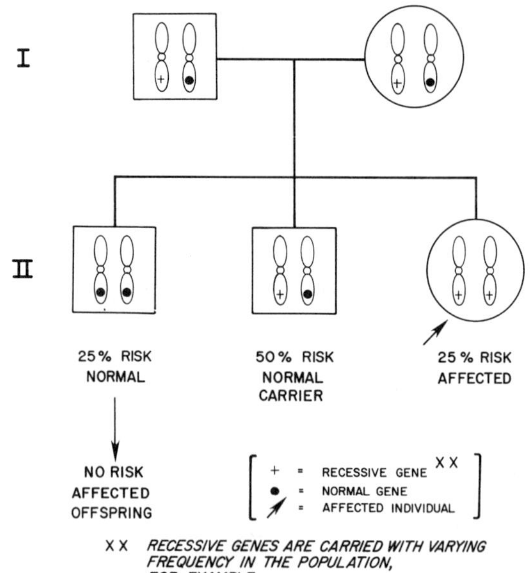

FIGURE 18-5. Recessive inheritance.

yolk sac endoderm to the mesonephric ridge where they interact with other cells to form the gonad (future ovary or testis).

Control over Mitotic rate. The size of particular structures as well as their form is to a large extent the consequence of control over the rates of cell divisions. The control of this mechanism is not yet understood.

Interaction between Adjacent Tissues. Such interactions are essential features in morphogenesis. For example, the optic cup (eye) induces the development of the lens from the overlying ectoderm; the urethral bud induces the development of the kidney from adjacent metonephric.

Adhesive Association of Like Cells. In the development of a structure such as a long bone, the early cells tend to aggregate closely in condensation, a membrane comes to surround them, and only later do they resemble cartilage cells. The association of like cells can be dramatically demonstrated by admixing liver and kidney cells in tissue culture and observing them reaggregate with their own kind.

Hormonal Influence over Fetal Development. Androgen effect is one example of a hormonal influence over morphogenesis, in this case, that of the external genitalia. Normally, the individual with a Y chromosome has testosterone from the fetal testicle which induces enlargement of the phallus, closure of the labis minoral folds to form a penile urethra, and fusion of the labioscrotal folds to form a scrotum. Prior to eight weeks of gestation, the genitalia appear female in type and will remain so unless androgenic hormone is present.

CRITICAL PERIODS OF DEVELOPMENT

The three essential stages of human prenatal development are those of the *ovum*, the *embryo* and the *fetus*. Following fertilization, implantation occurs approximately within the next seven days. The period of the ovum lasts from fertilization until establishment of the primitive villi by about 12 to 14 days of gestation. During this critical period the fertilized egg begins to divide by cleavage into smaller cells, termed blastomeres. In humans, the cleavage divisions are always mitotic, i.e., each daughter cell receives the full double assortment of chromosomes, one set from each parent. These cell divisions occur without much enlargement, the conceptus being dependent on the cytoplasm of the ova for most of its nutritional and metabolic needs. By seven to eight days, the early placenta is functioning both to nourish the embryo and to maintain the pregnancy via its endocrine functions. A major number of genetic and chromosomal abnormalities are spontaneously aborted during this period of the ovum.[3]

The next stage is the embryonic stage which includes the principal events of organogenesis (formation of organs) and lasts until a crown-rump length of approximately 32 mm. is reached by about 54 to 56 days of gestation. During this stage, the embryo is more susceptible to numerous adverse environmental agents which produce serious malformations.

ORGAN DEVELOPMENT

By the fourth week of gestation the embryo is almost straight and the external surface has conspicuous elevations (outline of body somites). The neural tube is closed except for the end nearest the head and part of the way down the "tail." By 24 days, the first (mandibular) and the second (hyoid) branchial arches begin to outline curvatures of the face which later become the upper and lower jaws. A very slight curve is produced in the embryo by the head and tail folds, and the heart has a large single chamber. The lung bud appears for the first time and the kidney and gut are but rudimentary.

Changes in the external appearance of the embryo from the fourth to fifth week are minor except perhaps for enlargement of the head. This is because the brain grows fairly rapidly during this time. Other external features which appear for the first time are the limb buds which by the end of the fifth week show regional differentiation in the uppers only. The heart begins to compartmentalize and the lung buds have branched to bronchi. By the sixth week the brain growth is so extensive as to cause it to bend over the front of the developing embryo. The gut is fairly well developed as are other organs of the abdominal cavity, namely the liver, pancreas, gallbladder, and spleen. By 37 days of age the upper limbs project over the front (area to be chest) and notches appear between the rays in hand plates indicating the future fingers. Although the legs are slower to develop, by now they show knee and ankle joints. It is during this time that the lip fuses in midline, however the palate does not close until the eighth or ninth week. By the seventh week the embryo has unquestionably human characteristics. The remaining 30+ weeks are devoted to organogenesis and growth of the fetus.

CONGENITAL MALFORMATIONS

Congenital malformations (often called "birth defects") refer to malformations present from birth. Although there is no connotation of heredity in the term, it is likely that both genetic inheritance and environmental factors, acting either directly on the fetus or indirectly through the maternal organisms, combine to produce or modify all congenital malformations. Despite considerable progress made in treatment and prevention of most infectious diseases, the number of children with congenital malformations has paradoxically increased. Given the differences reported among various countries, races, types of malformations, and methods of detection, a conservative appraisal shows an incidence of 2 to 3 per cent of all liveborn infants with one or more significant malformations at birth. However, many malformations are not discernible at birth and it is probable that statistics taken at the end of the first year would show this figure to be doubled.

From the data available on the action of teratogenic factors known to be implicated in congenital malformations a few basic principles have emerged:

1. *The stage of embryonic development determines the susceptibility to teratogenic factors, especially in the differentiating stage of the embryo.* The type of malformation produced, then, depends on which organ is differentiating most rapidly at the time of injury. The importance of age and structural specificity to the impact of environmental change has been demonstrated in experiments with rats maintained on a diet deficient in specific amino acids. Nelson and coworkers[4] found that in experimental animals abnormalities of the central nervous system and heart can be produced from days 7 to 9; skeletal, urinary, and cardiovascular abnormalities from days 9 to 11; and other skeletal anomalies from days 11 to 14.

2. *The effect of a teratogen depends on the genotype (genetic makeup).* This principle emerges from the differential susceptibility to the same teratogen observed among species, strains, and individuals. It is probable that the teratogenic agent accentuates the incidence of sporadically occurring defects. For example, when a strain of mice known to consistently produce skeletal abnormalities in approximately 2 per cent of their offspring was starved for 24 hours, skeletal defects increased to 22 per cent.[5]

3. *A teratogenic agent has a specific action at both tissue and cellular levels.* At the tissue level, it may exert its influence at one of three possible sites: the maternal tissue, the placenta, or the embryo itself. At the cellular level, a teratogen may act specifically on a particular aspect of cell

metabolism. Many teratogens produce a characteristic pattern of malformations when applied to a certain species at a specific stage of development.

4. *Many teratogenic agents have little or no pathologic action on the maternal organism.* As stated by Warkany, "so long as it was thought that a mother who appears healthy guarantees complete protection of the infant in utero, obstetrical care was considered adequate for the fetus."[8] However, since there is increasing evidence that the unborn child can be injured by agents well tolerated by the mother, this old belief cannot be upheld. One of the most dramatic examples of the differential sensitivity to drugs between mother and fetus is represented by thalidomide which is nontoxic for the mother but severely teratogenic or lethal for the fetus.

Let us expand this last example to review these concepts of teratogens. The embryo appears to be most sensitive to the effects of thalidomide between the third and eighth weeks after conception. A relatively small dose of the drug (therapeutic dose for mother) taken at this critical period in development is sufficient to cause malformations in the fetus. Some organs undergoing differentiation at this time and the resultant defects are: *head and associated structures*—absence (anotia) or reduced size (microtia) of the ears, facial palsy, clefts of lip or palate, or brain deformities; *limbs*—amelia (absence or malformations of legs or arms) or phocomelia (with or without reduction in number of fingers or toes); *heart*–atrial septal defects or ventricular septal defects. The actual pharmacologic action that produces these defects is unknown, but it is postulated that the drug acts as a metabolic inhibitor. It appears that drugs with molecular weight of 1,000 or less easily cross the placental barrier, and some of these may act upon fetal development in different ways and with different effects of varying intensity, e.g., fetal death, metabolic changes resulting in anatomic malformations, alterations in fetal growth and neonatal adjustment, as well as delayed postnatal effects.[7]

Malformations are divided into two general categories: those which represent a single, primary localized defect in morphogenesis in an otherwise normal infant, and those which represent multiple defects in one or more systems.

SINGLE DEFECTS

A single, localized defect in early development can upset the subsequent development of other structures and result in a baby with more than one anomaly at birth. A good example is the fact that failure of closure of the lip by 35 days of gestation may secondarily affect the closure of the palatal shelves at eight to nine weeks and result in both cleft lip and palate deformities. A primary defect of the neural groove, the structure destined to form the spinal cord and vertebra, can result in spina bifida or meningomyelocele which may also cause neurologic clubfeet, paraplegia, and bladder and bowel incontinence based on neurologic deficit. The most common single defects which occur in our population, each with an incidence of about 0.5 to 1 per 1,000 babies delivered, are defects of the neural groove (meningomyelocele), cleft lip with or without cleft palate, cleft palate alone, cardiac septal defects, dislocation of the hip, clubfeet, and pyloric stenosis. Together these comprise nearly half the number of defects recognized as serious in early life. Indirect evidence implicates polygenic inheritance, the combined effect of many minor gene differences, as the predominant mode of origin of these anomalies. The X or Y chromosome appears to contain at least some of the genes which exert an influence on the likelihood of these anomalies, none of which has an equal sex incidence. For example, pyloric stenosis is five times more likely to occur in the male,

TABLE 18-1. Recurrence Risk for Some Common Single Malformations*

Malformation	*Parents unaffected, have one child with defect: Risk for other offspring (%)*	*One of parents affected: Risk for any offspring (%)*
Cleft lip with or without cleft palate	4.9	4.3
Cleft palate alone	2.0	6.0
Club foot	2.8	
Anencephaly	3.4	
Meningomyelocele	4.8	
Dislocated hip	3.5 {Brothers 0.5, Sisters 6.3}	
Pyloric stenosis	3.2 {Brothers 4.0, Sisters 2.4}	Father affected 4.6 Mother affected 16.2

* From Smith.[8]

whereas dislocation of the hip is five times more likely to occur in the female. Part of the evidence favoring polygenic inheritance is the nonrandom occurrence of the same kind of defect in close relatives (Table 18-1). Although there are indications that environmental factors exert a role, no single environmental factor has yet been implicated as a common main cause of any one of the foregoing malformations. Hence, one must presently be very cautious about implying to a mother that any particular environmental factor during her pregnancy was responsible for a malformation in her infant.

MULTIPLE DEFECTS

Approximately 1 in 150 babies has multiple defects, and roughly half of them have a recognized clinical entity, a "syndrome." There are over 150 such syndromes, and with the exception of Down's syndrome (mongolism, trisomy 21) which has an incidence of 1:660 and XXY syndrome with an incidence of 1:500 males, no other syndrome occurs with a frequency greater than 1:3000.

With few exceptions, a clinical diagnosis of Down's syndrome or XXY syndrome in the neonatal period cannot be made on the basis of a single defect. Rather, the diagnosis depends on the total pattern of defect. Many minor anomalies, such as inner epicanthal fold of the eye, incomplete development (or flattening) of the upper part of the ear, or a single palmar crease on the hands, are nonspecific indicators of altered morphogenesis and may be found as features in several syndromes of widely variant origin. Genetic alterations, usually single gene mutations or chromosomal aberrations, appear to be the predominant cause of the recognized malformation syndromes. The majority of these gene defects, especially the autosomal-dominant, serious syndromes, represent a fresh gene mutation from unaffected parents whose recurrence risk is negligible. Occasionally (1 to 2 per cent of cases), chromosomal abnormalities are hereditary and one of the parents will be found to be a balanced translocation carrier with a high recurrence risk.

DETECTION OF GENETIC DISORDERS OF THE FETUS

A great deal of knowledge has accumulated recently on the natural history of many genetic disorders. In order to intervene for the prevention of these defects, early identification of the susceptible and/or affected parent is mandatory. The successful utilization of the technique of transabdominal aminocentesis for the detection and management of Rh disease has demonstrated the feasibility and safety of intrauterine diagnosis.

Amniocentesis now has been performed over 1,000 times, collectively, in numerous major centers during the fifteenth to twentieth weeks of pregnancy for the management of genetic high-risk patients. During these weeks there is approximately 150 to 200 cc. of amniotic fluid. The cellular material found in this fluid is derived from the amnion and fetus. These cells can be used for sex chromatin analysis which is useful for the management of pregnancies in women who carry X-linked recessive disorders such as hemophilia and muscular dystrophy. The chromosomes in the unborn fetus can be analyzed and cellular enzymes can be studied. The disorders which call for application of this new technique are rare, but the results for individual pregnancies at risk are overwhelmingly successful.

REFERENCES

1. National Foundation—March of Dimes: *Standardization in Human Cytogenetics.* Paris Conference, 1971 VIII:7, 1972.
2. Watson, J. D. and Crick, F. H. C.: Nature (London) 171:737, 1953.
3. Arakaki, D. T. and Waxman, S. J.: *Chromosome abnormalities in early spontaneous abortions.* J. Med. Genet. 7:118, 1970.
4. Nelson, M. W., et al.: *Multiple congenital abnormalities resulting from transitory deficiency of pteroylglutomic acid during gestation in rats.* J. Nutr. 56:349, 1955.
5. Runner, M. N.: *Inheritance of susceptibility to congenital deformity: Metabolic clues provided by experiments with teratogenic agents.* Pediatrics 23:245, 1959.
6. Warkany, J.: *Congenital malformations and pediatrics.* Pediatrics 19:725, 1957.
7. Smithells, R. W.: *Drugs and Human Malformations, Advances in Teratology*, vol. 1. Logas Press, London, 1966.
8. Smith, D. W.: *Patterns of Human Malformations.* W. B. Saunders, Philadelphia, 1970.

BIBLIOGRAPHY

Carter, C. O.: *An ABC of Medical Genetics.* Little, Brown and Company, Boston, 1969.

Dunn, L. C.: *A Short History of Genetics.* McGraw-Hill, New York, 1965.

McKusick, V. A.: *Human Genetics*, ed. 2. Prentice-Hall, Englewood Cliffs, 1969.

Smith, D. W.: *Recognizable Patterns of Human Malformations.* W. B. Saunders, Philadelphia, 1970.

Strickberger, M. W.: *Genetics.* Macmillan, New York, 1968.

Sturtevant, A. H.: *A History of Genetics.* Harper and Row, New York, 1965.

19 *Transport of Essential Elements in Fetal-Neonatal System*

SUK KI HONG, M.D., Ph.D.

The fetus is completely dependent on an aqueous environment provided by the mother for the supply of oxygen and nutrients which are transferred across the placenta. This requires a special circulatory system and a unique system for gas exchange which is similar to the gill of the fish. At birth, the newborn infant is suddenly removed from this dependence on the mother and dramatically adjusts to extrauterine life by establishing pulmonary respiration. The infant initiates many other anatomic and physiologic readjustments within minutes, hours, days and months to achieve a completely independent life.

CARDIOVASCULAR FUNCTIONS

FETAL CIRCULATION

The heart in all vertebrates is formed by the fusion of two symmetrically developing tubes, which in turn evolve from the splanchnic mesodermal cells in humans after approximately two weeks of gestation. This fusion is complete in three to four weeks, when the heart is a single tube within a tube. From the fifth to seventh weeks, a series of developments occur to form the four chambers which characterize the human heart. However, it should be pointed out that the two atria continue to communicate through the foramen ovale which is situated in the interatrial wall (septum secundum) and is covered by a flap-like valve (septum primum). Since the right atrial pressure is greater than the left atrial pressure, blood flows from right to left in these chambers of the fetal heart. At birth, the two atrial pressures become equal so that the septa secundum and primum are kept in contact and eventually fuse together. Likewise, the pulmonary artery and the aorta communicate with each other during fetal life, in this case via the ductus arteriosus, a vessel which is obliterated after birth. The fetal heart attains its permanent structural features two months prior to birth.

Because the fetus must maintain the blood flow to the placenta in order to obtain oxygen and nutrients, and to remove carbon dioxide and other waste products, the circulatory system of the fetus has several unique features, such as the presence of the foramen ovale and the ductus arteriosus. The fetal blood reaches the placenta via the two umbilical arteries and returns to the fetus via the umbilical vein. Some of the oxygenated blood in the umbilical vein passes through the liver and is conveyed to the inferior vena cava. However, a significant portion of this oxygenated blood bypasses the liver and enters the inferior vena cava directly through the ductus venosus. Thus, the blood in the inferior vena cava is an admixture of the well-oxygenated blood (80 per cent HbO_2) carried by the ductus venosus, the less well-oxygenated blood of the hepatic veins, and the very poorly-oxygenated blood (26 per cent HbO_2) returning from the lower limbs and the abdominal wall. Nevertheless, this admixture is relatively well-oxygenated (67 per cent HbO_2) compared with the blood in the superior vena cava (31 per cent HbO_2) which drains from the head and upper limbs.

The blood from the superior vena cava passes directly into the right ventricle through the right atrioventricular orifice. However, the blood from the inferior vena cava divides into two streams, one (approximately one third) directed into the right ventricle and the other (approximately two thirds) into the left atrium through the foramen ovale. This unique arrangement assures that the more-oxygenated blood enters the systemic circulation.

The less well-oxygenated blood entering the right ventricle is distributed to the lungs in small quantity (approximately 30 per cent of right cardiac output) by the pulmonary arteries and returned from the lungs to the left atrium via the pulmonary veins. This is because of the high pulmonary vascular resistance of the fetal lung, partially due to its limited degree of expansion. The greater portion of the right cardiac output is shunted into the descending aorta by way of the ducus arteriosus. Approximately 25 per cent of the blood flow through the descending aorta is distributed to the lower limbs and the viscera of the abdomen and pelvis. The remainder (75 per cent) is conveyed to the placenta via the umbilical arteries.

As shown in Table 19-1, the relative volume of blood flow through the placenta via the umbilical arteries is 55 per cent compared with only 12 per cent through the lungs. Thus, both the placenta, which can be viewed as a relatively "low-resistance circuit," and the lungs, which can be viewed as a "high-resistance circuit," are in parallel with the fetal tissues.

TABLE 19-1. Relative Volume of Blood Flow through Main Vessels in the Fetus*

Vessels	*Blood Flow (%)*
Total cardiac output	100
Left cardiac output	58
Right cardiac output	42
Ascending aorta	15
Descending aorta	73 (including 30% from the ductus areriosus)
Pulmonary artery	12
Umbilical artery	55
Foramen ovale (shunt from right to left atrium)	46

* Based on data of Dawes, Mott, and Widdicombe.[14]

It is generally agreed that the fetal heart begins to beat (about 65 beats per minute) at approximately the fourth week after conception, before the development of the conducting system. The heartbeat increases to 140 per minute before birth. Fetal heart sounds become strong enough to be heard by the eighteenth week. It is difficult to evaluate the performance of the fetal heart, especially during the early stages of development. The most widely used approach is electrocardiographic (ECG) evaluation, which is used as a means of early detection and treatment of intrauterine cardiac disturbance. It is of interest to note that between 4 and 10 weeks the ECG wave pattern is the reverse of the adult ECG pattern, indicating a reverse in the relative cephalocaudal position of ventricle and atrium between embryo and adult.

CIRCULATORY ADJUSTMENTS AT BIRTH

Toward the end of intrauterine life, fetal circulation is potentially self-sufficient and the lungs have reached a degree of development compatible with their future postnatal role. Upon delivery, the umbilical circulation through the placenta is arrested and, at the same time, the lungs expand. The arrest of the umbilical blood flow resulting from the constriction of the umbilical vessels decreases the amount of blood flowing in the inferior vena cava. As stated earlier, the umbilical blood flow represents as much as half of the entire combined ventricular output. Therefore, the removal of this huge vascular bed at birth must sharply increase the systemic arterial blood pressure and, at least for an interval of readjustment, decrease the right atrial pressure due to the reduced blood flow through the inferior vena cava. On the other hand, the onset of respiration suddenly changes the volume and physical state of the lungs with an equally abrupt reduction of pulmonary vascular resistance and a proportionate increase of pulmonary blood flow. The result is a rise in the left atrial pressure and a further lowering of the right atrial and right ventricular pressures. The combination of these events reverses the pressure difference across the valve (septum primum) covering the foramen ovale, thereby closing this passage (Fig. 19-1). It is generally accepted that the relatively complete "functional closure" of the valve of the foramen ovale takes place within an hour after birth. The valve fuses over the foramen ovale within a few months to years after birth.

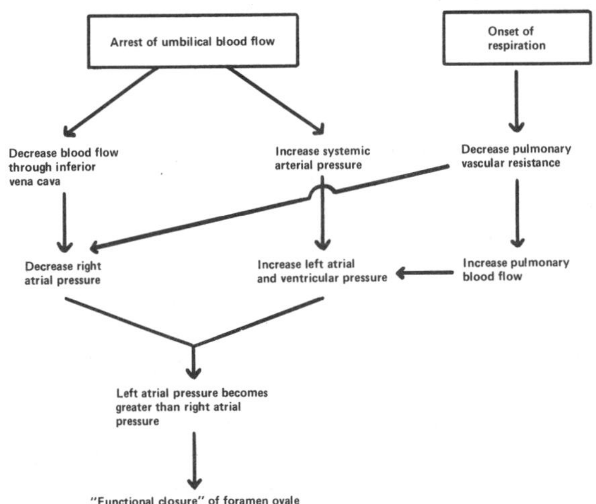

FIGURE 19-1. Chain of events leading to the closure of the foramen ovale after birth.

The second important adjustment of the cardiovascular system after birth is the functional closure of the ductus arteriosus. Unlike the foramen ovale, the ductus arteriosus has no valve to respond passively to pressure changes arising elsewhere, yet it appears capable of constricting sufficiently to reduce or prevent the flow of blood through this "fetal shunt" within hours after birth. Exactly how this closure is brought about is not clearly understood. One widely accepted view is that the closure of the ductus arteriosus essentially depends upon the direct vasoconstrictor effect of increased oxygen tension in the blood, an event that is not mediated by neurogenic or humoral mechanisms.[1] Thus, any interference with blood oxygenation might contribute to the maintenance of a patent ductus arteriosus. Compared with the rapid closure of the foramen ovale at birth, the closure of the ductus arteriosus is relatively slow. It may remain patent for hours or days after birth in some apparently normal infants. The flow through it during this time reverses to go from the aorta to the pulmonary artery and lungs. This flow is the consequence of the aortic pressure becoming much greater than the pulmonary arterial pressure after birth, and could provide a shunt of several hundred milliliters of blood per minute.[2] A permanent patent ductus arteriosus is seen in one in every 2,000 to 3,000 infants.

Pulmonary vascular resistance decreases from an assumed fetal value of 8,000 to 550 dyne-seconds per cm.$^{-5}$ within a few hours after delivery. It further decreases to the adult level by six months of age. Such a dramatic reduction in pulmonary vascular resistance at birth is associated with mechanical factors related to expansion of the alveoli, and possibly to changes in the geometry of the pulmonary vessels. In addition, the increase in oxygen tension also contributes to this lowering of pulmonary vascular resistance. Consequently, faulty oxygenation of the blood may result in high pulmonary vascular resistance and patency of the ductus arteriosus, and possibly, the foramen ovale.

The systemic arterial pressure initially falls, probably due to the change in direction of ductus arterious blood flow from the aorta to the pulmonary artery. It then recovers and slowly increases. The mean aortic pressure in infants 2 to 28 hours old is 56 ± 8 mm. Hg. With the rise in arterial blood pressure, there is a simultaneous fall in heart rate. The magnitude and duration of the reduction in heart rate (a fall of 10 to 30 beats per minute on the first extrauterine day) depend largely on the onset of effective breathing and adequate blood oxygenation. Once these are accomplished, the heart rate increases again but usually remains somewhat below fetal levels. The concomitant decline in body temperature has also been considered a cause of this initial heart rate reduction. The average cardiac output is approximately 550 ml. per minute. The neonatal ECG essentially resembles the fetal ECG. Compared with the adult, the duration of the P wave and the P-R interval are much shorter in the fetus and neonate, suggesting a faster atrial depolarization and conduction through the atrioventricular node. The amplitude of the waves is also smaller in the newborn and the infant than in the adult.

RESPIRATORY FUNCTIONS

FETAL RESPIRATION

The site of respiratory gas exchange in the fetus is the placenta. Here the venous blood in the umbilical artery gains oxygen and loses carbon dioxide before leaving via the umbilical vein as oxygenated blood. The fetal lungs do not participate in gas exchange although respiratory movements commence at the end of the first trimester. The basic process of gas exchange across the placenta is strictly a diffusion which transfers a gas in proportion to the difference in partial pressure. According to Fick's law of diffusion:

$$\text{Amount of gas transferred} = \text{diffusion constant} \times \frac{\text{surface area}}{\text{thickness of membrane}} \times \text{time} \times \text{partial pressure difference}$$

Placental permeability is relatively low until 8 to 12 weeks of gestation due to the small surface area and great thickness of the membrane. From 12 to 32 weeks of gestation, the surface area increases while the membrane becomes thinner and hence the placental permeability progressively increases. However, the permeability decreases somewhat during the last two months due to deterioration of the placenta. In addition to these morphologic changes, the placenta is a metabolically active tissue which constantly consumes oxygen at a high rate. Due to these and other complications, it is very difficult to clearly evaluate the process of gas exchange across the placenta, and there are many conflicts concerning the quantitative aspects of gas exchange.

During normal pregnancy, the average oxygen partial pressure (Po_2) of blood on the maternal side of the placenta (intervillous space) is estimated to be approximately 40 mm. Hg compared with 30 mm. Hg for blood leaving the placenta and returning to the fetus (umbilical vein). The best estimate of Po_2 of blood in the umbilical arteries is approximately 20 mm. Hg. Thus, gas equilibration between fetal and maternal circulation does not seem to be achieved during passage through the villous capillaries of the placenta. In the lung of a normal man at rest, gas equilibration takes place well before the blood has passed the full length of the alveolar capillary. Reasons for such a lack of gas equilibration across the placenta are not clear. Possible explainations include the presence of real diffusion barriers, or an artifact arising from 1) uneven distribution of placental blood flow, 2) possible differences in the directions of flow on either side of the placenta, or 3) the oxygen consumption of the placenta. Whatever may be the reason, this inadequate gas equilibration is demonstrable even for carbon dioxide, which is 20 times more diffusible than oxygen. The estimated carbon dioxide partial pressure (P_{CO_2}) of blood in the umbilical vein is 42 mm. Hg compared with 37 mm. Hg in the intervillous space. The P_{CO_2} of blood in the umbilical arteries is approximately 46 mm. Hg.

Although the degree of reliability of estimated values for partial pressures of various gases in the fetal blood has been questioned, it is generally agreed that the P_{O_2} of blood perfusing various organs is much lower in the fetus than in the mother. As discussed previously, oxygenated blood leaving the placenta via the umbilical vein is mixed with less-oxygenated blood before it reaches the left heart and hence the P_{O_2} of blood in the aorta is expected to be somewhat lower than 30 mm. Hg. Such a low P_{O_2} is not compatible with life in the adult, but seems to be sufficient in the fetus. Evidently, fetal blood carries sufficient amounts of oxygen even at such a low P_{O_2}. Indeed, actual measurements indicate that the oxygen content of fetal blood at P_{O_2} of 22 mm. Hg is 10.6 vol. % (ml. per 100 ml. blood), which is about 3 vol. % higher than that of adult blood at comparable P_{O_2}. In other words, the fetal blood has a higher oxygen carrying capacity. This is attributed to the higher affinity of fetal hemoglobin for oxygen and the higher concentration of hemoglobin in fetal blood.

The fact that fetal hemoglobin has a higher affinity for oxygen is illustrated in Figure 19-2. The HbO_2 dissociation curve of fetal blood is quite similar in shape to that of adult blood but

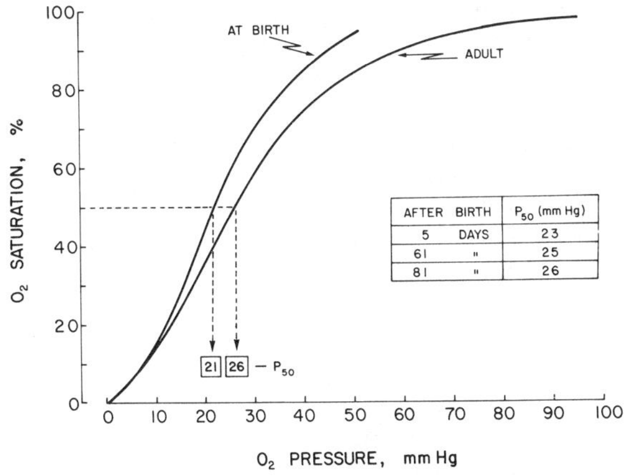

FIGURE 19-2. Oxygen dissociation curves of adult and fetal hemoglobin. (Based on data in *Biologic Handbook—Blood and Other Body Fluids.*[19])

is shifted to the left of the adult curve. This means that in fetal blood more oxygen molecules are bound to hemoglobin at a given level of P_{O_2}. In adult blood, 50 per cent of hemoglobin in the blood is bound to oxygen at P_{O_2} of approximately 26 mm. Hg. (This is expressed as P_{50} = 26 mm. Hg.) However, the P_{50} for fetal blood at the time of birth is approximately 21 mm. Hg. This difference in P_{50} between adult fetal blood may seem small but it could provide 10 to 30 per cent more oxygen for the fetus depending upon the level of P_{O_2}. This unique HbO_2 dissociation curve of fetal blood is due to the different chemistries of the fetal and adult hemoglobin molecule. The heme portion of fetal hemoglobin (hemoglobin F) is the same as that of adult hemoglobin (hemoglobin A), but the arrangement and composition of the globins (and perhaps the linkage between globin and heme) are apparently different. The two hemoglobins have the same molecular weight but have different solubilities, amino acid compositions, and other characteristics. However, it should be noted that some hemoglobin A is present in the blood of the fetus from 5 to 6 months of gestation onward, and there is a small amount (0.5 to 1 per cent) of hemoglobin F in the blood of normal adults. It is generally agreed that a relatively higher proportion of hemoglobin is in the F than in the A form in premature infants compared with term infants. On the average, the blood of a normal term baby has 85 per cent hemoglobin F content, compared with 65 per cent in the postmature baby. Hemoglobin F is gradually replaced by hemoglobin A beginning in the latter half or third of fetal life. However, there are many unanswered questions concerning this transition. Biologically, it is also of great importance to know how the organism can make one type of hemoglobin during fetal life and then replace it with another type after birth. Teleologically, fetal hemoglobin is an adaptation to the relative hypoxia of intrauterine life and is an aid to the transplacental passage of oxygen.

The concentration of hemoglobin in the blood at birth is approximately 18 g. % compared with approximately 15 g. % in normal adults. This also accounts for an estimated 20 per cent increase in the capacity of blood to carry oxygen at a given level of PO_2 in the fetus and neonate.

Despite these advantages of fetal blood for carrying oxygen, the oxygen content of arterial blood is only about 10 vol. % compared with nearly 20 vol. % in the adult. This is primarily due to the extremely low PO_2 of fetal blood.

Both PCO_2 and the CO_2 content of the fetal blood before or at birth are slightly greater than those of the maternal blood. However, the difference is not of sufficient magnitude to warrant further discussion.

RESPIRATORY CHANGES AT BIRTH

For more than a century, the argument has raged whether the fetus does, indeed, make respiratory movements in utero which are merely interrupted by the birth process, or whether the first extrauterine gasp for air represents the infant's "first breath."

At delivery, the newborn infant is removed from its warm, moist environment where its weight was supported by surrounding fluid. It is squashed and squeezed in its passage through the birth canal and thrust into a cool environment where it is assaulted by light, noise, and tactile sensations. The first act of the newborn in extrauterine life is to establish breathing in order to gain oxygen and lose carbon dioxide. The exact mechanisms responsible for the onset of breathing are still a matter of debate but are generally ascribed to reflexes and a number of environmental stimuli (such as touch or coldness) acting synergistically on the respiratory centers in the central nervous system. In general, respiratory function is established in two steps: the first consists of the initial gasp for air (within 6 to 10 seconds after birth) and the second involves the maintenance of rhythmic breathing activity which is qualitatively similar to that of the adult. Recently, it has been pointed out that the surge of thyroid activity in the newborn may lower the threshold of the respiratory center, thus increasing brain excitability and, in turn, rendering the respiratory center more sensitive to incoming stimuli.[3] In the past, changes in blood gas tensions (PO_2 and PCO_2) and pH have also been implicated in the onset and establishment of normal rhythmic respiratory movements. Moderate fetal hypoxemia (low PO_2) or hypercapnia (high PCO_2) induced by giving low oxygen or high CO_2 mixtures to the mother seems to have little effect of respiratory activity, whereas severe hypoxemia may cause premature gasping or ultimately depress pre-existing respiratory activity. During normal labor and delivery, PCO_2 rises while PO_2 and pH fall.[4] However, these blood gas changes normally do not incite gasping respirations until shortly after birth. There seems to be inhibition of chemoreceptor activity until that time. Newer studies have demonstrated that incoming cold and tactile stimuli accompaning birth activate or sensitize the chemoreceptors in the aortic and carotid body by way of the sympathetic nervous system. The effect of the relatively small changes in blood gases are then magnified and contribute significantly to the onset and establishment of rhythmic respirations by way of chemoreceptor impulses going to the respiratory center.

One of the first obstacles the infant must overcome at birth is the presence of liquid in the lungs. This fluid was once thought to be aspirated amniotic fluid, but this view has recently been disproved. It now appears that the lung fluid is formed within the alveolar spaces by a process of ultrafiltration, active secretion, or a combination of both.[5] Due to the high resistance of this fluid, extreme forces are required to open the alveoli for the first time. During the first inspiration, the lungs do not expand until the intrathoracic pressure reaches −40 cm. H_2O, and only 40 ml. of air enters the lungs as the pressure increases to −60 cm. H_2O. Similarly, about +40 cm. H_2O of pressure is needed to deflate the lungs during the first expiration. It takes approximately 40 minutes after birth for breathing to become normal. Removal of this fluid appears to be quite rapid since the functional residual capacity of the lungs rises to a near normal value of 25 to 30 ml. per kg. body weight within 15 minutes. It should be noted that normally this fluid contains a high concentration of lipid called surfactant (a surface-active material capable of reducing the surface tension forces at the air-fluid interface in the alveoli) without which the alveoli would collapse and respiratory distress would develop. This occurs in hyaline membrane disease which is extremely common in premature babies and those born of mothers who have type A, B or C diabetes mellitus.

Various respiratory functions of the newborn during steady state breathing are shown in Table 19-2. The vital capacity, inspiratory capacity, and total lung capacity per kg. body weight are approximately 20 per cent smaller in the newborn than in the adult. However, there is no significant difference in the values for residual volume, expiratory reserve volume, and functional residual capacity per kg.

TABLE 19-2. Comparison of Lung Volumes in the Newborn and Adult*

	Newborn (2.5 kg.)		*Adult (72.5 kg.)*	
Lung Volumes	*ml.*	*ml./kg.*	*ml.*	*ml./kg.*
Residual volume	35	14	1,190	6
Expiratory reserve volume	35	14	980	14
Inspiratory capacity	105	42	3,790	52
Vital capacity	140	56	4,780	66
Total lung capacity	175	70	5,970	82
Functional residual capacity	70	28	2,180	30

* Newborn values based on data of Cook et al.,[15] adult values based on data of Comroe et al.[16]

body weight between the newborn and the adult. These findings suggest that the inspiratory muscle is not able to function fully at birth. Since the metabolic demand per kg. body weight is nearly twice as high in the newborn as in the adult, pulmonary ventilation is expected to be correspondingly higher in the newborn. As shown in Table 19-3, this is accomplished not by increasing the tidal volume but by increasing the rate of breathing. Pulmonary ventilation is twice as high in the newborn as in the adult, thereby maintaining a comparable level of ventilatory equivalent regardless of age. This means that in the newborn the work of breathing must be higher and

TABLE 19-3. Comparison of Pulmonary Ventilation and Gas Exchange in the Newborn and Adult*

	Newborn	*Adult*
Tidal volume, ml./kg.	6	7
Respiratory rate/min.	40	15
Minute volume, ml./min./kg.	240	105
Dead space ventilatin, ml./min./kg.	88	33
Alveolar ventilatin, ml./min./kg.	152	72
Oxygen consumption, ml./min./kg.	6	3
Ventilatory equivalent (min. vol./O_2 consump.), ml./100 ml.	0.04	0.35

* Newborn values based on data of Cook et al.[15] and Dawes,[17] adult values based on data of Comroe et al.[16]

the efficiency of alveolar ventilation lower. In the adult, the resting rate of respiration is maintained at about 15 per minute, since the work of breathing is minimal at this rate. It is possible that, given the particular resistances of the newborn infant's lung, the work of breathing is likewise minimal at the respiratory rate of about 40 per minute in the infant.

Associated with the onset of breathing at birth is the filling of pulmonary capillaries with blood. Moreover, the diffusion of gas across the alveolar-capillary membrane appears to be satisfactory in the newborn. The oxygen saturation of hemoglobin is somewhat low (50 to 60 per cent) during the first 5 to 10 minutes after birth, and then increases rapidly to 90 per cent. The PCO_2 of arterial blood is soon maintained at about 35 mm. Hg.

Although the issue is still disputed, it appears that certain respiratory reflexes such as the Hering-Breuer inflation and deflation reflexes, coughing and tactile-respiratory reflexes are well developed at birth. This is also true of Head's paradoxical reflex which causes a gasp when the lungs are quickly expanded.

In clinical practice, any use of oxygen raises certain questions of safety. It is now accepted that exposure of premature infants to high oxygen concentrations can induce oxygen damage to the eyes, characterized by retinal vascular changes which may be followed by permanent blindness. Oxygen concentrations that maintain PO_2 between 50 to 80 mm. Hg are considered reasonably safe for small premature infants.

HEMATOLOGY

BLOOD VOLUME

Although a considerable portion of the total blood volume is in the placenta and umbilical vessels during fetal life, neither the amount nor the percentage of the total volume have been measured during human fetal life. According to indirect measurements, the placental circuit contains 125 to 150 ml. of blood at the moment of birth, which can be compared with a total blood volume of approximately 300 ml. in the term baby a few hours after birth. The average blood volume of the newborn is estimated to be 85 ml. per kg. body weight, consisting of 41 ml. of plasma and 44 ml. of red blood cell mass. Typical adult values are 78 ml. per kg. body weight for the blood volume, and 48 ml. and 30 ml. for plasma and red blood cell mass, respectively. Thus, the newborn has a greater blood volume (about 10 per cent) and red blood cell mass (about 20 per cent) and a smaller plasma volume (about 20 per cent) than the adult, when expressed per kg. body weight. The premature infant has a greater blood volume (approximately 108 ml. per kg. body weight) than the mature infant, largely due to a greater plasma volume (approximately 62 ml. per kg. body weight) rather than the red blood cell mass.

ERYTHROCYTES AND HEMOGLOBIN

Although the fundamental purpose of fetal hematopoiesis is the development of the type and number of blood cells suitable for life after birth, this process may be altered to some extent by the conditions of intrauterine oxygen supply. As discussed previously, the PO_2 of arterial blood is quite low in the fetus, and thus, if anything, the fetus is exposed to some degree of hypoxia. This hypoxic condition may be aggravated as activity of the developing fetus increases. The nucleated erythrocyte begins to form in yoke sac and mesothelial layers of the placenta at about the third week of gestation. At about the fourth week, the non-nucleated erythrocyte begins to form in the fetal mesenchyme and in the endothelium of the fetal blood vessels. At about the sixth week, the liver begins to participate in hematopoiesis. The spleen and other lymphoid tissues also begin forming blood cells at about the third month, after which the bone marrow begins to take over the hematopoietic function. After three months of fetal life, the erythrocyte count is approximately 1.1 million per mm.[3], the hemoglobin concentration is 9.3 g. %, and the hematocrit is about 25 per cent. It is interesting that at this stage the erythrocyte is more than twice as large (about 200 μ^3) as the adult cell (about 80 μ^3), and that approximately 20 per cent of erythrocytes at this stage are reticulocytes. During the rest of fetal life, the erythrocyte count, hemoglobin concentration, and hematocrit ratio increase while the size of erythrocytes and percentage of reticulocytes decrease continuously until birth. At birth, the erythrocyte count (and hence, the hemoglobin concentration and hematocrit ratio) is 10 to 15 per cent higher than the adult level. This may result from a temporary stimulation of hematopoiesis due to the limited oxygen supply during the last one to two months of gestation.

As shown in Figure 19-3, the erythrocyte count (5.7 million per mm.[3] at birth) decreases to 4.5 million per mm.[3] by 2 to 4 months after birth and then gradually increases again to the adult level. Similar trends are observed for the hemoglobin concentration and hematocrit ratio. Thus, between 2 months and 2 years of age, the infant seems to go through a stage of slight anemia. At birth, reticulocytes account for approximately 5 per cent of the total erythrocytes present. The size of the erythrocytes also decreases continuously after birth for 4 months. The hemoglobin concentration in the erythrocyte (38 g. per 100 ml. erythrocyte at birth) decreases continuously to 33 g. per 100 ml. erythrocyte at 2 years of age.

This postnatal recession is not necessarily a sign of inadequate blood production, and the resultant fall in hemoglobin content should not be considered a handicap with which the newborn infant is forced to begin life. Actually, the previous rapid rate of blood formation appears to cease because the stimulus for production is removed. The improved oxygenation made possible by pulmonary respiration suddenly removes the stimulus to red cell formation.[6] In addition, the life span of blood cells from newborns appears to be considerably shorter than the life span of blood cells from adults.

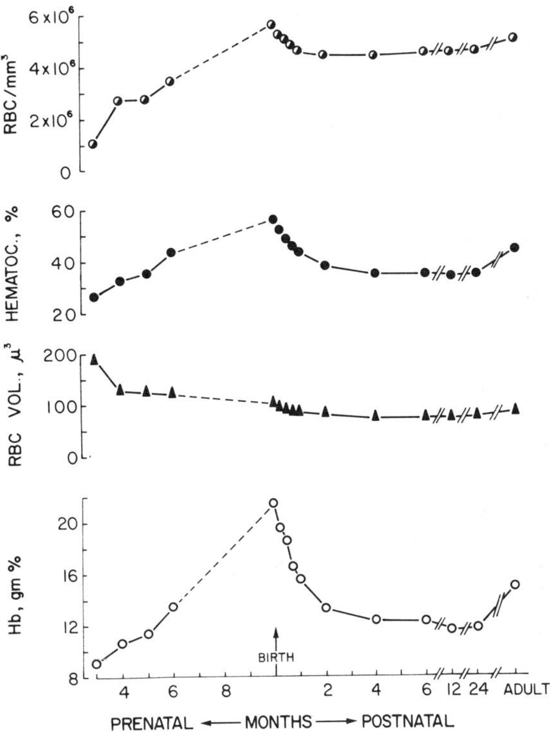

FIGURE 19-3. Various hematologic data obtained before and after birth. (Based on data in *Biologic Handbook—Blood and Other Body Fluids.*[19])

LEUKOCYTES

It is generally accepted that the total leukocyte count is elevated to about 18,000 per mm.[3] blood at birth, and further increases to about 23,000 per mm.[3] at 12 hours of age. Subsequently, the leukocyte count decreases to about 11,000 per mm.^{3} within 2 weeks and is maintained at this level for at least 2 years. Such a high leukocyte count at and immediately following birth is ascribed mainly to a high polymorphonucleocyte count which accounts for 60 to 70 per cent of the total leukocytes at birth, but only about 35 per cent 2 weeks after birth. Other leukocytes do not show any consistent change after birth.

The total leukocyte count of the premature infant is lower than that of the term infant. Moreover, the circulating blood of premature infants has a larger proportion of immature leukocytes than that of term infants. Little is known of the leukocyte in fetal blood. These differences are probably due to changes in the bone marrow activity, but there is no clear explanation concerning the mechanism. Teleologically, however, the observed leukocytosis at birth may be interpreted as a rapid, temporary adjustment of the defense mechanism upon sudden transition from sterile intrauterine life.

BLOOD COAGULATION

The platelet count at birth appears to be within the usual adult range, although it tends to increase slowly during the following six months. However, the prothrombin time is usually prolonged in the newborn, especially during the first two to four days. This is related to changes in the level of prothrombin, which is reduced in umbilical cord blood (though the prothrombin level of maternal blood may be elevated) and definitely tends to decrease further between two and four days after birth. The level of proconvertin undergoes changes similar to those in the level of prothrombin. In this connection, it is important to note that vitamin K administered to the mother before birth or to the newborn prevents the fall of prothrombin and proconvertin levels after birth. The fibrinogen level of the blood appears to be normal in the newborn infant.

RENAL FUNCTIONS AND BODY FLUID

RENAL STRUCTURE AND FUNCTIONS

The number of nephrons increases throughout gestation, reaching the full component of 822,000 by birth. The developmental changes occur gradually. Nephrons in all stages of development can be found in the fetal kidney until 35 weeks of gestation. In general, by 11 to 13 weeks, 20 per cent of the nephrons are relatively mature in morphologic terms; by 16 to 20 weeks, the proportion increases to 30 per cent; and at 35 weeks, all the nephrons have morphologic characteristics of the adult type. However, the dimensions of different sections of the nephrons as well as the relative growth of one section over another or with respect to the whole nephron, still change significantly after birth. For example, the proximal tubular length and the glomerular diameter are known to increase progressively from birth to adulthood. In general, the population of proximal tubules is less uniform in size in immature kidneys than in those of children older than 3 to 5 years and adults. It is also important to note that the loop of Henle is not fully differentiated until after birth.

Consistent with the anatomic immaturity of the glomerular membrane in the fetus and newborn, the glomerular filtration rate (as measured by inulin clearance, C_{IN}) during these periods (about 30 ml. per minute per 1.73 m.^{2}) is below that of the adult, but increases rapidly so that by the first week of life it is one half of the adult value. It attains the adult level (about 125 ml. per minute per 1.73 m.^{2}) within the first year of life. The characteristically low glomerular filtration rate of the developing kidney is partly due to the arterial pressure, which increases less than 50 per cent during the first year of life. This is in contrast to the glomerular filtration rate, which increases fourfold to fivefold. The renal plasma flow (as measured by para-aminohippurate clearance, C_{PAH}) is also low in the developing kidney: approximately 150 to 200 ml. per minute per 1.73 m.^{2} in the newborn, compared with 650 ml. in the adult. Several reports indicate that the filtration fraction (C_{IN}/C_{PAH}) is higher in the newborn, suggesting a greater reduction of renal blood flow than of glomerular filtration rate. However, the implication of low glomerular filtration rate in the newborn must be evaluated carefully in light of evidence which indicates a heterogeneity of glomerular functions. It appears that the juxtamedullary glomeruli are more functional early in development when those of the cortex are functionally limited. This means that as more and more of the cortical glomeruli become functional the glomerular filtration rate of the whole kidney would increase.

Detailed assessment of tubular functions in the developing kidney is difficult because appropriate experimental techniques are not readily available. The available data indicate that the percentage of the glomerular filtrate reabsorbed by the tubules is lower in the immature kidney than in the mature kidney. For example, whereas about 75 per cent of the filtered urea is excreted by the newborn, only 50 per cent is excreted by the adult. The poor tubular function in the developing kidney is more clearly illustrated by lower values of maximal glucose reabsorption (Tm_G) and PAH secretion (Tm_{PAH}). In the newborn, Tm_G is 60 mg. per minute per 1.73 m.^{2} (350 mg. in the adult) and Tm_{PAH} is 25 mg. per minute per 1.73 m.^{2} (75 mg. in the adult). The low value of Tm_G observed in the newborn cannot be fully accounted for by the low glomerular filtration rate. It takes about one year for these low values of Tm_G and Tm_{PAH} in the newborn to attain the adult levels. Tubular function is usually less well developed than glomerular function at birth. Strangely enough, the tubular reabsorption of amino acids seems to be well developed in the newborn when appropriate corrections are made for the low glomerular filtration rate. Similarly, the fractional reabsorption of the filtered sodium chloride (i.e., the percentage of sodium chloride in the filtrate reabsorbed by the tubule) in the newborn is comparable to that in the adult. The latter conclusion is based on the fact that the newborn infant has as low a sodium chloride clearance as the adult. However, this does not necessarily mean that the intrinsic reabsorptive capacity of the tubule for sodium is the same for both the newborn and the adult. As stated earlier, the glomerular filtration rate in the developing kidney is very low and hence the transit time (time needed for the filtrate to flow through the entire length of tubular structure) is expected to be longer than in the adult kidney. Since the tubular reabsorption of sodium is limited by the concentration gradient and the time, the low intrinsic reabsorptive capacity of the kidney in the newborn could be compensated by the high transit time for reabsorption, thereby maintaining the fractional reabsorption of sodium at a level comparable to that of the adult kidney.[7] The tubular reabsorption of bicarbonate and phosphate, and the tubular secretion of hydrogen ion and ammonia are also lower in the developing kidney than in the adult kidney.

It may be possible to increase the tubular function in the newborn to the adult level. Hirsch and Hook[8] reported that the tubular secretion of PAH in the newborn could be enhanced by treating the mother with penicillin prior to delivery. Since penicillin is secreted by the tubule by the same process as PAH, the above finding could mean that penicillin enhances the development of the existing tubular transport process or the synthesis of new enzyme proteins responsible for organic acid (such as PAH) transport. This observation may also help to explain why the tubular functions are generally low in the newborn. Many tubular transport systems are active and thus require metabolic energy supply and participation of specific enzymes. Therefore, it has been proposed that the poor tubular function in the newborn may be due to inadequate development of related enzyme systems. Many studies support this hypothesis. For example, the levels of sodium-potassium-activated adenosine triphosphatase, which appear to be involved in the active transport of sodium, are almost absent in the rabbit at birth but approach the adult level by 5 weeks of age. In addition, the activities of carbonic anhydrase (involved in hydrogen ion secretion) and glutaminase (involved in ammonia secretion) are low at birth but increase rapidly during early postnatal life. In this connection, it is of interest to note that enzymatic activity in the medullary tubules of the newborn is remarkably high compared with the adult, suggesting that the poor development of tubular functions in the cortex may be counterbalanced to some extent by the overdevelopment of tubular functions in the medulla.

One of the most important functions of the kidney in man is to conserve water. This is accomplished by excreting a hypertonic urine with the help of antidiuretic hormone (ADH) which increases the water permeability of the collecting duct. In dehydrated or ADH-treated subjects, the reabsorption of water from the collecting duct lumen into the interstitium is determined by the osmotic gradient across the collecting duct wall. Maximal osmolarity of urine is approximately 1,200 to 1,400 mOsm./l. in the adult. Since plasma osmolarity is about 300 mOsm./l., the maximal urine to plasma osmolar ratio is approximately 4.0. In contrast, infants during the first weeks after birth rarely concentrate their urines much above 600 mOsm./l. In fact, most urine collected within the first 48 hours is considerably more dilute than this, even when no water has been given. However, improvement is rapid and the maximal urine osmolarity increases to nearly 1,000 mOsm./l. by the eleventh day. This inability of the neonatal kidney to concentrate urine is not due to an insufficiency of ADH, for the newborn is known to produce ADH in response to various stimuli such as dehydration or an increase in plasma osmolarity. It may be that the newborn kidney is less sensitive to ADH than that of the adult. In fact, the magnitude of increase in urine osmolarity to a given dose of ADH is much lower in the newborn than in the adult. However, the reasons underlying the purported insensitivity of the neonatal kidney to ADH are not clear. One reason could be an inadequate response of the collecting duct wall to ADH. As stated earlier, ADH increases the water permeability of the collecting duct wall, possibly by stimulating the activity of adenyl cyclase in the membrane and thus increasing the intracellular concentration of cyclic adenosine monophosphate which somehow enhances water permeability. Many enzyme systems are not fully developed in the newborn, and it is possible that the adenyl cyclase system may also belong to this group. The second possibility is that the collecting duct is sensitive to ADH but the osmotic gradient across the collecting duct wall is less in the newborn than the adult. As mentioned earlier, the loop of Henle is not fully developed at birth. Thus, the kidney of the newborn is not equipped with a countercurrent system as efficient as that in the adult, and thus fails to build up an adequate medullary osmotic gradient. Actual measurements of medullary osmolarity indicate that this is the case. However, another important reason for the lower medullary osmotic gradient in the newborn is that the high anabolic state results in the low rate of urea excretion, which in turn limits the magnitude of medullary osmotic gradient. When an infant is fed urea, or a high-protein diet, a marked increase in concentrating ability occurs.

The ability to eliminate excess amounts of water or salt is another important function of the kidney. When the adult ingests a certain amount of water, the ADH system is inhibited as a result of the reduction in plasma osmolarity and water reabsorption in the collecting duct is suppressed, thereby temporarily increasing the urine flow. This phenomenon is called *water diuresis* and is characterized by a reduction of urine osmolarity to a level well below 300 mOsm./l., often 50 to 70 mOsm./l. The amount of extra urine output is equivalent to the amount ingested and the response usually lasts for 90 to 120 minutes. The newborn does not have this diuretic response to water loading.[9] Although there is some diuresis, this subsides before 50 to 60 per cent of the water load is excreted and the extent of reduction in urine osmolarity is much less than in the adult. Even after five days of age, although the diuretic response of the infant is comparable to that of the adult in terms of the degree of urinary dilution, the rate of urine flow lags.[10] It usually takes about one month before the infant can eliminate a water load as efficiently as the adult. Similarly, the newborn is not able to eliminate a salt load as efficiently as the adult. For example, following administration of hypertonic saline, both the rate of diuresis induced and the volume of urine excreted are much lower in the infant than in the adult.

As discussed previously, the glomerular filtration rate is very low in the newborn and this may be responsible for the inability to eliminate a given water or solute load. However, the actual mechanisms of this phenomenon are not fully understood. It is true that salt-retaining hormones, such as aldosterone, are present in relatively high concentrations in the newborn and induce sodium chloride reabsorption in situations in which the adult kidney would excrete it.

In summary, to quote Adolph: "Renal systems show independent maturations of several excretory activities and of several modes of arousal of those activities. Each activity matures according to its own schedule of development and, at present, no common onset can be found."[11]

BODY FLUID VOLUME AND COMPOSITION

As shown in Table 19-4, at 5 months of gestation (fetal weight of approximately 200 g.) the total body fluid represents approximately 87 per cent of body weight, and the major portion is extracellular fluid. As the fetus grows, both the total body fluid volume and extracellular fluid volume decrease progressively while the intracellular fluid volume increases. This process continues after birth, more or less leveling off at the age of 1 to 3 years. Not shown in this table is the phenomenon of *postnatal weight loss* occurring immediately after birth. This weight loss, mainly due to the fluid loss after birth, is essentially limited to the 72 hours following birth, and averages about 7 per cent of body weight. The material lost consists of meconium, water (as urine prenatally and postnatally formed, and insensible water loss from the lungs and skins), some vernix caseosa from the body surface, the occasionally vomited amniotic fluid swallowed before or during birth, and the fat, protein, glycogen, and glucose consumed for energy.[12]

TABLE 19-4. Body Fluid Volume (per cent Body Weight) as a Function of Age*

Age	*Total Body Fluid*	*Extracellular Fluid*	*Intracellular Fluid*
Fetal			
5 months	87	62	25
7 months	83	56	27
10 months	75	40	35
Postnatal			
3 months	70	30	40
6 months	67	28	39
1 year	65	25	40
3 years	65	23	42
10 years	62	22	45
Adult	65	20	45

* Based on data of Friis-Hansen.[18]

The decrease in extracellular fluid volume and the concomitant increase in intracellular water during development are the result of the relative growth and expansion of the cells that occupy a proportionately larger part of the body as the organism grows. It is also possible that the increase in the intracellular fluid volume with age may reflect the intracellular increase in nondiffusible proteins and other osmotically active substances within the cell. The high volume of extracellular fluid early in development has been taken to indicate low renal control during this period and possible lack of response of volume receptors and/or osmoreceptors.

The concentrations of sodium and chloride are essentially the same in the serum of the immature fetus and the term infant as in the adult. However, the concentration of potassium in the serum of the immature fetus is about 10 mEq. per liter, compared with 6 and 5 in the term infant and adult, respectively. Since the extracellular fluid volume per unit body weight is considerably larger in the infant than in the adult, the above findings mean that the distribution of potassium in the fetal body is quite different from that in the adult. For some reason the fetal cell seems less able than the adult cell to maintain its potassium against the concentration gradient. The intracellular sodium concentration is approximately 50 mEq. per liter in the fetus at 5 months and 25 in the term infant, compared with 10 in the adult. These findings suggest that the sodium-potassium-activated adenosine triphosphatase is not fully developed in the fetus, and as a result, the distribution of sodium and potassium across the cell membrane is different from that in the adult. The concentrations of bicarbonate and proteins in the serum are slightly lower in the immature fetus than in the adult, but are close to adult values in the term infant. In contrast, the serum concentration of divalent ions (calcium and magnesium) do not appear to undergo such marked changes during the transition from fetal life to adulthood. The serum concentration of inorganic phosphorus is subject to a great deal of variation depending upon either the ease with which the delivery is made or the nutritional state of the infant. For example, when delivery has been easy, phosphorus concentration may scarcely rise, whereas if the baby has been subjected to trauma or anoxia, the resultant starvation and injury to cells may lead to a marked increase in phosphorus concentration.[13] In addition, the phosphorus concentration declines in infants who are breast fed, but increases continually in infants fed cow's milk. The concentration of urea and other nonprotein nitrogenous compounds is maintained in the newborn at a level similar to that in the adult.

Serum iron is low (20 to 40 μg. %) during the first 6 months of gestation but rises significantly during the last 3 months to reach a level of 160 μg. %. However, in the first 24 hours after birth, the iron level decreases to about 50 μg. % and then rises again during the next 2 weeks. The significance of these complicated changes is not fully understood.

ACID-BASE BALANCE

During fetal life, acid-base balance is largely controlled through the placenta by the maternal lungs and kidneys. However, indirect evidence indicates that the hydrogen secretory mechanisms and ammonia-producing system are present in the fetal kidney, although at a low level of efficiency. In the first days of life, urine is rarely acidic and the average pH is 7.0. However, during the first 10 days the urine pH decreases continuously to reach the adult level of about 5.0. This reduction in urine pH following birth is not accompanied by other changes known to normally control the elimination of hydrogen ions. For example, the phosphate-excretion and ammonia-producing systems are not well developed in very young (one week old) infants. In other words, the urine pH could be lowered soon after birth, but the amount of hydrogen excreted per unit time seems to be rather low.

The above findings suggest that the developing kidney is not able to eliminate the fixed acid load which is continuously produced by tissue and delivered to the kidney for excretion. This is indeed the case, as shown by the low bicarbonate concentration and pH in the plasma of infants relative to those found in advance stages of childhood. Thus, the newborn seems to be in a state of slight metabolic acidosis. Measurements of blood P_{CO_2} in the newborn indicate approximate values of 34 to 35 mm. Hg for arterial blood and 37 to 38 for venous blood. These are about 5 mm. Hg lower than the corresponding values in the adult. It has been proposed that these findings suggest a relative hyperventilation, perhaps in response to metabolic acidosis.

REFERENCES

1. Moss, A. J., Emmanouilides, G. C., Adams, F. H. and Chuang, K.: *Response of ductus arteriosus and pulmonary and systemic arterial pressure to changes in oxygen environment in newborn infants.* Pediatrics 33:937, 1964.
2. Smith, C. A.: *The Physiology of the Newborn Infant*, ed. 4. Charles C Thomas, Springfield, 1975.
3. Timiras, P. S.: *Developmental Physiology and Aging.* Macmillan, New York, 1972.
4. Engström, L., et al.: *The Onset of Respiration.* Association for the Aid of Crippled Children, New York, 1966.
5. Adams, F. H., Fijiwara, T. and Rowsham, G.: *The nature and origin of the fluid in the fetal lamb lung.* J. Pediatr. 63:881, 1963.
6. Smith: op. cit.
7. Capek, K., et al.: *Regulation of proximal tubular reabsorption in early postnatal period of infant rats.* Proceedings of the XXIV International Congress of Physiological Sciences, 1968, p. 72.
8. Hirsch, G. H. and Hook, J. B.: *Maturation of renal organic acid transport: substrate stimulation by penicillin.* Science 165:909, 1969.
9. McCance, R. A., Naylor, N. J. B. and Widdowson, E. M.: *The response of infants to a large dose of water.* Arch. Dis. Child. 29:104, 1954.
10. Barnett, H. L., et al.: *Renal water excretion in premature infants.* J. Clin. Invest. 31:1069, 1952.
11. Adolph, E. F.: *Origin of Physiological Regulations.* Academic Press, New York, 1968, p. 89.
12. Smith: op. cit.
13. Timiras: op. cit.
14. Dawes, G. S., Mott, J. C. and Widdicombe, J. M.: *The foetal circulation in the lamb.* J. Pediatr. 126:563, 1954.
15. Cook, C. D., et al.: *Apnea and respiratory distress in the newborn infant.* New Engl. J. Med. 254:562, 1956.
16. Comroe, J. H., et al: *The Lung–Clinical Physiology and Pulmonary Function Tests*, ed. 2. Year Book Medical Publishers, Chicago, 1962.
17. Dawes, G. S.: *Foetal and Neonatal Physiology—A Comparative Study of the Changes at Birth.* Year Book Publishers, Chicago, 1968.
18. Friis-Hansen, B.: *Changes in body water compartments during growth.* Acta Pediatr. (Suppl. 110) 46:1, 1957.
19. Altman, P. L. and Dittmer, D. S. (eds.): *Biological Handbook–Blood and Other Body Fluids.* Federation of American Societies for Experimental Biology, Washington, 1971.

BIBLIOGRAPHY

Adolph, E. F.: *Origin of Physiological Regulations.* Academic Press, New York, 1968.

Dawes, G. S.: *Foetal and Neonatal Physiology—A Comparative Study of the Changes at Birth.* Year Book Publishers, Chicago, 1968.

Patten, B. M.: *Human Embryology.* McGraw-Hill, New York, 1968.

Smith, C. A.: *The Physiology of the Newborn Infant*, ed. 4. Charles C Thomas, Springfield, 1975.

Timiras, P.S.: *Developmental Physiology and Aging.* Macmillan, New York, 1972.

Willams, P. L. and Wendall-Smith, C. D.: *Basic Human Embryology.* J. B. Lippincott, Philadelphia, 1966.

UNIT 5

THE PRENATAL PERIOD

20 Application of Psychosocial Concepts

ANN L. CLARK, R.N., M.A.

THE FAMILY

A study of childbearing must begin with a focus on the family since maternal and child health care nursing is family-centered. A *family* is defined as *a unit of interacting persons whose central objective is to create and maintain a common culture and to promote the physical, mental, and social development of each member.*

Family structure has changed over the ages. In America, until recently the typial family was known as an *extended family*, and consisted of a number of generations living within one household. Today the typical American family consists of a mother, father, and one or more chldren. This *nuclear family*, as it is termed, most often lives in a family dwelling of its own. The extended family (grandparents, aunts, uncles, cousins) may live nearby or they may live many hundreds of miles away.

In the latter half of the twentieth century we are seeing some drastic changes in family life, some of which seem to threaten the very concept of marriage and family living. The family has traditionally performed certain functions:

Reproduction
Care and protection of children
Socialization of children
Economic production of family goods and services
Recreation
Love and emotional support.

Other agencies have increasingly taken over some of these functions. Schools, government, and industry have moved in to supersede the family.[1] However, in three areas of traditional family life there has been a minimum of intrusion: reproduction, child care, and the meeting of affectional needs. Even in these areas, family planning and the culture's attitudes toward family size and population growth intrude upon reproduction. Many mothers, even of very young children, are employed, thus changing the manner in which child care is being managed. The day-care center is a new institution. Thus, love remains as a function that truly justifies the institution of marriage and family—or does it? There are those who believe that marriage is obsolete. Barth writes:

> Marriage, if you think about it, is now no more than a ceremonial vestige of a by-gone era. It was a useful accommodation to the time when a woman had no means of gaining a livelihood save as a temporary or permanent companion to some man, when pregnancy seemed a nearly inescapable consequence of that relationship and when, from the man's point of view, a woman was an almost indispensable household appurtenance or possession.[2]

He suggests that a license, authorizing a man and woman to live together, is no longer a business of the government (religious solemnization of the pact would be up to the couple).

Dissatisfaction with the traditional family structure, or perhaps inability to cope with it, has caused thousands to set up counter-culture family structures. But these, too, are not new. The commune is as old as antiquity, it is merely new for twentieth century America. In these groups, children grow up, not in nuclear families, but in clusters, and a number of adults may assume some responsibility for the child care community.

Doubts about conventional family life have also led to the growth of another phenomenon: the single-parent family. Society has modified its ostracism of the unmarried woman raising her child. This has reduced her feeling that she should have an abortion, give the child up, or marry to "give the child a name," the latter often ending in disaster for all. Other forms of the single-parent family are due to paternal abandonment, death, or divorce. Liberalized adoption laws also make it possible for single men and women to become parents.

Re-examination of the traditional family and the desire to try other forms have also produced the trio marriage. Such households consist of one husband and two wives or one wife and two husbands. Chores, child care, and other family responsibilities and needs are shared. There are even larger groups functioning in a similar manner. However,

> Such eccentric arrangements obviously have no meaning for the vast majority of people, except perhaps as symptoms of an underlying malaise. Thus while sociologists and anthropologists make their plea for reordering the social structure, most are more immediately concerned with removing—or at least alleviating—the stresses of the nuclear family.[3]

For nurses, structural changes within the family are significant, since most types of families will have contact with nurses during the childbearing phase of life. The nurse needs to identify these various family units; not to label them, but to understand their methods for meeting the functions of the family as outlined earlier (reproduction, care and protection of children, socialization of children, economic production of family goods and services, recreation, and love and emotional support).

FAMILY STRENGTHS

In all types of families it is important to assess for family strengths. Family strengths keep the unit from disorganizing and are necessary components in the resolution of crises which every family must face. It is important to recognize these strengths and utilize them fully. According to Otto,[4] family strengths include:

> Ability to provide for the physical, emotional and spiritual needs of a family (includes food, shelter, utilization of space, provisions for family health, the giving of love and affection, understanding and trust, providing an environment of honesty and integrity).
>
> Ability to be *sensitive* to the needs of all family members.
>
> Ability to communicate effectively (includes depth of feelings and emotions as well as communication of ideas, concepts, beliefs and values).
>
> Ability to provide support, security, and encouragement (especially important is the encouragement to seek new areas of growth, to develop creativity, imagination, and independent thinking).
>
> Ability to initiate and maintain growth-producing relationships and experiences within and without the family.
>
> Capacity to maintain and create constructive and responsible community relationships in the neighborhood, school, town, local and state government.

Ability to grow with and through the children.

Ability for self-help and ability to accept help when appropriate.

Ability to perform family roles flexibly (to fill in and assume another's role when necessary).

Mutual respect for the individuality of family members.

Ability to use crisis or seemingly injurious experience as a means of growth.

Concern for family unity, loyalty, and interpersonal cooperation.

This framework can assist the nurse in obtaining an improved and comprehensive understanding of the family in terms of some clearly distinguishable strength dimensions. It is a further dimension of assessment useful to the nursing process.

Although, as discussed earlier, there is a swelling of voices against state licensing of marriages, these same voices are raised to demand that certain qualifications be evident and that a license be issued before a cohabiting couple are allowed to introduce a new member into society. Barth states:

> When a man and a woman decide they would like to reproduce, they ought to be required to . . . obtain a license or permit to do so. Such a license should not be granted quite as casually as marriage licenses have been issued in the past. Exacting qualifications ought to be set for parenthood. . . . These applicants ought to be required to prove emotional maturity, good health and financial responsibility . . . the new member of the community would have a good start in life . . . with a happy home and loving parents.[5]

Mead[6] suggests a "two step marriage" for young people. The first step would in effect be a trial marriage during which the young people would agree not to have children. If a stable relationship develops and the couple decide to have children, a second license would be obtained.

American family structure will undoubtedly undergo additional changes in the future. However, at present, we are still the most married and home-oriented nation in the modern world. In the 1960s, the number of U. S. families grew at a greater rate than the population. Eighty-seven per cent of Americans live in families that include both parents. Although the divorce rate is rising, so is the rate of remarriage among divorced people. Thus, the nuclear model will remain the basic family structure in the United States for some time.[7]

The family picture comes into focus when all members of the family and other persons intensely involved in the family's affairs are viewed as bound together as parts of the whole. Behaviors, thoughts, and feelings expressed by any part of the whole affect the state of the whole. Changes in one part of the whole are followed by changes in other parts.

The control concept of this theory is the undifferentiated *family ego mass.* This is a conglomerate emotional oneness that exists in all levels of intensity. Each person is confined in a network of interlocking relationships.

The family must be viewed as consisting of many different kinds of subsystems. Examples include the social system, cultural system, "games" system, communication system, and biologic system (reproduction). It is important for nurses to understand the components of these systems, for changes or "breakdowns" of any family system will influence the way the family handles stress and crisis. The childbearing experience always involves the maturational crisis of childbearing and often situational crises as well. Nurses must assess the "state of health" of all systems in order to take appropriate action. Indeed, without this assessment nursing actions may be very inappropriate.

SOCIAL CHANGES

There are many social changes which affect

the contemporary family. Some of those most relevant to childbearing and childrearing are discussed here.

As stated previously, we are a nation of nuclear families. This means that the same family unit lives in somewhat of a vacuum. Since the extended family relationships are less intense, more of the needs of all members must be satisfied by the nuclear family. This increases the physical and emotional demands made on each member. For example, there are fewer people available to help with household and child-care duties, and fewer cues on ways to cope with stress are available to family members.

The community also makes many demands on family members which draw on their time. This leaves less time for the family to be together. Thus, what may be good for a community may not necessarily be good for a specific family.

Work obligations limit the amount of time that the father is able to spend with his family. There is also considerable pressure on him to move up in business. The mother, too, is changing due to more liberal views on the woman's role. More mothers are working outside the home and thus are less available to their children. Women feel less fulfilled by homemaking and more dissatisfied with the role of housewife. For the first time in history, they can control conception and even do so without their husband's knowledge.

Marriage is becoming an association of complementary equals. A new kind of sexual companionship is developing in marriage. Authority patterns are changing both in family life generally and in childrearing. No longer is the father the uncontested authority with the wife and children carrying out his commands.

FAMILY DEVELOPMENTAL TASKS

Families grow through predictable stages in the family life cycle. As the family grows, each member must assume additional roles in order to successfully relate. The component parts of the role are known as developmental tasks of an individual.

The family life cycle begins with the *establishment phase*. The couple assume the roles of husband and wife and each must master the developmental tasks in a complementary manner and resolve conflicting possibilities. It is important that they suceed at these tasks for each family must successfully achieve the developmental tasks of each phase in order to move on to the next phase. The remainder of this chapter pertains to the second phase in the family life cycle, the *expectant phase*.

The developmental tasks of the expectant family according to Duvall[8] are:

1. Reorganizing house arrangements to provide for the expectant baby.
2. Developing new patterns for getting and spending income.
3. Re-evaluating procedures for determining who does what and where authority rests.
4. Adapting patterns of sexual relationships to pregnancy.
5. Expanding communication system of present and anticipated emotional constellation.
6. Reorienting relationships with relatives.
7. Adapting relationships with friends, associates, and community activities to the realities of pregnancy.
8. Acquiring knowledge about and planning for the specifics of pregnancy, childbirth, and parenthood.
9. Testing and maintaining a workable philosophy of life.

Each of these developmental tasks involves role preparation on the part of the expectant parents.

All roles are learned. Most are learned unconsciously through the process of growing up in a family. We come to "know" what is expected of us in a given role by the verbal and nonverbal cues we detect. We also learn, in a similar manner, how our role partner should respond. These roles must be complementary and reciprocal if family harmony is to be maintained.

The role of the expectant mother is different from that of the expectant father, both physiologically and psychologically. This chapter focuses on the psychologic adaptation to pregnancy and the preparation for parenthood.

PREGNANCY AND THE FAMILY

The ego mass of a family binds it in such a way that there is an emotional oneness. This response is acutely revealed when a woman becomes pregnant.

> Intermeshed with every woman's own personal drama is another which is found in the reactions she creates within her tiny segment of society—her family. Her open and subtle indications of acceptance, ambivalence, or rejection of her condition inevitably stirs up responses and repercussions among her family, relatives, and friends. They, in turn, set up reactions within the individual woman, which are indeed consequent to the reactions she perceives among her key reference group.[9]

Thus, it is necessary to explore the impact of pregnancy on individuals within a family. We need to know more about a mother's response to pregnancy and the etiology of that response. We need to know how the husband is affected, how the siblings are affected, and even what effects may be transmitted to the fetus. Finally, we need to know what differences the nurse can make in the life of the expectant family and how she can use the process of nursing to protect, nurture and stimulate.

PREGNANCY AND THE WOMAN

FEMININE IDENTITY

> Adequacy and pride in . . . femininity provides the expectant mother with a foundation for accepting the pregnancy and the integration of the new maternal identification. Conversely, lack of confidence in . . . feminine identity and . . . consequent inability to freely enjoy a potentially pleasant reality may find expressions in negative and unpleasant fantasy.[10]

Positive and negative attitudes about pregnancy have a number of causative factors, but basically, for a positive attitude to be present, the expectant mother must be comfortable with her sexuality.[11] Pregnancy may be entered with many fantasies and concerns not only about femininity and feminine functions but specifically about being pregnant and becoming a mother. This may cause considerable suffering and account for anxiety during the pregnancy.

The enlarged breasts and increasing size of the abdomen may be an embarrassing demonstration of the woman's sexuality. Women vary greatly in their feelings about their changing body image (Fig. 20-1). Some are proud of their gravid body, others are uncomfortable with it or even ashamed of it. The reflections of others, particularly the husband, also influence the woman's feelings about this change. Toward the end of pregnancy women frequently feel heavy and ungainly. They become impatient with their bodies. They may view their bodies as grotesque and yearn to return to their former size and shape.

Women facing motherhood think deeply about their ability to love a child and be loved by a child. They are concerned about how the coming of a child will change their life and their relationship with other family members, particularly the husband. If there is another child in the family, they may feel guilty about breaking that special bond with the older child by the addition of a new member. They may worry about sibling rivalry and their ability to cope with it in a manner which has growth potential for the child.

Feminine identity has further opportunity to develop through the mothering endeavor.[12]

The pregnancy itself may be a stimulus to the development of a positive feminine identity, since this identity formation continues well into maturity. Moreover, pregnancy assists many women to accept their physical bodies and functions and to bring about a better adjustment in sexual intimacies.[13]

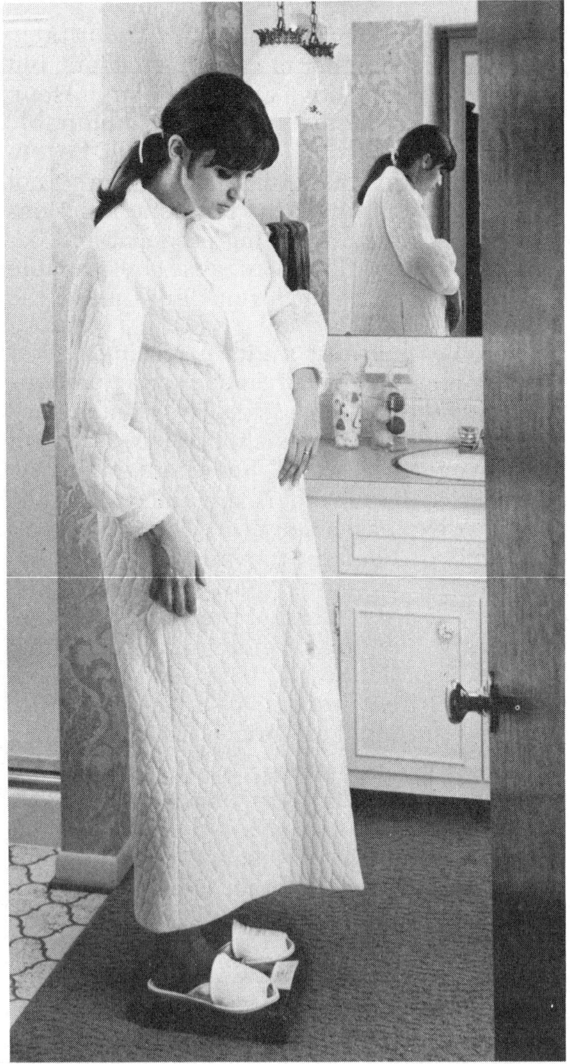

FIGURE 20-1. During pregnancy, a woman's body image changes. (Courtesy of Ross Laboratories.)

FACTORS INFLUENCING THE RESPONSE TO PREGNANCY

Pregnancy represents a clear turning point in a woman's life. It is unquestionably a stressful time requiring much adaptation. Whether or not maturation is the outcome of the adaptation, the psychologic and physiologic changes of pregnancy make a woman a mother, and once a mother the individual can never again be single.[14] Pregnancy has been called the fulfillment of the deepest and most powerful wish of a woman, an expression of fulfillment and self-realization, a creative act.[15] But is it? Is it always? May it not be different for different women? May it not be different for the same woman at different points in her life? Let us examine the various factors which influence a woman's response to pregnancy.

Personality

Although pregnancy provides physical evidence of belonging to the female gender, the psychologic aspects of being pregnant are not so obvious.[16] Virtually all who have studied the emotional reactions of women to their pregnancies agree that:

1. Women have *both* positive and negative attitudes toward their pregnancies
2. All women experience increased anxiety and tension during pregnancy.[17]

Women's reactions to pregnancy, labor, and motherhood are determined by many factors. They are based on the woman's life experiences and her characteristic mode of reacting to life. Her degree of maturity, particularly her level of psychosexual development, makes her the kind of person she is and determines the way she perceives herself as a person.

Her own mothering experiences as a child and her relationship with her mother will greatly influence her response to being a mother. Studies indicate that a higher perceived similarity with one's own mother results in better adaptation to pregnancy as well as a better sexual adaptation in general.[18]

Social Factors

Social factors also affect the acceptance of pregnancy. A family accustomed to an income from two salaries may now find it necessary to manage with only one salary. At the same time, they must assume added expenses and may not view a pregnancy with enthusiasm. Medical expenses, maternity clothing, and equipment for the infant's care can be a heavy burden on a family having their first baby and an increasing burden as each new child is added. Young parents, particularly the father, become anxious about managing and worry about the future. This anxiety has impact on the expectant mother and other family members.

There are also pressures from society and the extended family pertaining to adequate housing, equipment for child care, and so forth. The pressure of "keeping up with the Joneses" is an added stressor for some families.

Cultural Factors

Culture shapes a woman's reactions and behaviors concerning pregnancy and motherhood. Many cultures implicitly recognize the needs of pregnant women and structure specific roles and reciprocal roles of other family members so that behavior is accepted and extra demands of the expectant mother are satisfied.[19]

Many cultures encourage, or even pressure, young people to reproduce. The American culture, until recently, made it clear that people who marry should plan to have children and women who did so were accorded certain rights and privileges during their pregnancies. We now seem to have made an about-face. The message is now "don't overpopulate." Some women are already feeling guilty about becoming pregnant, particularly if they already have one or two children.[20] Women who have been raised with the conviction that childbearing and childrearing are component parts of feminine identity may well be in conflict. The culture is now suggesting that having children may not be the most fulfilling route to an effective and creative life. This will influence many women's feelings about becoming pregnant.

The desire to have children does not necessarily accompany the biologic capacity to become pregnant and bear a child. Even statements by the expectant mother that she wishes to be pregnant may not reflect her true feelings. She may be caught in a cultural and emotional current imposed upon her by demands of society and intimate relationships (with husband, parents, friends, etc.). The unwillingly pregnant woman is often pushed into the position of accepting with her own words what her feelings reject.[21] Many women hide their feelings not only because they conflict with their own value system, but also because they fear condemnation if they admit rejection of their pregnancy.[22]

Marital Relationship

The basic relationship within a marriage is another factor which influences a woman's feelings about becoming pregnant. Where there is love and mutual support between husband and wife, a pregnancy may not only be accepted but planned and anticipated with pleasure. Where these elements are missing, the pregnancy is likely to be viewed as a disaster.

Today when young people marry they usually set some goal concerning the number of children they desire, how they wish them spaced, and at what age they would like to complete their family. Modern methods of conception control make these realistic, possible goals. A pregnancy that does not fit the family's goals may well be viewed as less than desirable. A pregnancy occurring after the age of 35 to 40 is particularly distressing to many families. Added to the stress of this unexpected event is the statistical possibility of some genetic aberration in the developing fetus. Today many parents are knowledgeable of these facts and their fear is an added stressor.

Psychologic Responses

It is believed that many of the emotional manifestations of pregnancy are physiologically induced. They are the result of major hormonal and general metabolic changes occurring during pregnancy. Progesterone secreted in large quantities by the corpus luteum and later by the placenta is said to be responsible for the increased energy used by the woman for introversion during pregnancy.[23] Others suggest that a shifting of the id-ego relationship is responsible for the emotional changes. Caplan[24] believes that this shift in intrapsychic equilibrium (occurring in the second and third trimesters and continuing for four to six weeks after delivery) permits old, repressed conflicts and fantasies to surface to the conscious level with a minimum of anxiety. He feels that this permits the possibility of achieving a better solution to conflicts and a resolution of guilt feeling resulting in greater maturity on the part of a woman. Women do spend considerable time in introspection. They feel passive and think deeply about themselves and the baby within them. This interversion in effect causes women to withdraw from the family, not because they care less about them, but because they spend more time thinking about themselves. This behavior, occurring when a woman needs the most affection and consideration, may bring retribution, retaliation, and general family disequilibrium.

During all stages of pregnancy, women have alterations in their moods. They experience greater heights of joy and deeper moods of despair. They may shift from one mood to another with alarming rapidity. Unless it is understood as normal and not a forerunner of a psychic disorder, this behavior may upset the expectant mother and other members of the family. Other mood changes include emotional lability, irritability, and sensitivity. The alterations of moods observed in pregnant women are not surprising when one considers the fact that to be pregnant is to be committed in a direction that may not be entirely desirable.[25]

Women have increased needs for love and affection during pregnancy. These needs are not always met by sexual activity. What the woman does find gratifying is a demonstration of love through protection and concern about her (Fig. 20-2) and through assistance with her household responsibilities. Caplan[26] speaks of this as "charging of the battery" and warns that nourishment of this kind is as necessary as vitamins and proteins. Its importance is twofold. In addition to its gratifying aspect to the self concept it is also a necessary prerequisite to maternal love.

The concept of conflict is useful in understanding some of the responses to pregnancy. The wish for a child (goal) and the wish to continue a fulfilling career or social role (goal) may indeed conflict. There may also be deep-seated conflicts that may be reviewed simply because of the pregnancy (e.g., mother-daughter conflicts). A wish-fear conflict may also be operative. For example, remaining safe when faced with a powerful threat of danger (goal) versus the dream of motherhood (goal) may be the two opposing forces.

It must be remembered that a woman's attitude toward the pregnancy changes over the nine month span. The timing of the pregnancy is "all wrong" for the majority of women. Even when a pregnancy is planned, there is no assurance that conception will follow sexual relationships. When it does occur, it always seems to carry an element of surprise. A baby may indeed be in the plans of a couple, but the future suddenly projected into the present pulls the woman off balance. There are always current plans to be completed and expenses to be met. At first, the finality of a pregnancy is rejected by a large percentage of women. Caplan[27] found this to be true for 80 per cent of the women in his study. Feelings of grief (loss), anger, shame, and some guilt were also frequently felt. These negative attitudes are toward the pregnancy, not toward the baby at this point. Although some women, perhaps most women, feel fulfilled during a pregnancy, many do not, and some harbor considerable resentment of the "intrusion" into their lives. Of the women who begin pregnancy with negative feelings, most, if not all, begin to plan for the baby once quickening has occurred. Indeed, some women whose normal narcissistic personality is oriented towards themselves experience a sensual pleasure in the fetus and its movements. Those who are unable to develop a positive feeling toward the fetus may go through pregnancy visualizing it as a depersonalized foreign body.

Toward the end of pregnancy, when fetal movements cause sleeplessness and generalized or specific discomfort, negative feelings again increase to a certain degree. Some women describe the baby as "causing trouble already," "pushing me around," or "kicking my husband out of bed."

Some women have an intense fantasy life with the fetus. The mother's perception of her infant is important to the future mother-infant relationship. Fantasies may be so strong that they are carried over into post-delivery phase. It is not good for a mother to be so attached to her "dream child" that she is unable to see the real child, for only by recognizing reality can she build a dependable relationship and meet the needs of the child. The child that was dreamed of as *always* a boy or *always* a girl may find himself or herself in an unreceptive home if he or she does not meet that require-

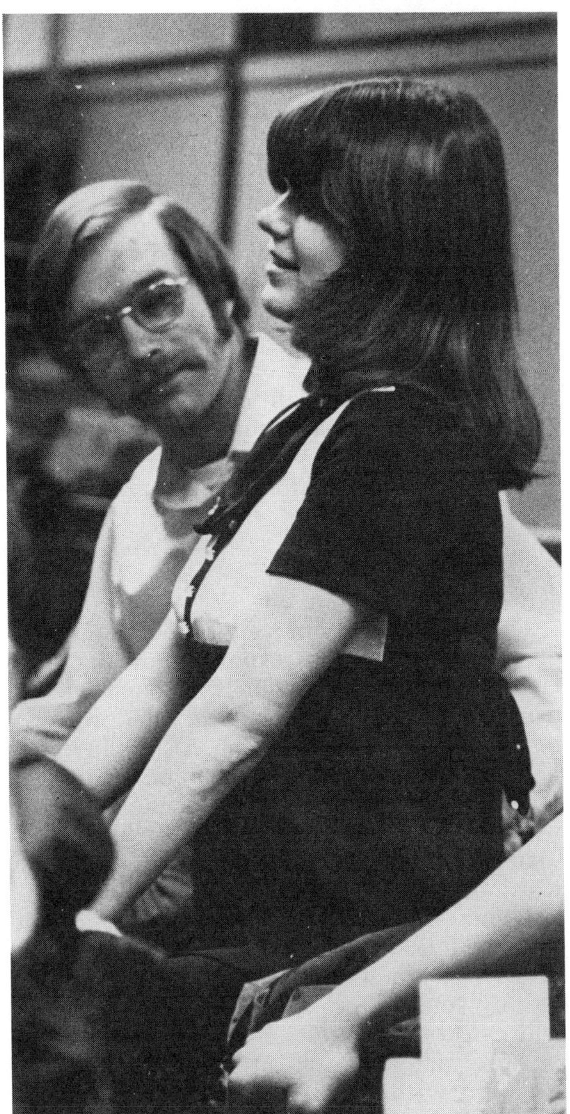

FIGURE 20-2. Women need demonstrations of concern for them by others during pregnancy. (Photograph by Alva Thomas.)

ment. Indifference to a specific sex is a good sign for a healthy mother-infant relationship.[28] Many cultures prefer a male child, particularly as the first-born. This cultural expectation may be an added stressor for the mother.

The newborn is a helpless, demanding individual—a bundle of uncontrolled responses. This may be threatening to the expectant mother who has spent a lifetime attempting to gain control of her own responses to life. A woman who constantly daydreams about a mature child or an adolescent may be unready to mother a neonate. Moreover, dreaming of a child with certain qualities or gifts may indicate that the expectant mother is already planning to meet some of her own unrealized ambitions through her child.

Sexual Responses

There may be some alterations in sexual desires and sexual responses during pregnancy. For some women freedom from the fear of becoming pregnant, coupled with an increase in pelvic congestion, results in better performance. Some women experience orgasm for the first time during pregnancy. Other women find that being pregnant reduces their sexual desires. In addition, many couples worry about the appropriateness of sexual intercourse during pregnancy. There is a good deal of folklore that is not based on facts. Moreover, much medical advice is not based on any scientific rationale. Fears that coitus will cause an abortion, be responsible for infection, or precipitate labor need to be explored with couples. Fear understandably affects sexual performance. The specific focus of fear (often described as "subconscious holding back") seems to center on the avoidance of orgasm (which tends to evoke an image of releasing the fetus). The fear may represent a kind of biologic protective mechanism.[29] It is also postulated that emotional reactions, such as concern about one's sexual attractiveness or fear of harming the fetus, can be translated into physiologic changes leading to a diminished level of sexual desire and erotic arousal during pregnancy.[30]

A study of sexual adjustments[31] reveals that pregnancy has a generalized adverse effect on sexual responses. Frequency of coitus, sexual desire, and eroticism decline during the first trimester, increase somewhat during the second trimester and early third trimester, but remain below the prepregnant baseline. The reasons given for these changes were:

- Fear of harming the fetus
- Breast tenderness
- Sex not satisfying due to modified positions or restriction of movements
- Fear of premature labor
- Vaginal numbness
- Pain on penetration
- Physical discomforts (tiredness, sleepiness, heartburn, nausea).

Sexual performance improved greatly after the pregnancy, ultimately surpassing the prepregnant level. However, in the early puerperium there was anxiety about the resumption of relations. The new mothers also experienced some perineal and breast discomforts. Fatigue and the physical discomforts reduced both the desire and frequency of sexual activity.

What advice can the nurse safely give to an expectant couple? First, it is important for the nurse to investigate her own feelings regarding the discussion of sexual responses with others. Modesty must give way to a mature approach to fulfilling this role. In a study by Quirk and Hassanein[32] only 4 per cent of expectant mothers had been advised about coitus by nurses and 66 per cent had received *no* information from any health professional concerning sexual responses and sexual behavior. Since coitus promotes a feeling of closeness between partners and helps to satisfy certain dependency needs in pregnant women, such as the increased need for nurturance,[33] discussion of sexual responses and behaviors should accompany other anticipatory guidance.

What are the facts? For example:

Does pregnancy necessarily make sexual relations uncomfortable?

Yes. For many couples the usual female supine position becomes uncomfortable. Couples should be counseled to try other positions such as side by side position, rear entry position, and female on top position.

Does coitus cause uterine contractions?

If coitus results in orgasm, uterine contractions do occur. Moreover, in self-manipulation to orgasm (without coitus), even more pronounced contractions are experienced.[34]

Does the orgasm cause premature labor?

There is no linear relation between sexual activity in late pregnancy and premature birth for the large majority of women.[35]

Does coitus cause bleeding in the later stages of pregnancy?

Some postcoital spotting may result from direct contact between the erect penis and the vasocongested predelivery cervix.[36]

Is coitus responsible for infections?

The prohibition of coitus during the latter part of the third trimester to protect the mother and child against infection is a residual of preantibiotic days in medicine and can largely be negated.[37] A competent cervix and intact membranes provide adequate protection against infections in the healthy pregnant woman.

Therefore, although advice about coitus during the third trimester of pregnancy should be individualized, coitus can generally be encouraged. Free sexual expression is usually helpful unless specifically contraindicated.[38] Contraindications appear to be limited to

ruptured membranes
incompetent cervix
spotting or bleeding
deeply engaged presenting part.

Fears

The expectant mother faces some realistic fears during pregnancy. Although no one can promise her a comfortable pregnancy, safe labor, or a baby free of defects, one can give the woman an opportunity to talk about her concerns and compare them with scientific facts.

Most women fear the pain of labor, although preparation (knowledge and physical readiness) for the event reduces this fear. Many women fear the operative procedures (episiotomy, forceps delivery, cesarean section) that may accompany the experience. Some women fear the administration of anesthesia. The majority of women fear the possibility of being alone during labor or of experiencing labor without a supporting person who is significant to them. Every woman seems aware that, even today, a woman occasionally loses her life during childbirth. Some women fear that this will happen to them.

Fund-raising drives to combat certain chronic and acute illnesses (cystic fibrosis, crippled children, muscular dystrophy, etc.) usually focus on defects occurring during the prenatal period and early childhood. They have increased expectant parents' fears for the safe outcome of their pregnancy. Moreover, low self concept on the part of either parent may be responsible for concerns about malformations. Some expectant mothers have vague concerns about their expected child, others focus on very specific defects. Some family histories include certain hereditary facts and defects such as sickle cell anemia, cleft lip and palate, Tay-Sachs disease, and so forth. Expectant parents from such families are understandably fearful. Many mothers will not readily share these concerns while they are actually pregnant. It is as though putting the fear into words will cause it to happen. Some things which women fear can be deleterious to their unborn child, but many of them are not valid. Those that result from "old wives tales" could be dispelled if they were shared with health workers.

Many women state that they feel unusually vulnerable during their pregnancy, particularly during the last trimester. Sometimes women prefer to leave the security of their home only with their husband. When the husband leaves for work they worry about his safety, and they display undue anxiety over other people's driving habits when they travel by car.

ALTERED STATE OF CONSCIOUSNESS

Pregnancy can be the epitome of a positive growth experience. Colman and Colman[39] view this experience in the light of an altered state of consciousness. Rubin[40] speaks of the "cognitive style of pregnancy." There is undoubtedly an altered style or state of perceiving events during pregnancy. Tart[41] defines an altered state of consciousness as "qualitative alteration in the overall patterning of mental functioning such that the experiencer feels his consciousness is radically different from the 'normal' way it functions."

"Pregnancy is an altered state of consciousness largely because it plunges the individual's awareness from its secular pursuits into profound involvement in universal processes."[42] Many of the psychologic responses to pregnancy have been discussed previously, e.g., mood swings, over-reacting to the world, obsessions, feelings of vulnerability, phobic feelings, and sensitivity. The Colmans continue, "it is that state in which each of us began, warm, protected, merged with another system whose reassuring rhythms, whose very life blood, sustained us."[43] Now the woman is repeating that cycle in becoming a mother. It is said women undergo some identity confusion in relation to their own mother. It is also suggested that the physical union with the fetus

> can be experienced as a mystical transpersonal state. The "I" is no longer alone. It is submerged in a larger and more meaningful system . . . as a pregnant woman . . . our physical and psychological status may predispose . . . us to ideas and confusion which we would not feel at other times.
>
> We know that pregnant women do become confused about who is the baby and who is the mother. This complicated and basically irrational confusion is generally quite normal. In fact, it seems to be a part of a healthy psychological progression through pregnancy.
>
> . . . .
>
> The ecstatic states of consciousness that so many strive toward . . . are potentially presented in a remarkably pure form in pregnancy, where merger is not only a subjective experience but a physical reality. The union of two creates the undifferentiated dyad of mother-fetus. This blending is unique to pregnancy but related to other altered states of consciousness in which the individual experiences himself at one with something other than himself. If we bury this potential in banal routine and in technology which has no meaning to the subject, we will be turning our backs on the prototype of profound human experience.[44]

What a beautiful way to relate the joyous moments many women experience during pregnancy!

Pregnancy may result in a related altered state of consciousness in both the man and the woman.

> Pregnancy may be the first occasion in a marriage when the partners realize the extent to which they are interdependent, psychologically, socially, and economically. The baby is literally a representation of the physiological union of the two into one. As such, it is a mystical symbol of their love. Life, however, has to be lived on a practical as well as a mystical plane. The merger may feel like a trap. One of the main tasks of

pregnancy is to reconcile the identity confusions and prepare for the smooth functioning of the family after the birth.[45]

TRANSACTIONAL ANALYSIS
OF A PREGNANT COUPLE*

MAN	WOMAN	
lover	lover	— adolescent, cultural overlay
husband	wife	— adult give and take interacting
father	mother	— primitive ideas from childhood

While interactions and confusions of these three levels are inevitable, there may be a dynamic tension rather than an irresolvable conflict. The role/person dichotomy can productively be worked on during pregnancy, when new roles are emerging and a new identity is being forged.

*From Colman, A. and Colman, L.: *Pregnancy as an altered state of consciousness.* Birth and Family 1:8, 1974, with permission.

CRISIS OF PREGNANCY

Pregnancy is to be regarded as a period of increased susceptibility to crisis. Factors operating on the biological plane in the expectant mother interact reciprocally with factors in her psychological functioning and in the interpersonal relationships of her family group, and this equilibrium is constantly affected by the interplay of social, cultural, and economic forces between the family and its external social and physical environment. . . . How this upset of balance of forces is resolved may have a lasting effect in any area of the functioning of the mother and her family and in particular may determine in large degree the quality of her future mental health and that of her baby, her husband and her other children.[46]

Since pregnancy is a transitional time in the individual's life, poised between the former childless life and the subsequent irreversible state of parenthood,[47] it is a life crisis of great impact. It is a time when an individual is more open to her inner resources, her dreams, and her fantasies. Pregnancy precipitates stress which is inherent in all areas—in the endocrinologic changes, in activation of unconscious psychologic conflicts pertaining to the factors involved in pregnancy, and in the interpsychic reorganization of becoming a parent.[48] It has an inherent disruptive factor, temporarily impairing an individual's usual capacity to cope with changing environmental stresses. It is often accompanied by a heightened state of tension and unpleasant affective reactions.[49]

ANXIETY

Some form of anxiety is always present during pregnancy.[50] Anxiety arises from unmet expectations related to one's needs. Many goals, desires, wishes, anticipations, and acquired needs related to prestige, status, esteem, and self views may not be met by pregnancy and expected motherhood. Indeed, pregnancy often results in new needs which may not be met.

This chapter has focused on many of the behaviors which indicate that anxiety is being experienced. Pregnancy anxieties can be seen in psychosomatic complaints and behaviors. Some examples may be excessive eating, food cravings, sleeplessness, fainting, and nausea and vomiting. Anxiety can be seen in demands for the sick role, in slavishly following certain regimes related to pregnancy, and in excesses of joy, fear, and secrecy. It may be observed in those who seek prenatal care on the first day of a missed menstrual period, or in the delay of seeking prenatal care. Over-concern about possible bleeding, fetal abnormality or death, and fear of hospitalization may indicate anxiety. Somnolent detachment (see often in early weeks of pregnancy), apathy, anger, irritability, or restlessness may be the cues indicating that energy is being expended to cope with anxiety. Deutsch states that:

> in this profound psychic life there are manifestations of lurking fear of death that remains uninfluenced by the conquest of civilization . . . whatever personal or universal human guilt feelings feed these fears, one has the impression that something profound and primitive lies at the bottom of this.[51]

There are studies which show a relationship between anxiety during pregnancy and difficulty of labor,[52] in the development of colic in the neonate,[53] and on the emotionality of children.[54] In a study by Burnstein and colleagues,[55] it was shown that women who have known someone who delivered an abnormal child or someone who has had a miscarriage have statistically higher anxiety scores than women who have not known such persons.

A woman who displays anxious behavior needs opportunities to "talk out" the anxiety-producing antecedents and recognize that the discomfort she is experiencing and the behavior she is manifesting are created by anxiety. Not only is the mother's mental health at stake but also the welfare of the entire family unit.

LOSS

Pregnancy may be viewed as a balance-type scale, with "gains" on one side of the scale and "losses" on the other. For most women the scale would tend to tip one way and then the other since there is much ambivalence during the nine months. There are gains for most women during pregnancy. Special foods are offered, a special place to sit is indicated, a supporting arm is offered, special concern is focused on her physical care, all of which indicate that someone cares. But even for these women, the losses may outweigh the gains. Any number of conditions may make the pregnancy undesired—she may be the sole support of her family, she may be unmarried, her health may make this pregnancy a risk for her. As Rubin states, "if other wishes are important and have to be abandoned in favor of the child, there is cause for regret and the regret for what might have been can persevere."[56] Loss, grieving, and the coping mechanism to handle the loss may be observed during pregnancy even though the feelings may not be expressed in words. The somatic distress, hostility, anger, and other changes in the woman's ordinary pattern of relating to others may indicate that loss is being experienced. Referring back to Chapter 10 of this book, Beniolel provides guidelines for assessing loss and coping behavior:

> Reactions [to loss] are determined by several interacting elements: the special meaning of a relationship which is gone, the degree to which the relationship is replaceable, the level of personal and social disruption that is produced by the loss, . . . and the availability of adaptive capacities and coping resources for responding to the effects of the change.

PREGNANCY AND THE MALE

A man responds in many different ways to the news that he is to become a father. His ego is enhanced by the event since it confirms his virility. However, he, like his mate, is now faced with a developmental crisis. How he responds to expected fatherhood depends upon the psychic tools and defense mechanisms inherent in his personality. His repertoire of past experiences and the environment in which the pregnancy is progressing influence the manner in which he copes with expectant fatherhood.

Fatherhood *forces* adulthood on the male, unless he denies paternity. Society now expects him to fulfill a mature, responsible role. He is to make whatever sacrifices are necessary to care for his wife and his child. Gone are his carefree days.

The man may experience anxiety as he anticipates the future economic burden. He may resent the added responsibility of fatherhood. He may be concerned about his ability to fulfill the role.

Pregnancy may evoke some physiologic responses in the male similar to those the pregnant woman is experiencing. Men have been known to gain weight, experience nausea and vomiting, and have abdominal bloating and intestinal distress which disappear after the birth of the baby.[57] These changes presumably result from the intense meaning that the pregnancy has for an individual and the profound identification of the man with the woman.[58] Caplan[59] states that men identify with their wives partly because as little boys rivalry was felt and because little boys fantasize about having children, just as little girls do.

Many men say that they were unprepared for the "lack of glamour that pregnancy brings." They express concern about the steady reduction in the amount of attention they receive and the demands of their pregnant wife. These demands are confusing to most husbands who wonder if their wives are ill or well, and whether the demands are necessary or are some hostile response to them and to the pregnancy. With his sexual gratification diminishing, or eliminated entirely, he recognizes that he is playing a progressively secondary role in the life of his wife. He is alarmed by her fatigue, introversion, and "nest building." He begins to feel competitive with his own child.

He may also feel some guilt and apprehension about having gotten his mate pregnant. He may feel that he has put her life in jeopardy and fear the responsibility which would result should misfortune occur.[60]

PREGNANCY AND THE FETUS

Can the mother's emotional life have an effect on the fetus?

It has been demonstrated that hormones can cross the placenta. Where there is excessive production of adrenal corticosteroids due to stress, an overdose may be hypothesized as affecting the developing fetus.[61] An expectant mother's emotional life may affect her food intake, posture, smoking, and consumption of alcohol and drugs.[62,63] All of these may affect the fetus. Ferreira[64] states that careless exposure to "accidents" by fast driving and other behavior may be an overt attempt by the expectant mother to take her own life and the life of the fetus.

In studies conducted over a number of years it has been demonstrated that emotional disturbances and severe fatigue in the expectant mother during the last stage of pregnancy were associated with an increase in activity of the fetus in utero and in disturbances such as irritability, gastrointestinal disorders, higher than average heart rate, vasomotor irritability, and changes in the respiratory pattern in the newborn.[65]

For centuries women believed that the unborn child could be influenced positively or negatively by the way a woman conducted her life during pregnancy. Prenatal maternal influences were considered superstition and relegated to the dusty shelves of history more than a half century ago. With a hard core of scientific studies the belief has begun to make a dignified re-entry.[66]

THE EXPECTANT GRANDMOTHER

The mother-daughter relationship has considerable impact on the expectant mother—preparing her or not preparing her for the task of mothering. Conflicts arising from her experience of being mothered may have left emotional scars with resulting feelings of ambivalence, guilt, anger, and remorse. Some of these are resolved when a woman faces motherhood herself.

The expectant grandmother is also affected by her daughter's first pregnancy. The pregnancy transforms her daughter into a coequal. Competition may result as the daughter now attempts to prove that she is a better mother than her own mother has been. The expectant grandmother may have difficulty in accepting her new role. She may resent the aging that is implied. She may feel anger at her daughter for this maturational phase which has been thrust on her. Differences in her daughter's experience with pregnancy may be viewed with jealousy.

If the mother-daughter relationship has been a mutually supportive one, the daughter often turns to her mother, sharing feelings and seeking advice. Indeed, the frequent telephone calls and visits to mother may be upsetting to the husband. An assessment of mother-daughter relationships provides valuable information.

THE ROLE OF NURSING

Chapter 1 introduced the process of nursing which is used throughout the book. This prenatal chapter begins the application of that process, and this particular section centers on the psychologic implications of pregnancy.

Psychologic functioning and physiologic functioning are not two separate orders of phenomena, but rather two aspects of an interacting unit. Presumably an influence described as psychologic is ultimately reflected in physiologic terms.

Faced with the responsibility for planning the nursing care for an expectant mother in an expanding family, the nurse must determine:

1. What is the impact of pregnancy on this woman and on her family? What are her conflicts over accepting the pregnancy and the mothering role and what coping strategies is she using?
2. How well are the tasks of pregnancy being accomplished?
3. What acts on the part of the nurse would be protective, nurturing, and stimulating?

ASSESSMENT FOR PREPREGNANT LIFE EXPERIENCES

The first part of this chapter alerted the reader to the numerous causes and the multiplicity of responses that relate to being pregnant or being a member of a pregnant family. The impact of pregnancy on an individual has as much to do with past life experiences as it does with the present situation. The nurse will be most helpful to the expectant family if her data collection includes many of these prepregnant details. It is not to be interpreted that this is the "first order of business," for the nurse must develop a trusting relationship with her patient before much of this information will be shared.

Some of the possible problem areas concerning developmental tasks and the process of daily living that should be explored are:

- Conflicts about sexual identity
- Lack of mothering
- Mother-daughter conflicts
- Loss of a significant person
- Conflicts involving separation from parents
- Difficulty with maturational steps of puberty
- Marital or family difficulties
- History of pseudocyesis, infertility, abortion, prolonged difficult labor, birth of a defective child.

DEVELOPMENTAL TASKS OF PREGNANCY

Next, we must view the pregnancy itself as a *developmental task*. This task, like other developmental tasks, has subtasks to be accomplished in order for the experience to be integrated into the total life process. Pregnancy and childbirth lend themselves well to an examination of these progressive steps for there is an outward and visible aspect to the inward and hidden phenomena. Using skillful interviewing techniques and a good system of recording, it should be possible for all members of the health team to be kept aware of the disequilibrium being experienced by the expectant mother and coordinate their efforts in helping her to resolve it. This is very important, for successful coping with the critical tasks of pregnancy is reflected in the psychologic health of the woman. Successful resolution of each task prepares her to cope with future tasks. When such critical tasks are not resolved, the whole family may well suffer. When they are resolved, the woman completes pregnancy with growth, self-esteem, and autonomy.

The nurse has a primary role with respect to assisting women to deal with the psychologic tasks of pregnancy. Unless the nurse is available and fills the role of protecting, nurturing and stimulating the expectant mother, there is every chance that this important support will not be available to women.

The psychologic timetable of pregnancy presented in the tasks which follow must not be viewed as a precise instrument, for the themes overlap.[67] However, it is very useful in assisting the nurse to recognize, or even anticipate, which individuals may be vulnerable to undue stress. In addition, nursing assessment explores the coping behavior manifested, the state of disequilibrium, and the support system available to the individual. All of these are "keys" to nursing intervention.

The four tasks of pregnancy are:

1. Pregnancy validation
2. Fetal embodiment
3. Fetal distinction
4. Role transition.

Task 1. Pregnancy Validation

Task

To ascertain if pregnancy is a reality. To accept the reality of pregnancy and its implications.

Responses (verbal and nonverbal behavior, fantasies and dreams, activity to be expected)

Surprise at the possibility of having conceived.

Ambivalence and rejection may likely be the first response, followed by a conflict of wanting and not wanting.

Unpleasant symptoms of pregnancy may exaggerate the ambivalence.

Physiologic responses (somnolence, nausea, vomiting, fatigue, lack of appetite) bring about decreased activity.

Strange fantasies and dreams about the unknown, unforeseen, unfelt organism growing inside the body.

Thoughts turn inward and focus on "self," not on a baby (it is unreal as yet).

Reassesses the signs and symptoms of pregnancy over and over (missed menstrual period, breast changes, etc.).

Seeks prenatal care as a validating tool.

Feels special, as though housing a secret.

Begins to decide with whom and how she will share the news.

Reduces sexual activity.

Feels fearful if had previous unpleasant experiences related to childbirth or knows of others who did.

Nursing Assessment

Inquires into the meaning of this pregnancy to the life of the individual and her family.

Encourages expression of feelings both positive and negative.

Assesses symptoms of pregnancy, particularly the discomforts which may exaggerate the ambivalence.

Inquires as to who has shared in the knowledge of the pregnancy and their response to this disclosure.

Explores any changes in interprersonal relationship with the family, coworkers, others.

Recognizes degree of anxiety exhibited.

Nursing Intervention

Encouraging the expression of feelings helps the individual obtain a better perception of what being pregnant means to her and where she can obtain the needed assistance and support. The verbalization can be expected to reduce the tension. It permits the nurse to help the individual to look at the alternatives to being pregnant and to make some basic decisions about the future. The nurse's attention to the woman's feelings denotes respect and enhances her self view. The expressions of pride, blame, guilt, and so forth need to be expressed. The nurse may encounter strong responses to the pregnancy, such as anger, helplessness (crying), joy—indeed almost any behavior can be expected and should be encouraged and accepted.

The nurse focuses on the optimal task achievement (to accept the reality of pregnancy and its implications) and directs her patient toward this goal. She examines the support system (husband, family, friends, health care system, and others) and helps the patient to use it for improved mental health. When partial or complete adequate task achievement has been accomplished, the nurse reinforces that achievement.

The nurse intervenes to reduce some of the stressors, particularly the physical discomforts (nausea, vomiting, lassitude, etc.), and to tell her patient of the time limitation that can be anticipated.

The nurse should remember that this task must be satisfactorily accomplished before she can expect her patient to move on to the next task. It is therefore inappropriate at this time to try to focus the woman on the fetus, her changing role, labor and birth, and so forth.

The nurse should always keep in mind that referral to professional colleagues may be a most appropriate nursing action. The above nursing actions can be expected to help prevent a developmental crisis. When situational crises are based on deep structural changes in personality, education (logic) may not be the answer. To avoid maladaptive or neurotic solutions to task achievement, professional referral should be considered.

Task 2. Fetal Embodiment

Task

To incorporate the fetus into the body image. To shift in dependency and identity relationships with the husband and with mother.

Responses (verbal and nonverbal behavior, fantasies and dreams, activity to be expected)

Turns inward (identity diffusion) with greater openness to the inner world. There is silent introspection.

Depends on husband to make more of the day-to-day decisions.

Notices changes in the body. Likes most of them but at times is ambivalent about the changes.

Buys maternity clothing.

Anxiety is reduced. Period of calmness sets in as pregnancy is accepted.

Reviews conflicts with own mother and her quality of mothering.

Reviews loss (what must be given up) and responds to it, depending upon its importance.

Becomes more physically active.

Seeks new acquaintances (pregnant

women and recent new parents).

Dreams shift from self to others.

Sexual activity somewhat improved but still lower than prepregnant level.

Tends to increase food intake in the interest of the fetus.

Shows some concern over possible loss of fetus through miscarriage.

Nursing Assessment

Inquires into any changes in interpersonal relationship between self and significant others (especially husband, children, mother).

Reviews body changes and response to these changes.

Observes for anxious manifestations.

Inquires about mothering. Discusses what is considered relevant for this decade and what is not. Listens for and encourages discussion of own mothering.

Discusses balance between what is to be lost (given up) by this pregnancy and what is to be gained.

Inquires as to physical activity (sleep, nutrition, general well-being).

Observes any change in dress (maternity clothing) and whether this is needed because of physiologic changes or has preceded that need.

Notes who is the person most often referred to in conversation (that person is important).

Ascertains husband's response to mood changes and sexual activity.

Nursing Intervention

Physical care, including both prenatal medical care and self-care related to good grooming, is an indication that the woman feels good about herself as a pregnant woman. Education related to care of the expectant mother's needs is appropriately begun during this period. Good body mechanics are reviewed.

The discussion of mothering will help the woman to confront the conflicts she may have experienced in her own childhood. She can be helped to manage the feelings of love, hate, frustration, satisfaction, and rebellion that are a part of every mother-child relationship.[68] These feelings are very relevant to this task of pregnancy.

Mood swings and sexual response may be changing relationships within the family. The nurse needs to relate why changes are occurring and how they can be handled. In terms of anticipatory guidance, the nurse should review with the family another response that will soon surface—dependency. She should work toward establishing a family communication system to deal with all of these changing relationships.

Anxiety should be relatively low during this period. If anxious behavior is observed, further data collection should be performed and nursing intervention planned.

Permitting the woman to listen to the fetal heartbeat (after the twentieth week of pregnancy) and to talk about fetal movements (after quickening) may also be positive nursing actions.

Task 3. Fetal Distinction

Task

> To view the fetus as an individual being, separate from self. To formulate personally relevant, unique mothering identity, separate and apart from own mothering.[69]

Responses (verbal and nonverbal behavior, fantasies and dreams, activity to be expected)

Conceptualizes fetus as an individual with a personality.

Outwardly relates with the fetus, indicating it is truly separate.

Searches for cues as to what the baby will be like.

Buys baby supplies.

Tries to interest husband in participating in the events (feeling fetal movements, attending classes, reading, purchasing infant supplies, naming the baby).

Shows concern for husband's assumption of new role as father, and his dependability.

Searches for welcomed responses of others for her coming child.

Takes an active interest in children, watches their activity.

Fantasizes and dreams about babies.

Tries out names for the new baby.

Shows interest in learning to care for self and baby (reads, seeks classes, asks questions).

Accepts body image, not as a deformity but as a "full with life" feeling.

Preoccupation with own mother fades (has already reviewed and cast out negative or unacceptable behaviors, and accepted respected and valued behaviors).[70]

Sexual activity decreasing.

Reduces independence, becomes more dependent on others in the family, seeks expression from others that she is loved.

Better control of food intake since the baby now "shows."

Anxiety low now that danger of miscarriage is past.

Nursing Assessment

Explores knowledge of child care and activities related to obtaining such information.

Inquires about purchase of layette.

Discusses fantasies related to fetus.

Inquires about desired sex and name for the baby.

Explores the value of the baby.

Discusses parents "valued" maternal behavior.

Observes mode of dress and interest in grooming.

Reviews dependent behavior and response of others to her dependent needs.

Explores husband's response to introversion and changes in sexual activity (if any).

Explores husband's transition in roles and behavior.

Inquires about relationships with mother.

Nursing Intervention

The expectant mother is (or should be) ready to talk about her coming baby and focus on his needs. Expectant parent eduction will now appropriately focus on bathing, feeding, clothing, and so forth. Maternal behavior can now be explored and the mother can be warned that maternal attachment takes time and matenal feelings do not usually surge forth at birth. The "value" of this child, as seen by the parents, is important. This is the value *to* the parents (i.e., what the baby can do *for* the parents shoud be of concern). Fantasies about the baby let the nurse know if the expectant parents' concept of a baby is realistic. This indicates the degree of readiness to care for a small, helpless infant. A scale for the determination of maternal feeling may be administered at this point.

There may be some family disequilibrium since the mother (usually the giver) is now making personal demands to be taken care of (i.e., showing dependency). The nurse appropriately intervenes to help others in the family understand what is occurring, why it is occurring, the universality of the occurrence, and the importance of supporting the mother at this time.

She helps the couple find alternative ways for sexual gratification if this is becoming a problem for the family.

The nurse's observation helps her to assess the feminine, maternal, wifely task achievement and to reinforce observed adequate achievement.

Task 4. Role Transition

Task

To prepare to give up the fetus, to experience labor and birth, and to mother the infant.

Responses (verbal and nonverbal behavior, fantasies and dreams, activity to be expected)

Anxiety increases due to approaching labor, the fear of losing control, and concerns about the arriving baby.

Feels dependent.

Feels vulnerable to harm.

Pride of fulfillment mixed with dread of empty feeling.

Some nostalgia for special prerogatives of pregnancy that have begun to be taken for granted.

Body image almost discontinuous with usual physical state.

Impatient with unwieldy body.

Experiencing frequent urination, insomnia, shortness of breath.

Fantasizes mothering role and the "unknown."

Increased energy. Aware of time limitations, that labor may interrupt the completion of a task.

Annoyed and frustrated with any time on her hands.

Vicariously tries out new role of mother (sets up equipment, prepares "nest," cares for children of others).

Dreams are filled with babies, children, and births. These dreams reflect reality of being prepared for soon to occur events.

Makes plans for the home while being hospitalized. Prepares the other children for the changes.

Anxious interest in knowledge of labor and birth experience.

Decides on method of infant feeding.

Sexual activity low or discontinued.

Nursing Assessment

Explores expectations of labor experience, knowledge base, feelings about pain, support desired, and preparation.

Inquires about preparation of home (for hospitalization and for infant) and preparation of children.

Inquires about plans to feed infant.

Explores expectations of early weeks as a new mother.

Explores plans for assistance in the home after the hospitalization.

Identifies community resources for families—public health nursing, child health services, social welfare, homemaking services, and so forth.

Explores plans for husband support during the childbearing experience.

Explores father's plans for participation in parenting.

Nursing Intervention

A thorough discussion of labor and birth is appropriate during this stage of pregnancy. Learning relaxation and controlled breathing is useful. Although the discussion of labor will be anxiety-producing, the anxiety can be worked through and acts as a sort of "emotional vaccination." Orientation to the hospital routine reduces future tensions. Observation of a neonate better prepares the parents to accept their coming child—not as a rosy cherub, but as a normal infant.

Physical discomforts such as sleeplessness, pelvic pain, and shortness of breath should be dealt with so that a minimum of stressful experiences accrues. They will multiply in labor and need to be kept to a minimum.

Information related to infant feeding should

be furnished so that the mother may make a decision based on facts and in keeping with her desires. Once the decision is made, further information to help her succeed in this first task of mothering is furnished.

Changes in roles and in the home are realistically reviewed. Parents should be helped to plan changes in the other children's routines with a minimum of stress. Parents need to be warned of the fatigue and conflicts that may accompany the early weeks of parenthood and helped to find ways to reduce and cope with these experiences.

Although the above tasks of pregnancy carry with them feelings of stress and anxiety as inevitable consequences of the rapid changes taking place, it would be a mistake to leave the reader with the impression that anxiety is the root experience. On the contrary, for many women the overwhelming sense is that of ecstasy.[71] We would therefore like to share with you a passage from Colman and Colman's *Pregnancy, the Psychological Experience*[72] and refer you to this entire book. It is a classic! Figure 20-3 illustrates the beginning of this passage.

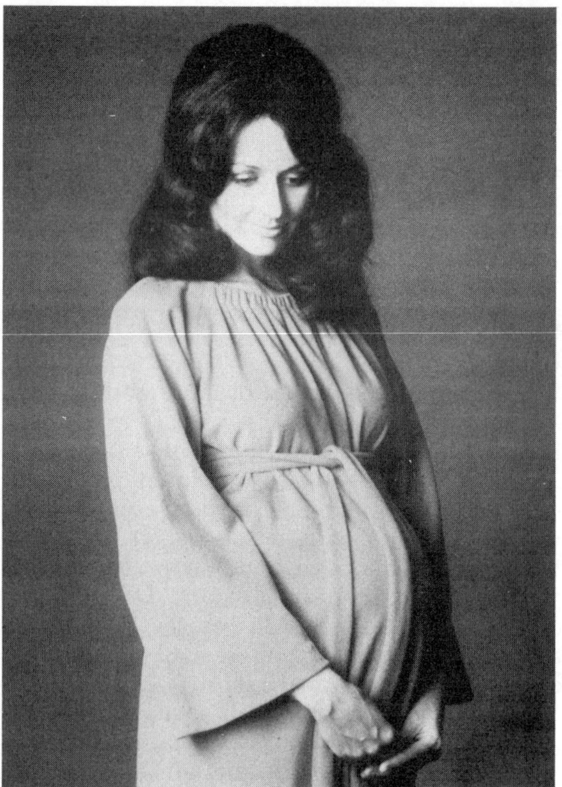

FIGURE 20-3. Many women experience a feeling of ecstasy during pregnancy. (Courtesy of Lederle Diagnostics.)

> Finally, in the ninth month, a woman reaches one of the most beatific phases of human existence. She acquires a physical form which has stimulated not only art but worship throughout the ages. Her smile may surpass the Mona Lisa's. Her presence will affect everyone in the room. Friends may pat her tummy in greeting, or ask to sit next to her to enjoy her radiance. She may be teased, but in a loving way, as if everyone were trying to participate vicariously in what she is doing. She may not fit the *Playboy* image of femininity, but she will epitomize another kind of womanly beauty. Men will see her as a full, rich vessel. Some may say that their image of the most beautiful scene in the world is that of a woman 8½ months pregnant running across an open field. Photographers and painters have captured this state best when they show the pregnant woman standing serenely at a window, emphasizing the extent to which their experiential world is taking place on the inside, but with a reminder that it is on the brink of making the transition, of passing through the window into the world beyond.

If this is too "sugar coated" for you, read on. There are many more stressors to cope with and many more opportunities for the nurse to protect, nurture, and stimulate the expectant and expanding family. Fortunately, however, the end result is, for most families, a happy culmination of dreams. Nursing can help to make that difference.

REFERENCES

1. Hill, R.: *Interdisciplinary workshop on marriage and family research.* Marriage and Family Living 8:21, 1951.
2. Barth, A.: *Permit to Reproduce Urged.* Arizonia Republic, December 27, 1969, p. 34.
3. Time: *Family life style.* December 28, 1970, p. 38.
4. Otto, H. A.: *Criteria for assessing family strengths.* Canada Mental Health 6:107, 1966.
5. Barth: op. cit.
6. Mead, M.: television interview.
7. Time: op. cit.
8. Duvall, E.: *Family Development.* J.B. Lippincott, Philadelphia, 1962, p. 159.
9. Stone, A. R.: *Cues to interpersonal distress due to pregnancy.* Am. J. Nurs. 65:88, 1965.
10. Warrick, L.: *Femininity, sexuality, and mothering.* Nurs. Forum 8:212, 1969.
11. Caplan, G.: *Concept of Mental Health and Consultation.* U. S. Government Printing Office, Washington, D.C., 1959, p. 47.
12. Shainess, N.: *Psychological problems associated with motherhood.* In Arieti, S., et al. (eds.): *American Handbook of Psychiatry, vol. III.* Basic Books, New York, 1966, p. 52.
13. Falicov, C. J.: *Sexual adjustment during first pregnancy and post partum.* Am. J. Obstet. Gynecol. 117:991, 1973.
14. Nadelson, C.: *Normal and special aspects of pregnancy.* Obstet. Gynecol. 41:611, 1973.
15. Deutsch, H.: *Psychology of Pregnancy, Labor and Puerperium,* in Greenhill, J. P.: *Obstetrics,* ed. 13. W. B. Saunders, Philadelphia, 1965.
16. Nadelson: op. cit., p. 613.
17. Richardson, S. A. and Guttmacher, A. F.: *Childbearing–Its Social and Psychological Aspects.* Williams & Wilkins, Baltimore, 1967, p. 3.
18. Nilsson, A., Uddenberg, N. and Alongren, P. E.: *Parental relations and identification in women with special regard to para-natal emotional adjustment.* Acta Psychiatrica Scandinavica 47:57, 1971.
19. Caplan, G.: *Psychological aspects of maternity care.* Am. J. Public Health, 47:25, 1957.
20. Colman, A. D. and Colman, L. L.: *Pregnancy: The Psychological Experience.* Herder and Herder, New York, 1971, p. 169.
21. Ferreira, A. J.: *Prenatal Environment.* Charles C Thomas, Springfield, Ill., 1969, p. 136.
22. Caplan: op. cit., p. 26.
23. Bibring, G.: *Some considerations of the psychological processes in pregnancy.* Psychoanal. Study Child 14:113, 1959.
24. Caplan, G.: *Principles of Preventive Psychiatry.* Basic Books, New York, 1964.
25. Ferreira: op. cit., p. 131.
26. Caplan, G.: *Concepts of Mental Health and Consultation.* Department of Health, Education and Welfare, Washington D.C., 1959, p. 49.
27. Ibid.: p. 58.
28. Ibid.: p. 66.
29. Falicov: op. cit., p. 998.
30. Falicov: op. cit.
31. Ibid.
32. Quirk, B. and Hassanein, R.: *The nurse's role in advising patients on coitus during pregnancy.* Nurs. Clin. North Am. 8:501, 1973.
33. Caplan, G.: *Psychological Aspects of Pregnancy.* In Lief, N. I. (ed.): *The Psychologic Basis of Medical Practice,* Harper and Row, New York, 1973, p. 441.
34. Masters, W. H. and Johnson, V. E.: *Human Sexual Response.* Little, Brown and Co., Boston, 1966, pp. 141–168.
35. Solberg, D. A., Butler, J. and Wagner, N. N.: *Sexual behavior in pregnancy.* N. Engl. J. Med. 288:1098, 1973, p. 1102.
36. Masters and Johnson: op. cit., p. 166.
37. Ibid., p. 167.
38. Neubardt, S.: *Coitus during pregnancy.* Medical Aspects of Human Sexuality 7:197, 1973.
39. Colman, A. D. and Colman, L. L.: *Pregnancy as an altered state of consciousness.* Birth and Family, 1:7, 1973.
40. Rubin, R.: *Some cognitive aspects of childbearing.* In Bergersen, B. S., et al. (eds.): *Current Concepts in Clinical Nursing, vol. 2.* C. B. Mosby, St. Louis, 1969, p. 327.
41. Tart, C. T.: *Scientific foundation for the study of altered state of consciousness.* J. Transpersonal Psychology 2:93, 1971.
42. Colman and Colman: *Pregnancy as an altered state of consciousness,* op. cit.
43. Ibid.
44. Ibid.
45. Ibid.
46. Caplan: *Psychological aspects of maternity care,* op. cit.
47. Colman and Colman: *Pregnancy: The Psychological Experience,* op. cit., p. 170.
48. Bibring: op. cit., p. 116.
49. Stoeckle, J. D., et. al.: *The quality and significance of psychological distress in medical patients.* J. Chronic Dis. 17:964, 1964.
50. Pleshelte, N., Asch, S. S. and Chase, J.: *A study of anxieties during pregnancy, labor, the early and late puerperium.* Bull. N. Y. Acad. Med. 32:436, 1956.
51. Deutsch, H.: *Psychology of Women, vol. 2.* Grune and Stratton, New York, 1945.
52. Davids, A., De Vault, S. and Talmidge, M.: *Anxiety, pregnancy and childbirth abnormalities.* J. Consult. Psychol. 25:74, 1961.

53. Lakin, M.: *Personality factors in mothers of excessively crying (colicky) infants.* Monogr. Soc. Res. Child Develop. 22:64, 1957.
54. Sontag, L. W.: *War and the fetal-maternal relationship.* Marriage & Family Living, 6:1, 1944.
55. Burstein, I., Kinch, R., Stern, L.: *Anxiety, pregnancy, labor, and the neonate.* Am. J. Obstet. Gynecol. 118:195, 1974.
56. Rubin, R.: *Cognitive style in pregnancy.* Am. J. Nurs. 70:506, 1970.
57. Trethowan, W. H.: *The couvade syndrome.* Brit. J. Psychiatry 111:57, 1965.
58. Colman and Colman: *Pregnancy as an altered state of consciousness,* op. cit., p. 8.
59. Caplan, *Psychological Aspects of Pregnancy,* op. cit., p. 60.
60. Howells, J. G. (ed.): *Modern Perspectives in Psycho-Obstetrics.* Brunner and Mazel, New York, 1972, p. 87.
61. Grimm, E. R.: *Psychological and social factors in pregnancy, delivery and outcome.* In Richardson, S.A. and Guttmacher, A.F. (eds.): *Childbearing—Its Social and Psychological Aspects.* Williams & Wilkins, Baltimore, 1967, p. 35.
62. Ibid.: p. 37.
63. Ferreira: op. cit., p. 135.
64. Loc. cit.
65. Grimm: op. cit., p. 35.
66. Ferreira: op. cit., p. 131.
67. Colman and Colman: *Pregnancy: The Psychological Experience,* op. cit., p. 33.
68. Ibid.: p. 40.
69. Colman and Colman: *Pregnancy as an altered state of consciousness,* op. cit.
70. Ibid.
71. Ibid.: p. 58.
72. Ibid.: p. 59.

BIBLIOGRAPHY

Caplan, G.: *Psychological aspects of maternity care.* Am. J. Public Health 47:25, 1957.

Colman, A. D. and Colman, L. L.: *Pregnancy: The Psychological Experience.* Herder and Herder, New York, 1971.

Ibid.: *Pregnancy as an altered state of consciousness.* Birth and Family 1:7, 1973.

Duval, E.: *Family Development,* ed 4. J. B. Lippincott, Philadelphia, 1971.

Erikson, E.: *The problem of ego identity.* J. Am. Psychoanal. Assoc. 4:56, 1956.

Josselyn, I. M.: *Cultural forces—motherliness and fatherliness.* Am. J. Orthopsychiat. 26:264, 1956.

Pavenstedt, E. and Bernard, V. W. (ed.): *Crisis of Family Disorganization.* Behavioral Publications, New York, 1971.

Pleschelte, N., Ash, S. and Chase, J.: *A study of anxieties of pregnancy, labor, and the puerperium.* Bull. N. Y. Acad. Med. 32:436, 1956.

Richardson, S. A. and Guttmacher, A. F.: *Childbearing—Its Social and Psychological Aspects.* Williams & Wilkins, Baltimore, 1967.

Rubin, R.: *Cognitive style in pregnancy.* Am. J. Nurs. 70:502, 1970.

Schoenberg, B., et al.: *Loss and Grief.* Columbia University Press, New York, 1970.

Sexual Relations During Pregnancy and the Post Delivery Period. SIECUS Study Guide No. 6. Sex Information and Education Council of the U. S., New York, 1967.

Solberg, D. A., Butler, J. and Wagner, N. N.: *Sexual behavior in pregnancy.* Obstet. Gynecol. Survey 28:704, 1973.

Strickland, M. D.: *Environmental influences on the fetus.* In Anderson, E. H., et al. (eds.): *Current Concepts in Clinical Nursing, vol. 4.* C. B. Mosby, St. Louis, 1973.

21 Application of Physiologic Perspectives

ANN L. CLARK, R.N., M.A.

During the 40 weeks of gestation, a new human being is conceived, grows to a state of viability, and is born. This complex process occurring within the mother's body has profound effects on her physiologic system and on her feelings and behavior, as we have seen in the preceding chapter.

The growth of the fetus and the maternal changes are progressive and predictable. The nine months of gestation are divided into three trimesters, each consisting of three months. Early and continuous health supervision beginning in the first trimester is important to the good health of the mother and is of great consequence to the fetus and neonate. Health supervision consists of ongoing assessment of maternal physical and emotional health, fetal health, and education of the mother for self-care. It also includes communication with the expectant parents to help them understand the changes that are occurring in their lives and to prepare for the role changes both for themselves and for other members of the family.

Pregnancy is a *normal* physiologic process. However, there are many physiologic adjustments the mother's body must make. A healthy body can be expected to make these adjustments with a minimum of stress. Nevertheless, it is a stress. Each organ of the body and the total structure are called upon to exert themselves to a greater degree. Pregnancy involves multiple readjustments to living and some discomforts. Health problems which may normally be of little consequence may have considerable impact on the pregnant womans physiology and on the developing fetus. The fetus is particularly vulnerable during the earliest phases of its development when basic organ structures are being established. Women who enter pregnancy with poor nutritional status or acute or chronic health problems are in jeopardy during pregnancy, and their unborn child is also in jeopardy. Thus, prenatal assessment and prenatal self-care should begin as early in pregnancy as the first missed menstrual period.

The traditional "routine care" that varied little from woman to woman unless complications developed is now giving way to very different types of clinics. Studies[1,2] indicate that clients whose pregnancies can be expected to be uneventful can be identified. Likewise, high-risk mothers can be determined very early in pregnancy and special consideration can be given to their health and the health of their fetuses. Thus, priorities based on individual and family needs can be ascribed and health personnel can be more appropriately used. High-risk prenatal patients are usually cared for by the obstetrician, using other health care personnel (e.g., social workers, nutritionists, and public health nurses) as appropriate.

Today, more and more clinics and medical

groups are providing prenatal care using an interdisciplinary team. This constitutes a much better utilization of health personnel. The patient is usually seen by the physician on her first prenatal visit. The medical history is taken and the physician performs a complete physical examination, including a pelvic estimation. In some clinics the nurse-midwife or the maternal health nurse practitioner may be the first person to see the patient and make the assessment. If it is predicted that the patient will have an uneventful prenatal course, the patient is assigned to the "nurse clinic." Some of these clinics are known as maternity continuity clinics in which the patient sees the same nurse practitioner at each prenatal visit.[3] The obstetrician is the consultant to the nurse practitioner whenever she feels the patient needs his expertise. When this occurs, the patient, depending on her health problem, may be assigned to the physician-conducted clinic, or returned to the nurse's care after a medical regimen is prescribed. Ideally, a nurse-physician conference is held when the patient reaches 32 weeks of gestation and another when she approaches full term. The nurse practitioner assumes responsibility for assessing the expectant mother's psychosocial, physical, and informational needs. She makes judgments concerning the physical normalcy of her patient, cares for the minor discomforts of pregnancy, and plans for the educational needs of her patient. She provides anticipatory and supportive guidance. She no longer fills the conventional managerial role, but becomes the health professional with primary responsibility for the delivery of health care to specific patients within the institutional setting and extended into the home.

A type of nurse clinic is described by Kowalski.[4] In this clinic there are several "two-nurse teams" which care for a "case load" of expectant and laboring mothers. One of the two nurses sees the expectant mother at each prenatal visit and in a continuous care pattern also supports her during her labor experience. After delivery the nurses make rounds to their patients and the new infants. They share significant data with the nurses on the postpartum and nursery units and contribute to the nursing care plan as appropriate.

When the staff includes nurse-midwives, they assume full responsibility for their patients, including their deliveries, unless a patient develops a complication. The physician is always accessible to the nurse-midwife as a consultant.

PRENATAL ASSESSMENT

The initial prenatal assessment consists of 1) the interview, 2) the history, 3) the physical examination, and 4) the laboratory tests. All of these will be discussed in detail.

THE INTERVIEW

In addition to the mainly physiologic facts obtained from a medical history, the many various psychosocial influences on a woman and her family are an extremely important aspect of pregnancy and must be considered when planning prenatal care. This information can be obtained by conducting a patient profile interview.

This prenatal interview, if it is to be successful, must be based on mutual trust and confidence. Nurses, due to their educational background in interviewing, counseling, and teaching, are the most logical individuals within the health team to do the interview. Some clinics have prepared a form which the patient may complete prior to the initial interview (Fig. 21-1). This can be helpful to the nurse and to all the health team, but nurses should be vocal in their insistence that the prenatal interview is a logical and essential aspect of nursing practice.

Patients and nurses meet each other with a lifetime of experiences which they each carry with them into an initial interpersonal relationship such as an interview. Nurses need to

INDIVIDUALIZED OBSTETRICAL QUESTIONNAIRE

The information you provide is confidential and will become a permanent part of your medical record. Please fill it out as completely and as accurately as you can.

Date__________ Birthdate___________ Age_____ Name____
Last First Maiden

Address____ Phone_______________ ____________

Your occupation__________________ Birthplace_________________ Race_________________________

Circle where appropriate: Single Married Widowed Divorced Separated
Year of marriage_____________ Husband's name________________________________ His age________
Education: Circle highest grade completed: Elementary K-8 High 9-12 College 1-4 More

	YES	NO	COMMENTS
Menstrual History: EDC________________			
Date of FIRST day of last menstrual period?______________			
Was it different from other menstrual period?	( )	( )	
Are your menstrual periods: shorter than 25 days?	( )	( )	
longer than 33 days?	( )	( )	
Obstetrical History:			
What is your ideal non-pregnant weight?_____ Present_____ Height_______ BP_____			
How many times have you been pregnant before?_____ Any miscarriages?____ Caesarian?_____			
Where did you have your last baby?________________________________			
What was the weight of your largest baby?____ lbs.____ oz. Smallest baby?____ lbs.____ oz.			
What are the sexes of your children? Male________ Female________			
How long was your longest labor?_____ hours. Your shortest labor?_____ hours.			
Are there twins in YOUR side of the family?	( )	( )	
In those pregnancies <u>not</u> resulting in a live baby:			
Did any end before 5 months?	( )	( )	
Did any end after 5 months, but before going into labor?	( )	( )	
Did the baby's death occur during labor?	( )	( )	
Did the baby's death occur after labor?	( )	( )	
Have any of your children been born with problems?	( )	( )	
Defects	( )	( )	
Deformaties	( )	( )	
Jaundice	( )	( )	
Other than delivery, were you hospitalized during any of your other pregnancies?	( )	( )	
Did you have any of the following problems during your other pregnancies?			
High blood pressure	( )	( )	
Sugar or protein in the urine	( )	( )	
Swelling of face, feet, or fingers	( )	( )	
Anemia (low iron, low blood count)	( )	( )	
Other problems	( )	( )	
Did you have any of the following problems after other pregnancies?			
Fever or infection	( )	( )	
Blood clots	( )	( )	
Depression	( )	( )	
Other problems	( )	( )	
Do you have any of the following problems now?			
Nausea--vomiting	( )	( )	
Constipation	( )	( )	
Burning with urination	( )	( )	
Headaches	( )	( )	

FIGURE 21-1. A personal prenatal assessment. (Courtesy of Kaiser Medical Center.)

	YES	NO	COMMENTS
Troublesome vaginal discharge	( )	( )	
Problem with your eyes	( )	( )	
Ankle or leg swelling	( )	( )	
Vaginal bleeding	( )	( )	
Other	( )	( )	
Have you been ill since becoming pregnant?	( )	( )	
Colds or "Flu"	( )	( )	
Measles	( )	( )	
Others	( )	( )	
Have any birth defects occured in your family?	( )	( )	
Past History:			
Have you ever had or been treated for the following?			
An operation	( )	( )	
Serious illness	( )	( )	
Sexual problems	( )	( )	
Veneral Disease	( )	( )	
Heart Disease	( )	( )	
Rheumatic Fever	( )	( )	
High blood pressure	( )	( )	
Transfusion	( )	( )	
Varicose Veins	( )	( )	
Tuberculosis	( )	( )	
Asthma	( )	( )	
Pneumonia	( )	( )	
Ulcers	( )	( )	
Jaundice or Hepatitis (liver infection)	( )	( )	
Gall Bladder Disease	( )	( )	
Diabetes	( )	( )	
Thyroid problems	( )	( )	
Bladder infections (Cystitis)	( )	( )	
Other problems	( )	( )	
Have any member of your family had (or do they have) any of the conditions mentioned in the above question? (Father, mother, brothers, sisters,etc)	( )	( )	
Do you feel you have emotional problems such as:			
Depression or tension	( )	( )	
Difficulty sleeping	( )	( )	
Are you having marital difficulties?	( )	( )	
Was this pregnancy unexpected?	( )	( )	
Are you allergic to any medicines?	( )	( )	
Are you taking any prescribed medicines?	( )	( )	
Have you used any medicines or drugs during this pregnancy including LSD, speed, or marijuana?	( )	( )	
Has there been any change in your general health during the last year?	( )	( )	
If you have completed your desired family size with this pregnancy, are you interested in a permanent method of contraception such as:			
Vasectomy	( )	( )	
Tubal Ligation	( )	( )	

Please circle if you want more information about any of the following:

Labor and Delivery   Anesthesia   Breast Feeding   Personal Hygiene

Good diet during pregnancy   Contraception (Family Planning)   Childcare

Other____________________________________

________________ Date

________________________ Signature

be cognizant of how those experiences relate to the reciprocal communication that follows. Interest, concern, warmth, and friendliness on the part of the nurse interviewer help to assure that a trusting relationship will follow.

Initiating the Interview

Every interview should take place in an area where privacy is insured. Telephones, interruptions, and overheard voices of others intrude upon the interview and are detrimental. There are some basic considerations which convey the respect one holds for another individual. The patient should be told the interviewer's name and the position she holds in the health facility. She also needs to know the purpose of the interview and its benefits to her, her child, and her family. She should understand that the interview is an opportunity for her to talk about herself, her pregnancy, and her coming baby so that she and members of the health team can formulate the best possible plan of prenatal care for her. It is preferable not to suggest that you will discuss "problems," since no one wishes to be seen as an individual who has problems he cannot resolve.

The use of the client's name helps her to retain her sense of identity and personal worth, even in a strange, anxiety-producing setting. The interviewer should know and use her patient's name. Expectant mothers should never be called by a number, by labels such as "mother" or "dear," by last name or first name only, or without a proper title.

The expectant mother has a right to confidentiality. The nurse should inform the woman that the information she shares with her will be used only in her own interest.

The time limitation on an interview should be shared with the patient. This allows the patient to decide how she would like to use the time. However, time schedules cannot be rigidly set since some patients may not need all the time allowed while others may need much more. The nurse's analysis of the manner in which the patient utilizes the time available will help her to understand her patient.

The interview must be structured so that the focus is on the client and not on the nurse. Some clients will try to switch the focus to the nurse. It is understandable that at some point the patient may ask, "Do you have any children?" However, if she then tries to focus on the nurse's children, her labor, or other aspects of her life, the nurse must try to understand what is occurring in this relationship. Has the client just been introduced to or relating something that is anxiety-producing, so that she feels a need to "switch off"? Does she manifest anxiety in other ways? The client may be attempting to establish some kind of a peer relationship with the nurse. However, in order to be therapeutic, the interview must remain a warm nurse-client relationship. It is the nurse's responsibility to refocus the interview on the client.

The client must be free to tell her story in a nonthreatening, permissive atmosphere where her life style and behavior will not be criticized or condemned. Expressions of empathy and praise provide encouragement during the interview when used appropriately and sincerely.

Obtaining Relevant Data

The patient profile is the basic component of the interview. The nurse needs to know the patient's age, marital status, and the family constellation. She also needs to know the significant others in her patient's life and how they can be relied upon to help her cope with pregnancy and childrearing.

In terms of housing, she needs to know who lives in the same household and their relationship to her patient. She needs to understand the size of the home and housing arrangements, such as who buys the food and who prepares the meals. She needs to learn the sources of income and the adequacy of that amount.

She needs to obtain information about the community and the neighborhood in which the family resides. Cultural beliefs, values, and practices related to childbearing and childrearing influence the kind of prenatal care that should be arranged for the woman. The nurse needs to know something of the life style of her client. Information related to her sexual partner, and her use of alcohol, tobacco, and drugs must be considered in her prenatal care.

Knowledge of the educational and employment background of the client will help the nurse to select an appropriate approach and vocabulary. Moreover, recognition of her place in the business world is ego-supportive.

Listening

Concentration on what the woman is expressing demonstrates the nurse's respect for her and her feelings. Expectant mothers need to be given time to think things out and to express themselves. The nurse must be able to wait during pauses and to tolerate silences. Some silences ultimately become nonproductive and the nurse, through experience, will learn when to intervene.

Nonverbal Communication

The nurse must be as observant of nonverbal communications as she is of the words spoken. Gestures, facial expressions, posture, and tone of voice all speak loudly of what the patient is feeling. The nurse should validate these communications with her patient. Apparent incongruences between verbal and nonverbal communication should be explored further.

Problem-Solving and Teaching

When a problem is identified, the nurse needs to collect all possible data related to the problem. She needs to understand exactly how the problem is seen by the patient. Important aspects of the problem are when it began, how it has changed activities of daily living, what she has tried to do about it, what results followed, and what other ideas the client has for overcoming the problem.

The nurse will often need to use questions to help the patient tell her story. Rather than closed questions which elicit "yes" or "no" answers, open questions should be asked so that the expectant mother can clarify her situation. For example,

Closed question:	Are you upset about being pregnant?
Open question:	Many women find that a new baby is arriving at an inopportune time, how is it with you?

Questions must be nonthreatening and not seen as prying. The nurse should not collect data out of curiosity. She should collect only that data which can be useful in understanding her patient.

If the nurse needs additional information on a particular aspect of the problem, she may focus the interview by saying, for example, "Can you tell me more about how you felt when. . . ."

Clarification and restatement are used until the nurse is sure she understands the problem completely. Indicating that the problem is understood before all the facts are obtained will only close off the discussion. If the nurse says "I understand" or "I see what you mean," the patient, particularly if she knows the nurse does not have all the data, will feel that the nurse has limited concern for her. Examples of clarification and restatement include "Are you telling me that. . . ." and "Did I understand you to say that. . . ."

All problems or needs, as identified by the patient or suggested by the data the patient shares, should be acknowledged. It is not easy at first to determine priorities. The interviewing nurse must remain keenly aware of all that is occurring in the session. She must determine the relative importance of each problem and decide whether it should be explored in the present interview or at a later date.

In helping the expectant mother to solve a problem, the nurse keeps her from wandering from topic to topic, and helps her remain goal-directed until some resolution is reached. If an impasse occurs, the nurse can help her to explore alternatives by posing appropriate hypothetical questions, such as "What would happen if. . . ."

When patients ask specific questions, the answers must be based on sound scientific knowledge, be of sufficient depth to help the individual, and be at her level of understanding. The nurse will not necessarily have all the answers, but she can obtain the answers or make appropriate referrals. Indeed, the best judgment may be to refer the patient to another professional.

THE HISTORY

History-taking is an important component of the diagnostic assessment and can be an excellent instrument for building a trusting relationship with the expectant mother. The components of the history are:

- A. Subjective data
    - 1. Initial prenatal history
        - a. Family history of health problems
        - b. Past medical history
        - c. Menstrual history
        - d. Obstetric history
        - e. Sexual and marital history
        - f. Contraception history
        - g. Progress of this pregnancy
        - h. Immunication
    - 2. Interval prenatal history
        - a. Updating of medical history, medical problems, minor disturbances
- B. Objective data
    - 1. Physical examination

Initial Prenatal History

Most history-taking begins with a *chief complaint.* This may seem a strange term to be using in maternity care, however it is an accurate term. The patient's chief complaint is usually amenorrhea. In obstetrics this chief complaint would be written "last menstrual period" (LMP). The interviewer would also elicit other information to assist in making the determination, such as:

Frequency of urination
Breast changes (tingling, heaviness, presence of colostrum)
Nausea and vomiting.

These subjective symptoms are only presumptive signs of pregnancy since that they could be caused by conditions other than pregnancy. They are, however, an *elaboration of the patient's chief complaint.*

The prenatal history now begins to vary somewhat from a medical-surgical history. A *family history of health problems,* significant to every patient, has particular importance for both the mother and her infant. It is important to know all of the family history but special interest is focused on diseases and events in which heredity appears to be a contributory factor such as diabetes mellitus and pregnancy-induced hypertension. The family history should include such items as:

Multiple pregnancies
Cardiovascular diseases
Diabetes
Tuberculosis
Epilepsy
Congenital abnormalities
Hereditary diseases
Mental, emotional, and psychiatric problems.

The *past medical history* of the patient is also of particular significance. Some conditions may have impact on the present pregnancy; others, presently resolved, may be activated by the pregnancy. The past medical history includes:

- Heart disease
- Urinary tract disease
- Hypertension
- Rheumatic triad (polyarthritis, carditis, chorea)
- Asthma
- Tuberculosis
- Venereal diseases
- Ulcers
- Varicose veins
- Diabetes
- Thyroid dysfunction
- Phlebitus
- Psychic disorders
- Jaundice or hepatitis
- Epilepsy
- Drug sensitivity
- Allergies
- Blood dyscrasia
- Blood transfusion
- Surgery
- Accidents
- Gallbladder disease.

The *menstrual history* of the expectant mother is important to this pregnancy. It should record:

- Date of onset of menses
- Interval, duration, and amount of flow
- Associated symptoms and medical management
- Date of last menstrual period and its characteristics
- Date of quickening
- Estimated date of confinement
- Menstrual disorders
- Gynecologic disorders.

The *past obstetric history* has some predictive value for the outcome of this pregnancy. Complications that arose during pregnancy, labor, and the puerperium are carefully noted, and a summary of the records is obtained. Likewise, neonatal problems related to the birth process and any growth and development problems of children in the family are recorded. The following items are explored:

- Problems related to infertility
- Full-term deliveries (date of delivery, weight of infant, length of labor, type of delivery)
- Premature deliveries (cause, if known; weight; developmental pattern of child)
- Multiple births
- Abortions (month of gestation attained; cause, if known)
- Voluntary interruptions of pregnancy (month of gestation; method used)
- Stillbirths (cause, if known)
- Children living (ages, any developmental problems)
- Maternal complications
- Isoimmunization (RhoGAM given)
- Fetal and neonatal complications.

The *sexual and marital history* will be reviewed with the patient. Problems related to sexuality may be present at the onset of pregnancy or may be precipitated by pregnancy. Consultation may be sought by the expectant parents, and anticipatory guidance should be a part of prenatal care. The following aspects should be explored:

- Age of onset of sexual activity
- Frequency and timing of sexual relations
- Libido
- Changes in pattern of sexual activity since pregnancy
- Marital difficulties.

A history of the use of contraceptives should also be obtained. Families who seek further assistance following the present pregnancy may wish guidance in different methods or may decide to undergo a permanent method of sterilization. Such plans should be made prior to the date of delivery. The *contraceptive history* should include:

Methods of contraception used
Acceptance or rejection of the method
Whether use was consistent or sporatic
Was this pregnancy an outcome of contraceptive failure
Goals in relation to the family size.

The *present pregnancy history* usually focuses on pathophysiology. These items are important because they may be symptoms of or actual pathologic conditions which place the mother and/or her infant in jeopardy. The present pregnancy history includes:

Gastrointestinal symptoms
Headaches, dizziness, visual disturbances
Edema
Abdominal pain
Urinary tract symptoms
Bleeding
Fatigue
Symptomatic vaginal discharge
Immunizations
  Diptheria
  Tetanus
  Oral polio vaccine
  Other
Sleep patterns
Taking of prescribed medication
Self-medication
Mantoux or chest roentgenogram (date and result).

Interval Prenatal History

The expectant mother is seen by the physician or the nurse at specified intervals during her pregnancy. Usually, until the seventh month of pregnancy the mother is given an appointment every month. During the seventh and eighth months of pregnancy she is seen every two weeks and during the ninth month she is seen weekly. At each of these visits her ongoing prenatal record is updated.

Discomforts and disturbances which are minor in a medical sense may be major stressors for the expectant mother and may occur at any time during pregnancy. These include:

Heartburn	Urinary frequency
Constipation	Puritus
Leg cramps	Bleeding from nose or gums.
Backache	
Dependent edema	

The nurse must be able to perform data collection and analysis relating to these or other symptoms. The following technique* is used:

1. *What is the chief complaint of the patient?* This is a brief statement of the complaint of the patient. The onset and duration of the symptom are included in the statement. It refers to a concrete complaint, avoiding the use of diagnostic terms or names of a disease. It uses the patient's own words as nearly as possible.
2. *What in the patient's profile on personal history, habits, family situation, or life situation may have relevance to her diagnosis?* (This does not include past history or family history at this point.) Examples: sleep habits, diet, exercise, hobbies, alcohol, tobacco, caffeine, nonprescription drugs, medication therapy, living environment, adequacy of income. Be sure to include any *recent* changes in her profile.
3. *What are the basic components of the present problem?* This includes an elaboration of the chief complaint, a history of the present problem from the time of onset, a full description of the current status of the problem, and a summary of

* *Programmed Instruction. Patient Assessment: Taking a Patient's History.* Am. J. Nurs. 74:293, 1974, was used, with permission, as a guide in developing this technique.

significant "positives" (conditions found) and "negatives" (conditions not found).

4. *Are there other chief complaints that are apparently unrelated?* If yes, each of these complaints should be reviewed separately and recorded as in steps 1, 2, 3, above. Use a paragraph for each complaint.

To analyze the chief complaint(s), the following steps are taken:

1. *The onset.* When and how it began, was it a sudden onset, or did it build up? What were the predisposing and precipitating factors to the onset? Record in the following manner:
   date of onset
   manner of onset
   precipitating or predisposing factors.
2. *Further data.* What are the *characteristics* of the complaint, how did the patient feel just prior to the event? Did climate, work load, personal crisis, etc. seem to precipitate the event? Is physical exertion, fatigue, toxin, allergens, or environment in any way involved in the onset of the complaint? Where is it located? How intense are the symptoms? Do the symptoms remain constant or come and go? Record the characteristic of the complaint in the following manner:
   character
   location and radiation (of pain)
   intensity
   timing
   aggravating and relieving factors
   associated symptoms.
3. What is the *course since the onset?* Were there one or more recurrent attacks? Is it daily, periodic, or continuously chronic in character? What is the duration of the attack? Are there temporal relationships to the bodily functions? If any drug, rest, exercise, diet, or psychotherapeutic measure was taken, did it alleviate, suppress (mask), or introduce any toxic symptom that overshadows the original symptom? Record this analysis in the following manner:
   pattern of incidence
   progress
   effect of therapy.

An example of this technique using a frequently encountered stressor is:

1. Onset

   The patient, a 24-week-pregnant woman, complains of "itching and burning" in the perineal area of "several days" duration. Over the past week she has been increasingly aware of irritation around the vulva and anus.

   She is married and has continued sexual relations with her husband about once a week. She denies use of any "hygienic" deodorants. She does not complain of dysuria. She wears pantyhose.
2. Characteristics

   The irritation at present is persistent. She has a profuse greenish vaginal discharge. The symptoms have disturbed her sleep and are usually aggravated by urination and after sexual relations. She admits to frequent scratching of the parts.
3. Course since onset

   The patient has washed the vulval area with soap and water several times daily and applied bath powder to the area. She has discontinued using nylon undergarments. She does not feel the treatment has in any way helped to ameliorate the condition. She feels depressed and is concerned that she may have "contracted some dreadful disease." She is also concerned that she will be thought of as someone who does not keep herself clean, which she denies.

Use of this technique for data collection and analysis provides a sound foundation upon which to base the planning, implementation, and evaluation of appropriate nursing actions to manage or resolve complaints.

INITIAL PHYSICAL EXAMINATION

The expectant mother should receive a complete physical examination when she first presents herself for care. Women often have little or no medical supervision during their childbearing years, except when they are pregnant. It is therefore important that the physical examination be a thorough one and include:

E.E.N.T.	Lungs
Thyroid	Abdomen
Teeth	Extremities
Heart	

Examination of the breasts, abdomen, and pelvis takes on special importance during pregnancy. They are an integral part of the initial as well as subsequent physical examinations and are discussed separately here.

Breast Examination

The examination (inspection and palpation) is begun with the patient sitting on the examining table with her arms extended upward and then brought down by her sides. Inspection should note any asymmetry in size, shape, or contour of the breasts and any puckering or dimpling of the skin of the breasts. Each nipple is gently rolled between the fingertips to see if there is any discharge from the nipple. (Colostrum is expected to be present after 16 weeks of pregnancy.) The patient then assumes a recumbent position. The breast tissue is palpated between the fingers and the chest wall, starting at the sternum and working in small circular motions toward the nipple, then around the nipple line, the lower part of the breasts, the outer part of the breast, and the upper part of the breast. All tissue of the breast is reviewed in this manner. The

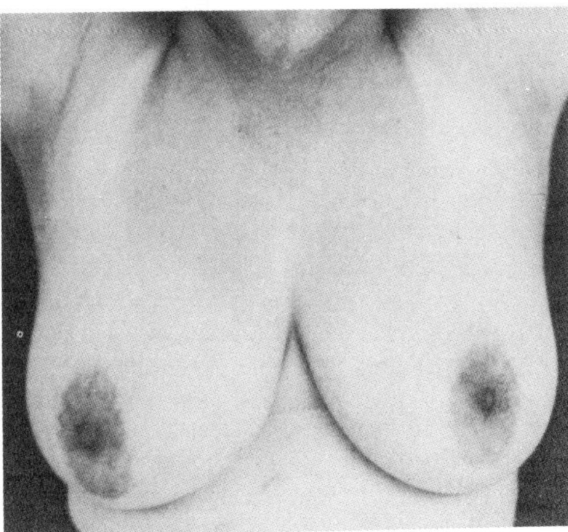

FIGURE 21-2. The patient tenses her pectoral muscles for inspection. (From Snodgrass, W.: *Fundamentals of Family Practice.* F. A. Davis, Philadelphia, 1975, with permission.)

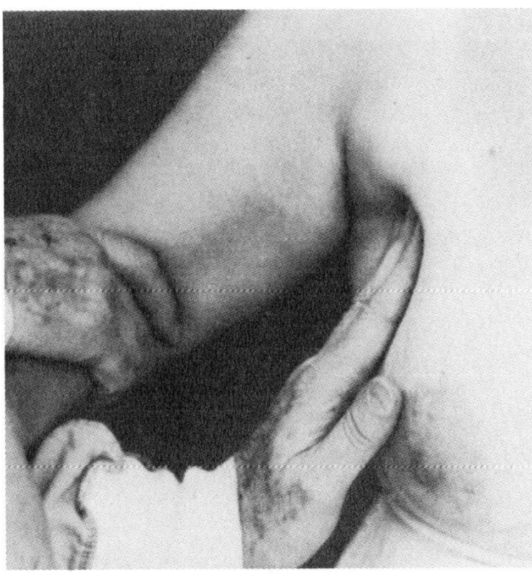

FIGURE 21-3. While the patient rests her forearm in your arm, palpate the axilla for enlarged nodes. (From Snodgrass, W.: *Fundamentals of Family Practice.* F. A. Davis, Philadelphia, 1975, with permission.)

axilla is palpated with the tips of the fingers while the patient raises her arm and then lowers it against the chest wall (Figs. 21-2 to 21-6).

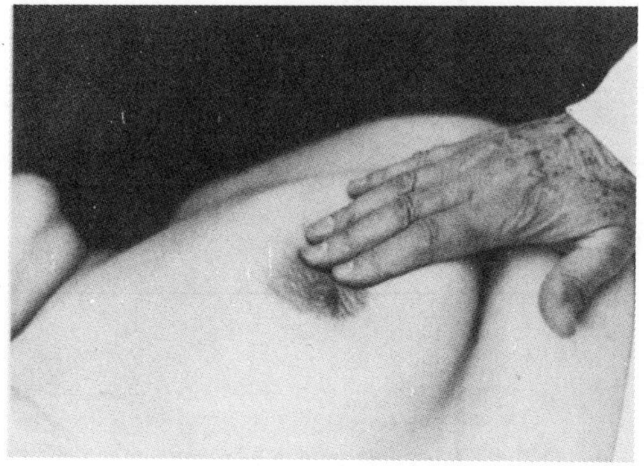

FIGURE 21-4. Palpate the breasts for tumors. (From Snodgrass, W.: *Fundamentals of Family Practice.* F. A. Davis, Philadelphia, 1975, with permission.)

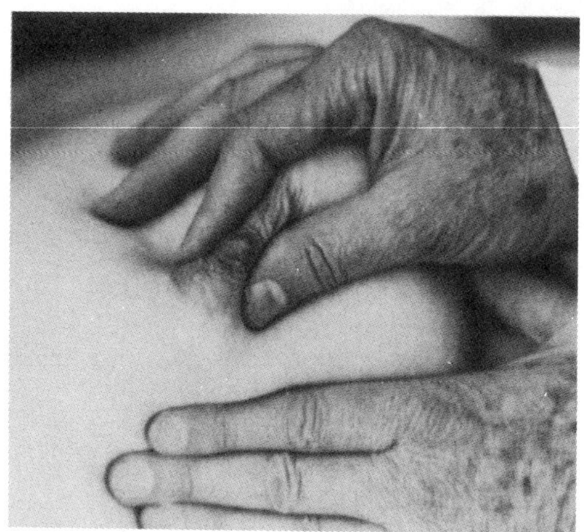

FIGURE 21-5. Milk the nipple to express secretions. (From Snodgrass, W.: *Fundamentals of Family Practice.* F. A. Davis, Philadelphia, 1975, with permission.)

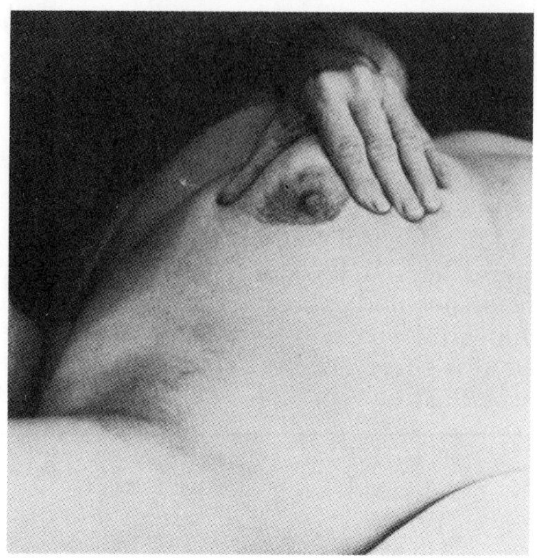

FIGURE 21-6. The patient should learn to inspect her own breasts. (From Snodgrass, W.: *Fundamentals of Family Practice.* F. A. Davis, Philadelphia, 1975, with permission.)

Abdominal Examination

Prior to the examination, the nurse should explain the procedure to her patient and secure her cooperation. The patient should totally undress and be clothed in a gown which opens in the front. She should also empty her bladder.

The examination begins with the patient in a recumbent position. The abdomen is inspected for scars and striations, and the contour is noted. Diastasis of the rectus muscle or an umbilical hernia will be obvious if the patient raises her head and coughs. The abdomen is palpated for the height of the fundus. This is palpable after 13 weeks of pregnancy. This measurement is recorded and used as a guideline for all subsequent measures. It helps assure that fetal development is normal.

The fetal outline can be ascertained by 30 weeks of gestation. Palpation is done with the full length of the fingers and the palms, not with the fingertips.

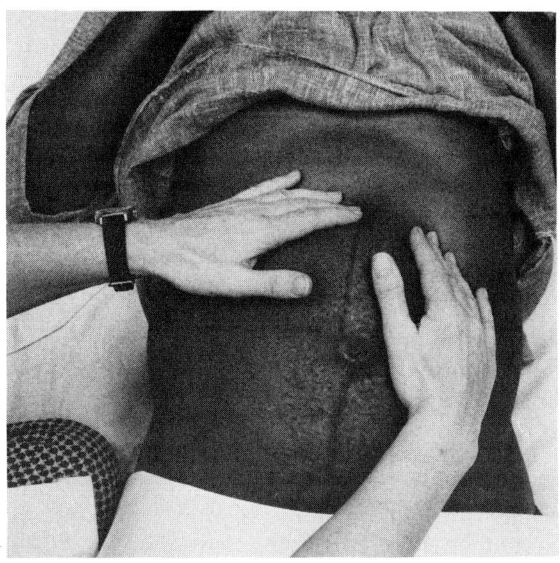

FIGURE 21-7. Palpating the fundus of the uterus. (Photograph by Robert Goldstein.)

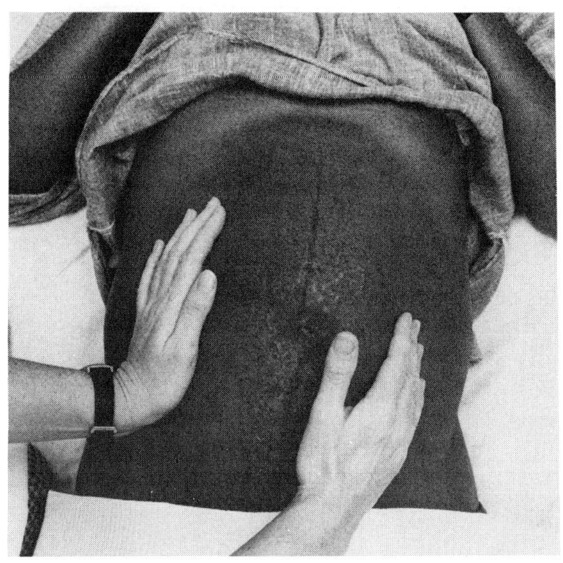

FIGURE 21-8. Palpating for the spine and small parts of the fetus. (Photograph by Robert Goldstein.)

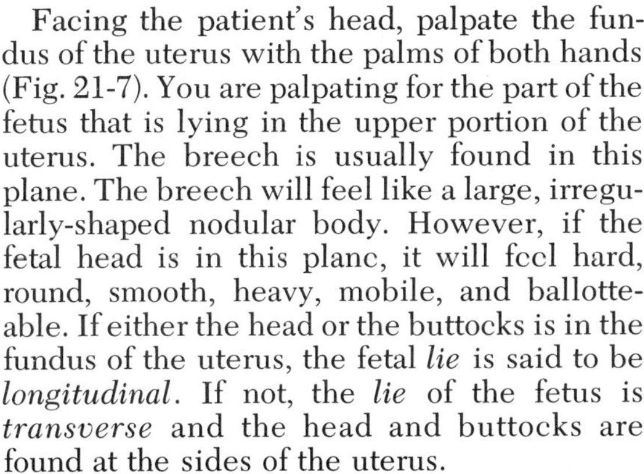

Facing the patient's head, palpate the fundus of the uterus with the palms of both hands (Fig. 21-7). You are palpating for the part of the fetus that is lying in the upper portion of the uterus. The breech is usually found in this plane. The breech will feel like a large, irregularly-shaped nodular body. However, if the fetal head is in this plane, it will feel hard, round, smooth, heavy, mobile, and ballotteable. If either the head or the buttocks is in the fundus of the uterus, the fetal *lie* is said to be *longitudinal*. If not, the *lie* of the fetus is *transverse* and the head and buttocks are found at the sides of the uterus.

Now palpate the uterus, with one hand on each side of the uterus, to feel the fetal spines. A firm continuous resistance on one side, and small parts (knees, feet, arms) on the other side should be felt (Fig. 21-8). Finally, facing the patient's feet, palpate the lower uterine segment using one hand on either side of the uterus (Fig. 21-9). If the fetal head is felt, it

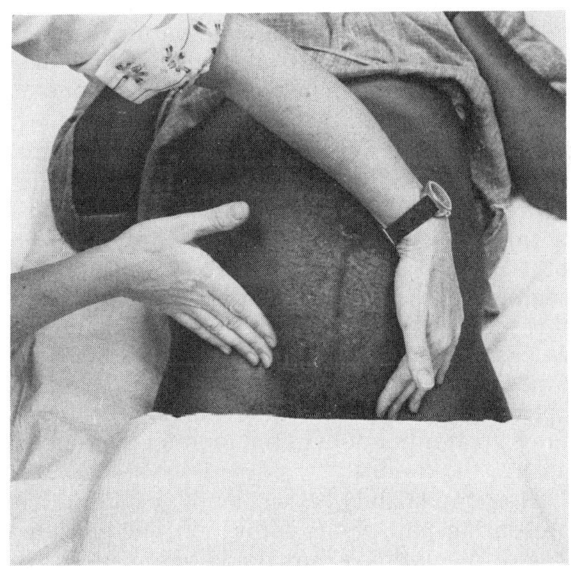

FIGURE 21-9. Palpating the lower uterine segment. (Photograph by Robert Goldstein.)

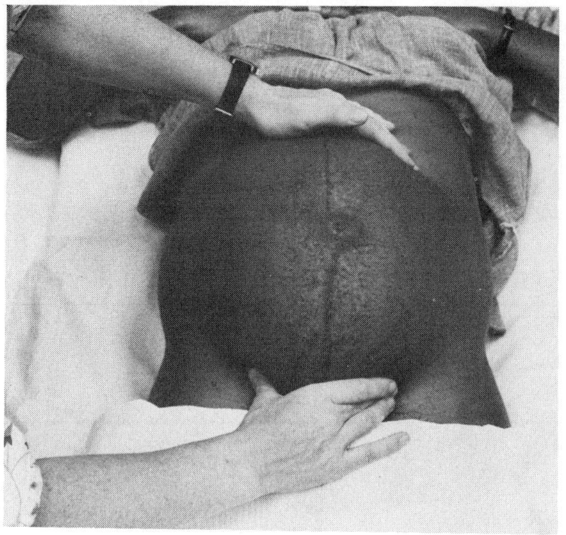

FIGURE 21-10. Palpating for engagement of the presenting part. (Photograph by Robert Goldstein.)

will be hard, round, and smooth. Using the fingers of both hands, the head can usually be felt higher on the side opposite the fetal spine because the head is usually flexed and the occipital part of the head is not as prominent to palpation.

Until 32 weeks of gestation the large amount of amniotic fluid in relation to the fetus and the uncrowded environment within the uterus permit the fetus to float more freely. The breech may be found in the lower uterine segment, although the fetal head usually is in this segment (an occipit presentation). After 32 weeks of gestation the fetus, if it has been in breech presentation, will usually turn, simply because the more movable part of the fetus finds greater freedom in the roomier part of the uterus, the fundus.

At approximately 38 weeks of gestation the presenting part of the fetus will become engaged. When this occurs the largest transverse diameter of the biparietals of the fetal head has passed through the pelvic brim. Using both hands, point the fingers downward and inward. Dip the fingers downward into the pelvis and exert pressure to determine how firmly the presenting part is engaged (Fig. 21-10). Now place the fingers of both hands on either side of the fetal head. If the fetal head has descended through the pelvic inlet it will not be possible to reach the lower part of the head. The examining fingers when pushed downward over the lower abdomen will slide over that portion of the head proximal to the biparietal plane (nape of the neck) and diverge. Conversely, if the head is not engaged the examining fingers can easily palpate the lower part of the head and hence will converge.[5] The engagement of the head can also be ascertained by rectal or vaginal examinations.

The fetal heart tone is now checked. It cannot be heard by fetoscope until 20 to 24 weeks of gestation. It can be heard earlier than this if a Doptone is available. The presentation, position, and fetal heart rate are recorded.

Pelvic Examination

The client is placed in lithotomy position with her feet in stirrups and buttocks well over the edge of the table with a drape over the thighs and abdomen. The client is asked to spread her legs wide apart. A good light is positioned so that a thorough examination can be made.

The external genitalia are inspected (Fig. 21-11). The clitorus, prepuce, urethral meatus, labia minora and majora, perineal body, perineal skin, and anal sphincter are examined for discoloration and lesions. The ducts of the Bartholin's glands are normally not palpable. If they are cystic or abscessed a mass will be felt. Pressure should be exerted over the mass to see if a purulent discharge can be expressed.

The labia are separated and the fourchette and hymen are examined for evidence of old lacerations and scarring. The patient is requested to bear down. Any protrusion into the vagina or loss of urine from the urethra should be noted.

Further pelvic assessment is now delayed until a cytologic (Papanicolaou) smear can be taken. Smears may also be taken for gonorrhea and, where indicated, for vaginal trichomoniasis or moniliasis. A speculum of appropriate size is lubricated with warm tap water (never lubricating jelly) and carefully inserted to cause as little patient discomfort as possible. Tissues of the anterior portion of the vagina are especially sensitive. However, the perineum can be markedly depressed without undue discomfort. The closed speculum is therefore pressed toward the perineal floor as it is slowly introduced. Once the speculum is in place it is opened and "locked." The patient should be instructed to breathe deeply. The comforting hand of the attendant may be reassuring, and the examiner should not be so engrossed in the procedure that the woman and her feelings are forgotten. Communication with her is important. She will be particularly

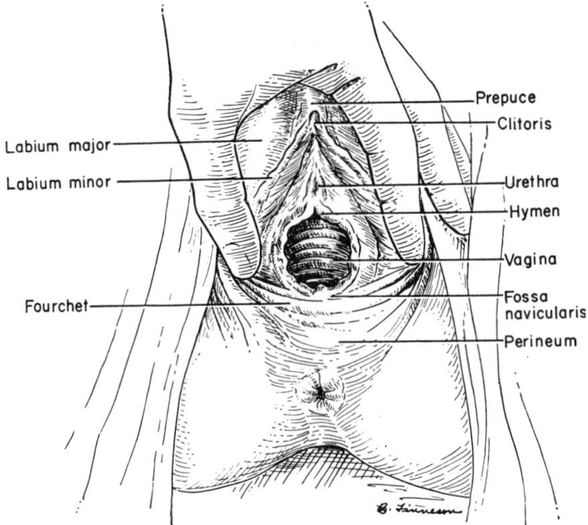

FIGURE 21-11. External genitalia. (From Bryant, R. D. and Overland, A. E.: *Woodward and Gardner's Obstetric Management and Nursing.* F. A. Davis, Philadelphia, 1966, with permission.)

interested in what is being accomplished by the examination. The cells are collected from the cervical canal, cervix, and vaginal vault by one of several methods—by scraping, by using a cotton swab, or by aspiration. The cells are *immediately* spread on a slide, "fixed" using a solution of equal parts of ether and grain alcohol, and left open to dry.

The cervix will be bluish (Chadwick's sign) due to the pregnancy, 2 to 3 cm. in diameter, and covered by multilayered squamous epithelium. Before the speculum is removed, the cervix shoud be inspected for erosions, hypertrophy, and lesions. As the speculum is slowly removed, the perineum again depressed and the vaginal canal is inspected.

The pelvic examination is now continued using bimanual palpation. The index and middle fingers of the right hand are lubricated and gently introduced into the vagina. The hand is positioned such that the back of the hand is toward the floor and the finger pads are facing the anterior vaginal wall. The left hand is placed flat over the lower abdomen. Care is taken not to use pressure against the sensitive urethra. As the fingers pass through the vagina, firmness, induration, tenderness, and cystic or tumorous masses are noted. Soft bulging of the anterior wall of the vagina indicates a cystocele. Soft bulging the posterior wall of the vagina indicates a rectocele.

The cervix is now identified—a round, convex protrusion with a central dimple. During pregnancy there is a marked softening in the consistency of the cervix (Goodell's sign). Note any nodules or lacerations.

Using pressure on the abdomen, attempt to feel the uterus between the two hands. Separate the two fingers in the vagina so that one is on each side of the cervix and attempt to outline the uterus. Note the contour, position, size, mobility, and consistency. The lower uterine segment becomes softened by the second month of gestation (Hegar's sign). Palpate for any protrusions (myomas) on the surface of the uterus.

Identify the ovaries, using *gentle* pressure on each side of the cervix to push up and back while at the same time pressing the right hand, which is on the abdomen just medial to the anterior superior iliac spine, toward the fingers in the vagina. Note the size, shape, mobility, and any enlargement (over 5 cm) of each ovary. If pregnancy is advanced, it may not be possible to identify the ovaries. However, a gentle attempt should be made in case there is any abnormal mass present.

Rectovaginal exploration is performed with the index finger in the vagina and the middle finger in the rectum. The anus is inspected for hemorrhoids and fissures and the rectum for any herniation and masses.

Pelvimetry

Pelvic measurements are, at times, done early in pregnancy, but many obstetricians believe that accurate measurements are difficult to obtain at that time. Moreover, the examination may cause considerable discomfort to the patient. This carries the added disadvantage of encumbering a trusting relationship when a woman leaves the examining room feeling the examiner has not been gentle with her. Some women may be so disturbed by the experience that they decide to have a minimum of contacts with the health system, thereby reducing the effectiveness of the prenatal care.

When the measurements are taken in the third trimester, the pelvic tissues are more pliable and relaxed and the examination can be done with less discomfort and more accuracy.[6] The examination should be repeated just prior to term so that a more accurate evaluation of fetopelvic accommodation can be made (i.e., relationship between size of presenting part of the fetus and size of the maternal pelvis). It is important that the size of the pelvis be accurately estimated so that any suspected pelvic disproportion can be recognized.

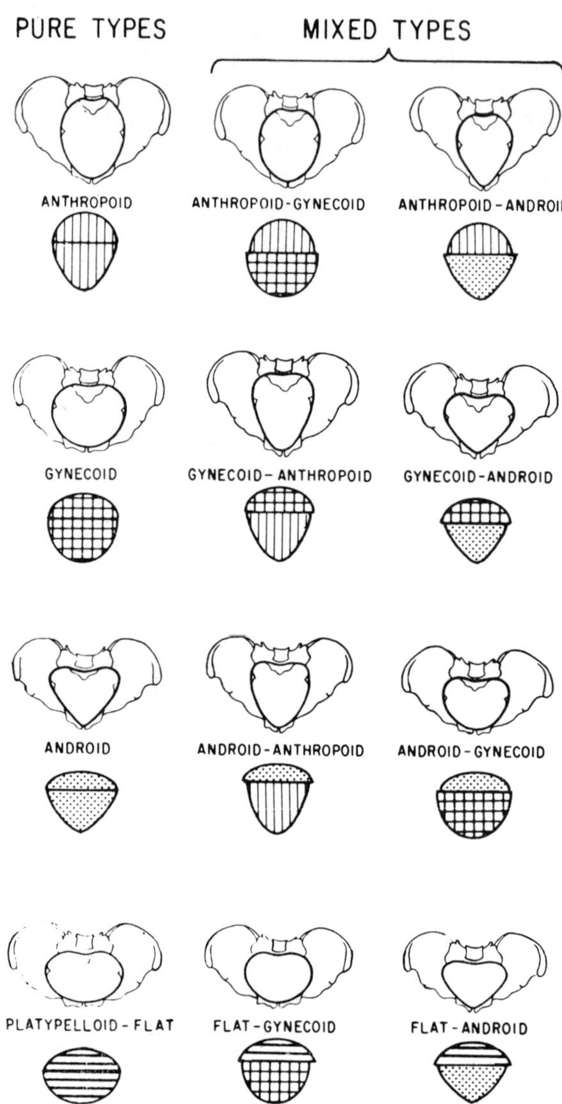

FIGURE 21-12. Female pelvis. Parent and mixed types. Posterior segment may conform in shape to one standard type and the anterior segment to another to produce mixed forms. In classifying the mixed forms the first term indicates the shape of the dominant posterior segment and the second term the shape of the anterior segment. (From Bonica, J.: *Obstetric Principles and Practice of Analgesia and Anesthesia*. F. A. Davis, Philadelphia, 1972, with permission.)

Pelves are classified according to the shape of the brim (inlet) (Fig. 21-12). The typical female pelvis, found in 30 per cent of women, is known as a *gynecoid* pelvis (gyne meaning woman). The inlet of this pelvis is almost a complete circle except for the slight indentation due to the bulge of the promontory of the sacrum.

The typical male pelvis is called the *android* pelvis (andro meaning man). Its brim is wedge-shaped or beak-shaped so that it is long from front to back and narrow transversely. It is an undesirable pelvis for delivery since it is funnel-shaped. Both the inlet of the pelvis and the outlet may not be large enough to facilitate the birth. Only 3 per cent of women have this type of pelvis.

The majority of women have pelves with characteristics of both these types (*gynecoid-android*). They have female characteristics but exhibit some male features.

Still other women, less than 15 per cent, have *anthropoid* pelves. The brim in this type of pelvis is oval, with the transverse diameter being less than the anterior-posterior diameter.[7]

The bony *pelvic girdle* is made up of four bones (Fig. 21-13):

the sacrum
the coccyx
two innominate bones.

They are connected by four important joints:

two sacroiliac joints
the sacrococcygeal joint
the symphysis pubis.

The landmarks shown in Figures 21-14 and 21-15 make the examination of the pelvis more meaningful.

There is a clear demarcation within the pelvis, the *linea terminalis*, which is the anatomic boundary between the false pelvis above and the true pelvis below. The measurement of the true pelvis is of greater importance in assessing the adequacy of the pelvis.

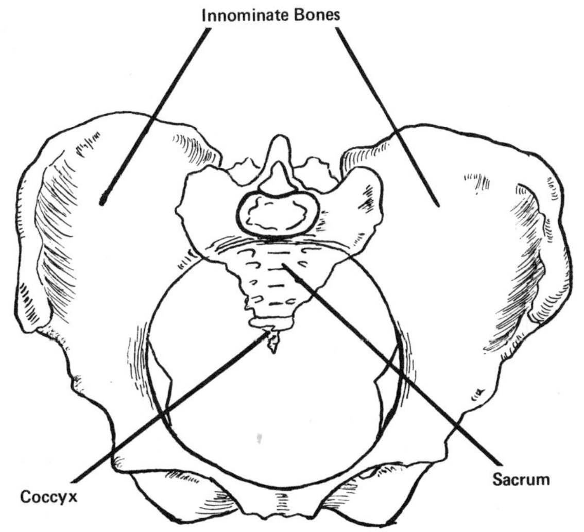

FIGURE 21-13. Bones of the pelvis. (Drawing by Caroline Affonso.)

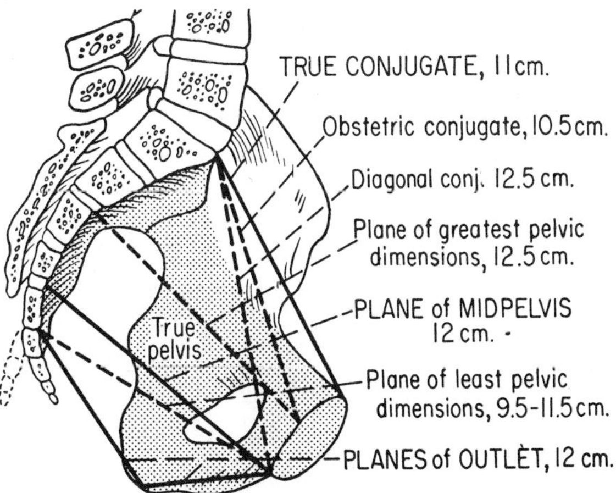

FIGURE 21-14. Sagittal view of pelvis showing important anteroposterior diameters (solid lines and large letters) and subordinate diameters. (From Bonica, J.: *Principles and Practice of Obstetric Analgesia and Anesthesia.* F. A. Davis, Philadelphia, 1972, with permission.)

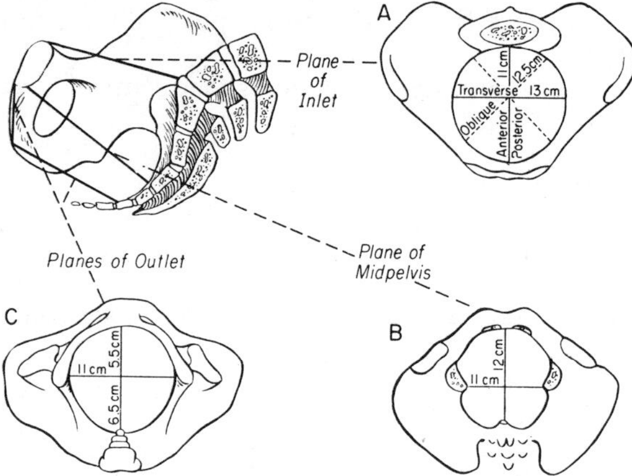

FIGURE 21-15. Planes and diameters of the pelvis. *A*, Superior plane of obstetric inlet, bound posteriorly by the promontory of the sacrum, laterally by the iliopectineal line and anteriorly by the rami of pubic bones and the upper margin of the symphysis pubis. *B*, Midpelvic plane bound posteriorly by the sacrum near the junction of the 3rd and 4th sacral vertebrae, laterally by the ischial spines and anteriorly by the inferior aspect of the symphysis. *C*, Inferior plane or obstetric outlet composed of two triangular components: the *posterior* is bound behind by the sacrococcygeal joint, laterally by the sacrotuberous ligament and anteriorly by the bi-ischial diameter, the *anterior* component is bound by the bi-ischial diameter behind, the inner margin of the pubic arch laterally and by the inferior margin of the symphysis anteriorly. The floor of the pelvic outlet is composed of the soft tissues of the perineum and the structures making up the urogenital diaphragm. (From Bonica, J.: *Principles and Practice of Obstetric Analgesia and Anesthesia*. F. A. Davis, Philadelphia, 1972, with permission.)

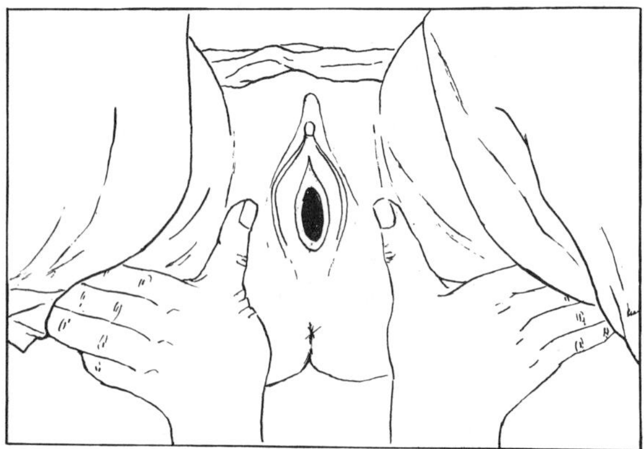

FIGURE 21-16. Estimating the pubic arch. (Drawing by Caroline Affonso.)

Pelvimetry should be performed using a step by step procedure.

The *subpubic arch* is an important landmark. It must conform to the round shape of the fetal head as it extends during its birth process. The *pubic arch* (Fig. 21-16) is recorded as:

narrow
average
wide.

For *palpation of the pubic arch*, the vagina is entered with two fingers, the index finger and middle finger. It is more comfortable for the patient if the middle finger is introduced first, followed by the index finger. The *ischial spine* on one side is located. By pronation of the examining fingers, the fingers pass to the opposite spine, following the conformation of the pelvic soft parts.[8] The maneuver is repeated several times in order to reach an estimation of adequacy (Fig. 21-17). This examination also gives more information about the subpubic arch as one notes any resistance to the examining fingers as they search for the spine. The ischial spines are recorded as:

not prominent
average
prominent or sharp.

The interspinous diameter is recorded as:

narrow
average
wide.

Next the *sacral tip* and *coccyx* are identified. The coccyx should be freely movable and not fixed, or forward (Fig. 21-18). An estimation is made of the measurement from the sacral tip to the under aspect of the symphysis pubis[9] (Fig. 21-19). The sacral tip and coccyx are recorded as:

forward
average
backward.

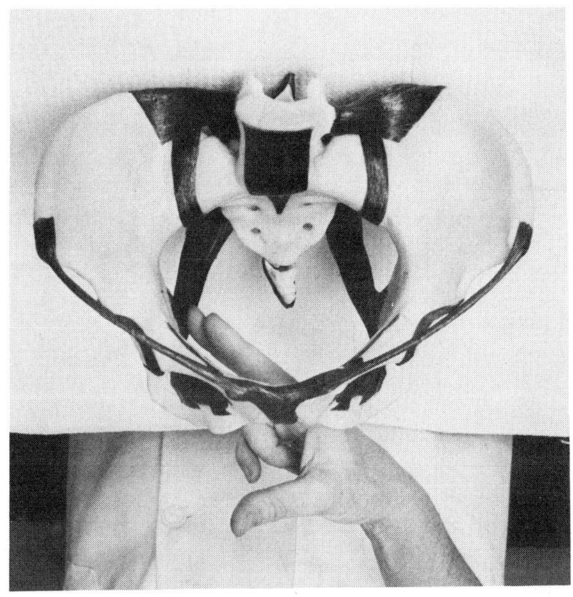

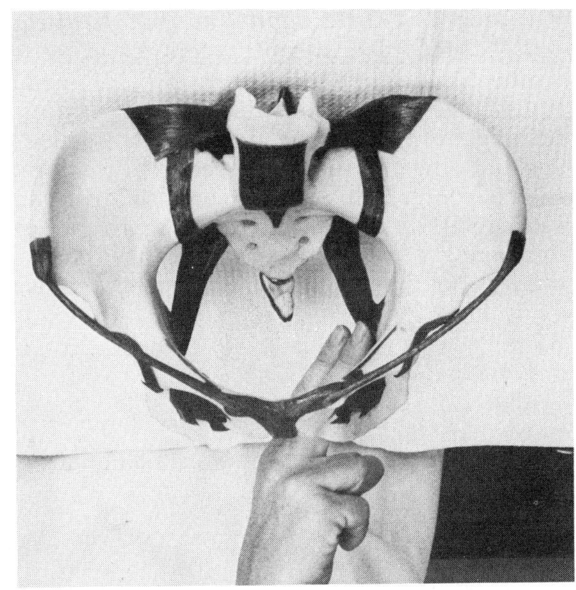

FIGURE 21-17. Estimating the ischial spines. (Photograph by Robert Goldstein.)

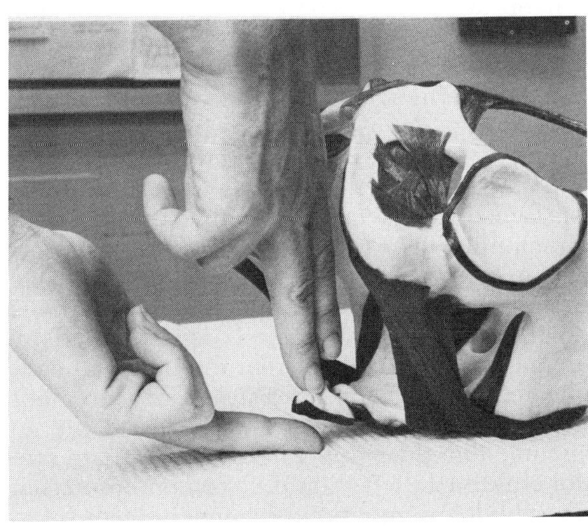

FIGURE 21-18. Checking the flexibility of the coccyx. (Photograph by Robert Goldstein.)

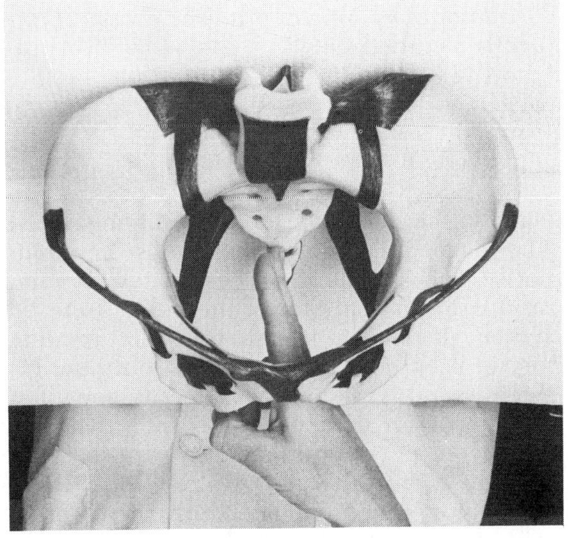

FIGURE 21-19. Estimating sagittal space to sacral tip. (Photograph by Robert Goldstein.)

The length of the *diagonal conjugate of the outlet* is recorded in centimeters.

The distance between the level of the sacral tip and the interspinous diameter may be estimated by placing one finger on the spines and the other on the sacrococcygeal platform in the center. This maneuver also gives an estimation of the length of a sacrospinous ligament.[10] The *lower sacrum,* with respect to the level of the ischial spines, is recorded as:

low
average
high.

The length of the sacrospinous ligaments is recorded as:

short
average
long.

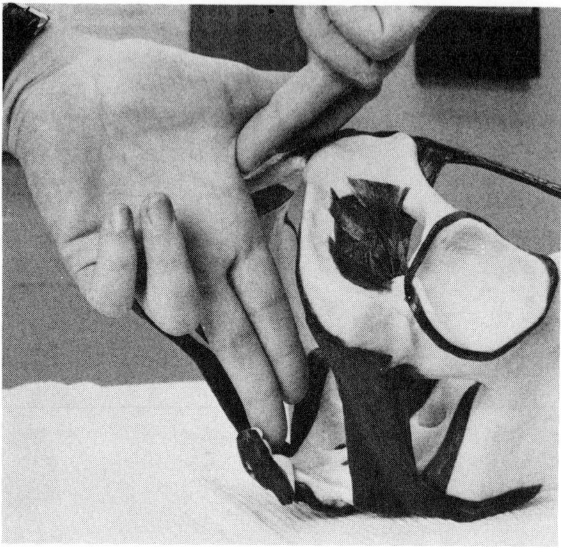

FIGURE 21-20. Measuring the diagonal conjugate. (Photograph by Robert Goldstein.)

The anterior surface of the sacrum is then methodically palpated upward and its vertical and lateral curvature is noted. This gives some picture of the pelvic depth. The *sacral curvature* is recorded as:

average
straight or flat
marked.

Finally, the *diagonal conjugate* is measured. The diagonal conjugate is the most important pelvic measurement. It estimates the anterioposterior diameter of the pelvis from the symphysis pubis in front to the sacral promontory in back. In a normal pelvis, only the last three sacral vertebrae can be felt without pushing upon the perineum. In a markedly contracted pelvis, the anterior surface of the sacrum is readily accessible.[11] The sacral promontory is approximated with the tip of the middle finger. The point where the symphysis pubis touches the index finger is marked with the finger of the other hand (Fig. 21-20). The fingers are withdrawn from the vagina, and the distance between that mark and the tip of the middle finger is measured with the pelvimeter. An alternative method is to use a fixed wall measuring device. The measurement you have just taken is the *diagonal conjugate* which measures the distance from the *outer* surface of the symphysis pubis to the sacral promontory. The *true conjugate* (or anterioposterior conjugate of the inlet) is the distance from the *inner* surface of the symphysis pubis to the sacral promontory. It is estimated by deducting 1.5 to 2 cm. from the diagonal conjugate. If the diagonal conjugate measurement is greater than 11.5 cm., it is justifiable to assume that the *pelvic inlet* is of adequate size for childbirth.[12] It should be remembered that the pelvic examination is somewhat painful to the patient. She should be helped to understand what the examiner is assessing, that the discomfort will only be momentary, and that her relaxation and cooperation will help the

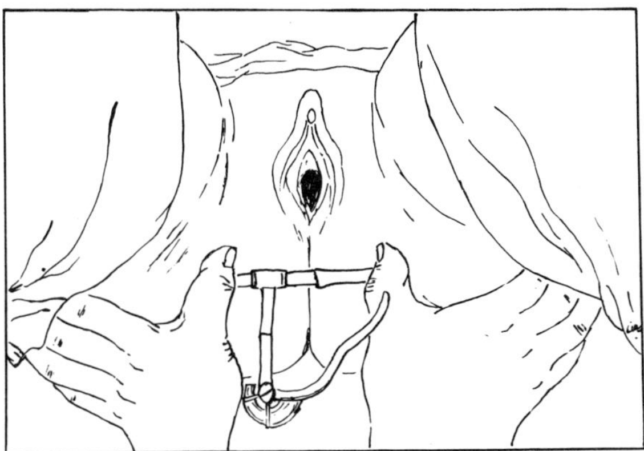

FIGURE 21-21. Measuring the transverse diameter of the outlet using a Thom's pelvimeter. (Drawing by Caroline Affonso.)

examiner to complete the evaluation with greater speed.

The second most important dimension accessible for clinical measurement is the *transverse diameter of the outlet*. This is the distance between the *ischial tuberosities*. The measurement is made with a Thom's pelvimeter (Fig. 21-21) or it may be estimated using a closed fist placed between the protrusions of the ischial tuberosities. A measurement over 8 cm. is considered normal.[13]

Clinical estimation of the *midpelvic capacity* by direct measurement is not possible. Contracture in this region is suspected if the ischial spines are quite prominent, if the sidewalls of the pelvis are felt to converge, or if the concavity of the sacrum is very shallow. However, roentgenograms are necessary to adequately measure the midpelvic region.

The external diameters of the pelvis are measured using a pelvimeter. The *interspinous diameter* is the distance between the outer edges of the anterior superior iliac spines, approximately 25 cm. (Fig. 21-22). The *intercristal diameter* is the distance between the outer edges of the most prominent portions of the iliac crests, approximately 28 cm. (Fig.

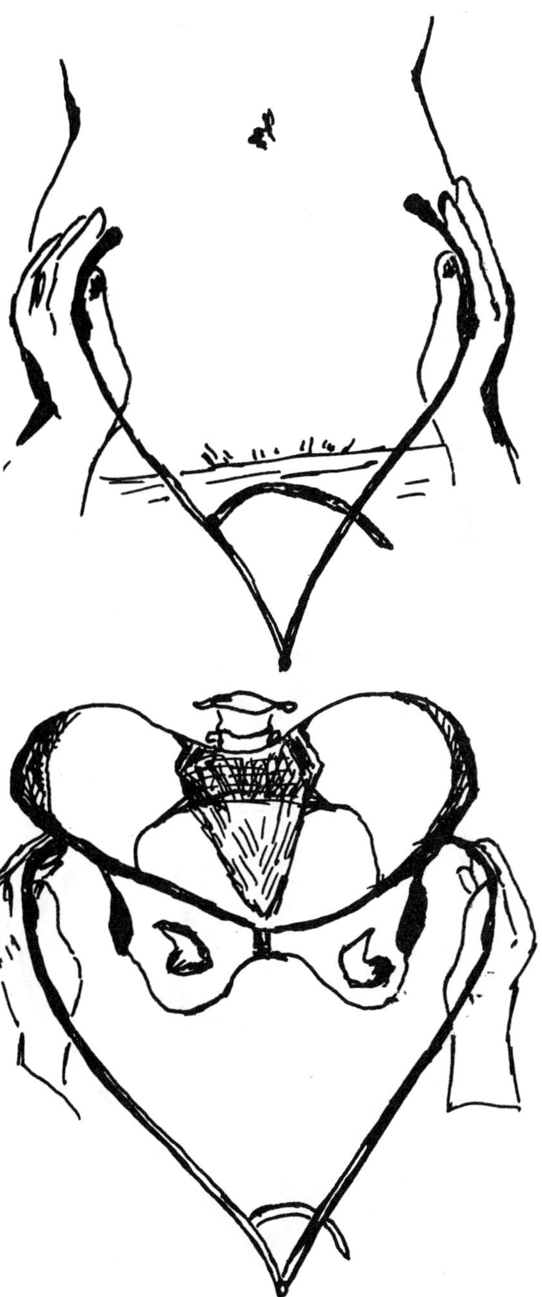

FIGURE 21-22. Measuring the interspinous diameter. (Drawing by Barbara Herman.)

21-23). The *external conjugate* is the distance from the undersurface of the spinous process of the last lumbar vertebra to the upper margin of the anterior surface of the symphysis pubis, approximately 20 cm. (Fig. 21-24).

The nurse will need a period of clinical experience with a preceptor in order to develop skill and accuracy in assessing the pelvis.

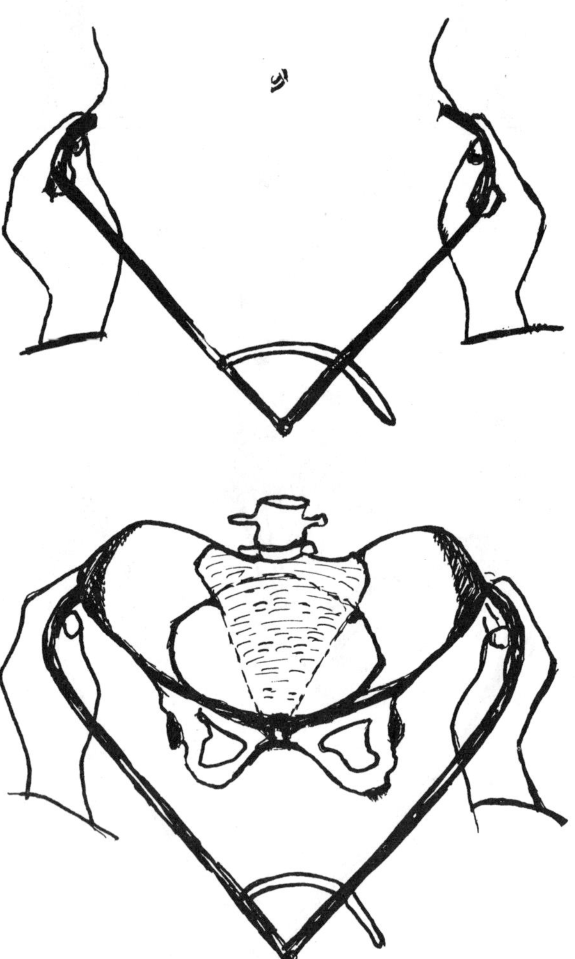

FIGURE 21-23. Measuring the intercristal diameter. (Drawing by Barbara Herman.)

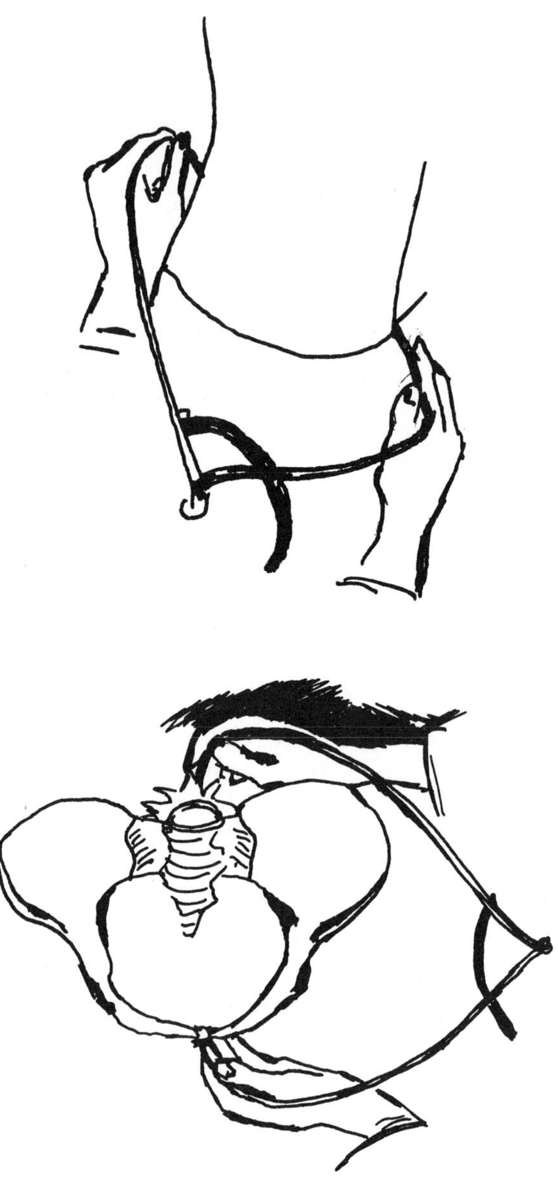

FIGURE 21-24. Measuring the external conjugate. (Drawing by Barbara Herman.)

LABORATORY TESTS

In order to protect the health of the mother and her infant, a number of laboratory assessments are utilized.

1. Hemoglobin or hematocrit should be ascertained at the first prenatal visit. The well-being of the woman and her fetus depends on a hemoglobin of more than 12 g. per 100 ml. (80 per cent). If it is abnormally low at any time, further hemotologic evaluations and appropriate therapy are indicated.
2. The Rh factor and blood type should be obtained. If the mother is Rh^-, her mate's Rh factor should be obtained. Unless both are Rh^-, in which case the fetus would also be Rh^-, antibody titer assays should be done on the expectant mother at 24, 28, 32, and 36 weeks of gestation. The expectant mother should also be titered for miscellaneous atypical antibodies.
3. A serology test for syphilis is usually mandated by state law. The presence of syphilis in the mother is a serious complication since the microorganisms cross the placenta and infect the fetus. The fetus may be born with congenital syphilis or be seriously ill. Syphilis may also cause intrauterine death. Fortunately, if the disease is discovered and treated prior to five months of gestation, danger to the fetus is reduced.
4. Papanicolaou cervical smear to rule out cervical cancer and to check for atypical (precancerous) cells.
5. Cervical smear to rule out gonorrhea. If the patient has a gonorrheal infection at the time of delivery the infant's eyes could become infected causing opthalmia neonatorum which results in blindness.
6. Cervical smear to rule out trichomoniasis and candidiasis where indicated by excessive, irritating vaginal secretions. It is important to bring candidiasis under control prior to delivery both for the patient's comfort and to avoid monilial infection of the mucous membranes (thrush) of the fetus.
7. Blood pressure as a baseline.
8. Clean-catch (midstream) urine specimen to check for the presence of glucose and albumen.
9. Weight as a baseline and for detection of toxemia of pregnancy.

ONGOING PHYSICAL EVALUATION

At each prenatal visit the expectant mother should be assessed for the following:

1. Growth of the Uterus and Estimation of Fetal Size.
   It is important to measure and record the size of the uterus, including the height of the fundus, at each prenatal visit. During the first two months of pregnancy the gravid uterus remains in the pelvic cavity. By 13 weeks of pregnancy the fundus of the uterus rises out of the pelvis and can be palpated just above the symphysis pubis. Measurements of the fundal height are now made and recorded. Table 21-1 shows the relationship between fundal height and fetal age. The fundus reaches the lower border of the um-

TABLE 21-1. Relationship of Fundal Height to Fetal Age

Linear distance, symphysis to fundus (cm.)	*Estimated fetal age (weeks)*
26.7	28
30.0	32
32.0	36
37.7	40

bilicus at 20 weeks and the tip of the sternum at 36 to 37 weeks. Two weeks prior to term the presenting part of the fetus sinks into the pelvis and becomes engaged. This is a rather sudden descent in the primigravida and a slower process in the multigravida. After engagement the fundal height is lower than it was at 38 weeks.

Fundal measurements in conjunction with other evaluations give some indication that the fetus is alive and growing in a normal manner.

If the fundus is higher than anticipated, one might suspect the following:

- multiple pregnancies
- hydramnios (excessive amniotic fluid)
- hydatidiform mole (cystic degeneration of chorionic villi)
- concealed hemorrhage such as an abruptio placenta
- errors in estimating the fetal progress
- ovarian or uterine tumors.

If the fundus is lower than anticipated, one might suspect:

- intrauterine death
- placental insufficiency
- fetal abnormality
- abnormally small amount of amniotic fluid
- errors in estimating the gestation.

2. Fetal Heart Tones (FHT).

   Fetal heart tones can be heard by 20 weeks of pregnancy, even earlier with a Doptone, and are checked during each prenatal visit after that. The heartbeat can be heard best through the anterior shoulder of the fetus, (thus the importance of palpating the fetal outline first). The rhythm of the heart is regular, with normal rates of 120 to 160 beats per minute. Very slow or accelerated heart rates are usually indicative of fetal distress; however, the degree of intensity normally varies from time to time as the fetus changes position in utero. The maternal heartbeat may, at times, be mistaken for the fetal heartbeat. The two can be differentiated by keeping a finger on the maternal pulse while counting the FHT.

3. Weight.

   Measurements of weight gain are helpful in assessing fetal development and to some degree maternal nutrition and maternal health. During pregnancy a considerable amount of new tissue is added to the mother's body. Breast tissue, uterine musculature, blood plasma, protein, and tissue fluid contribute to increased weight. The fetus, amniotic fluid, and placenta also add to the mother's total weight. The main increase in weight occurs during the second half of pregnancy. It should not be less than ½ pound (0.22 kg.) per week nor more than 2 pounds (0.9 kg.). Weight gain should not exceed 5 pounds (2.25 kg.) in any month. Total weight gain for an average woman should approximate 25 per cent of her nonpregnant weight—28 pounds (12.5 kg.).[14]

4. Blood Pressure.

   Blood pressure is not expected to rise or fall from its normal baseline during pregnancy. It is checked and recorded at each prenatal visit and, based on the first blood pressure reading, any changes should be noted. If the pressure is elevated, have the patient rest 20 minutes and retake it. The elevation could be due to excitement. A systolic pressure of approximately 140 and a diastolic reading of approximately 90 are considered upper limits, beyond which pathology is suspected. However, blood pressure readings below 140/90 may still be elevated for those individuals whose baseline blood pressure is normally low. Elevated blood pressure readings in conjunction with other data may be indicative of developing toxemia of pregnancy.

5. Urinalysis.

   Urine is examined at each visit during the prenatal period. Because the danger of preeclampsia progressively increases as term approaches, more frequent observations, including urinalysis, are indicated during the third trimester of pregnancy. Urinalysis should include measurement of specific gravity (1.017 to 1.020 normal) and testing for albumin (proteinuria). The amount of albumin found in the urine is recorded as: trace, 1^+; small amount, 2^+; moderate amount, 3^+; and large amount, 4^+. The urine is also examined for glucose and a microscopic examination is done for casts and white blood cells. If bacteria or leukocytes are found in a clean-catch urine sample, a urine culture should be taken. Any urinary infections are treated with proper antibiotics or urinary antiseptics to prevent pyelonephritis of pregnancy. This condition is often responsible for premature delivery.[16]

6. Edema.

   It is not unusual for pregnant women to develop edema of the lower extremities. It is usually absent in the morning but increases as the day progresses. The large amounts of progesterone and estrogen secreted by the placenta adversely affect kidney tubular function and influence the production of edema.[15] However, edema of the hands or face and pretibial edema are not normal. Evaluating any edema is an important part of every prenatal visit.

7. General physical appearance.

   The expectant mother's general appearance and demeanor should be assessed at each prenatal visit. Mannerisms, facial expressions, posture, and so forth give some indication of the mother's general well-being. Changes may be indicative of either physiologic or psychologic alterations.

SPECIAL ASSESSMENT

Certain assessments, made first when the client presents herself for prenatal care are again assessed as pregnancy progresses:

1. Hemoglobin is checked again at 32 weeks of gestation.
2. Serology and smear or culture for gonorrhea are checked at 36 weeks of gestation.
3. Pelvic assessment is done by 30 weeks of gestation and repeated at the time of fetal engagement at or about 38 weeks of gestation.

A tine test is often used as an initial screening for tuberculosis. In many prenatal clinics a chest roentgenogram of the pregnant woman is routinely done. The danger of radiation to the fetus after the first trimester is considered to be small, especially when the mother's abdomen is shielded. This slight risk is balanced against the possible benefit of detecting a previously unrecognized condition. It has been variously estimated that from 2 to 8 per cent of all cases of pulmonary tuberculosis have been diagnosed for the first time in expectant mothers.[17]

THE RECORD

Each agency has their own method for recording the history, the physical examination, and other pertinent information. Examples of such records for the initial physical examination and ongoing physical evaluation are shown in Figure 21-25. Cumulative assessment forms for family planning and for the prenatal, intrapartal, and postpartal periods are shown in Appendices 2 and 3.

PHYSICAL EXAMINATION

Type Skin B.P.

E.E.N.T. Thyroid

Glasses Not Palpable

Teeth Breasts Nipples

Adequate Repair Need Attention Small Med. Large C.C.M. Good Poor Inverted

Heart Lungs

ABDOMEN: Scars Masses: Striae H.F. Position F.H.T. +

PELVIS: Sacral Curve Sidewalls

D.C. B.T. P.S. Normal Flat Normal Converging

Spines Coccyx Pubic Arch

Blunt Sharp Prominent Normal Forward Normal

VAGINAL:

Perineum Vagina Cervix

Adequate Poor Nulliparous Parous Erosions Lacerations

Fundus

Anterior Retroverted Size in Wks. Soft Firm Symmetrical Irregular

Adnexa

Negative Husb. RH Group

RECTUM:

EXTREMITIES

LABORATORY: HCT HGB RH: Blood Group: Serology: (Date) Cytology

Edema Varicosities GMS. % Neg. Neg.

REMARKS

Vitamins:

Iron:

Laxative:

Other ℞ :

Chest X-ray:

Immunization:

Diet Advised

Low Caloric Salt Poor Normal Preg.

Milk

Glasses per Day

NOTES:

FIGURE 21-25. A sample prenatal record. (Courtesy of Kaiser Medical Center.)

HAWAII PERMANENTE MEDICAL GROUP
Kaiser Medical Center
Honolulu, Hawaii

CLINIC:

RECORD OF VISITS

E.D.C. ______________________

No. Preg.	F.T. Del.	Mid-Trim. Losses	Early Abs.	No. Living Children	Neonatal Deaths

Largest baby lb. oz.	Longest labor hrs.
Smallest baby lb. oz.	Shortest labor hrs.

QUICKENING: ______________

Weeks of Preg.	Date	Wt.	B.P.	Fundus	Pos.	Sta.	F.H.T.; Q	Urine Alb.	Urine Sugar	Edema	Complaints, Treatment, Tests

Obstetrician:
Pediatrician:
Anesthesia:
Nursing: Yes No
General Remarks:

RH Factor - Pos.
Neg.
32 Wk. Hgb.____Hct.___
Rubella:
Susceptible________
Immune__________

Family Planning____
Lamaze___________
Registered: Yes____

95077 3/69

PROTECTING THE PRENATAL CLIENT

THE BREASTS

The mammary glands need special care during the period of pregnancy both to insure cleanliness and to prepare them for nursing the infant. Under the influence of estrogen, progesterone, and prolactin, the breasts undergo changes in preparation for nourishing the baby. Enlargement due to growth of the secretory ductile system requires that the breasts have special support. This support is needed to maintain proper alignment, retain their shape, aid in correct body alignment, and prevent backache. The breasts are composed of modified and enlarged skin glands embedded in the superficial fascia, a fatty membranous covering underlying and attached to the skin. They have neither bone support of their own, nor voluntary muscles with which to control their motion at will.[18] Thus, a well-fitted maternity brassiere is needed by most women during pregnancy to support the three pound increase in size and weight. The support should have the following features:

- Wide adjustable straps
- Adjustable size to permit continued enlargement
- Smooth interior to prevent irritation and constriction
- Uplift support so that the breast is held up and in, on top of the chest.

If the woman plans to breast feed, the brassiere should open in the front and be constructed in such a manner that disposable pads can be inserted to absorb excess milk due to leakage.

Colostrum forms in the breast as early as 16 weeks of pregnancy. The colostrum may be colorless, milky, or yellowish-orange and the leakage of small drops of the fluid is normal. This leakage plus sebum which is formed by the follicles of Montgomery's glands may, if not carefully removed, form crusts around the nipple. If this occurs, they may be softened with hydrous lanolin and then removed as a part of the daily bath. The breasts should be bathed with soap and water daily; however, soap should not be used on the nipple itself since it tends to cause dryness. Clear water and a rough washcloth will suffice.

Special care of the breasts and nipples during pregnancy reduces the risk of cracked, sore, and bleeding nipples during breast feeding. The nipples can be toughened for nursing by using a rough turkish towel for drying purposes. Work from the outer aspect of the breast toward the nipple, then grasp the nipple between the thumb and forefinger, pull it out firmly but only until it is slightly uncomfortable, never painful, and roll it between the fingers for a few seconds.

Beginning in the eighth month of pregnancy, hand expression of colostrum from each breast is recommended by many physicians and by La Leche League International. Expressing colostrum daily keeps the milk ducts open and thus facilitates free drainage of milk from the ducts and decreases discomfort when lactation occurs. The following technique is suggested by La Leche League:

> Wash your hands. Cup the breast in your hand, placing your thumb above and the forefinger below the breast at the edge of the dark area (areola) and simply squeeze the thumb and finger together. Don't slide the finger or thumb out toward the nipple. Don't worry if nothing comes out the first few times you try it. You'll get the knack soon. Rotate your hand slightly back and forth several times in order to reach all the milk ducts, which radiate out from the nipple. You may only get a few drops at first, but that is sufficient.[19]

The size of the breasts has nothing to do with their adequacy to produce sufficient nutrition for the infant. However, the nipple does have to be prominent enough for the infant to grasp. If the nipple is flat or inverted, special care should be given to the nipple during the third trimester of pregnancy. The nipple is composed of erectile tissue which becomes more prominent when stimulated. Thus the flat nipple can readily be stimulated to become erect for the infant's grasp. The inverted nipple presents a greater problem since it tends to fold in on itself. It can usually be everted by placing down-and-out thumb pressure on both sides of the nipple and then gently rolling the nipple between the thumb and index finger. This should be done several times daily. It is also possible for the woman with an inverted nipple to wear a Wollwich nipple shield in which the nipple is pushed forward through the circular opening in the base of the shield and protected from pressure of the brassiere.

THE SKIN

The integumentary system is more active during the period of pregnancy. Daily bathing is encouraged both as a hygienic practice and because the skin assumes an added role in the elimination of waste products produced by the growing fetus. Tub baths and showers are now acceptable health practices. However, the expectant mother should be warned that her center of gravity has changed and she is in greater danger of losing her balance and sustaining physical injury as she gets in and out of the tub.

The stria over the enlarged abdomen and on the sides of the breasts of some women cannot be prevented, thus no treatment is suggested.

DENTAL CARE

The expectant mother is prone to increased hypertrophy and irritation of the gums. Her teeth are also susceptible to pain due to the increased hyperemia from the increased blood volume. Pregnancy does not aggravate tooth decay, and the teeth will not be decalcified by the demands of the fetus. It is important that the mother understands that the teeth of the developing fetus are being formed from the nutritional components of her diet. The pregnant woman should have a dental check-up and removal of plaque from her teeth early in pregnancy. It is generally agreed that dental repair and even extractions, preferably under local anesthesia, can be undertaken during pregnancy. Dental roentgenograms and extensive dental work should not be undertaken without consultation with the person supervising the prenatal care.

TRAVEL

There are no restrictions on travel during pregnancy provided it does not cause undue fatigue. Airline travel permits more personal mobility and is frequently less fatiguing. However, airlines do have restrictions on how late in pregnancy one may travel by air. Their concern is related to the problems which would arise should labor occur during the flight. If it is necessary for the expectant mother to travel by car for long distances, she should stop at intervals and walk for brief periods to improve the circulation. In every mode of travel the woman should stretch her legs and flex and contract the leg muscles to improve circulation. Short excursions can and should be encouraged for they broaden her horizons and keep her from feeling confined.

In automobile travel the expectant mother *should* use the lap and chest belt equipment in the car. Although the belt may cause injury to the gravid uterus and to the fetus,[20] it does reduce maternal injury by preventing ejection and by limiting secondary impact with the interior of the vehicle. Table 21-2 shows the results of a study on maternal and fetal mortality in automobile accidents.

TABLE 21-2. Maternal and Fetal Mortality in Automobile Collisions*

			Fetal Deaths with Maternal Survival						
Group	*Total Collisions*	*Fetal and Maternal Deaths*	*Number of mothers surviving*	*Abruptio placentae*	*Maternal shock*	*Unknown cause*	*Hyaline-membrane disease*	*Total*	*Total Fetal Deaths*
Lap-belt restraint	24	1 (4.2%)	23	1	0	2	0	3 (13.0%)	4 (16.7%)
No restraint	166	13 (7.8%)	153	5	3	2	1	11 (7.2%)	24 (14.4%)

* Pregnancy > 12 wk.
(From Crosby,[21] with permission.)

EXERCISE, REST, AND RECREATION

Pregnancy need not be an indication for curtailing most forms of exercise which the expectant mother enjoys. Even the more strenuous sports, for women who are somewhat skilled in them, such as tennis, swimming, and golf, can be continued through pregnancy as long as the woman feels able. However, strenuous exercise in which body balance is greatly involved, such as skiing, diving, horseback riding, and surfing, should be discussed with the physician. Walking in the open air is excellent exercise and should be part of the daily regimen. Gardening and homemaking activities can likewise be continued, although now that body balance has changed body mechanics should be modified. A discussion of appropriate body mechanics appears later in this chapter. All activities to which a person is accustomed are appropriate and can be continued providing excessive fatigue is avoided.

Sleep is a psychophysical phenomenon essential for the maintenance of both physical and emotional health. From the beginning of pregnancy there is an increased need for sleep, presumably due to increased metabolic requirements. If sleep deprivation is added to the cumulative stresses of pregnancy, it may affect the woman's personality functioning as well as her adaptive responses.

There are several reasons why the pregnant woman may experience periods of insomnia. Some of them are psychosocial and pertain to conflicts and anxieties related to pregnancy and impending motherhood. There are, however, a number of physiologic changes which intrude upon the woman's ability to sleep. Fetal activity and skeletomuscular changes produce strain and discomfort, particularly during the later part of pregnancy. The increasing abdominal pressure also makes it difficult to sleep.

Eight hours of sleep daily are needed by the expectant mother and a rest period in the afternoon is also beneficial. However, prior to suggesting a particular pattern of rest and sleep it is important to explore the woman's usual patterns and her other family responsibilities. A therapeutic trusting relationship will be endangered if the nurse makes recommendations to a busy mother or employed woman to which she cannot adhere. It is possible to help her make adjustments in her schedule that will assist her to get the needed rest and relaxation (Fig. 21-26). One suggestion is "Never stand when you can sit, and never sit when you can lie."

Toward the end of pregnancy, when the gravid uterus makes sleeping more difficult, the woman should be encouraged to experiment with extra pillows to support her head. One small pillow under the uterus, while resting in a side-lying position, may provide greater comfort.

Recreation, always an important component of healthful living, assumes even greater significance during pregnancy. Women experiencing their first pregnancies often find time on their hands if they leave their jobs to await the birth of their babies. Women with other children may feel trapped by home and child care responsibilities. It is important, when at all possible, that some time be set aside for pleasurable family activities. Moreover, every woman needs some time just for herself, to utilize in whatever way she prefers. It is important that these aspects of life be reviewed not only as they relate to the period of pregnancy, but also as they relate to the early period of parenthood.

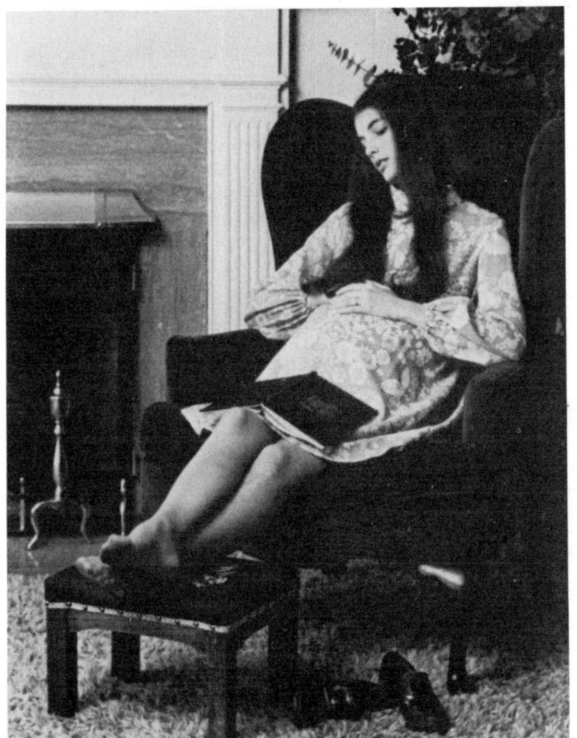

FIGURE 21-26. Sitting with feet elevated aids in relaxation and improves circulation. (Courtesy of Ross Laboratories.)

RELAXATION AND CONTROLLED BREATHING

Learning to relax is important to the expectant mother. She will also find relaxation useful during the labor experience and certainly during the fatiguing months in the early puerperium. Some people seem to be able to achieve relaxation without special training but the majority achieve relaxation by learning *progressive relaxation.* In order to appreciate the feeling of total relaxation, it is essential to experience tension in different groups of muscles. To practice progressive relaxation, the expectant mother should assume a relaxed position, lying on one side with the head, but not shoulders, resting on a pillow and all joints flexed with no part of the body supporting any other part. The lower arm is placed behind the back and the upper arm is bent forward to rest upon the supporting surface. The upper leg is bent at the hip and the knee is brought forward to rest upon the supporting surface. The lower leg is flexed at the knee and placed behind the upper knee. In this position the enlarged abdomen rests gently on the supporting surface and all joints are flexed and relaxed.

Relaxation is learned by first tensing a portion of the body and then consciously relaxing it. Starting with the toes, the expectant mother bends them up gently, and then lets them drop loose. Next the ankles are bent forward, and then relaxed. The muscles of the hips are contracted by sliding each knee toward the abdomen a fraction of an inch and then relaxing. The abdomen is "sucked in" and then relaxed. The buttock muscles are tightened, then relaxed. The shoulders are hunched together and then relaxed. The face is screwed up, and then relaxed, allowing the chin to drop and the tongue to rest, relaxed, not pressing against the roof of the mouth. Then with eyes closed concentrate only on normal breathing—slowly in and out. Complete relaxation will usually be followed by sleep in a short time.

After the expectant mothers learns progressive relaxation, she can tighten her whole body and then go limp and loose, "like a rag doll." This is the position the woman should assume (either side) during labor. It facilitates relaxation and makes it possible for someone to apply sacral support during the labor contractions. It prevents hypotensive syndrome and thereby increases oxygenation to the uterus, placenta, and fetus.

BODY MECHANICS

There is a necessary change in posture as pregnancy progresses (Fig. 21-27). The upward extension and gradual enlargement of the gravid uterus cause displacement of the small intestines, transverse colon, and occasionally the liver and kidneys. The abdominal muscles become stretched and the diaphragm assumes a higher position, particularly during the last trimester. With the abdomen protruding forward there is a downward inclination of the pelvis. In the later part of the pregnancy, the sacroiliac joints and the fibrocartilage of the symphysis pubis become more relaxed. Unless a woman learns to carry her body in proper alignment, her forwardly tilted pelvis increases the curvature of her spine. This alignment does not permit the weight to be transferred directly through the bodies of the vertebrae and part of it falls on ligaments and muscles. The result is a backache and overstretched muscles.

It is preferable to teach good body mechanics early in pregnancy so that discomfort can be avoided. Moreover, an attractive posture improves the woman's body image and her general outlook on pregnancy.

Pelvic tilting is taught in the following manner. As the pelvis is rocked forward, the buttock muscles are tightened and the buttocks are tucked under. The abdominal muscles are likewise tightened. When the woman experiences back fatigue, she gently and slowly rocks the pelvis back and forth; and then with the head held high, shoulders back and rib cage lifted, she will be able to comfortably go about her work.

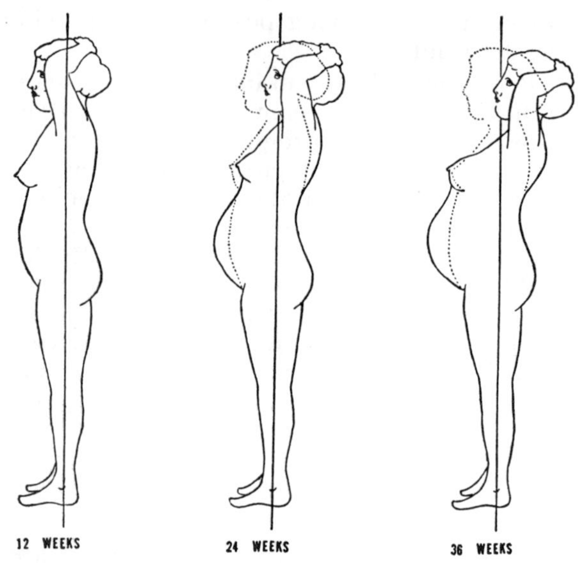

FIGURE 21-27. Changes in posture during pregnancy. The first figure and the subsequent broken line figures represent the posture of the nonpregnant woman and the woman in early pregnancy before the growth of the uterus and its contents affects the center of gravity. As pregnancy advances the head and shoulders are thrown backward to counterbalance the anterior protrusion of the abdomen which results from the enlarging products of conception. (From Bonica, J.: *Principles and Practice of Obstetric Analgesia and Anesthesia.* F. A. Davis, Philadelphia, 1972, with permission.)

This posture is maintained when walking, sitting, squatting, and climbing stairs. Moderate or low heels give a broad base of support and cause less inclination of the pelvis. If the work surface is low, the knees are bent, not the back. When is it necessary to pick up something from the floor or to work at floor level, leg muscles should be used to lower the body, and the woman should assume a squatting position. Sitting tailor fashion for periods during the day has the added advantage of promoting the slight natural enlargement of the pelvis at the joints, and of stretching the perineum and the thigh muscles, all helpful in terms of preparation for labor.

NUTRITION

Nutrition is of such great importance to both the mother and the developing fetus that a separate chapter has already been devoted to a detailed discussion of this subject. See Chapter 17.

CLOTHING

Considerable attitudinal changes have occurred during the latter half of the twentieth century with relation to the pregnant shape and its exposure. No longer do women avoid being seen in public during their pregnancy. For the most part, they now proudly display their gravid figures and look forward with anticipation to buying and wearing their new maternity clothes (although admittedly they become weary of them before their pregnancies are completed).

Two events have caused this more healthy attitude. Maternity clothes, once two-piece Mother Hubbards, have given way to very attractive maternity fashions. This has had considerable effect on women's feelings about being attractive and well groomed. Moreover, contemporary attitudes about sexuality are more free and open, so that fewer women feel ashamed of their protruding abdomens.

Maternity clothing should be functional as well as attractive. Restricting bands around the body should be avoided. Hose must not be supported by garters or stretch bands on kneehigh hose which restrict the venous circulation of the lower extremities and predispose or aggravate varicose veins. These veins are already somewhat constricted by the pressure of the gravid uterus, thus slowing return circulation. Hose can be held up by a special, inexpensive garter belt or the expectant mother can wear maternity pantyhose.

Good abdominal musculature does not require a special supportive girdle during pregnancy. However, if the woman is accustomed to such a support she may be more comfortable with a maternity girdle. The garment will not disguise her pregnant figure, but it may help prevent discomfort.

Shoes should provide adequate support. The expectant mother has an increased need for such support due to the increased weight she is carrying. The heel should not be more than 1½ inches high since heels tend to increase lordosis of the spine and complicate posture and balance.

BOWEL FUNCTION

Increases in steroid metabolism promote bowel sluggishness by suppressing smooth muscle motility. This may also be increased by taking oral preparations of iron. The resulting constipation may be aggravated by displacement of the intestines by the gravid uterus. Constipation also aggravates hemorrhoids. Bowel function can often be maintained by ensuring a liberal water intake, by exercise, and by intake of generous amounts of fruits and vegetables. Mild laxatives may be used to secure a daily evacuation of the bowel. Stool softeners, milk of magnesia, prune juice, and bulk-producing substances are generally acceptable. Enemas and strong cathartics are to be avoided.[22]

SPECIAL PRECAUTIONS TO PROTECT MOTHER AND FETUS

EMPLOYMENT

Many women wish to work during part or all of their pregnancy. However, many agencies have restrictions on the length of time an expectant mother may be employed. These are discriminatory, often illogical, and unnecessarily restrictive for many women unless they are exposed to noxious substances or are in danger of falling. Many working women find that when they relinquish their work they have time on their hands and feel bored and out of the mainstream of life.

Generally speaking, if the woman is happy in her position, the work is not overtiring, and her pregnancy is progressing normally, she should be permitted to continue work. Positions which require manual labor should be relinquished as soon as they cause undue fatigue. However, that recommendation should not be made before sufficient data has been collected to understand the importance of employment to her.[23] It may be possible for the woman, whose income is necessary for the family's support, to be transferred to a position less physically demanding.

SMOKING

More than a decade of research has shown that cigarette smoking has a deleterious effect on the developing fetus and on the outcome of the pregnancy in other ways.[24] There is, as yet, no satisfactory explanation of how cigarette smoking affects the fetus. It is known that blood flow to the placenta is slowed due to vasoconstriction of the placental vessels. Carbon monoxide blood levels in women (and men) who smoke are increased twofold and 5 to 6 per cent of available hemoglobin is combined with carbon monoxide.[25] Hemoglobin has a greater affinity for carbon monoxide than for oxygen; consequently there is less oxygen available for the fetus. In addition, it has been proposed that there is a direct effect of the nicotine on the fetus. Whatever the etiology, the following facts are clear:

1. Infants of smoking mothers weigh less than infants of nonsmoking mothers in each gestational age. Indeed, there is a twofold increase in prematurity and the weight difference is in direct proportion to the number of cigarettes smoked.[26] See Tables 21-3 and 21-4.
2. The neonatal mortality rate for single live births of "low birth weight" are substantially and significantly lower for infants of smoking than nonsmoking mothers.[27]
3. There is a slight increase in abortion rate found in smokers, but no significant increase in stillbirths, major fetal anomalies, or maternal complications. There is some suggestion of an increase in the incidence of premature rupture of membranes in smokers.[28]

TABLE 21-3. Average Weight of Newborn Infants According to Mothers' Smoking History

Smoking History	*Number of Mothers*	*Average Birth Weight*	
		grams	*pounds*
Nonsmokers	1,043	3,320	7 lb. 5 oz.
All Smokers	957	3,091	6 lb. 13 oz.
Less than 10 per day	260	3,205	7 lb. 1 oz.
10–20 per day	395	3,090	6 lb. 13 oz.
21–30 per day	264	2,970	6 lb. 8¾ oz.
Over 30 per day	38	3,190	6 lb. 13¾ oz.

(From Zalriski,[26] with permission.)

TABLE 21-4. Percentage of Premature* Births According to Mothers' Smoking History

Smoking History	*Number of Mothers*	*Number of premature births*	
		Number	*Per cent*
Nonsmokers	1,043	40	3.83
All Smokers	957	95	9.93
Less than 10 per day	260	17	6.54
10–20 per day	395	36	9.11
21–30 per day	264	38	14.39
Over 30 per day	38	4	10.53

* Premature = <2,500 grams.
(From Zalriski,[26] with permission.)

Women who smoke should make every effort to discontinue the habit when they become pregnant. Expectant mothers often have an aversion to a number of tastes and odors during early pregnancy, so it may be possible for them to break the habit permanently at that time. However, psychosocial factors may produce such tensions for the woman that she finds an increased need to smoke. Advice should follow, not precede, appropriate assessment of what smoking does for the patient and the extent of her habit. Any reduction in cigarette smoking can be expected to improve the outcome for the fetus.[29]

ALCOHOL

Alcohol ingested by the expectant mother quickly enters the blood stream and crosses the placenta to reach the fetus. However, moderate consumption of alcohol has not been shown to produce pathologic changes in the mother or the fetus.[30] The caloric value of alcohol is high but it contains no food value for the expectant mother. Therefore, when taking a nutritional history, it is important to obtain data about alcohol consumption.

Chronic alcoholism has been shown to have profound effects on the fetus, increasing the risk for both prenatal and postnatal growth and developmental failures.[31] Alcoholism often results in poor prenatal nutrition in terms of both caloric intake and necessary components of the diet. Infants of chronic alcoholic mothers show retarded development using standard evaluation tools such as Gesell and the Denver Development Evaluations. It is theorized that the infants are victims of ethanol toxicity. Many are born with malformations of the heart, head, face, and extremities.

Infants of alcoholic mothers show the same kind of acute alcohol withdrawal symptoms as do their mothers. In a study by Nichols,[32] the clinical appearance of agitation, sweating, tremors, and seizures was identical in the infant and mother. The agitation in the infant was followed by lethargy and severe hyperbilirubinemia.

PICA

Pica is the practice of ingesting nonfood substances, such as starch, clay, charcoal, ashes, dirt, and plaster. This practice is as old as man and occurs in all parts of the world. In America it is influenced by some of our subcultural patterns, religious beliefs, and economic contingencies and is often practiced during pregnancy.

The expectant mother needs an increased iron intake for new and additional hemoglobin synthesis and the increase in plasma volume. Furthermore, one of the greatest demands made on the maternal physiology by the fetus is that for iron. Research indicates that pica has a direct relationship to the development of anemia in the mother, with a resulting higher incidence of perinatal casualties.[33,34] It is unclear whether iron absorption is reduced due to pica as supported by Minnich and colleagues,[35] or whether the intake of products such as laundry starch merely provided large amounts of calories and no iron.[36] Either way, the normal biophysical changes and adaptations of pregnancy in the presence of pica may place an undue burden on the maternal organs and systems to the extent that malfunction or inability to cope with these additional factors occurs. It is possible that metabolic adaptations in the presence of pica are inimical to the development of the fetus. Since the adaptability of the human organism to stress situations is dependent upon and augmented by the reserve store of essential elements, deficiency of essential elements as well as pica may contribute to malfunction.[37]

The widespread pica practices reported in the literature and the subsequent poor outcomes have implications for nutritional assessment and expectant parent education.

DRUGS AND DRUG ABUSE

Drugs taken by a woman during her pregnancy may adversely affect the developing embryo and fetus. These drugs are known as teratogens. It was long believed that the placenta was a barrier to the transmission of most, if not all, harmful substances and that fetal abnormalities were of genetic origin. We now know that this is not true. Although the placenta appears to protect the fetus from the effects of some agents, it is a relative rather than an absolute barrier. Every drug given to the mother by any route can eventually be found in the fetus in some quantity as soon as placentation is established. The greatest danger of drug-induced malformations is during the first trimester of pregnancy. Such vital structures as the brain and heart have begun formation before the average woman realizes her menstrual period is late or has been missed (Fig. 21-28).

Sunday	Monday	Tuesday	Wednesday	Thursday	Friday	Saturday
Last Normal Menstrual Period					6	7
8	9	10	11	12	13	Ovulation
Ferti-lization	16	17	18	Blastocyst Implantation Begins		
22	23	24	25	Implantation Complete		28
First Missed Menstrual Period				Brain and Heart begin to form		

FIGURE 21-28. Menstrual and embryonic timetable. (From Am. J. Nurs. 66:1304, 1966, with permission.)

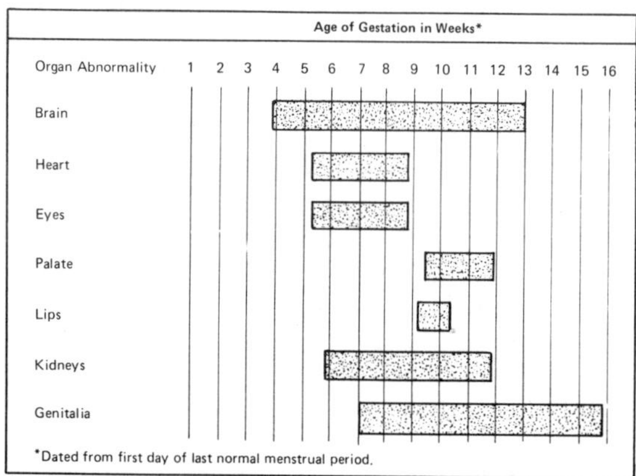

FIGURE 21-29. Teratogenic timetable for human beings. (From Am. J. Nurs. 66:1305, 1966, with permission.)

The time when developmental errors occur due to any etiology is related to the morphologic mechanism. Although almost all organogenesis occurs during the first few months of pregnancy, any single organ may undergo its critical development during a relatively short period of time (Fig. 21-29).

There are other factors which influence the degree to which a drug crosses the placental barrier and causes fetal damage.[38]

1. The higher the molecular weight of the drug, the lower the diffusibility or rate of transfer.
2. Two agents administered simultaneously may in some instances enhance the teratogenic effect and in other instances decrease the expected teratogenic effect.

In addition to acting as teratogens, drugs may also have other deleterious effects on the fetus and neonate. The effects of some maternal medications are shown in Table 21-5.

When any medication is administered during pregnancy, the advantages to be gained should clearly outweigh any risks inherent in its use. Most pregnant women require iron, folic acid, and vitamin supplements and some may require phenobarbital. All of these medications can be postponed until after the period of organogenesis. Even then, phenobarbital may have a deleterious effect on the fetal liver. Immunizations should be delayed until after pregnancy is completed. Live virus should never be utilized during any part of pregnancy.

Women should be warned that they should not take nonprescription drugs without first discussing their use with the physician or health personnel responsible for their prenatal care.

Other drugs to be considered are those generally known as "street drugs." There is an increased incidence of drug abuse among the American public, including women and girls who are or may become pregnant. According to current estimates there are between 500,000 and 600,000 heroin addicts in the United States. All addictive drugs affect the infant, and the infant will demonstrate withdrawal symptoms shortly after birth. In heroin addiction, there is a direct correlation between the length of maternal addiction and the symptoms of the infant at birth. An increase maternal intake of the drug will bring about an increase in symptoms of withdrawal.[40] Methodone and barbiturates also cause congenital addiction with acute withdrawal symptoms.[41,42]

There have been reports of infants born with multiple deformities to mothers who smoked marihuana and took multiple drugs including lysergic acid diethylamide (LSD). However, it is not possible to draw a definite association between the maternal use of these drugs and the development of anomalies in the infant. There is some evidence that LSD may induce birth defects in experimental animals, but these findings are not conclusive.[43]

The use of street drugs should be avoided to safeguard the fetus and neonate and to prevent harmful effects on the mother's physiology and her cognitive awareness relating to her life situation.

TABLE 21-5. Some Maternally Administered Drugs That Can Adversely Affect the Fetus and Newborn

Maternal Medication	*Effects on Fetus and Newborn*
Drugs to control epilepsy	Low levels of coagulation factors II, VII, IX, and X
Vitamin K analogues in excess	Hemolysis and kernicterus
Bishydroxycoumarin (Dicumarol)	Hemorrhage
Ethyl biscoumacetate (Tromexan)	Hemorrhage
Sodium warfarin (Coumadin)	Hemorrhage
Salicylates in large amounts	Neonatal bleeding
Sulfonamides	Kernicterus
Nitrofurantoin (Furadantin)	Hemolysis insusceptible fetuses, kernicterus
Tetracyclines	Inhibition of bone growth, staining of deciduous teeth
Potassium iodide	Goiter
Propylthiouracil	Goiter
Methimazole (Tapazole)	Goiter
Ammonium chloride	Acidosis
Reserpine	Stuffy nose, obstructed breathing
Morphine or heroin chronically	Addiction, withdrawal symptoms
Androgens	Masculinization
Some progestins	Masculinization
Tolbutamide (Orinase)	Neonatal hypoglycemia
Chlorothiazide	Thrombocytopenia
Quinine	Thrombocytopenia
Cephalothin (Keflin)	Positive direct Coombs test

(From Hellman and Pritchard,[39] with permission.)

COMMON PHYSIOLOGIC STRESSES

There are a number of so-called minor discomforts of pregnancy that are usually the result of normal physiologic changes due to the pregnancy. Many of these do not require therapy, and others can be alleviated by relatively simple measures. However, all require explanation and reassurance because many women will be unable to assess the seriousness of any particular symptom.

NAUSEA AND VOMITING

Nausea and vomiting are among the earlier symptoms of pregnancy, occurring to some degree in about 50 per cent of all pregnant women. Some women only experience them upon arising, while others experience them at any time during the day. The sight of food, motion, or certain odors may seem responsible for the feelings of nausea. In some instances, nausea and vomiting are persistent and dehydration and ketosis develop. This condition is termed *hyperemesis gravidarum* and is a serious complication of pregnancy.

There are many theories on the etiology of nausea during pregnancy but the exact mechanism has not yet been proved. Possibly hormonal changes of pregnancy are the cause. Serum gonadotropin rises in early pregnancy at precisely the same period that nausea and vomiting occur (6 weeks) and then it falls at the point when nausea and vomiting subside (12 weeks). Changes in the physiology of the gastrointestinal tract during pregnancy include increases in gastric acid and pepsin. The acids in the stomach are in inverse proportion to the level of urinary gonadotropin. Thus, gastrointestinal and endocrine functions *probably* induce the process which leads to nausea and vomiting of pregnancy.[44]

Many authorities believe that emotional factors contribute to the severity of the nausea and vomiting. The extent to which women react to pregnancy with nausea seems to be largely determined by their emotional stability and their adaptability to whatever mental stress is imposed by the pregnancy.

Although treatment for nausea and vomiting is seldom totally successful, some of the discomfort and unpleasantness can be reduced. Conditions that tend to precipitate the nausea should be eliminated. If cooking certain foods causes nausea (e.g., some women complain of cooking meat), perhaps the husband or someone else in the family can prepare this part of the meal.

Such simple remedies as eating a piece of dry toast or sipping a hot drink prior to arising may be sufficient to give relief. Small, frequent, carbohydrate-rich meals, dry crackers, and elimination of greasy foods from the diet may be effective. Some women find that drinking ginger ale, cola, or lemonade is helpful. By trying various remedies, the expectant mother may find one that is effective for her.

Sometimes antiemetic drugs are necessary. However, drugs should be avoided at this time if at all possible since fetal organogenesis is proceeding rapidly.[45] Dimenhydrinate (Dramamine 50 mg.) taken upon arising and repeated every four hours, as long as symptoms persist during the day, has been found to reduce nausea and vomiting. Meclizine (Bonine) and meclizine with pyridoxine (Bonadoxin) have been widely used and provided some benefit.[46] In any event, nausea and vomiting almost always disappear by the fourth month of pregnancy.

HEARTBURN (PYROSIS)

Heartburn is probably due to relaxation of the cardiac sphincter to the stomach plus relaxation of the lower end of the esophagus. The pressure of the gravid uterus and the decreased gastrointestinal motility also play a role, causing regurgitation of stomach contents into the esophagus and a burning feeling in the esophagus accompanied by an unpleasant taste. Heartburn resulting from these causes can be relieved by the administration of antacids such as aluminum hydroxide, magnesium trisilicate, or magnesium hydroxide, either alone or in combination (e.g., Amphojel, Gelusil, Maalox, and milk of magnesia).[47] The pregnant woman should be warned against taking antacids containing sodium, such as sodium bicarbonate, since the excess sodium can be responsible for retention of fluids in tissue.

In some instances heartburn persists throughout pregnancy, becoming increasingly severe. There is almost constant and often severe heartburn. The pain may radiate into the neck. It is increased in the supine position, after eating, and upon bending and straining.[48] These patients are probably suffering from hiatus hernia. Since barium studies cannot safely be performed during pregnancy, the patient is treated symptomatically. She will find some comfort by sleeping propped up with several pillows, eating her evening meal 3 to 4 hours before retiring, and avoiding bending and straining.

BACKACHE

Many pregnant women complain of backache and pelvic discomfort. Most of these symptoms result from muscular fatigue and strain due to the changes in body balance caused by the gravid uterus. Others are due to the softening of ligaments and pelvic joints caused by the steroid hormones. Pressure on nerve roots (causing nerve pain and cramps) and muscle spasm (causing backache) are the results.

When the pelvic joints and ligaments are relaxed due to endocrine changes, the bones of the pelvis are less stable. The sacroiliac joints and the symphysis pubis have considerable play, giving rise to the waddling gait of pregnancy. Weight-bearing functions are performed by the ligaments and this may cause painful sacroiliac strain, usually affecting one side more than the other.

Treatment is not always as effective as would be desired. The patient is taught to do the pelvic tilting exercise. Heat, analgesics, and rest are prescribed. It may be necessary for the woman to wear a supporting girdle. Steps to avoid back pains should be part of early prenatal care. Good body mechanics should be taught and should be reinforced as pregnancy progresses. Shoes should offer sufficient support and the heels not be so high as to increase the spinal curvature.

LEG CRAMPS

Painful spasms of the gastrocenemius muscles are likely to occur whenever a pregnant woman lies flat and stretches her legs with her toes pointed. The spasms are believed to result from an imbalance of the calcium/phosphorus ratio in the body and from the pressure of the gravid uterus on the nerves supplying the lower extremities.

Drinking large quantities of milk or taking dicalcium phosphate predisposes to muscular tetany as a result of the excessive amount of phosphorus absorbed from them. High amounts of phosphorus depress rather than elevate the diffusible serum calcium. Paradoxically, the ingestion of excessive quantities of milk may produce the tetany by lowering the content of ionized calcium.

The condition is corrected by 1) reducing the milk intake to one pint per day and prescribing calcium lactate to elevate the ionized calcium level in the plasma, or 2) continuing to drink one quart of milk daily and prescribing aluminum hydroxide gel which will trap the dietary phosphorus in the intestinal tract.

The expectant mother should be taught to avoid lying in the prone position and to point with the heel rather than the toe. When a painful spasm occurs, it can be relieved by simultaneously forcing the toes upward and placing pressure on the knee to straighten the leg (Fig. 21-30).

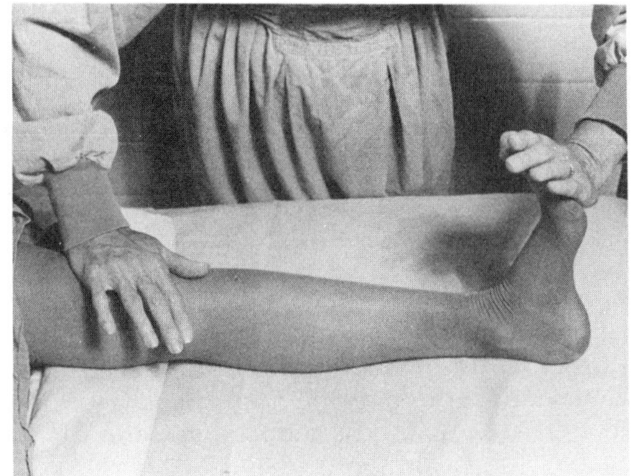

FIGURE 21-30. Relieving painful leg cramps.

SHORTNESS OF BREATH

The gravid uterus ultimately rises in the abdomen to the point that it encroaches upon the excursions of the diaphragm, causing overall discomfort and a constant sense of pressure under the ribs. This is particularly troublesome at night since it often interferes with sleep. Although it is one more stressor of the third trimester and for that reason alone must not be ignored, it will help the expectant mother to know that neither her life nor the life of the fetus is being compromised. Considerable relief will be experienced when lightening occurs and the fetal presenting part engages into the pelvis. In the meantime, sitting up, preferably in a straight chair, during the day and sleeping propped up with several pillows at night will give some relief. The head of the expectant mother's bed may be elevated by placing some large object, such as a suitcase, under the mattress.

Whenever shortness of breath becomes particularly stressful, it can be relieved by lying on the back with the arms extended above the head. This position stretches the thoracic cavity to its maximal and allows the fullest possible expansion of lung tissue. After a few minutes, relief will be obtained. It will then be possible to change to the side position, relax, and fall asleep. Intercostal (deep chest) breathing may also give some relief.[49]

PRURITUS AND VAGINAL DISCHARGE

There is a normal increase in the amount of vaginal secretions from the cervix and vagina during pregnancy. This is due to the increased vascularity of the cervix and the increased mucus formed by the cervical glands. Moreover, desquamation from the cervix and transudation through the vaginal walls is increased. The acidity is reduced and the pH is raised.

During pregnancy, vaginal secretions may be milky or yellowish in color. Since the increased moisture of the perineum and vulva and the change in pH facilitate the growth of organisms in the vagina, prophylactic care should be taken. Cleanliness of the area, loose absorbent (cotton) undergarments, and the use of bath powder are helpful. The woman should be warned not to sit for long periods of time.

The four types of organisms which may cause increased vaginal discharge (leukorrhea) with subsequent intense pruritus during pregnancy are Trichomonas vaginalis, Candida albicans, Neisseria gonorrhoeae, and Herpes vaginalis.

Trichomonas vaginalis

Trichomonads are oval-shaped, mobile, protozoal organisms with several flagella, and are found in 20 to 30 per cent of all pregnant women (Fig. 21-31). They cause symptoms and are usually responsible for vaginal discharge, vulval irritation, itching, and dyspareunia (painful sexual intercourse). Urinary frequency and dysuria may also occur. The vaginal secretions are profuse, of various colors, and frothy in nature. Small bubbles are typically seen in the posterior fornix. Small, punctate, hemorrhagic

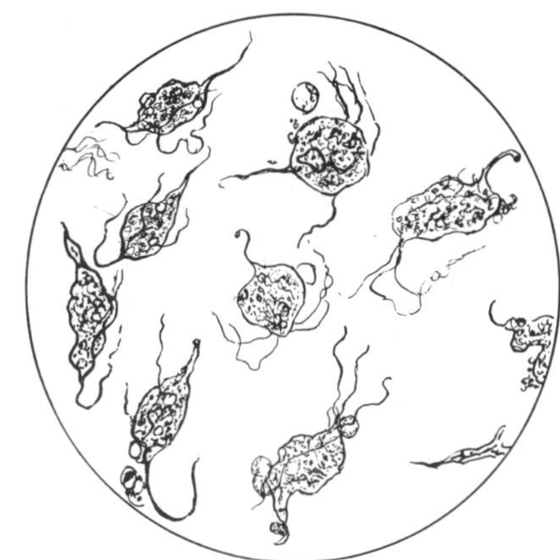

FIGURE 21-31. Trichomonads.

areas are seen on the cervix and vagina, giving the tissue a "strawberry" appearance.[50] Trichomonads are easily seen by microscopic examination of a drop of the discharge in isotonic saline.

In the nonpregnant state, metronidazole (Flagyl) is an effective treatment, but it is said to be contraindicated during the first half of pregnancy[51] since it crosses the placenta and enters the fetal circulation. However, the drug has been prescribed during pregnancy to hundreds of women and no adverse effects have been found in the fetus.[52] The medication is given in doses of 250 mg. three times daily for 10 days. Vaginal tablets are also available, but they are less effective and usually unnecessary if oral medication is given. Relief of symptoms is at least partially achieved within a week and is usually complete by two weeks. Good results with a single course of treatment may be expected in over 90 per cent of women, and in the remainder further relief may be obtained from a second course.[53]

The male urinary tract may also harbor the trichomonad but with few symptoms. It is therefore important that the woman's sexual partner also be treated at the same time she is, in order to eradicate the infection from both individuals and prevent reinfection.

Vaginal douches of a mild vinegar and water solution will not eradicate the infection but will offer the expectant mother considerable relief from the itching and burning. The douche solution consists of 2 quarts of warm water to which 3 tablespoons of vinegar have been added. The following precautions should be taken:

1. Hand bulb syringes must never be used. (Several deaths from air embolism have followed their use.)
2. The douche bag should be placed not more than two feet about the level of the hips to prevent high fluid pressure.
3. The douche nozzle should be inserted no more than three inches into the vagina.
4. The labia are held firmly around the douche nozzle, allowing the solution to fill the vagina and reach all the rugae, and then released quickly to flush out the debris.
5. The expectant mother can take a vaginal douche while seated on the toilet.

It is important that these directions be written, as well as be verbally explained, in a manner which the expectant mother can understand so that they will be followed effectively and safely.

Candida albicans

The effects of glycosuria on the vaginal acidity of the pregnant woman create favorable conditions for yeast, such as monilia, to flourish (Fig. 21-32). It can be cultured in 25 per cent of all women at term. The monilia can be easily identified microscopically in a hanging drop saline preparation or by smearing the exudate on Nickerson's medium and keeping it at room temperature for one week.

The patient complains of vulval irritation, itching, urinary frequency, dysuria, and dyspareunia. The vulva is often edematous and

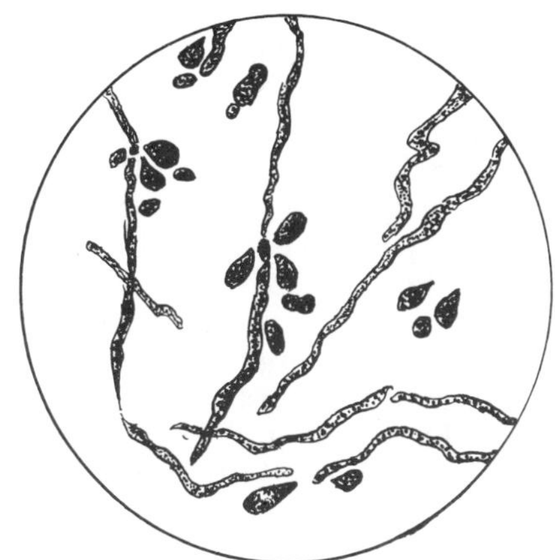

FIGURE 21-32. Monilia.

indurated. The vagina is dry, pale, and somewhat cyanotic, with accentuated rugal folds and patches of thick, tenacious exudate suggesting cottage cheese.

The infection is treated by nystatin (Mycostatin), an antibiotic against fungi. Vaginal tablets of 100,000 U. are ordered twice daily for two weeks. In addition, the use of vaginal creams containing gentian violet or the use of 1 per cent aqueous gentian violet, on a daily basis, may be necessary. The patient should be warned to wear a pad and protect her clothing from the gentian violet, for it causes a permanent stain. If the external vulva is edematous and irritated, the patient may apply KY jelly to the area or bathe the area with a solution of sodium bicarbonate.

Neisseria gonorrhoeae

Gonococcus infection may be a source of profuse purulent cervical and vaginal discharge. The urethral glands around the urethra and cervix may be seen to be infected upon speculum examination. A culture or a smear is taken. A smear of the purulent discharge stained with Gram's stain will reveal biscuit-shaped intracellular diplococci. This infection can be successfully treated with penicillin (480,000 U. of procaine penicillin in doses of 240,000 U. in each buttock), and it is most important that the infection be eradicated prior to delivery to protect the infant's eyes during passage through the birth canal. Moreover, the disease can be further spread to the uterine cavity during the puerperium. All patients who have had the disease should undergo another culture or smear following the treatment and again at 36 weeks of gestation to be certain they are free of the disease. It is very important that this disease be reported to the local Department of Health so that all contacts can be followed up and treated.

Herpes vaginalis

A herpes simplex type of eruption may appear on the vulva. The vesicular rash, a very painful condition, usually follows a sensory nerve path. The vaginal pain and dysuria are accompanied by the sudden onset of vaginal discharge. Simple or multiple vesicles are followed by shallow ulcers on the cervix and vulva. The virus can be cultured from these lesions. The cytologic smears show enlarged nuclei with inclusions.[54]

It is treated with photosensitive proflavin (dye red) in a 1:500 solution followed by exposure to fluorescent light for 15 minutes on two occasions. The lesions will heal within a 24-hour period.

Women with primary herpetic infections at the time of delivery should be delivered by cesarean section and the infant should be isolated from the mother and other infants. The infant is in serious jeopardy since the virus can attack his visceral organs, cardiorespiratory system, or central nervous system.

Recent studies have indicated that herpetic infections of the female genital tract are caused more frequently by herpes virus Type II rather than the Type I virus implicated in oral herpetic infections. There is also evidence suggesting that Type II herpes virus infection is associated with an increased incidence of carcinoma of the cervix.

Women who have had herpes vaginalis infections should be followed with cytologic smears for possible early detection of cervical carcinoma.

Additional Considerations

It must be emphasized that the woman may be infected with more than one of the above vaginal and vulval infections, making the treatment even more complicated. There are also other causes of pruritus that should be explored, such as pediculosis pubis, varicosities of the vulva, threadworms, whipworms, and local applications of deodorants.

Complaints of pruritus should not be taken lightly. It can interfere with sleep, may be a source of secondary infection due to scratching, and may give rise to serious mental depression.[55]

HEMORRHOIDS AND VARICOSITIES

Varicosities of hemorrhoidal veins are a frequent occurrence during pregnancy, causing swelling and pain. They may appear first during pregnancy, or small hemorrhoids already present may be exacerbated due to the pregnancy. The development of hemorrhoids during pregnancy is due to increased pressure on the hemorrhoidal veins by the gravid uterus, causing obstruction of venous return. The tendency toward constipation is also a causative factor. Thrombosis of a vein may occur causing considerable pain. Even considerable bleeding may occasionally occur. The painful edema may be treated by ice packs and topically applied anesthetics, suppositories, or ointments. Warm soaks and a stool softener are also effective. The thrombosed hemorrhoidal vein can be treated in the office or clinic by a simple incision and evacuation of the blood clot. Most hemorrhoids become asymptomatic shortly after delivery and surgery is usually not necessary unless there is persistent bleeding. Explaining this to the mother will help relieve her fears.

Varicosities occur in about 20 per cent of all pregnant women and tend to become more prominent with each successive pregnancy. There appears to be some familial predisposition to the development of varicosities.

Veins which were previously normal may become varicosed as early as the fourth week, a time when uterine pressure cannot conceivably play any part in their formation. One explanation of this early onset is the increased vascularity of the pelvic organs which leads to turgescence of all the tributary veins of the pelvis. A probably accessory cause is the generalized atony of unstriated muscles including those of the vein wall, a physiologic attribute of pregnancy.[56]

Varicosities cause the expectant mother to complain of lower extremity pain, particularly by the end of the day. She also complains of the cosmetic blemishes of the veins. Varicose veins are usually not treated by surgical means or by the injection method during pregnancy, but they should be treated following pregnancy. It may be necessary to convince the expectant mother to seek such treatment since the veins will improve once pregnancy is ended, only to return, with more distressing symptoms, in her next pregnancy.

The veins are supported by wearing elastic stockings. The stockings should be full length and should be put on before arising in the morning. Varicose veins can be drained, thus giving some relief, by assuming the following position: the woman lies on the floor or her bed, raises her legs, and rests them against the wall in a right angle position.

Some women develop varicose veins of the vulva and perineum and these, too, cause aching and heaviness in the affected parts. They may become a serious complication should they hemorrhage during labor. Vulval varicosities are treated by application of a foam rubber pad suspended across the vulva by a belt around the waist. These varicosed vessels can be drained and temporary relief obtained by elevating the hips on a pillow.

Information on the avoidance of varicosities should be part of expectant parent education. The expectant mother should:

- Avoid tight restricting garments and round garters.
- Avoid constipation.
- Sit with feet flat on the floor, avoid crossing the legs.
- Avoid standing for long periods of time. Use sitting and recumbent positions as much as possible.
- Sit with legs elevated whenever possible.
- Wear support hose if necessary to stand for extended periods.

HIGH-RISK ASSESSMENT

Careful assessment and research studies indicate that certain women and certain families can be expected to present unusual biopsychosocial problems related to reproduction and parenting. Recently the term *high-risk* has been used to signify a group of women and their infants who may be in jeopardy. Placing such individuals in facilities where their health care and opportunities for guidance are given top priority can be expected to improve their chances for favorable outcomes.

When a large number of women receive care in one facility, it is very important to identify the population which is at risk. When these individuals are so identified, services can be directed to them and professional time can be used in the most appropriate manner.

This section explores high-risk families in relation to predicting the perinatal outcome for both the mother and infant.

INDEX SCORING

Certain events occurring before and during the prenatal and intrapartal periods can adversely influence the outcome of pregnancy. Index scoring of these events forces attention to the importance of being able to select, on an objective basis, those women who need special medical care and those who need special nursing care.

Among the factors which determine high risk are:

- Age under 16 or over 40.
- Parity—primigravida or gravida of five or over.
- Past obstetric history of multiple abortions, low-birth-weight infants, fetal and neonatal death, congenital anomalies, or birth injury.
- Chronic diseases such as hypertension, heart disease, diabetes, syphilis, severe anemia, thyroid imbalance, malnutrition, marked obesity, chronic tuberculosis, chronic urinary tract infection, sickle cell anemia, and isoimmunization to the Rh factor.
- Familial diseases or traits such as Down's syndrome and Tay-Sachs disease.
- Reproductive system disorders, such as myomata uteri, history of previous cesarean section, and contracted pelvis.
- Nervous or emotional problems.
- A disrupted marital unit or single-status unfavorable environment.
- Serious accidents, violence, rape, or surgery.
- German measles during the first trimester of pregnancy.
- Toxemia of pregnancy.
- Recurrent or serious bleeding.

An example of one such health index is shown in Figure 21-33.

There are also high-risk pregnancy screening systems which are based on a prospective analysis of prenatal, intrapartal, and neonatal factors. They have been developed to predict perinatal morbidity and mortality. One such system reported by Hobel and colleagues[57] clearly shows that there is a positive correlation between the incidence of high-risk neonates (scores $\geq$ 10) and an increasing risk score in the prenatal and intrapartal periods. Data from this study is recorded on coded forms for subsequent data processing by a computer. Patients are "screened" on the initial visit, at 30 weeks, 35 weeks, and 39 weeks of gestation.

The various factors and scoring* are:

Maternal Factors	*Score*
I. Cardiovascular and renal	
1. Moderate to severe toxemia	10
2. Chronic hypertension	10
3. Moderate to severe renal disease	10

*From Hobel et al.,[57] with permission.

COLORADO MATERNAL HEALTH INDEX

PART I

PATIENT'S NAME ____________ PLACE OF INTERVIEW ____________

ADDRESS ____________ INTERVIEW DATE ____/____/____

PATIENT'S AGE ____ YRS. (at last birthday)

Para ________ Gravida ________ Race-ethnicity ________

PART II

1) MARITAL STATUS
- ☐ (2) Married
- ☐ (2) Widowed
- ☐ (2) Separated
- ☐ (5) Divorced
- ☐ (2) Never Married

2) AGE OF PATIENT
- ☐ (1) Under 20
- ☐ (1) 20 – 24
- ☐ (3) 25 – 29
- ☐ (3) 30 & over

3) RELIGION
- ☐ (0) Catholic
- ☐ (3) Protestant
- ☐ (6) L.D.S.
- ☐ Other (specify)

4) WEIGHT/HEIGHT RATIO
- ☐ (0) Under 1.75
- ☐ (3) 1.75 – 1.99
- ☐ (2) 2.00 – 2.24
- ☐ (4) 2.25 & over

5) PULSE
- ☐ (3) Under 80
- ☐ (1) 80 – 89
- ☐ (4) 90 & over

6) SYSTOLIC B.P.
- ☐ (0) Under 100
- ☐ (2) 100 – 109
- ☐ (1) 110 – 119
- ☐ (10) 120 & over

7) PULSE PRESSURE
- ☐ (0) Under 40
- ☐ (5) 40 – 49
- ☐ (7) 50 & over

8) BLOOD TYPE
- ☐ (1) A
- ☐ (4) B
- ☐ (3) O
- ☐ (2) Other

9) RH OF PATIENT
- ☐ (2) Positive
- ☐ (8) Negative

10) HEMATOCRIT
- ☐ (6) Under 35
- ☐ (3) 35 – 39
- ☐ (1) 40 & over

11) PREV. ABNORMAL PREG.
- ☐ (1) None
- ☐ (1) One
- ☐ (3) Two & over

12) KIDNEY TROUBLE
- ☐ (8) Yes
- ☐ (2) No

13) PREV. BABIES WITH NEWBORN MORBIDITY
- ☐ (7) Yes
- ☐ (2) No

RISK INDEX (Summation of Part II) ☐

RISK STATUS (Based on Parts II & III)

- ☐ HIGH RISK (Index of 35 or more or Condition in Part III Present)
- ☐ MODERATE RISK (Index of 26-34)
- ☐ LOW RISK (Index or 25 or less)

PART III

- ☐ CANCER OF WOMB
- ☐ DIABETES
- ☐ GERMAN MEASLES (During 1st Trimester)
- ☐ ACUTE URINARY TRACT INFECTION
- ☐ TOXEMIA
- ☐ PREVIOUS HIGH BLOOD PRESSURE

PART IV

NURSE'S OBSERVATIONS & OTHER HISTORY

- ☐ SERIOUS ACCIDENT, RAPE, VIOLENCE
- ☐ PREVIOUS MULTIPLE PREGNANCIES
- ☐ SERIOUS CARDIAC DISORDER
- ☐ THYROID DISTURBANCE
- ☐ TUBERCULOSIS
- ☐ VENEREAL DISEASE
- ☐ PSYCHIATRIC CONDITION
- ☐ GENETIC PROBLEM
- ☐ X-RADIATION OF ABDOMEN
- ☐ SMOKING 2 OR MORE PKGS. CIGARETTES/DAY
- ☐ USE OF HARMFUL DRUGS
- ☐ CONTRACEPTIVE USE
- ☐ LESS THAN 2 YEAR INTERVAL SINCE LAST PREG.
- ☐ MULTIPLE SOCIO-ECONOMIC PROBLEMS
- ☐ PREVIOUS DYSTOCIA
- ☐ RECURRENT BLEEDING

REMARKS:

PART V

CURRENT PREGNANCY OUTCOME

MOTHER: ☐ FAVORABLE ☐ UNFAVORABLE

COMMENTS: ____________

INFANT: ☐ FAVORABLE ☐ UNFAVORABLE

COMMENTS: ____________

FIGURE 21-33. Colorado Maternal Health Index. (Courtesy of the Colorado Department of Health.)

4. Severe heart disease, Class II–IV	10
5. History of eclampsia	5
6. History of pyelitis	5
7. Class I heart disease	5
8. Mild toxemia	5
9. Acute pyelonephritis	5
10. History of cystitis	1
11. Acute cystitis	1
12. History of toxemia	1
II. Metabolic	
1. Diabetes ≥ Class A-II	10
2. Previous endocrine ablation	10
3. Thyroid disease	5
4. Prediabetes (A-I)	5
5. Family history of diabetes	1
III. Previous histories	
1. Previous fetal exchange transfusion for Rh	10
2. Previous stillbirth	10
3. Post-term > 42 weeks	10
4. Previous premature infant	10
5. Previous neonatal death	10
6. Previous cesarean section	5
7. Habitual abortion	5
8. Infant > 10 pounds	5
9. Multiparity > 5	5
10. Epilepsy	5
11. Fetal anomalies	1
IV. Anatomic abnormalities	
1. Uterine malformation	10
2. Incompetent cervix	10
3. Abnormal fetal position	10
4. Polyhydramnios	10
5. Small pelvis	5
V. Miscellaneous	
1. Abnormal cervical cytology	10
2. Multiple pregnancy	10
3. Sickle cell disease	10
4. Age ≥ 35 or ≥ 15	5
5. Viral disease	5
6. Rh sensitization only	5
7. Positive serology	5
8. Severe anemia (< 9 Gm. Hgb)	5
9. Excessive use of drugs	5
10. History of TB or PPD ≥ 10 mm.	5
11. Weight < 100 or > 200 pounds	5
12. Pulmonary disease	5
13. Flu syndrome (severe)	5
14. Vaginal spotting	5
15. Mild anemia (9-10.9 Gm. Hgb)	1
16. Smoking ≥ 1 pack per day	1
17. Alcohol (moderate)	1
18. Emotional problem	1

Intrapartal Factors	*Score*
I. Maternal factors	
1. Moderate–severe toxemia	10
2. Hydramnios or oligohydramnios	10
3. Amnionitis	10
4. Uterine rupture	10
5. Mild toxemia	5
6. Premature rupture of membrane > 12 hr.	5
7. Primary dysfunctional labor	5
8. Secondary arrest of dilation	5
9. Demerol > 300 mg.	5
10. MgSO > 25 Gm.	5
11. Labor > 20 hours	5
12. Second stage > 2½ hours	5
13. Clinical small pelvis	5
14. Medical induction	5
15. Precipitous labor < 3 hours	5
16. Primary cesarean section	5
17. Repeat cesarean section	5
18. Elective induction	1
19. Prolonged latent phase	1
20. Uterine tetany	1
21. Pitocin augmentation	1
II. Placental factors	
1. Placenta previa	10
2. Abruptio placentae	10
3. Post-term > 42 weeks	10
4. Meconium stained amniotic fluid (dark)	10
5. Meconium stained amniotic fluid (light)	5
6. Marginal separation	1
III. Fetal factors	
1. Abnormal presentation	10

2. Multiple pregnancy	10
3. Fetal bradycardia > 30 minutes	10
4. Breech delivery total extraction	10
5. Prolapsed cord	10
6. Fetal weight < 2,500 grams	10
7. Fetal acidosis pH ≤ 7.25 (Stage I)	10
8. Fetal tachycardia > 30 minutes	10
9. Operative forceps or vacuum extraction	5
10. Breech delivery spontaneous or assisted	5
11. General anesthesia	5
12. Outlet forceps	1
13. Shoulder dystocia	1

Neonatal Factors	*Score*
I. General	
1. Prematurity < 2,000 g.	10
2. Apgar at 5 minutes < 5	10
3. Resuscitation at birth	10
4. Fetal anomalies	10
5. Dysmaturity	5
6. Prematurity 2,000-2,500 g.	5
7. Apgar at 1 minute < 5	5
8. Feeding problem	1
9. Multiple birth	1
II. Respiratory	
1. RDS	10
2. Meconium aspiration syndrome	10
3. Congenital pneumonia	10
4. Anomalies of respiratory system	10
5. Apnea	10
6. Other respiratory distress	10
7. Transient tachypnea	5
III. Metabolic disorders	
1. Hypoglycemia	10
2. Hypocalcemia	10
3. Hypomagnesemia or hypermagnesemia	5
4. Hypoparathyroidism	5
5. Failure to gain weight	1
6. Jitteriness or hyperactivity with specific causes	1
IV. Cardiac	
1. Major cardiac anomalies which require immediate catheterization	10
2. CHF	10
3. Persistent cyanosis	5
4. Cardiac anomalies not requiring immediate catheterization	5
5. Murmur	5
V. Hematologic problems	
1. Hyperbilirubinemia	10
2. Hemorrhagic diathesis	10
3. Chromosomal anomalies	10
4. Sepsis	10
5. Anemia	5
VI. CNS	
1. CNS depression > 24 hours	10
2. Seizures	10
3. CNS depression < 24 hours	5

AMNIOCENTESIS

The structural chemical components and activity of the cells shed by the fetus and found in the amniotic fluid can provide information regarding fetal high-risk and genetic abnormalities.[58–60] Amniocentesis is the procedure whereby amniotic fluid is removed from the uterine cavity by the insertion of a needle through the abdominal wall, into the uterus, and through the amniotic sac. The procedure is usually performed at approximately the 14 weeks of gestation, by which time a sufficient volume of amniotic fluid has formed. It may be done initially or repeated later in pregnancy when later development of the fetus is being assessed.

The following fetal conditions may be studied through the cellular components and supernatant fluid components of the amniotic fluid:

Rh isoimmunization
Fetal maturity
Respiratory distress syndrome dangers
Inborn errors of metabolism
Fetal genetic abnormalities
Fetal sex
ABO blood grouping

Amniocentesis is indicated for prenatal diagnosis in the following conditions:

1. Chromosome disorders
   a. Parent with chromosome mosaicism (e.g., G trisomy).
   b. Parent with balanced translocation (e.g., D/G, G/G).
   c. Pregnancy in women age 40 years or over.
2. Biochcmical disorders
   a. Both parents heterozygotes for autosomal recessive disorder (e.g., Tay-Sachs disease).
   b. Mother a known or suspected carrier of a sex linked disorder (e.g., hemophilia).
   c. Previous affected child from same parentage.[61]

Late in pregnancy amniocentesis may be used to assess fetal growth to ascertain disparities between gestational age and fetal size. It is also useful to assess fetal size when pregnancy is to be terminated, but should be done prior to the onset of labor by induction or cesarean section. The following changes occur in the amniotic fluid late in pregnancy:

1. Bilirubin pigment disappears from amniotic fluid rather abruptly at approximately 36 weeks of fetal life.
2. Creatinine levels increase in the amniotic fluid with fetal age. Maturity of the fetus is assumed to have been attained when the creatinine reaches 2 mg. per 100 ml.
3. Cylotogic examination of amniotic fluid in the latter part of pregnancy can measure the number of fat staining cells. A fat cell count of less than 2 per cent of the total cells present is encountered prior to 36 weeks of pregnancy or when the fetus weighs less than 2,500 grams. After that period the number of fat cells increases. When they comprise 20 per cent or more of the total cells examined, the fear of prematurity is no longer a consideration.

Amniocentesis does have some limitations. The technique requires great skill to culture the cells. The expertise of those who interpret the findings is critical. The time needed to culture the cells may limit the usefulness of the procedure. The biochemical analysis of fetal cells may take as long as 30 days to perform and it may be necessary to repeat the amniocentesis two or three times if the cultures do not grow. The time lost may make any decision about terminating the pregnancy useless, since the pregnancy may be too advanced to terminate. However, when cells are successfully cultivated, chromosome analysis can be achieved in 99 per cent of the specimens. The current cost of the procedure is about $200, but the cost may be reduced as it becomes more popular and less expensive ways are found to perform the analysis. In addition, facilities for doing the studies are limited. Women are advised to locate such a facility early in pregnancy, or even better, before becoming pregnant. The following voluntary agencies maintain listings of diagnostic and consultation centers:

The National Genetics Foundation
250 West 5th Street
New York, New York 10019

The National Foundation—March of Dimes
1275 Mamaroneck Avenue
White Plains, New York 10602

There are some risks to the procedure. Several researchers have estimated that 1 per cent of all amniocentesis procedures are responsible for spontaneous abortions. Other possible fetal complications include trauma, infection, and later disturbances in the child's development. A small number of fetal and placental punctures have been cited and have resulted in anemia or death of the fetus. Possible maternal complications include bleeding, infection, and Rh sensitization resulting from fetal bleeding into the maternal circulation. With the advent of ultrasonic detection devices to locate the placenta and fetus, the risk to mother and fetus is considerably reduced.

Moral issues may also arise from the use of this diagnostic procedure. For example, should a woman expose herself and her fetus to the risk of amniocentesis if she does not intend to terminate her pregnancy in the event that a severe abnormality is discovered? (As yet, there is no method to modify the natural history of fetal abnormalities). Is it valuable enough to outweigh the possible emotional effects of the outcome? Also, there is always the basic moral issue concerning voluntary interruption of pregnancy.

The prenatal detection of genetic disorders adds a new dimension to genetic counseling. Parents no longer need to be content with an empirical risk figure but may be in a position to know definitely what risk is involved.[62] Unfortunately, therapy today is restricted to the termination of pregnancy when severe mental deficiencies or death in early infancy is inevitable. If the decision is made to carry the pregnancy to term, the diagnosis has the advantage of alerting the medical team to deal with the problem.

The nurse, although not performing the amniocentesis herself, plays a vital role in supporting the patient during the procedures. Women will be anxious due to the necessity of the procedure and the procedure itself. The nurse must be knowledgeable about the technique and able to discuss it with her patient. Her presence will give the woman a greater sense of security. The nurse will assume responsibility for assessment and for aspects of physical care. Assessment includes monitoring the fetal heart, monitoring vital signs, and observing for manifestations of anxiety.

Nurses are becoming more responsible for some aspects of genetic counseling and must keep aware of recent and ongoing research in this area.

PULSED ECHO ULTRASOUND (SONAR)

Ultrasonic echo sounding or sonar has recently been added as a diagnostic technique to assess fetal growth and to make other critical assessments of maternal problems. The technique employs intermittent or pulsed sound waves of very high frequency, above the range of animal hearing. These are projected from a crystal, under directional control, as beams of very small quantities of energy. Echoes of these sound waves are picked up from the junctions or interfaces between tissues of different physical properties, and these echoes are detected by the same crystal that propagates the original ultrasonic beam. The echo signals are then displayed upon the face of a cathode ray tube or screen so that a two dimensional picture of the intrauterine contents is built up progressively on the screen as the ultrasonic scanning beam traverses the abdomen. Time-exposure Polaroid photography is used to convert a transient image into a permanent record.[63] When two definite points can be identified, e.g., the biparietal eminences, it is possible to measure the distance between them. The patient experiences no discomfort from the procedure, except for the inconvenience of having some contact medium such as olive oil applied to the skin. The interpretation of ultrasonic pictures cannot be compared with roentgenograms.

Roentgenograms show the projected surface of the structure being examined, while ultrasonic pictures give a cross-sectional view. It is now possible to use ultrasonic pictures for many of the diagnostic procedures usually accomplished by roentgenograms, thereby eliminating the necessity of exposing the mother and fetus to radiation. This method achieves a new dimension of visualizing normal and pathologic structures which were previously inaccessible.[64]

Ultrasound may be used to ascertain whether the individual is actually pregnant. By having the patient fill her bladder completely, the very early products of conception can usually be seen by the fifth week of pregnancy. The appearance may confirm the diagnosis of pregnancy before the tests for gonadotropin in the urine are positive.[65] If the ovum is arrested in its development and a "blighted" ovum forms, or if a hydatidiform mole forms, this can be diagnosed by sonar. After 14 weeks of gestation the fetal head has developed to the extent that it cannot be missed by careful screening, and between 14 and 16 weeks of gestation the placenta can be detected. After 20 weeks of gestation it is possible by biparietal cephalometry to follow the growth of the fetal head. This is especially useful when there is concern about fetal maturity due to maternal disease, or when menstrual history is uncertain so that the estimated date of confinement cannot be assured. This technique is most useful in caring for women who relate an obstetric history of previous underdeveloped fetuses and those who have diseases known to interfere with intrauterine development, such as hypertension, chronic renal diseases, toxemia, and diabetes. Figure 21-34 compares an ultrasonic photograph of the fetus in the vertex position with one of the fetus in the breech position.

Ultrasonic echo sounding can also be used to diagnose other obstetric and gynecologic problems which may place the patient in the high-risk group. Early in pregnancy an ectopic pregnancy or an incomplete abortion can be diagnosed. Hydramnios can also be determined. Twins can easily be visualized. Ovarian tumors and other pelvic masses which might interfere with the process of delivery can be diagnosed. Ultrasonic localization of the placenta is useful in diagnosing placenta previa and as a prerequisite to amniocentesis.

The nurse can assure the pregnant woman undergoing a sonar study that neither she nor her baby will be harmed. She will be anxious that such a diagnostic procedure is necessary, but may well be assured of a better outcome based on this and other methods of assessment. The nurse's presence will help allay anxiety.

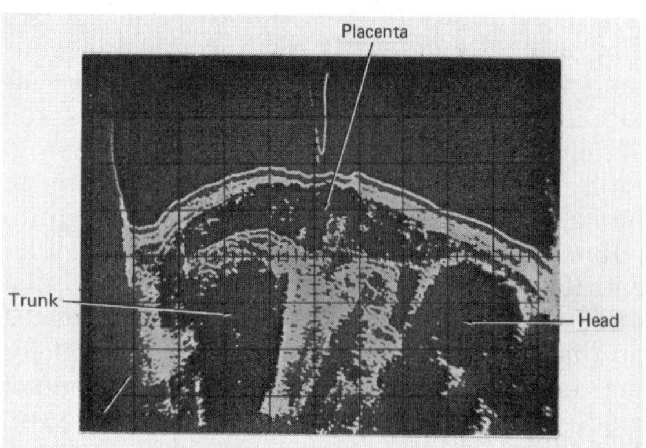

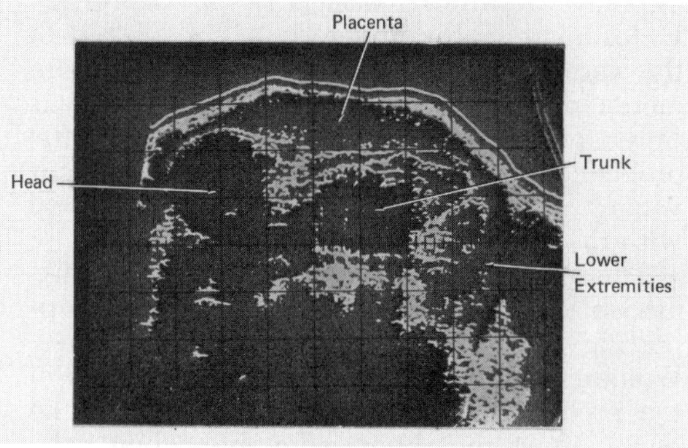

FIGURE 21-34. *Left,* Ultrasound photograph of a fetus in the vertex position. *Right,* Ultrasound photograph of a fetus in the breech position. (Courtesy of Samuel Cheney.)

FETAL PULSE DETECTOR (DOPTONE)

New equipment is constantly being developed to assist health professionals in monitoring mothers and infants and in assessing their risk status. One example is the Doptone, a fetal pulse detector which uses the ultrasonic beam. By transmission and reception of ultrasound, the motion of organs and blood within the pregnant uterus are detected. It can be used to detect fetal life as early as 12 weeks of gestation, to monitor the fetal heart tones during pregnancy and labor, and to localize the placenta. Localization of the placenta is valuable for amniocentesis and for making a differential diagnosis when vaginal bleeding occurs during pregnancy.

URINARY ESTRIOL

When maternal disease processes impinge on the developing fetus, it is often essential to know when the fetus has reached a stage of maturity in order to guarantee a greater chance of survival outside the uterus. One of the most useful such laboratory tests is a study of the expectant woman's 24-hour urinary estriol excretion.

Estriol is produced by the placenta. Because it represents the metabolic activity of both the fetus and the placenta, a significant drop in estriol production may indicate serious dysfunction in either or both.[66]

Urinary estriol excretion usually increases as pregnancy progresses and correlates reasonably well with the weight of the fetus. Twenty-four hour estriol excretion curve studies are useful in identifying the fetus at risk.

Except in pregnancy with an anencephalic fetus, urinary excretion of estriol of less than 3 or 4 mg. per day during the third trimester of pregnancy indicates fetal death or some severe difficulty. There are factors apparently unrelated to the fetoplacental unit that also result in decreased urinary estriol. One of these is acute pyelonephritis. Therefore, a single measurement considerably outside the normal range must be verified.

Incomplete 24-hour urine collections may affect serial estriol determination. The nurse must be very explicit in her instructions to the expectant mother when this determination is being made. The mother can best cooperate when she appreciates the purposes of the tests and the important decisions to be reached based on the test results.

REFERENCES

1. Rubbelke, L. and Waller, M. V.: *Maternal Health Index — A Nursing Aid to Decision of Priority of Service.* ANA Clinical Conference. Appleton-Century-Crofts, New York, 1969, p. 175.
2. Hobel, C. J.: *Prenatal and intrapartum high-risk screening.* Am. J. Obstet. Gynecol. 117:1, 1973.
3. Grimm, L. M.: *Maternity continuity clinic.* Am. J. Nurs. 73:1723, 1973.
4. Kowalski, K.: *"On call" staffing.* Am. J. Nurs. 73:1725, 1973.
5. Hellman, L. M. and Pritchard, J. A.: *Williams Obstetrics,* ed. 14. Appleton-Century-Crofts, New York, 1971, p. 303.
6. Taylor, E. S.: *Beck's Obstetrical Practice,* ed. 8. Williams & Wilkins, Baltimore, 1966, p. 133.
7. Smout, C. F. V.: *An Introduction to Midwifery.* Williams & Wilkins, Baltimore, 1962, p. 21.
8. Steer, C. M.: *Moloy's Evaluation of the Pelvis in Obstetrics,* ed. 2. W. B. Saunders, Philadelphia, 1959, p. 49.
9. Ibid.: p. 53.
10. Ibid.: p. 54.
11. Hellman: op. cit., p. 299.
12. Ibid., p. 305.
13. Ibid.
14. Garrey, M. M., et al.: *Obstetrics Illustrated.* Williams & Wilkins, Baltimore, 1969, p. 23.
15. Taylor, S.: *Essentials of Gynecology,* ed. 3. Lea and Febiger, Philadelphia, 1965, p. 344.
16. Ibid., p. 105.
17. Mattax, J. H.: *The value of routine prenatal chest x-ray.* Obstet. Gynecol. 41:243, 1973.
18. Wiedenbach, E.: *Family Centered Maternity Nursing.* G. P. Putnam, New York, 1967, p. 210.
19. *The Womanly Art of Breastfeeding.* La Leche League International, Franklin Park, Illinois, 1958, p. 29.
20. Rubovits, F. E.: *Traumatic rupture of the pregnant uterus from "seat belt" injury.* Am. J. Obstet. Gynecol. 90:828, 1964.

21. Crosby, W. M. and Costiloe, J. P.: *Safety of lap-belt restraint for pregnant victims of automobile collisions.* N. Engl. J. Med. 284:632, 1971.
22. Danforth, D. N.: *Textbook of Obstetrics and Gynecology.* Harper & Row, New York, 1966, p. 273.
23. Clark, A. L.: *Leadership Technique in Expectant Parent Education.* Springer, New York, 1973, p. 35.
24. Mukshy, R., Murphy, J. and Martin, F.: *Placental changes and maternal weight in smoking and nonsmoking mothers.* Am. J. Obstet. Gynecol. 106:703, 1970.
25. Underwood, P., et al.: *The relationship of smoking to the outcome of pregnancy.* Am. J. Obstet. Gynecol. 91:270, 1965.
26. Zabriskie, J. R.: *Effects of cigarette smoking during pregnancy.* Obstet. Gynecol. 21: 405, 1963.
27. Yerushalmy, J.: *Mother's cigarette smoking and survival of infant.* Am. J. Obstet. Gynecol. 88:505, 1964.
28. Underwood: op. cit., p. 273.
29. Ibid.
30. Hellman: op. cit., p. 342.
31. Ulleland, C., et al.: *The offspring of alcoholic mothers.* Pediatr. Res. 4:474, 1970.
32. Nichols, M. M.: *Acute alcohol withdrawal syndrome in a newborn.* Am. J. Dis. Child 113:714, 1967.
33. Laufer, B.: *Geophagy Field Museum of Natural History, Anthropological Series, Publication 280, No. 28,* Chicago, 1930.
34. Dunston, B. N.: *Pica practice: its relationship to hemoglobin level and perinatal casualties.* Nurs. Science 1:33, 1963.
35. Minnich, V., et al.: *Pica in Turkey. Effect of clay upon iron absorption.* Am. J. Clin. Nutr. 21:78, 1969.
36. Talkington, K., et al.: *Effect of ingestion of starch and some clays on iron absorption.* Am. J. Obstet. Gynecol. 108:262, 1970.
37. Dunston: op. cit., p. 35.
38. Little, W. A.: *Drugs in pregnancy.* Am. J. Nurs. 66:1303, 1966.
39. Hellman: op. cit., p. 342.
40. Zelson, C., et al.: *Neonatal narcotic addiction: 10 year observation.* Pediatrics 48:178, 1971.
41. Rajegowda, B. K., et. al.: *Methadone withdrawal in the newborn infant.* J. Pediatr. 81:532, 1972.
42. Bleyer, W. A. and Marshall, R. E.: *Barbiturate withdrawal syndrome in a passively addicted infant.* J.A.M.A. 221:185, 1972.
43. Bogdanoff, B., et al.: *Brain and eye abnormalities possible sequelae to prenatal use of multiple drugs including LSD.* Am. J. Dis. Child 123:145, 1972.
44. Browne, J. C. and Dixon, G.: *Browne's Antenatal Care,* ed. 10. Williams & Wilkins, Baltimore, 1970, p. 158.
45. Ibid.: p. 157.
46. Hellman: op. cit., p. 344.
47. Ibid.: p. 345.
48. Browne: op. cit., p. 320.
49. Ziegel, E. and Van Blarcom, C.: *Obstetric Nursing,* ed. 5. Macmillan, New York, 1966, p. 142.
50. Danforth: op. cit., p. 859.
51. Garrey: op. cit., p. 102.
52. Perl, G.: *Metronidazole treatment of trichomoniosis in pregnancy.* Obstet. Gynecol. 25:273, 1965.
53. Danforth: op. cit., p. 858.
54. Nahmias, A. J., Josey, W. E. and Naib, Z. M.: *Neonatal herpes simplex infection. Role of genital infection in mother as source of virus in the newborn.* J.A.M.A. 199:164, 1967.
55. Browne: op. cit., p. 298.
56. Ibid: p. 229.
57. Hobel: op. cit.
58. Nitowsky, H. M.: *Prenatal diagnosis of genetic abnormality.* Am. J. Nurs. 71:1551, 1971.
59. Nadler, H. L. and Gerbie, A.: *Present status of amniocentesis in intrauterine diagnosis of genetic defect.* Obstet. Gynecol. 38:789, 1971.
60. Hiatt, B.: *Research and diagnosis in human genetics.* Research News, Office of Research Administration, University of Michigan, 23:15, 1973.
61. Nitowsky: op. cit., p. 1555.
62. Nadler: op. cit., p. 795.
63. Donald, I.: *Sonar study of prenatal development.* J. Pediatr. 75:326, 1969.
64. Thompson, H. E.: *The clinical use of pulsed echo ultrasound in obstetrics and gynecology.* Obstet. Gynecol. Surv. 23:903, 1968.
65. Donald: op. cit., p. 327.
66. Tracht, M. E.: *The laboratory in the problem pregnancy.* Consultant 13:119, 1973.

BIBLIOGRAPHY

Assessment of Sexual Function: A Guide to Interviewing. Vo. 8, Report No. 88, 1973.

Danforth, D. N.: *Textbook of Obstetrics and Gynecology,* ed. 2. Harper & Row, New York, 1971.

Hellman, L. M. and Pritchard, J. A.: *Williams Obstetrics,* ed. 14. Appleton-Century-Crofts, New York, 1971.

Hiatt, B.: *Research and Diagnosis in human genetics.* Research News, Office of Research Administration, University of Michigan, 23:15, 1973.

Hobel, C. J.: *Prenatal and intrapartum high-risk screening.* Am. J. Obstet. Gynecol. 117:1, 1973.

Kon, J. K. and Cowie, A. T.: *Milk: The Mammary Gland and Its Secretion, vol 1.* Academic Press, New York, 1961.

Rugh, R. and Lamfrum, S.: *From Conception to Birth.* Harper & Row, New York, 1971.

Taylor, E. S.: *Beck's Obstetrical Practice,* ed. 9. Williams & Wilkins, Baltimore, 1971.

22 Expectant Parent Education

ANN L. CLARK, R.N., M.A.

Including *Preparation for Childbirth with the Psychoprophylactic Method for Painless Childbirth* by Flora Hommel, R.N., B.S.

Almost without exception, conducting classes on preparation for parenthood has come to be accepted as a role of nursing. To date there are far too few classes for expectant parents and far too few young people are enrolled in such groups. Although classes, as a form of preparation for parenthood, are not the only way people learn to prepare for the role changes, they are a needed community facility. Today more and more young people in America are growing up in small nuclear families where their opportunities to see and practice child care are limited and where opportunities to compare their parents' practices with those of others are virtually nonexistent. Moreover, when young people begin their families they most often establish nuclear families far removed from their own families, thus limiting available support and guidance.

Today's economy also presents problems. In the majority of families both adults are employed outside the home. Employed grandmothers and other female relatives are less available to assist with childrearing even in a crisis. Employed assistance in the home is not financially possible for many families and is also very difficult to obtain in most communities.

On the brighter side, some preparation for family living classes are being offered in the more progressive high schools. Somehow, the all important responsibility for bearing and rearing children has not been given the importance it deserves and, indeed, requires. Young people are encouraged to expend much more energy on problems outside the family. The ability to drive a car or to type are skills one would be sure to master before they were needed. Learning to parent has no such priority.

Nurses who conduct expectant parent classes are cognizant of the many unrealistic expectations young people have concerning pregnancy, labor, and childrearing. Unmet expectations engender anxiety, frustration, and conflict. Many of these feelings can be and are avoided and the stressors minimized through anticipatory guidance and knowledge provided by expectant parent classes.

The author teaches expectant parent classes using the leadership technique method.[1] Some of the experiences, in terms of parental expectations, as well as the method will be shared with the reader throughout this chapter.

Expectant parent education is an awesome responsibility as well as a joy. Sharing the experience of expectant parenthood is a special privilege and provides the nurse with insight into the feeling tone of this era of life. Learning the expectations, sharing the feelings, and exploring the interest areas of expectant parents is the focus for developing the course content and planning the method of presenting that content. The following are some of the various expectations that members of one class held at the time they joined the class.

Expectations of labor
- The pain is like a stomach ache, what makes it hurt?
- The place where you give birth will be noisy with screaming women.
- They won't let you eat anything.
- Stressful!
- I will be anxious not knowing what to expect.
- It hurts. I'm expecting a lot, but not the worst pain.
- A lot depends on who is with you.
- Some have easy times, others are different.
- It depends on how you are built.
- There is some pain involved. I've been told it's like a menstrual cramp—I get them.
- It's important what attitude you go into labor with. If you scream, you tighten the muscles more. If you breathe proper, it eases things.
- I can't imagine, I'm frightened.
- Beautiful.
- I think beside the pain, there must be a lot of joy.
- You don't have any control, scarey.
- It's a natural process, there is nothing you can do about it.
- Overwhelming. I'm scared stiff.
- You forget it after the experience is over.
- Hardest job you ever have to do, you have to work.
- The afterbirth is the most painful, I hear.
- I hear women go all out of character.

Expectations immediately after birth
- Happy child is born and it is all over.
- Tired.
- Groggy.
- Worried, fear that something still is not right with the baby.
- Ashamed of myself.
- So proud and happy.
- Might not want to care for the baby, want to relax and sleep.
- Friendly feeling gone, empty feeling.

Expectations of the newborn and his needs
- Proud and happy, I hope.
- Depends on whether it's a boy.
- Cry and cause us a lot of sleepless nights.
- Demand a lot. I don't want to spoil him.
- Will be sorta misshaped.
- It will feel kind of strange, take time to learn to love him.
- Shaken by the reality, the responsibility of caring for a helpless baby.
- We've had stitches, we may have feelings of maternal rejection.

The above examples are only a small sample of the expectations and concerns this class shared with the author, but they are enough to give some idea of the content needed. Expectant parents come to these classes with high motivation for assistance and reassurance about the task which lies ahead.

APPROACHES TO EXPECTANT PARENT EDUCATION

There are a number of different approaches to expectant parent education. Classes are one approach. They should be sponsored by some well-recognized community agency and organized and taught by nurses with special preparation to do so. The philosophy of parent education and the objectives to be attained must be clearly defined, for they will guide the course development and the selection of the parent educator.

The classes may be held at appointed times, with preregistration of a group that stays together throughout the series. On the other hand, they may consist of an open group where individuals waiting for prenatal clinic appointments come for one or for the series of

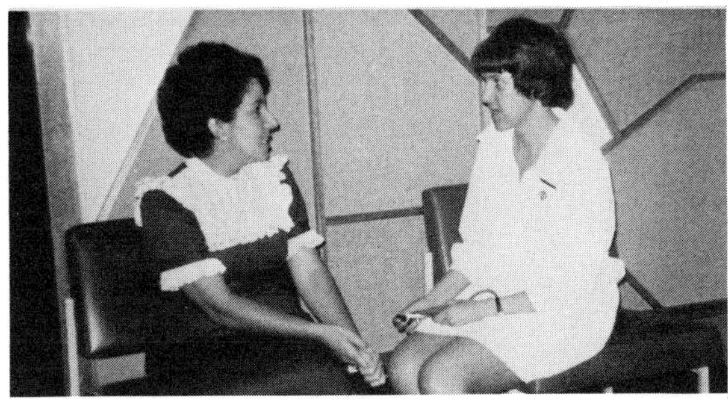

FIGURE 22-1. Clinic bench instruction may be the only way to reach some expectant mothers.

classes, and where there is constant turnover with new members joining and other members withdrawing as they reach their delivery dates.

Discussion or instruction may also be held informally on clinic benches for women who will not take advantage of more formal classes[2] (Fig. 22-1). One such class is carried out in a clinic using role playing by nursing students to spark group discussion.

Some multimedia instruction can be planned for waiting rooms of clinics or physicians offices. This consists of a slide and tape communication technique which gives information on prenatal self-care and on infant care. However, it provides none of the advantages of a group discussion or even of having individual specific questions answered.

Mass media in the form of booklets, pamphlets, and television programs offer needed information for expectant women. The extent to which they do so is discussed later in this chapter.

There is also the "one to one" method of expectant parent education.

FORMAL CLASSES

When formal classes are planned the decision must be made as to type—didactic planned course, leadership technique method, or a combination of the two. The preplanned, didactic course has a set curriculum with time for questions and answers at the end of each class. The leadership technique method allows class members to decide the course content, with leadership provided by the parent educator (Fig. 22-2).

Some classes are planned for expectant mothers only and are held during the day, others are for expectant parents and are held in the evening. Some classes are for adolescents only. Some classes prepare for labor and delivery only. They include the process of labor and delivery, body mechanics, relaxation, and controlled breathing. Some courses plan one husband-only evening or one wife-only class during the series.

LEADERSHIP TECHNIQUE

Leadership technique classes presuppose that the group leader has:

1. Knowledge of the subject. She knows contemporary maternal and child care. She keeps up with the research in this area.
2. Knowledge of group technique.
3. Self insight. She is comfortable with her own sexuality.
4. Knowledge of the variety of ethnic, income, and social levels of persons who attend expectant parents classes. She is aware of maternity practices in her community.

The nurse will be better able to teach classes for expectant parents using the leadership technique method if she believes that:

1. Expectant parents are rational people, capable of determining what their needs are.
2. Each expectant family is unique and the baby they are about to bring into the world is likewise unique.

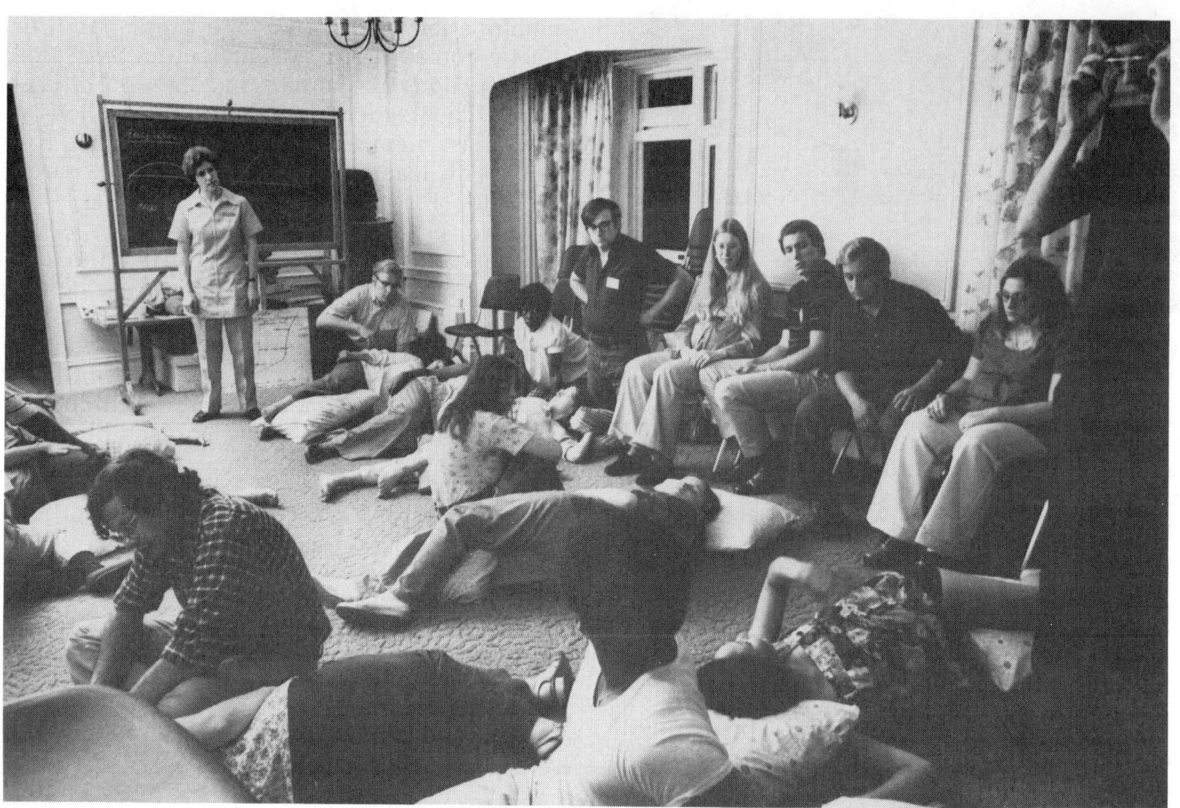

FIGURE 22-2. Group classes led by expectant parent educator (nurse). (Photograph by Robert Goldstein.)

3. Expectant parents want to be good parents and the most appropriate way she can help them is to permit them to become active partners in determining how they wish to approach labor, birth, and parenting.
4. Sharing feelings helps individuals to recognize that others too share the same feelings and ultimately one's feelings of being different, unworthy, or alone can be reduced.
5. Verbalization with a group of interested, supportive persons increases one's sense of personal worth.
6. Anxiety must be reduced if learning is to take place.
7. A group method of problem-solving can help individuals to improve their problem-solving skills which in the long run will better serve parents throughout all the years to follow.

ASPECTS OF LEADERSHIP

The nurse in a leadership role in expectant parents classes is an active member of the class. Sometimes she acts as the leader of the group, sometimes she simply supports whatever member of the class is leading the discussion (Fig. 22-3).

She creates an atmosphere for learning and helps individuals to find their way into the group process.[3]

She guides the discussion, giving it form and direction by helping parents identify their concerns, relate them to the interest of the whole group, clarify them, and explore their meaning.[4]

She deepens the discussion by making explicit the undertones of meaning and emotional responses that are implied.[5] She supports, uses empathy and sympathy, and offers "strokes" as appropriate.

She puts the content into a broader framework by relating experiences to basic knowledge, thereby reducing fears by examining them realistically in the face of scientific knowledge.

She adds information which the expectant parents do not have. She clarifies assumptions and corrects errors.

She encourages the expression and honest exploration of different points of view, without taking sides, so parents can make their own choices based on personal preference.[6]

She sets an example in her acceptance of each member of the class by indicating that they are someone to be listened to with respect.[7] Life styles and approaches to life situations are accepted with a nonjudgmental attitude.

She responds freely and spontaneously to the group's requirements, but keeps in mind certain basic knowledge which each individual needs in order to avoid the unexpected that engenders anxiety. She finds ways to arouse exploration of all needed topics before the series ends.

She makes audiovisual aids available to the group to clarify, to emphasize a point, and to create discussion.

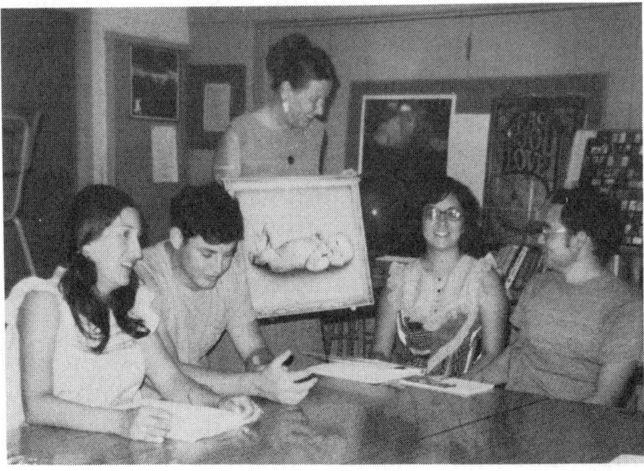

FIGURE 22-3. The nurse in a leadership role is an active member of the expectant parent education class.

CONTENT

Whether the expectant parent educator uses the group leadership technique described above or a preplanned curriculum, the content knowledge base which all expectant parents will find useful during pregnancy and during the early period of parenthood remains the same. All expectant parents will wish to:

Understand what is happening to their bodies and to their lives (physiologically, psychologically, and sociologically).

Understand how each partner can support the other to reduces and facilitate coping.

Be prepared for the labor experience, both emotionally and physically.

Recognize the needs of their infant at birth and develop skill to meet those needs.

Understand the complexities of family interplay and how to keep communications open.

Move into the new roles and new relationships precipitated by the addition of a child to the family with a minimum of anxiety, conflict, and frustration.

With these interests, concerns, and needs in mind the expectant parent educator can begin to develop course content. Many nurses decide to wait until the first class and involve the members in the course planning. Regardless of the method of instruction, almost all expectant parent programs include some or all of the following content,[8] although not necessarily in this order:

- I. Human Reproduction
  - A. Heredity (biologic inheritance)
  - B. Anatomy of reproduction
    - 1. Male
    - 2. Female
  - C. Conception and the intrauterine process
    - 1. Fetal development
- II. Maternal Health
  - A. Psychologic changes inherent in pregnancy
  - B. Physiologic changes in pregnancy prenatal hygiene
  - C. Body mechanics during pregnancy
- III. Nutrition for the Family
  - A. Nutritional needs during pregnancy
  - B. Nutritional needs for the new mother
  - C. The nursing mother
- IV. Labor and Childbirth
  - A. Premonitory signs of labor
  - B. Labor
  - C. Preparation for labor
    - 1. Relaxation
    - 2. Controlled breathing
  - D. Emotional implications to labor
    - 1. The hospital experience
  - E. Control of pain in childbirth
- V. The Newborn Infant
  - A. Birth and its meaning to the neonate
  - B. The newborn, his physical properties
  - C. Needs of the newborn
    - 1. The baby bath
    - 2. Formula making and bottle feeding
    - 3. Technique of breast feeding
- VI. Family Relationships
  - A. Physiological changes during puerperium
  - B. Psychological aspects of puerperium
    - 1. Mother-infant attachment
  - C. Parent-infant relationships
  - D. Triadic relationships
  - E. A baby in the home
- VII. Family Planning

LOGISTICS

Discussion-type classes, even those in which members are free to ask questions and share information, need to be kept small. There is no place for classes of more than 50 individuals in expectant parent education. Twenty members, or 10 to 12 couples, is an appropriate group for leadership technique classes.

The class period should be limited to 90 minutes and a break should be provided during the session. Shifts in activity, such as viewing a film, doing exercises, and working in small groups, are helpful to keep interest alive.

Comfort must be of prime importance. A large table and comfortable chairs provide the most convenient type of seating to facilitate communication. In this arrangement, name cards can be placed in front of each individual so that names can be used during the session. Good ventilation, rest room facilities, and adequate visual aid equipment are essential. If the course includes exercises, equipment will be needed—or the parents could supply their own beach mats and pillows.

Audiovisual aids, appropriately used, can add valuable realistic information. The film should be selected on the basis of the group's needs and desires. It should be an aid to learning and not the focus of the class. Proper selection and use of the film are mandatory. A prior review, during which the instructor notes important points to be explained prior to the showing and for discussion following the presentation, is valuable. Certain aspects of some films will cause anxiety and tension. These can be offset by prior explanation, thus providing a better vehicle for learning. Feedback after the showing will help the instructor evaluate its usefulness. Some useful films and their sources are:

Generation to Generation. McGraw-Hill Text Films, 330 W. 42nd Street, New York, N. Y. 10036

Human Reproduction. McGraw-Hill Text Films, 330 W. 42nd Street, New York, N. Y. 10036

Birthday. Pomes and Popcorn, Box 22169, Cleveland, Ohio 44122

Journey with a Friend. Pomes and Popcorn, Box 22169, Cleveland, Ohio 44122

Labor and Childbirth. Medical Arts Productions, Inc., P.O. Box 4042, Stockton, Calif.

Normal Birth. Medical Arts Productions, Inc., P.O. Box 4042, Stockton, Calif.

Not Me Alone. Polymorph Films, Inc., Boston, Mass.

The Management of Breast Feeding. University of Washington, Audio-Visual Services, Seattle, Wash. 98105

Planned Families. Allend'or Productions, Inc., 3449 Cahuenga Blvd., W. Hollywood, Calif.

The Newborn. Johnson & Johnson, New Brunswick, N. J. 08903

Talking about Breast Feeding. Polymorph Films, Inc., 331 Newbury Street, Boston, Mass. 02115

The First Two Weeks of Life. Rental: American Journal of Nursing Co. Film Library. % Association—Sterling Films, 600 Grand Ave., Ridgefield, N. J. 07657

Maternity Care: Medical Examination during Pregnancy. % Association—Sterling Films, 600 Grand Ave., Ridgefield, N. J. 07657

Maternity Care: Personal Care during Pregnancy. % Association—Sterling Films, 600 Grand Ave., Ridgefield, N. J.

If the class is composed of couples, the instructor may want to consider setting aside an evening for a separate class for husbands only and/or wives only. An expectant fathers-only session might include the following subjects:

- Coaching in labor
- Aspects of fatherhood
- Providing a relaxed environment for nourishing the mother-infant relationship
- Expression of feelings about choice of methods of feeding the infant
- Sexual adjustment during pregnancy and after the birth
- Coping with the moods of pregnancy.

Some time should be set aside in each class series to discuss the role of mass media in the lives of expectant and new parents. Much material presented on television and in the press is confusing, conflicting, and anxiety-producing. Programs or publications viewed or read by class members during the series can be explored as part of the discussion.

Members of the class should know something about the nurse's professional background and about each other.

The instructor needs to know as much as possible about the composition of her class in order to further interpersonal relationships.

Family Name ____ Husband's Name ____ Wife's Name ____

Address (full) ____

Tel. No. ____ If no answer call ____

Physician's Name and Address ____

Going to ____ Hospital. Date Baby Due ____

WIFE	HUSBAND
Age ____	Age ____
First Baby: Yes ____ No ____	First Baby: Yes ____ No ____
Education: H.S. ____ College ____	Education: H.S. ____ College ____
Degrees ____ Major ____	Degrees ____ Major ____
Work Experience ____	Occupation ____
Sex & Age of other children, if any ____	Sex & Age of other children, if any ____

FIGURE 22-4. Registration card for expectant parent class.

Information should be obtained concerning culture, age, family consultation, occupation, education, trimester of pregnancy, and work experience. This also helps the nurse present material on an appropriate level and at an appropriate time. Figure 22-4 shows an example of a form for obtaining this information.

It is the author's experience that some topics never seem to be introduced by class members and yet, when introduced by the instructor, are of obvious interest and concern to the members. Examples include sexual relations, sexual appetites, and sexual problems arising from the pregnant state. The instructor can keep a list of these topics and plan for their introduction in some manner.

There are many excellent pamphlets and booklets published by the U. S. Department of Health, Education and Welfare, State Departments of Health, food and drug companies, and others. These are often free or cost very little. If they are used judiciously, they can be a valuable adjunct to the wealth of knowledge that the parents are assimilating. Some suggestions follow:

Prenatal Care. Superintendent of Documents, U. S. Government Printing Office, Washington, D. C. 20402
Infant Care. Source listed above
Your Baby's First Year. Source listed above
Breast Feeding Your Baby. Source listed above
How Does Your Baby Grow? Gerber Baby Foods, Fremont, Michigan
Preparation for Childbearing, ed. 3. Maternity Center Association, New York, N. Y.
How a Baby Grows. Johnson & Johnson, New Brunswick, N. J. 08903
The Womanly Art of Breast Feeding. La Leche League International, Franklin Park, Illinois
Modern Methods of Birth Control. Planned Parenthood—World Population, 810 7th Avenue, New York, N. Y. 10019
Becoming a Parent. Ross Laboratories, Columbus, Ohio 43216
Useful Facts for the Father-To-Be. Source listed above
Discovering Parenthood. Source listed above
Feelings of Conflict in New Parents. Source listed above
The Phenomena of Early Development. Source listed above

EVALUATION OF RESULTS

The instructor will want to evaluate the outcomes of her classes from time to time. Research indicates that education for parenthood is not of the value desired,[9] but there are also some optimistic views.[10] Booklets and leaflets given to some expectant or new parents without some accompanying discussion apparently are of little or no worth.[11–12] Empirically, nurses have long been aware of the difference in response that couples prepared for the experience of labor exhibit. Another more recent example is the behavior of new mothers in the attachment process when the Nurse's Modification of the Brazelton Assessment Tool is used with new mothers.

CRITIQUE OF SALIENT SITUATIONS

The author has found two methods that help her to assess her program and make adjustments and improvements. One needs the participation of a colleague who critiques the salient situations in a class.

> A salient situation is when the interaction process has a particularly significant effect upon a succeeding situation. Any time the leader or a participant speaks, the group's interaction is affected to some extent. On certain occasions, the nature of the person's behavior, rather than the content of what he says, has the more significant effect on the group's movement. Some situations will be considered salient purely because of the

nature of the interaction process; others, because of both the nature of the process and the character of the content.[13]

The form used to critique the class follows:

I. Critique of each salient situation observed
   1. What did the leader do in the situation? (interpret, lecture, explain, change subject, ignore lead, miss point, ask questions, refer back to group, praise, joke, other)
   2. What factors determine this type of intervention?
   3. In your opinion, was this appropriate behavior for the leader?
   4. Was the information accurate? Complete?

II. Description of each participant's behavior in each situation
   1. Was the salient relevent or irrelevant?
   2. Glancing about the table and listening to the comments of members, what was the reaction of other class members to the situation? (hostile, friendly, anxious, noncommital, poised and self-assured, not listening, "lost")

III. Of the entire class
   1. How near did it accomplish its objective to
   a. Communicate factual information?
   b. Stimulate the participants to plan and to think, so that they may enter into this new role with sound expectations?

EXPECTATION ⇄ OUTCOME

The second method used to evaluate the outcomes of a class deals with 1) expectations held by class members before the class, 2) their expectations following the class, and 3) what the actual experience was for the new parents. Since one of the objectives of the program is to minimize anxiety by exploring many aspects of childbearing and childrearing experiences, the above evaluation is mandatory.

Prior to the first class, individuals complete a form related to expectations. They repeat this process at the end of the series. Within a month of the birth of the infant, the instructor calls the mother and discusses specific aspects of the pregnancy, labor, and parenting experiences. The questions to be explored concerning expectations are:

1. What do you expect the last three to four weeks of your pregnancy will be like?
2. How do you expect labor to begin? What feelings do you expect to have?
3. What do you expect labor will be like for you? How will you respond to labor and what will be your feelings about those responses?
4. What do you expect your baby to look like, act like? What are the demands he will make on you and how will you feel about those demands?

A FAMILY STUDY

This is a brief description of one couple's expectations, the final outcome, and the evaluation of the efficacy of an expectant parent session.

Martha and Eugene are 28 and 30 years of age, respectively. Martha, a Caucasian, holds B.S. and M.A. degrees in library science. She has been both a librarian and a teacher. Eugene, a Japanese-American, has had two years of technical school training and is an engineering assistant. This will be their first child.

Pregnancy

When classes began Martha said, "I expect

to be waddling around staying home due to fatigue by the end of pregnancy. Perhaps having indigestion, too." Eugene said, "I expect her to be moody and demanding because of her condition."

They completed the classes two weeks prior to her estimated date of confinement. Martha was experiencing some shortness of breath, but she was still doing private tutoring and felt as energetic as she had throughout her pregnancy. Martha ascribed her changing attitude to the classes. She said, "I learned I didn't have to fulfill a sick role, even when I become this large. I also learned how to relieve the shortness of breath so I could get some sleep at night." Eugene described his wife as "bouncy and full of life as ever. Whatever discomfort she may have she bears well and without complaint." Both believed that the demonstration of body mechanics helped Martha very much. They both recognized that some of the discomforts of late pregnancy were still possible and they felt they would understand them if they should occur.

Labor

Martha shared with the class her fear of labor. "I'll be scared, really nervous when it starts. I'm afraid of a long laborious labor. I guess I could endure it if someone could reassure me that it would be short. I hope I don't end up screaming my head off. Controlling my emotions in front of people is pretty important for me." Eugene said, "I expect she'll cry a lot and cuss me out. The only way I can see myself helping would be as a moral support."

At the end of the class series Martha wrote: "My powers of concentration are limited, but with my husband's assistance in the labor room, I hope to be able to draw on the breathing techniques we learned. Since I know what is happening and will have my husband's support, I hope to be able to remain relaxed. I know I will feel ashamed if I let my pain get to me." Eugene wrote: "With her attitude toward her pregnancy so far, and the enthusiasm she shows toward learning what to do during labor to help, she will have a minimum of problems whether the labor is short or long. Easy or hard, I think she will give her best." Both ascribed the change in expectations to knowledge of the mechanics of labor and to the relaxation and controlled breathing techniques they had learned. They both displayed confidence. The classes, however, had not been successful concerning Martha's expectation of behavior in labor. She was still concerned about self-control.

Martha first described her labor as only being two hours long, but in recounting the event it was obvious it had been more than seven hours in length. She felt she had been able to follow through with the controlled breathing quite well. Her husband had been a great coach. He had also been very helpful in reducing the back discomfort through sacral support and back rubs. She felt proud of her performance and said both the doctor and her husband said she did "great." The classes were evaluated by Martha as having been the key to a "controlled" labor and birth.

The Newborn

Martha and Eugene both hoped the child would be a boy, although a healthy child of either sex would be welcomed. They were vague about what a neonate looked and acted like. Martha said, "It will be sweet, I can't wait" and Eugene said, "I haven't any idea."

At the end of the class Martha wrote, "I know now my child may likely be a bit misshapen. He will probably cry a lot and make a lot of demands on us. I hope we can figure out what he's trying to tell us. I'll do my best." Eugene wrote, "I expect we'll lose a lot of sleep. Life won't be the same, that's for sure. But at least we now know something about what he will need, how he will tell us and also more about how we may feel about him. We expect our love for him to grow." Both agreed that the classes had given them a realistic expectation of what a newborn was like. They now had some skills to care for him and were more confident. They understood that relationships with a baby develop slowly.

Martha did experience loss of sleep during the first month and felt continuously fatigued. The infant had "fussy" spells every night (midnight to 3 A.M.). Her breast feeding went very well. She did not tub bathe the infant for the first two weeks of life, but finally felt strong enough and confident enough to do so, with the support of her husband. Classes prepared Martha for a successful breast feeding experience. The bathing instructions were helpful, but lack of self-confidence (plus fatigue) prevented her from utilizing the tub bath for a period of time. Although the couple expected an unstructured home life with a new baby, they still were not fortified with how to manage a baby who slept during the day and cried at night.

Resume

Martha and Eugene avoided much anxiety through attending expectant parents classes. Body mechanics kept Martha feeling well throughout the entire pregnancy. Stress concerning the impending labor was reduced, leaving her with vital energy to attend to the activities of daily living. She was insulated against other outcomes of the pregnancy should they occur.

Labor was made more comfortable through knowledge of the process and self-help remedies. Her husband was a good support. Both surmounted the experience with dignity and pride. Martha was still vulnerable to any labor which might have caused her to cry out. ("I know I will be ashamed if I let my pains get to me.") Her Oriental husband may also have expected her to be stoical (this was not validated, however). Had conditions arisen in labor over which she had no control (posterior position, cervical dystocia, etc.), she was aware that her best effort had been demonstrated and it is believed she would have been ready to accept the outcome in a way that would not have been ego destructive.

She was aware of the possibility of delayed maternal emotions and could accept this in herself. She related, "You know that discussion in class about not loving your baby right away? My husband brought it up last night. We agreed you don't love them right away—it's grown on us—and it makes sense. We really didn't know him. It helped us not to expect too much at first."

Learning the technique of infant care did not mean that the parents would have sufficient confidence in themselves to perform. The delayed infant bath was a good example of this. There seems as yet no way to "insulate" parents through expectant parent education against all the fatigue and anxiety that the early weeks of parenthood bring. The classes are realistic in that they help the expectant parents to recognize the stress that they may expect and to make some plans for coping with it.

PREPARATION FOR LABOR

All over the world, since time immemorial, neurologists, physiologists, psychologists, psychiatrists, philosophers and poets have sought the answer to "What is pain?"[14] Over the last two decades a number of nonpharmacologic methods of reducing or abolishing the pain of childbirth have evolved. Special programs have developed to prepare expectant parents for the labor experience. Not only have many women benefited by experiencing pain relief, but the practices also brought other concomitant benefits. Support during labor took on new meaning when nurses, husbands, and specially-trained *monitrices* provided special comfort and coaching for the laboring woman. The labors of "prepared" women tend to be shorter. The neonate is delivered without the noxious assault of drugs given the mother during labor, and thus is in an improved physical condition to begin life outside the uterus. Perhaps most importantly, new parents derive a sense of accomplishment by *participating* in the birth of their child through prepared parenthood. The experience was ego-building and emotionally nourishing, especially for the new father. It helped to produce mutual sharing, interdependence, and gave greater meaning to the marriage.

The nomenclature of these methods have varied over time and from country to country. In each method the important factor is the psychologic one and for this reason they are known as *psychoprophylactic* techniques. Essentially, all psychoprophylactic techniques for painless childbirth are based on the Pavlovian concept of conditioned reflex training which enables a patient to block painful sensation by providing a center stimulus at the appropriate time.[15]

You will hear the term *natural childbirth* also used. This system was begun in England by Grantly Dick-Read. He believed that pain in childbirth was a psychologic response rather than a physiologic one, its presence being produced by fear, apprehension, and tension. Programs using this method concentrate on re-education, relaxation, and controlled breathing to produce a labor with a minimum of discomfort.

Inevitably, aspects of one method have been combined with those of other methods of pain relief by psychophysical methods. There are now multitudinous variations in techniques. Here is a partial list of programs you may find in use here and in Europe:

Psychophysical Childbirth Preparation
Psychoprophylaxis
L'accouchement sans Douleur
Hyponosis Training
Natural Childbirth
Read Method
Childbirth without Fear
Educated Childbirth
Prepared Childbirth
Autogene Training
Hypno-Suggestive Method
Lamaze Method
Childbirth without Pain
Education for Labor
Scientific Relaxation for Childbirth
L'accouchement Naturel
Bradley Method

As may be inferred from these designations, emphasis is variously placed on educational preparation, psychologic preparation, exercises, breathing, relaxation, and support in labor. There is also great diversity of opinion as to the appropriate pharmacologic assistance required. Some clinics are liberal in this respect and depend upon the laboring women to make choices, others are not.[16]

In spite of the dissimilarities, there are many similarities among the various methods. The remainder of this chapter provides a detailed discussion of the psychoprophylactic method for painless childbirth.

PREPARATION FOR CHILDBIRTH WITH THE PSYCHOPROPHYLACTIC METHOD FOR PAINLESS CHILDBIRTH*

Major, minor or even complete differences in prepared childbirth methods and techniques will be found from community to community. There is no "right" way. Different teachers may find their own methods. A major consideration should be to avoid rigidity (be flexible) since the student learns best *not* by rote, but by using her brain to figure out the best way to achieve the goal. However, under-

* This section written by Flora Hommel.

standing widely accepted techniques and particularly the principles on which they are based, nurses will be able to adapt the techniques and to support the couple effectively. Contradictions between what has been learned in classes and what actually occurs in the labor and delivery experience could be detrimental to the woman's childbirth experience.

Nurses who enter the field of maternity nursing, particularly those who become active in the preparation of parents for labor and/or who support them in labor, will want to familiarize themselves with the four classic works of Bonstein, Karmel, Lamaze and Vellay (see bibliography). Moreover, the concept of Pavlov's conditioned reflex theories will be of importance. Some of the early and ongoing childbirth education programs (Read, Thoms, Goodrich, Millere and Bradley) may also be of interest.

Early in the pregnancy, with the permission of the woman's physician, the prospective parents enroll in a course in which the following is taught in six (one and one-half hour) classes.

First. The principles on which the Method is based. The principles explain the probable causes of pain including poor psychological conditioning of the woman, physical or emotional tension, reduction of oxygen supply, and how these can be dealt with; also, comfort and health measures for pregnancy. Where possible, this class, in contrast to the remaining five classes, should be conducted in a large group of about 50 or more couples and should take place early in a woman's pregnancy.

Second. Relaxation, preferably called neuromuscular control or disassociation, necessary for conditioned reflex activity and to promote good circulation to the working uterus.

Third. The normal mechanism of the first stage of labor. Introduction to breathing patterns to be used during labor. This class offers facts to offset a lifetime of misinformation, ignorance and social and cultural conditioning which, if not corrected, becomes a deterrent to normal labor.

Fourth. Special breathing techniques used during the first stage of labor, another superimposed conditioned reflex activity which also provides the working uterus with necessary oxygen. Discussion of the sensations of the first stage is included.

Fifth. The normal mechanisms of the second or birth stage of labor—the exciting and satisfying stage. A short discussion about the newborn and the third stage of labor is included in this class.

Sixth. How to put together the information taught in the preceding five classes—a general review.

A special review class has been established for those who have already attended the above series for a previous birth.

In most communities, classes are held in the evenings so that the majority of husbands can participate. Many programs will include other classes dealing with related topics, such as the physiology of pregnancy, hygiene, infant care, and so on. But because there are excellent classes in many hospitals, Red Cross, La Leche, etc. we have eliminated these related aspects and have adopted the Psychoprophylactic (Lamaze) Method for Painless Childbirth, and will use it in this chapter.

Psychoprophylaxis means, "mind prevention of pain in childbirth." While the following concepts are not totally scientifically substantiated, empirical evidence of their success in the form of thousands of birth experiences, both abroad and in this country, supports them.

How Psychoprophylaxis Can Prevent or Modify Pain

Conditioned Reflexes

The main principle upon which psychoprophylaxis is based is that the majority, if not all, of pain in normal childbirth is created by conditioned reflexes. By conditioning, we have all experienced a sensation without the actual physical stimulus being present. In a similar way that a person may experience the feeling of being tickled from a person across the room saying, "I'm going to tickle you," and we can "taste" a lemon by watching another person suck on one, so might the woman feel pain from past conditioning. Consider the woman who has heard all of her life that childbirth is pain: She has heard it in tales she has been told, stories she has read, movies she has seen, even in religious concepts.

We must replace the conditioned "childbirth is pain" with "childbirth is a joyful experience; it is work with a relaxed body and a controlled breathing pattern." *Conditioning* is as important as the techniques used in the method. Both are necessary for an effective outcome.

Tension—Physical and Emotional

A second principle of psychoprophylaxis recognizes that both physical and emotional tension can divert the flow of blood from the actively contracting uterus to other parts of the body. As an example, swimming following the eating of a meal can divert the blood supply needed for digestion to the muscles used in swimming with resulting cramps or soreness (physical tension). Fear can divert the blood supply from the internal organs to the extremities, readying the body for "flight." Again, cramps or soreness can result (emotional tension).

You will learn that the woman entering labor without adequate preparation tends to be both physically and emotionally tense. While it is possible for many women to be taught physical relaxation at the time of labor, most women require training to be able to completely relax. To be most beneficial, the actual training to relax should be in advance of labor. To remove emotional tension, prior conditioning and clear understanding are necessary, though again, information, definitions, and on-the-spot reassurances are also helpful.

Nutrition for the Working Uterus

Assuming now that we have an adequate blood supply going to the uterus of a conditioned woman, it is necessary to see that the blood supply carries adequate nutrition for the working muscle. Therefore, a third principle of pain relief in psychoprophylaxis relates to the supply of glucose and oxygen. The woman who is reasonably healthy (not diabetic or with other problems affecting sugar metabolism) will have enough glucose to supply energy to the working uterus. Oxygen, however, necessary to metabolize the glucose as well as the lactic acid (product of metabolism, and not stored as is glucose) must be supplied in an ever-increasing quantity during labor. The nurse who has had the opportunity to observe the untrained woman in labor will note her tendency to hold her breath, even as the contractions become longer, stronger, and closer, when *more* oxygen is required, not less. It would appear that a simple solution of teaching the woman on-the-spot correct breathing and the use of oxygen by mask would suffice. But again, conditioning plays an important role and makes earlier learned breathing preferable. It might be well to note here that with the development of various methods for childbirth preparation this author cautions against experimenting with "new breathing techniques" without adequate clinical observation.

Position of the Fetus

The presentation and position of the fetus is an important aspect in the origin of pain during labor and delivery. It has been generally agreed that anterior vertex (head) presentations are "normal" and that posterior vertex position and breech presentations are "abnormal." We find a variance with this belief when applied to the woman experiencing labor using the psychoprophylactic method.

When the fetus is in a L.O.A. (left occiput anterior) or R.O.P. (right occiput posterior) labor will progress as expected. Moreover, L.S.A. (left sacral anterior) and R.S.P. (right sacral posterior) cause little difference in the progress of labor. Usually at the start of the second stage of labor, the woman's efforts at pushing will rotate the posterior position to an anterior one and the breech presentation, L.S.A. and R.S.P., in a prepared patient seldom present problems at delivery. However, we have noted with R.O.A. (right occiput anterior) and L.O.P. (left occiput posterior) and their breech counterparts R.S.A. (right sacral anterior) and L.S.P. (left sacral posterior) most, if not all, of the following can be observed.

1. Frequent and long bouts with false labor accompanied by nagging backache.
2. Spontaneous leaking of membranes prior to actual labor onset.
3. Labor contractions starting three to five minutes apart with indefinite start and finish, the woman feeling they last longer than can be actually observed.
4. Contractions lasting longer (50 to 60 seconds as opposed to 20 to 30 seconds) at the start of labor so that by the end of labor they feel like one continuous contraction.
5. Severe backache and low abdominal cramping which does not completely disappear between contractions.
6. Long labor.

We suspect that these unpleasant sensations and responses to labor are caused by pulls and pressures from internal structures such as the large intestines and from uterosacral and other ligaments. Preparation in the form of conditioning can do much to assist the woman through this more difficult labor. Positioning of the woman, during the labor, in a left Sims' position helps to remove some of the pressures and decreases the distress.

Posture during Pregnancy

Poor posture in pregnancy and poor muscular tone can create or add to backache during labor. Postural exercises and back exercises can do much to prevent or eliminate such problems.

Inhibition

Another tool of psychoprophylaxis is inhibition, distraction or blocking, for the relief of pain. Forces of inhibition can be either positive or negative for the woman in labor. If her entire concentration is on the sensations from the uterus, they may be perceived as pain. However, if her brain is actively concentrating on her activities and the processes, she may be able to remove the perception of painful stimuli.

Methods of Training and Practicing Psychoprophylactic Method

Practice is most effective when:

1. The expectant mother realizes her primary objective is conditioning the mind (psychoprophylaxis) and secondary objective is learning to use her body effectively.
2. She realizes why she is doing what she is doing and knows what to expect and which techniques to use throughout labor.
3. It is done two or three times daily and is of short duration, 10 to 15 minutes each period, 20 to 60 minutes per day.
4. She frequently receives monitoring (checking and directing) preferably from the expectant father.

5. Braxton-Hicks contractions are used for conditioning response.

6. The expectant mother's mind is alert for good inhibition and her body is not fatigued (*not* at the end of a long day).

7. Done in various positions and under various conditions or distractions, so that adaptation to various hospital conditions will be easier.

Neuromuscular Control and Relaxation

By analyzing the term "neuromuscular control," the nurse will "recognize that relaxation is the work of the brain conveying itself as a negative effect from a motor point of view. Muscular relaxation is thus an active phenomenon and not a passive one as far as the brain is concerned,"[17] as stated by Lamaze in *Painless Childbirth*. In order to respond with complete relaxation of all muscles, two things are necessary—proprioception and establishment of reflexes. To accomplish these, the expectant mother will practice tightening a small part of her body, trying to feel the muscles involved for proprioception, keeping all other parts as relaxed as possible, and then consciously release that part of the body. Repeating this will establish reflexes.

An example would be to first tighten the hand, while the wrist, shoulder, back are completely relaxed. She should repeat this two or three times and then go on to tightening a different part of the body (still relaxing all other parts), and then relax. In a few days, she will become familiar with nearly all of her voluntary muscles. It should be emphasized that this procedure (tightening and relaxing) is *not* done during labor or you may find the woman tightening and relaxing during the actual labor contractions. In the meantime, the expectant father should be taught to check for tenseness, realizing that relaxed muscles offer no resistance—the relaxed part is heavy and should resume its original position when released. After the expectant mother has practiced the exercise for several days and begins to feel confidence in her ability to release each muscle on command of her husband or herself, she will proceed to disassociation—isolating one part of the body from all others—so that during labor she can separate uterine activity from voluntary muscular activity.

In this exercise, the woman will tighten a large part of her body, such as her entire arm, while the rest of her body remains completely relaxed. She then proceeds to relax various muscles of that part of the body, in this case shoulder, upper arm, lower arm, wrist, hand. When disassociation has been mastered in that manner, still more mental control can be accomplished by the following exercise. The woman will tighten two specified parts of her body, such as right arm and left leg, and upon command will switch to two other parts, left arm and right leg. The monitor (husband) must make sure that only those parts specified are tense and check for immediate relaxation when commanded to be relaxed. Disassociation is then advanced so that a part of the body will be maintained in activity (substituting for a contraction in the woman's mind), while all other parts of the body are to be relaxed. A continuous rhythmic movement of one part of the body can be used for this purpose. For example, the woman will move her foot side to side, metronome fashion, while her monitor will check her hand for relaxation, perhaps moving it in a different fashion from her foot movement to see if she can maintain relaxation of the hand while not disturbing movement of the foot. This gives the woman some realization of how difficult it will become to relax the body completely while the uterus is contracting during labor.

Kegal Exercises

The nurse should familiarize herself with

exercise for control of the perineum (see Chapter 27). It is important for good muscle tone and control of gynecologic and urologic problems as well as for enhancement of sexual pleasure. I would strongly recommend the reading of *The Key to Feminine Response in Marriage* by Ronald M. Deutsch (see bibliography).

Particular emphasis in the practice of all of the above should be placed on the following:

1. Each time a muscle is contracted the woman should ask herself (or be asked):
   How does it feel?
   Where is it felt?
   Is any other muscle contracted?
   When relaxed, how does it feel? Different?
2. Are all parts of the body being considered?
   Muscles of the face, neck, upper abdominal muscles, back, hips, buttocks, and particularly perineal muscles.
3. Can the woman recognize the frequency of "chain reactions"?
   Do the muscles of her calves, thighs, buttocks, back, neck and shoulders become involved or tight?

Massage during Labor

Effleurage

This is a light, rhythmic stroking over the abdomen to be done with complete release of all but the hands, and in rhythm with the breathing during all first stage contractions. The main purpose is to provide another conditioned reflex activity and is therefore best accomplished by the woman herself. It is also found to have an extremely soothing effect on what might be interpreted as "crampy" feelings and may serve the purpose of another tool of inhibition. It can be done by the monitor or *monitrice*, to be discussed later in this chapter. The nurse should note that many women will perceive of effleurage as a narcissistic or even masturbatory activity, perhaps not on the conscious level, and may therefore reject this extremely helpful tool. The nurse's attitude may help overcome these feelings.

Effleurage is accomplished by placing the hands above the pubic area (lower abdomen) and with fingers spread apart, using all fingertips touching the abdomen, stroking upward and outward toward the hip crests, then toward the center of the abdomen and downward to the starting point. Some women may prefer to limit the area to just the lower abdomen. The lightest possible brush stroke is used. Tiny circular strokes in rhythm with breathing may be preferred, and greater pressure can be exerted.

Back Massage

If backache is present during labor, pressure can be applied in several ways, obviously it is preferable to have the monitor or monitrice exert pressure to avoid tensing on the part of the woman. A towel or ice-pack may be placed under the patient's back to provide pressure or she may lie on her own fists.

When the massage is provided by another, the woman lies on her side, a preferable position to relieve backache and to speed labor. While the monitor or monitrice places the heels of both hands on either side of the spine and exerts pressure. The woman can indicate how much pressure is comforting. If the woman is lying on her back, one hand is placed in the small of the back, finger tips on one side of the spinal column, heel of the hand on the other and gentle pressure is exerted during the contraction.

Pressure on the Lower Abdomen

If cramping is strong in the low abdomen,

the woman may prefer constant pressure in that area, perhaps gently lifting the abdomen upward.

Breathing

Once the woman has mastered neuromuscular control, she can go on to learn breathing techniques. Emphasis should be placed on the fact that neuromuscular control is the most difficult to accomplish during labor and breathing techniques become easier in labor, and are not as critical to a better experience. This can be impressed upon the woman by requiring that she add breathing techniques to the relaxation. Besides the two or three short practice sessions already established, breathing techniques can be practiced at other times throughout the day, perhaps while watching television or while doing chores. Each breathing technique should be practiced starting at 20 to 30 seconds duration, increasing by 5 seconds each day until 60 seconds is reached, or until dizziness is felt, whichever is sooner. The dizziness is caused by extra oxygen not needed in practice. It will not occur during labor as the oxygen will be required at that time.

As each breathing technique is mastered (along with complete relaxation) effleurage should be added.

Headstart and Ending Breaths

Each time a breathing technique is used, in practice or in labor, it is *begun* and *ended* with a very deep breath in through the nose, to get a headstart on or put an end to a contraction.

Slow Deep Chest Breathing

This is used during contractions of early, mild labor. A headstart breath is taken, then throughout the contraction, a breath is taken in through the nose slowly and deliberately, slightly deeper than normal breathing, and let out through the mouth. Even rhythm at approximately 10 to 15 breaths per minute should be maintained. Ribs should expand sideways when inhaling. Shoulders, arms, abdomen should remain relaxed. At the end of a contraction, an ending breath is taken.

Candleblowing

This may be substituted for slow deep chest breathing for early, mild labor. In this type of slow breathing, after taking headstart breath, inhale through the nose, only the amount of air that would be inhaled in a normal breath, then exhale through the mouth with pursed lips and with sufficient force to bend (but not blow out) the flame of a candle if it were 12 to 18 inches away, blowing out *more* than normal exhalation and taking approximately four times as long as the inhalation. Then take an ending breath.

The rate will be between 10 to 15 breaths per minute. The abdomen and rest of body should be completely relaxed throughout. The woman will not be inhaling deeply, but she will be getting more oxygen because she replaces more of the "stale" air in her lungs than with a normal breath.

Panting

This is rapid, shallow, or light chest breathing. It should be used when slow, deep or candleblowing is no longer sufficient to maintain comfort, usually when the cervix is 3 to 4 centimeters dilated. A headstart breath is taken starting with between 40 to 60 breaths per minute, or one breath per second, and increasing the speed as labor progresses so that by 6 or 7 centimeters dilated the expectant mother would be panting about 120 breaths per minute. Each contraction ends with an ending breath. Either nose or mouth breathing can be used, however during labor most women find mouth breathing easier.

To reduce dryness, the woman should put her tongue on the roof of her mouth behind her upper teeth. Sips of water or ice chips should be offered between contractions. Hard candy, suckers, chewing gum (removed during contractions) may help moisten mouth. Abdomen and shoulders should remain relaxed (motionless); tightening of back and chest muscles may cause them to move. Inhalation and exhalation should be equal in quantity or a buildup or emptying may occur, making breathing irregular and difficult.

Accelerated-Decelerated Breathing

Occasionally the panting breathing may be altered as labor progresses so that with each contraction it begins slowly, picking up speed as contraction reaches peak and slowing down as contraction subsides. Should this technique be used, it is most important to control the rate and depth of breathing at the peak, for there is a strong tendency to breathe either so fast that no oxygen gets to the lungs to be exchanged, or so heavily that too much energy is exerted on the breathing and hyperventilation may occur.

Modified Panting or Panting with Blowing

Transition breathing

This breathing is used during transition when contractions are very intense and/or to counteract the reflex desire to push before the cervix is completely dilated. Beginning with a headstart breath, panting is done as described above. When the urge to push is felt, the woman will blow out firmly, rather forcefully. At first, the pushing reflex is infrequent, however as the reflex becomes more constant during the contraction, it is desirable to set up a pattern of panting and blowing, such as seven panting breaths to each blowing breath, or five panting breaths to each blowing breath. Women should be instructed, however, to maintain at least four panting breaths between each blowing breath to avoid hyperventilation.

Hyperventilation

Panting should be quiet to reduce dryness and to keep from heavy breathing which could cause hyperventilation. Usually the only symptoms, in a controlled and monitored parturient, would be tingling of fingers and hands, and perhaps around the mouth. In more severe cases, stiffness in fingers, hands, and feet might occur. These symptoms could also indicate a lack of circulation to the extremities during uterine activity. This can be checked by having the woman, between contractions, flex her hands to draw circulation to them. Hyperventilation occurs *less* frequently in the trained parturient than in the nontrained parturient. Should it occur, the nurse should first correct the woman's breathing, and second, recognizing that its cause is the exhalation of too much carbon dioxide, have the woman stop breathing for 10 to 20 seconds between contractions or breathe in a paper bag until the symptoms disappear. The administration of oxygen is also helpful.

Techniques for Second Stage Expulsion

Expectant mothers are taught positions, patterns, and release of the pelvic floor. They need not exert force during practice as this will be easily accomplished during the actual labor.

Primipara

In most hospitals a large part of the second

stage is accomplished in the labor room with only approximately 15 minutes in the delivery room. The woman may be propped slightly with a pillow under her head and shoulders which can be raised by her monitor or monitrice during the pushing.

One or two headstart breaths (two if there is time) are taken, then a deep inhalation which should be held to maintain pressure from the diaphragm for about 20 seconds. As this breath is being held, the woman raises her head and shoulders and starts to tighten the upper abdominal muscles. Then she brings her knees up and back toward her shoulders, taking hold of something with her hands and pulling to tighten the abdominal muscles, at the same time releasing buttocks, perineum, legs and feet. The most efficient, and when given a fair chance, most comfortable position for women in the labor room (where the primipara does most of her pushing) is with the arms on the outside of the legs, elbows out, hands on the inside of the ankles, thumbs down. Or she may hold her knees or thighs, making sure her elbows are out.

The eyes should be open, mouth and throat closed, back and shoulders rounded. When the woman can no longer hold her breath (about 20 seconds), she puts her head back enough to blow out the air, inhales again, holds her breath again, all the while continuing to push. At the end of a contraction an ending breath or two is taken, with complete relaxation. When transferred to the delivery room, the same procedure is followed.

Multipara

It is well to have the multipara practice just as the primipara, in case she is requested to push in the labor room or before stirrups are adjusted in the delivery room, or if she is allowed to give birth without the stirrups. Most multiparas who are practicing psychoprophylaxis should be transferred to the delivery room as soon as the reflex to push is definitely established (prior to second stage). Legs or feet are usually placed in stirrups in a comfortable position, and the nurse should see that handles are set toward the foot of the delivery table with the woman's hands on or near them. If wrist straps are used, they should be very loose and used as a reminder rather than a restraint.

Birth

More doctors are cooperating with women who do not wish to have routine episiotomies, but even if an episiotomy is performed, it should be as minimal as possible so that the baby's head is not being born too rapidly or with too much force. Therefore, most doctors advise their patients to stop pushing with the last one or two contractions for greater control. The most effective means of limiting the push at this period is by rapid panting.

Second stage of labor can be considerably shortened and damage to perineal muscles prevented by proper pushing technique. The perineal muscles must remain relaxed, while the force to propel the infant through the birth canal come from the uterine and abdominal muscles.

Bearing down (pushing) prior to the complete dilitation of the cervix, and improper pushing technique during the second stage of labor can be damaging to the perineal muscles. In later life this damage can result in the development of a cystocele or a rectocele. With proper pushing technique there is less danger of lacerations of the perineal tissues even without the "routine" episiotomy. The damages can also be prevented, as noted before, by teaching women how to do Kegel exercises.

Understanding Is Key

According to the couples who have been through classes, one of the most valuable aspects of preparation for childbirth is a total understanding of the birth process, which I believe adds to conditioning. A nurse working with any parturient will of course want to make sure that she understands the processes of labor, including the contractions and their functions, dilitation of the cervix, descent of the presenting part, rotating, etc. I would refer the reader to the chapter on labor and delivery in Dr. Vellay's *Childbirth Without Pain*. Teaching, of course, should be accomplished at the level of understanding of the individual. At present it would appear that the majority of people attending preparation for childbirth classes have had more formal education and have done reading outside of suggested class reading; however, this is rapidly changing in many communities and it may be difficult for the teacher to adapt to the diversity in her classes. In the actual labor experience a good monitrice or hospital staff nurse should remember that the couple, no matter what their social, cultural, or economic background, is capable of absorbing a great deal of information providing she can establish a good rapport and a meaningful communication system with them.

Experiences with many women in labor have taught me some facts that do not usually appear in print. If they do, they bear repeating.

1. Labor seldom starts with rupture of membranes (if it does, the nurse might be watching for poor position of the baby) or a bloody show or mucus plug discharge.
2. Contractions will not always start far apart (25 to 30 minutes or so) and/or be clock regular. As a matter of fact, many labors will progress perfectly normally without contractions ever becoming completely regular or even in a pattern of regularity. More reliable information to determine true as opposed to false labor would be that contractions almost always will become longer, stronger, and closer together.
3. Frequently when a woman is told the contractions will become stronger, she interprets that it will be painful. She must be reminded that as with other muscles, such as the biceps, the uterine muscle can work very hard without causing pain.
4. When a woman lies on her side during labor, the interval between contractions might be slightly greater, but contractions may be more effective.

REFERENCES

1. Clark, A. L.: *Leadership Technique in Expectant Parent Education*, Springer, New York, 1973.
2. Beebe, J. E., Pendleton, E. M. and King, E.: *Bench conferences in a large obstetric clinic*. Am. J. Nurs. 68:85, 1968.
3. Auerbach, A.: *Parents Learn through Discussion*. Wiley, New York, 1968, p. 161.
4. Ibid.
5. Ibid.
6. Ibid.
7. Ibid.
8. Clark: op. cit., p. 1.
9. Brim, O. G.: *Education for Childrearing*. Russell Sage Foundation, New York, 1959.
10. Hereford, C. F.: *Changing Parental Attitudes through Group Discussion*. University of Texas, Austin, Texas, 1963.
11. Downs, F. S. and Fernbach, V.: *Experimental evaluation of a prenatal leaflet series*. Nurs. Res. 22:498, 1973.
12. Brooks, M. S., et al.: *Reaction of mothers to literature on childrearing*. Am. J. Public Health 54:803, 1964.
13. *Educational and Research Pilot, Project Parent Education*. Nursing Staff Education, Visiting Nurse Service of New York.
14. Buxton, C. L.: *A Study of Psychophysical Methods for Relief of Childbirth Pain*. W. B. Saunders, Philadelphia, 1962, p. 17.
15. Ibid.: p. 15.
16. Ibid.: p. 16.
17. Lamaze, F.: *Painless Childbirth*. Pocket Books, New York, 1972.

BIBLIOGRAPHY

Adams, M.: *Early concerns of primagravida mothers regarding infant care activities*. Nurs. Res. 12:72, 1963.

Anthony, E. J. and Benedek, T.: *Parenthood, Its Psychology and Psychopathology*. Little, Brown & Co., Boston, 1970.

Applebaum, R.: *The modern management of successful breast feeding*. Child and Family 9:61, 1970.

Benedek, T.: *Parenthood as a developmental phase*. J. Am. Psychoanal. Assoc. 7:389, 1959.

Benson, L.: *Fatherhood—A Sociological Perspective*. Random House, New York, 1968.

Bonstein, I.: *Psychoprophylactic Preparation for Painless Childbirth*. William Heinemann Medical Books, London, 1969.

Bowlby, J.: *Separation anxiety: a critical review of the literature*. J. Child Devel. Psych. 1:251, 1960.

Ibid.: *Separation anxiety*. Int. J. Psychoanal. 41:89, 1960.

Ibid.: *Grief and mourning in infancy: Early childhood*. Psychoanal. Study Child. 15:9, 1960.

Brody, S.: *Patterns of Mothering*. International Universities Press, New York, 1956.

Buxton, C. L.: *A Study of Psychophysical Methods for Relief of Childbirth Pain*. W. B. Saunders, Philadelphia, 1962.

Cameron, J.: *A design for a new maternity system*. In Duffy, M. et al. (eds.): *Current Concepts in Clinical Nursing, vol. III*. C. V. Mosby, St. Louis, 1971.

Chabon, I.: *Awake and Aware: Participating in Childbirth through Psychoprophylaxis*. Delacorte Press, New York, 1966.

Clark, A. L.: *The beginning family*. Am. J. Nurs. 66:802, 1966.

Countryman, B. A.: *Hospitalized care of the breast-fed newborn*. Am. J. Nurs. 71:2365, 1971.

Crow, R. M.: *Why my babies are bottle fed*. Am. J. Nurs. 71:2367, 1971.

Deutsch, R. M.: *The Key to Feminine Response in Marriage*. Random House, New York, 1968.

Disbrow, M.: *Any woman who really wants to nurse her baby can do so???* Nurs. Forum, 2:39, 1963.

Engel, G. L.: *Grief and grieving*. Am. J. Nurs. 64:93, 1964.

Falicov, C. J.: *Sexual adjustment during first pregnancy and post partum*. Am. J. Obstet. Gynecol. 117:991, 1973.

Gordon, R. E., Kapostins, E. E. and Gordon, K. K.: *Factors in postpartum emotional adjustment*. Obstet. Gynecol. 25:158, 1965.

Grossman, E.: *Helping mothers to nurse their babies*. Child and Family 5:3, 1966.

Hogenboon, P.: *Man in crisis: The father*. J. Psychiatr. Nurs. 5:457, 1967.

Hommel, F.: *Twelve years experience in psychoprophylactic preparation for childbirth*. Psychosom. Med. Gynaecol. S. Karger, London, 1972.

Ibid.: *Nurses in private practice as monitrices*. Am. J. Nurs. 69:1446, 1969.

Horney, K.: *Feminine Psychology*. W. W. Norton, New York, 1967.

Howells, J. G. (ed.): *Modern Perspectives in Psycho-Obstetrics*. Brunner/Mazel, New York, 1972.

Jacobson, G. F., Strickler, M. and Morley, W. E.: *Generic and individual approaches to crisis intervention*. Am. J. Public Health 58:338, 1968.

Karmel, M.: *Thank You, Dr. Lamaze*. Doubleday, New York, 1965.

Klaus, M. H.: *Human maternal behavior at the first contact with her young*. Pediatr. 46:187, 1970.

Klaus, M. and Kennell, J.: *Mothers separated from their newborn infants*. Pediatr. Clin. North Am. 17:1015, 1970.

Klaus, M., et al.: *Maternal attachment: importance of the first post-partum days*. N. Engl. J. Med. 286:460, 1972.

Kon, J. K. and Cowie, A. T.: *Milk: the Mammary Gland and Its Secretion, vol. 1*. Academic Press, New York, 1961.

Lamaze, F.: *Painless Childbirth*. Pocket Books, New York, 1972.

LeMasters, E. E.: *Parenthood as crisis*. in Parad, H., (ed.): *Crisis Intervention*. Family Service Association of America, New York, 1965.

Liebenberg, B.: *Expectant fathers*. Child and Family 8:265, 1969.

Lidz, T.: *The Person*. Basic Books, New York, 1968.

Menninger, K.: *The Vital Balance*. Viking Press, New York, 1963.

Meerloo, J. A. M.: *The psychological role of the father*. Child and Family 7:102, 1968.

Montagu, A.: *Touching: The Human Significance of the Skin*. Columbia University Press, New York, 1971.

McBride, A. B.: *The Growth and Development of Mothers*. Harper & Row, New York, 1973.

Newton, N.: *Nipple pain and nipple damage*. J. Pediatr. 41:411, 1952.

Newton, N. and Newton, M.: *Psychologic aspects of lactation*. New Engl. J. Med. 277:1179, 1967.

Porter, C.: *Maladaptive Mothering Patterns: Nursing Intervention*. In *A. N. A. Clinical Sessions, 1972*. Appleton-Century-Crofts, New York, 1972.

Richardson, S. A. and Guttmacher, A. F. (eds.): *Childbearing Its Social and Psychological Aspects*. Williams & Wilkins, Baltimore, 1967.

Rugh, R. and Lamdrum, S.: *From Conception to Birth*. Harper & Row, New York, 1971.

Schaefer, G.: *The Expectant Father, His Care and Management*. Postgrad. Med 38:658, 1965.

Shainess, N.: *Motherhood: a tempering experience*. Child and Family, 4:3, 1965.

Spaulding, M. R.: *Adapting postpartum teaching to mother's low income style*. In Bergersen, B., et al. (eds.): *Current Concepts in Clinical Nursing, vol. II*. C. V. Mosby, St. Louis, 1969.

Vellay, P.: *Childbirth without Pain*. Dutton, New York, 1971.

Williams, B.: *Sleep needs during the maternity cycle*. Nurs. Outlook 15:53, 1967.

The Womanly Art of Breast Feeding. La Leche League, Franklin Park, Illinois.

UNIT 6

THE INTRAPARTAL PERIOD

23 Application of Psychosocial Concepts

DYANNE D. AFFONSO, R.N., M.N.

Including *Monitricing* by Flora Hommel, R.N., B.S.

The role of nursing during the experience of labor and birth is enhanced through an understanding and appreciation of what the experience means to the individuals involved. To achieve this, the nurse must be able to apply knowledge of the psychosocial impact the experience has on the childbearing family.

IDENTITY AND SELF

Some childbearing families emerge from the intrapartal experience with a sense of awe, ecstasy, and elation. They express "exhilaration about birth" and refer to it as a "miracle producing life." From these families we may hear comments such as:

> It was the most beautiful day of my life. I couldn't believe I could give life—I brought the baby into the world.
>
> That blackish object became bigger and suddenly there was a head, and then a face with eyes, nose, mouth. Before I could put the pieces all together, the entire body was there. Imagine, right before your eyes! I just laid there feeling like a million, you know—feeling good about yourself.
>
> I suppose it was the happiest moment of my life. Just to be there with ____ and see the baby at the very moment it was heralding into the world. I was so proud!

For such families, labor and birth is an experience which enhances the self. What are the ingredients necessary for such positive dimensions on the self? Some contributing factors are categorized below:

I. Childbirth is viewed as a *meaningful event*.
   A. The role of culture or society emphasizes childbirth as a significant life activity, providing positive input in terms of expectations and roles.
      Example: Children may be valued and producing them brings status and prestige. Women may receive special benefits of exemption from responsibilities and husbands may receive increased attention for asserting their masculine physiologic functions. Childbirth is viewed as a normal function for women and there is less emphasis on discomforts or dangers inherent in it.
   B. Attitudes of the individuals reflect a belief that self-fulfillment can occur through childbirth.
      Example: Labor is viewed as a time of creativity and production of new life. There is no conflict with one's feelings about being feminine or masculine. Men and women feel

good about their roles (including their sexual relationship) and are willing to accept the responsibilities of parenthood. Negative feelings by either husband or wife regarding the impact of childbearing on the body image are minimal. For example, a woman does not become preoccupied with the gravid uterus distorting her contour and the husband does not grieve the loss of his "shapely wife." In essence, pregnancy and labor do not not threaten the couple's good feelings about their concepts of self or their relationship with each other.

II. *Expectations* and *goals* about childbirth are *realistic* and *attainable*.

A. There is a realistic perception of the event.

Example: The woman, husband, and family members have an understanding of the labor process. Preparation for childbirth is usually valued and educational classes are attended. Husband and wife both share an enthusiasm about new knowledge gained and take pride in performing the preparatory exercises in anticipation for the real event. The woman, husband, and family reinforce feelings that the event may include discomforts but are prepared to deal with them when they occur.

B. Personal goals are realistic and not in conflict with the events occurring or the goals of others.

Example: Scott and Sheri J. prepared for labor through the Lamaze method. They both expressed a desire to achieve relaxation and pain relief through the exercises and breathing learned. They had strong desires that Scott support his wife and be present throughout the labor and delivery. They practiced diligently prior to labor and felt ready for the real event. The medical and nursing management reinforced a mutual respect for the couple's desires. Thus, the labor was experienced with minimal need for analgesia and the couple's goals were attained.

C. The woman's ideal expectations become her actual performance during labor and delivery.[1]

Example: Mary L. practiced her Lamaze exercises diligently weeks before labor. She also kept telling herself that medications would be all right to use should she find herself unable to maintain control. During labor she obtained relief through her breathing exercises. However at 6 cm. dilatation she asked for medication, which she promptly received, and was able to continue controlled breathing through the rest of the process.

III. There is *positive feedback* to all participating in the process.

A. Recognition and positive feedback.

Women should receive positive feedback for their efforts to cope with labor. They need to know that their energies are not wasted and their attempts to help themselves are recognized. They need to feel that the health professionals realize that they are in a "challenging situation."

B. Support to families and friends.

Husbands, friends, and others in attendance with the woman should also receive positive reinforcement for their participation in the process. They need to feel that their attempts to help are significant and valuable.

C. Communication among health professionals.

Feedback should also be given

among the health professionals. Everyone should be made to feel that their involvement contributes to the progress and healthy outcome of the labor experience. Unfortunately, sharing among health professionals usually focuses on negative aspects. For example, everyone hears about the mishandling of a situation but rarely about a situation that is managed very well.

Unfortunately, not all labor experiences are regarded as pleasant. It is not unusual to hear negative comments such as:

> I never want to go through *that* again! I'm happy with one child and don't intend to take *that* risk again. I never was so frightened as in labor. I thought I wasn't going to make it.
>
> I never ever had such feelings in my entire life. I almost thought I was going to die. They kept telling me to push when I was already pushing as hard as I could. I just wanted to give up!
>
> After seeing my wife suffer I don't think we'll plan to have any more children. I really wonder if having a child is worth all that trouble.

As a counterpart, let us explore the same categorization of factors, but this time as they create a *negative* impact on the self.

I. The meaning of the event.
  A. Childbirth viewed as a stressful period.
     Example: Sometimes childbirth is viewed as a period of stress or an undesirable activity due to dangers to the individual and society. This can relate to cultural mores, input from mass media, and attitudes of the individual. For example, a culture may emphasize the presence of dangers to the mother and baby from forces more powerful than the self. Therefore, supernatural forces are sought to ward off evil spirits. A culture may also view childbirth as a mysterious event. Mystery breeds fears because the individual must resort to his own fantasies. Mass media may also contribute to stress by emphasizing population control for ecologic considerations. Individuals who engage in childbearing may receive negative feedback.
  B. Society reinforces the negative aspects concerning childbirth.
     Example: In the United States, more attention is given to stories emphasizing the "horrors of labor." When women discuss their experiences, those who had long, difficult labors usually receive more attention than those who had short, uncomplicated labors. In these story sessions, details of the experiences are frequently distorted.
  C. Negative attitudes toward the feminine role in the reproductive process.
     If motherhood is not a desired role, labor can be very threatening. Sensations to the perineum, the stress of contractions, fatigue, nausea, and vomiting, can make the woman feel a threatened loss of physical attributes she values about her body. If she values her physical appearance, she may be upset that during labor she cannot tend to her usual routines to ensure a "pretty face," such as use of makeup and combing her hair.

II. Expectations, ideals, goals versus reality.
  A. A desired goal is not realized.
     Example: Some women and their husbands desire labors which allow them to be actively involved in the process. They hope to achieve a

sense of mastery over the reproductive experience. In contrast, other couples may desire labors in which they are dependent upon others. Their participation is minimal and they see themselves as observers and recipients of care. If the expectation for the desired role is not realized, feelings of disappointment and defeat may arise and lower self-esteem.

B. Desired goals or expectations are in conflict with those defined by others and the health professionals.

Examples: 1) A woman may desire to turn on her side or sit up but is restricted to the supine position. 2) A husband may desire to witness the delivery but is permitted only in the labor room. 3) A woman may request the presence of a friend or relative but only her husband is permitted.

C. Goals and expectations are unrealistic.

Example: Mary M. prepared for labor through the Lamaze method and her goals focused on a labor with minimal analgesia. Everything appeared congruent with her goals until her amniotic membranes ruptured and the fetal cord prolapsed. A cesarean section was indicated. Mary insisted that she could deliver vaginally and became aggressive and hostile as she was being prepared for surgery. Her anxiety increased and she became uncontrollable. Medications were given to sedate her. The conflict arose when she rigidly adhered to her goals and failed to incorporate other alternatives should complications arise.

III. Detrimental feedback patterns given to the laboring family.

A. Negative feedback.

Example: Tom and Amy C. are expecting their first child. Although they haven't attended formal classes, they gained knowledge about labor through reading. They are excited and confident about being able to handle the labor situation. Amy approaches 4 cm. dilatation and becomes restless and irritable. She moans softly and requests medication for pain relief. The nurse tells her that the doctor is busy and she'll have to wait until he returns. The nurse also states, "It is too early for medications anyway." Half an hour later, Amy cries out during the peak of a contraction. The nurse quickly enters the room and scolds her for making noise and disturbing others. She also tells Amy she should try harder to "control herself." Amy apologizes for her behavior and clings to her husband. Time passes and Amy continues to have difficulty coping with the contractions and expresses fear of losing control. Tom finally goes out to ask the nurse for something to help his wife. He is told that the doctor is detained and no medications can be given without his order. When the doctor arrives, Tom and Amy are both panic-stricken due to fears that no assistance would be given to help them continue the labor process. They were made to feel that their behaviors were inappropriate. Their calls for help were ignored and they were made to feel that they should "do better" in coping with the situation. This generated feelings of guilt, anxiety, and anger. Thus, their attempts to help themselves become less effective.

B. Inadequate or incomplete feedback.

Example: Kimo and Malia K. are

expecting their third baby and feel confident due to positive experiences with the last two labors. During the active phase of labor, the doctor decides to use a monitoring device. Since this is the couple's first experience with such a device, they both have numerous questions about it. However, the doctor has other priorities and appears perturbed by their questions. He manifests his feelings in his nonverbal behaviors and his only comment is, "Later, I'll explain later." He leaves and the nurse enters. Kimo and Malia ask, "Is something wrong?" The nurse responds, "Didn't the doctor tell you?" as she checks the equipment. They ask again if anything is wrong. The nurse hesitates and then responds, "No, not really. We have many of our patients on monitors these days." She then leaves. When the doctor and nurse return, Malia cries, "Take it out. I don't want this in me." Meanwhile, the monitor has become disassembled because of her increased restless activity.

This example illustrates the effect of inadequate feedback as well as conflicting messages given by verbal and nonverbal behaviors of the staff. The doctor and nurse failed to realize the impact of their nonverbal behaviors. As verbal interactions with the staff decreased, the couple became increasingly more sensitive to nonverbal cues for feedback. The lack of interaction caused them to imagine that there were dangers in their situation. They had no means to explore reality and to validate their perceptions with someone. Therefore, the situation became highly threatening.

This by no means completes the influencing factors which contribute to how the labor experience can strengthen or weaken the self concept. What is important for health professionals is an appreciation that labor and birth are not merely a series of processes by which the uterus expels its contents. The experience creates an impact on the individuals. This impact deserves attention because it can enhance or impede future growth and development of the family.

ROLE THEORY

During labor there are certain variables which have implications for the concept of role as presented in Chapter 4. First, it is important to examine role expectations versus role performances. Role expectations may be defined by culture, the event, and the individual's perception of desired behaviors. For example, culture may dictate that labor is an event to be experienced with the least manipulation or interference from others. Thus, women are expected to assume an independent role in meeting their own needs during labor. In contrast, some women prefer to be dependent and exhibit this dependency by frequent demands and inability to make even minor decisions. Role expectations may be defined by the setting. In the United States this is usually a hospital, an environment associated with illness. Therefore, it is not uncommon to see the sick role as an expectation from the staff for women in labor. The very routines that hospitals impose, such as bedrest, exemption from responsibilities, and various other restrictions, reinforce this role. If role expectations coincide with the expectations of the woman and her family, there is harmony. However, more often than not, role strain or conflict occurs due to discrepancies between role expectations and role performances. Let us examine situations in the labor experience which can affect role expectations and performances. The principles are adapted from Lum's discussion of role theory in Chapter 4.

Principle: The individual attempts to behave and tries to get others to behave toward him in ways consistent with his self concept.

A woman may expect to assume an active role during labor with learned measures to relax and achieve comfort. She expects to be involved in decisions affecting use of analgesia or anesthesia. She also expects the doctors and nurses to respect her need to remain as independent as possible. Role strain occurs when her own behaviors do not live up to her expectations to exhibit control of the situation and when the environment does not reinforce her attempts to be independent. Role strain may also occur when the husband, family, or staff are unable to manifest behaviors congruent with their perceptions of their roles (as good husband, mother, doctor, or nurse).

Principle: Role strain can arise if the role does not allow use of skills and abilities, is not suited to one's personality, or does not meet one's needs.

During labor, men and women may not be able to utilize learned skills or coping. The husband may find himself displaced by staff members, use of mechanical devices, or effects of analgesia. He may be asked to leave the room during routines. These disruptions may interfere with his role expectation and performance to support his wife. This creates frustration and feelings of unfulfillment regarding his role. The woman may also be affected by these disruptions. While she is trying to assume a comfortable position, or concentrate on breathing during a contraction, someone may decide to ask a question or perform a procedure. Unfortunately, during labor there is little coordination among the priorities defined by the woman, the husband, and the health professionals. The result can be role strain for all.

Principle: Role expectations need to be clearly defined to avoid different interpretations or uncertainty of what is expected.

Typically, during labor men and women are uncertain of what behaviors are permitted or prohibited in the setting. This frequently is due to different attitudes and expectations from members of the health team. For example: Clara, a 20 year old primipara, is in latent labor. She makes comments that she doesn't handle pain well and is a dependent person when it comes to meeting her own needs. She rings her call bell frequently and makes numerous requests of wanting things done. The day-shift nurse recognizes Clara's behaviors as indicative of dependency and increased anxiety. She meets Clara's needs by responding to her requests and making attempts to be present with her as much as possible. When the evening-shift nurse arrives, Clara finds that all her previously accepted behaviors are now provoking anger and aggression from the nurse. She is reprimanded for childish behaviors and "not acting her age." She is also threatened verbally that her labor will be long if such behaviors continue.

Another factor for consideration is the emergence of new roles. For the couple experiencing their first labor, new roles of parenthood must be established. Behaviors indicative of mothering or fathering may not be clearly evident. They may not have had life experiences, such as exposure to newborns, to help prepare them for the new role. Therefore, before and after delivery, there may be increased anxiety about what is expected to nurture the newborn.

Principle: Role behavior is learned behavior. Reference groups provide the standard or model for the new behaviors to be learned. They also provide feedback regarding the progress in the learning of a new role.

With the impact of a mobile society, men and women may find themselves with limited role models from which to learn behaviors related to labor and parenthood. Women may not have mothers, aunts, or grandmothers readily available to teach the role expectations. With couples moving farther from their extended families, reference groups may consist of total strangers. If so, time will be needed to establish a trusting relationship with these individuals before learning can occur. Circumstances may not always permit this and a couple may be faced with the reality of being parents before adequate preparation for the new responsibilities has occurred. Consideration of current trends to control population growth as they affect parental role readiness may also be significant. It is hypothesized that couples will have fewer available role models (aside from their parents) as zero population growth programs become more attractive. Finally, feedback is essential in the learning process. Praise and criticism provide incentives as well as guidelines in the progress of learning. During labor and early parenthood, there is the danger of receiving minimal, negative, or no feedback regarding one's role performance. This will decrease motivation for learning which in turn will lower the self-esteem and affect role performance.

ANXIETY

Observations and clinical studies investigating attitudes and reactions during labor reveal that anxiety is not uncommon during this time.[2-5] Women express vague feelings of apprehension as well as specific fears and concerns for themselves and the baby during labor.[6,7]

Anxiety is not always a detrimental force. At mild and moderate levels, it is an effective stimulant to action. It makes the individual more alert, responsive to the environment, and serves as a signal for the body to mobilize its resources against perceived dangers and threats. At mild levels, anxiety enhances learning because the person can hear, see, attend, and retain with greater efficiency. However, when anxiety is increased to severe and panic levels, it immobilizes problem-solving attempts. During labor, anxiety can increase rapidly as stressors multiply with time and progress of labor. Therefore, assessment of the level of anxiety is essential to guide actions which will prevent it from going out of control and impeding labor progress.

SOURCES

The hospital environment may be a source of anxiety during labor. A woman is forced to leave her home, family, and friends. In effect, she leaves an environment where she can predict communication patterns, is conditioned to expect certain norms of behavior, and has a sense of security because there is no mystery concerning expectations from her. The hospital environment presents a different experience. Its physical structure alone communicates an awesomeness which minimizes the significance of the individual. Its organization is complex and often overwhelming, as validated by admission procedures and lengthy directions to locate its various services. Other factors which may cause stress are: new faces; strange professional language; unfamiliar sounds and smells; hospital routines such as the perineal preparation, enema, and intravenous therapy; and equipment such as monitors, glaring lights, and needles.

Anxiety and fear during labor arise not only from physical stressors, but also from unmet expectations, desires, or images. For example:

1. The onset of labor may occur before or after the expected date of confinement. Mothers often state that they weren't prepared to go into labor or were frustrated and discour-

aged because they were weeks past due. Fathers and siblings are also affected by an early or late EDC. Their activities and commitments may be altered. Children may become tired of waiting for the new arrival because the gestational period may seem like years according to their perception of time. Another stressor is that preparation for the baby may be incomplete. The family may be without "essentials" to nurture the newest member.

2. Events in the labor process may not occur as expected from past experiences, cultural conditioning, or influences from mass media. For example, a woman may anticipate that contractions will be regular before the rupture of her membranes. If the reverse occurs, she may perceive this event as indicating danger or abnormality. Another example is the multipara who expects the sequence of events in labor to occur as in her previous labor experiences. When new sensations are felt or the length of labor differs, she may become anxious that something is wrong. Cultural conditioning through stories heard from family and friends may also generate anxiety. When events do not occur in the manner described by others, the woman may feel that she must deal with some unknown or mysterious event. The multipara has the advantage of previous labor and delivery experiences, but the primipara must cope with an unknown experience. Mass media also affect one's expectations. The events in labor may not occur as seen on TV, or described in a book.

One's degree of knowledge also influences expectations about labor. Lack of knowledge or misconceptions generate mystery and fantasies. Individuals may misinterpret normal activities in the labor process as indicative of danger. Anxiety is contagious and fears may be reinforced by both the laboring woman and her family and friends. The inappropriate application of knowledge may also generate anxiety. For example, a woman and husband may enter labor with extensive knowledge and preparation. However, they may adhere to a rigid plan of expecting their labor experience to coincide exactly with what they learned. This rigidity may create anxiety since any deviation is viewed by them as an abnormality or complication.

Fears during labor focus on fear for self and fear for the baby.

Fear for Self. Women frequently express fears about being injured, mutilated, or even dying during labor. Husbands also express these concerns for their wives, especially when contractions become stronger and their wives become more uncomfortable. For example:

> John and Mary M. entered labor in anticipation of their first child. When routine admission procedures were completed, John quickly asked why his wife needed an IV. "Is something wrong? Is she going to need blood?" he asked in an anxious voice. Mary appeared to be tolerating labor well until her contractions became stronger and closer at 3 minute intervals. She progressed to 7 cm. dilatation at which time she made the following comments indicating fears of being injured. "Are you sure the baby can come out without tearing me. Is everything all right? I feel like my back and bottom are beginning to split apart."

Fear for the Baby. Fears of injury, abnormality, complications, and death can also be directed toward the baby. It is not uncommon for mothers and fathers to ask repeatedly during labor, "Is the baby all right?" This question may be asked even after nurses and doctors have repeatedly stated that the fetal heartbeat is strong and everything appears to be going well. These fears may also be manifested in indirect approaches such as repetition of a common theme with verbal denial of concern. For example:

> Susan: Nurse, I had a friend whose baby had trouble breathing because the cord was around its neck.

Nurse: Yes, sometimes that can happen. Are you concerned that it could happen to your baby?
Susan: No, not really.

Five minutes later.

Susan: I read something about babies needing help to be born and they use forceps to pull them out. Doesn't that injure them in some way?
Nurse: (After explaining the use of forceps for delivery and reassuring Susan about precautions to protect the baby.) Are you concerned about the use of forceps for your delivery?
Susan: No, I'm not afraid of forceps. If it's needed, it's needed.

Half an hour later.

Susan: Nurse, I haven't felt my baby move in the last half hour. It's always been so active and suddenly it's not moving. Something must be happening! Something must be wrong!

It is important to appreciate the wide variations in the manifestation of anxiety and fear during labor. It is essential to help the person identify what she or he is feeling, when such feelings began, and what precipitated them. This allows the "unknown" to become "known" and steps to reduce anxiety, as discussed in Chapter 9, can be implemented.

SENSORY ALTERATION

Different kinds of sensory alteration (see Chapter 7) may occur during the labor experience. The type of sensory alteration is determined by an assessment of the the person's usual quality and quantity of sensory input. This section examines factors which can increase the likelihood of creating sensory alterations of deprivation or overload during labor.

SENSORY OVERLOAD

Physiologic Phenomena

During the first stage, sensations from vaginal secretions, ruptured membranes, frequency of contractions, and changes in the cervix can increase sensory stimuli. The second stage is frequently seen as a period of overcharge or bombardment due to events inherent in the delivery process.[8] Increased stimuli arise from descent and rotations of the baby, urge to bear down, and discomforts from the intensity of the contractions.

Environment

A concomitant increase in sensory input occurs with preparation for delivery, such as frequency of vaginal examinations, transfer to the delivery room, and manipulations to aid in the delivery process. The atmosphere during delivery is usually intense, the number of individuals present and the procedures to be performed increase, and the staff are moving faster. The third stage brings increased stimuli with manipulations to deliver the placenta and control maternal bleeding. When delivery is over a woman may feel tired and relieved that she has completed the process. Just as she looks forward to getting some rest, the environment continues its increased sensory input. Now numerous assessments are to be done, such as vital signs, state of the fundus and bladder, and lochia flow. Increased stimuli may also continue from other patients in the room and visitors.

Inability to Recognize or Receive Meaningful Input

Inappropriate Conversations. The staff may discuss the patient's condition in her presence or within her range of hearing. These discussions are usually in medical language and are confusing or incomprehensible to the woman and her husband. The conversation may be about another patient but the woman relates the discussion to herself. She then becomes very anxious about overheard comments which are inconsistent with her situation. An even more detrimental example is the staff's conversations on irrelevant topics, such as their social activities. This not only confuses the woman, but forces her to cope with extra sensory stimuli which further depletes her energy reserves.

Strange Procedures and Equipment. A couple may have received explanations on the purpose and need for a monitoring device, but has become confused in attempts to interpret the auditory stimuli of beeps, or the visual stimuli of flashing lights.

Stimuli Occurring so Rapidly that Synthesis into a Meaningful Whole is Inhibited. For example, doctors and nurses are frequently heard giving a "dissertation" about a procedure or aspect of the labor process. Detailed explanations are given in one session. They then expect that since the facts were given, the patient understands. However, sensory overload has inhibited learning. Instead of understanding, the person is more anxious due to uncertainty about the new facts.

A couple may be bombarded by unanticipated events which occur suddenly during labor. These may arise from complications or abrupt changes in plans for management. If a complication occurs, it elicits a series of unanticipated events such as the use of monitoring devices and decisions for rapid delivery. During such situations, time is usually of such importance that safety and protective measures take priority over helping the individual assimilate the increased sensory input. Therefore, explanations may be sacrificed or given so hastily that the couple becomes more confused as to exactly what is occurring and why.

The progress of labor may occur so rapidly that the reality of the situation does not have its impact. A woman, usually a multipara, may be admitted in active phase of labor and after a perineal preparation and an enema, may progress to transitional or second stages. She may still be integrating the reality that her labor is actually here. Suddenly, she is bombarded by rituals in preparation for delivery, such as transfer to the delivery room, administration of an IV, rapid and forceful contractions, and the hurried pace of the staff. She may not realize what is happening and be overwhelmed by the multitude of events.

SENSORY DEPRIVATION

Interruption of Usual Activities to Meet Needs

The numerous restrictions imposed by bedrest, nothing by mouth, lack of visitors, and inability to rest can leave the woman with a sense of inability to meet her own needs. A decrease in one's usual patterning for stimuli occurs.

Loss of Identity

Upon admission, a woman is usually stripped of her personal belongings. Her physical claims indicative of her identity are removed. To compound this, she may be referred to by a number or other label instead of by name. This may also occur to the husband or other visitors. The consequences of this "identity-stripping phenomenon" are feelings of isolation or separation from the environment. The woman or husband may begin to feel that they are undeserving of attention from others, and feelings of loneliness and rejection emerge.

Decreased Sensory Stimulation

Visual stimuli are restricted to the color, lighting, and objects in the labor room. Auditory stimuli may involve input from one's own voice, or be restricted to the voices of the staff or other patients. Other auditory stimuli may be available through music piped into the room. However, even with this, the choice for tone and volume is restricted because the staff makes the decision as to the type of music to be played. Olfactory stimuli are limited to the smells of the hospital, which may not enhance feelings of comfort and peacefulness. Tactile stimulation is determined by input from the staff, husband, or other visitors. The amount and type of contact should be compatible with the woman's wishes. If not, simple acts such as stroking, rubbing, and patting can be a source of discomfort and anxiety. When desired, touching acts during labor promote comfort and decrease feelings of abandonment. Kinesthetic stimulation is also affected by the labor experience. Restriction in movement and positioning may make muscles tense and rigid, directly affecting the woman's ability to relax and achieve comfort. The detrimental effects of decreased sensory stimuli increase proportionately with the length of the labor. When labor is rapid, the impact is less because the effects are transitory. However, when labor is prolonged, limited stimuli may cause manifestations of disorientation, anxiety, and even panic.

Social Isolation

During labor there is a reduction or elimination of meaningful interactions with others. Labor involves separation from one's family and the individual enters an unfamiliar environment. In this strange setting the norms for communication patterns may be unknown or different from one's own patterns. Feelings of isolation and loneliness are normal when one cannot feel secure in communicating his needs to others. Hopefully, a significant person, such as a husband or mother, can be present with the woman during labor. However, even in these instances, the usual communication patterns between the individuals may be restricted. Lack of privacy and frequent interruptions may inhibit the content and style of communication. Social isolation may also occur as a result of the environment and behaviors by the staff. The setting may present situations that do not permit regular attendance by others. Staffing shortages may leave the woman unattended for periods of time. The attitudes and values of the staff also are influencing factors.

Feelings of separation or isolation can be felt even in the presence of verbal communication. This occurs when staff talk about or around the person instead of *with* the person. Usually this is done through the use of highly technical language which is incomprehensible to the person. It is also important to understand that restriction of direct verbal communication increases the meaningfulness of nonverbal forms. Therefore, staff must value the importance of recognizing and handling their negative feelings about the patient before they are manifested unconsciously through some nonverbal behavior. In dealing with feelings of isolation for the woman in labor, planned approaches must provide pleasurable sensory input not merely from verbal stimuli, but also through integration of stimulation through tactile, visual, and kinesthetic means.

BEHAVIORAL RESPONSE

The nurse needs to understand that certain factors affect behavioral response to sensory alterations. This section explores significant factors during labor.

Conditioning to Certain Types of Sensory Stimuli. For example, some women may be conditioned to expect tactile stimulation in their interactions with others. Touching acts convey a feeling of being loved, accepted, and sense of worth to these individuals. When touching acts are not provided in interactions with the staff, the opposite feelings of hate, rejection, and insignificance may be felt.

Influence of Anxiety on Perception of Reality. Women who are highly anxious during labor show more intense discomfort with the multitude of stimuli from bodily sensations. They may even have visual and auditory imagery and disorganization in their thought processes.

Degree of Enclosure and Restraints. These include such factors as restrictions on movement and positioning, size of the room, curtains constantly drawn, doors kept closed, use of restraints on extremities, and single room occupancy. When these factors exist during labor, some women may become more anxious because they feel trapped or imprisoned, even though they are aware that their room is easily accessible to others. Women frequently state that they feel as if the walls are closing in.

Permitted and Forced Tasks. A task may serve as a distractor from boredom and source of sensory input. For example, women who are concentrating on breathing techniques may react less to feelings of deprivation when left alone because they are oriented to a stimulus. However, when the woman is *forced* to perform a task, the consequences are sensory overload and stress. For example, forcing a woman to bear down when she is extremely fatigued or has no sensations to bear down may make her feel more anxious due to the burden to meet the demands expected from her. It appears that the tasks a woman initiates on her own while in labor are more effective in helping her to adapt to sensory alterations. The nurse's role is then to coach her to perform the task and support her efforts.

PAIN

The subject of pain during labor is discussed in detail in Chapter 25. Therefore, though it is necessary to include a certain amount of material on the physiologic aspects of pain, the discussion presented here focuses on the psychosocial factors which influence the perception of pain.

There is physiologic validation for a pain experience during labor. Uterine contractions stimulate pain receptors by:

- Myometrial anoxia creating an ischemic state during contractions
- Stretching of the cervix
- Pressure on the nerves
- Traction on tubes, ovaries, peritoneum, and supporting ligaments
- Pressure on urethra, bladder, and rectum
- Distention of muscles of pelvic floor and peritoneum.

Pain pathways during labor have been documented by various researchers such as Bonica.[9] Pain perception during labor is augmented by factors such as:

- Frequency, intensity, and duration of uterine contractions
- Fatigue
- Lack of sleep
- Decreased nutritional intake
- Anxiety and fears.

In the experience of pain, there is an association in the brain to identify sensations which are interpreted as painful. This is called nonbodily pain, or *interpretation of pain*. Interpretation of pain by a woman in labor is influenced by her life experiences, such as:

- Past and present hospitalizations and injuries
- Childhood pain experiences
- Previous labors
- Cultural norms regarding pain and labor
- Psychosexual development of the person.

In the same manner that a child associates a needle with pain, a woman may recollect events which evoked feelings of pain. She may feel pain with the mere sight of a needle or by being told that a procedure will be done. Cultural norms influence expectations, acceptance, reactions, and coping with pain. A woman may or may not exhibit pain reactions during labor depending on whether or not this is viewed as "acceptable" behavior. When these cultural norms are prohibited or interfered with, anxiety is generated which augments pain. The psychosexual development of the woman concerns her attitudes and adaptation to femininity and its roles and expectations. Pain interpretation is affected by feelings toward the feminine parts of the body (breasts, genitalia) and other factors associated with being a woman, such as motherhood. Negative feelings augment pain. This is especially applicable during labor when there is an increased emphasis on the feminine parts of the body in terms of manipulation and exposure.

Pain elicits feelings of anxiety and fear. In working with anyone in pain, it is important to appreciate the cyclical relationship between anxiety and pain. The rationale for this cycle is that anxiety generates tension which augments pain perception by intensifying the pain impulses which reach the brain. Pain impulses are described as moving in circuits that set off reverberating activity and increase the excitability of the cells in the cerebral cortex.[10] This intensifies the response to pain, which in turn may increase the anxiety level, setting up the vicious circle. The fear of pain is ranked second only to the fear of death, and pain is often associated with death.[11] Death fears during labor have been described by Deutsch.[12] They are usually manifested in the late phase of labor as contractions increase in intensity, frequency, and duration. These fears should not be ignored or minimized.

Anxiety and pain also cause feelings of helplessness, not only for the woman but also for others. The husband and staff may feel a sense of nervousness or apprehension about their ability to help control pain. The impact of anxiety on the pain experience is vitally important and cannot be negated if the management of pain is to be successful.

The physiologic reactions to pain are similar to the autonomic reactions to stress. These include diaphoresis, hyperventilation, increased heart and respiratory rates, dry cracked lips, tense muscles, restlessness, and irritability. These reactions impose additional discomforts and prolong the labor process. Tense muscles can inhibit cervical dilatation and the descent of the baby. Hyperventilation and increased heart rate can interfere with maternal oxygen–carbon dioxide exchange, thereby affecting oxygenation of the fetus.

Consideration must also be given to ethnic and cultural differences among reactions and coping mechanisms. Culture defines whether childbirth is an event in which pain is expected and accepted. It dictates behaviors which acknowledge or deny the presence of pain during labor. Culture may also define the cause for pain and the degree to which it is a threat to the woman. For example, an exploratory study[13] investigating attitudes toward pain and labor in a specific culture in Hawaii indicated that culture may determine that the cause of pain during labor be unknown and mysterious. Women from these cultures were seen to be very frightened, even to the point of expressing fears about the possibility of death during labor. They viewed labor as a long, fearful process in which suffering was unavoidable. They felt there were limited resources that a woman could employ by herself to cope with the pain. Rather, supernatural forces were called to help. It was not uncommon to find these women praying during contractions. Most of these women had little knowledge or preparation for labor which perpetuated the attitude of mystery. This attitude was even expressed by multiparas who had experienced labor before but still had no understanding of the process. At times, the cultural norms for responses and coping with pain of labor were misinterpreted by the staff, leading to judgmental labeling of the women. For example:

> Women were noted to be very quiet and had minimal verbal interactions with the staff. They did not ask questions, make requests, or voice their concerns or need. In spite of their minimal verbal communication, they manifested nonverbal behaviors indicative of anxiety and pain. They were seen lying in bed in fixed, rigid positions, or tossing and turning restlessly. During contractions they manifested tense muscle reactions in hands, feet, neck, and face. Hyperventilation and diaphoresis were commonly seen. The staff labeled these women as "doing well" because they weren't "asking for anything." The staff then decreased their interactions with these women and focused on others they perceived as needing more help. These women were also labeled as "good patients" because they "did not bother the staff or others." When interviewed, these women expressed their biggest fear to be that of being left alone. When asked what they expected from the staff, the reply was a simple "just to be with me," or "not to leave me alone." Ironically, the very thing they valued from the staff—*presence*—was denied because the staff perceived that no help was needed because they were "doing so well."

There may be conflict between the patient's cultural norms and the staff's norms regarding acceptable responses to pain during labor. Moans or chants may be viewed as a cultural necessity by the woman, but be prohibited by the staff. It is not uncommon to see women reprimanded for making such noises during labor. They sometimes are labeled negatively as "acting like a baby" or "aggressive and hostile." These comments may even be written in the woman's chart. The effects are devastating! New personnel arriving at the change of shift may form judgments merely from the "labels" seen in the chart or heard during the nursing report. This perpetuates the lack of effectiveness in the management of pain during labor.

LOSS

During labor, the experience of loss may be seen in three forms:

1. Loss of a valued object or person
2. Loss of expectations or values
3. Loss of some aspect of the self

The concept of loss during the labor experience is usually associated with the threatened loss of the baby. However, this is not the most frequent type of loss manifested. Many times an experience of loss occurs when expectations are unmet or a valued aspect of the self is removed or threatened. This discussion examines these less obvious aspects of the experience of loss.

LOSS OF EXPECTATIONS OR VALUES

Prior to labor, a woman, her husband, and family all develop expectations about their forthcoming childbirth experience. These may focus on fantasies about the baby's appearance and behaviors, sex of the baby, events during labor and delivery, and expectations concerning the self and others. A sense of loss occurs when these expectations are not fulfilled. The intensity of the loss is frequently associated with the amount of time the lost expectation or value has been held. However, this may not always be the rule and is open for challenge. For example, a father who has desired and expected a male child during his wife's entire pregnancy is speculated to feel more grief over the birth of a female than one whose desire for a male began during the last trimester of pregnancy. Likewise, the extent to which a mother has developed fantasies about her unborn child will determine her sense of loss. The earlier the fantasies, and the more detailed and specific they become, the greater the loss when reality presents a different newborn. Another area frequently overlooked concerns expectations about events during labor and delivery. A woman who expects her membranes to break spontaneously, medications for pain relief, and a saddle block anesthesia will feel a sense of loss if these events do not happen. The father who expects to be present with his wife and comfort her through learned techniques will suffer a sense of loss if his efforts are interfered with or do not produce the desired results. It is speculated by this author that a sense of loss due to unmet expectations is experienced more frequently than we realize during the labor experience. This area has major implications in planning effective care for the woman and her family during labor.

LOSS OF SOME ASPECT OF THE SELF

This type of loss is manifested when there is removal of a desired aspect of one's self system. During labor this frequently relates to body image, self-esteem, roles, communication patterns, and activities of daily living.

Loss of Body Image. After delivery, it is not unusual to hear a woman express grief over the loss of her expanded figure. She may even make comments about losing bodily sensations which she has come to enjoy during her pregnancy. For example, one mother frequently touched her abdomen during the fourth stage of labor and stated:

> It feels so strange. So flat! It doesn't feel like me anymore. I really do miss that big hump. I use to enjoy feeling the baby move and kick. It made me feel so alive to have something in there. Now there's nothing. I really am going to miss all those good feelings.

Loss can also be directed to the body image in the form of losing control over bodily functioning. This is frequently seen in the second stage with increased bearing-down sensations. Spontaneous bowel movements or urination may generate feelings of losing control over one's eliminative functions. This fear about control over bodily functions can also be felt when uncontrollable chilling or shaking occurs after the delivery of the baby.

Loss of Self-Esteem. Loss of self-esteem can be devastating to a woman in labor! She loses trust and confidence in herself and is left with an experience that is unfulfilling and incomplete. Loss of self-esteem is usually interrelated with the following:

- Losing control over coping with the situation
- Negative or no feedback about one's behaviors
- Unmet expectations.

It is not uncommon for women and their supporters to have feelings of losing control over the situation at one time or another during the labor process. The physiologic activities of labor, pain, anxiety, and sensory alterations contribute to feelings of being overpowered by a force bigger than the self. Frequently this feeling occurs during transition or second stage when fatigue is paramount and energy for coping is diminished. The woman may lose control in coping with one or two contractions and then generalize the loss to the entire labor process. Her coping behaviors, such as moans and screams, may not be acceptable to the staff. She may receive negative feedback or be forced to abandon these behaviors making her vulnerable to losing control. Women and their husbands may be well prepared for labor, having practiced newly learned resources. However, when the environment does not support the use of these new coping measures, a sense of losing control over the situation is felt. A sense of loss is usually related to self-esteem when one is made to feel that behaviors are not legitimate or acceptable.

Loss of Roles. Loss may also be associated with the removal of one's status or role. Confinement for labor brings a halt to responsibilities and privileges afforded because of one's career role. The woman who enters labor is usually not given recognition for her career status. Rather, she is viewed simply as another woman in labor. Sometimes pregnancy brings a special role for a woman by increased attention and sanctions. This may be terminated when attention is directed to the newborn after delivery. For example, the first questions visitors usually ask focus on collecting information about the baby instead of the woman. Husbands may also be affected by this redirection of attention to the baby. He may feel displacement of significance in his wife's world as the baby's needs become paramount. Role loss is also manifested in the redirection from being independent to dependent. Restrictions on the ability to make judgments will do this.

Loss of Communication Patterns. Labor may interfere with one's ability to interact with others. Anxiety, pain, and other stimuli create obstacles in the ability to communicate and establish relationships with others. A woman and her husband may find it difficult to respond to questions clearly or to express their feelings and concerns. Crying behaviors indicating a sense of helplessness may lead the staff to label the person as childish or regressing. Aggressive-hostile behaviors over frustrations of not being able to communicate clearly may lead to labels of being uncooperative and belligerent.

Consideration should be given to the relationship the woman has developed with her fetus. Some women develop an intimate, close, symbiotic relationship in which they feel a unity with their fetuses. Delivery brings an abrupt end to this symbiosis. Suddenly there is a separate individual, apart from one's self.

Loss of Patterns to Meet Bodily Needs. During labor one's eliminative, ingestive, and sleep patterns are drastically altered. The woman and her husband may feel helpless, isolated, and anxious.

A significant nursing implication arises from knowledge of the various manifestations of loss during labor. Nurses need to plan care that will help the woman and her family work through the grief for the perceived loss. This is best done in the postpartal period. To do it during the intrapartal period would be overloading the patient; the priority then is to move her through the completion of the actual labor and birth process.

CRISIS

The preceding sections have presented variables indicating that the intrapartal period is a time of increased stress. This increased stress predisposes the childbearing family to crisis.[14–17] Stress is cumulative and appears to reach a climax with the approaching labor and delivery. Emotional stress as well as physical stress must be considered. Klein states:

> A pregnant woman brings to the experience of labor all her structural, physiologic, and psychological assets and liabilities. Particularly since the physiology of labor is largely under the domination of the parasympathetic division of the nervous system, the role of emotional factors is important.[18]

Anxiety is a major cause for psychologic stress as stated by Derschimer:

> Mystery makes labor appear as a ghostly function and is approached in terror.[19]

The crisis of labor and birth is not necessarily detrimental. Caplan states that crisis is a turning point in one's life because through it better problem-solving approaches emerge.[20] In essence, crisis provides an opportunity for better mental health. Whether crisis will weaken or strengthen the family is dependent upon the process by which it is resolved.

ROLE OF THE NURSE

When applying the psychosocial concepts to nursing the woman in labor, there are two major goals:

1. To nurture the woman and significant other during labor and delivery so that they can cope optimally during the experience
2. To stimulate the woman and significant other so that they will emerge from the labor experience with a strengthened self system and family unity.

The first step towards attaining these goals is identification of significant factors which will provide information about the impact that labor is predicted to have on the individual. Assessment allows the nursing care to be relevant to the individual's perception of the experience.

SIGNIFICANT FACTORS FOR ASSESSMENT

These factors have been previously discussed but are presented again to emphasize their importance.

Expectations and Perception of Labor. Data should be collected about the woman's expectations of her behaviors during labor and those of the hospital staff and others. Nurses should seek answers to questions such as:

What do you expect labor to be like for you?
Did you have any preparation for labor?
Were there any stressful events which happened to you before your labor began or during your pregnancy?
Do you anticipate any discomforts during labor? If so, how do you plan to handle them?
Can you tell me what you know or have heard about labor?
Do you have any goals, specific wishes, or desires, which you hope to achieve during labor?
What do you expect the staff and others to do to help you during labor?

Meaning of the Labor Experience. Data on the attitudes and values of the labor experience are important because such meanings and purposes as defined by culture, mass media, and the individual can be a means of support or a source of additional stress during labor. Questions for consideration are:

Is labor viewed as a life-threatening event or a means of self-fulfillment and attainment of desired goals.
What is the cultural meaning or significance of labor?
Is there support or conflict of the individual's ascribed meaning of labor compared with that of the hospital or the culture?

Factors Which Increase Stress and Threaten the Self during Labor. Information should be obtained concerning the following:

Knowledge and understanding of the labor process
Concerns and fears
Awareness and understanding of events to occur in the hospital
Degree of discomforts and disruption of daily patterns prior to onset of labor
Attitudes toward the pregnancy and the labor.

Such data helps the nurse identify other stressors which will impose upon the uncontrollable physiologic stressors inherent in labor. This aids in predicting the amount of stress with which a woman must cope. It also provides cues which enable the nurse to anticipate the effects of anxiety and tension earlier in the labor process.

Support System Desired and Available during Labor. Data to obtain are:

What are plans or expectations in regard to coping?
Who is desired for attendance during labor and what is expected from them?
Are situational supports available?

SKILLS FOR DATA COLLECTION

To effectively collect data on the above factors, certain knowledge and skills are needed. The nurse must be able to obtain data through verbal interaction using interviewing skills, through awareness of nonverbal behaviors using observational skills, and through identification of optimum time periods when such skills should be used during the labor process.

Use of good interviewing techniques should begin with the first contact between the nurse and the expectant family. The nurse may begin by asking how the woman is feeling and what she expects labor to be like for her. Such broad, general questions allow the woman to direct the interaction to whatever area she feels is important. The nurse can then seek clarification and further explanations about specific data. It is important to appreciate that good interviewing creates a favorable climate for the sharing of feelings. The nurse should introduce herself, show respect by addressing the person by name, and lower anxiety through anticipatory guidance.

Interviewing during labor should be a continuous process since stimuli from contractions may not permit an uninterrupted session in which feelings can be shared. The nurse must be able to identify opportunities which lend themselves favorably to interviewing. For example, a woman may be eager to share her feelings while the nurse is performing routines such as checking vital signs. The woman should not be stopped or interrupted from doing so. The nurse should not expect or force women to respond to questions during contractions when all energies are directed toward coping with stress.

The ideal time for interviewing is during the latent phase of labor. Stresses are minimal and anxiety is at a mild level, making the woman more alert and responsive. At this healthy arousal level, the woman can focus on others as well as herself, and her ability to communicate has not been altered as will usually happen when labor progresses.

Good observational skills should be employed throughout the entire labor process. For some individuals, verbal communication is very stressful so they exhibit their reactions through nonverbal behaviors, such as gestures, facial expressions, and body position. This is especially true of individuals from another culture who enter an American hospital. They may not be able to speak the language and cultural norms may de-emphasize the use of verbal forms of communication. Also, in times of stress, the ability to communicate verbally may be hindered.

What is the nurse looking for as she observes nonverbal communication patterns? One area is the autonomic reactions to stress and pain, such as increased breathing and heart rate, dilated pupils, diaphoresis, and tense muscles. The nurse should observe for any behavior indicative of a response. This is important because possible significance may be attached to the stimuli which caused the reaction. For example:

> A 27 y./o. Korean woman, unable to speak English, is in active labor, 5 cm., 0 station. This will be her third child, but the first to be born in an American hospital. She is very quiet during labor and makes no verbal comments. She appears to be oblivious to the environment as well as the contractions. However, the nurse noted the following

behaviors indicating possible stress:

Tense, rigid position, unchanged since admission an hour ago
Blank facial appearance, staring fixedly at the ceiling, eyes open wide
Feet must be tense because the sheet is held taut against them
Hands tightly gripping the sides of the bed.

This woman made no response to the staff's verbal comments when they asked if she was in pain and wanted medications for pain relief. The nurse remained with her continuously for 15 minutes during which time she stroked the woman's arms gently and sponged her forehead with a cool towel after each contraction. After this 15 minutes, it was noted that the sheet was no longer raised tightly against her feet. No verbal interaction took place between the nurse and the woman. However, the woman made her first reaction since admission over an hour ago—she changed her position!

NURSING ACTIONS

After assessment, the nurse is ready to identify her purposes more specifically. This will direct the planning and implementation of actions for nursing care. The following are suggested categories for nursing actions in nurturing and stimulating the woman in labor and her family:

1. Creating an environment which communicates trust and security
2. Meeting the informational needs of the individuals
3. Promoting of relaxation and comfort
4. Providing a support system
5. Facilitating the immediate maternal-infant claiming process
6. Integrating the labor experience into a meaningful whole.

It is hoped that the following discussions provide a stimulus for new and creative approaches while working with a woman in labor instead of merely carrying out routines. Nothing is relevant unless it is directed to the needs and perception of the individual concerned. Therefore, the reader is encouraged to investigate new approaches and be prepared to utilize more than one set of actions based upon assessment and constant search for new knowledge.

Developing Trust

A sense of trust and security minimizes perceptions of dangers or threats during labor. It also increases confidence in the ability to handle and maintain control of the labor situation. To establish trust, interaction between the nurse and the patient is essential—no mechanical device can do it. Actions which promote trust must begin with the initial interaction. It is worth remembering that first impressions are lasting. The nurse should convey a feeling of respect by addressing the person by name and introducing herself and stating that she is her nurse. It is important at this initial contact to be observant for signs of stress and to be a good listener. The woman and/or husband may be sharing crucial assessment data spontaneously due to their excitement or anxiety over the possibility of being in labor. Nurses should not be so preoccupied with collecting routine information that they inhibit these valuable unsolicited comments. Nurses need to assess the priorities at this initial interaction. Unless labor progress is rapid or complications are present, routine questioning can be done later. Therapeutic listening also involves uninterrupted attention. This should be conveyed by nodding or other nonverbal cues rather than verbal interjections. Attention is also provided by maintaining some eye to eye contact while listening. These little behaviors provide feedback acknowledging that the expressed feelings are genuine and significant to the listener.

Trust also develops by decreasing anxiety and fears. The following are suggested approaches. First, the nurse should be aware of the presence of anxiety. Cues indicating anxious feelings may be bodily discomforts such as tossing, turning, and tense muscles. The woman may also state her anxious feelings verbally. Second, the nurse should help the woman identify the cause for stress and tension. Feelings of anxiety are vague and undefined, usually generalized to everything. One way to identify the cause for anxiety is to have the woman identify the event or events which occurred just before tension was felt. Third, the nurse should help eliminate stressors or facilitate coping with them. When anxiety and fears are caused by fantasies or lack of knowledge, the nurse provides input through teaching. When anxiety arises from doubts about the ability to maintain control of one's behaviors, the nurse can point out the woman's ability to make labor progress. When anxiety originates from unmet expectations, the nurse manipulates the situation to allow reality to come as close as possible to the expectations. Fourth, nurses need to appreciate that anxiety increases the need to be sustained by another human being. Feelings of helplessness lead to dependency and to the fear of being abandoned or isolated.

Stressful stimuli increase as labor progresses, making the woman more anxious or fearful. Thus, the need to be with another human being increases with labor progress. The nurse can meet this need by "simply being there." But exactly where is there? Nurses need to value how they position themselves next to the patient. When the nurse is at the foot of the bed, she may not be seen or felt to be close by. This may also cause feelings that the nurse is looking at or more interested in the perineal area instead of the woman herself. However, when the nurse is near the woman's face, eye contact can be provided to communicate the reality of human presence. The effects of the presence of the nurse have been attributed with achieving results similar to the administration of analgesics, such as 100 mg. of Demerol.[21] While the nurse is with the woman, she can provide tactile and verbal stimuli to indicate a caring attitude. Use of gentle touch such as stroking, patting, or rubbing, can convey kindness and compassion. Use of firm touch, such as a hand on the shoulder or holding hands firmly during contractions, conveys a sense of "I am really here to help you. I will not abandon you." Verbal stimuli should be used judiciously. Rapid, loud, high-pitched voices by nurses can communicate excitement, anxiety, and tension. A slow, hardly audible, monotone voice can convey disinterest or a lack of importance to the situation. The nurse should use her judgment and convey confidence and control of the situation through her voice. A trusting relationship will communicate that the nurse understands what the woman is experiencing and cares enough to help her complete the labor and birth.

Meeting Informational Needs

Another category of nursing actions provides knowledge to meet the learning needs of the woman and husband during labor. Essential to this objective is assessment of the teaching-learning needs of the persons involved. Data should be collected about what the individuals know about the physiologic process, sensations to be felt, and the rationale for the mechanisms of labor. Teaching allows clarification and correction of misconceptions and also prepares the woman for future phases of labor (Fig. 23-1). Effective teaching approaches also provide a feedback process by which women and men can seek further clarification through questions. Teaching during labor is not an easy task. Consideration must be given to the effects of such factors as anxiety upon the couple's ability to learn. The nurse

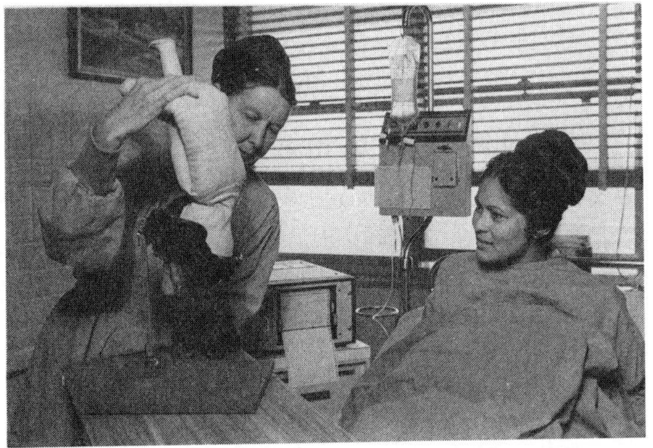

FIGURE 23-1. The nurse meeting the teaching-learning needs of the woman in labor.

must appreciate when content can best be presented for optimum retention and learning. It is a fallacy to assume that once content has been presented, it has been learned. Repetition and reinforcement of previous teachings are necessary during labor. The author has developed a guideline by which content can best be presented at different phases in the labor experience.[22] The following is an elaboration of this primary guideline.

Latent Phase. Latent phase is an excellent period for assessment of learning needs. Anxiety enhances learning. The person can observe, describe, and analyze—all essential components to good learning. Data are easily collected because the woman can express her needs clearly. Content should include:

- Description and rationale for the physiologic mechanisms of labor
- Bodily sensations to be felt
- Expectations to be made upon the woman during labor
- Measures by which the woman can best help herself.

Active Phase. Active phase (4 to 7 cm.) stressors increase at this time and anxiety rises. Content should include:

- Reinforcement of the rationale for stressors to minimize the threats they evoke
- Rationale for limitations such as bedrest and nothing by mouth to increase their acceptance
- Reinforcement of previous teachings because fatigue and confusion increase with the elevated anxiety level
- Preparation for the next phases (transitional and second stages).

The woman needs to know that demands to push or pant may occur. Teaching approaches toward the end of this phase should be made in short sentences or phrases to increase retention.

Transitional and Second Stages. Now the individual's perceptual field is greatly narrowed and learning is difficult. Teaching should be done in brief sessions using short phrases. Only essential content should be presented and should focus on immediate events, such as answering questions and reinforcing how she can cope with one contraction at a time. It is best not to introduce new content at this time because new learning is inhibited by the increased anxiety. Nurses are cautioned to consider the elements of fatigue, irritability, and pain, and not to overwhelm the woman with content.

In any application of teaching-learning principles, the use of audiovisual programs enhances the presentation and increases retention. Nurses are encouraged to use available pamphlets and demonstration models, and to create and develop new programs. An innovative approach is a self-learning program which can be used by patients whose anxiety level is conducive to learning. This allows the nurse more freedom to work with more patients instead of being confined to presenting content to just one individual. Nurses can then spend their time seeking more feedback from the women.

Promotion of Comfort and Relaxation

The discomforts of labor lead to difficulty with relaxation, which creates muscle tension. This results in spasms which can cause cramps, fatigue, and interference with feelings of well-being. Thus, muscle tension can augment the existing pain experience, and oppose the progress of labor by prolonging it. Therefore, the rationale for implementing actions which provide comfort and relaxation is to minimize muscular stress, which will decrease pain perception and facilitate the progress of labor. Suggested nursing actions to achieve this are:

1. Hygienic Measures
   Oral hygiene to combat dry mucous membranes
   Cleansing after nausea and vomiting
   Body and facial sponges to relieve discomforts from diaphoresis
   Perineal cleansing to combat discomforts from secretions
   Linens dry and taut to decrease friction on the skin caused by wrinkles and wetness
   Proper fitting clothing.
2. Combat Effects of Immobility (Confinement to Bed)
   Proper anatomical positioning to relieve muscular stress from pressure on bony prominences. All parts of the body should be supported and joints slightly flexed (Fig. 23-2).
   Back rubs and change of position to stimulate circulation and combat muscle fatigue due to decreased movement which retards blood flow.
3. Minimize Adverse Environmental Stimuli
   Control glaring lights
   Decrease traffic flow and noise
   Organize care to decrease disturbances from routines such as checking vital signs
   Draw curtains to provide privacy
   Adequate room temperature and ventilation.
4. Conscious Relaxation Methods
   Relaxation enables the woman to obtain maximum benefit from the rest periods between contractions to reduce fatigue and increase her energy. This allows her to return to the task of labor refreshed and revitalized. A discussion of

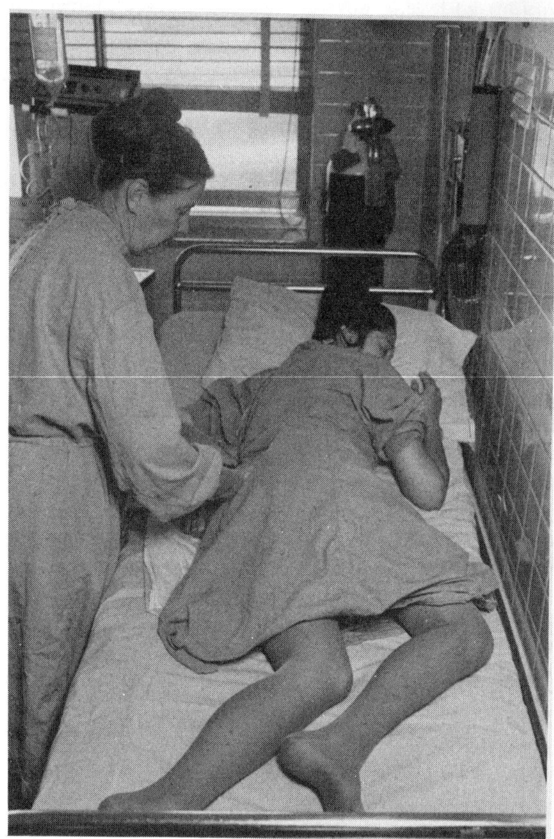

FIGURE 23-2. Proper anatomic position for promoting relaxation while lying on the side.

relaxation methods was presented in Chapter 21.

5. Management of Pain

Nursing seeks to manipulate variables which affect pain perception, pain interpretation, and reduction of effects from pain reactions. Theoretical support for nursing's unique goals can be found in Melzack and Wall's *gate control theory on pain.*[23] This theory conceptualizes that a "gating mechanism" based on the excitation and inhibition of nerve fibers determines whether pain impulses are transmitted or blocked along the transmission route through the spinal cord to the brain. Melzack and Wall theorize that the pain gate is open when small fibers are activated with little activity in the large fibers, and when nerve fibers descending from the brain stem and cerebral cortex are not stimulated. They propose that several inhibitory mechanisms can be activated to close the gate for pain. Examples are:

(a) Stimulation of large cutaneous afferent fibers which are close to the skin surface. Such actions as rubbing, patting, vibrating will achieve this.

(b) Cerebral processes should be activated to stimulate the many neural areas of the brain such as the thalamus, cerebral cortex, and brain stem. Melzack and Wall propose that cerebral activities involving sensory-perceptual (awareness), motivation-affect (emotional), and cognitive (intellectual) skills help to alter such variables as pain perception, interpretation, and reactions. How do such cerebral activities influence pain? Cognitive skills delve into past and cultural experiences to provide meaning to the pain experience. Motivation-affect processes identify the degree of unpleasantness affecting the suggestion and anticipation of pain. Sensory-perceptual skills explore the frequency, intensity, duration and location to influence anxiety, attention and tolerance of pain impulses.

The beauty of the gate control theory is it provides nursing with theoretical support to validate goals which penetrate beyond the realm of pharmacologic interventions. We now have a theoretical basis to support such actions as exploring a person's anxieties and fears; assessing for cultural norms; exploring past pain experiences; and, finally, our unique approaches in the therapeutic use of self through such actions as allowing expression of feelings, giving explanations, use of touch, and eye to eye contact.

When working with the pain experience for a woman in labor the following actions help nurses to achieve their goals:

a. Distraction

Distraction is a means of providing sensory input in an attempt to decrease concentration on pain. It contributes to pain relief by eliciting responses incompatible with pain responses, and reducing anxiety associated with the pain.[24] For example, a woman in labor is unlikely to cry out during a contraction if she is concentrating on another activity such as doing an exercise. Also, input for distraction stimulates the central control system (cerebral processes) thereby inhibiting the pain gate in the gate control theory. Engaging in an activity makes her less occupied with the threat of pain as she anticipates another contraction.

Stimuli for distractors can take many forms. Auditory stimuli can be provided through music, chantings, or other desired sounds. Visual stimuli can be provided through pictures or other images, as well as reading. Stimuli can be combined into an audiovisual medium such as television. Other audiovisual stimulation can occur through involvement in a task with others, such as a game of cards. Unfortunately, most of these stimuli are not available to the woman confined in the hospital in labor. There are many reasons for this, such as economics and the danger of promoting infection. However, most of these are not valid and result from the lack of value placed on distraction as an effective pain reliever.

There are certain principles to enhance the use of distraction. According to McCaffery[25] these are:

(1) The stimuli or set of stimuli used must be compatible to the individual
(2) The longer the pain, the greater the variety of distractions
(3) When one is very frightened about his pain, or feels severe pain, distraction is attained by first getting the person's attention and then providing a simple, quick stimuli.

What does this mean to the nurse? First, what type of stimuli will interest the woman long enough for her to attend and concentrate? Second, simple stimuli are more effective distractors during latent phase when pain is at a lower intensity. However, as pain increases with labor progress, more complex stimuli may be needed to keep attention away from intense sensations created by the stronger contractions. Also, after hours of laboring, a woman in active phase may be fatigued by the monotony of simple stimuli. The use of different distractors is demonstrated in the Lamaze method. There are three different types of rhythmic breathing for the various stages of labor. A breathing technique is replaced by another when it begins to lose its effectiveness. Third, distraction is less effective when a very anxious person is perceiving intense pain. In such situations, distractors should be short and simple.

Nurses should make more deliberate attempts to provide sensory input for distraction from pain. During the latent phase of labor, distraction is an especially appropriate measure for pain relief because effects of contractions are not so intense and it may be too early in the labor process for medications.

b. Cutaneous Stimulation

Cutaneous stimulation involves sensory input from touch as a mode for pain relief. One rationale for its effectiveness relates to the gate control theory in which the large fibers are stimulated to close the gate. Another rationale relates to the phenomenon of extinction which means the perception threshold for a sensory stimulus is higher when another is being applied. Thus, pain is better tolerated when another stimulus is applied below the intensity to produce discomfort. One of the most vivid examples of cutaneous stimulation during labor is providing sacral pressure during contractions. The palm of the hand is placed in the lower curvature of the back and firm, constant pressure is exerted evenly during the contraction. The nurse should always assess if sacral pressure is relieving pain; if not, it should be discontinued as it can be an additional source of discomfort. Other forms of cutaneous stimulation for pain relief during labor are:

(1) Effleurage or rhythmic, soft rubbing of the abdominal area in a circular fashion. This is also an effective distractor.
(2) Cool, moist cloth or the cool hand of the nurse to areas of the skin which are hot. This is also a distractor and a means of providing comfort.
(3) Back rubs to enhance relaxation.
(4) Holding the woman's hand firmly during contractions to decrease her anxiety or fears of being abandoned during the pain. It also is a means of meeting dependency needs which result from feelings of helplessness in trying to ease the pain of labor.
(5) Women may at times rub or hold the

area which hurts. Usually during labor, women are seen doing this to the area near the symphysis pubis and the lower back.

Cutaneous stimulation is an effective nursing measure during labor not only because it relieves pain but also because it provides the woman with the presence of the nurse.

c. Pharmacologic Agents

The rationale for the use of analgesics is that they exert a depressing effect on the central nervous system (primarily the sensory cortex and thalamus) and thereby dull the perception of pain. Certain influencing factors need to be valued by the nurse when drugs are used for pain relief during labor. These are identified along with the nursing implications in the following:

(1) Analgesics given before or at the beginning of a pain experience will act both at the cortical and thalamic level.

Cortical action modifies the interpretation of stimuli as painful while thalamic action decreases the perception of pain. Maximum effect of a drug in terms of longer action is achieved when depressing effects are exerted on both cortical and thalamic levels of the brain.

Nurses need to identify behaviors indicative of the presence of pain during labor. The presence of pain should be acknowledged as legitimate and its management should not be ignored. The nurse may need to seek medical orders for drugs instead of merely waiting for the doctor to initiate such action. The waiting period can increase the pain for the woman as her contractions become stronger. This will only minimize the action and duration of the medicine when given.

(2) Analgesics given during the latent phase of labor can depress contractile patterns of the uterus and prolong labor.

Other measures to relieve pain should be utilized during latent phase to avoid interference with the body's attempt to regulate the contractile patterns. The use of drugs at this phase is usually indicated in two situations. One is when the latent phase is prolonged (six hours or more) and rest is needed to allow the body to continue through the labor process once the effects of the drug wear off. The other situation is when a very anxious woman needs medication to control her through sedation.

(3) Depressant effects to the fetus are greater when systemic analgesics are administered close to delivery (within two hours).[26]

It is a good rule to avoid the administration of analgesics within two hours before delivery. The nurse can advocate this by sharing data indicative of labor progress, such as the frequency and intensity of contractions. Nurses should also question medical orders which call for the administration of analgesics within this time period.

(4) Is the person conditioned to handling pain through the use of medications?

Use of medication may be the only way a person knows of relieving pain. If so, it should not be withheld without the patient being involved in the decision. When medications are limited during the latent phase, the nurse needs to reinforce the rationale for such actions. This will decrease anxiety which may emerge when one is told no medications will be given. Nurses also need to follow through with any promise made about giving medications. Frequently the nurse may state she will return to give a drug but is either distracted or forgets to do it.

Another factor to consider is that conditioning the woman to the use of medications for pain relief may result from the actions of the hospital staff. Too often, patients receive attention only when they demonstrate pain reactions, such as pleas for help, moaning, tossing, irritability. Attention may be given through negative remarks by the nurse, but nonetheless, the patient gains the presence of the nurse. Therefore, nurses are cautioned not to pattern the need for medications by providing attention only for pain behaviors or only during the administration of drugs.

(5) Safety actions should be implemented to protect the mother and fetus from depressant effects of the drugs.

In addition to the basic precautions pertaining to the use of any drug, the following are unique to the labor setting:

(a) Fetal heart tones should be checked after a drug is given. Assessment is recommended immediately after the drug is given. This provides guidelines for immediate as well as late reactions to effects of depression.

(b) The mother's blood pressure and pulse rate should be checked after any drug is given. Regional analgesia such as pudendals, paracervicals, and epidurals, have the hazard of creating maternal hypotension. Therefore, any woman receiving such measures should have her blood pressure monitored a minimum of two to four times after such techniques. If hypotension occurs, several actions are warranted:

Change her position from supine to lateral

Immediately elevate the legs to decrease venous pressure and increase peripheral circulation

Increase intravenous fluids

Administer oxygen by face mask at 6 to 8 liters per minute if there is no response to position changes

Report the patient's hypotensive status to the physician immediately.

(6) Use of drugs does not eliminate the pain source during labor. It merely dulls the perception to the sensation of pain.

It is essential that nurses do not state that no pain will be felt once a drug has been given. Anxiety increases when the woman realizes that the discomforts from contractions are not stopping as she had been led to anticipate by the nurse. Rather, the nurse should explain that the use of drugs will help the woman to better tolerate the discomforts.

d. Other Measures

Other means of providing pain relief during labor are:

Provision for comfort and relaxation

Behavior therapy

Hypnosis

Psychoprophylactic methods

Promotion of relaxation and general comfort contributes to pain relief by reducing physical strain which may lead to fatigue. Fatigue enhances pain by depleting energy available to cope with discomforts. Nursing actions to provide relaxation and comfort have been discussed in the preceding section.

Behavior therapy is used to denote a form of treatment or teaching-learning process that employs the principles of classical and operant conditioning.[27] In its use with the labor patient, the main principle which applies is the fact that a behavior will occur more frequently when it is consistently followed by a reward. Therefore, when the nurse is trying to teach the woman new ways to handle the pain of labor, positive reinforcement for coping efforts is essential. For example, when a woman breathes correctly during a contraction, the nurse gives encouragement with comments such as, "Good, that's it, keep it up. You're doing well." After the contraction is over the woman should be rewarded for her efforts with comments such as, "You did very well. You worked hard during that contraction." Nurses need to be cognizant of which behaviors they are reinforcing. If the woman is attended only when she cries for help or is restless and irritable, then these undesirable behaviors will continue. Remember, attention can be provided in negative ways such as reprimands or labeling of the woman. When women and their husbands are doing well, do not leave them unattended because "they don't need any help." The nurse still needs to visit the couple to provide reinforcement for their good efforts of handling the pain.

In the use of hypnosis for pain relief during labor, results depend upon the patient's susceptibility to suggestion and the nature of the suggestions made.[28] It requires the talents and skills of a person prepared and trained in hypnosis. The role of the nurse is to support its use and provide positive reinforcement when it is effective.

Psychoprophylactic methods also provide a means for achieving pain relief during childbirth. The following section describes the role of the monitrice during psychoprophylactic preparation for childbirth.

Monitricing*

As Dr. Lamaze wrote, "Childbirth without pain is attained above all by teamwork." The monitrice acts as a coach-assistant during labor and birth. Specially trained in the Method and qualified as a Registered Nurse (in the United States), her attendance is an integral part of the birth team and one of the reasons for the greater success of this Method.

While the term "monitrice" has come from the French, or Lamaze program for Psychoprophylaxis, there is no reason why a nurse could not function as a *monitrice* with every woman in labor. Of course, her task will be made much easier when she is dealing with a prepared woman, but many of the techniques and much of the information will be of invaluable assistance to the non-prepared parturient as well. I believe that special training in monitricing should be an integral part of every labor and delivery nurse's training and certification is available through the Childbirth without Pain Education Association.

Specifically, the monitrice interprets the changes unique to each labor, reminds each woman of all that was taught during the Method classes, and suggests appropriate adaptations to be made as the labor progresses (Fig. 23-3). Her presence gives reassurance to the couple, helping them more easily adapt to the unfamiliar surroundings and activities.

* By Flora Hommel.

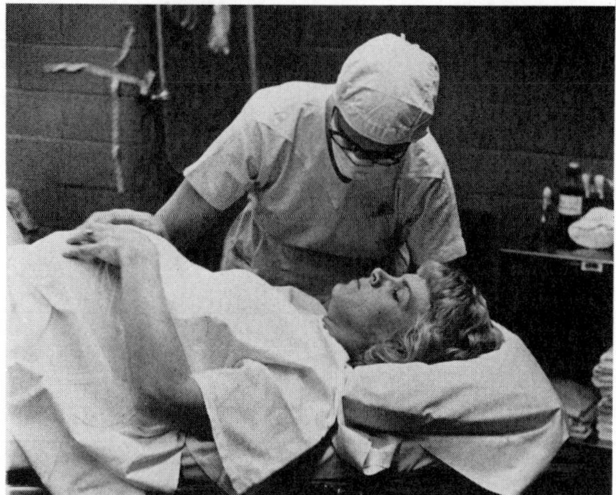

FIGURE 23-3. The nurse-monitrice acts as a coach-assistant during labor and birth. (Courtesy of Flora Hommel.)

The husband or father of the child is always considered to require the same kind of support as the woman, but will not be referred to throughout this section. It is generally preferable that the woman's mother *not* be allowed because of poor and negative conditioning. If, however, the mother or another person is permitted in the labor and delivery areas, great care must be taken to make sure negative conditioning is not reinforced by that person.

The monitrice will probably want to remind the woman of much of what has been previously discussed in this chapter.

Progress of effacement, dilatation, and descent are not usually uniform and regular throughout labor and plateaus may be reached for periods during labor while contractions progress. The woman must therefore not be allowed to become discouraged.

One such plateau may occur at about 3 to 4 centimeters of dilatation. Most labors seem to take a sharp turn which can be noted by the fact that prior to this period most women are excited and self-confident, but now they become anxious and concerned. Frequently at this point, artificial rupture of membranes is done by the doctor to speed up labor. The monitrice may note that this is a period when most non-prepared women request analgesics. Informative and encouraging words from the monitrice at this point can be critical to establish a calm and reassuring atmosphere. She should spend some time at this point helping the woman to adjust to this period in her labor. One of the most effective means is to help the woman take one contraction at a time, not worrying about future contractions. We often hear a psychoprophylactically prepared woman say at this point in labor, "I think I am going to need some medication." When we question her, we find she is not in pain, but is anticipating it, setting up a cycle of fear which leads to improper handling of contractions, which more importantly reinforces negative conditioning. Then once the adjustment has taken place, support from a monitrice is usually less crucial and perhaps not even required for most women until the period of transition.

The period of transition (from first to second stage) which normally starts around 7 centimeters of dilatation is usually the most difficult part of labor. The monitrice can remind the parturient that contractions are now at their apex and will not get longer, stronger, or closer. She should also help with comfort measures with many of the symptoms the woman is likely to experience and remind her of her adaptation. The woman should be reminded that she is on the top of the mountain, and once this part is over it will be downhill all the way.

The following are symptoms which may be perceived by the woman and/or the monitrice, not necessarily in order of importance:

1. Urge to push.
2. Backache. Relieved by pressure and perhaps by position change, cold or warm application.
3. Pressure of rectal area. She must not obey the reflex to hold in. This is pressure of baby, not bowel movement.
4. Trembling. It cannot be controlled. It may begin with labor and be a constant

stressor. Usually it occurs during the transitional period when the woman is 6 to 8 centimeters dilated. It may be due to a very rapid labor, although the etiology is unclear.

5. Sleepiness. May be from being awake for an extended period of time, but also because of increased body workload.
6. Mood changes. Keep perspective. She may exhibit any or all of the following behavior: irritability, meanness, crankiness, grouchiness, particularly toward husband (she may not notice, but he will). She will be less intelligent and seem dopey. She may feel panic or a desire to escape. She may have a loss of inhibitions, such as throwing off her clothes with the heat.
7. Stomach upset. Loud burps, as opposed to retained earlier ones, nausea and vomiting (like trembling this may occur all through labor).
8. Perspiration. The woman has been getting warmer with increased work of uterus, and is now *hot*. Relief is from cold washcloth on face.
9. Cold feet. Due to all circulation in uterus and upper body. A blanket may be placed over feet.

The monitrice should have the following perspectives. Time is the greatest enemy of good labor. Fatigue, both physical and emotional, is very detrimental. A normal primipara may take 24 hours, a multipara 12 hours. The woman should count on a long labor. Labor very often starts soon after retiring. She should count on this as well. The nesting reflex, like a bird hurriedly building a nest before laying her eggs, may be present and if followed will most certainly cause fatigue.

Help the woman work with the present during labor. She must not worry about the future. Let it take care of itself and it will! Deal with one contraction at a time. Make her proud of what she has done, not what she will do.

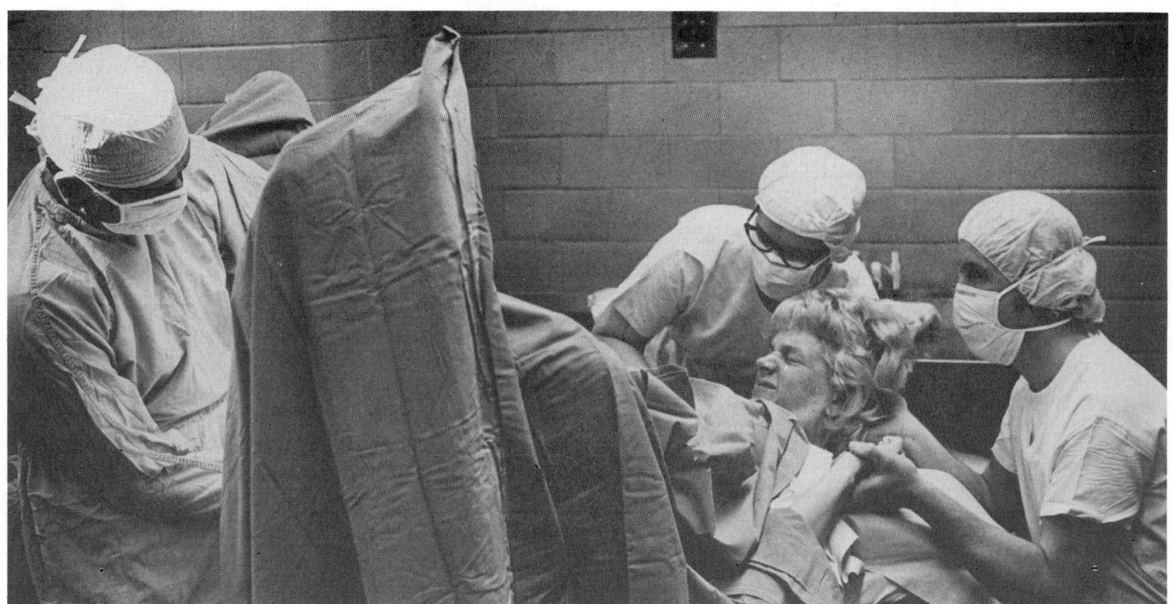

FIGURE 23-4. Woman receiving support during the second stage of labor. (Courtesy of Flora Hommel.)

The woman should be encouraged to trust her doctor, act as the patient's advocate. Interpret to the staff what the woman is attempting to accomplish and that she has medical cooperation and encouragement to do so.

The woman is working to get the best possible experience. If things do not work as planned or expected, she will still have achieved success. It will still be better than it would have been.

Progress in labor is not steady. There are plateaus. The woman must not be allowed to become discouraged.

Encouragement during this trying and difficult part of labor is made easier by reminding the parturient of what she is about to experience, e.g., a very good, satisfying and if psychoprophylactically prepared, painless period of the labor.

It is most helpful to move the multipara into the delivery room at the first strong reflex pushing contraction of transition. Psychoprophylactically prepared parturients generally go very quickly from this point on and moving earlier may allow delivery room preparation to be accomplished before the woman starts to push. Support from the monitrice in moving from labor room to delivery room is critical.

The second stage of labor is generally easier for the parturient and the husband and monitrice's job generally becomes less strenuous also. They maintain their effective support by reminding the woman of a good position for pushing (elbows out and head and shoulders raised) and by encouraging her efforts (Fig. 23-4).

The husband should be allowed and encouraged to assume as much coaching of his wife as is practical. If the husband is to be present in the delivery room, he should be properly gowned early in the second stage. He is positioned at his wife's head where he can continue to support her head and shoulders, and offers emotional support. In this position, they will be together as their child is born (Fig. 23-5).

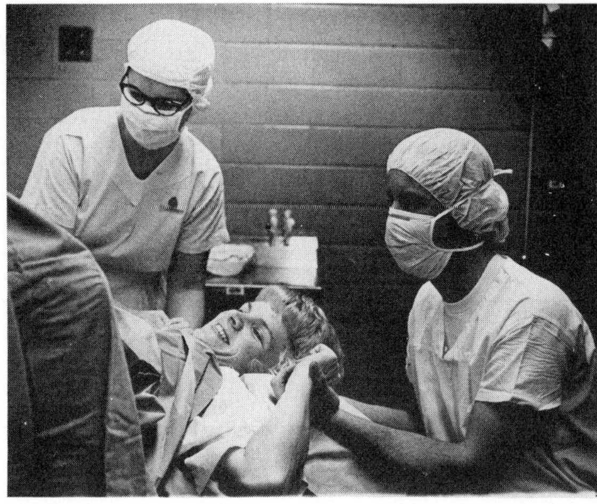

FIGURE 23-5. Husband providing support and encouragement to his wife as their child is delivered. (Courtesy of Flora Hommel.)

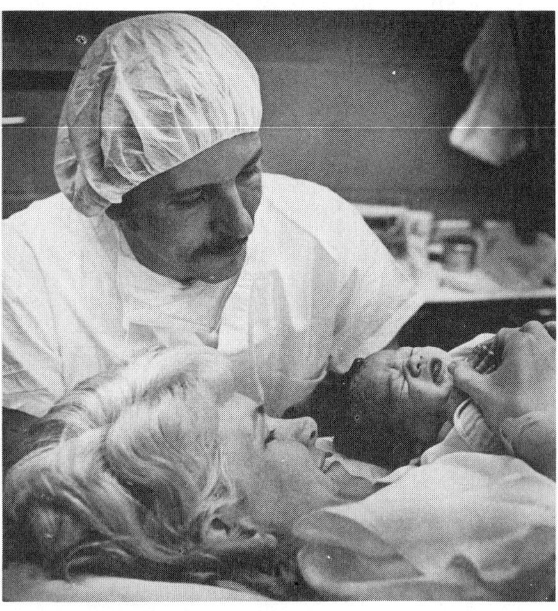

FIGURE 23-6. Success is the best experience labor will allow. (Courtesy of Flora Hommel.)

During the delivery the monitrice reminds the woman to stay relaxed, to pant and not to push. It may be necessary for her to breathe with the woman as she attains effective control during the birth.

Success is the best experience labor will allow (Fig. 23-6).

The Support System

A support system is a means of providing help because there is difficulty in handling the situation by one's self. When support is available, a woman (and husband or significant other) can emerge from labor with a sense of well-being, accomplishment, and a stronger self concept.

Supportive Role of the Nurse

Nursing provides support by developing a *helping relationship*. This relationship has two significant characteristics, as defined by Rogers[29] and Barrett-Lennard.[30] These are identified and applied to nursing in a labor-delivery setting as follows:

1. Empathy and Understanding
   Actions which help the nurse to be supportive through empathetic understanding are:

   Recognition of verbal and nonverbal behaviors indicative of stress and anxiety. Nurses need to appreciate subtle, nonverbal cues indicating stress and pleas for help. These may be more prevalent in foreign-born and highly anxious individuals who have more difficulty communicating their needs verbally.

   Exploration of stressors and pleasurable experiences during labor. The purpose here is to reduce stimuli which are stressful and to increase those which are pleasurable. Nurses need to help women identify and acknowledge their concerns and fears, and proceed to reduce them when possible. Assessment of the anxiety level is also important to determine if it is facilitating or inhibiting adaptation to labor. Nurses are cautioned not to be so preoccupied with stressors that they fail to reinforce stimuli which are pleasant and significant in helping the woman to continue through labor. Assessment for pleasant stimuli should explore what the woman feels happy or excited about during her labor.

   Defining who and what behaviors are perceived as supportive. It is imperative to assess who the woman desires for support. Hospitals usually allow husbands to be present. However, a woman may prefer a friend, relative, or the montrice because she feels they are better qualified to help. Women should also be asked what they expect from these persons and from the doctors and nurses. This will facilitate efforts to have reality and expectations coincide.

   Communicate to the woman and husband that their behaviors are legitimate and acceptable. This can be done verbally through comments such as, "It's all right. You're doing well." Verbal encouragement should be given from the beginning to the end of the labor. Women need to receive positive feedback on their performance periodically during labor. Nonverbal acceptance is conveyed by use of gentle touch, tone of voice, facial expressions, and the degree of physical closeness of the nurse. At times, coping behaviors are misunderstood and lead to negative labels, reprimands, or attempts to make one feel guilty or ashamed of the behaviors. Nurses can become advocates for the woman by explaining the significance of these behaviors and protecting the woman against interference with them.

2. Respect and Caring

   This implies that care is given regardless of the woman's reactions and that nothing is expected in return. It also means that help is provided through the availability of a human being and not a mechanical device. Actions which help the nurse to communicate care and respect are:

   Address woman and significant other by name
   Orient all to environment, staff, and procedures
   Acknowledge their behaviors as acceptable and significant
   Recognize their desired role of either independence or dependence
   Meet physical needs for comfort and safety without request
   Keep all informed of the status of the labor process
   Meet teaching-learning needs through explanations, demonstrations, and provision of feedback
   Allow participation in decisions
   Follow through with any commitments, such as promises of when the nurse will return
   Therapeutic use of self by the nurse—increase contact time proportionately with the anxiety level, and use touch and voice effectively to communicate that help is deserved and available.

Supportive Role of the Significant Other

Nurses have a responsibility to help other persons give support to the woman during labor. It is not unusual to find the husband off in a corner, far away from his wife, feeling tense and anxious. He may demonstrate his anxiety by aggressive or hostile comments, such as, "Why isn't anyone helping her?" Nurses must be aware that such behavior is significant and not retaliate with anger. The nurse can help the husband to approach his wife and also teach him measures which will help the woman relax and be more comfortable. Teaching is enhanced through demonstrations by the nurse. This allows the couple the benefits from the presence of the nurse for evaluation and feedback. Positive reinforcement and encouragement to ventilate feelings will communicate a sense of caring for the couple as a team.

Sometimes it is difficult to predict responses when a person watches a loved one experience stress and pain. The desire to escape and outbursts of anger are not uncommon when feelings of helplessness increase. The nurse needs to be observant of this person's reactions. Increased anxiety may result in unrealistic commands and demands on the woman in an attempt to be more forceful in the perceived helping role. A husband may scold his wife when she is not able to complete a breathing exercise as he commanded. The nurse should intervene to protect the woman from such demands through explanations and encouragement that she is doing a great job and trying very hard. Sometimes a husband becomes so anxious that he can no longer perform simple supportive acts, such as holding his wife's hand. Nursing intervention is to remove him from the situation in such a way as to protect him from "losing face" in front of his wife and suffering the effects of a threatened self concept. Removal can be done graciously by suggesting that he take a break to eat or drink something and relax for a while. The nurse then replaces him in the supportive role to prevent feelings of desertion on his part as well as the woman's. As soon as possible, the nurse should discuss the situation with him in private. She should encourage him to express his feelings about his behavior as well as that of his wife.

Facilitating the Immediate Maternal-Infant Claiming Process

One of the most significant events a woman must cope with during the final phase of the labor experience is to integrate the reality of producing a child. The woman may need to have concrete evidence that the baby is really present and to explore the newly produced being in an attempt to test reality against one's expectation and fantasies. Nurses can facilitate this process in the delivery room as soon as the baby is born. Every attempt should be made to allow the woman to see, touch, and listen to the baby. This process should be void of judgmental comments frequently made by the staff, such as, "Here is your cute girl," or "You're lucky, she's a healthy girl." Such comments may inhibit the woman's spontaneous expression of how she perceives the baby at this initial contact. She may not view the baby as being "cute" but may be unable to share her true feelings for fear of reprisals. Women should also be allowed to explore their newborns through touch and/or sight, as they desire at that time. Too often, the staff will present a tightly wrapped baby with just a head visible. This may not seem like a whole, complete baby and may make it difficult for the woman to convince herself that she did produce a complete baby. The mother may also be concerned about missing parts of the body unless she can see them for herself. The nurse should listen carefully to the mother's initial verbal comments. If she expresses concerns about the baby's color, activity, or cry, the nurse can offer explanations immediately to prevent fears about abnormalities. This facilitating process should occur at the pace the mother sets by her degree of willingness and interest in the baby. Nurses should not impose the baby on the mother. Fatigue, preoccupation with events during delivery, and grieving over a child of the undesired sex are factors which inhibit this claiming process. In such cases, nursing intervention should focus on the mother and her feelings, instead of the new baby.

Integrating the Labor Experience Into a Meaningful Whole

Assisting the woman and family to find meaning in the labor experience is another significant nursing goal. We are all products of our past and present life experiences and their impact affects our present and future growth and development. It has been stated that growth is possible with healthy resolution of a crisis situation because the individual gains better intellectual understanding of his situation and is able to identify his feelings, coping patterns, and available situational supports. It is imperative for nurses to value this concept because after childbirth a woman is forced to face the responsibilities of multiple roles as defined by society, such as woman, mother, wife, and career woman. She is better able to meet these multiple demands when she has ego integrity from a sense of achievement and worth rather than ego disintegration due to feelings of shame, guilt, and low self-esteem. Therefore, nursing actions must help mothers to integrate the entire labor experience into a meaningful whole. Women need to be encouraged to express their feelings about their behaviors and have their questions answered. If feedback is withheld she may resort to fantasies or distortions about her perceived behaviors. When feedback is given it should emphasize the positive aspects and thus enhance the self concept instead of minimizing its importance. Nurses must understand that the process of integrating all the pieces of the labor experience occurs over a time period and women may ask repeatedly for feedback already given by the nurse. Patience and the ability to communicate without judgmental overtones, either verbal or nonverbal, is essential. In situations in which the mother has no one available to talk to or is reluctant to express her feelings to another person, suggest that she write her experiences down in any form she desires and/or record them on a tape recorder. These means will allow her to read her words or hear herself as often as needed to help her integrate the experience.

Coping Behaviors

Appropriate nursing actions during the labor experience depend on the recognition and assessment of coping behaviors. Table 23-1 presents a guide which was developed to help nurses recognize behaviors reflecting adequate and inadequate coping during the various phases of labor.[31] Adequate coping behaviors are those which do not interfere with the labor process but facilitate the woman's movement into another phase. Less desirable are behaviors resulting from increased anxiety which create physical and psychologic fatigue and interfere with labor and the process of maternal adaptation. Appropriate nursing actions are suggested to reinforce or modify behaviors.

TABLE 23-1. Recognition of Coping Behaviors during Labor

Latent Phase (0–3 cm.)
Impact of Stressors: Minimal
Contractions not intense in frequency or duration
Anxiety level usually mild; enhances perception, learning, and problem-solving
Increased anxiety usually develops from stressors in environment, distorted perceptions of labor, and expectations unmet

Behaviors	*Significance*	*Role of Nurse*
Adequate Coping Behaviors		
1. Healthy use of defenses Smiling, laughing, crying Increased activity, appears hyperactive Talkative, spontaneous verbal expression a. Volunteers information freely b. Asks questions Able to focus on others besides self (husband, children)	These are attempts to release the surge of energy generated by excitement or relief about being in labor. Increased energy can be a preparatory stimulus for the forthcoming labor and birth. Verbal expressions help to integrate the reality of what is happening. Focus on others reasserts the significance of the event to individuals viewed as supportive.	Listen, do not minimize her comments; do not interrupt her spontaneity. Give her your attention and provide eye contact.
2. Desires to exert an independent role Able to meet essential bodily needs (can go to the bathroom instead of using bedpan) Wants to be included in decision-making (desires to be given choices instead of commands) Seeks information about status of her situation (wants to be informed of events happening	Independence reaffirms confidence in the self to maintain control. The ability to meet one's needs and to make decisions is the validation that one is not helpless.	Allow her to participate in her care; allow her to make decisions. Provide her with positive feedback regarding her progress. Prepare her for anticipated procedures.
3. Able to utilize previous coping patterns (e.g., use of rocking brings comfort from pain, crying brings feelings of relief, rationalization eases tension.)	Familiar coping behaviors have previously been tested to prove their effectiveness. Tension is released as these measures continue to bring the expected relief from discomfort.	Do not interfere with her efforts to cope, e.g., do not ask questions while she is using controlled breathing during a contraction.

TABLE 23-1. *Continued*

Behaviors	*Significance*	*Role of Nurse*
4. Able to initiate newly learned techniques independently and is motivated to continue their use (e.g., breathing and relaxations techniques are done well without the need to be stimulated or reinforced by others).	Confidence and trust increases as one utilizes measures for relief without undue tension or strain on the self.	Praise her when you see her do things successfully. Tell her you're proud she is in control of her situation.
Less Desirable Coping Behaviors (relate to impact of increased anxiety)		
Preoccupation with isolated details such as contractions, time, procedures, or fears Increase in perception of dangers and threats. This leads rapidly to fears for the self, baby, and of the unknown Use of defense mechanisms which further distort perceptions from reality and increase feelings of helplessness in attempts to cope (e.g., aggression, hostility, fantasizing, withdrawal)	Perceptual disturbances augment the stress of stimuli making the labor situation seem insurmountable to cope with. Increased discomforts are perceived which make further demands on energy available for coping.	Assessment: What are anxiety-producing factors? Major sources in the latent phase are factors in the environment such as procedures and behaviors of the staff. Remain with patient as much as possible until anxiety is at a lower level.

Active Phase (4–7 cm.)
Impact of Stressors: Contractions intensify pain experience
Increased fatigue
Situation of mind is ready to tackle the problem but body had decreased energy for coping

Behaviors	*Significance*	*Role of Nurse*
Adequate Coping		
1. Decreased responsiveness to the environment Less talking, activity decreases, becomes serious and determined, preoccupation with the self and the labor process, communication patterns become more reactions and responses instead of initiation of interactions	Attempt to redirect energy towards coping instead of nonessential activities as talking, laughing, etc.	Do not expect woman to initiate conversations with you as she did previously. Provide "quiescence" environment.
2. Dependency needs manifested Frequent demands, complaints, or obsequious behaviors Decreased ability to meet essential bodily needs	Feelings of increased helplessness creates the need to be sustained by another human being. Dependency is a means of receiving help as well as maintaining human contact with others.	Meet those requests and demands as courteously as possible. Don't retaliate with aggression.
3. Behaviors indicate stress and a desire for its relief, especially in terms of anxiety and pain Autonomic reactions to stress (↑ heart rate, ↑ respirations, dilated pupils, diaphoresis)	The increased anxiety is an attempt to prepare the body for a fight or flight against the stressors. However, it intensifies sensations of discomforts and pain. There is a need for help in decreasing or eliminating stressful stimu-	Relieve additional discomforts from such reactions by using: Facial sponges Dry clothing Back rubs Straighten sheets

TABLE 23-1. *Continued*

Behaviors	*Significance*	*Role of Nurse*
Skeletal muscle reactions (grimaces, facial expressions, gripping bedrails, rigid positioning) Restlessness, agitation, frequent changes in position Verbalizations indicating fears, suffering, and pleas for help	li. Verbal and nonverbal behaviors are a means of communicating pleas.	Stay with patient as much as possible.
4. Decreased ability to implement coping actions Concentration on coping may decrease or be hindered by the multitude of stressors (may begin a breathing exercise but have difficulty completing it) Becomes a "follower" instead of initiator (easier to be reminded as to what to do instead of having to recall)	With stress accumulating over a period of time, fatigue and tension inhibits cognitive thought processes. This will deteriorate efforts to problem-solve. An important need is to receive feedback from others in recognition of coping efforts.	Do not make demands on woman. Do not ask her to make major decisions on her own. Example, This is not the best time to ask what type of anesthesia she prefers for delivery.
5. Anger and aggression may appear Vulgar verbalization Physical assaults on others Demoralizing others	Means to depreciate others in an attempt to protect the self. The blame and anger for feelings of losing control are placed on others instead of the self.	Allow the behaviors; do not take it as a personal assault on you; do not retaliate.
Less Desirable Behaviors (perpetuate cognitive disturbances as well as feelings of isolation and abandonment)		
Fantasy, regression, denial	Attempts to escape by denying the reality of the stressors.	Remain with patient. Reorient her to reality in terms of person, place, time (who she is, where she is, what is happening). Give her a sense of worth: Positively reinforce her; no behavior should be reprimanded Tell her she can complete the process; you'll help her to do it
Withdrawal	Increases feelings of isolation leading to a sense of worthlessness or insignificance.	
Depression	Lack of confidence and feelings of hopelessness about one's ability to complete the labor process.	

Transitional and Second Stages (8 cm. to birth of baby)
Impact of Stressors: Fatigue and exhaustion predominant
Forced participation by women, either to push or pant for controlled delivery

Behaviors	*Significance*	*Role of Nurse*
Adequate Coping Behaviors		
1. Withdrawal from the environment Less responsive to questions Decreased ability to attend to events or engage in lengthy conversations	The woman has been working hard for a period of time and must still face the task of delivery. Therefore, coping behaviors reflect a more deliberate at-	Let her rest between contractions. Make no demands on her. Praise her participation through efforts to "push or pant."

TABLE 23-1. *Continued*

Behaviors	*Significance*	*Role of Nurse*
Decreased interest in making decisions, usually stating, "It doesn't matter," when her opinions are sought Less awareness of stimuli, even those which are stressful Frequent dozing between contractions—periodic sleep Episodes of amnesia between contractions	tempt to conserve energy. Also, activation and responses to stress cannot continue indefinitely. As time goes on, the body cannot sustain the fight or flight reactions and responses to stress diminish. This is manifested by decreased response to stressful stimuli. The stimuli which arouse the woman back to awareness of her environment are contractions.	
2. Aggressive behaviors such as clawing, physical assaults, fighting back, uncooperative	Desperate attempts to prevent pain and loss of control. To protect the self, anger and aggression are redirected to others.	Accept such behaviors.
Less Desirable Behaviors Panic, uncontrollable behaviors. Withdrawal to the point of not responding even to strong commands on physical stimuli Verbal expressions of "giving up" "I can't go on" "I won't make it through"	Feelings of a loss of control lead to hopelessness and desires to abandon coping behaviors. Death fears may elicit panic-type behaviors as an attempt to fight off the possibility of dying.	Remain with patient. Get her attention and communicate that she is not alone. Communicate a sense of progress, that all hope is not lost. Must reduce anxiety level.

Third and Fourth Stages (delivery of the placenta to immediate stabilizing period post-delivery)

Impact of Stressors: Stress diminishes returning to a state resembling latent phase.
If a normal delivery has occurred, fears for the self and baby are eliminated.
If complications occurred, situational crises will impose upon the existing stress.
Coping behaviors are similar to those in latent phase. Once again the woman can be seen talking, laughing, crying, and focusing on others besides the self. She becomes more alert and responsive.

Two significant events to cope with emerge in these stages.
1. The reality of producing a child must be faced.
2. The entire labor experience must be integrated into a meaningful whole.

Behaviors	*Significance*	*Role of Nurse*
Adequate Coping Behaviors 1. Confirm the reality of producing a new baby Attempts to see, touch and listen for sounds by the baby Questions the behaviors and appearance of baby Seeks reassurance from others that baby is normal and healthy	Efforts to validate that the baby is really present. Exploration through touch and questions is a means to test reality against one's expectations and fantasies.	Allow woman to have contact with baby in delivery room through sight, touch, breast feeding or anything else she requests. Answer questions about newborn confidently.
2. Integrate the entire labor into a meaningful experience Frequent questions about performance and events which occurred	This process allows data collection about events and behaviors during labor. It helps clarify or provide "missing pieces" of the experience which	Listen; answer questions. Give opportunity to express self, such as, "What was labor and delivery like for you?" Tell her she

TABLE 23-1. *Continued*

Behaviors	*Significance*	*Role of Nurse*
Dreams and preoccupation with the labor Spontaneous and frequent expression on feelings about labor Frequent recall of events remembered vividly Rationalization or apology for coping behaviors when they are perceived as less than desirable Frequent repetition of the above may occur.	were forgotten or confusing. Now the the woman can evaluate and make judgments concerning her performance during labor. When the conclusion is positive, this increases respect and confidence in the self, allowing a woman growth and development through labor. When the reverse occurs, labor is threatening to the self. Women manifest a need to express themselves and may do so to anyone available, e.g., cleaning lady, technicians, nurses, doctors, visitors. Repetition allows reorganization of content until it becomes meaningful to the woman. It also allows her to hear herself. This helps her to synthesize and accept the event that has occurred.	doesn't need to apologize for her behaviors. Don't get upset when she repeats her stories or asks the same questions. If you can't be with her make the following suggestions: Write feelings down Record feelings on a tape recorder (These suggestions are also helpful when she's home and may have a need to express herself.)

REFERENCES

1. Colman A.: *Psychological state during first pregnancy.* Am. J. Orthopsychiatry 39:795, 1969.
2. Pleshette, N., Asch, S. and Chase, J.: *A study of anxieties during pregnancy, labor and late puerperium.* Bull. N. Y. Acad. Med. 32:436, 1956.
3. Kartchner, F.: *A study of the emotional reactions during labor.* Am. J. Obst. Gynecol. 60:19, 1950.
4. Lane, V. and Williams, B. (eds.): *Parents' Perceptions of Pregnancy, Labor and Delivery.* Project in Nursing Education and Research, Southern Regional Educational Board, Georgia, 1966.
5. Shainess, N.: *Psychologic experience of labor.* N. Y. State J. Med. 2923, 1963.
6. Affonso, D., *Response to pain in the experience of labor in a specific culture of Hawaii.* In *Impact of Culture and Childbearing and Childrearing.* University of Hawaii, Honolulu, 1975, p. 89.
7. Delmendo, D.: *Exploration of attitudes toward labor in the postpartum and non-pregnant woman.* Unpublished undergraduate honors thesis, University of Hawaii, Honolulu, 1966.
8. Botella-Jose, L.: *Obstetrical Endocrinology.* Charles C Thomas, Springfield, Ill., 1961. pp. 118- 119.
9. Bonica, J.: *An atlas on the mechanisms and pathways of pain in labor.* What's New 217:16, 1960.
10. *Programmed Instruction on Pain—Part I.* Am. J. Nurs. 66:1099, 1966.
11. McCaffery, M.: *Nursing Management of the Patient with Pain.* J. B. Lippincott, Philadelphia, 1972, p. 5.
12. Deutsch, H.: *Psychology of Women, vol. I.* Grune and Stratton, New York, 1945, p. 203.
13. Affonso: op. cit.
14. Pleshette: op. cit.
15. Deutsch: op. cit.
16. Caplan, G.: *Psychological aspects of maternity care.* Am. J. Public Health 47:25, 1957.
17. Larsen, V.: *Stresses of the childbearing year.* Am. J. Public Health 56:32, 1966.
18. Klein, H., Potter, H. and Dyk, R.: *Anxiety in Pregnancy and Childbirth.* Paul Hoeber, New York, 1950.
19. Derschimer, F.: *Influence of mental attitudes in childbearing.* Am. J. Obst. Gynecol. 31:447, 1936.
20. Caplan: op. cit.
21. Allen, S.: *Nurse attendance during labor.* Am. J. Nurs. 64:74, 1964.
22. Affonso, D.: *Assessment of pain during labor.* In Anderson, E., et al. (eds.): *Current Concepts in Clinical Nursing, vol. IV.* C. V. Mosby Company, St. Louis, 1973.
23. Melzack, R. and Wall, P. D.: *Gate control theory of pain.* In Soulairac, A., et al. (eds.): *Pain.* Proceedings of the International Symposium on Pain organized by the Laboratory of Psychophysiology, Faculty of Sciences, Paris, 1967. Academic Press, London, 1968, p. 29.
24. McCafferty: op. cit., pp. 121-125, 139, 189.
25. McCafferty: ibid.
26. Danforth, D. (ed.): *Textbook of Obstetrics and*

Gynecology, ed. 2. Harper and Row, New York, 1971, p. 587.
27. McCaffery: loc. cit.
28. Ibid.
29. Rogers, C.: *The Characteristics of a Helping Relationship*. Canada's Mental Health Supplement, March, 1962.
30. Barrett-Lennard, G. T.: *Significant Aspects of a Helping Relationship*. Canada's Mental Health Supplement, No. 47, July-Aug., 1965.
31. Affonso, D.: *Coping Behaviors during Labor*. In Clinical Conference Papers 1973. American Nurse Asso., Kansas City, 1975, p. 124.

BIBLIOGRAPHY

Affonso, D.: *Assessment of pain during labor*. In Anderson, E., et al. (eds.): *Current Concepts in Clinical Nursing, vol. IV*. C. V. Mosby, St. Louis, 1973.

Ammon, L. L., et al.: *Expressions of hostility in early labor*. Matern.-Child Nurs. J. 2:215, 1973.

Bardon, D.: *Psychological implications of provision for childbirth*. Lancet 2:555, 1973.

Bonica, J.: *An atlas on the mechanisms and pathways of pain in labor*. What's New 217:16, 1960.

Botella-Jose, L.: *Obstetrical Endocrinology*. Charles C Thomas, Springfield, Ill., pp. 118, 119, 1961.

Bradley, R.: *Father's presence in delivery rooms*. Psychosomatics, 3:474, 1962.

Brown, W. A., et al.: *Prenatal psychological state and the use of drugs in labor*. Am. J. Obstet. Gynecol. 113:598, 1972.

Ibid: *The relationship of antenatal and prenatal psychologic variables to the use of drugs in labor*. Psychosomatic Med. 34:119, 1972.

Burnstein, I., et al.: *Anxiety, pregnancy, labor and the neonate*. Am. J. Obstet. Gynecol. 118:195, 1974.

Buten, J.: *A Philosophy of Labor and Delivery Nursing*. In Anderson, E., et al. (eds.). *Current Concepts in Clinical Nursing*. C. V. Mosby, St. Louis, 1973.

Cassidy, J. E.: *A nurse looks at childbirth anxiety*. J. Obstet. Gynec. Nurs. 3:52, 1974.

Danforth, D. (ed.): *Textbook of Obstetrics and Gynecology*, ed. 2. Harper and Row, New York, 1971.

Estey, J.: *Natural childbirth—word from a mother*. Am. J. Nurs. 69:1453, 1969.

Farill, A.: *Adolescent in labor*. Am. J. Nurs. 68:195, 1968.

Friedman, D.: *Parturiphobia*. Am. J. Obstet. Gynecol. 118:130, 1974.

Goetsch, C.: *Fathers in the delivery room—helpful and supportive*. Hosp. Top. 44:104, 1966.

Haase, M. N.: *Giving supportive care during labor: A rewarding experience for nurse*. Hosp. Top. 49:47, 1971.

Hellman, L. M. and Pritchard, J. A.: *Williams Obstetrics*, ed. 14. Appleton-Century-Crofts, New York, 1971.

Hoff, J.: *Natural childbirth—how any nurse can help*. Am. J. Nurs. 69:1451, 1969.

Hommel, F.: *Natural childbirth—nurses in private practice in Monitrices*. Am. J. Nurs. 69:1446, 1969.

Horan, J. J.: *"In vivo" emotive imagery: A technique for reducing childbirth anxiety and discomfort*. Psychol. Rep. 32:1328, 1973.

Kartchner, F.: *A study of the emotional reactions during labor*. Am. J. Obstet. Gynecol. 60:19, 1950.

Keaveney, M. E.: *Supporting the Lamaze patient in labor*. Nurs. Care 6:15, 1973.

Kemp, J.: *The dignity of labour*. Nurs. Times 66:1436, 1970.

Klein, H., Potter, H. and Dyk, R.: *Anxiety in Pregnancy and Childbirth*. Paul Hoeber, 1950.

Kopp, L. M.: *Ordeal or ideal—the second stage of labor*. Am. J. Nurs. 71:1140, 1971.

Lane, V. and Williams B. (eds.): *Parents' Perceptions of Pregnancy, Labor, and Delivery*. Project in Nursing Education and Research, Southern Regional Educational Board, Georgia, 1966.

Montgomery, E.: *Coping with pain—felt or fancied*. Midwives Chronicle 83:248, 1970.

Newton, N.: *Childbirth and culture*. Psychology Today 4:74, 1970.

Passim, J.: *The nursing challenges of obstetric anxiety, ectasy, and the nurse's role*. Superv. Nurse 3:36, 1972.

Pleshette, N., Asch, S. and Chase, J.: *A study of anxieties during pregnancy, labor, and the early and late puerperium*. Bull. N.Y. Acad. Med. 32:436, 1956.

Post, J. A.: *Expectations and reality in the expected day of confinement of a primigravida*. Matern.-Child Nurs. J. 1:87, 1972.

Price, H. V.: *Programmed instruction on pain—part I*. Am. J. Nurs. 66:1099, 1966.

Rich, O.: *How does the patient use the nurse during labor*. In Duffey, M., et al. (eds.): *Current Concepts in Clinical Nursing, vol. III*. C. V. Mosby St. Louis, pp. 189–193, 1971.

Turbeville, J.: *Nurses' role in intrapartum care*. Hosp. Top., 50(6):85, 1972.

Tyron, P.: *Assessing the progress of labor through observation of patients' behavior*. Nurs. Clin. North Am. 3:315, 1968.

Ibid.: *Use of comfort measures as support during labor*. Nurs. Res. 15:109, 1966.

Van Muiswinkel, J.: *Support in labor*. Matern.-Child Nurs. J. 1:273, 1972.

Winget, C., et al.: *The relationship of the manifest content of dreams to duration of childbirth in primiparae*. Psychosom. Med. 34:313, 1972.

24 *Maternal-Fetal Accommodation*

Dyanne D. Affonso, R.N., M.N.

The accommodation of the maternal host and the fetus in preparation for birth involves a series of processes called *parturition*. Parturition, synonymous with the term labor, is defined as the series of events by which the products of conception (fetus, amniotic fluid, placenta, and membranes) are separated and expelled from the uterus into the vaginal canal and out of the maternal body. The following terms are used in reference to the person experiencing this process:

Parturient: The woman in labor

Parous: Having given birth, vaginally or abdominally, at or beyond 20 weeks of gestation

Parity: Refers to the number of above deliveries, whether live birth, single or multiple, stillbirth, vaginal or cesarean section

Nullipara: A woman who has had no deliveries at or beyond 20 weeks of gestation

Primipara: A woman who has had one delivery at or beyond 20 weeks of gestation

Multipara: A woman who has had more than one delivery at or beyond 20 weeks of gestation

Gravida: Refers to the total number of pregnancies, regardless of the result of the pregnancy, e.g., abortion

To illustrate the use of these terms, let us examine a patient who has had one abortion, delivered a viable male, had one ectopic pregnancy, and delivered viable twins by cesarean section. After the abortion she was gravida 1, para 0. Delivering the viable male added both a gravida and a parity, resulting in gravida 2, para 1. The ectopic pregnancy added another gravida but no parity, resulting in gravida 3, para 1. The viable twins via cesarean section added one more pregnancy and one parity, despite the multiple births. Thus, this woman's obstetric history is gravida 4, para 2.

THEORIES OF ONSET OF LABOR

Explanations regarding the cause for the onset of labor are varied and remain largely theoretical assumptions. Several theories relate the onset of labor to *myometrial stimulating agents*. These are substances which cause the myometrial muscle of the uterus to contract. One such substance is oxytocin, a hormone which is believed to increase just before the pregnancy comes to term and initiate labor due to its contractile activity on the myometrium.[1] Another source of myometrial stimulating activity relates to the estrogenic hormones. It is known that estrogen production reaches a maximum before labor. Progesterone, a hormone which blocks the myometrial contracting activity, diminishes before labor and thus allows estrogen dominance which stimulates contractions.[2] Another more recently discovered stimulant of myometrial activity is a substance called prostaglandin. One of the actions of this substance is stimulation of smooth muscles to contract, especially in the myometrium and gastrointestinal tract.[3]

Another group of theories focuses on the stretching of the uterus. It is believed that any hollow organ, such as the uterus, tends to contract and empty itself when distended. With progression of pregnancy, uterine distention increases and becomes the stimulus for the onset of labor.[4] This theory has given some basis to the earlier onset of labor with multiple pregnancies and polyhydramnios.

PREPARATION FOR LABOR

There are certain phenomena which occur prior to the onset of labor as preparation for the process. These include:

Lightening. This refers to the settling of the presenting part of the fetus into the maternal pelvis. It usually occurs two to four weeks prior to labor in the primigravida but may not occur until labor begins in the multigravida. The presenting part of the fetus does not merely fall into the pelvis but assumes this position through uterine myometrial contractile activity pulling against the pericervical axis and supports. Lightening is a subjective sensation felt by women, and can occur gradually over a period of days or suddenly with a perceptible thud. The woman is usually aware of its occurrence because it is accompanied with ease in breathing due to lack of pressure by the uterus upon the diaphragm. Increased urinary frequency and constipation also occur due to the increased pelvic pressure.

Braxton Hicks Contractions. These are rhythmic tightenings of the uterus (contractions) which are irregular in frequency, intensity, duration, and are usually painless. However, they may become increasingly painful with succeeding pregnancies in the multipara. Braxton Hicks contractions become prominent in the last six weeks of pregnancy in the primigravida but may begin as early as the sixth month in the multipara. They occur as part of the preparatory changes for labor. With time, these contractions become better coordinated to effect changes in the cervix.

Cervical Effacement. This is the process whereby the cervix becomes soft and thin (Fig. 24-1). The cervix is usually thick and rigid prior to effacement and cannnot be dilated forcibly without tearing. Contractions of the uterine myometrium pull the cervix upward resulting in the thinning of the cervix's dense fibrous connective tissue, making it shorter, softer, and more pliable (Fig. 24-2). In the primigravida, effacement usually precedes dil-

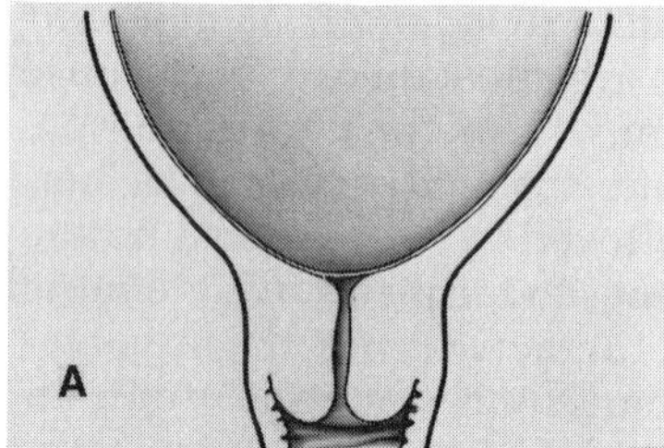

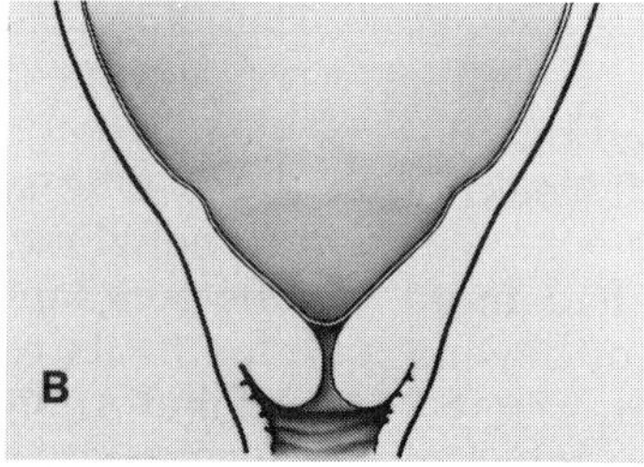

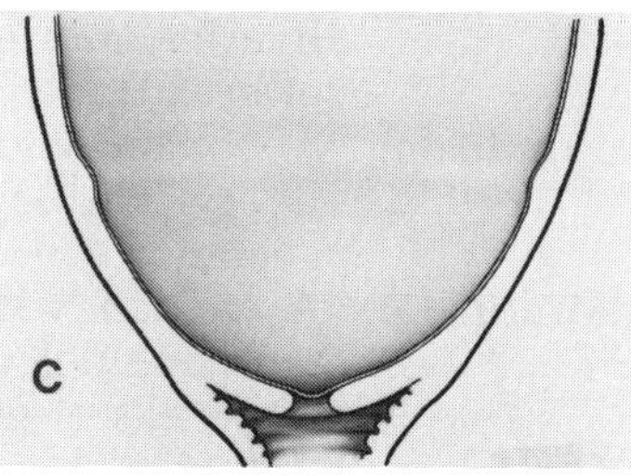

FIGURE 24-1. Cervical effacement. *A*, Thickness and length of the cervix before effacement. *B*, Cervix becomes shorter as uterine contractions pull the fibers upward. *C*, Cervix is soft and thin (completely dilated) and ready for dilatation. (Courtesy of Ross Laboratories.)

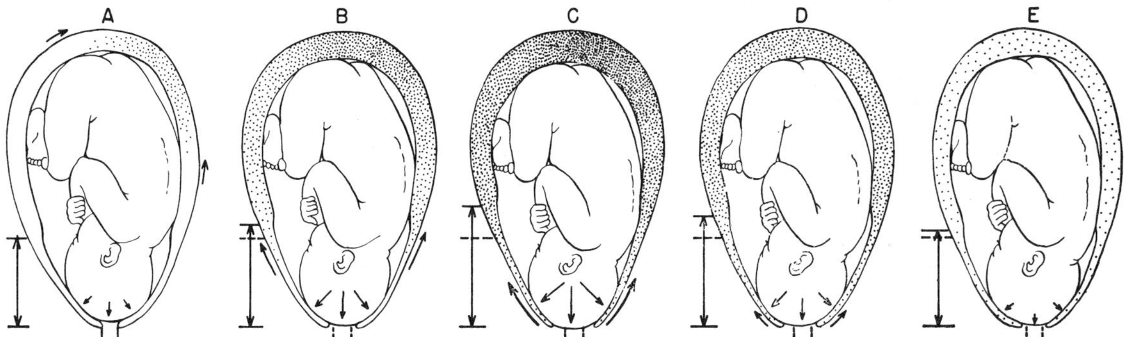

FIGURE 24-2. Frontal sections of the uterus corresponding to successive stages from the beginning to the end of a uterine contraction. The dotted area indicates the part which is contracted and the density of the dots represents the intensity of the contraction. The arrows at the head of the fetus show the pressure exerted by the head on the cervix. The arrows on the outside of the uterus indicate the traction exerted by the contracted parts, while the vertical arrows indicate the length of the lower uterine segment. Note that as the intensity of the contraction increases the length of the segment increases and the cervix becomes dilated. With a regression of the contraction these changes regress, but not to the original point. As a result, the upper segment remains shorter and thicker than before the contraction, while the cervix becomes more effaced and dilated and the lower uterine segment becomes thinner and longer. The upper segment shortens without losing its ability to contract (brachystasis) and the lower segment lengthens without changing its tension (mecystasis). (From Bonica, J.: *Principles and Practice of Obstetric Analgesia and Anesthesia.* F. A. Davis, Philadelphia, 1972, with permission.)

atation, often occurring in the beginning phase of labor. In the multigravida, the cervix may be slightly dilated before complete effacement occurs. This is attributed to the cervix never returning to its completely closed, prepregnant state once delivery has occurred.

Increased Vaginal Secretions. These are due to the congestion of the vaginal mucous membranes.

Presence of Bloody Show. This is blood in the vaginal secretions due to the rupture of the superficial blood vessels by the increased pelvic pressure.

Increased Backache and Sacroiliac Pressure. This is due to the relaxation of the pelvic joints by the hormone relaxin.

Frequency of Urination. This is caused by pressure of the presenting part of the fetus on the bladder, especially when lightening has occurred.

Weight Loss of One to Three Pounds. This is due to fluid loss as the result of electrolyte shifts produced by changes in estrogen and progesterone levels.[5]

STAGES AND PHASES OF LABOR

The complex processes of labor can best be understood in terms of the physiologic activities occurring during the various stages and phases.

STAGES OF LABOR

There are four stages of labor. The *first stage, stage of dilatation*, begins with the onset of regular uterine contractions and ends with the complete dilatation of the cervix. The completely dilated cervix is 10 cm. in width. The main goal is the shortening, thinning, softening (effacement) and opening (dilatation) of the cervix. The *second stage, stage of expulsion or delivery*, begins with the complete dilatation of the cervix and ends with the birth of the baby. The main goals are descent of the presenting part lower into the pelvis and fetal rotations or maneuvers to accommodate his body (usually the head) to the defined

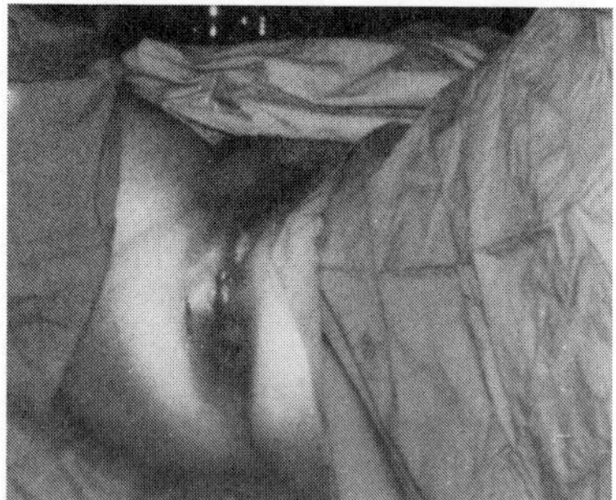

FIGURE 24-3. Second stage of labor. Note bulging of the perineum. The anus is dilated and the labia are being forced apart. (Courtesy of Dennis and Judi Christopherson.)

passage of the pelvis and out through the vaginal canal (Fig. 24-3). The *third stage, placental stage,* begins after the complete birth of the baby and ends with the delivery of the placenta. The goal is the separation and expulsion of the placenta.

The *fourth stage, immediate recovery period*, begins after the expulsion of the placenta and lasts for at least one hour. This first hour is critical in assessment of the body's immediate reactions and adaptation to the events of labor and delivery. The goal is to prevent uterine atony which predisposes to hemorrhage and infection. Some extend the fourth stage until that time, when the woman stabilizes her vital signs, especially blood pressure readings, and her uterus remains contracted and lochia flow is not heavy. Until these stabilizing signs are manifested, the woman may be viewed as being in the fourth stage of labor, regardless of amount of time since completed delivery.

PHASES OF LABOR

There are three distinct phases of labor, all occurring during the first stage. The phases supply important data to predict whether or not a woman is making normal progress in labor. They are also useful in predicting the patient's ability to cope with the multitude of stressors, such as pain and anxiety, so that intervention can be appropriately implemented.

The first phase, the *latent phase*, begins with the onset of regular contractions and heralds the beginning dilatation of the cervix usually resulting in 2 to 3 cm. of dilatation. It constitutes the longest phase of labor in which effacement is completed and dilatation is established. During this phase patients are usually happy and eager to be in labor. They are comfortable and can relate well to the environment. The average duration of this phase is 8.6 hours for primigravidas and 5.3 hours for multigravidas[6] (Fig. 24-4).

The next phase is called the *active phase* in which dilatation is accelerated until the cervix is almost completely dilated, resulting in 8 cm. of dilatation. Uterine contractions are now stronger, last longer, and come at frequent intervals. These contractions make possible a maximum rate of dilatation in this phase. The patient may feel nauseated and may vomit. She becomes increasingly restless, her breathing is labored with a tendency toward hyperventilation, and she is uncomfortable. The contractions now become a pain source and a major stressor for the patient. The average length of this phase is four hours for a primigravida and two hours for a multigravida.[7]

When the patient is 8 cm. dilated she enters the *transitional phase*. This is a very difficult time for most women. She may be fatigued and exhausted from the previous hours of labor. Her face may be flushed, with beads of perspiration due to the increased basal metabolic rate of the body and dissemination of heat and waste products via the skin. She may complain of shaking, chills, nausea, and vomiting, probably due to reflex stimulation from the uterine contractions. She may feel as if she needs to defecate due to increased pressure of the presenting part on the large intestine and colon stimulating the urge to defecate. She is restless and in the height of her pain experience because the uterine contractions stretch, distend, and put pressure upon the surrounding structures of the uterus and perineum. During this

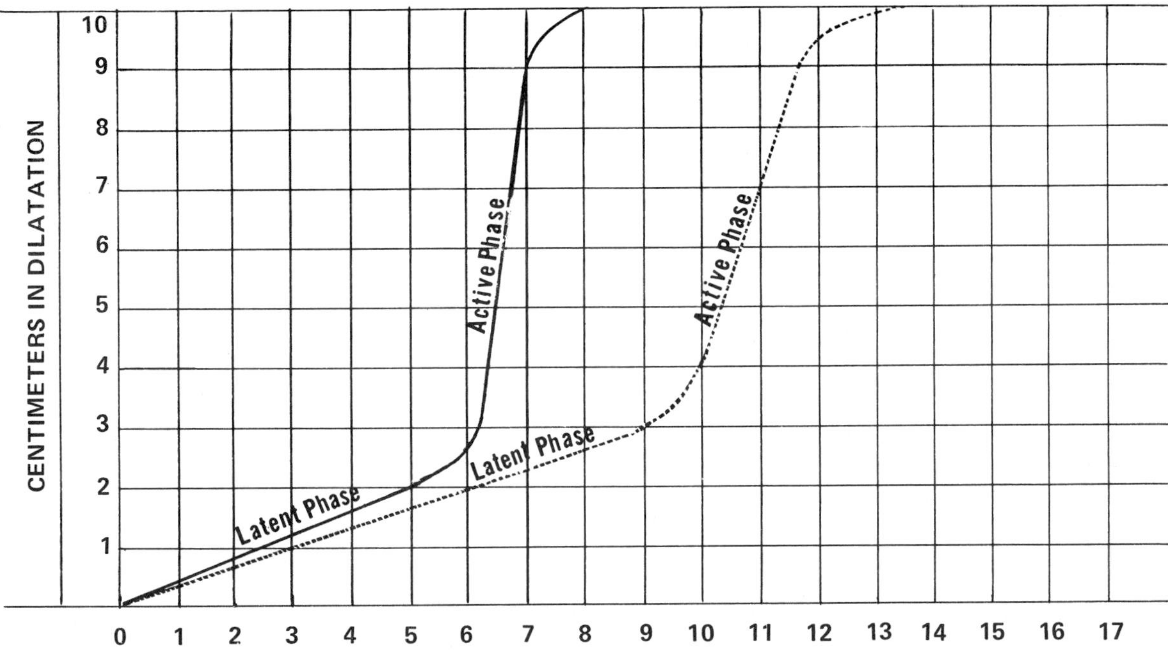

FIGURE 24-4. Graphic analysis of labor utilizing Friedman's curve. The mean labor duration for primigravadas is shown by the dotted line, and the mean for multigravidas is shown by the solid line. (Modified from Bryant, R. and Overland, A.: *Woodward and Gardner's Obstetric Management and Nursing.* F. A. Davis, Philadelphia, 1964.)

phase the cervix becomes a part of the lower segment of the uterus due to shortening and thickening of muscle fibers under the influence of uterine contractions. The average length is .9 hour for a primigravida and .2 hour for a multigravida.[8] The shortness in time does not negate that anxiety, exhaustion, and pain may contribute to the fear of death becoming a reality during this phase.

THE PHENOMENA OF LABOR

The two major variables which allow the uterus to expel its contents are fetopelvic relationships and uterine contractions.

FETOPELVIC RELATIONSHIPS

The accommodation between the *fetal passenger* and the *maternal passage* during birth is termed the fetopelvic relationship. The fetus goes through a series of maneuvers in order that its body parts align in a favorable manner to pass through a relatively immobile passageway.

The maternal pelvis consists of four bones united by four joints. During pregnancy the joints of the pelvis are relaxed by a hormone known as relaxin, allowing the pelvis to become more mobile and expandable. The passage of the pelvic cavity is divided vertically into three areas, the inlet, the midplane, and the outlet. They are important because each is bounded by borders which will limit passage of the fetus. Ideally, the widest presenting part of the fetus will fit into the widest diameter of the pelvis.

The presenting part of the fetus may be the head, buttocks, or shoulders. The head is the

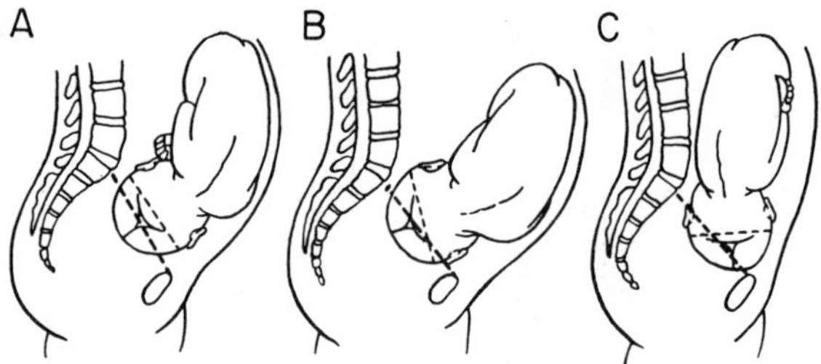

FIGURE 24-5. Synclitism (*A*) and asynclitism (*B* and *C*). *A*, Sagittal suture of the fetus lies exactly midway between the symphysis and sacral promontory. *B*, Sagittal suture is close to the sacrum and the anterior parietal bone is felt by the examining finger—anterior asynclitism or Nägele's obliquity. *C*, Posterior parietal presentation or posterior asynclitism or Litzmann's obliquity. (From Bonica, J.: *Principles and Practice of Obstetric Analgesia and anesthesia.* F. A. Davis, Philadelphia, 1972, with permission.)

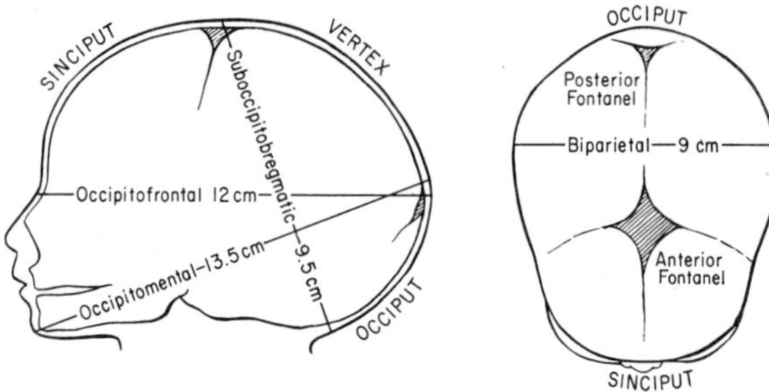

FIGURE 24-6. Diameters of the fetal skull. (From Bonica, J.: *Principles and Practice of Obstetric Analgesia and Anesthesia.* F. A. Davis, Philadelphia, 1972, with permission.)

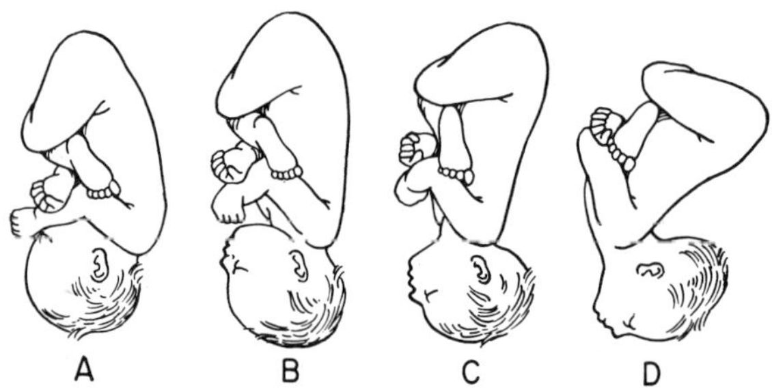

FIGURE 24-7. Attitudes of the fetus in *A*, vertex, *B*, sinciput, *C*, brow, and *C*, face presentations. (From Bonica, J.: *Principles and Practice of Obstetric Analgesia and Anesthesia.* F. A. Davis, Philadelphia, 1972, with permission.)

largest, least compressible, and most frequently presented part of the body (Fig. 24-5). Once the head is born, rarely is there delay or difficulty with the expulsion of the rest of the body. The fetal head, like the maternal pelvis, consists of bony parts which can aid or hinder the journey of birth. It is made up of seven bones which are thin, poorly ossified, easily compressible, and separated by sutures. This permits the bones to overlap under pressure, modifying the shape of the head to better fit the pelvis. This process is known as molding. The diameters of the fetal head vary according to the degree of flexion or extension of the fetal head (Figs. 24-6 and 24-7). These measurements are important because they determine the amount of space available between the fetus and the pelvis.

The following terminology is used to describe the fetopelvic relationship.

Lie is the relationship of the long axis of the baby to the long axis of the mother. There are two lies: *longitudinal* which is normal, and *transverse* which is uncommon and threatens the possibility for vaginal delivery.

Presentation refers to the presenting part of the fetus, i.e., that part which can be touched by the examining finger in the vagina. There are three major presentations: head, known as cephalic or vertex, which occurs in approximately 95 per cent of the cases; *breech or buttock* which occurs in approximately 5 per cent of the cases; *shoulder* which is rare and complicates vaginal delivery.

Station refers to the level of the presenting part in the pelvic midplane (Fig. 24-8). When the presenting part is at the level of the ischial spines the station is referred to as zero and indicates engagement. Levels above the ischial spines refer to a minus station, the numerals refer to centimeters above the spine, such as −1, −2, −3. Levels below the ischial spine refers to a plus station, such as +1, +2,

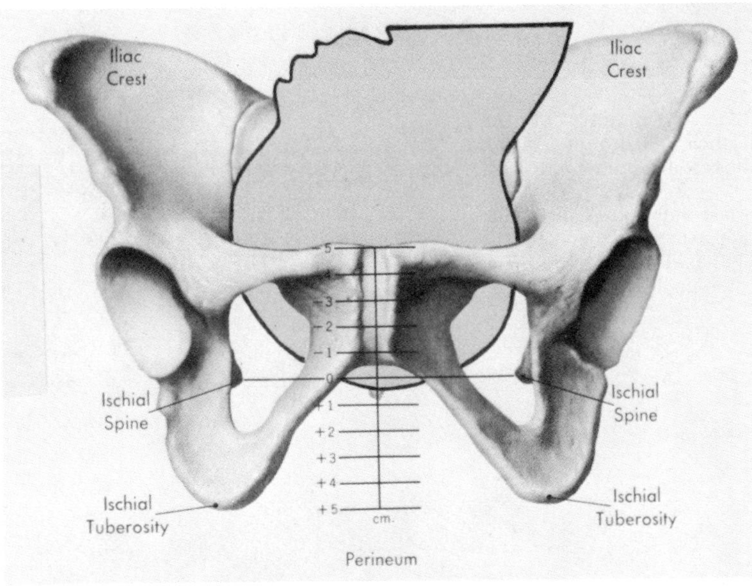

FIGURE 24-8. Stations of the presenting part. (Courtesy of Ross Laboratories.)

+3, and indicate passage onto the perineal floor. The station gives important data to indicate adequacy of fetopelvic accommodation for descent of the fetus and vaginal delivery.

Position of the presenting part of the fetus refers to the position of a specific bodily structure (usually a bone) which is presenting into the pelvic passage. In cephalic presentations this structure is the occiput with flexion, frontum (forehead) with partial extension, and mentum (chin or face) with complete extension of the head. In buttock or breech presentations the point of reference used is the sacrum regardless of flexion or extension of the hips and knees. In shoulder presentations the structure used is the scapula. The structure assumes a position to the front (anterior), back (posterior), or sides (trasnsverse) of the maternal pelvis, and may also be slightly to the right or left. In defining position, the following abbreviations are used:

Right	R
Left	L
Occiput	O
Mentum	M
Sacrum	S
Scapula	Sc
Anterior	A
Posterior	P
Transverse	T

Table 24-1 lists the positions of the fetus in various presentations. The position affects the length of labor. Transverse and posterior positions result in longer and more painful labors because a greater degree of fetal rotation is essential for delivery.

Figure 24-9 illustrates the relationship between the fetus and maternal pelvis in terms of accommodation of each other's diameters for birth. The maneuvers made by the fetus are known as the cardinal movements for the mechanism of labor. The mechanisms of labor for various positions are shown in Figures 24-10 to 24-13.

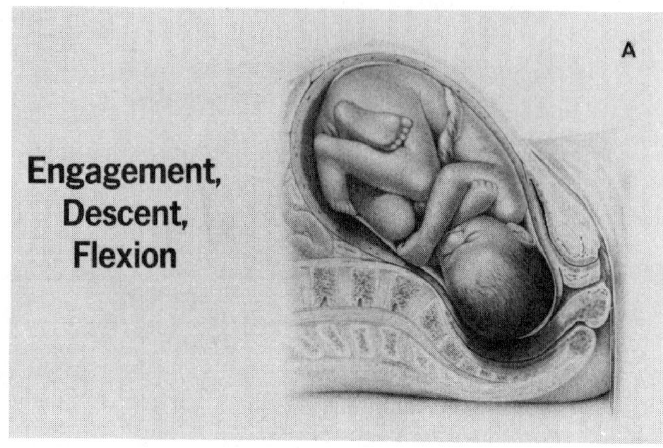

FIGURE 24-9. Cardinal movements of the mechanism for normal labor (left occipitoanterior position). (Courtesy of Ross Laboratories.)

A, The presenting part descends and engages into the midpelvis transversely to accommodate the largest diameter of the pelvis. Flexion of the head allows presentation of the smallest skull diameter into the pelvis.

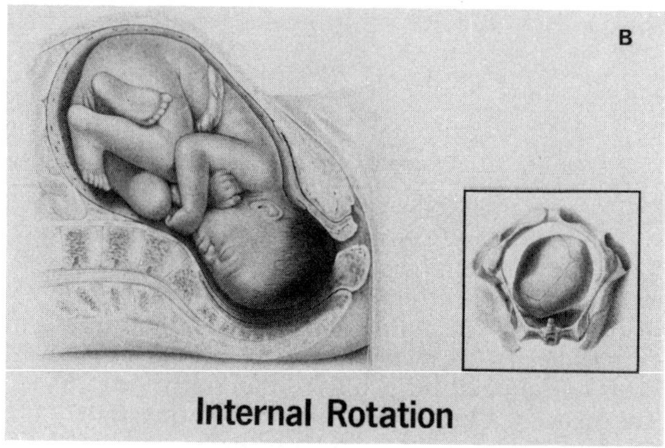

B, Internal rotation occurs when the head reaches the pelvic floor. It involves alignment of the head with the maternal anterioposterior diameter which is the pelvic outlet's largest diameter and direction of least resistance.

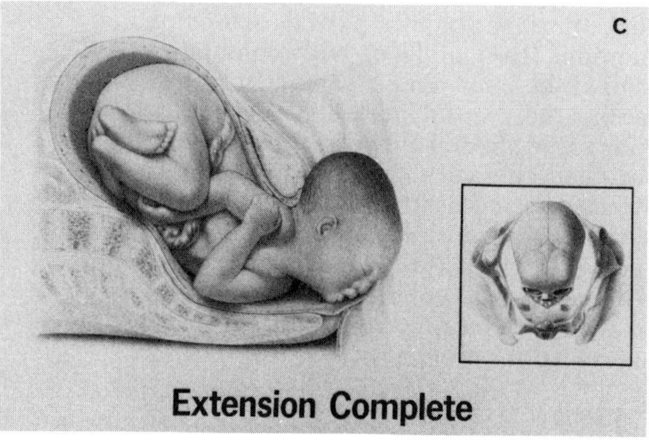

C, Extension allows the fetal head to negotiate the pelvic curve (pubic arch) and to distend the vulva and perineum. Completion of extension results in birth of the head.

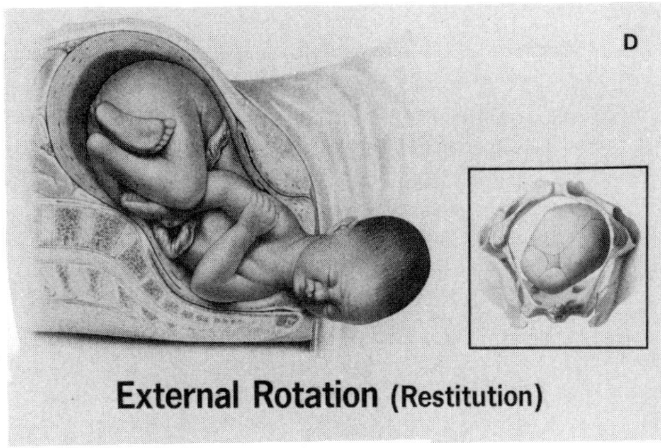

D, External rotation involves two manipulations after the head is born. The first process is called restitution and involves the head turning to realign itself in a normal relation to the position of the shoulders which are engaged in a transverse diameter of the pelvic inlet.

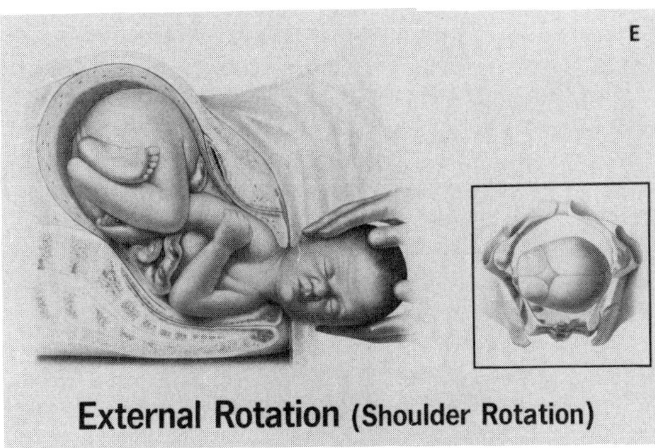

E, The other phase to complete the external rotation process involves rotation of the shoulder. After the head is born and the shoulders are on the pelvic floor, the anterior shoulder swings toward the pubic arch (symphysis pubis) causing the head to rotate in the same direction.

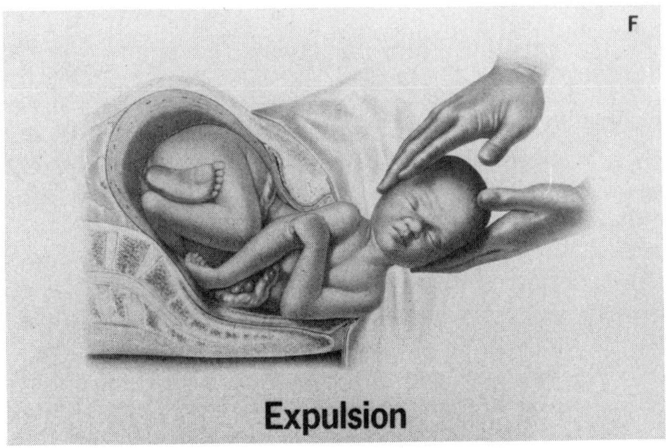

F, Expulsion or birth of the baby involves the posterior shoulder pushing forward over the perineum, rapidly followed by the birth of the anterior shoulder. After the shoulders, the rest of the body (which is smaller) slips out easily, completing the birth.

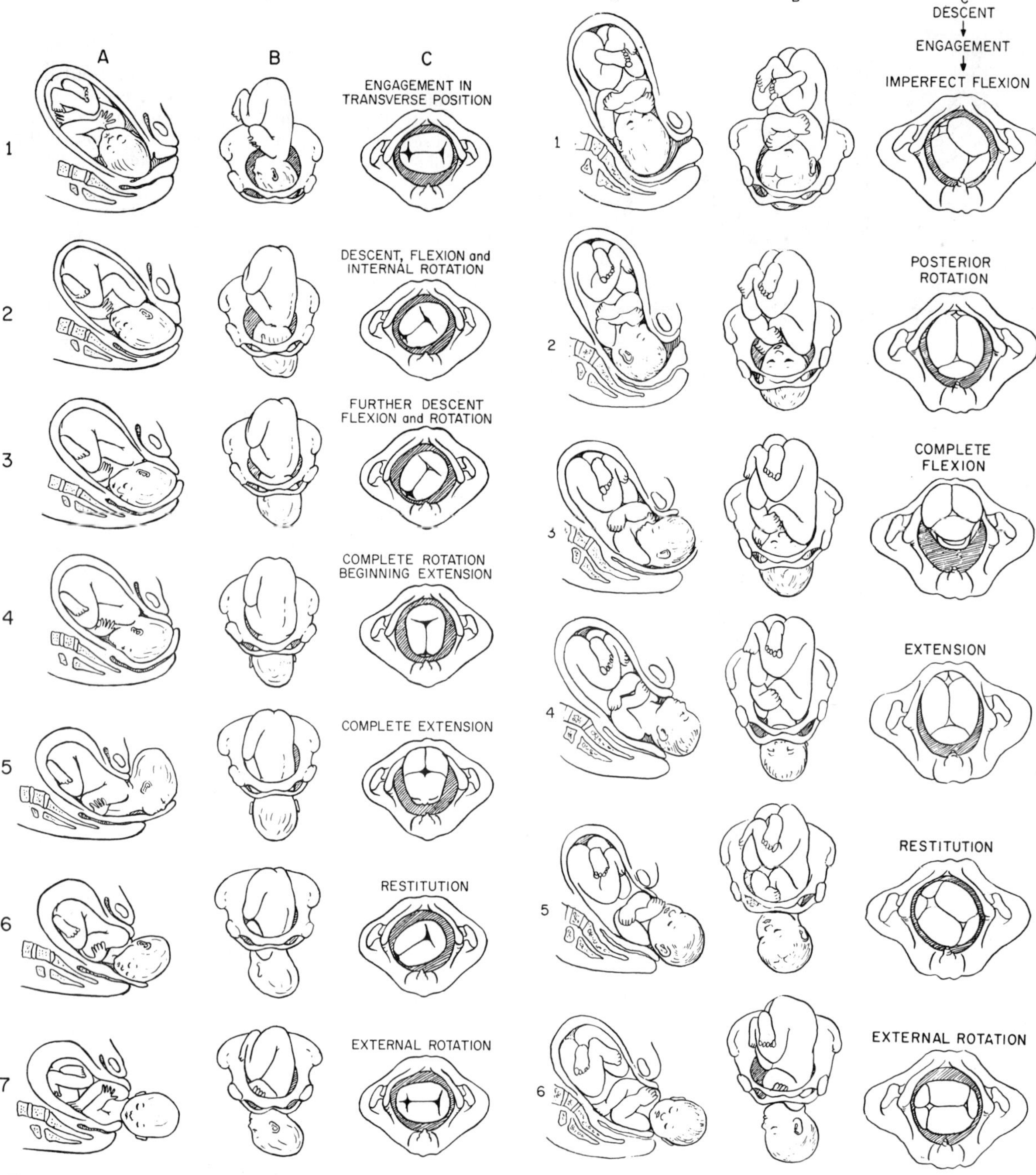

FIGURE 24-10. Mechanism of labor for the left occipitoanterior (LOA) position. (From Bonica, J.: *Principles and Practice of Obstetric Analgesia and Anesthesia.* F. A. Davis, Philadelphia, 1972, with permission.)

FIGURE 24-11. Mechanism of labor for the left occipitoposterior (LOP) position. (From Bonica, J.: *Principles and Practice of Obstetric Analgesia and Anesthesia,* F. A. Davis, Philadelphia, 1972, with permission.)

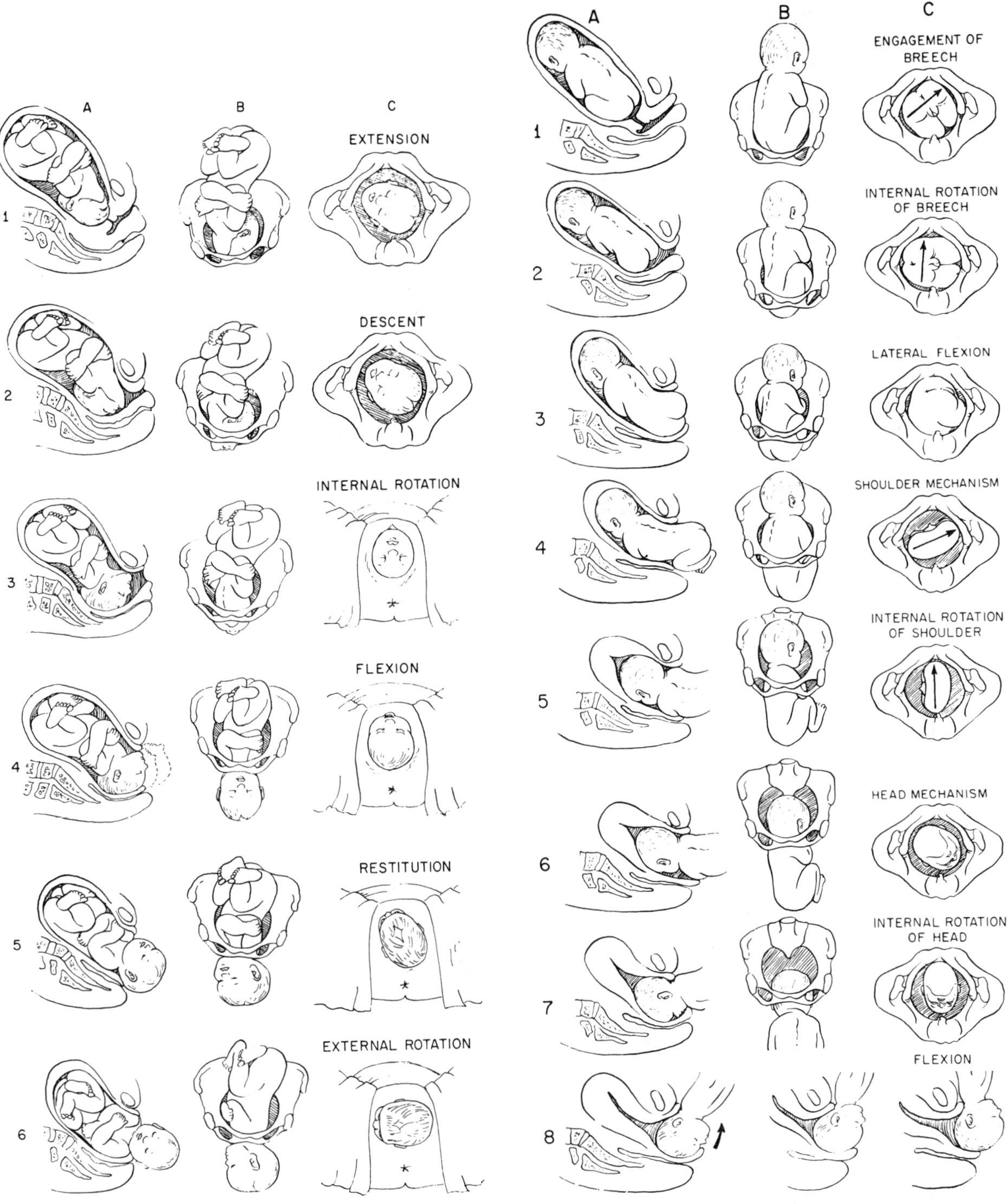

FIGURE 24.12. Mechanism of labor for the right mentoanterior (RMA) position. (From Bonica, J.: *Principles and Practice of Obstetric Analgesia and Anesthesia.* F. A. Davis, Philadelphia, 1972, with permission.)

FIGURE 24-13. Mechanism of labor for the right sacroanterior (RSA) position. (From Bonica, J.: *Principles and Practice of Obstetric Analgesia and Anesthesia.* F. A. Davis, Philadelphia, 1972, with permission.)

TABLE 24-1. Positions of Fetus in Utero*

Position	Abbreviation
Vertex Presentation (point of designation—occiput):	
Left occiput anterior	LOA
Right occiput posterior	ROP
Right occiput anterior	ROA
Left occiput posterior	LOP
Right occiput transverse	ROT
Left occiput transverse	LOT
Occiput anterior	OA
Occiput posterior	OP
Breech Presentation (point of designation—sacrum):	
Left sacroanterior	LSA
Right sacroposterior	RSP
Right sacroanterior	RSA
Left sacroposterior	LSP
Sacroanterior	SA
Sacroposterior	SP
Left sacrotransverse	LST
Right sacrotransverse	RST
Face Presentation (point of designation—chin [mentum]):	
Left mentoanterior	LMA
Right mentoposterior	RMP
Right mentoanterior	RMA
Left mentoposterior	LMP
Mentoposterior	MP
Mentoanterior	MA
Left mentotransverse	LMT
Right mentotransverse	RMT
Transverse Presentation (point of designation—scapula of presenting shoulder):	
Left scapuloanterior	LScA
Right scapuloposterior	RScP
Right scapuloanterior	RScA
Left scapuloposterior	LScP

* From *Taber's Cyclopedic Medical Dictionary*, ed. 12. F. A. Davis, Philadelphia, 1973, with permission.

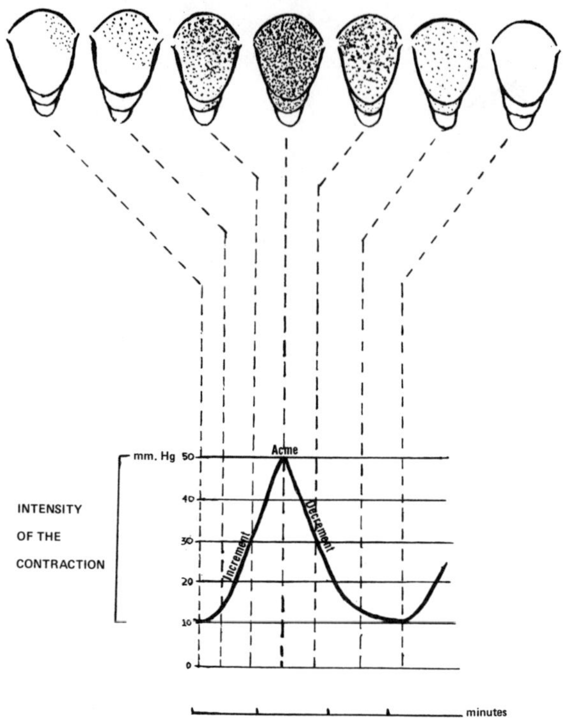

FIGURE 24-14. Fundal dominance in a contraction. Note how the contraction originates in the cornual area and propagates over the entire fundus, working down into the lower segment. This also provides a pattern in intensity as illustrated by the increment, acme, and decrement phases. (Modified from Caldeyro-Barcia, R. and Poseiro, J.: *Physiology of the Uterine Contraction.* Clin. Obstet. Gynecol. 3:386, 1960.)

UTERINE CONTRACTIONS

Uterine contractions during the labor process provide the source of energy for the:

Cervix to efface and dilate
Fetus to engage and rotate
Placenta to separate and be expelled
Uterus to regain its normal muscle tone after the trauma of pregnancy and birth.

Characteristics

Fundal Dominance. Contractions are initiated in the fundus (top) and radiate over the body of the uterus towards the cervix. This phenomena is known as *fundal dominance* (Fig. 24-14). The rationale for fundal dominance is that the concentration of myometrial cells is greatest at the fundus as contrasted to the lower portion which has less concentration of myometrium. Thus, the greatest contractile force occurs at the fundus.

Rhythmic Pattern. Each contraction has three phases: *increment*, the period in which intensity increases; *acme*, the point when the contraction is at its strongest; *decrement*, the period of decreasing intensity (see Fig. 24–14). These patterns indicate that contractions have intensity and duration which means they will become stronger in force and last longer as labor progresses. These patterns also imply a downward propagation of the contraction with descending force due to fundal dominance.

Intermittency or Frequency. In spite of the increase in intensity, frequency and duration, contractions are not a constant occurrence. There must be an interval between them. The rationale for this is to allow the fetus and uterine cells to accommodate the vasoconstriction or compression of circulation by the uterine contractions. Contractions which are assessed to be constant indicate pathology and deserve medical attention immediately.

Sensations of Pain or Discomfort. There are many theoretical bases for contractions becoming a pain source. Contractions cause stretching of the cervix, traction upon the peritoneum and supporting ligaments, pressure upon the urethra and bladder, distention of the soft tissues, ischemia of the uterine cells, and pressure on nerve ganglia adjacent to the cervix and vagina. The pain experience for the patient in labor does have physiologic validation. Further discussion on this concept is found in Chapter 25.

Effects

The effects of productive uterine contractions are manifested in clinical changes as labor progresses. First, *effacement* occurs due to the upward traction by the contracting uterine muscle. The cervix becomes soft and thin. As one contraction succeeds another, the lower portion of the myometrium is pulled upon by the overwhelming component of the fundus with the result that the lower portion becomes thinner and thinner as labor progresses. This is the process of *dilatation*.

Uterine muscles have a property of *brachystasis* which refers to the progressive shortening and thickening of the muscle fibers with each contraction. This results in the thickening and shortening of the fundus and the thinning and widening of the lower, less muscular portion of the uterus. The result is *descent*, the process by which the fetus is literally forced to go in one direction—downward—because there is less room at the top. Another effect of uterine activity is the loosening of the amniotic sac from the decidual lining with possible breakage from the increasing pressure. This is known as *spontaneous rupture of the membrane* when it occurs due to uterine contractions.

CLINICAL PICTURE OF LABOR

In the first stage of labor, the cervix effaces completely and dilates to 10 cm. Mild contractions which may have begun as much as 20 to 30 minutes apart with short duration will progress to approximately every 2 or 3 minutes, last between 47 to 80 seconds, and be strong in intensity. The presenting part should engage effectively into the pelvis at a 0 station and progress downward to a plus station. The amniotic membranes may rupture, if not, the physician may artificially break them, a procedure known as amniotomy. The uterine contractions cause vasoconstriction which is manifested clinically by a slight decrease in fetal heart rate and increased maternal blood pressure during the contraction. Seconds after the contraction is over, there should be compensation of the maternal-fetal systems to a normal fetal heart rate and maternal blood presure. Other clinical manifestations are increased blood-tinged vaginal secretions, stretching or bulging of the perineum, increasing pain, discomfort, anxiety and fatigue. Medical intervention focuses on proper fetal-maternal monitoring, pain relief with pharmacologic or regional anesthesia, and assessment for labor progress to predict vaginal delivery.

The second stage of labor focuses on the passage of the presenting part through the vaginal canal and the birth. The woman can be seen bearing down with uterine contractions to provide intra-abdominal pressure to aid in

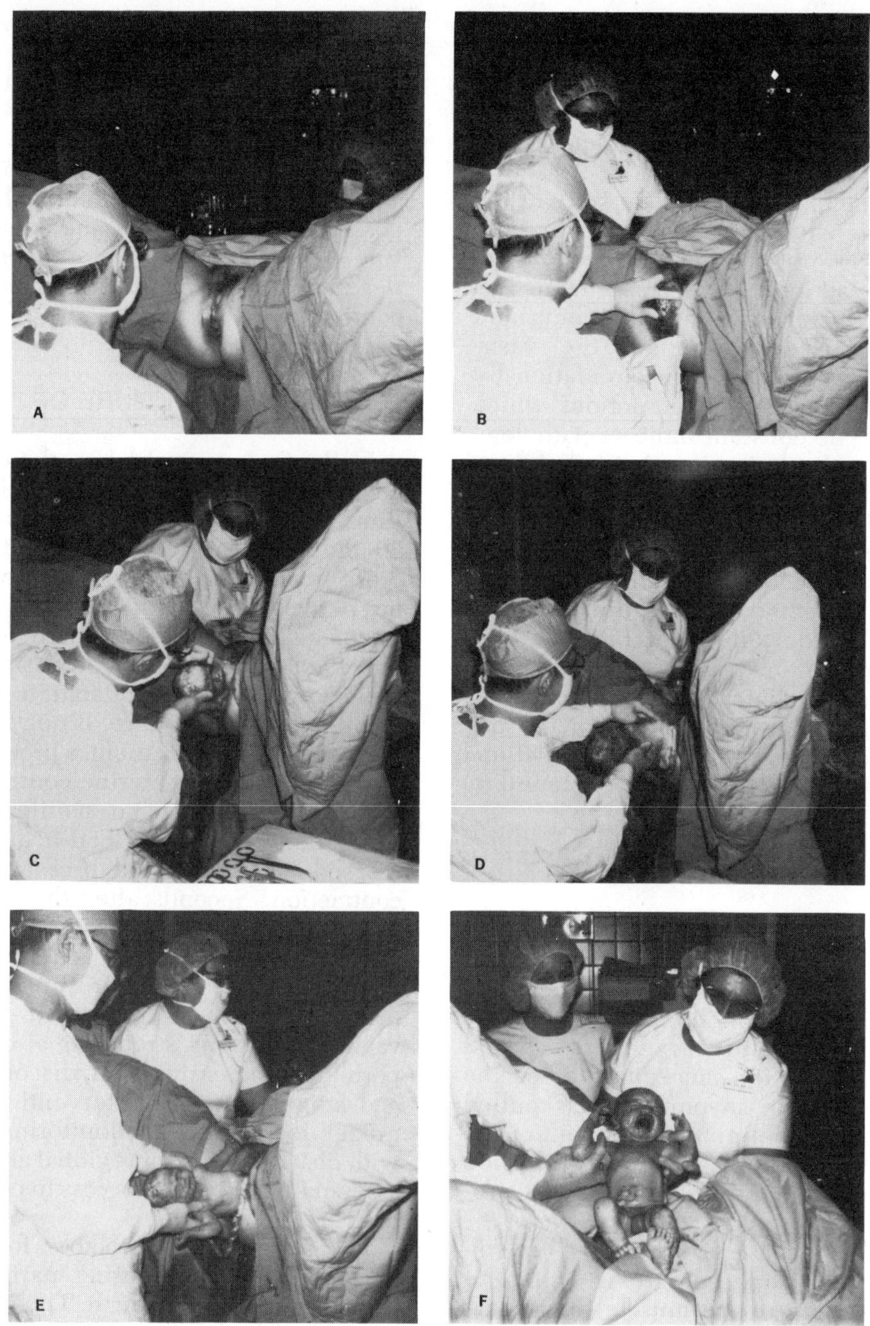

FIGURE 24-15. *A-F*, Spontaneous delivery. (Courtesy of Dennis and Judi Christopherson.)

the expulsion process. Increased bloody show will be present. Patients are usually exhausted and may be slightly amnestic in an effort to conserve energy. Medical management focuses on assessment for the delivery process, anesthesia or analgesia for delivery, manual stretching of the vagina or performance of an episiotomy (surgical incision to widen the perineum) to protect the perineum from damage during delivery, and establishment of a patent airway in the baby (Fig. 24-15)

The third stage is concerned with the separation and expulsion of the placenta. First, a slow, progressive separation of the placenta from the uterine wall occurs. The rationale for separation is the sudden decrease in the size of the uterine cavity once the fetus is expelled. Since the placenta is noncontractile, it cannot alter its surface area and thus separates. After separation, blood accumulates behind the placenta and the uterus rises in the abdomen. Firm uterine contractions begin and the placenta is expelled. A rising, *contracting, firm* uterus indicates placenta separation and impending explusion. A rising, *noncontracting, soft* uterus may indicate intrauterine bleeding. The placenta should not be manually forced to expel until it has separated completely in order to reduce the risk of retained fragments which may lead to hemorrhage. Medical management for this stage consists of assessment of placental separation, ascertainment of complete expulsion of total placenta and membranes, assessment of maternal laceration and source of bleeding, and management to control maternal blood loss with pharmacologic and other means. This third stage contains the greatest maternal risk due to the dangers related to excessive blood loss. Manipulations to control the bleeding increase the hazards of infection.

The fourth stage focuses on the body's physiologic reactions in adapting to the trauma of labor and birth. Uterine contractions continue to maintain control over bleeding from the site of placental separation from the uterine wall. Thrombosis gradually develop within the open sinuses. Medical intervention during this stage centers on enhancing the contractile ability of the uterus. This is achieved through oxytocic medications such as Ergotrate, Pitocin, and Methergine. These are given intravenously or intramuscularly some time between the delivery of the baby's anterior shoulder and immediately after the placenta is expelled. Preference is dependent upon the physician. The American College of Obstetrics and Gynecologists recommend that the postpartum patient be under constant observation by an experienced nurse who will check the woman every 15 minutes during the first hour for uterine atony, hemorrhage, deviations in blood pressure and pulse, and other complications.[8]

A phenomenon which occurs frequently during this stage is chilling. Women may feel chilling sensations any time from delivery to this immediate recovery period. The entire body may shake uncontrollably for some time (usually no longer than 15 minutes). This chilling may be frightening and frustrating for the woman. Although it is a common and normal manifestation, the rationale for its cause is not completely understood. Several hypotheses have been proposed.[9-12] These focus on theories relating to a sudden release of introabdominal pressure after the uterus is empty with delivery, muscular exertion creating disequilibrium in body temperature, reactions from the fatigue and exhaustion caused by the stress of labor, and sensitization of the maternal system to the fetal blood.

Assessment for adaptation during this phase includes the following categories:

- Fundus
  - location (height)
  - consistency (contracted-firm, or uncontracted-soft)
- Perineum
  - episiotomy site (intact? swelling? discoloration?)
  - development of a hematoma (signs of swelling, ecchymosis, tenderness or pain upon slight touch to the area)

Lochia
 color, amount, odor
Vital Signs
 temperature, blood pressure, pulse, respirations
State of Hydration
 provision of fluids and food
Fatigue and Exhaustion
 provision for rest and sleep

Nursing actions in these categories are discussed in detail in Chapter 26.

REFERENCES

1. Reynolds, S. and Hendricks, C.: *Physiology of uterine contractions and onset of labor.* In Danforth, D. (ed.): *Textbook of Obstetrics and Gynecology*, ed. 2. Harper and Row, New York, 1971, p. 498, 519.
2. Ibid.
3. Berger, S.: *Other aspects of the endocrine physiology of the female reproductive tract.* In Danforth, D. (ed.): *Textbook of Obstetrics and Gynecology*, ed. 2. Harper and Row, New York, 1971, p. 148.
4. Guyton, A.: *Textbook of Medical Physiology*, ed. 4. W. B. Saunders, Philadelphia, 1971, p. 985.
5. Reynolds
6. Friedman, E.: *Graphic analysis of labor.* Am. J. Obst. Gynecol. 68:1568, 1954.
7. Ibid.
8. The American College of Obstetricians and Gynecologists: *Standards for Obstetric-Gynecologic Hospital Services.* Chicago, 1969, p. 42.
9. Hellman, L. M. and Pritchard, J. A.: *Williams Obstetrics*, ed. 14. Appleton-Century-Crofts, New York, 1971, p. 471.
10. Jaamen, K. E. U., Jahkola, A. and Perttu, J.: *On shivering in association with normal delivery.* Acta Obstet. Gynecol. Scand. 45:383, 1966.
11. Goodlin, R. C., O'Connell, L. P. and Gunther, R. E.: *Childbirth chills: are they an immunological reaction?* Lancet 2:79, 1967.
12. Clausen, J.: *The fourth stage of labor.* In Clausen, J., et al. (eds.): *Maternity Nursing Today.* McGraw-Hill, New York, 1973, p. 529.

BIBLIOGRAPHY

Buxton, R. S. J.: *Maternal respiration in labour.* Nurs. Mirror 137:22, 1973.

Caldeyro-Barcia, R., et al.: *Effect of position changes on the intensity and frequency of uterine contractions during labor.* Am. J. Obstet. Gynecol. 80:284, 1960.

Ibid.: *Physiology of the uterine contraction.* Clin. Obstet. Gynecol. 3:386, 1960.

Case, L.: *Ultrasonic monitoring of mother and fetus.* Amer. J. Nurs. 72:725, 1972.

Friedman, E.: *The functional division of labor.* Am. J. Obstet. Gynecol. 109:274, 1971.

Friedman, E. A., et al.: *Computer analysis of labor progression. 3. pattern variations by parity.* J. Reprod. Med. 6:179, 1971.

Gabert, H. A., et al.: *Effect of ruptured membranes on fetal heart rate patterns.* Obstet. Gynecol. 41:279, 1973.

Humphrey, M.: *The influence of maternal posture at birth on the fetus.* J. Obstet. Gynaecol. Br. Commonw. 80:1075, 1973.

Karim, S. M.: *The role of prostaglandins in parturition.* Proc. R. Soc. Med. 64:10, 1971.

Kopp, L. M.: *Ordeal or ideal–the second stage of labor.* Am. J. Nurs. 71:1140, 1971.

Laros, R. K., et al.: *Amniotomy during the active phase of labor.* Obstet. Gynecol. 39:102, 1972.

Lasater, C.: *Electronic monitoring of mother and fetus.* Am. J. Nurs. 72:728, 1972.

Lorincz, R.: *Danger signs in the first stage of labor.* Hosp. Med. 6:115, 1970.

O'Gurek, J., Roux, J. and Newman, M.: *Neonatal depression and fetal heart rate patterns during labor.* Obstet. Gynecol. 40:347, 1972.

Oxorn, H. and Foote, W.: *Human Labor in Birth*, ed. 2. Appleton-Century-Crofts, New York, 1968.

Poppers, A.: *Overventilation during labor.* Bull. Am. Coll. Nurse-Midwif. 13:4, 1968.

Price, H. V.: *Onset of labour: A pediatrician's view.* Arch. Dis. Child 47:675, 1972.

Ibid.: *Programmed instruction on pain–part I.* Am. J. Nurs. 66:1099, 1966.

Reed, B., et al.: *Management of the infant during labor, delivery, and in the immediate neonatal period.* Nurs. Clin. N. Amer. 6:3, 1971.

Rice, G.: *Recognition and treatment of intrapartal fetal distress.* J. Obstet. Gynecol. Neonat. Nurs. 1:15, 1972.

Scheff, J., et al.: *Uterine blood flow during labor.* Obstet. Gynecol. 38:15, 1971.

Schifrin, B. S.: *Fetal heart rate monitoring during labor.* J. Am. Med. Assoc. 221:992, 1972.

Schulman, H., et al.: *Maternal acid-base balance in labor.* Obstet. Gynecol. 37:738, 1971.

Smith, B. A.: *The transition phase of labor.* Am. J. Nurs. 73:448, 1973.

Turnbull, A. C., et al.: *Endocrine factors in the onset of labor.* Proc. R. Soc. Med. 63:1095, 1970.

Walker, D. W., et al. *Temperature relationship of the mother and fetus during labor.* Am. J. Obstet. Gynecol. 107:83, 1970.

Williams, B. and Richards, S. *Fetal monitoring during labor.* Am. J. Nurs. 70:2384, 1970.

25 *Pain during Labor**

TOSHIO J. AKAMATSU, M.D.
JOHN J. BONICA, M.D.

In recent years there has been an impressive surge of interest in obstetric anesthesia by patients, physicians, and nurses. This trend is exerting social and professional pressure on physicians and nurses to provide the parturient with better and more widespread pain relief during childbirth. Parturients have been made aware of the benefits of good obstetric analgesia through the news media and have come to expect it just as they have come to expect painless surgery and painless dentistry.

A thorough understanding of the nature of pain and especially its relationship to childbirth is a sine qua non for proper management, teaching, and understanding the pain associated with parturition. The initial part of this chapter is devoted to general concepts of pain which serve as a framework for the details regarding the pain of parturition. This is necessary since, although it is generally acknowledged that childbirth is usually associated with pain and suffering to some degree, there still exist misconceptions about the nature of labor pain.

CURRENT CONCEPTS OF PAIN

Although pain has classically been considered a purely sensory experience, its uniqueness among the sensations experienced by humans differentiates it from other sensory experiences. At times pain becomes overwhelming, disrupts ongoing activity, and may lead to personality changes. Therefore, although the original noxious stimulus may be the same for all individuals the associated sensations, which include emotional reactions, affect the state and the psychophysiologic reactions result in a loss of "sameness" as a result of those modifying influences. This means that the reactions to a given stimulus vary not only among individuals, but in the same individual at different times. The reaction depends entirely on what the sensation means to the individual in view of his past experiences, as well as his present attitude, judgment, mood, and emotional status, and the importance or significance he assigns to it.

NEUROPHYSIOLOGIC ASPECTS

Among the sensory systems pain is unique in that it not only involves discriminative capacities to identify the onset, duration, location, intensity, and physical characteristics of the stimulus, but also includes motivational, affective, and cognitive functions leading to the private experience of the stimulus. Moreover, pain is profoundly modified by

*This project was supported by USPHS Grant GM #15991.

pyschologic and pathologic conditions of the central or peripheral nervous system that can alter the intensity.

Nerve impulses conducted by pain fibers are essential for pain sensation. These peripheral nerve fibers synapse with neurons in the dorsal spinal gray matter activating an ascending system in the ventral lateral spinal cord and then project to the medial brain stem, hypothalamus, thalamus, and limbic forebrain structures subserving the motivational-affective dimension of pain. Impulses in the larger nerve fibers ascend in the dorsal spinal cord and activate central posterolateral thalamic and cortical neurons providing spatial-temporal discriminative capacities. These two parallel systems together form the neural basis for somatic pain.

The magnitude and effect of the reflex responses to pain depend on the intensity, duration, and site of the stimulus. With increasing intensity or prolonged stimulus, the responses persist and may add to the physiopathology. These autonomic reflex responses cause alteration of function in the gastrointestinal and genitourinary tracts, bronchial constriction, muscle spasm, and vasospasm. All of these in turn create new stimulation which adds to the reflex disturbances.

At this point "gate control" activity has two important therapeutic implications: 1) pain can be controlled in some situations by increasing large fiber functions such as those initiated by massage or tactile stimulation during labor, and 2) pain can be modified by maximizing central control factors by means of specific training as in childbirth education, using suggestion, distraction, and behavioral conditioning.

PSYCHOLOGIC ASPECTS

Factors which affect pain experience include: 1) Attention or perception may contribute to increasing or decreasing the pain. Suggestion is a potent method of controlling tension to decrease the pain behavior, particularly in acute pain such as childbirth pain. 2) Anxiety or the subjective feeling of fear coupled with the increase in autonomic reflex responses influences the pain experience. In this way interpersonal conflicts, threats of failure, stress of parturition, decision conflicts, and neurosis contribute to the pain threshold. 3) Rewards for suffering, especially when successive, lead to the development of behavior habits which may form sequential patterns of behavior. Since both the parturient and her supervisor interact with the environment for rewards and modify ongoing behaviors to maximize rewards and minimize losses, the patient may experience more rewards for being in pain than she received in her normal routine. This is especially true when the patient is frustrated and generally dissatisfied with the status of her pregnancy. 4) Other factors which are important psychologic influences include depression, hysteria, early conditioning, social and cultural factors, and drug abuse.

When an antepartum pain problem originates and is noted to have large psychologic influence, counseling should focus on three factors: 1) helping the parturient develop insight into her problems, 2) developing alternative, healthy ways to meet these problems, and 3) identifying determinants of factors supporting pain behaviors in order to disrupt their mechanism.

NATURE OF PAIN DURING CHILDBIRTH

For many centuries normal childbirth has been considered a painful experience. More recently, this view has been disputed by those who claim that pain is not an inherent part of the physiologic process of childbirth but rather a product of social, cultural, and emotional influences. Ethnologic studies, however, show that childbirth is a painful process in all societies including primitive societies and also in subhuman primates and lower animals. The obvious conclusion is that while emotions play an important role in childbirth, the pain of childbirth must be considered an integral part of the physiologic process.

MECHANISMS OF LABOR PAIN

The pain of labor, like pain in general, may produce significant mental and physical effects which on occasion prove harmful to the parturient. These effects are interrelated with some of the physiologic alterations produced by the process of labor and the psychosomatic effects produced by the resulting emotional reaction.

As evidenced by laboratory and clinical observations, most data suggest that the pain during the first stage of labor is primarily due to the dilatation of the cervix with distension, stretching and possible tearing of the structure. Additionally, contraction of the uterus and stretching of the lower uterine segment contribute to the pain of childbirth. During the end of the first stage of labor and in the second stage of labor, stretching and distension of the birth canal and perineum by the presenting part produces the severest pain of labor. This is largely due to the stretching, tearing, and hemorrhage within the fascia, skin, subcutaneous tissues, and other somatic structures which are extremely pain-sensitive. Other factors contributing to the pain of childbirth include tension and torsion of supporting ligaments of the uterus and adnexa, parietal peritoneum, and the structures they envelope, and pressure upon adjacent organs, especially nervous structures during abnormal presentation.

PATHWAYS OF LABOR PAIN

Laboratory and clinical studies reveal that the pain of the first stage of labor, which is primarily due to dilatation of cervix, travels by way of the sensory pathways which accompany the sympathetic (efferent) nerves and pass in sequence through: 1) the uterine plexus, 2) the pelvic (inferior hypogastric) plexus, 3) the middle hypogastric plexus, 4) the superior hypogastric plexus, 5) the lumbar and lower thoracic sympathetic chain, 6) the white rami communicantes associated with the tenth, eleventh, and twelfth thoracic nerves and first lumbar nerve, 7) the formed spinal nerve, and then pass through the posterior roots of these nerves to enter the spinal cord. Typical of visceral pain, the pain from the uterus and cervix is referred to the dermatomes supplied by the spinal cord segments and includes the lower abdominal wall and the skin over the lower lumbar spine and upper sacrum. With intensity of stimulation, there is spread to segments above and below these segments so that pain is felt in the upper thighs, midsacral area and umbilical region.

The pain of the second stage of labor is produced primarily by distension of the lower birth canal and perineum, and is conveyed by sensory fibers which are components of the pudendal nerves. These fibers enter the spinal cord via the posterior roots of the second, third, and fourth sacral nerves. Since this pain arises from superficial structures, it is well localized to the perineum and adjacent regions and is associated with an uncontrollable "bearing down" urge.

Additional pain may occur with passage of the placenta and contraction of the uterus. These impulses, like those which occur during the first stage of labor, pass by way of the sensory nerves and enter the spinal cord through the thoracic and lumbar nerves. Discomforts from traction on other pelvic structures, including the ovaries, fallopian tubes, and ligaments, are conveyed by sensory nerves associated with the various plexuses. These reach the midportion of the lumbar sympathetic chain and proceed centrally into the spinal cord along with the nerves of the uterus and cervix.

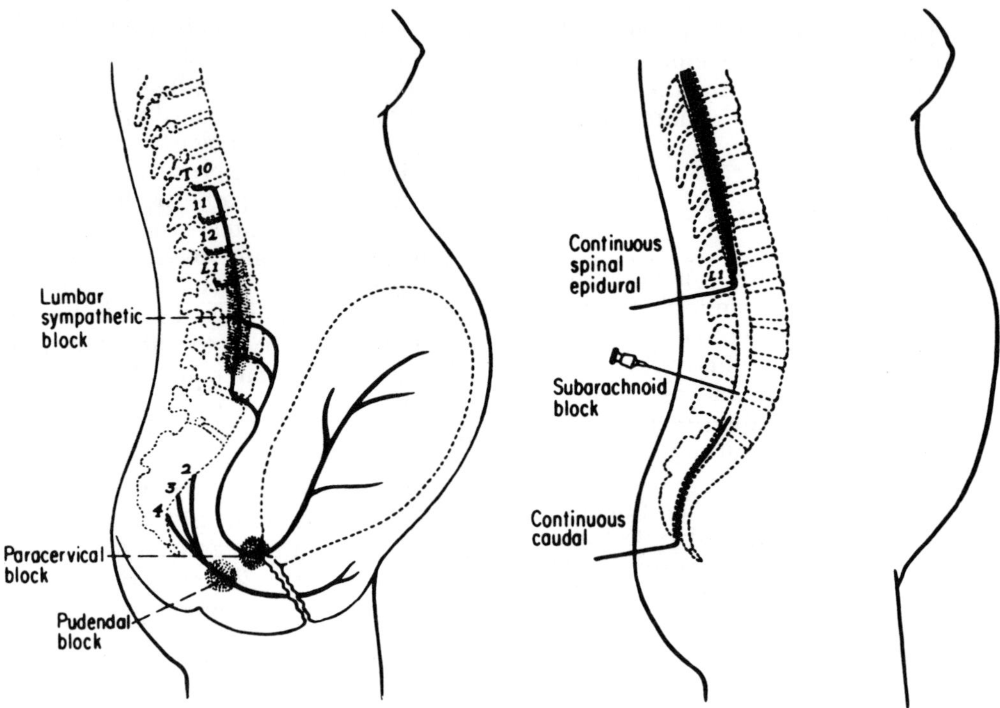

FIGURE 25-1. Pathways of parturition pain and regional techniques used to relieve it. (From Bonica[2] with permission.)

Pharmacologic interuption of the various pain pathways may be produced by using specific nerve block techniques and local anesthetics (Fig. 25-1). The duration, intensity of block, and selectivity (motor or sensory) can easily be determined by the technique or local anesthetic utilized to produce the nerve block.

OBSTETRIC ANALGESICS, ANESTHETICS AND RELATED DRUGS

Currently, many drugs and techniques are available to provide relief of childbirth pain. The methods used vary from one area to another and from one country to another, depending upon the culture, medical personnel, facilities, and other psychologic and professional factors. For proper clinical application, each of these drugs and techniques must be evaluated from four interrelated viewpoints:

1. Analgesic potency or other therapeutic efficacy
2. Side effects on the mother
3. Side effects on the fetus and newborn
4. Side effects on labor

Table 25-1 contains a critical evaluation of the drugs and techniques in common use based on these four viewpoints. In applying this information to a particular patient, it is important to realize that these effects are modified by the changes produced by pregnancy

TABLE 25.1. Pharmacology of Obstetric Analgesia-Anesthesia*

Agent or Technique	*Optimal Dose or Concentration*	*Therapeutic Effect*	*Side Effects on Mother*	*Effects on Labor*	*Placental Transfer*	*Effects on Fetus and Newborn*	*Remarks*
Sedatives							
Barbiturates	100 mg IM 50 mg IV	Sedation and sleep	None with OD† mild depression with overdose	None with OD; slowing with excessive doses given prematurely	Rapid; within 30–60 seconds of IV and 3–5 minutes of IM	None with OD; depression with overdose	Useful during early (latent) phase of labor
Ataractics	Dose varies with drug	Sedation and tranquility; antiemetic	None, except hypotension and extrapyramidial signs with some	None	Same as above	Same as above	Same as above; Useful in combination with narctoics
Diazepam (Valium)	15–20 mg IM 10 mg IV	Sedation, amnesia	None with OD				
Scopolamine	0.3 mg IM	Amnesia & sedation	None alone, but respiratory depression when combined with barbiturates	None	Same as above	May produce minimal depression	Best avoided because of side effects
Analgesics							
Narcotics	Dose varies with drug	Analgesia; sedation, euphoria; decrease of anxiety	Mild respiratory and circulatory depression and delay in gastric emptying	None if properly used (OD) during active phase; retarded if given too early	Same as above	Mild depression with OD; severe depression with overdose	Effective analgesics for moderate to severe pain in 75–90% of paturients
Psychologic Analgesia	Intense preparation during pregnancy and reinforcement during labor	Analgesia & amnesia in 20%; partial relief in another 50% mood and behavior improved	None studied in gravida; deleterious effects seen only when technique fails	None		None; condition of fetus better than with other methods of analgesia	Of benefit to all patients, but must be complemented with other analgesics in most parturients
Inhalation Analgesia	40% N_2O 0.3–0.5% methoxyflurane, trilene	Complete or partial analgesia in 75–90% without loss of consciousness	None with proper administration	None with OD; with depression with deep anesthesia	Rapid transfer	None	Better analgesia than narcotics
Bilateral Paracervical Block	5–10 ml each side	Block of uterine pain → analgesia during labor	None if properly executed; systemic toxic reactions with convulsions and neonatal depression if excessive dose of drug used	Transient depression of contractions, but no effect on labor	Rapid transfer of local anesthetic to fetus	Bradycardia in 5–30%, neonatal depression with complications	Simple and can be done by obstetrician; analgesia during labor, but no perineal anesthesia. Combined with pudendal or saddle block
Bilateral Pudendal Block	5–10 ml each side	Analgesia in perineum	Same as bilateral paracervical block	Loss of bearing down reflex	Same as extradural block	None except with complications	Same as above
Disassociative (ketamine)	25 mg IV	Analgesia, amnesia	None with proper administration	None	Rapid	Depression with overdose	Simple but easy to overdose

* Modified from Bonica.[1] † OD = optimum dose.

TABLE 25-2. Summary of Obstetric Analgesia-Anesthesia Techniques*

Phase of Pregnancy	Degree of Discomfort	*Primary Technique of Analgesia-Anesthesia*: Systemic Sedatives Analgesics	Inhalation Analgesia-Anesthesia	Regional Analgesia-Anesthesia	Psychologic Analgesia
Pregnancy	Emotional reactions Mild discomfort	Psychologic preparation of the gravida. Inform patient about various types of analgesia-anesthesia. Reassure about proper selection of best method. Instruct how to bear down.			Intense preparation for psychologic analgesia
First Stage a) *Latent Phase* Onset of labor ↓ progress to ↓ 3 cm cervical dilation	Usually mild pain Unprepared patient has fear and anxiety → may complain of moderate or severe "pain"	Good nursing care—avoid food and fluids Psychologic support—reassurance, sympathy, suggestion, information, companionship Pharmacologic sedation: 1. Barbiturate—100 mg IM or 50 mg IV after admission routine completed 2. Repeat in 1 or 2 hours 3. Add ataractic if barbiturate insufficient 4. Give small dose of narcotic *only* if discomfort severe or latent phase prolonged 5. If admitted in evening and progress slow, give 100 to 150 mg barbiturate by mouth to assure sleep			Reinforce psychologic analgesia ↓ Sedative may be needed
b) *Active phase* 3 cm cervical dilation	Moderate uterine pain	Narcotic or Narcotic-Ataractic or Narcotic-Narcotic Antagonist: IV q 1 to 2 hours or IM q 2 to 4 hours or continuous infusion	Narcotic alone or in combination as described in column on left		↓ Narcotic often needed but in smaller doses than with other methods
progress to	progress to	↓	continued until late first stage		↓
10 cm cervical dilation	Severe uterine pain	Paracervical block or Trilene analgesia →	Inhalation analgesia		↓
Second Stage a) *Early*	Severe uterine pain Moderate perineal pain	Pudendal anesthesia			Reinforce psychologic analgesia Narcotics may be necessary
b) *Delivery* Spontaneous or Forceps	Severe perineal pain Perineal relaxation required	Perineal anesthesia		Ketamine IV 25 mg just prior to delivery	Perineal anesthesia with pudendal block desirable
Third Stage a) *Delivery of placenta* b) *Perineal repair*	Minimal uterine pain Perineal analgesia required	←			Maintain perineal analgesia
Fourth Stage	Little or no discomfort	↓	Emergence from anesthesia		

* Modified from Bonica.[2]

and labor and the pathophysiology of any obstetric or medical complication present. The many agents and techniques which are being used can arbitrarily be included in four categories which are summarized in Table 25-2. It deserves re-emphasis that each of these methods has its own specific indications and that the advantages, disadvantages, and limitations of each method vary under different conditions. To obtain best results with obstetric analgesia and anesthesia, it is essential for the obstetric team to adhere to certain basic principles. The objective is to provide optimal relief of pain to the mother without unusual risk to her or her infant. The sine qua non of obstetric anesthesia should be safety for mother and child. It is the primary mission of the administrator of the agent or technique to select and employ them in such a manner as to cause the least degree of disturbance to the bodily functions of the mother and none to those of the infant. How effectively this responsibility is discharged depends primarily upon one's current knowledge, judgment, skill, and experience—these are far more important than the specific drug or technique used.

Currently there is no analgesic agent or technique which offers such superior advantage over others that it can or should be used in all cases. Therefore, the patient should never be forced to accept a method unless unusual circumstances exist which preclude the use of all other methods. The type of analgesia and anesthesia must be tailored to the needs of the individual patient. There are many factors which must be considered in the selection of methods that will provide the best results:

1. Physiologic status, psychologic makeup, and desire of the mother
2. Condition of the infant during labor and at the time of delivery
3. Experience, skill, and practices of the person who is to perform the delivery and where it will be done (hospital, home, or elsewhere)
4. Most importantly, the competence and skill of the administrator as well as the facilities available to him or her.

High quality analgesic and anesthetic management requires observance of the Five Cardinal C's: communication, coordination, cooperation, courtesy, and (sometimes) compromise by every member of the obstetric team.

REFERENCES

1. Bonica, J. J. (ed.): *Obstetric Analgesia and Anesthesia.* Springer-Verlag, Berlin, 1972.
2. Bonica, J. J.: *Principles and Practice of Obstetric Analgesia and Anesthesia.* F. A. Davis, Philadelphia, 1972.

BIBLIOGRAPHY

Akamatsu, T. J.: *Advances in obstetric anesthesia.* In Fabian, L. W. (ed.): *Decade of Clinical Progress.* Clinical Anesthesia Series, F. A. Davis, Philadelphia, 1973.

Bonica, J. J.: *The Management of Pain.* Lea and Febiger, Philadelphia, 1953.

Bonica, J. J.: *Principles and Practice of Obstretric Analgesia and Anesthesia.* F. A. Davis, Philadelphia, 1972.

Bonica, J. J. (ed.): *Obstetric Analgesia and Anesthesia.* Springer-Verlag, Berlin, 1972.

Casey, K. L. : *The neurophysiologic basis of pain.* Postgrad. Med. 53:58, 1973.

Halpern, L. M.: *Analgesics and other drugs for relief of pain.* Postgrad. Med. 53:91, 1973.

Melzack, R. and Chapman, C. R.: *Psychologic aspects of pain.* Postgrad. Med. 53:69, 1973.

Merskey, H. M. and Spear, F. G.: *Pain: Psychological and Psychiatric Aspects.* Bailliere, Tindall and Cassel Company, London, 1967.

Petrie, A.: *Individuality in Pain and Suffering.* University of Chicago Press. Chicago, 1968.

Soulairac, A., Cahn, M. and Charpentier, J.: *Pain: Neurophysiological and Psychophysiological Basis of Pain.* Academic Press, New York, 1968.

26 Assessment and Support during Labor

DYANNE D. AFFONSO, R.N., M.N.

This section focuses on suggested approaches to achieve a primary nursing goal: *Protection and safety of the maternal-fetal systems to ensure a healthy outcome.* Actions to protect the fetus are discussed separately from those which protect the mother only because it helps to organize the content. This does not negate the interrelationship between the maternal and fetal systems. It is not possible to identify every action which will achieve the above goal because new techniques and knowledge are constantly emerging. Thus, many presently unknown nursing approaches are probable for the future. The reader is encouraged to participate in their discovery.

FETAL ASSESSMENT

To ensure the safety and protection of the fetus, the nurse must understand the various means by which data are collected about the welfare of the fetus during labor. Assessment may include:

1. Fetal heart rate patterns
2. Status of membranes
3. Fetal capillary blood sampling.

FETAL HEART RATE PATTERNS

The heart rate of the fetus responds to stress by accelerating or decelerating. The normal fetal heart rate is considered to be between the limits of 120 to 160 beats per minute. Levels less than 120 beats per minute are considered bradycardia and rates greater than 160 beats per minute are considered tachycardia. Thus the heart rate gives an indication of the fetus' tolerance to the stress of labor and birth. Various techniques for assessment of the fetal heart rate are discussed below.

Intermittent Auscultation

This method involves listening to the fetal heartbeat with a fetal stethoscope and counting the beats for a fraction of or a full minute between contractions. The number obtained is multiplied by the appropriate factor to yield a value of beats per minute. For example, if the fetal heart rate of 15 seconds is 35, this is multiplied by four (the factor to yield a one minute reading) and the fetal heart rate would be 140 per minute. In addition to the rate, the rhythm is also assessed for regularity and depth. The disadvantages of this method include errors in counting rate, difficulty in hearing the heartbeat during contractions when assessment is most crucial, and no provision of a *continuous* heart rate pattern to obtain a baseline norm; only profound, prolonged, and serious heart rate deviations can be identified. Thus, this method is not reliable in the recognition of fetal distress, although it is still the most practical and frequently used method for assessment.

How does the nurse locate the fetal heart sounds when using intermittent auscultation?

It has been stated that a fetoscope is not the best way to assess heart rate patterns but is still the most frequent device used by majority of nurses. Therefore, the nurse must be able to locate the point on the mother's abdomen which will allow the best audible heart sounds (Fig. 26-1).

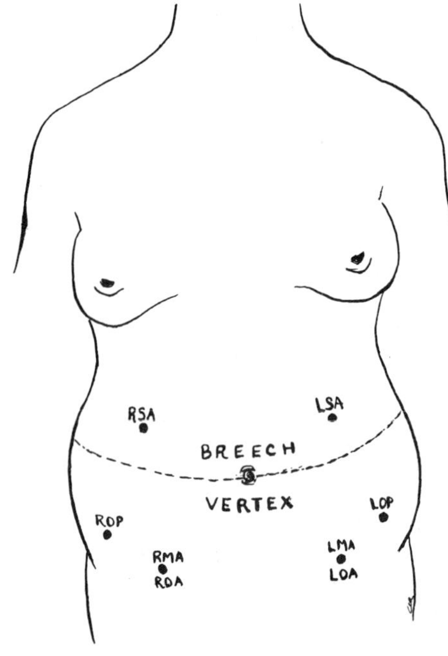

FIGURE 26-1. Areas where the fetal heartbeat can best be heard in various presentations, positions of the fetus. (Modified from Danforth.[1])

The heart sounds are usually heard in the lower quadrant of the mother's abdomen, below the umbilical area. The point of location is determined by the position, presentation, and lie of the fetus. For example, in a breech presentation heart sounds are located above the umbilical area (upper quadrant of the abdomen).

Fetal heart sounds are best transmitted through the back or chest of the fetus, depending on which lies closer to the uterine wall. Assessment for the fetal back can be done by abdominal palpation. Location of the fetal back will eliminate hit-and-miss attempts of placing the fetoscope all over the maternal abdomen. It also helps to prevent anxiety which may arise when the woman senses the nurse's difficulty. Too often the nurse cannot locate heart sounds audible enough for assessment of the rate and rhythm.

The sounds of a normal fetal heartbeat are regular in rhythm, like the ticking of a clock. However, the nurse may hear other sounds in her attempts to assess the heart rate. These may be:

1. A soft murmur known as the uterine bruit resulting from passage of blood through the dilated uterine vessels. It is synchronous with the maternal pulse.
2. A hissing sound, known as the funic souffle which is produced by the rush of blood through the umbilical arteries. It is similar to the fetal pulse and has the same significance as the fetal heartbeat.[1]

Continuous Auscultation

Continuous listening to the heartbeat can usually be done with an ultrasonic device which amplifies the heart sounds. The Doptone or Doppler ultrasonic sensor is a small, battery-operated unit which attains this (Fig. 26-2). It is superior to a stethoscope and can be applied during transportation of a patient for diagnostic work-up, anesthesia, or transfer to the delivery room. It involves no discomfort to the patient. Its disadvantages are limitations during strong uterine contractions, lack of a printed record of the heart rate patterns or

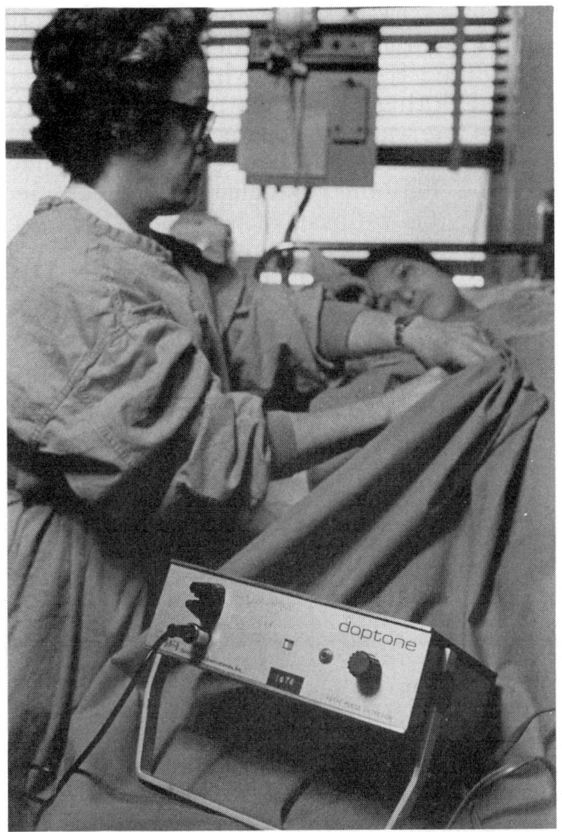

FIGURE 26-2. Monitoring the fetal heart rate with the Doptone device.

uterine contractions, loss of heart sounds with fetal movement, and lack of effectiveness for monitoring over an extended period.

Indirect Continuous Monitor (Cardiotocograph)

This method records the fetal heart sounds simultaneously with the frequency and duration of uterine contractions. Separate transducers in capsules are mounted with elastic straps on the woman's abdomen and translate abdominal tension and fetal heart sounds into electric signals which are recorded on a strip chart. This instrument records changes in the abdominal contour as perceived externally. Therefore, the readings may reflect changes in position such as those from coughing or vomiting and should not be interpreted as intrauterine pressure readings. A major advantage of this method is its easy application by personnel other than a physician because it requires no internal manipulation. Its disadvantages are frequent repositioning of the sensor with maternal or fetal position changes which interrupt the readings, discomforts from the abdominal straps, and interruption of effectiveness due to bearing down efforts in second stage or a low station. Also, this method works best with the patient in a supine position which may not be the most comfortable position for the woman.

Direct Monitoring (Corometric)

This is a method of recording the intrauterine pressure of the labor pattern and the fetal heart rate pattern through internal measurements. A small electrode, clipped to the presenting part of the fetus, yields a continuous recording of the heart rate on a graph and

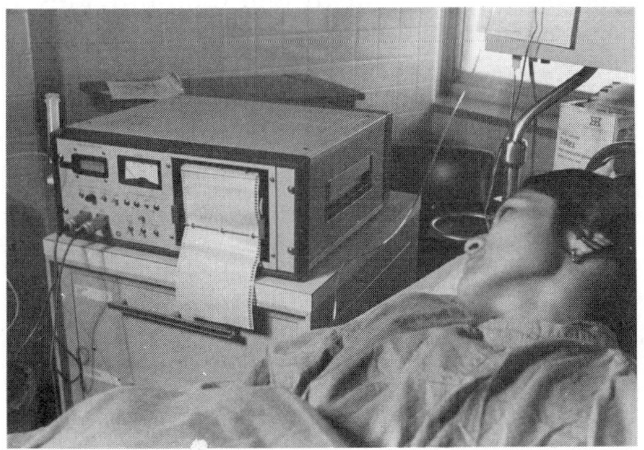

FIGURE 26-3. Direct monitoring of fetal heart rate and uterine contractions with the Corometric device.

meter and also provides the fetal electrocardiograph on an oscilloscope (Fig. 26-3). Recording of the intensity of the uterine contraction is done with a catheter filled with saline which is placed in the uterine cavity. The saline acts as a transmitter of uterine pressure to a transducer which converts the uterine pressure into millimeters of mercury. Monitor strips record the quality of the uterine contractions and fetal heart rate patterns simultaneously. The advantage of this method is its optimum effectiveness in continuous recording unaffected by maternal-fetal position changes or fetal descent during second stage. Its limitations are the need for skilled personnel to apply the equipment, ruptured membranes are necessary, and the presenting part must be low enough for placement of the electrode.

INTERPRETATION OF FETAL MONITORING DATA*

With the use of the stethoscope only, evaluation of fetal heart rate (FHR) is restricted usually to the interval between contractions, yielding information unfavorable for detection of abnormal FHR responses. It is during the contraction that the fetus is under stress and information on its heart rate then provides an accurate measurement of its response to the stress.

It is important that we then think about the continuous monitoring of fetal heart rate, and divide the fetal heart rate into two basic components:

1. Baseline FHR: FHR in the absence of or in between contractions
2. Periodic FHR: Changes in FHR associated with uterine contractions.

* This section is based on the research of Hon,[2] and was adapted from the work of Bednar[3] on his interpretation of the significance of Hon's work.

Baseline FHR levels are evaluated at 10-minute intervals and are described by designating the FHR range in which the baseline is located during the major portion of the 10-minute interval. If the change in baseline FHR exceeds 10 minutes, it is considered a new baseline. Periodic FHR changes are classified primarily on the basis of waveforms, and secondarily on the timing relationship between the beginning of a uterine contraction and the onset of FHR changes. Since periodic FHR changes are usually short-lived and closely related to uterine contractions, their transitory nature is implied.

The terms "bradycardia" and "tachycardia" are limited to *baseline FHR changes only*, so that an increase in FHR to a new baseline level is described as a "rise," while a decrease is described as a "fall." Thus the terms "bradycardia," "tachycardia," "rise," and "fall," are limited to descriptions of baseline FHR. Comparable terms for periodic FHR changes are referred to as "acceleration" and "deceleration."

Baseline FHR levels which are higher than normal appear to be influenced largely by the maturity of the fetal autonomic nervous system, maternal fever, and fetal hypoxia.

Tachycardia, a baseline fetal heart value greater than 160 beats per minutes which persists for at least two complete cycles, can be further divided into degrees:

1. Moderate—160 to 179 beats per minute
2. Severe—180 beats or more per minute.

Clinically, the significance of fetal tachycardia *alone* is difficult to assess. However, if it is present with late deceleration (which is discussed later) it is thought to be an ominous sign of fetal compromise. Also, moderate tachycardia and acceleration (a phenomenon of periodic FHR changes) occur in a relatively high percentage of breech presentations. Its full significance is not yet known.

Bradycardia, persistent FHR levels below

120 beats per minute, also can be divided into degrees:

1. Moderate—120 to 90 beats per minute (usually not significant)
2. Marked—89 to 70 beats per minute (often associated with progressive acidosis)
3. Severe—less than 70 beats per minute.

These perisistently low levels are not as commonly seen as are high levels. Those which occur repeatedly during the prenatal course may be associated with congenital heart lesions.

Another important characteristic of the baseline FHR is the degree of short-term FHR fluctuations which gives it varying degrees of irregularity. In the infancy period of the continuous monitoring technique, this irregularity was felt to represent fetal compromise. However, with more and more experience gained, it is now felt that FHR baseline irregularity appears to be an important indicator of the state of the nervous mechanisms controlling the heart, and may prove to be a sensitive indicator of a healthy condition. Often a *lack* of this irregularity indicates a number of possibilities:

1. Immature nervous control mechanisms
2. Use of drugs—autonomic drugs, tranquilizers, narcotics, anesthetic agents
3. Chronic fetal distress.

Periodic FHR changes are those associated with uterine contractions and have no counterpart when stethoscopic monitoring of the fetus is used. These are classified primarily on the basis of waveforms, and secondarily on the timing relationship between the beginning of a uterine contraction and the onset of the FHR changes. These periodic changes are identified by either an increase or decrease in FHR when the uterine contraction (stress) is applied to the intrauterine fetus. Increase in the periodic FHR is called *acceleration*, while decrease in periodic FHR is called *deceleration*.

Periodic FHR changes are thought to be due to the mechanical effects of a uterine contraction applied directly to the fetus and umbilical cord, or indirectly to the intervillous space by decreasing blood flow.

Acceleration is, by definition, an increase in FHR concomitant with uterine contractions. Its full significance in regard to fetal outcome is by no means clear at this time. Our understanding of deceleration patterns is much greater. However, we do know that presence of acceleration alone has not been associated with poor clinical outcomes or significant changes in fetal acid-base status.

The mechanical energy of a uterine contraction may cause fetal stress in at least three ways:

1. By application of pressure directly to the fetal body, usually vertex
2. By occlusion of the umbilical cord
3. By impeding venous outlfow from and arterial inflow to the intervillous space.

Deceleration can be categorized for purposes of definition as:

1. Early
2. Late
3. Variable.

How have these terms been derived? What significance does each have regarding the outcome of labor? This is what I will now briefly attempt to discuss. Identification of FHR deceleration patterns is based on five factors:

1. Shape of FHR pattern versus shape of uterine contraction
2. Time-relationship of onset of FHR deceleration to beginning of uterine contraction
3. Time-relationship of lowest level of FHR deceleration to the peak of uterine contraction

4. Range of FHR deceleration
5. Ensemble characteristics of FHR deceleration.

Early deceleration is thought to be due to *fetal head compression.* It is of uniform shape, reflects the shape of the associated intrauterine pressure curve, and has its onset early in the contracting phase of the uterus. *Late deceleration* is thought to be due to *acute utero-placental insufficiency* as a result of decreased intervillous space blood flow during uterine contractions. It is also of uniform shape and also reflects the shape of the associated intrauterine pressure curve. Its onset occurs late in the contracting phase of the uterus. *Variable deceleration* is thought to be due to *umbilical cord compression.* It is of variable shape, does not reflect the shape of the associated intrauterine pressure curve, and its onset occurs at a variable time during the contracting phase of the uterus.

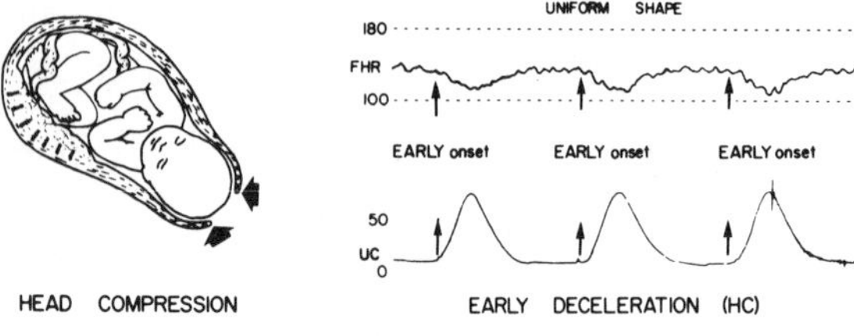

FIGURE 26-4. Early deceleration pattern. (From Hon[2] with permission.)

Let us now dissect each of these three types of deceleration more fully to appreciate just how and why each may occur. *Early deceleration* is a uniform pattern whose shape reflects the shape of the intrauterine pressure curve (Fig. 26-4). Its onset is early in the contracting phase, and is thought due to application of mechanical forces of uterine contractions to the fetal vertex by the dilating cervix.

What are some other characteristics of early deceleration?

1. FHR usually does not fall below 100
2. Duration of deceleration usually less than 90 sec.
3. Usually associated with baseline FHR in normal range
4. Not affected by maternal hyperoxia
5. Markedly modified by atropine administration
6. Usually not associated with changes in fetal acid-base status.

Caldeyro-Barcia and associates[4] using external monitoring techniques have recently demonstrated a marked increase in the number of early deceleration patterns *after* artificial rupture of membranes. Prior to rupture of membranes they suggest that occurrence of early decleration is extremely rare. On the basis of the condition of the neonate at delivery, and fetal biochemical and infant follow-up studies, this FHR pattern was felt to be innocuous. Most important of course is to clinically distinguish early from late deceleration, since both of the patterns are uniform and reflect the shape of the uterine contraction.

The FHR pattern of *late deceleration* is a uniform pattern whose shape reflects the shape of the associated intrauterine pressure curve (Fig. 26-5). Its onset occurs late in the contracting phase of the uterus. It is thought to indicate acute uteroplacental insufficiency due to decreased intervillous space blood flow as the result of impeded venous outflow from

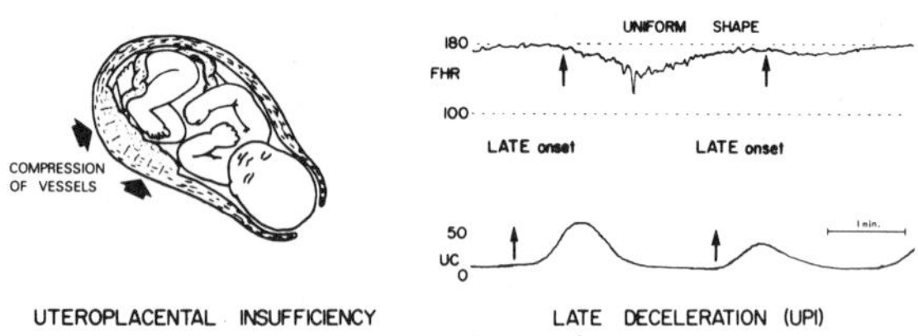

FIGURE 26-5. Late deceleration pattern. (From Hon[2] with permission.)

and arterial inflow to the intervillous space by the contracting uterus.

What are some of the other characteristics of late deceleration?

1. Usually less than 90 sec. duration
2. Usually associated with baseline FHR in top normal or tachycardia range
3. Markedly altered by maternal hyperoxia
4. Partially modified by atropine administration
5. Associated with fetal acidosis, when persistent or severe.

What are the major factors which lead to decreased maternal-fetal transfer of metabolic substances essential for fetal survival? If there is a decrease in maternal-fetal transfer of oxygen, the fetus will first become hypoxic; if the hypoxia is more than momentary, this will be followed by acidosis, hypercapnea, and electrolyte disturbances. There are indications that hypoxia resulting from decreased maternal-fetal transfer stimulates peripheral and central vagus mechanisms. If prolonged, hypoxia may have a direct effect on the myocardium and possibly on the conduction system of the heart. Certain portions of late deceleration are blocked by atropine administration and others are not; the former thought to be due to vagal reflex action, while the latter are thought to be the result of depression of the myocardium. Fetal beat-to-beat arrhythmias, gross FHR irregularity, and passage of meconium are not unusual simultaneous events.

In discussing how to alleviate *late deceleration* we know that the treatment of late deceleration in the normal uncomplicated obstetrical patient is largely prophylactic. It can usually be avoided by careful maintenance of maternal blood pressure within normal limits and by careful infusion of oxytocics for medical induction of labor, if this is being done. In patients with medical complications, extreme care must be used with agents such as conduction anesthesia which may produce maternal hypotension, and oxytocic agents which may increase uterine activity. The injudicious use of such agents may further decrease intervillous space blood flow in a situation in which maternal-fetal exchange is already compromised, and may prove disastrous to the fetus.

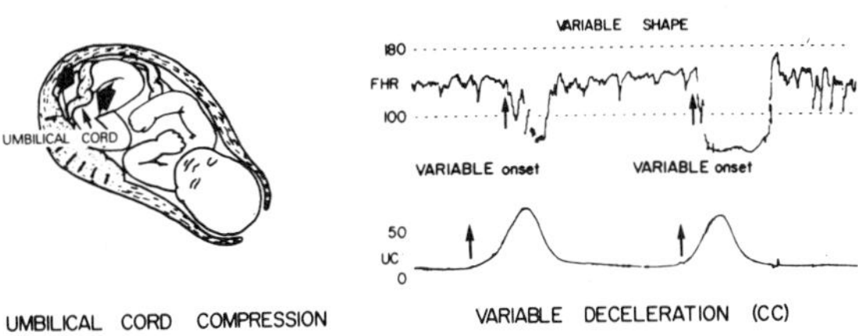

FIGURE 26-6. Variable deceleration pattern. (From Hon[2] with permission.)

The FHR pattern of *variable deceleration* is extremely important in clinical obstetrics, because it is said to be the type of deceleration found in approximately *90 per cent* of patients diagnosed as having fetal distress. It has various waveforms whose shapes do not reflect the shape of the associated intrauterine pressure curve (Fig. 26-6). Its onset occurs at *variable* times in the contracting phase of the uterus and unlike early and late deceleration which occur in groups with consecutive contractions, variable deceleration may be quite sporadic.

Studies of human and animal fetuses indicate that the mechanisms underlying variable deceleration are probably those due to *umbilical cord occlusion.* It is thought to be initiated by a strong vagal stimulus which could be due to factors other than transitory umbilical cord occlusion. Even so, during labor and delivery, it is imperative to equate variable deceleration with umbilical cord occlusion. May I make one point very strongly—even though there is no obvious cord complication at the time of delivery, this does not mean that during labor significant occlusive factors were not present on the umbilical cord.

What are some of the other characteristics of variable deceleration?

1. FHR usually falls below 100 and is frequently as low as 50 to 60
2. Duration of deceleration varies from a few seconds to minutes
3. Usually associated with baseline FHR in normal or low normal range
4. *It is markedly altered by maternal position or fetal manipulation*
5. Does not appear to be altered by maternal hyperoxia
6. Altered by atropine administration to fetus or mother
7. Not associated with fetal acidosis unless frequent and prolonged
8. Extremely common at the time of uncomplicated vertex delivery

Combined FHR Deceleration Patterns. While it is usual to see a single type of FHR deceleration pattern at a given time during labor, the possibility of a combination of two or even three patterns exists since a single uterine contraction is capable of evoking all three types of FHR deceleration patterns.

When mild forms of combined patterns exist, identification of separate patterns is relatively easy. However, when more marked deceleration patterns exist, visual identification can be tremendously difficult, if not impossible. If positive identification of the combined pattern cannot be made, the deceleration pattern is termed *indeterminate.*

Diagnosis of Acute Fetal Distress. Acute fetal distress may be defined as a compromise in fetal well-being which is related directly to the recurring stress of uterine contractions or umbilical cord complications. It is important to realize the difference between chronic fetal distress, which may be considered as a condition where chronic uteroplacental insufficiency exists before the beginning of labor, and acute fetal distress, a condition where uteroplacental function may be normal in the antepartum period.

There appear to be two major mechanisms for acute fetal distress:

1. Umbilical cord complications
2. Excess uterine activity—that exceeding fetal margin of reserve.

With the use of continuous monitoring techniques, I feel significant numbers of cesarean sections done previously for "fetal distress" can indeed be avoided.

STATUS OF AMNIOTIC FLUID AFTER RUPTURE OF MEMBRANES

The passage of meconium in the amniotic fluid after rupture of the membranes, when the fetus is in the vertex position, usually accompanies fetal distress such as hypoxia. Passage of meconium is thought to occur as a result of increased peristalsis and relaxation of the anal sphincter induced by anoxia.[5] However, the major disadvantage of this method for assessment is that the passage of meconium alone does not warrant a diagnosis of distress. It gives no indication of the severity of stress upon the fetus. Information provided by this method may be received too late for life-saving measures to be implemented.

FETAL CAPILLARY BLOOD SAMPLING

This method involves withdrawal of fetal blood into a capillary tube from a small skin nick in the presenting part, usually the scalp or buttock. The fetal blood is taken for measuring pH, oxygen pressure, and carbon dioxide pressure. Fetal pH values normally decline during labor from 7.30–7.35 to 7.20–7.25.[6] The pH indicates the acid-base balance of the body and is related to the distribution of electrolytes which affect cellular functioning. This technique is most helpful in evaluation of infants known to be at risk for fetal hypoxia from such conditions as toxemia, postmaturity, maternal diabetes, and older primigravidas. Imbalances lead to grave and fatal consequences. When two successive pH samples from a fetus are below 7.20, immediate delivery is indicated or fetal death from acidosis may occur. The advantage of this method is that early recognition of acidosis allows immediate intervention through abdominal delivery or umbilical injection of a buffer solution soon after birth of the infant. Its disadvantages are the high cost for skilled personnel and equipment, the cervix needs to be dilated to obtain blood samples, and strict aseptic techniques must be employed.

OTHER TECHNIQUES

Amniotic Fluid Studies. The amniotic fluid reflects numerous metabolic processes, primarily of the fetus but also of the placenta and mother. Certain of these chemical metabolic by-products found in the amniotic fluid vary with advancing age of the fetus and therefore are the best indices of fetal maturity.

Creatinine is a by-product of protein metabolism, especially muscle protein. It is one of the best indicators of fetal maturity. Creatinine concentrations greater than 1.8 mg. per 100 ml. in the amniotic fluid are found after 36 weeks of gestation. Any value less than this figure indicates that gestational age is less than 36 weeks.

Lecithin is a lipid substance produced in the lung and secreted into the amniotic fluid. Its concentration correlates well with the degree of fetal maturity. A sudden increase at approximately 35 to 36 weeks of gestation indicates that the fetus is now ready for extrauterine life where his own lungs must take over the task of gas exchange. The amount of lecithin in the amniotic fluid is contrasted with the amount of sphingomyelin to give the L:S ratio. When this ratio is greater than 2:1 the lungs are considered mature and there is little likelihood that the infant will develop respiratory distress syndrome.[7] The foam test is a simplified version of the same determination.

Nonradiologic Assessment of Fetal Size. Ultasound is a technique whereby intermittent sound waves of a very high frequency (above hearing) are directed from a crystal to the uterus and its indwelling fetus, and "bounced back" to the same crystal. These echos which bounce back are also sound waves but are altered due to the differing physical properties of the various tissues through which they have passed. The width of the fetal head (biparietal diameter) and also location of various parts, including the placenta, can be determined. A biparietal diameter of 9 cm. indicates a gestational age of approximately 37½ weeks. This procedure is stated to carry virtually no danger to the fetus or to the mother.[8]

Radiologic Assessment of Gestational Age and Size. The more frequent use of amniocentesis and diagnostic ultrasound should diminish if not completely replace the need for x-ray examination of the fetus. The major roentgenographic indices of age are certain ossification centers in the distal and proximal femoral epiphyses. The distal femoral epiphysis should be visible by 36 weeks of gestation and the proximal femoral epiphysis by 38 weeks. Fetal length can be calculated by measuring the lumbar spine and comparing the length with tables prepared by Fagerberg and Roonemaa.[9]

Oxytocin Challenge Test (OCT). In certain situations, when there is suspicion that fetoplacental well-being is threatened, the obstetrician may elect to give the mother and fetus a "trial run" or "rehearsal" for the labor experience. The objective is to simulate labor by administering a dilute concentration of oxytocin intraveneously (usually 5 units per 500 cc. D5/W), and to simultaneously assess uterine contractions and fetal heart rate patterns with a monitoring device. The fetal heart rate is studied in its response to uterine contractions. A negative test will result in no periodic late decelerations. A positive test as reflected by deceleration patterns indicates that the fetus is compromised by mild contractions and thus may not be able to withstand the stress of labor. The OCT results can determine whether a vaginal or abdominal delivery is indicated for the best interest of fetal welfare.[10]

The OCT is usually given at weekly or biweekly intervals, from approximately 34 weeks of gestation until delivery. The test is conducted in a hospital environment where monitoring equipment is available and may last anywhere from one to several hours, depending upon how long it takes to produce regular contractions. It is not uncommon to witness a mother who is near term go into spontaneous labor after stimulation with an OCT. It is important for the nurse to appreciate that these women will experience similar sensations during the test as women in early labor. Therefore, nursing care to women undergoing a OCT should also include the nurturance and protection the nurse would give to a patient in labor.

NURSING ACTIONS TO PROTECT THE FETUS

Knowledge of the various methods mentioned above for assessing the fetus is a prerequisite for nursing actions but not an end in itself. Nurses need to interpret the data obtained into a meaningful diagnosis and engage in a decision-making process to implement necessary actions without prolonged deliberation. Time is usually of the essence during fetal distress and lack of recognition of significant findings and indecisiveness in actions may have grave consequences. Therefore, the nurse needs to know crucial times when the fetal heart rate should be assessed:

During contractions to assess fetal tolerance to the stress

During progress of labor to another phase and as contractions become stronger

After any procedure, such as amniotomy or administration of analgesics, anesthetics, or oxytocics

When complications arise, such as toxemia or diabetes.

Assessments of the fetal heart rate pattern should increase proportionately with the progress of labor. The following are suggested minimum intervals for checking the heart rate in the various phases of labor:

Latent Phase: minimum of every hour
Active Phase: minimum every half hour
Transitional-Second Stage: minimum of every 15 minutes.

Nurses should engage in casefinding women who are potential candidates for complications such as the development of toxemia during labor. Prenatal records provide clues to anticipate the occurrence of fetal distress and thus identify patients who should have priority for fetal monitoring.

Diagnosis of uterine hyperactivity should be reported immediately because it decreases the perfusion of the intervillous space and retards fetal oxygenation. Women who receive oxytocic infusions should be watched closely for uterine hyperactivity. If it occurs, the infusion should be discontinued or decreased immediately, as directed by the physician.

Other nursing actions related to the fetus are discussed in Chapter 31.

MATERNAL ASSESSMENT AND NURSING ACTIONS

Assessment to ensure the safety of the mother during labor is just as important as safety to the fetus because effects on one system have consequences for the other.

CONTRACTIONS

Contractile activity of the uterus creates stress for the mother as well as for the fetus. Maternal arterial pressure rises during contractions, probably owing to an increase in peripheral resistance.[11] Increase in peripheral arterial resistance means increase of the force opposing the moving of blood.[12] It creates an elevation of arterial blood pressure, thus impairing oxygenation of cells. To ensure the safety of the mother from such effects, the nurse must assess contractile patterns during labor and monitor maternal blood pressure to ascertain the system's tolerance to stress.

The following technique is suggested as a way to assess uterine contractions when electrical monitoring equipment is not available:

1. Place *fingertips* gently on the fundus
2. As a contraction begins, pressure (tension) will be felt under the fingertips
3. The intensity felt will increase, reaching a peak in hardness at the acme of the contraction, and will then slowly diminish
4. Contractions should begin in the fundus; if they begin elsewhere (mid-abdomen or lower quadrant), it may indicate pathology and should be reported immediately.

Intensity. The intensity of a contraction is usually stated as weak or mild, moderate, or strong. The author once heard an obstetrician make the following comparison:

Weak Contractions: You can indent your fingers into the abdomen freely; similar to what the tip of your nose feels like.

Moderate Contractions: Your fingers indent slightly, but you can feel some tension under them; similar to the area between your nose and upper lip.

Strong Contractions: Your cannot indent your fingers into the abdomen; you feel firm tension.

Some institutions use a number code for the intensity. Whatever the assessment tool, everyone on the health team should use the same assessment tool to ensure consistency.

Frequency and Duration. The frequency pattern is measured in minutes and reflects the interval between one contraction and the next. The duration pattern is measured in seconds and tells how long the contraction lasted, from its onset to its end. Here is a typical record illustrating this assessment of contractions:

Time of Onset	*Duration*
8:55 a.m.	35 seconds
9:10 a.m.	35 seconds
9:25 a.m.	35 seconds

Nurses' notes reflect this pattern with such comments as: contractions every 15 minutes, 35 seconds, and moderate.

Uterine hyperactivity, manifested by abnormal contractions which become constant instead of intermittent, should be reported immediately. Elevated blood pressure readings, especially the diastolic which reflects the degree of peripheral arterial resistance, should also be reported immediately.

PHYSIOLOGIC STATUS

Hyperventilation, an increase in the rate and depth of breathing, is not uncommon during stressful periods. It causes loss of carbon dioxide leading to respiratory alkalosis. Consequences of this for a patient in labor are dizziness or fainting which can compromise the uteroplacental exchange system. Hyperventilation can be corrected by having the woman hold her breath for a few moments or having her rebreathe exhaled carbon dioxide by breathing in a paper bag (Fig. 26-7).

Measures to combat maternal *hypotension* should be known to nurses. Monitoring maternal blood pressure is essential to establish a baseline norm. Any woman receiving conduc-

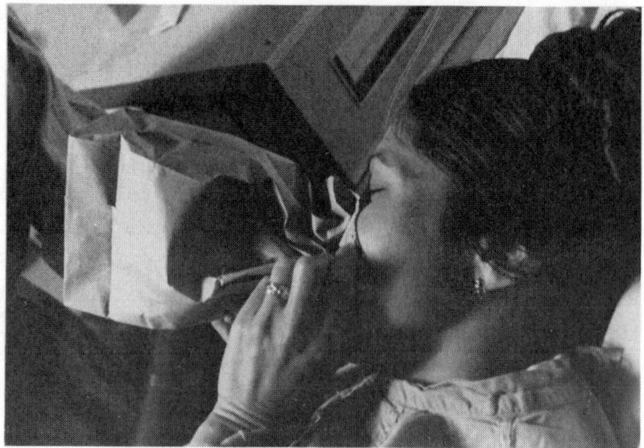

FIGURE 26-7. The effects of hyperventilation can be reduced by having the woman rebreathe exhaled carbon dioxide by breathing in a paper bag.

tion anesthesia, such as a saddle, caudal, or pudenal block, is susceptible to hypotension. The hypotension is the result of sympathetic nerve block and systemic toxic reactions resulting from excessive and rapid absorption or excessive dosage of the drug. Blood pressure readings should be taken at least every half hour during active labor. Crucial periods for assessment are:

After administration of analgesics or anesthetics
After administration of oxytocics
When contractions become stronger and more frequent (to assess the body's tolerance to the stress).

When women are found to be hypotensive, several actions are warranted. Change her position from supine to lateral. This removes pressure from the gravid uterus on the inferior vena cava which is retarding the flow of blood. Elevate her legs to decrease venous pressure and improve peripheral circulation. Increase the intravenous fluid intake in an attempt to increase the fluid volume of the circulatory system. These measures raise the maternal arterial pressure, increasing the intervillous space blood flow and thus increasing fetal oxygenation. Administration of oxygen by tight face mask at 6 to 8 liters per minute may also be indicated if there is no favorable response to maternal position changes.

Nurses also need to know what to do when a diagnosis of *variable deceleration in fetal heart rate pattern* is made. Because the cause is attributed to umbilical cord compression, measures to alleviate the pressure must be implemented immediately. Maternal position change again is a priority. Trendelenburg, knee-chest, or Sims side-lying are appropriate positions to relieve perineal pressure on the cord. Oxygen administration may be indicated to increase the fetal oxygen reserve which has been reduced. Instruct and coach the woman to slow down her breathing, especially during contractions.

TOLERATION OF PHARMACOLOGIC AGENTS

Women should be observed for systemic reactions to any drug received, regardless of the route of administration. Some reactions to local anesthetics are presented in Table 26-1 and treatment measures are described in Table 26-2.

ELIMINATIVE NEEDS

With the numerous stimuli from cervical dilatation, descent of the fetus, and stretching of the perineum, the urge to urinate may be decreased. A distended bladder impedes labor by hindering descent of the fetus and predisposes the woman to urinary stasis and infection. Thus, women need to be assessed for signs of bladder distention, and offered the bedpan or reminded to try to void at regular intervals. All means to encourage voiding, such as upright positioning, running tap water, and pouring water over the vagina, should be

TABLE 26-1. Summary of Signs and Symptoms of Systemic Toxic Reactions from Local Anesthetic Drugs*

Central nervous system effects
- A. Stimulation of
  - 1. Cerebral cortex → excitement, disorientation, incoherent speech, convulsions
  - 2. Medulla
    - a. Cardiovascular center → increased blood pressure and pulse
    - b. Respiratory center → increased respiratory rate and/or variations in rhythm
    - c. Vomiting center → nausea and/or vomiting
- B. Depression of
  - 1. Cerebral cortex → unconsciousness
  - 2. Medulla
    - a. Vasomotor → fall in blood pressure and rapid or absent pulse (syncope)
    - b. Respiratory → variations in respiration and/or apnea

Peripheral effects
- A. Cardiovascular (syncope)
  - 1. Heart → bradycardia, i.e., depression from direct action of local anesthetic agent on myocardium
  - 2. Blood vessels → vasodilatation from direct action of local anesthetic agent on blood vessels

Allergic responses
- A. Skin → urticaria, etc.
- B. Respiration → depression ("clinical anaphylactic shock")
- C. Circulation → depression ("clinical anaphylactic shock")

Miscellaneous reactions
- A. Psychogenic
- B. To other drugs, e.g., vasoconstrictors

* Adapted from Moore, D. C.: *Regional Block,* ed. 4. Charles C Thomas, Springfield, Ill., 1967.

employed. However, when a diagnosis of distention is made and measures to encourage voiding are unsuccessful, the bladder should be emptied by catheterization or other means immediately, rather than retard labor progress and increase the hazards of infection.

PROTECTION FROM DEHYDRATION

Women in labor may have an intravenous

TABLE 26-2. Summary of Active Treatment of Systemic Toxic Reactions from High Blood Level of Local Anesthetic Agent*

While following measures apply specifically to toxic reaction from high blood level of local anesthetic agent, they are general principles to resuscitation and are applicable to any reaction which may progress to shock.

1. Be sure airway is clear. If patient becomes unconscious, establish clear airway with oropharyngeal airway or preferably cuffed endotracheal tube.
2. Clear vomitus from pharynx, larynx, trachea. If cuffed endotracheal tube is in trachea and cuff inflated when vomiting occurs, no emergency exists. Vomitus may be cleared from mouth and pharynx when time permits—cuffed endotracheal tube prevents vomitus from entering tracheobronchial tree. If endotracheal tree is not in place when the patient vomits, a true emergency may exist—vomitus must be cleared from mouth.
3. Administer oxygen. Oxygen administration should be performed with bag and mask apparatus and inadequate respirations supplemented.
4. Start intravenous fluids. This is essential part of initial treatment of reaction and should be done when first signs of reaction occur, because it assures the physician a means of intravenous administration of drugs even if reaction progresses to cardiovascular collapse.
5. Stop convulsions
   - a. Administer oxygen, for oxygen alone may stop convulsion.
   - b. If oxygen alone does not stop convulsion, use intravenous injections of succinylcholine, 2 ml. (40 mg.) and oxygenate parturient. If convulsions recur after succinylcholine is dissipated (6 to 8 minutes), repeat dose. Then, if convulsions recur, give d-tubocurarine 3 to 5 ml. (9 to 15 mg.).
   - c. If muscle relaxants are not available or anesthetist is not familiar with their actions and uses, give small amounts of short-acting barbiturate, thiopental 50 mg. at ½ to 1-minute intervals. In obstetrics a single dose of succinylcholine and oxygenation is preferred. A barbiturate should not be used unless convulsions are persistent. It merely adds to depression of both parturient and fetus.
6. Raise blood pressure. When peripheral vascular collapse starts, immediate steps to raise blood pressure to approximately preoperative level must be taken—use vasoconstrictor drugs.
7. Institute manual systole. If cardiac arrest or fibrillation occurs, closed manual systole (cardiac massage) must be rapidly instituted.

* From Moore, D. C.: *Regional Block,* ed. 4. Charles C Thomas, Springfield, Ill., 1967, with permission.

kept open not merely for administration of drugs but also to replenish needed body fluids. Labor is hard work and the body needs to replenish its energy supply.

PROTECTION FROM ASPIRATION OF VOMITUS

Vomiting during the active phase of labor is not uncommon and women should be positioned to facilitate its drainage, e.g., turning on the side or lowering the head. This prevents dangers from aspiration of vomitus. To minimize vomiting, oral intake is usually restricted.

PROTECTION FROM ACCIDENTS AND ADDITIONAL PAIN SOURCES

During labor, women become preoccupied with themselves and/or their contractions. They may lose awareness of their environment through drowsiness or brief amnesia. Environmental safety should be provided through:

- Use of siderails
- Footstools for high beds
- Adequate lighting
- Uncluttered passageways for women with bathroom privileges.

Leg cramps are a frequent source of additional pain. They may result from poor anatomical positioning during the long hours of labor, or rigid positioning maintained by patients with high anxiety. Proper positioning and relaxation techniques can prevent muscle cramps. However, should they occur, the nurse can stop the cramp by extension of the leg and dorsiflexion of the toes.

Leg cramps, as well as trauma to leg vessels, may occur through improper use of the stirrups during delivery. Important points to consider when using stirrups are:

- Both legs should be elevated simultaneously
- Legs should be spread apart wide enough for good visualization of the *perineum* (not merely the vulval area)
- Both legs should be raised to the same height and spread apart to the same degree
- Support should always be maintained under the knee (A good way to check for this is to place your hand under the knee and if the ligaments feel rigid and hard, there is undue tension on the leg muscle from improper support.)
- Always bring the legs down from the stirrups simultaneously and slowly to prevent muscle spasms.

PROTECTION AGAINST INFECTION

Guidelines should be employed in judgments regarding when asepsis should be instituted and maintained. *Asepsis should be the rule for any procedure which involves the penetration of the skin or entrance into a body cavity of the paturient* (e.g., IV's, intrauterine procedures). The woman should be protected from contact with infectious staff and patients.

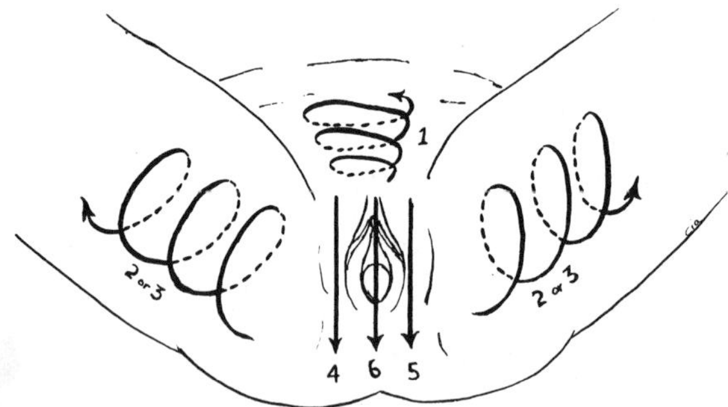

FIGURE 26-8. Proper technique for aseptic preparation of the perineum for delivery.

One area in which asepsis is frequently sacrificed for convenience or routine is the perineal preparation for delivery. All too often nurses merely "wash off" the area in the most expedient manner for the nurse. The area to be scrubbed includes the vulva, lower thighs, and perineum. It should be scrubbed in the following manner (Figure 26-8). The rationale for the precedure of preparing the perineum is the principle of asepsis: work away from the area desired to be the cleanest, without retracing previous motions. Thus, area 1 involves an upward movement, areas 2 and 3 involve outward movement and areas 4, 5, and 6 involve downward movements. When delivery is imminent, time may allow only scrubbing of the area from the vagina to perineum (motions 4, 5, 6).

Another factor for consideration is that susceptibility to infection increases proportionately with time-elapse from the rupture of the amniotic membranes. Thus, women who have had early or prolonged ruptured membranes should have temperature readings at least every two hours, even if not in active labor.

PROTECTION FROM ANXIETY DUE TO FETAL MONITORING*

The fetal monitoring device adds stress, such as:

- Implication that baby might be in jeopardy
- Fear of the machine itself
- Fear that movement will dislodge the leads or harm baby
- Fear of instrumentation
- Anxiety about any fluctuations of "beeps," during contractions or at other times.

A thorough explanation of the monitor is essential (Fig. 26-9).

- What it is
- Why it is being used
- How it is to be applied
- Explanation of the "beeps" and tracings.

* This section was prepared in cooperation with Col. Mary Fowler, ANC Tripler Army Medical Center, Honolulu, Hawaii, who has since retired.

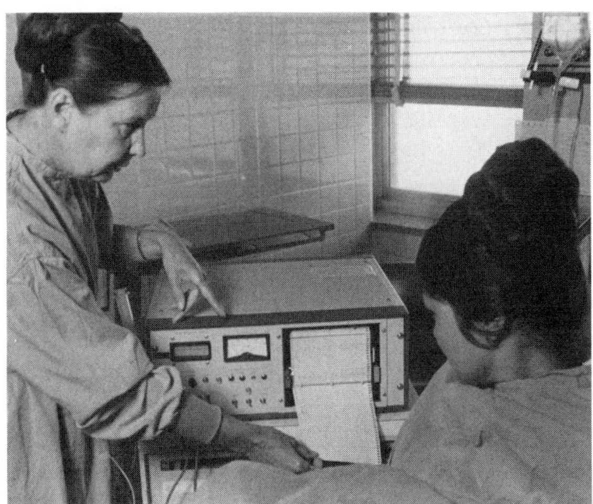

FIGURE 26-9. The woman in labor is given explanations regarding electrical monitoring devices.

Remember, the patient who does not understand English is exposed to additional sources of stress when on a monitor.

In addition to the care usually given, doctors and nurses must not let the machine come between them and the patient. It is easy to become so involved with the monitor that the patient is almost forgotten. When central monitoring stations are set up, it is even easier to forget the patient. Sometimes the husband is so fascinated by the monitor that he, too, forgets his wife. Remember, the woman needs to feel that attention is given to her as a person and not as a by-product of the equipment.

Relief of pain or assisting to successfully cope with pain and discomfort may become a greater need for patients on the monitor. Added anxiety and fear of moving increases discomfort. Comfort measures and medication may be needed more frequently. The monitor also registers the strength of the contraction. It is important to remember that you cannot equate the strength of the contraction with the individual's perception of pain. Accept the patient's behavior! Preservation of her ego is very important. Patients should not be classified as "good" or "bad." Don't tell her that her contractions are not *that* strong. Help her to relax with breathing techniques, positioning, or back pressure. Bodily cleanliness, lip care, wiping face, and speaking quietly and calmly are as essential as with any other labor patient.

Don't give false assurances, but give factual information which is easily comprehensible at her level. Use of diagrams and analogies to daily life experiences can be helpful.

PROTECTION FROM ELECTRICAL HAZARDS

With the increased use of electrical devices, there is the risk of accidental exposure of the patient, as well as others in the environment, to electrical shock from equipment and techniques being used. Because the nurse is the member of the health team who provides continuity of care, it is imperative that nurses have knowledge of electrical safety. Also, in times of crisis, it is the nurse who frequently organizes essential equipment. Inservice instruction by the hospital's electrical department is recommended. Some key safety points[13] are:

1. Cords: Avoid kinking, heat, moisture, draping on pipes and plumbing, placing on wet floors and surfaces. Inspect periodically for wear and evidence of breaks in third grounding wire. Avoid use of extension cords.
2. Plugs (power cords): Use *three-prong type* only (the third prong allows for grounding) in the vicinity of the patient. Never break off third prong.
3. Wires (grounding):
   a. Associate good electrical grounding with equipment, not the patient. Grounding to *equipment* allows current flow a safe path to "drain off," whereas ground connection to the *patient* makes the patient's body the current pathway.
   b. Connect wires to a single common ground point to ensure that all are at same electrical potential.
   c. Be sure all metal surfaces in a room are grounded.
4. Noise from Equipment or Its Scope Trace: May indicate warning sign of possible electrical problems such as loose or dry electrodes, defective cable, or hazardous current levels. Have equipment checked.
5. Tingling Sensations from Equipment or Patient when Touched: Warning sign of leakage of current indicating presence of high levels which can produce ventricular fibrillation if it contacts the heart. *Urgent*—unplug equipment not necessary to life support immediately, notify doctor and hospital electrical services.
6. You—the Nurse: Think of yourself as part of the electrical equipment surrounding the patient. Avoid touching the equipment with one hand and the patient with the other as you may electrically bridge the two. It is a good practice not to touch metal surfaces or electrical devices when you adjust controls, attachments, or handle the patient with the other hand.
7. "Routines:" The only routine is to have all electrical equipment checked and dated to ensure rechecking within a reasonable time.
8. Electrical equipment should not be "banged around" while being moved as electrical short-circuiting can result when in use.
9. All equipment should have routine safety checks by the hospital's Department of Electrical Services and the date should be indicated to insure rechecking within a reasonable time.

EMERGENCY DELIVERY BY THE NURSE*

The nurse may find herself responsible for

* Adapted from Clark.[14]

the care of the mother and her infant during the delivery phase under several conditions:

Precipitous delivery prior to the physician's arrival in the hospital
Precipitous delivery in the home, in a public place, or in the emergency room
Delivery during a natural disaster
Delivery during a man-made disaster such as warfare.

When the delivery occurs in the hospital, there is sufficient equipment to safely manage the delivery and care for the neonate. However, in the home or in a public place, the nurse needs to consider the equipment she can quickly assemble. She will need the following minimum equipment:

Newspaper to protect the bed, covered with heavy plastic or other waterproof material
Absorbent bath towels
Solution of water and liquid soap, clean washcloth
Cord ties (2) of heavy cord, new shoelace, or other stout material
New razor blade, a scissors, or a sharp knife
(The ties and the scissors or knife must be boiled for five minutes for protection.)

The nurse must remember that her patient may experience undue anxiety when her expectations are not met. For most women, to deliver in a strange environment without her physician will be an additional stressor. Confidence on the part of the nurse will help allay these feelings. The nurse should remember that 95 per cent of all women can bring their babies into the world normally and sustain their children. The nurse's responsibility is to assist the *mother* to deliver her infant and to protect each of them from harm.

The steps of the delivery follow:

1. As the head begins to crown, have the mother pant. Support the perineum and allow the head to be delivered between the contractions. This action will protect the infant's intracranial structure and minimize the danger of perineal laceration.
2. As soon as the head is delivered, support it with one hand and quickly wipe mucus and fluid away from the nose and mouth.
3. Feel about the neck for the cord. It will usually not be present. If it is, and is loose, slip it over the head or push it down over the shoulders. If it is too tight to remove, it will be necessary to tie or clamp it in two places and cut between the ties.
4. Wait for the next contraction (there is no rush), allow the anterior shoulder to be born and then the posterior one. Support the baby's body as it is being born. Grasp the baby by the feet and hold it up, head down, allowing the mucus and fluid to drain out. Remember, there is a mother present who no doubt is much more anxious than you. Hold the baby up for her to see, and with enthusiasm, tell her what a good job she has done.
5. Place the infant on the mother's abdomen and wait for the placenta to be delivered (15 to 30 minutes). Do not pull on the cord.
6. If you have sterile cord ties and scissors, knife, or new razor blade, tie the cord 4 to 6 inches from the baby's body with a double knot ligature and sever between the ties. If no sterile equipment is present, leave the placenta attached until they can be obtained. There is no danger in doing so. If necessary, baby, cord, and placenta can be wrapped together. Aesthetically, this may not be too acceptable, but it is safe.
7. Wrap the baby, and if necessary, cord and placenta, in whatever is at hand, and put the infant to breast. This will aid the uterus to contract and minimize uterine bleeding.
8. Observe the uterus closely to see that it

remains contracted. If it does not, massage the fundus to cause it to contract and then hold the uterus between your two hands.

9. Do not separate the mother and infant, for they need the haven of comfort they will find in each other.
10. The mother should be offered nourishing fluids and rest for several hours. However, if necessary, she can arise and with her infant go to a place of greater safety.

The infant born under these circumstances will, if he is normal and vigorous, very likely cry spontaneously. His two great needs for the moment are an open airway and warmth. If he does not cry within one minute, remove all mucus present from the mouth with your finger and then apply mouth-to-mouth resuscitation, using small puffs of air from your mouth (not lungs) approximately 20 times a minute. Avoid unnecessary or harmful methods of resuscitation such as spanking, anal dilatation, and compression of the chest.

Every nurse should be cognizant of the statutes of her own state governing medical practice, nursing practice, and midwifery practice. There are very few laws that cover a nurse delivering a baby in an undeclared emergency, and few court decisions involving the nurse have been published in law reports. In any event, the nurse is expected to act as a prudent practitioner.

REFERENCES

1. Danforth, D. (ed.): *Textbook of Obstetrics and Gynecology*, ed. 2. Harper and Row, New York, 1971, p. 271.
2. Hon, E. H.: *An Atlas of Fetal Heart Rate Patterns.* Harty Press, New Haven, 1968.
3. Bednar, J. A.: Unpublished paper presented at Tipler Army Medical Center, Honolulu, Hawaii, 1973.
4. Caldeyro-Barcia, R., et al.: *Effects of maternal hypotension on the fetus.* Am. J. Obstet. Gynecol. 92:847, 1965.
5. Towell, M.: *Influence of labor on the fetus and the newborn.* Pediatr. Clin. North Am. 13:576, 1966.
6. Williams, B. and Richards, S.: *Fetal monitoring during labor.* Am. J. Nurs. 70:2384, 1970.
7. Smith, D. W.: *Patterns of Human Malformation.* W. B. Saunders, Philadelphia, 1970.
8. Donald, I.: *Sonar as a method of studying prenatal development.* J. Pediatr. 75:326, 1969.
9. Fogerberg, J. and Roonemaa, J.: *Radiological determination of foetal length by measurement of lumbar spine.* Acta Obstet. Gynecol. Scand. 38:333, 1959.
10. Ray, M., et al.: *Clinical experience with the oxytocin challenge test.* Am. J. Obstet. Gynecol. 114:1, 1972.
11. Towell, op. cit.
12. Beland, I.: *Clinical Nursing: Pathophysiological and Psychological Approaches.* ed. 2. Macmillan, New York, 1970, p. 427.
13. *Using Electrically-Operated Equipment Safely with the Monitored Cardiac Patient.* Hewlett-Packard Company, Waltham, Massachusetts, 1970.
14. Clark, A. L.: *Childbirth during disaster.* Nursing World 12:15, 1959.

BIBLIOGRAPHY

Alderman, M. M.: *How fetal monitoring helps during labor and delivery.* Patient Care 7:47, 1973.

Allen, S.: *Nurse attendance during labor.* Am. J. Nurs. 64:74, 1964.

Bond, S.: *Reevaluating positions for labor–lateral versus supine.* J. Obstet. Gynec. Nurs. 2:29, 1973.

Brown, W. A., et al.: *The relationship of antenatal and prenatal psychologic variables to the use of drugs in labor.* Psychosom. Med. 34:119, 1972.

Brunner, J.: *Hazards of electrical apparatus.* Anesthesiology 28:396, 1967.

Buten, J.: *A philosophy of labor and delivery nursing.* In Anderson, E., et al. (ed.): *Current Concepts in Clinical Nursing.* C. V. Mosby, St. Louis, 1973, p. 179.

Buxton, R. S. J.: *Maternal respiration in labour.* Nurs. Mirror 137:22, 1973.

Caldeyro-Barcia, R., et al.: *Effect of position changes on the intensity and frequency of uterine contractions during labor.* Am. J. Obstet. Gynecol. 80:284, 1960.

Crawford, J.: *Physiological and behavioral cues to disturbances in childbirth.* Bull. Am. Coll. Nurse-Midwif. 14:13, 1969.

Farill, A.: *Adolescent in labor.* Am. J. Nurs. 68:195, 1968.

Friedman, E.: *Labor: Clinical Evaluation and Management.* Appleton-Century-Crofts, New York, 1967.

Ibid: *An objective method of evaluating labor.* Hosp. Prac. 5:82, 1970.

Greenhill, J. P.: *Obstetrics*, ed. 13. W. B. Saunders, Philadlephia, 1965.

Greiss, F.: *Obstetric anesthesia.* Am. J. Nurs. 71:67, 1971.

Haase, M. N.: *Giving supportive care during labor: A rewarding experience for nurse.* Hosp. Top. 49:47, 1971.

Hellman, L. M. and Pritchard, J. A.: *Williams Obstetrics*, ed. 14. Appleton-Century-Crofts, New York, 1971.

Hoff, J.: *Natural childbirth–how any nurse can help.* Am. J. Nurs. 69:1451, 1969.

Hommel, F.: *Natural childbirth–nurses in private practice as monitrices.* Am. J. Nurs. 69:1446, 1969.

Horan, J. J.: *"In vivo" emotive imagery: A technique for reducing childbirth anxiety and discomfort.* Psychol. Rep. 32:1328, 1973.

Humphrey, M.: *The influence of maternal posture at birth on the fetus.* J. Obstet. Gynecol. Br. Commonw. 80:1075, 1973.

Karim, S. M.: *The role of prostaglandins in parturition.* Proc. R. Soc. Med. 64:10, 1971.

Kartchner, F.: *A study of the emotional reactions during labor.* Am. J. Obstet. Gynecol. 60:19, 1950.

Keaveney, M. E.: *Supporting the Lamaze patient in labor.* Nurs. Care 6:15, 1973.

Kemp, J. : *The dignity of labour.* Nurs. Times 66:1436, 1970.

Kopp, L. M.: *Ordeal or ideal–the second stage of labor.* Am. J. Nurs. 71:1140, 1971.

Laros, R. K., et al.: *Amniotomy during the active phase of labor.* Obstet. Gynecol. 39:102, 1972.

Lasater, C.: *Electronic monitoring of mother and fetus.* Am. J. Nurs. 72:728, 1972.

Lorincz, R.: *Danger signs in the first stage of labor.* Hosp. Med. 6:115, 1970.

Luckner, K. *Fetal heart rate monitoring: The nurse's role as facilitator.* In Anderson, E., et al. (eds.): *Current Concepts in Clinical Nursing, vol. 4.* C. V. Mosby, St. Louis, 1973, p. 194.

Montgomery, E.: *Coping with pain–felt or fancied.* Midwives Chronicle 83:248, 1970.

O'Gureck, J., Roux, J. and Newman, M.: *Neonatal depression and fetal heart rate patterns during labor.* Obstet. Gynecol., 40:347, 1972.

Oxorn, H. and Foote, W.: *Human Labor in Birth*, ed. 2. Appleton-Century-Crofts, New York, 1968.

Passim, J.: *The nursing challenges of obstetric anxiety, ectasy, and the nurse's role.* Superv. Nurs. 3:36, 1972.

Poppers, A.: *Overventilation during labor.* Bull. Am. Coll. Nurs-Midwif. 13:4, 1968.

Reed, B., et al.: *Management of the infant during labor, delivery, and in the immediate neonatal period.* Nurs. Clin. N. Am. 6:3, 1971.

Rice, G.: *Recognition and treatment of intrapartal fetal distress.* J. Obstet. Gynecol. Neonat. Nurs. 1:15, 1972.

Rich, O.: *How does the patient use the nurse during labor?* In Duffey, M., et al. (eds.): *Current Concepts of Clinical Nursing*, Vol. 3. C. V. Mosby Company, St. Louis, 1973, p. 189.

Riffel, H. D., et al.: *Effects of meperidine and promethazine during labor.* Obstet. Gynecol. 42:738, 1973.

Sasmor, J., et al.: *The childbirth team during labor.* Am. J. Nurs. 73:444, 1973.

Scheff, J., et al.: *Uterine blood flow during labor.* Obstet. Gynecol. 38:15, 1971.

Schifrin, B. S.: *Fetal heart rate monitoring during labor.* J. Am. Med. Assoc. 221:992, 1972.

Schulman, H., et al.: *Maternal acid-base balance in labor.* Obstet. Gynecol. 37:738, 1971.

Smith, B. A.: *The transition phase of labor.* Am. J. Nurs. 73:448, 1973.

Turbeville, J.: *Nurses' role in intrapartum care.* Hosp. Top. 50:85, 1972.

Turnbull, A. C., et al.: *Endocrine factors in the onset of labor.* Proc. R. Soc. Med. 63:1095, 1970.

Tyron, P.: *Assessing the progress of labor through observation of patients' behavior.* Nurs. Clin. North Am. 3:315, 1968.

Ibid: *Use of comfort measures as support during labor.* Nurs. Res. 15:109, 1966.

Van Muiswinkel, J.: *Support in labor.* Matern.-Child Nurs. J. 1:273, 1972.

Walker, D. W., et al.: *Temperature relationship of the mother and fetus during labor.* Am. J. Obstet. Gynecol. 107:83, 1970.

Williams, B. and Richards, S.: *Fetal monitoring during labor.* Am. J. Nurs. 70:2384, 1970.

UNIT 7

THE POSTPARTAL PERIOD

27 Maternal Adaptation to the Childbirth Process

ANN L. CLARK, R.N., M.A.

The period from the termination of pregnancy by means of labor until the reproductive system returns to its normal state is known as the *puerperium*. Within six weeks almost all of the growth changes,which took nine months to develop, are terminated and reversed. Although it is not accurate to say that the maternal system completely returns to its prepregnant state, the female body does make surprising adaptations to the childbirth process.

IMMEDIATE POSTDELIVERY PHASE

Following birth, the new mother undergoes some unique experiences. Unless analgesia and anesthesia have been excessive, the mother is promptly wide awake and euphoric. She exclaims about her new child, her flat abdomen, and her state of hunger. She may experience a chilling sensation within the first postpartal hour. This chilling condition can be expected to occur more frequently when regional anesthesia has been used or when an operative delivery has been necessary. Its etiology is unclear, but it correlates with the appearance of fetal blood cells in the maternal plasma and according to McLennon,[1] may represent a fetal-maternal transfusion reaction.

After the mother has been assured that her infant is well and after her mate has visited, she feels fatigued and will sleep for an extended period if she is undisturbed. This is the body's way of compensating for the activity of labor. It gives the body cells the time required to restore themselves.

CLINICAL MANIFESTATIONS OF THE PUERPERIUM

UTERINE ADAPTATIONS

Immediately following delivery of the infant and expulsion of the placenta, the uterus weighs about 1,000 g. (2.2 lb.). Its walls are 4 to 5 cm. thick and literally collapsed together. The myometrium, under the influence of the hormone oxytocin, is contracted, compressing the blood vessels of the uterus, particularly over the placental site, and reducing the blood loss. The uterus rapidly begins to involute by means of dimunition of the myometrial cells by the process of autolysis which breaks down uterine muscle protein, especially the greatly increased volume of connective tissue collagen and elastin, into simple compounds that are absorbed and eliminated in the urine. The mechanism and control of this process are not clearly understood. The superficial layers of the decidua become necrotic and are discharged in the vaginal flow. One week after delivery the uterus weighs 500 g. (1.1 lb.), and only 350 g. (11 oz.) a week thereafter.

The new endometrium begins to form from a base of the fundi of the uterine glands. Within 21 days the entire endometrium, except the placental site, is restored to a prepregnant state. The placental site takes as long as six weeks to regenerate by a process known as exfoliation, an undermining of the placental site by the growth of new endometrial tissue leaving no scar on the uterine lining.

At the time of delivery, the fundus of the uterus is approximately at the level of the umbilicus. The uterus on external palpation feels about the size of a large grapefruit and is very firm. On the first postpartal day the fundus is one fingerbreadth above the umbilicus due to filling of the bladder, and then slowly begins to involute at the rate of one fingerbreadth a day. On the tenth postpartal day it is nonpalpable through the abdominal wall.

In the primiparous patient the muscles of the myometrium normally remain contracted. The multiparous patient, on the other hand, experiences relaxation and contraction of the uterus which cause uncomfortable "after pains" for the first two or three days. These contractions are also enhanced by breastfeeding and may necessitate the administration of an analgesic.

The necrotic superficial layer of the myometrium and blood from the uterine sinuses at the placental site are excreted by means of a vaginal flow known as *lochia*. The total amount of lochia excreted over the first three weeks of the puerperium is approximately 225 g. The flow during the first three days is bright red and is known as *lochia rubra*. The lochia then changes to a pink or brown color and consists of erythrocytes, leukocytes, shreds of decidua, mucus from the cervix, and microorganisms. This is known as *lochia serosa*. The lochia gradually turns creamy white in color by the tenth day. It continues to be composed of decidual cells, mucus, and many microorganisms and is known as *lochia alba*.

Bright red lochia beyond the third postpartal day may indicate the retention of fragments of the placenta. Clots in the lochial flow are also abnormal. Lochia does not normally have an offensive odor. A putrid odor may indicate an infection. All of these conditions should be investigated.

CERVIX

The cervix following delivery is bruised, soft and succulent, and frequently has some small lacerations. Two fingers may be easily introduced into the cervix at first, but changes occur quickly. In 18 hours it shortens, hardens, and regains its form. At the end of one week the cervical opening is barely 2 cm. wide. New muscle cells develop and the lacerations heal. The cervix never quite returns to the prepregnant state. The external os will always remain somewhat wider and the lacerations will leave visible depressed scars.

VAGINA AND PELVIC FLOOR

The vagina gradually recovers from the great distension caused by delivery. It diminishes in size but never quite returns to the nulliparous condition. The vaginal mucosa is thin due to estrogen deprivation. Rugae begin to reappear by the third week.

Following delivery the supportative tissue of the pelvic floor is infiltrated with bloody serum and the muscle fibers are often torn or overstretched. Although the pelvic floor never quite regains its former tone, it does regain considerable tone by six months after the birth.

PERINEUM

The perineum is edematous following the birth. If an episiotomy or a repaired laceration is present, there will be tenderness and considerable resistance on the part of the parturient to ambulate freely. Occasionally, blood escapes into the connective tissue beneath the skin of the perineum or under the vaginal mucosa due to injury to a blood vessel without laceration of the external tissue and forms a large hematoma. The hematoma will be seen as a tense fluctuant, painful mass. This condition is very painful and may constitute a serious loss of blood. Prompt intervention is required.

VASCULAR SYSTEM

Several hours after delivery the cardiac load will be found to be substantially increased. This appears to be due to changes in uterine blood vessels and a return of the uterine blood to the general circulation. Within one week after delivery the blood volume returns to the prepregnant level.

VITAL SIGNS

An elevation in temperature is not expected following delivery unless dehydration is considerable or an infection is present. Puerperal morbidity is defined as any temperature above 38° C. (100.4° F.) on any two postpartal days excluding the first 24 hours. It is generally believed that engorgement of the breasts is not responsible for a temperature rise.

Bradycardia is common following delivery. Rates of 50 to 70 per minute are normal. The cause is uncertain but the horizontal position, decreased nutritional and fluid intake, and increased loss of body fluids from the skin and uterus may combine to produce the slow pulse. It is not to be considered an untoward symptom.

The postpartal blood pressure is generally not changed. A few women do show hypertension following delivery, but except in pathologic situations, it returns to normal within two months.

INTESTINAL TRACT

Except for early nausea which may accompany general anesthesia, the appetite of the parturient is usually ravenous. Food and fluids are required to replenish the bodily resources utilized during labor. The parturient may resume a well-balanced diet of 2,500 to 3,000 calories and fluid intake to satisfy her needs.

Increased tympany is normal due to slight intestinal paresis. Constipation is a common problem due to a relaxed lower bowel, lack of food and fluids during labor, and overstretched abdominal and perineal muscles. Hemorrhoids or a painful episiotomy will also inhibit bowel action.

URINARY TRACT

The parturient experiences diuresis for the first two to five days due to increased output by the kidneys. Sugar in the urine following delivery is common and is due to lactose forming in the mammary glands. Acetonuria is also common after a prolonged labor due to muscular activity and lack of nutritional intake. Proteinuria in the immediate postpartal period occurs in about 40 per cent of women but disappears by the third day.

Edema of the trigone of the bladder, the urethral orifice, or vulva, or a reflex spasm of the sphincter due to the perineal wound repair may cause an inability to urinate. In even more cases, the patient urinates a small amount but retains most of the urine. This condition is known as retention with overflow. It causes pelvic discomfort and the full bladder always displaces the uterus which usually rises toward the right side.

Dilatation of the ureters, a condition present during pregnancy, disappears in the early puerperium without residual problems.

SKIN

Striae, which are red during pregnancy, turn silvery and persist indefinitely.

The tone of the rectus muscle returns to a varying degree after the birth of the baby. However, some women are left with a midline separation of the rectus muscle (diastasis recti).

Excessive perspiration is a common phenomenon in the early puerprium. Many waste products from the work of labor and the many changes of the early puerperium are excreted via the skin.

WEIGHT

Immediate weight loss results from expulsion of the infant, placenta, amniotic fluid, and some tissue fluids. Other losses due to uterine involution can be anticipated. Nevertheless, the parturient will generally leave the hospital heavier than her prepregnant weight and with a protruding abdomen due to the slow return of the tone of the abdominal wall.

MENSTRUATION

The non-nursing mother may expect menstruation to return within six to eight weeks after delivery. Follicle-stimulating hormone will have stimulated the ovary to produce a mature ovum four to six weeks after pregnancy is terminated. The menstrual flow for the first few periods may be heavier than usual.

Nursing mothers experience anovulation for varying periods of time, some for as long as they lactate, others only until the second month after delivery. Presumably the cycle is inhibited during this time due to preoccupation of the adenohypophysis with the production of prolactin, reducing the rate of secretion of other gonadotropic hormones.

Lactation does confer a substantial degree of infertility on the woman, particularly if it is associated with amenorrhea, but it is generally not considered a very reliable method of family planning.

LACTATION

The changes in the ductile and lobular-alveolar systems of the breasts in preparation for lactation occur during the nine months of pregnancy. The thin yellowish fluid known as *colostrum* is present in the breasts from four months of gestation onward, and is available to the infant at the time of birth. Colostrum is composed of watery fluid and fat globules. It contains protein materials and salts but less fat and slightly less sugar than mature human milk. Colostrum continues to be secreted from the breasts for the first three or four days of the puerperium. It is believed to contain substances that give the infant a temporary im-

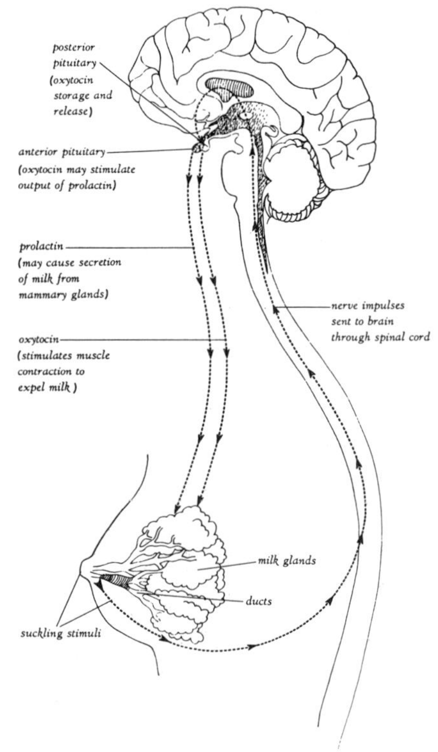

FIGURE 27-1. Mechanism of lactation. (Courtesy of *Merrell-National Laboratories.)*

munity to infectious diseases. It also has a laxative effect on the neonate.

The mechanism of lactation, the production and secretion of milk by the mammary glands, is a complex process involving many hormonal and neural factors. Lactation is established by the sucking of the infant (Fig. 27-1).

Just prior to lactation and as a precursor to it, the breasts may become heavy, hot, and painful, particularly in the primiparous patient. This is known as *engorgement*. It is not an overaccumulation of milk as is frequently believed, but represents an exaggeration of the normal venous and lymphatic engorgement of the breasts. During the period of engorgement, edema of the areola and tenseness of the breast make it difficult for the infant to grasp the nipple.

Within two to three days after delivery the breasts are filled with milk in place of colostrum. Once the inhibitory effects of estrogen and progesterone abruptly cease with the expulsion of the placenta, the adenohypophysis releases luteotrophic hormone which induces the continuous secretion of milk into alveoli in the milk glands of the breasts.

Once the infant begins to suckle, nerve impulses reach the hypothalmus. The neurohypophysis is stimulated to release oxytocin. Oxytocin then becomes the humoral efferent stimulus to the mammary gland. Its contractile effect on the myoepithelial cells which surround the alveoli of the milk glands forces the milk into the ductile system. The milk finally reaches the lactiferous sinuses, small reservoirs beneath the areola of the nipple, where it is available to the baby through the 18 to 20 openings in the nipple. This ejection mechanism is known as the "let down" reflex.

In addition to the hormonal and neural factors, a relaxed environment supports the lactation process. Disturbances such as pain, fright, anxiety, and other stressors may inhibit milk ejection.

REFERENCE

1. McLennon, C. E.: *Synopsis of Obstetrics*, ed. 8. C. V. Mosby, St. Louis, 1970, p. 192.

28 Application of Physiologic Perspectives

ANN L. CLARK, R.N., M.A.

CONTRACTION OF THE UTERUS

It is most important that the myometrium remain contracted in the early puerperium to minimize blood loss. Hemostasis is controlled at the placental site by local vasoconstriction of a well contracted uterine musculature. The body produces systemic oxytocin which acts on smooth muscles, causing contractility. At delivery this is usually supplemented by the administration of synthetic oxytocin e.g., Pitocin, Ergotrate, or Methergine. After delivery, the fundus of the uterus can be felt by palpating the abdomen. It should be at the height of the umbilicus, firm, and about the size of a large grapefruit. If the uterus is not firm, it should be promptly massaged by cupping the fundus with the hand and rubbing vigorously until it is contracted. It may be necessary to hold the uterus with both hands to keep it contracted. If the uterus is firm, however, it should not be massaged, since to do so may break up the blood clot which is forming over the placental site.

The nurse should be particularly observant of certain patients who are prone to hypotonic uterus. Contributing factors include:

Overdistended uterus due to large infant
Multiple birth
Polyhydramnios
Rapid labor
Unduly prolonged first or second stage of labor
Mulliparity
Prolonged general anesthesia
Toxemia of pregnancy

There are a number of causes for excessive vaginal bleeding; however, a relaxed fundus coupled with increased vaginal flow indicates uterine atony.

INVOLUTION

Each day the level of the fundus is checked and recorded. The position of the uterus is normally in the midline but will shift with a full bladder, usually misplacing the fundus up and to one side. To facilitate accurate measurement of the height of the fundus, the patient should empty her bladder and the head of the bed should be lowered so that the patient is in the supine position.

If the uterus is one fingerbreadth above the umbilicus, as it usually is on the first postpartal day, it is recorded I/U. As the uterus involutes, i.e., returns to nearly its prepregnant size and position, its descent is assessed and recorded daily (U/1, U/2, U/3, etc.). The nurse may use the period of observation to teach the new mother about the physical phenomenon which is occurring in her body. The mother will be particularly interested in how long her abdomen will protrude and what is causing the protrusion. Knowledge of the rearrangement of her abdominal and pelvic organs helps her to appreciate the changes and makes her more patient with the process.

UTERINE DISCOMFORT

Contractions of the uterus in the multiparous patient usually cause cramp-like pains which may make the early puerperium miserable and delay mother-infant adaptation. Analgesics such as Darvon 65 mg., or codeine 0.03 g. with aspirin 0.3 g. are usually ordered for the patient and left for the nurse to administer as necessary. These should be used unsparingly during the first two or three days postpartum to keep the mother comfortable. The nurse can control the degree of discomfort by anticipating the need and giving the medication just before the patient feels the discomfort. This reduces the amount needed and increases the effectiveness of the drug. Nursing actions should also include a thorough explanation of the physiologic etiology of the discomfort to the patient.

LOCHIA

The vaginal flow (lochia) should also be assessed and recorded daily. Lochia should be observed by loosening the back of the perineal pad with the patient turned on her side. Lochia is recorded by amount (profuse, normal, scant) as well as type (rubra, serosa, alba). Clots or tissue passed vaginally should be saved and clots should be checked for tissue. The tissue may be placental fragments left in the uterus. The size of the clot should be described and any tissue should be saved for the physician's inspection. If the lochia has an offensive odor, this should also be recorded and reported to the physician.

THE PERINEUM

A procedure and plan for teaching self-care of the perineum should be devised and taught to the new mother. Lochia should be removed from the vulva and perineum by washing both for aesthetic and hygienic reasons. The mother will feel more comfortable and the perineal suture line will heal more readily. The technique of perineal care varies from institution to institution. Generally speaking, it is becoming more simplified, but each procedure follows some basic principles. Cleaning from the front of the vulva toward the anus helps to protect the patient from entry of pathogenic organisms into the vagina. The equipment used should be clean. The area of the perineal pad that comes in contact with the body is not touched. The pad is placed on from front to back and removed from front to back.

EPISIOTOMY

Many patients will have an episiotomy (surgical incision in the perineum) or repair of a perineal laceration and this wound needs special care. It is often a source of extreme discomfort for the patient, making it difficult for her to rest or sleep and intruding upon the maternal-infant claiming process. The pain is due to the body's inflammatory response to the tissue damage. These responses are related to changes in the blood vessels and the mobile inflammatory cells. Following the perineal incision or laceration, there is a momentary vasoconstriction followed by prolonged vasodilatation with hyperemia. There is also increased capillary permeability, with fluid leaking out of the capillaries into the injured tissue. The tissue therefore becomes edematous. White blood cells migrate to the injured area where they phagocytize foreign bodies and cellular debris.[1]

Various treatments may be prescribed by the physician or instituted by the nurse to facili-

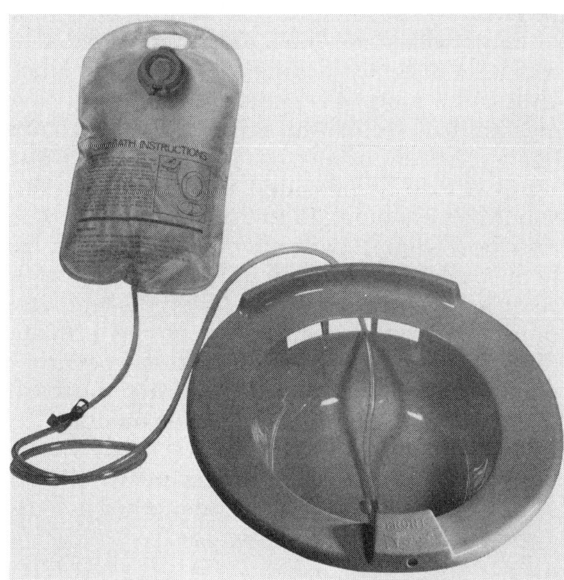

FIGURE 28-1. Sitz bath equipment. (Courtesy of Ipco Hospital Supplies.)

tate healing and increase the patient's comfort. Local applications of heat will increase vasodilation, thereby promoting healing. Heat may be applied by moist soaks to the perineum, by a heat lamp, or by a warm sitz bath (Fig. 28-1). After the patient returns home she may continue the treatment by using a portable sitz bath, her bathtub, or standing under a warm shower. Tension around the wound is undesirable since it is both uncomfortable and may cause wound disruption. One method of assisting the mother to find a more comfortable sitting position is to have her stand in front of the chair, one foot in front of the other, tighten her buttocks muscles, lower herself to a sitting position and then relax the buttock muscles. This relieves the strain of sitting on one buttock.

Tightening and relaxing the pelvic floor muscles facilitates better circulation to the area and promotes healing.

Local anesthetics may be applied by means of a spray, cream, or ointment. These surface anesthetics penetrate the sensory nerve endings and reduce responsiveness to sensory stimuli. They produce insensibility to pain by their depressant effect on the peripheral nerves.[2]

The local application of astringents, such as witch hazel, acts as a protein precipitant, causing shrinking of tissue and reduction of tissue swelling. A cotton flannel pad saturated with witch hazel and glycerine (Tucks) is used in many hospitals.

Analgesics or narcotic analgesics may be necessary to relieve the pain. Darvon 65 mg., Demerol 100 mg., or codeine 0.03 to 0.06 g. combined with aspirin 0.3 g. every four hours may be ordered.

A large hematoma, due to bleeding into the connective tissue beneath the skin of the perineum or under the vaginal mucosa, occurs frequently enough to warrant careful observation of the perineal area. If the patient complains of undue perineal discomfort during the first 24 hours, a hematoma is a likely causative factor. The nurse should not give the patient an analgesic without first examining the area under a good light to ascertain what is causing the patient's discomfort. If the patient has had saddle block anesthesia, she will not complain of pain, therefore the nurse must observe the area for a soft, fluctuating mass. Such observation may save the patient a considerable loss of blood, thereby hastening her recovery. If a hematoma is present, it should be promptly reported to the physician.

THE BLADDER

Monitoring urinary output of the postpartal patient is an important nursing function. Diuresis causes the bladder to quickly fill; however, the bladder may be insensitive to fullness. If allowed to become overdistended it will displace the uterus, interfering with the ability of the uterus to contract and control bleeding. Overdistention also causes considerable pelvic and back discomfort and could lead to cystitis.

The patient should be encouraged to empty her bladder within six hours of delivery and every six hours thereafter. The amount of the first voiding should be measured. If the bladder is only partially emptied, it will eventually appear above the symphysis pubis as a large, bulging, cystic mass.

If the patient has difficulty emptying the bladder, a warm, external, vulvar douche or the sound of running water may assist her. Catheterization should be avoided if possible due to the danger of contaminating the bladder and increasing susceptibility to infection. However, catheterization is generally considered less hazardous than an overdistended bladder with retention of urine.

During the catheterization procedure, edema and trauma of the vulvar area may make locating the meatus difficult. Gentleness on part of the nurse is essential. Patients are usually anxious about the procedure. Prior to catheterization the nurse should spend some time with her patient explaining the measures to be taken and permitting the patient to verbalize her concerns about not being able to be in command of this bodily function. The patient will be helped by knowing that the condition is of a temporary nature.

It is at times necessary for a retention catheter to be in place for a period of 24 hours. This procedure prevents distention of the bladder and gives traumatized tissues an opportunity to heal. Chemotherapy may be ordered by the physician as a prophylactic measure to avoid bladder infection. After the catheter is removed, it is again necessary to monitor the frequency and amount of voiding until the patient has control of the function.

FOOD AND FLUIDS

Some patients will arrive from the delivery suite with an intravenous still running. It is important that fluids by mouth be given promptly after the birth. They are needed to replace fluids lost during the activity of labor. Unless the mother is nauseated, she may have any kind of fluids she wishes. Some women desire hot tea, others cool fruit drinks. Fresh water should be provided and the new mother should be encouraged to drink freely. She may also be hungry, particularly if the labor has been prolonged. She may have a full diet as soon as she wishes. Many women feel very deprived by the restrictions of the prenatal diet. Food is a part of the "taking in phase"[3] and should not be limited during the early days of the puerperium. Besides meeting the physiologic need of restoring the body's cells, food may meet a psychologic need as well. Nutritional needs of the new mother are discussed in detail in Chapter 17.

SLEEP

Plans for the nursing care of postpartal patients must consider sleep needs. The physical activity and stress of labor have likely left the new mother's body cells depleted. A period of decreased activity is needed to reduce the muscle fatigue and restore the cells. The first period of uninterrupted sleep should be planned as soon as possible after labor is completed. Moreover, the new mother needs sufficient sleep each night during hospitalization if she is to return to her home ready to assume her increased responsibilities. Sleep will help relieve her of feelings of fatigue and give her a sense of well-being. Energy is required both for responding to stimuli and for repressing response to stimuli.[4] There are many sensory stimulations ahead for the new mother.

Due to the constant activity of a maternity department, the nurse must intervene to protect her patient from interruption so that she can obtain necessary sleep, otherwise the mother may return home with "sleep-hunger" which becomes one more contributing factor to postpartal depression. The nurse may take over one feeding, if the infant is fed formula, or it may be necessary to intervene in the maternity department's "routine" related to meals, baths, visitors, etc. so that the mother may rest uninterrupted. If the mother is unable to sleep, the nurse should assess her physical comfort, relieving pain and discomfort as necessary. Psychologic discomfort may also cause restlessness or sleeplessness. The nurse needs to set up a good communication system with her patient so that such concerns can be shared and nursing care can respond to psychologic needs. Sleeplessness and restlessness may be forerunners of depression and should not be ignored.

The use of sedatives, as ordered, may be needed to help the new mother get a good night's rest and feel refreshed. After the parents take the new infant home, lack of sleep usually becomes an increasing problem. It is therefore of utmost importance that the mother does not leave the hospital with a sleep deficit.

VITAL SIGNS

Blood pressure should be monitored beginning immediately after delivery. Since blood pressure is generally maintained at a normal level in the puerperium, a progressive drop in blood pressure may indicate excessive blood loss from the uterine sinuses. Elevation of blood pressure may be indicative of toxemia of pregnancy. Although the symptoms of toxemia usually occur during pregnancy, they have been known to occur in the puerperium. If the patient complains of a headache, the nurse should check the blood pressure before administering an analgesic.

Temperature, pulse, and respiration should be checked every four hours for the first two days and then once or twice daily for the remainder of the hospital stay. Temperature is taken orally, but is also checked rectally if it is elevated.

If the patient has an elevated temperature, the nurse should collect additional relevant data and report this to the physician also. For example:

Does the patient have any symptoms of upper respiratory infection?
Are there any painful or endurated areas on the breasts?
Are the nipples fissured?
Is there abdominal tenderness?
Is the uterus involuting normally?
Is the lochia normal?
Is there burning on urination?
Is the perineum healing?
Is there pain or swelling in the legs?
Is there pain in the back?
Have the bowels moved?

Some patients feel faint or lose consciousness when getting out of bed for the first time. A sudden change from a supine position to a sitting position can result in a sudden decrease in the supply of blood to the brain. This is upsetting to the patient, and is also dangerous in that the mother may be injured. The nurse should warn the patient to move her extremities slowly and rise gradually. She should be accompanied by an attendant when she first ventures from her bed, so that she can be protected from injury. Emergency call systems are usually installed in bathrooms of maternity departments, and the patient should be oriented to their use.

BOWEL FUNCTION

The second or third day of the puerperium may bring another concern for the new mother, that of constipation. Some physicians routinely order stool softeners, such as Doxicol 60 mg. or Colace or Doxinate 100 mg., on each night after delivery. These surface-active agents are inert chemicals which soften the stool by reducing the surface tension of the fecal content thereby permitting water and fatty materials to penetrate and make a more moist and bulky mass. In the postpartal patient they permit the stool to pass without undue strain on the perineal sutures and reduce further discomfort if the patient is also suffering from hemorrhoids.

Mild cathartics may be ordered by the physician on the evening of the second postpartal day. It may be necessary to administer a suppository, such as Ducolax, to stimulate the peristaltic contractions of the colon, or a small enema which would increase the intestinal fluid, bringing about peristalsis. A 100 ml. Fleets enema is frequently ordered for postpartal patients.

HEMORRHOIDS

Many women develop hemorrhoids during pregnancy and these often increase in size during the expulsive stage of labor. In the postpartal period the patient may be made uncomfortable by the pressure and a few patients experience considerable pain from large thrombosed hemorrhoidal veins. The patient may be reassured that the condition is usually a temporary one and surgery is usually not needed. However, vigorous nursing care is required to relieve the discomfort. Cold compresses of witch hazel, magnesium sulfate, and glycerine will bring about vasoconstriction. Topical analgesic sprays used several times daily, analgesia given by mouth, and warm sitz baths offer some relief, as they do for perineal suture discomfort. The patient is usually reluctant to have her first bowel movement, even though its delay increases thrombosed veins. The measures discussed previously for relief of constipation are helpful.

SKIN CARE

Excessive diaphoresis is experienced during the puerperium. Frequent bathing is necessary not only because it is refreshing and gives a sense of well-being, but to remove the waste products deposited on the skin. Many new mothers are anxious to take a shower and may usually be permitted to do so after the first postpartal day.

It is the opinion of the author that a woman should be given a bed bath by the nurse on the first postpartal day, unless, of course, the patient resists this kind of nurturient care. The bath serves several purposes. This type of supportative care begins to meet the new mother's dependency needs. These needs must be met before the mother moves on to giving care to her dependent child. Moreover, it helps the nurse establish a trusting relationship with the patient. It offers the nurse an opportunity to do a nursing assessment on which she can base much of the nursing care during the patient's stay in the hospital. It also affords the nurse an opportunity to teach the patient about her changing body and ways she can care for her body. Some of the things she may teach or make plans to teach at some other point in the patient's hospital stay are:

- How to cleanse the nipples and breasts (bathe first, do not use soap on the nipples).
- How to strengthen the pelvic floor muscles (contract and hold the muscles of the perineum several times a day).
- How to cleanse the perineal area and care for the perineal sutures.
- How to support the breasts.

The nurse may have ample time to explore the mother's feelings about labor, her conduct during the labor, her feelings about her new infant, and how she perceives the child will change her life and the lives of her husband and other children, if any. The nurse may use this period to explore the goals of the family in relation to the number of children desired and what information about conception control may be needed. She can assess the mother's experience in infant and child care and make plans to teach the mother what she needs to know about feeding and caring for her infant. She may explore other aspects of family life that may need further discussion, such as, problems with sibling competition, concerns about separation anxiety on the part of children at home, and sex education of the older children.

If the new mother is sent off to a strange shower for her first bath, not only does the nurse miss an important opportunity to gather valuable information for planning nursing care, but the mother is deprived of an important interpersonal relationship at a time when she may need it the most.

LACTATION

It is the mother who ultimately makes the decision on how she will feed her infant. Nevertheless, her culture, peers, physician, and husband will enter into this decision. It is not the role of the nurse to recommend a method, but rather to be knowledgeable about both breast feeding and bottle feeding so that she may effectively teach and support the woman in this first task of motherhood, regardless of which method is used.

BREAST FEEDING

The decision to breast feed one's child is influenced by many factors. Some focus on what is preferable for the infant, but more often the decision is based on identity and self concept.

The advantages of breast feeding are:

Economy
Convenience
Asepsis
Automatic adjustment to infant's need
Psychologic closeness
Benefit to involution.

Disadvantages and contraindications include:

Nipple or breast lesions
Pregnancy
Maternal illness
Mother's need to return to work
Mother's aversion to breast feeding.

The infant may be placed to breast and encouraged to suck immediately after birth unless the mother has had heavy sedation or deep anesthesia for the delivery. This sucking stimulates the mammary glands and promotes earlier secretion of milk. After the mother has had a sufficient period of rest the infant should be brought to her for breast feeding every three to four hours, or preferably, left with her if a rooming-in arrangement can be made available.

The mother should be instructed to wash her hands prior to feeding her baby and to cleanse the nipples with clear, warm water using a disposable washcloth or cotton pledgets. Soap should not be used on the nipples since it removes the protective skin oils and leaves the nipples susceptible to damage. If the nipple tends to be flat or a bit inverted, the mother should grasp the nipple between her thumb and forefinger and roll it gently to the right and to the left. This stimulates the erectile tissue and the nipple will become more prominent and available to the infant.

At first, most mothers can manage breast feeding better lying flat with only a pillow under her head and cradling the infant's head. She turns to the side to nurse, places the nipple between the index and third finger to make it more prominent (Fig. 28-2), and places the nipple near the infant's mouth to encourage him to "root" for the nipple. The mother should be cautioned not to place her hand on his cheek to guide him to the breast, for this only confuses him and he will automatically turn toward the hand and away from the breast. The infant should grasp not only the

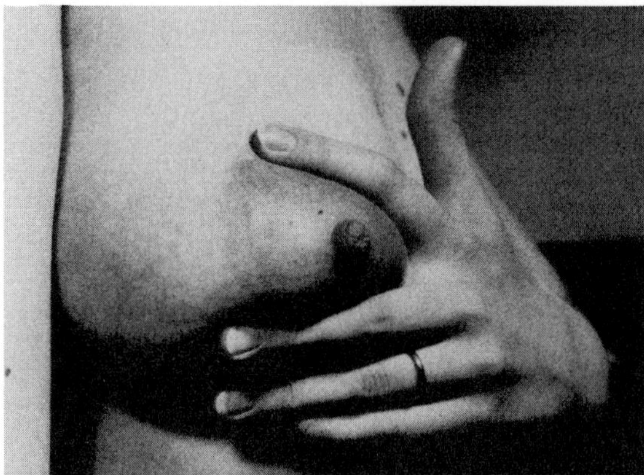

FIGURE 28-2. Pointing the nipple. (Courtesy of Ross Laboratories.)

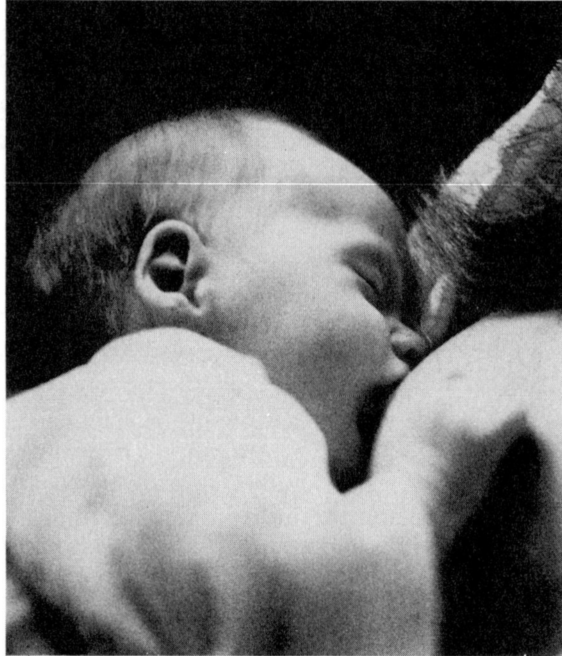

FIGURE 28-3. Proper position of infant's mouth on the breast.

nipple but also a considerable portion of the areola, for the lactiferous sinuses which hold the milk are in this area (Fig. 28-3). Moreover, sucking on the nipple alone may cause it to become tender or even macerated. If the mother's breast is soft and large the infant may bury his nose in it, making it impossible to suck and breathe at the same time. He will therefore cease nursing. The mother should be instructed to use one finger to compress the breast and permit free breathing for the infant. To remove the infant from the breast, the mother should use one finger in the corner of the infant's mouth to break the suction and again protect the nipple from damage. After some success with breast feeding and after the perineal area is less tender, the mother may wish to nurse her baby sitting upright in bed (Fig. 28-4) or in a comfortable chair with an armrest and a footstool so she can cuddle the baby to her body. After she returns home, she may wish to use the reclining position for one or two feedings a day in order to rest.

Many nursing mothers, even multiparas, need assistance during the early days of lactation. The mother needs encouragement from the nursing staff, as well as from her physician, husband, and other family members. The nurse can tell her when she is doing well and support her in other ways when success is not instantaneous. If the infant cries, help her to comfort him and then try again. The first few feeding sessions will be less tense if the mother is encouraged to use the periods to get to know her child, with less focus placed on success at the breast. Most of all, the mother needs a private, tension-free environment where she can enjoy her infant and the breast-feeding experience.

The length of the nursing period need not be limited since the sucking promotes the early secretion of milk. Almost every woman has some discomfort when the baby is put to breast the first few days after birth. This usually disappears as milk secretions begin and the baby becomes satisfied. In the course of a single feeding, discomfort is often felt only until the ejection reflex occurs.[5] Both breasts should be nursed at each feeding until lactation is well established, alternating the breast with which the mother begins each feeding. A safety pin on the brassiere strap will help the mother to remember which breast should be used to begin the next feeding. After lactation is well established the mother can nurse on one breast, alternating breasts for each feeding. The nursing period need not exceed 20 minutes, and often much less time is necessary

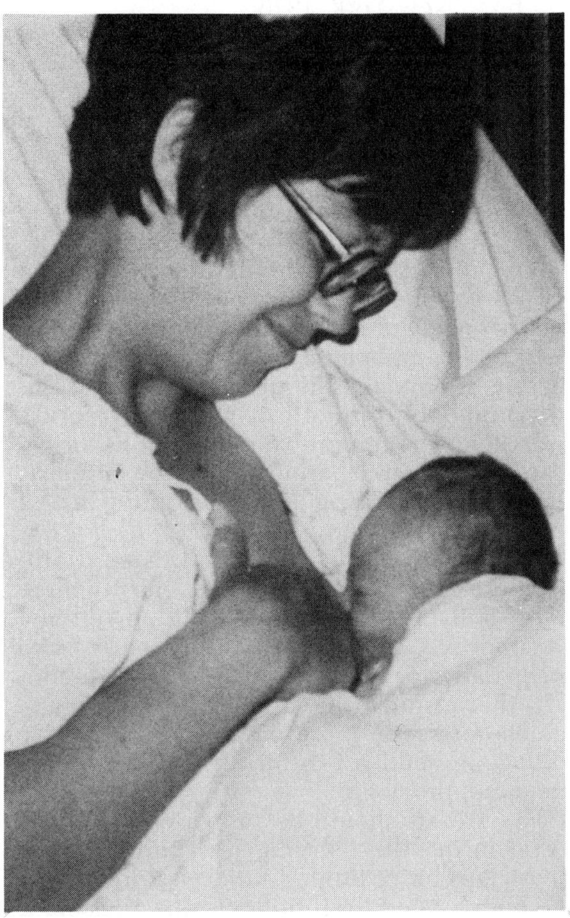

FIGURE 28-4. Mother sitting upright in bed to nurse.

if the supply is good, the milk flows freely, and the infant nurses vigorously.

Initially, some women have difficulty with the milk "let down reflex." Synthetic oxytocin nasal spray (Syntocinon) is sometimes ordered by the physician. The oxytocin acts specifically on the myoepithelial elements surrounding the alveoli of the breasts, causing them to contract and thus force milk into the larger ducts where it is more readily available to the infant. It is administered by spray into one or both nostrils two to three minutes prior to nursing.

If the nipples become painful, unmedicated hydrous lanolin may be used on the nipples after the nursing. Exposure of the sore nipple to a 25 watt light bulb at a distance of 8 to 12 inches for 10 minutes will also afford relief. The heat causes vasodilatation, thereby increasing blood supply to the damaged tissue and promoting healing.

Prelacteal, supplementary, or complementary feedings while lactation is being established will tend to reduce the sucking reflex at breast and should be avoided. Once lactation is well established, at about three weeks, the mother may leave a bottle of formula or hand-expressed breast milk with a trusted babysitter and enjoy an evening of relaxation away from home. The method of hand expression follows: Wash the hands, cleanse the nipple with tap water, grasp the areola with the thumb above and the index finger below, support the rest of the breast with the other fingers, and compress the areola deeply and firmly with the thumb and forefinger (Fig. 28-5). The expressed milk is collected in a cup or glass held with the other hand.

A good brassiere with wide shoulder straps, which lifts the breasts up and in, should be worn throughout the day and night. Nursing brassieres come with plastic pockets which hold disposable pads, useful when the breasts leak a bit as they frequently do during the initial stages of lactation. Leaking from the nipples may be controlled by pressure from

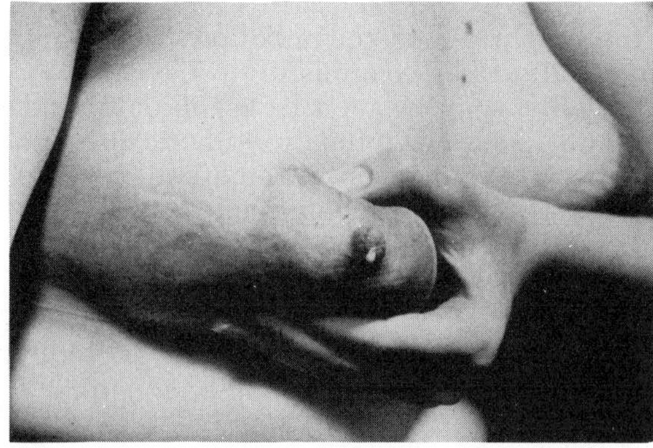

FIGURE 28-5. Manual expression of milk. (Courtesy of Ross Laboratories.)

the heel of the hand against the nipple.

Nutrition for the nursing mother is of considerable importance and is covered in detail in Chapter 17.

During the first few days at home the mother may experience a decrease in her milk supply and should be told of this possibility prior to discharge from the hospital. The mother can return to nursing both breasts at each feeding and increase the number of feedings. The increased sucking will cause an increased production of prolactin and the secretory ducts will adjust to the increased demand made upon them. There may be two other periods in the nursing experience when the mother's supply does not seem to meet the infant's increased demands due to his spurt of growth. This means that temporarily his appetite is greater than the milk supply. Again, she should nurse the infant as frequently as he demands it, even every hour or two, and the milk supply will increase to meet his requirements.

The professional nurse should be aware of the community facilities available to support breast-feeding mothers. Many communities have local chapters of the La Leche League, an organization composed of successful breast-feeding mothers who are available to give telephone advice to nursing mothers and who conduct meetings to support breast feeding. Several books which may be particularly helpful to the breast-feeding mother are:

The Womanly Art of Breast Feeding. La Leche League, 3332 Rose Street, Franklin Park, Illinois 60131

Newton, N.: *The Family Book of Child Care*. Harper and Row, New York, 1957

Instructions for Nursing Your Baby. ICEA Supplies Center, 208 Ditty Building, Bellevue, Washington 98004

Prayor, K.: *Nursing Your Baby*. Harper and Row, New York, 1973.

INHIBITING LACTATION

The mother who cannot or decides not to breast feed will need some medical and nursing intervention. Many physicians order testosterone enanthate and estradiol valerate (Deladumone OB). This intramuscular injection should be given just prior to the onset of the second stage of labor and should be given deep in the upper outer quadrant of the gluteal muscle following the usual precautions for intramuscular injection. This long-acting androgen-estrogen preparation inhibits the release of lactogenic hormone from the pituitary, thereby preventing lactation and painful breast engorgement.

Another therapy is to administer diethylstibestrol (Stilbestrol) 5 mg. one to three times daily for a total of 30 mg., or ethinyl estradiol (Estinyl) tablets 0.5 mg. one or two times daily for three postpartum days, gradually diminishing the dose to two 0.05 mg. tablets for seven more days. These synthetic estrogens act by inhibiting the lactogenic hormone, prolactin.

The breasts should be supported by a brassiere during this "drying up" period. Some physicians order limited fluids, but in view of the body's need for fluids it is questionable if fluid can be kept from the breasts during this period without dehydrating the body.

Analgesic drugs may be given the mother to relieve the pain, and ice caps on the breasts cause vasoconstriction and afford relief from the tension and throbbing of the breasts. The breasts should not be pumped and hand expression of milk should not be employed since both stimulate further secretion of milk.

CONCEPTION CONTROL

Recent studies show that ovulation may occur as early as 36 days postpartum in nonnursing mothers and 39 days in nursing mothers, although the average is much higher in both cases.[6] It is therefore appropriate that part of the nursing care should be assessment of the new mother's wishes about further children and how soon she wishes to conceive. It is possible that the woman may conceive before the six-week postpartum examination. This may not be a part of her plans and from a physiologic standpoint it is undesirable, thus nursing care should include a discussion of conception control.

Intrauterine Devices (IUD). The intrauterine device is a plastic or metal coil or loop that is inserted through a tube, using a plunger, into the uterine cavity. When the device is released into the uterus, the coil or loop springs back into its original shape. It needs no further attention, except to be sure it has not been expelled, and can safely be left in place for several years without removal. However, a visit to the physician each year for a thorough examination is essential. The device should be checked frequently to be sure it has not been expelled, at least every three to four days during the first month after insertion and after each menstrual period thereafter. The examination is accomplished by feeling for the bead-like appendage or the polyethylene suture which protrudes through the cervix.

The rationale for such devices controlling conception is not totally clear. It may be that the presence of the device speeds up the movement of the ovum through the Fallopian tube and into the uterus, thus preventing fertilization. Another theory is that fertilization does occur but that nidation of the fertilized ovum is prevented.

Although this method is not 100 per cent effective, the intrauterine device is among the most effective means of conception control. Once the device is removed, pregnancy usually occurs within three to four months.

Some women experience uterine cramping for a short time after insertion. The first few menstrual periods may be heavier and a little bleeding may occur between periods. These occurrences usually subside after the second or third menstrual period.

Oral Contraceptives (The Pill). There are several oral contraceptives. Those most commonly used involve the administration of tablets combining estrogen and progestin which alters the delicate balance between FSH and LH, thereby suppressing ovulation. Another regime, referred to as the sequential method, administers a synthetic estrogen daily for the first part of the menstrual cycle (15 or 16 days) to inhibit ovulation and is followed by a mixture of estrogen and progestin for a period of five days. Menstruation occurs three to five days after the last tablet is taken.

Both of these regimes prevent production of the ovum, so fertilization cannot occur. Oral contraceptives are reliable if directions are followed explicitly. If the medication is forgotten for one day, the pill should be taken as soon as remembered and the next pill also taken at the regular time, even if this means taking two pills close together. If two pills are forgotten, the two should be taken as soon as remembered and the next pill taken at the regular time. *However*, the patient should be advised to use some other additional method of conception control for the remainder of the cycle. If more than two pills are forgotten, the patient is advised to discontinue the regime, wait for the next menstrual period, and then start the next series of pills five days later. She should use some other form of conception control for the remainder of the cycle. It is also preferable to use a second method of conception control during the first month on the regime.

Some women experience side effects from the medication during the first two or three months. Some of these symptoms are similar to the early signs of pregnancy, e.g., nausea, breast tenderness, weight gain. Some women experience occasional mid-cycle spotting and increased menstrual flow, others have shorter periods and decreased flow. Occasionally, the menstrual period does not occur at all. All of these conditions are temporary and usually disappear after the pill has been taken for several menstrual cycles. The pill is generally not prescribed for the breast-feeding mother and some other form of conception control is advised.

Most women feel unusually well while on the medication. Premenstral tension usually disappears, and menstrual irregularity and discomfort are often relieved. The use of the pill allows many couples to enjoy sexual relations more fully because it frees them from fear of an unwanted pregnancy.

Diaphragm. The diaphragm is a flexible, cup-shaped device made of rubber which is inserted into the vagina in such a way that it covers the cervix and prohibits the sperm from entering the uterus. It is used in conjunction with a spermicidal cream or jelly which gives the protection of a chemical barrier. The diaphragm must be fitted by a physician, and the fitting checked every two years and after each pregnancy. Used properly, it is a highly reliable method of conception control.

The diaphragm may be left in place for as long as 24 hours. It should not be removed until six hours after intercourse, at which time a vaginal douche may be used if the woman wishes.

Condom. A thin, strong, rubber or latex sheath can be worn by the male as a highly effective method of conception control. Indeed, it is generally the method of choice during the puerperium. (The author is aware that some physicians suggest that their patients abstain from sexual intercourse during the puerperium; however, few families carry out this dictum.)

The sheath fits the erect penis and prevents the sperm from entering the vagina of the female. For added protection the woman may also use a contraceptive cream or jelly.

Chemical Contraceptives. Contraceptive creams, jellies, and suppositories act as powerful spermicides. These are not as reliable as other conception control methods described earlier but are successfully used by many couples. The spermicide should be inserted into the vagina no more than one hour before sexual intercourse, and each application is effective for one sexual contact only. If sexual intercourse is repeated, another application should be used. A vaginal douche should not be used for at least six hours following sexual relations; in fact, a douche is not necessary at all.

Rhythm Method. The rhythm method of conception control is based on abstention from sexual intercourse during the fertile period of the women's menstrual cycle. Lack of knowledge as to the exact length of the fertile period[7] and irregularities in the menstrual cycle make this an unreliable method. However, if this is the method of choice the woman should keep careful records of her menstrual cycle for several months and then seek the assistance of a family planning clinic or a physician in plotting her fertile and "safe" periods within the cycle. Computation of a safe period is complicated after delivery and during and after lactation.

Permanent Methods. Vasectomy for the male and tubal ligation for the female are permanent methods of conception control. Vasectomy is done on an outpatient basis. Tubal ligation is usually done within 24 hours after the delivery of the child; thus, the decision should be reached by the couple and necessary forms signed prior to labor and delivery.

Other Methods. Coitus interruptus, or withdrawal, is not an effective method of conception control. Vaginal douching following sexual relations is also not a reliable method of preventing pregnancy.

PREPARATION FOR CARING FOR THE NEONATE

New parents have many adjustments to make in the early stage of the expansion of the family. For a time the physical and emotional needs of the infant will seem to fill their every moment, crowding out their own needs. Any way in which the nurse can help to prepare the parents to meet these needs will reduce the stress and increase the joys of parenthood. Many expectant parents prepare themselves to meet the day to day physical needs of the infant by attending classes, reading, and caring for friends' or relatives' infants thereby developing some skills. Far too many parents come to parenthood poorly prepared even to bathe and dress the infant or to make formula. Indeed, some parents seem not to have considered that these skills will need to be learned, and are tense an anxious when they are faced with the reality.

In planning to help new mothers learn infant care skills, the nurse should begin by ascertaining what the mother already feels comfortable in doing. Previous experience with younger siblings, baby sitting, classes attended and the like, as well as the mother's own feeling of security or lack of it, will indicate to the nurse the appropriate point of entry for teaching infant care skills. The mother will learn best when perfection is not the goal, and when she is helped to recognize that the infant does not judge her and that he has no one with whom he can compare her. She will feel free to learn when the nurse helps her to problem solve rather than to "tell her" or to "show her." She will learn best when her nurse uses positive feedback at appropriate times.

THE BABY BATH

Bath time may be any time of the day convenient for the mother and comfortable for the infant. It is preferable not to bathe just prior to a feeding when the infant is hungry and restless, or just after a feeding when the infant is relaxed and sleepy. The bath time should be planned so that other activities will not interfere.

The bath is usually given in the kitchen, on a table or counter, or in the bathroom if it is large enough. The room should be free from drafts and about 75 to 80° F. All necessary equipment and a fresh set of baby's clothes should be at hand. Rings or other jewelry that may scratch the baby should be removed. A waterproof apron will protect the mother's clothes. The mother washes her hands, collects all equipment, and then brings the baby.

A suggested technique follows, but mothers should be encouraged to experiment and modify to find ways that are more convenient and offer more pleasure for both her and her infant.

The infant is ready for a tub bath as soon as the cord has fallen off and the umbilicus has healed, and as soon as the circumcision wound is healed. A sponge bath is given prior to that time.

Equipment

Tub or bathinette
Pad or folded blanket covered with a soft bath towel
Second soft bath towel
Soft wash cloth
Mild soap (Ivory, castile, baby soap, Dial, or Safeguard are acceptable choices)
Container of cotton balls
Powder *or* lotion *or* cornstarch (not essential, but may be used sparingly if the mother wishes)
Comb or soft brush
Container of alcohol for umbilical cord

Container of petroleum jelly and roll of 1″ gauze if infant has been circumcised.

Technique

1. Remove any outer garments so that the baby is in shirt and diaper.
2. Inspect the eyes. If necessary, clean each eye with the end of a clean washcloth dipped in clear water. Cotton balls may be used if the mother prefers.
3. Inspect nose. If necessary, clean with small wisps of cotton that have been rolled between the fingers. The cotton may be moistened with water if necessary. Frequently, the cotton will cause sneezing which brings further mucus.
4. Inspect ears. Clean with wisps of dry cotton.
5. Clean the face with clear water and pat dry.
6. Clean the shell of each ear, area behind the ears, and the neck with soap and water. Rinse and dry, paying special attention to the creases.
7. Approximately every three to four days, soap the scalp, making a lather with the hands. Pick up the baby, and hold football fashion over the tub to rinse. Use care not to get the soap in the eyes. Return to flat area and dry. The mother should have the "soft spots" (anterior and posterior fontanels) pointed out to her only to impress her with the fact that firm strokes on the infant's head cannot injure him.
8. Undress the infant. Soap the entire body using the hands or the washcloth. Work the soap well into the creases. The mother rinses her hands. Supporting the infant's head with the left arm she grasps the infant's left arm, supporting the buttocks with the right hand, she grasps the infant's left thigh and lifts the infant and then slowly lowers the infant into the bath water. She removes her right hand and permits the infant's buttocks to rest on the tub. She continues to hold the infant's left arm and support his head. The soap is rinsed from the infant and he is returned to the flat area and dried carefully, using a blotting motion.
9. The mother sprinkles cornstarch or powder on her hands and then applies it to the infant's skin. She may apply lotion instead, if she prefers.
10. The bath towels are removed and the infant is dressed in fresh clothing.
11. The hair is combed or brushed away from the scalp so air can circulate to the scalp, helping to prevent cradle cap.

Care of the Cord. The cord and umbilicus need no special care unless there is serous or blood-stained drainage. In this case saturate a cotton ball or a Q-tip with alcohol and cleanse around the folds in the area.

Care of the Circumcision Site. Cleanse the circumcision wound gently with cotton balls and clear, warm water. Cut a two-inch strip of 1″ gauze. Place a small amount of petroleum jelly on the gauze and wrap it around the penis leaving the tip of the penis uncovered. After five days the wound will have healed so that the penis may be cleansed with soap and water during the bath.

Care of the Vulva. Separate the labia and gently cleanse the area from front to back with cotton, soap, and water. Rinse and pat dry.

FORMULA PREPARATION

There are several methods of preparing the infant's formula. The terminal sterilization method is generally considered a safe, easily-learned procedure and is frequently preferred by the physician.

Equipment (Fig. 28-6)

Measuring pitcher (32 oz.) or a measuring cup and a mixing pitcher
6 to 8 bottles (8 oz.), nipples, and caps
Tablespoon measure and table knife if dry products are used
Can opener

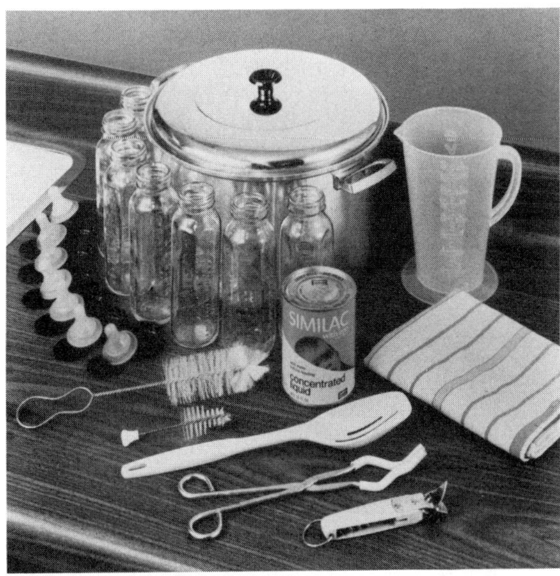

FIGURE 28-6. Formula equipment. (Courtesy of Ross Laboratories.)

Spoon for stirring
Bottle and nipple brush
Sterilizer
Formula ingredients as prescribed

Technique

1. Assemble all equipment and wash hands.
2. Wash all equipment with hot soapy water, rinse thoroughly, and allow to drain dry. Special care should be taken of the nipples. Clean with a nipple brush and force water through the holes. Salt may be sprinkled in the nipple and the sides rubbed together to thoroughly clean the inside of the nipple.
3. Measure the required amount of hot tap water.
4. Measure the required amount of carbohydrate (sugar, syrup, etc.). Level with the knife and add to the water. Stir until the sugar is completely dissolved (some specially prepared formulas will not need this step).
5. Cleanse the top of the can of milk with a cloth. Rinse under hot tap water.
6. Open the can, add the required amount to the other ingredients, and stir. (Any milk left in the can may be placed in a clean, covered container in the refrigerator and used the following day. Do not keep the milk more than one day.)
7. Pour the required amount of the formula mixture into all but two of the bottles. Fill the two empty bottles with water. The water is sterilized along with the formula and is used for drinking purposes.
8. Nipple (turn the nipple upside down in the bottle and cover with a disk), add the top or cap. Do not tightly cover the bottle with the top or cap, leave it loose so the steam can enter and circulate within the bottle.
9. Place all bottles (formula and water) in the sterilizer and add two inches of water to the sterilizer.
10. Cover the sterilizer with its lid, turn on the heat, and note the time when the water begins to boil. (A gentle boil is sufficient. Do not boil the sterilizer dry.)
11. After the water has boiled 25 minutes, remove the sterilizer from the burner but *do not remove the lid* of the sterilizer until the sides are cool enough to touch. (This step will prevent a film from forming on the top of the formula and clogging the nipple.)
12. When cool, remove the bottles from the sterilizer, tighten the nipple covers and refrigerate.

BOTTLE FEEDING

The mother removes the formula from the refrigerator prior to the feeding so the chill is removed. The formula may be fed at room temperature, or if the mother prefers, she may warm the bottle by placing it in a pan of hot water. The mother washes her hands before the feeding, and holds the infant in her lap with his head resting in the curve of her arm. Using a rocking chair is an excellent way for the mother and infant to enjoy each other during the feeding. All mothers prop some feeding and for very good reasons. No mother should be made to feel guilty for not holding her infant for *all* feedings. The bottle should be held at an angle so that the neck of the bottle is kept full of milk. In this way the amount of air swallowed by the infant will be minimized. However, all babies swallow some air with their feeding and need to be bubbled, often after each ounce. The infant may be held over the shoulder and gently patted on the back to bring up the air, or the mother may prefer to hold the baby upright on her lap, supporting the jaw and chest with one hand and gently patting the back with the other. It is not unusual for an infant to regurgitate part of a feeding and the mother should be made aware of this to allay anxiety.

EXERCISES

The new mother should be taught exercises to help her regain her body tone and strengthen her muscles (Fig. 28-7). Most mothers are unhappy with their excess weight gain and their protruding abdomen.

Some of simple exercises should be begun in the hospital as early as the first postpartal day. Some hospitals have daily, planned sessions with a physiotherapist, others have prepared a mimeographed sheet, complete with drawings, so that the mother may take her instructions home with her. The exercises which follow are not strenuous and can be accomplished in a 10-minute period each day. Within a short time the mother will notice that her abdomen and waistline have begun to become firm and the improved circulation will increase her energy and zest for living. The improved muscle tone will lessen strain and fatigue and, most importantly, her self concept will receive a boost.

First Day

1. Gluteal and pelvic floor exercise (to strengthen pelvic floor muscles, slim buttocks, and improve circulation to the pelvis)
   Position: On the back, arms at side, knees straight, legs crossed at the ankles.
   Exercise: Squeeze the buttocks together tightening the large muscles in the buttocks and the muscles of the pelvic floor (between the vagina and the rectum) as though you were checking a bowel movement and at the same time press the inner thighs together.
   Repeat: 10 times, twice daily.
2. Ankle exercises (to improve circulation in the extremities)
   Position: On back, legs straight
   Exercise: Lock knees, push toes toward end of bed, then bend ankles and push heels toward end of bed, toes pointed toward head.
   Repeat: 10 times, four times daily.
3. Head raising (to strengthen abdominal muscles)
   Position: On back without pillow, arms at sides.
   Exercise: Raise head so chin touches chest. Lower slowly.
   Repeat: 10 times, four times daily.

Second Day

4. Pelvic rock (to strengthen lower back and abdominal muscles)
   Position: On back, arms at sides, knees bent, feet flat.
   Exercise: Tighten buttocks and abdominal muscles. Rock pelvis anteriorly, flattening the lower back against the floor. Hold for a count of 10, then rock pelvis posteriorly, arching lower back.
   Repeat: 10 times, three times daily.
5. Partial trunk raising (to strengthen abdominal muscles)

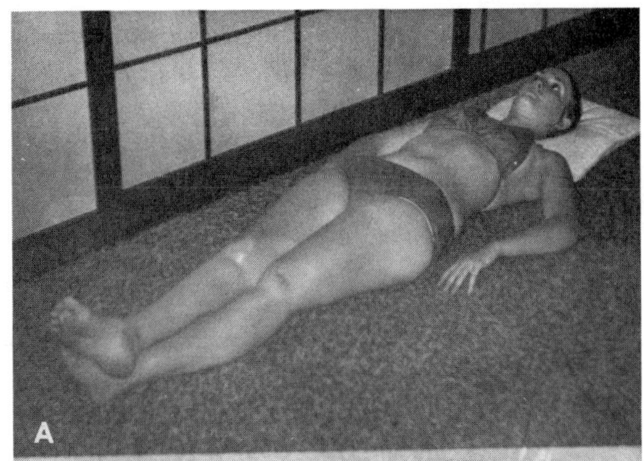

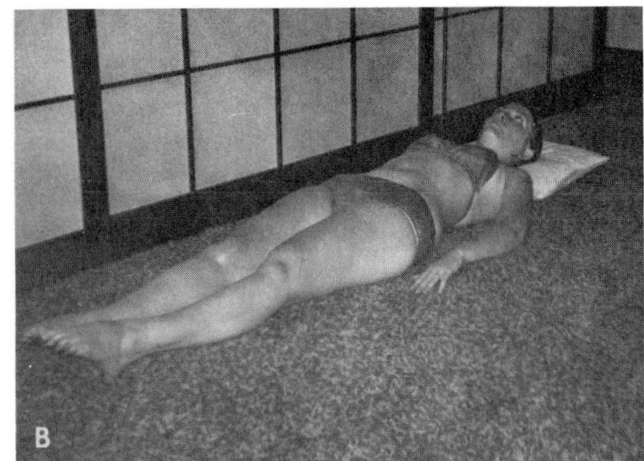

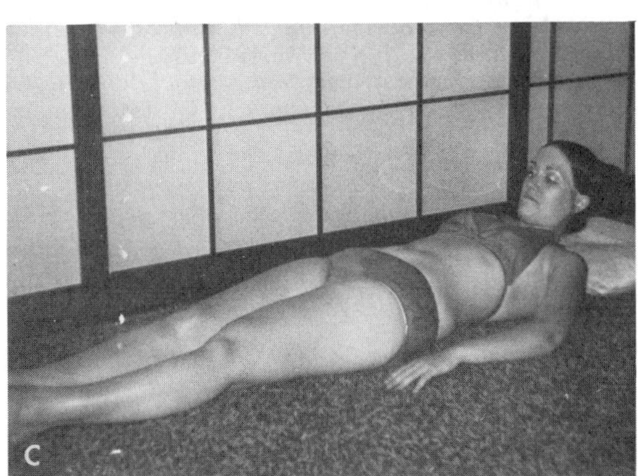

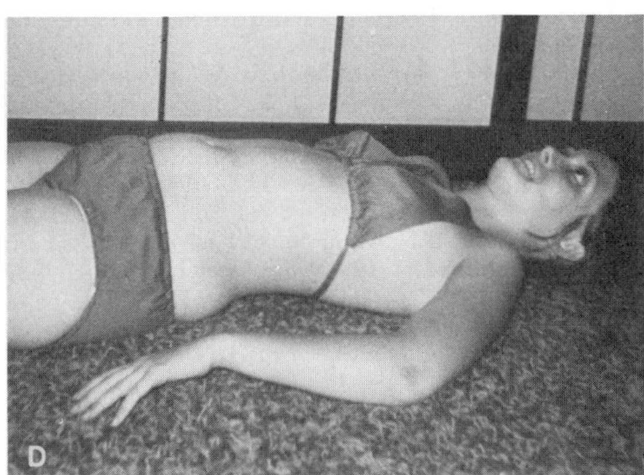

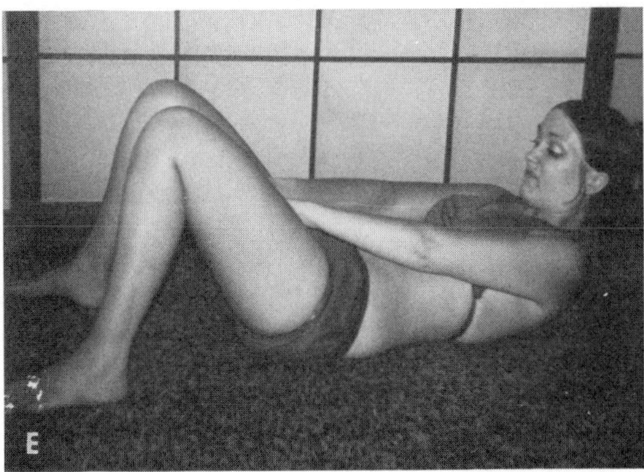

FIGURE 28-7. Exercises. *A*, Gluteal and pelvic floor exercise. *B*, Ankle exercise. *C*, Head raising. *D*, Pelvic rocking. *E*, Partial trunk raising.

Omit Exercise #3 and begin this exercise.

Position: On back, no pillow, arms at sides, knees bent, feet flat.

Exercise: Tuck chin on chest, raise head, then shoulders off the bed (or floor) and reach for the knees with outstretched hands. Each day advance forward as much as possible until a complete sit-up is possible.

Repeat: 6 to 10 times, three times daily.

REFERENCES

1. Nordmark, M. T. and Rohweder, A. W.: *Scientific Foundations of Nursing*. J. B. Lippincott, Philadelphia, 1967, p. 180.
2. Rodman, M. J. and Smith, D. W.: *Pharmacology and Drug Therapy in Nursing*. J. B. Lippincott, Philadelphia, 1968, p. 180.
3. Rubin, R.: *Puerperal change*. Nurs. Outlook 9:753, 1961.
4. Nordmark and Rohweder: op. cit., p. 134.
5. Newton, M. and Newton, N.: *The normal course and management of lactation*. Clin. Obstet. Gynecol. 5:59, 1962.
6. Perez, A., et al.: *First ovulation after childbirth: the effect of breast feeding*. Am. J. Obstet. Gynecol. 114:1041, 1972.
7. *Biology of Fertility Control by Periodic Abstinence*. WHO Technical Report Series No. 360. World Health Organization, Geneva, 1967.

BIBLIOGRAPHY

Adams, M.: *Early concerns of primagravida mothers regarding infant care activities*. Nurs. Research 12:72, 1963.

Applebaum, R.: *The modern management of successful breastfeeding*. Child and Family 9:61, 1970.

Eppink, H.: *Catherizing the maternity patient*. Am. J. Nurs. 75:829, 1975.

Murdaugh, A. and Miller, L. E.: *Helping the breastfeeding mother*. Am. J. Nurs. 121:465. 1975.

Newton, N.: *Psychologic differences between breast and bottle feeding*. Am. J. Clin. Nutr. 24:993, 1971.

Otte, M. J.: *Correcting inverted nipples—an aid to breastfeeding*. Am. J. Nurs. 75:454, 1975.

Perez, A., et al.: *First ovulation after childbirth: The effect of breastfeeding*. Am. J. Obstet. Gynecol. 114:1041, 1972.

Rubin, R.: *Puerperal change*. Nurs. Outlook 9:753, 1961.

Shulman, J. J.: *Contraceptive provisions in the immediate postpartum period*. Obstet. Gynecol. 40:403, 1972.

Tanner, L. M.: *In hospital care and post hospital follow up*. Clin. Obstet. Gynecol. 14:1124, 1971.

Thompson, M.: *Establishment of lactation*. Nurs. Forum 10:292, 1971.

Womanly Art of Breast Feeding, The. La Leche League, Franklin Park, Ill.

29 *Application of Psychosocial Concepts*

ANN L. CLARK, R.N., M.A.

CRISIS

According to Caplan,[1] a crisis is provoked when a person faces an obstacle to an important life goal that is, for the time being, insurmountable through utilization of customary methods of problem solving. A period of disorganization ensues; a period of upset, during which many different abortive attempts at a solution are made. Eventually some adaptation is achieved which may or may not be in the best interest of the person or of the family.

When a new member is added to the family, there is a forced reorganization of this small social system which amounts to a critical event or a crisis. Roles must be reassigned, status positions shifted, values reoriented, and needs met through new channels. In a study conducted by LeMasters[2] 83 per cent of new parents viewed the addition of the first child as a crisis event, forcing the couple to move from an adult-centered, pair-type organization into a child-centered, triad-group system. What often happens in this system, since a triadic relationship is more difficult to maintain, is that one parent, usually the mother, relates intensely to the infant and the father becomes isolated.

The study goes on to point out some of the reasons why, in our Western culture, this is so. One reason was that the parents, due to lack of knowledge and preparation for parental roles, had almost completely romanticized parenthood. The world of reality was something else again. The mothers reported negative feelings in adjusting to motherhood, for example:

- Chronic fatigue
- Extensive confinement to the home
- Curtailment of social contacts
- Lack of the satisfactions of outside employment
- Lack of income from employment
- Additional laundry
- Guilt over not being a "better" mother
- Long hours needed to care for an infant
- Decline in housekeeping standards
- Worry over personal appearance.

The fathers in this study also added their adjustment problems:

- Decline in sexual reponse of wife
- Economic pressures
- Worry about another pregnancy in the near future
- General disenchantment with the parental role.

Fortunately, all crises do not have negative outcomes. If the family can be helped to resolve the crisis in a healthy manner, the experience can be a constructive force for mental health. It can help the individuals in the family and the family itself to develop better problem-solving methods that will be useful as the family faces subsequent maturational and situational crises in the future.

ROLE BEHAVIOR

The family is a social system with a structure that is related to the functions to be performed by the family members. Statuses and roles are component parts of the structure, with roles channeling the behavior of individuals into specific statuses so that functions of the system are performed.[3] Behaviors and actions of a role are acquired, conditioned, reinforced learnings and are culturally determined.[4]

Role, sometimes referred to as the dynamic aspect of status, is the *minimal* behavior required of an individual to maintain a status or position. In addition to the minimal requirements, social values are reflected in delineating *ideal* role performance. Thus a person may maintain a role if he complies with those aspects which his culture indicates are requirements, but he may also fulfill the role so well that he is described as "ideal" or "perfect" in that role. All of these factors influence an individual as he or she faces taking on the new role of mother or father.

An individual usually learns something about a role he is to assume prior to assuming the role. The less role clarification he needs, the less will be the impact of the crisis of role change. In relation to the roles of mother and father, expectations of status and function are clarified in four ways:

1. Observation of parents, siblings, and peers enacting the role (role models)
2. Portrayals of the role in mass media
3. Role clarification by the mate (husband or wife)
4. Modifications of the role as a reciprocal framework established with the role partner (infant).

All of these role clarifications involve the possibility of disagreements and conflicts.

Role Models. Today, parents too often feel that there is a generation gap in relation to their parents' childrearing practices. A recent study by this author[5] indicates that many mothers do not believe that their own mothers' childrearing practices are relevant to the late twentieth century. They stated that there was lack of communication for the exploration of feelings and for learning about life. They felt that their parents had not found a workable balance between letting their children be independent and at the same time setting the necessary limits. Moreover, they felt that they had not been considered the unique human beings they felt they were. Perhaps the stress of our contemporary society has produced strains with resultant conflicts between the two generations. Mothers working outside the home, our extended educational system in which young people are dependent economically yet independent in all other aspects of growth and development, technical changes, rising cost of living, and shifting values in our society all contribute to confusion in parental role acquisition.

Mass Media. Mass media with their conflicting advice from "experts" and *ideal* role portrayals are not to be depended on as one readies oneself for the role of parent. The present generation of parents is the first to have been "plugged in" to mass media since they were old enough to be propped up before a television set. Conflicting advice leaves parents confused and anxious. This uncertainty takes its toll in terms of energy expended. Parental roles, especially that of the mother, are often portrayed in the "perfect" or "ideal" image. When parents cannot perform to fit this image, they re-examine their self concepts and often make modifications based on fantasy rather than on reality.

Mate's Expectations. Each man and woman comes to parenthood with an image of how they should perform and also how their mate should perform in his or her new role. Some of the conflicts in early parenthood result from the fact that the couple's images do not necessarily coincide. To compound the difficulty, the probability is great that each expectant parent thinks that they *agree completely*. Much to their disillusionment, disagreements occur. In a study done on the adaptation problems of the expanding family,[6] husbands expected their wives to know how to care for and quiet an infant. Wives did not find role reversal acceptable to them when they became temporarily dependent on their mate for assistance with chores of homemaking. Some husbands also resented the role reversal.

Role Partner's Feedback. The parent-infant relationship develops within a reciprocal framework. Each partner must receive a feedback of satisfactions, rewards, and gratifications if the relationship is to grow. Each parent has expectations of himself or herself, and expectations of the infant. Many expectations are based on fantasies and may differ greatly from the realities of parenthood and infancy. The mother may expect her infant to be a cuddly, warm infant. If it turns out that the infant is stiff and cries whenever she attempts to fondle him, she must modify her behavior as a mother to *this* small infant.

Cultural Influences. There are significant differences in the definition of family roles among subcultural groups within our society. The differences between feminine and masculine tasks may be more sharply drawn in some ethnic groups, even in today's society where roles seem to be less distinct and considerable overlapping occurs. It is important to be sensitive to ethnic influences on beliefs, values, and behavior reflected in role definition.

Socioeconomic positions also have implications for family roles. For example, women in the upper socioeconomic class are likely to place the role of wife above the role of mother. These women can rely on mother substitutes in the form of governesses or nurses to give care to their children. The middle-class mother tends to feel that her role as a mother takes precedence over her role as wife. Her peers would frown on any other behavior. In the lower-class family there is often considerable instability. Families may be incomplete. Women often need to work and often have inadequate substitutes to provide child care. The concept of a mother differs sharply from that in other strata of society under these circumstances.[7]

IDENTITY AND SELF CONCEPT

Femininity, masculinity, and a feeling of security in one's sexual role begin at birth and emerge as an evolving configuration. It is not fixed at the point of physical maturity. A person's sense of identity and the acceptance of a feminine or masculine role may be given an opportunity to develop and expand during the childbearing and childrearing experiences.

MOTHERLINESS

Mothering is a complex, more or less culturally determined, learned behavior; the many practical attitudes necessary to take care of infants and guide learning are facilitated by characteristic qualities of a woman's personality.[8] Mothering is defined for our purposes as acts of tender, warm behavior on the part of a woman in the interest of the child. It differs from other forms of warm, tender behavior in that it includes ability to love unconditionally. It is unique in that during one stage of the relationship one of the partners is a living, developing organism (the fetus) within the body of the other (the mother). Expressions of motherliness are the result of the mental apparatus modifying patterns originating via instinct. This instinct begins with the early memory traces and influences the personality as it develops. Maternal behavior has two resources which are tightly interwoven:

Female physiology
Personality development.

These two resources are further modified when a child becomes a part of the interaction and the mother gains experience and knowledge of childrearing.

Benedek[9] correlates the qualities of motherliness, in its developmental phases, with cyclic hormonal fluctuations. Following the expulsion of the ovum, the hormone progesterone is produced. Benedek describes the emotional state during the progesterone phase as a "quiet period." The woman's interest shifts from outside activities to her body month after month during her nonpregnant state and for prolonged periods during pregnancy. The pregnant woman commonly experiences a surge of well-being during the later half of pregnancy. The woman's resulting enjoyment of her pregnant body is due to the effects of progesterone. The somatic adjustment caused by this hormone is used by the psychic apparatus and becomes an active vehicle in the development of motherliness.

McFarland and Reinhardt describe the development of motherliness as:

> gradual transition from being the dependent one, protected and nurtured by a cherishing mother through the increasingly active and autonomous stages . . . to becoming the giving nurturing person.[10]

There are critical stages in the development of motherliness. The female child's identification with her mother is believed to be a critical first step in a woman's ultimate ability to meet her child's needs. Studies indicate a correlation between a mother's recall of the mothering she received and the solicitous care she gives her own infant, even as early as the second day of motherhood. Originally the mother-daughter relationship is a symbiotic one, in which the fetus and then the infant has a warm, continuous, intimate relationship with its mother. Later, the girl develops an object relationship with her mother. During adolescence the cyclic changes related to menstruation bring about changes in feelings and attitudes. The girl internalizes concepts of femininity and childbearing. It is important at this phase that the girl develops positive feelings toward the feminine sex and its functions.

Pregnancy, labor, and birth are also critical periods in the development of motherliness. During this time the woman may be particularly vulnerable due to increased dependency needs. There is a great need to experience love and affection. If it is not forthcoming the woman may not be able to express warmth for her child. It well may be true, as Gail has said, that:

> The maternal instinct is a comfortable male myth; a woman can only give freely if she is in a position where she does not feel deprived herself.[11]

Experiences during labor also play an important role in helping the mother to display acts of motherliness to her child. Mothers who have experienced warmth and bodily contact from a caring person during their labors are able to use their hands more readily and more effectively in comforting their infants.[12]

FATHERLINESS

Fathering is also a complex, culturally learned behavior which may be modified by contemporary society. Fatherliness consists of instinctive responses of empathy for the children as the man fulfills his ultimate goal as protector and provides for his family.[13]

The male child, like the female, goes through a gradual transition, first being the dependent one, protected and nurtured by a cherishing mother. This dependence on his mother aids in his development of empathy. His role model is his father and his goal is to be like his father. One way of achieving this goal is through paternity.

A man's self-esteem is partially dependent on his sexual potency but this is a means to an end, not an end in itself. His child is his link in the generation of man. Fatherhood assures his place in the continuity of mankind. Through his newborn child, he can project all his hopes for self-realization and fulfillment of his own ego aspirations.

SIBLING RELATIONSHIPS

The fetus lives a symbiotic existence within his mother until contractions of labor rudely disrupt this comfortable existence. He arrives in this world a helpless individual, indeed, one of the most helpless creatures to inhabit this earth. He knows and understands nothing of others or the world around him, feeling that he *is* the world. He is unable to separate a *not me* from a *me*.

Throughout infancy he is dependent upon others for his nurturant care and for help in developing his social role. Slowly he begins to recognize the boundary between himself and the rest of the world. A critical task and the central theme of infancy is related to his development of a sense of *trust*. The establishment of trust is basic to his ability to live with a sense of security and permits the child to move into the next phases of growth and development.

At about this point in time, as his early developmental tasks are being surmounted, the infant or child may well be faced with the necessity of sharing his comfort and his security with a sibling. Since so much is at stake, it is to be expected that the child will feel that the new infant is an intruder, as indeed he is.

Parents prepare their children for a new baby in the family in different ways. Some parents present the facts logically and include the many advantages and disadvantages of having a new baby in the family. They tell the child that a new baby will be fun at times, but at other times he will be a lot of trouble. He will cry, soil his clothes, and will need to be washed, fed, and taken care of. They tell the child that he may feel unhappy at times and that he should tell his parents when he feels that way. In this way they keep communications open and give permission for full expression of feelings.

Other parents tell the child they are bringing a new baby into the home so he will have a playmate. Still others state the newborn will be *his* baby. They may even say they love him so much they want to have another child just like him. These comments may confuse the child and will likely upset him more than the facts. The newborn cannot play in any way that could meet the older child's need. Role confusion ("your baby") will result from promising to convert a sibling into a possession. Since the parents cannot fulfill the promise, it will soon be an obvious untruth and a threat to the trust relationship. The child will soon question, "if they love me so much, how come they need someone else to love?"

Some parents still tell stork stories, or cabbage patch, garbage can, or Santa Claus stories. It might be useful to examine what these stories have to say about human dignity and human worth. Some parents do not even share the fact of an expected new infant with the child at all. Often they reason that their child is too young to understand. Sometimes they feel that it is inappropriate to do so, or that the questions that may follow the disclosure are too difficult to answer.

When the mother leaves the child to enter the hospital and then returns several days later with a new brother or sister, several undesirable situations may occur. The separation from the mother may bring about separation anxiety on the part of the child. There may follow a prolonged period when the child, fearful that his security will vanish again, will not permit his mother to be absent from his sight. He may increase his demands on his mother for services. He may regress in a developmental sense, e.g., return to wetting his bed and requiring to be fed. He may, due to his anger with his mother for leaving him, refuse to speak to her. This can be a crushing blow for his mother who has missed him as much as he has missed her. What occurs next will depend upon the insight his parents have into his behavior and how well they can use this knowledge to assist the child to work through his crisis.

Parents can expect that sibling competition will occur and can use these experiences to help their children learn to cope with the stresses of the competitive world in which we all must learn to live. Sibling rivalry too may well be present. If the parents cannot help their children to work this out in the home, the children will take their aggressions outside the home, complicating relationships with peers and having implications for school.

Sex education of children can find a natural place in the family with the addition of a new child. It provides an opportunity for the parents to help their children understand something of love, marriage, the origin of human beings, and the facts of birth.

LOSS

The concept of loss can be seen to apply to most, if not all, of the family members following the birth of a child, even when the infant is healthy and the mother is physically well. Some of these losses are necessary concomitants of growth and many of them are predictable. Whether the loss is a physical one or whether it involves some aspect of the self, it is unwanted and uncomfortable and the usual longing related to grief and grieving are present.

A person's response to loss depends upon the meaning of the loss, i.e., the value it holds for him, his own resources for coping with loss, and the environmental supports available. The function of grieving is to restore the ego equilibrium.[14] Perhaps the chronic fatigue observed in new parents is due not only to the extra work of caring for a new infant, but also to the process of grieving.

THE MOTHER

Loss of a Pregnant Body. Many women find comfort in their pregnant bodies. The complacency sets in late in the second trimester when the woman begins to feel a sense of introversion. She thinks about herself and the baby growing within her. One expectant mother patted her protruding abdomen and said, "It's my friend, I'll miss it." Women often state that they feel a sense of emptiness after delivery, and in a very real sense they have lost part of themselves in giving birth to the baby.

Loss of a Privileged Position. Pregnancy and the rewards and interest it brings to the expectant mother has been compared with a position on a pedestal. The supply of special food, special attention, etc., are all comforting experiences, ones not to be relinquished without regret. When the focus of attention shifts from the mother to the new infant, she feels a sense of loss. Even when there is elation and excitement, grieving can still be experienced. Grief work, however, is useful to the new mother when it is worked through. Former roles are relinquished when they are incompatible with the new role. The grief work appears to be a catalyst for the new role-taking operation,

Loss of a Model Figure. In the early puerperium the mother's loss of a desired slender shape may be experienced. Now she is neither obviously pregnant nor nonpregnant and shapely. Her abdomen may still be bulging and the skin stretched and flabby. Her weight may be 10 to 15 pounds above the normal and desired weight. Moreover, she now has no clothes that fit. Her maternity clothes are too familiar as well as large and ill fitting, and her usual wardrobe is too tight. She knows she doesn't look well and she grieves for her lost figure.

Loss of Control over Body Functions. Many new mothers have difficulty with their physiologic return to normal function. Inability to empty the bladder, have a bowel movement, or enter into activities of daily living are seen as losses. The mother has a great need to get her body back in its usual working order and may feel helpless, frustrated, and angry until this is accomplished.

Loss of Self-Control. Inability to control one's emotions may be particularly distressing to the new mother. Some mothers are concerned that they may become emotionally ill when they experience depression and periods of crying. One mother said, "How can I care for this baby when I'm such a baby myself?" This mother, like many others, was mourning her lack of self-control.

Loss of Self-Definition in Social Roles. Loss of independence is usually a part of early motherhood. This is particularly distressing when the mother has previously led an active social or professional life. Pride in one's work, with the feedback which enhances the ego, will be lost and grieved. This loss can be partially compensated for if there is sufficient feedback to the mother in her new role. Our culture tends to give lip service to the importance of the mother's role, but most mothers realize very little approval of their best effort. Indeed, what she often receives, if anything, is criticism.

THE FATHER

Fatherhood also involves many losses and the man may react to these in ways that are destructive rather than supportive.

In a new triadic relationship the father may become isolated while his wife and infant develop a duo relationship. He may feel that he is no longer important to his wife. There may also be a loss of sexual gratification. Moreover, the husband may lose many of his comfortable patterns of daily living. His sleep may be broken, his usual type of recreation may no longer be possible due to the cost or the time it would require him to be absent from his family. He may have to "make do" with hastily prepared meals rather than the specially prepared food that he has come to expect and to enjoy. All of these losses may cause grief and mourning.

THE SIBLINGS

There are many things in the immediate environment of the child upon which he depends for a feeling of security. Loss of his mother (due to hospitalization) and his home (if he is cared for by others during his mother's hospitalization) are the first of the losses the sibling may experience. His status in the family may seem to be lost as he observes his mother giving almost exclusive care to the newborn. He may further feel status loss as he seeks the gratification of closeness and support from an already fatigued mother. He may lose control and regress to an earlier infantile pattern of behavior.

The small child is often in a more vulnerable position than is the adult due to his limited capacity to cope with the loss. Unless his parents understand his problem, support him, and permit expressions of the loss, he will be unable to develop the coping power necessary for future use.

THE NEONATE

The newborn's loss may be viewed as a developmental loss. Birth itself constitutes the sudden loss of a safe and secure intrauterine life. The neonate loses the quiet, warmth, and snug fit of the fluid and amniotic sack about him. This is the beginning of many other predictable losses due to the growth and developmental processes of life.

SENSORY ALTERATION

Sensory overload and sensory deprivation may become problems for each member of the family during the puerperium.

Preliminary studies indicate that new mothers tend to experience varying degrees of depression in the six weeks following delivery, correlating with the degree of sensory alteration they experience. Women who report sufficient assistance and social stimulation manage the early days of motherhood with a minimum of depression.

The new mother can expect a great deal of sensory overload. For example:

- In the hospital
  - Physical discomfort
  - Broken sleep due to different sleeping arrangement and lack of quiet
  - Hospital routines such as early morning rituals—temperature taking, morning care, early infant feedings, breakfast
  - Scheduling of a day which leaves little time for rest periods
  - Visitors, telephone calls
  - Care of the infant while still trying to develop necessary skills
- At home
  - Excessive advice and assistance from family, friends, and neighbors
  - Demands of other children
  - Cultural expectations
  - Infant care
  - Lack of sleep
  - Fatigue
  - Social obligations

Examples of situations which cause sensory deprivation are:

- In the hospital
  - Symbiotic break
  - Separation from the infant (central nursery)
  - Interruption of communication with significant others
  - Reduced energy
  - Separation from husband and other children
- At home
  - Monotonous input due to environmental void
  - Lack of intellectual stimulation from adults
  - Lack of situational support in care of the infant and the home
  - Decreased energy

The new father experiences sensory alteration also, much of it due to the infant's schedule and his wife's concentration on the infant's needs. He will experience deprivation in such things as sleep, eating, sexual relations, social activities, and communication with his mate. He may experience overload by the demands made by his wife, his children, and others who are present in the home at this time.

The neonate may experience sensory deprivation due to isolation (lack of tactile and auditory stimulation) or sensory overload due to excessive handling by his parents or visitors. Additional overload may be caused by an anxious mother who tries to force him to eat. He may also be overdressed or insufficiently protected from the atmosphere.

Gordon, Kapostin, and Gordon[15] developed a rather simple preventive experiment which provides a method of reducing the present day problems related to some of the sensory alterations enumerated above. This kind of instruction can have a profound and lasting beneficial effect upon social adjustment and upon the mental and physical health of the family. It was seen as particularly effective in preventing postpartal emotional problems. Their suggestions are:

The responsibilities of motherhood are learned; hence, get informed.

Get help from husband and dependable friends and relatives.

Make friends of other couples who are experienced with childrearing.

Don't overload yourself with unimportant tasks.

Don't move soon after the baby arrives.

Don't be overconcerned with keeping up appearances.

Get plenty of rest and sleep.

Don't be a nurse to relatives or others at this period.

Confer and consult with husband, family, and experienced friends and discuss your plans and worries.

Don't give up outside interests, but cut down on responsibilities and rearrange schedules.

CONFLICTS

Conflicts deal with goals. Two or more goals may be equally desirable but are opposing and each competes for dominance. An individual may be unaware that he is experiencing conflict but is aware of the feelings which accompany it. Behavioral responses include hesitation, vascillation, blocking, and indecision. Conflict is a very uncomfortable state and takes its toll in terms of diminished energy. Thus, continuous fatigue may indicate conflict.

Conflict forces a choice that is often expressed in behavior that seems to others to be inappropriate for the situation. Interference with a goal or its related activity may cause aggressive behavior. If a desired goal is not achieved, frustration may be expressed in the form of anger.

When a new baby is added to the family, conflict may be experienced by the mother, the father, or the siblings. Conflicts may be categorized in this context as:

Idealized role vs. inadequacy or unwillingness to perform the role

Expectations vs. reality

Independence vs. dependence

Love vs. resentment

Self-realization through parenthood vs. preclusion of other personal opportunities.[16]

Examples of these types of conflicts have been presented throughout this chapter.

ROLE OF THE NURSE

IMMEDIATE POSTDELIVERY PHASE

The immediate postpartal period, which merges into the fourth stage of labor, is experienced differently by each new mother. On the surface, things do fit into a routine. There is the checking of vital signs, the physical care given to the mother and her infant, the reporting of vital statistics, and the charting. This tends to routinize birth and the puerperium. However, this day is far from a routine day for the new mother, the newborn infant, the new father, and other significant persons. It is a very unique day and the feelings that accompany it are unique feelings.

In relation to the new mother, there are a number of observations the nurse should make. How does the new mother respond to all that is occurring to and about her? In the psychosocial sphere the mother's feelings will be influenced by her personality, the length of labor, her feelings about the pain she has experienced and her response to it, the meaning this child has to her, the manner in which the nurses, physicians, and her husband have related to her during labor and the immediate postpartal period, and many other factors specific for her.

The new mother needs to be reassured that all is well with her infant and with herself. Her first response to her infant should be carefully observed, assessed, and recorded for other health professionals who will be responsible for her continued care.

Crying, which signifies a feeling of helplessness, may be one of the first responses, but the causative factors are not always the same. Some women who have been given considerable amounts of analgesia and/or anesthesia will not feel in command of the situation. Helplessness will be experienced in relation to herself and her physical body. On the other hand, if she experiences an overwhelming feeling of tenderness for the infant the tears may again signify helplessness, but for a different reason.

Most mothers have a feeling of relief that the labor is completed and the infant is safely delivered. They may respond to this with euphoria. The woman may laugh aloud and carry on a steady stream of chatter. The need for assurance that the infant is normal may be expressed in various ways and may be related to the fantasies she has experienced during pregnancy in relation to her baby. Most mothers ask if the baby is normal. A positive response on the part of the nurse or physician may be all that is needed. However, some mothers wish to check for themselves. Some mothers may wish to do so but are hesitant, either because they are unsure of the appropriateness of this behavior or are afraid of what they may discover. The nurse's assessment of the mother's behavior is vital, for here is the beginning of a complex reciprocal relationship between the mother and her child.

The mother should be permitted to state her own feelings about the sex of the infant and how she perceives the child without comments from the nurse. The statement "It's a beautiful boy" by the nurse or physician may not coincide with the mother's feelings at all. It may inhibit her from expressing her own feelings, and it is important to know what the mother is thinking. Once the mother has made her evaluation, the nurse may appropriately respond to the mother's pleasure and pride in her offspring. This kind of feedback reinforces the mother's own concept of self. The nurse should not counter the mother's expressions of disappointment in her child. Helping the mother to express what it is she is feeling by the use of communication expanders is more helpful to both the mother and the nurse. Once the nurse understands what is distressing the mother, she can better intervene in a therapeutic manner. Some things cannot be changed, but some things do change. For example, if the mother is concerned with the contour of the face and head due to the edema of birth, the nurse can reassure her that the infant's features will change in the next several days.

If the husband is present in the delivery suite, the nurse can make valuable observations concerning how he relates to his wife and to his new child. If the father is not present, the nurse should be sure he is notified of the event and reunited with his wife at the earliest opportunity.

WOMAN TO MOTHER ADAPTATION

Self Concept

Maturation into motherhood is a transitional period in a woman's life. Labor, the pinacle of the experience by which a childless woman becomes a mother, created a delicate balance between the positive factors which promote growth and the negative factors which promote regression. Every moment of joy, anticipation, creativity, and exhilaration was likely balanced by anxiety, ambivalence, loss, and fear.[17] What are the reactions to this experience and the developmental aspects of it? What implications does it have for nursing?

All women approach labor with certain expectations—expectations of what labor will be like, expectations of their response to it, expectations of how they will be cared for in labor. However, these expectations are mixed with uncertainties and anxieties, for unfortunately, many aspects of labor are not under control of the individual. Thus, there is the possibility that their expectations may not be met.

Once labor is over, each woman must integrate this critical life experience into her psyche, a process which begins even during the labor experience. The two basic aspects of the mother's concern about her labor experience are unmet expectations and unacceptable behavior.

Unmet Expectations. If the woman's expectations have not been met, anxiety can be expected both during labor and upon recalling the labor experience. A number of women experience severe and even panic stages of anxiety during the transitional and delivery phases of labor. The threatening and distressful feelings that accompany anxiety are perhaps partly offset by the physical activity of expulsion during labor (fight). However, she may feel a loss of control of her body as though some force greater than herself has taken over and is in full command.

Unacceptable Response. The woman will also recall her own behavior during the labor experience. One's identity needs to be preserved despite the vicissitudes of life. The concept of ego identity implies the attainment of a homeostasis of the self and it tends to resist radical change.[18] What impact does an experience such as labor have when one perceives she has not performed in an appropriate manner? How can the nurse help?

In an experience which is highly anxiety producing, the individual blocks out much of what is occurring in the environment and focuses only on the self. In so doing, one part of the experience may be "blown up" all out of proportion. Thus, in attempting to recall the labor experience, a woman may find that some aspects of the experience are missing and some can only be recalled in a vague manner. She may recall her own behavior as being unreal or even bizarre. This may cause anxiety as she feels a threat to her own impulses.

The ego contemplates and evaluates the self, but in doing so the ego considers the reaction of others. Thus, we achieve self knowledge only through contrasting ourselves in many ways with other selves, that is, self consciousness depends on social contrast.[19] The nurse can use this theory in helping her patient to correctly perceive her behavior in the context of the expectation of the culture (in this case the hospital environment). At this point, the woman needs someone with whom she can discuss the experience and the feelings that accompanied it. She needs to be helped to identify and understand the events that led to her anxious feelings and her resulting behavior. In helping her patient to understand the experience, the nurse communicates to her patient that *she* understands and accepts this behavior, thus acting in an ego-supportative manner to help her patient regain her ego identity. Rather than repressing those aspects of her behavior which she views as inconsistent with her concept of self, the patient can instead discard those *expectations* of herself which are unrealistic.

Nurses make a tremendous contribution to the individual and consequently to the family when they help a new mother work through the threatening experience of labor. If the opportunity is not provided, the anxiety will remain, become part of the psyche, and appear later, perhaps as a feeling part of another experience. If the opportunity is provided, the woman feels a sense of mastery of her most vital function, reproduction, in terms of ego identity, thus shaping her acceptance of herself and of her child.[20]

Dependence to Dependable

Dependent behavior, which has been discussed as an important aspect of pregnancy and labor, continues to be a necessary component of the early puerperium. Rubin[21] has described the phases of "taking in" and "taking hold" more sensitively than has perhaps any other author. The new mother's taking in needs consist of the following:

A therapeutic sleep
Food (quantity as well as quality)
The reality and the pieces that are component parts of her labor and delivery

To be cared for
To be cared about.

In the assessment process, the nurse caring for the new mother requires information about all of these aspects in order to judge their impact on the patient and the appropriate nursing actions to take.

Women enter labor in varying stages of rest or fatigue. Some have not slept well for many days due to anxiety, Braxton Hicks contractions, difficulty in breathing, general body discomfort, or other activities in the home, such as caring for an ill child, that have reduced their normal sleep pattern. Labors that are entered into during the day, after a restful night's sleep, are generally managed with less fatigue than are labors which occur during the night when the woman most needs her rest. Physical exhaustion after labor is also influenced by the length of time and the activity needed to deliver the baby. Factors to be assessed in order to plan for a vital period of sleep and inactivity include:

Sleep pattern during last two to three weeks of pregnancy
Sleep on night prior to labor
Time of day labor began
Length of labor
Feelings expressed by patient about lack of sleep and fatigue.

Labor is a physically demanding experience for most women, the degree depends on the woman's physical condition on entering into the experience, the length of labor, and the nutrients supplied during this period. In addition, food is usually associated with being mothered or being loved and thus has high psychologic value in fulfilling dependency needs. The nurse's assessment should include:

Appetite and food intake in past 24 hours
Length of labor
Presence or absence of nausea
Plan to breast or bottle feed.

Very few women bring a child into the world that is not also welcomed by other persons significant in her life. These significant others must be relied on to give the new mother love and affection and to show her that they care for her and will assume responsibility for seeing that she is cared for. The nurse has a responsibility to see that the communications of these persons are made available to her. Mail, gifts, flowers, telephone calls, and visits signify to the new mother she is cared about. The nurse has a responsibility to meet the dependency needs concerned with physical care and comfort. The assessment should include:

The husband's or mate's visits
Expressions of interest on the part of others—flowers, cards, visitors, or the lack of them
The manner in which the mother handles her passive dependency needs (i.e., accepted, rejected, caused anxiety).

Independence and autonomy replace dependency, usually prior to or at about the time the woman returns home. In the hospital environment she begins to get "organized." She sends gifts and floral arrangements home and has clothes for herself and the infant brought to the hospital. She is on the telephone ordering supplies from the store and lining up family, friends, or husband to make last minute purchases. She begins to think more specifically of the other children, planning gifts for them and how she will introduce the new child to them. She now wishes to be in command, independent, and the *dependable* one. Dependable in providing care for the dependent infant, and dependable as the homemaker once again.

The new mother is rather vulnerable at this stage. Frustrations and failures make her hypercritical and intolerant of herself.[22] She continues to need assistance in the home and if this is her first baby she will have many concerns over the care her new child requires. She has an inner drive for excellence which will cause conflicts.

Transitory Depression

Many new mothers experience transitory states of emotional distress during the puerperium. This is characterized by unexplainable sadness and frequent crying. It may occur in the hospital but due to early postpartal discharges it usually occurs after the new mother returns home. The depression is a reactive depression in that it is believed to be precipitated by environmental pressures, role changes, endocrine changes, and interpersonal conflict.

A study by Anderson[23] indicates that depression in the postpartal period is related to repression and to preconscious maternal identification. Self identification is reorganized following the birth of a child. When there is interlevel personality conflict with underlying aggression and a lack of identification with one's mother (on a preconscious level), transient depression may follow. Although such women are more vulnerable, all new mothers should be protected from low physical reserves and remarks and assistance that lower self-confidence and self-esteem. Nursing assessment should include:

- Physical reserves, particularly low Hgb., nutrition, and rest
- Insomnia
- Lack of self-confidence in the care of the infant
- Culture of the family
- Responses of the mother to her infant's behavior
- Amount and type of home help
- Sensory overload and sensory deprivation in the home.

Culture also appears to influence the occurrence of postpartal depression. Depression occurs more frequently in cultures which place a high value on both the privileges and responsibilities of the individual, and occurs less often in cultures in which the individual is de-emphasized in favor of the extended family.[24]

MOTHER-INFANT ADAPTATION

Nursing assessment of the mother-infant claiming process begins as soon as the woman has cognitive awareness that the pregnancy will lead to a baby, *her* baby. The symbiotic relationship in utero is an important part of the maternal-infant claiming process. Labor and birth break this symbiosis, which is then reestablished after the delivery. If the mother is unconscious during the delivery, it may be more difficult for her to bridge the gap from the fetus in utero to her own baby. The woman's response to the fact that she is a mother, her coping with the event, and the state of disequilibrium are important data needed by the nurse to help her understand the behaviors which she will continue to assess as the mother moves to claim the child and minister to its needs.

The following data will be useful to the nurse as she begins the assessment process upon which nursing actions will be based in the interest of mother-infant adaptation.

- Ages of mother and father
- Desire for this baby
- Acceptance of this baby (sex, physical attributes, and behavior)
- Fantasies during pregnancy and labor concerning this infant
- Response of mother to neonate when first presented to her in the delivery room
- Father's response to the neonate and the mother since the birth
- Any stressful experiences occurring to the

new mother or her family during pregnancy and labor, including state of disequilibrium caused and coping mechanisms used

Ethnic and socioeconomic group from which this family comes.

Some of this information may have been obtained previously and will be available to the nurse. Other parts of it can be obtained directly from the mother after a trusting relationship has been established.

Maternal Inspection

One of the mother's first needs is to be reassured that her infant is normal. Most expectant mothers are deeply concerned throughout pregnancy that their infants may not be normal. Some mothers are very fearful that their children will have some specific defect. The reasons for these fears are numerous. Some of them may involve the woman's concept of self. When a woman has matured with deep feelings of inferiority about herself, she will find it difficult to believe that she can give birth to a normal, healthy infant. What she says about "I" and her searching for what is wrong with her child when the child seems normal and healthy will give the nurse some insight into the etiology of the situation. Other women may have deep concerns about the care they have given themselves during pregnancy, fearing that some event caused damage to the developing infant. Inspecting the infant will help to dispel many of the mother's fears, although it will not necessarily eradicate those which are of deep psychologic etiology.

Re-establishment of the symbiotic mother-infant relationship after birth requires maternal task solution on three levels: physical, social, and psychologic. The nurse will see this problem solving begin as she presents the infant to the mother for inspection. The nurse's first act is to identify the infant as the mother's by whatever identification system the hospital uses. She then undresses the infant and carefully observes the mother as she inspects her infant and relates to it.

The mother, in examining the anatomy of her infant, will soon begin to relate it to herself, her husband, or another member of the family. How she views the child in this context is an important indication of how well the child has met her expectations, and since she produced the child, it also reflects her own self concept.

The mother's first tactile contact with her infant is exploratory and is usually made with the fingertips. Mothers seem to have an orderly progression in the way in which they explore the infant, although the speed with which they move from one mode of contact to another varies radically from one mother to another. According to Rubin,

> The rate of progression from one predominating form of touch or contact to another is dependent on how she feels herself in this particular function of her role, on how she perceives her partner's (the infant's) reciprocal response to her, and on the charter of the relationship at any given point. All these factors operate in determining the extent to which she dares permit herself to become progressively and more intimately involved.[25]

If one stops to think about it, it is acceptable social behavior to await some response on the part of another before we consider making tactile contact. The infant is a stranger in the beginning, thus the mother, after a tentative first approach to her child, awaits some response of his part (Fig. 29-1).

Some mothers make auditory contact with their infants very early and carry on a continual stream of chatter with their infants. Some of this verbalization can be viewed in the context of relating the infant to themselves, e.g., "It's okay, Mommy is here. You are all

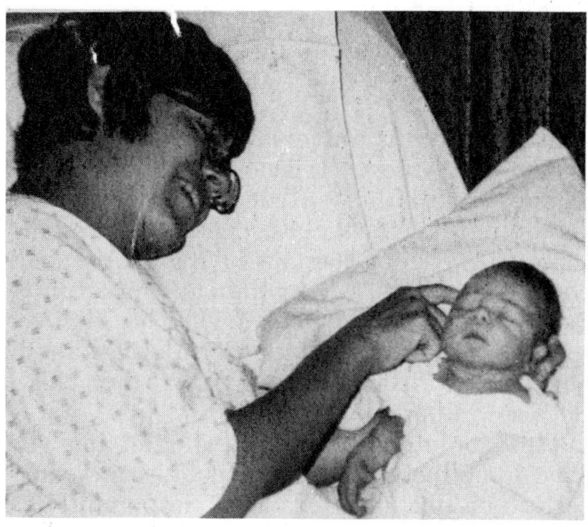

FIGURE 29-1. Maternal exploration.

right." Other comments are early attempts to relate the child to the world, e.g., "It's noisy in here today, isn't it?" On the other hand, some mothers are totally mute with their infants, perhaps feeling that it is foolish to talk to someone who cannot respond.

Mothers usually feel that the infant has not begun to relate to them in any meaningful manner until they have made eye to eye contact. You will observe mothers in the maternity wards moving their infant so they are "en face" with the child. If the infant does not or has not opened his eyes you may hear the mother say, for example, "Open your eyes, you haven't even looked at Mommy."

Mothers also progress in an orderly fashion through the stages of identifying their infant as a sexual being with a name, although again, each mother seems to move at her own pace. At first the mother may refer to the infant as "it" or "the baby." Later, the child is referred to as "she" or "he." The mother's identification may sometimes become confused. For example, a female child may be referred to as "he" if another young child in the family is a male. Still later, the mother begins to use the given name. Sometimes the mother uses the formal name, such as "John," but more often mothers use the familiar name, such as "Johnny." Mothers also label their children using words that may be significant to the developing mother-infant relationship. For example, "chow hound" or "sleepy head" may indicate her feelings about the way her infant is responding to her and perhaps something about her concept of self as well.

Malidentification and disclaiming behavior on the part of a mother may also be observed in the very early mother-infant relationship. Malidentification is the process whereby the mother identifies her newborn infant with negative, toxic, dangerous qualities which she experiences in herself and others.[26] Often these mothers have never felt pleasing to their mothers and have unsatisfactory marital relationships. Such stresses increase the possibility of toxic identification between the mother and her infant and may lead to infants and children who fail to thrive and who are battered children.

The nursing assessment should include:

How much does she touch the infant? What parts are touched? What parts does she not touch?

Does she use fingertips, hands, arm, and/or body in touching and holding the infant?

What kind of body contact does she permit? Is the infant held to the chest, to the face?

Does she attempt to hold the infant "en face" in order to relate to it?

If the infant yawns, grunts, coughs, sneezes, gags, or cries, how does she respond to this behavior?

Does she try to relate to it by making comments about opening the eyes, seeing her?

What are her questions about the infant's features or any marks or imperfections?

Does she relate to it by identifying it with herself, or other members of the family? Are these positive features or negative features?

Is the infant identified as "it," "she," "he," or does she have a name for the infant and use it?

Some nursing intervention will begin immediately as the nurse answers the mother's questions and explains any phenomenon related to the infant that seems appropriate. Following the inspection the infant is dressed at the bedside, returned to his crib, and the nurse continues her assessment and intervention by sitting down with the mother and talking with her in an unhurried manner.

Maternal Feelings

Full maternal feelings do not occur when the mother first sees her newborn child. Indeed, they may not occur before the third week of life and even then may be intermittent and brief. Physical discomfort may delay the mother's ability to relate to her infant in a meaningful manner, although some mothers are more able to subjugate their comfort for that of the infant than are others (Fig. 29-2). Until full maternal feelings are experienced, the mother may wonder about her maternal capacity and even the wisdom of having a child.[27] Mothers may feel guilty if they expect to feel an immediate warmth toward the infant and then find that they "like the baby" but have no real feeling of attachment for the child.

This information needs to be related to the new mother in order to allay her fears. What the nurse needs to know is how her patient does feel. The method of obtaining this information is through an interview statement which is nonthreatening, universal in scope, and opened-ended in character. For example:

> I know many people believe that a new mother feels instant love for her new child, but that isn't really the way most mothers feel at first. It takes some time, often weeks, to get that full maternal feeling. When you saw your son (daughter) just now, how was it for you?

This statement is universal in that it speaks of "many" and "most." It is nonthreatening since it does not indicate that the new mother should necessarily feel as society declares she should, i.e., "feel instant love." It is open-ended because it offers the mother an opportunity to express how she does feel. The feelings she expresses may include her feelings about herself as well as her response to her baby. Both are important.

This conference with the mother may be used to collect other useful data as indicated earlier in this chapter. Most importantly, a nurse-patient relationship is developing. The mother recognizes that here is a person who cares about her and her infant and can be depended on to help her in the days ahead.

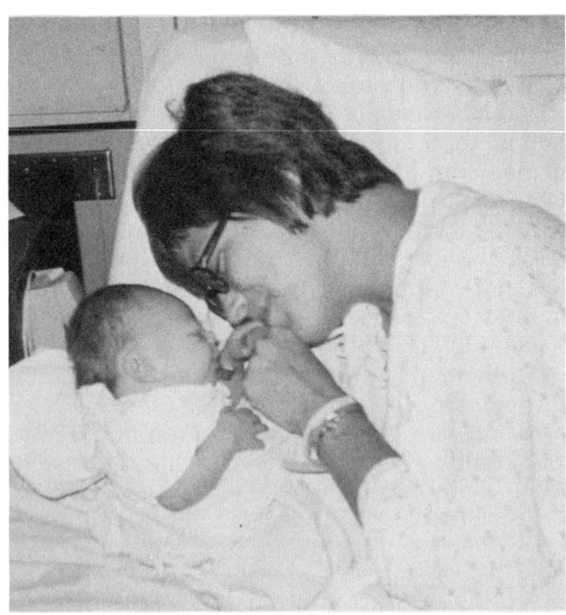

FIGURE 29-2. Maternal affection and tenderness in spite of discomfort.

Maternal Behavior

Mothering may be viewed as a series of developmental tasks. Each of these tasks must be resolved in an adaptive manner in order for further maturation to take place.[28] The degree of conflict which a mother experiences concerning child care depends upon the manner in which she resolves each of these issues. The social milieu is a potent force in her adaptation. The hospital is the environment in which she must first tackle these tasks. Thus, the nurse can be an important force in helping the mother toward successful maturation and is significant to the developing mother-infant relationship.

The first task of mothering is to develop skill in feeding the infant. The nurse can do much to change the environment so that the mother has a chance at "success" in this venture. An early discussion about the reasons for choosing breast or bottle feeding will be useful to the nurse. The nurse can reduce the pressure on the mother by explaining that most infants have to be taught how to suckle and that the infant's degree of wakefulness and interest in sucking depends to a considerable extent on the length of labor and the medication given the mother during labor.[29] The rooting reflex is explained and the mother is shown how to stimulate it by lightly touching the infant's cheeks and lips with the nipple (breast or bottle). The nurse should also explain to the mother that her infant is born with sufficient nourishment to support the body processes for the first day or two and that she need not be overly concerned if he seems very sleepy and unresponsive to the feedings offered. Making the first few visits of the infant to the mother a "getting to know you" experience will permit the mother to begin to relate to her child without the pressure to be immediately successful at feeding. The nurse utilizes the available support systems to facilitate the feeding process. Seeing that the infant is available to the mother when he is awake, helping her to keep the infant awake during the feeding, and seeing that she is physically comfortable when caring for the baby are appropriate nursing actions (Fig. 29-3).

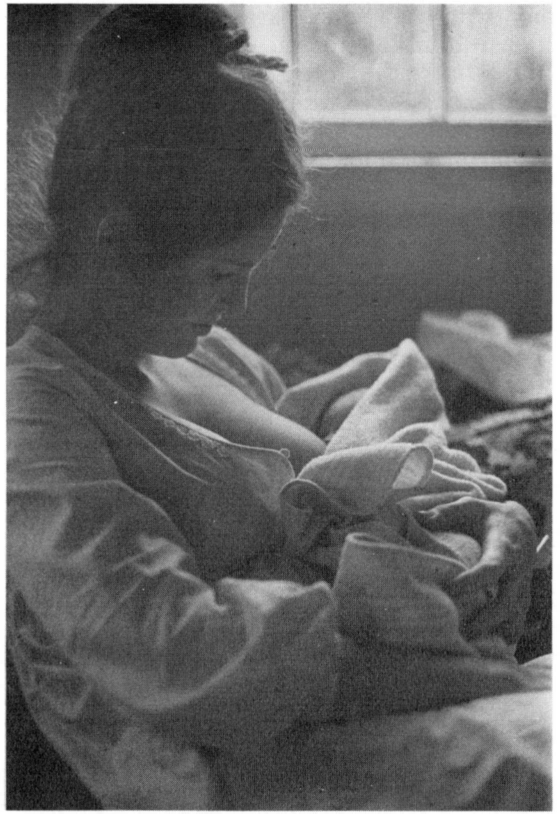

FIGURE 29-3. Helping the mother develop skill in feeding her infant promotes the mother-infant relationship. (Photograph by Richard Schwartz.)

The mother needs freedom to touch and to comfort her infant. The nurse should be available to the mother for support, to teach, and to answer the numerous questions mothers ask.

Positive feedback from a number of sources helps the mother gain confidence in herself. Although the nurse plays an important role in the development of maternal self-confidence, the response of the infant is most important. The mother-infant relationship is initiated by the mother, but she searches for some response from her infant. According to Robson and Moss[30] the release of human maternal feelings appears to depend largely on the infant's capacity to exhibit behaviors characteristic of adult forms of social communication. The nurse should help the mother understand the behavior of a newborn infant. All babies regurgitate feedings at times, they have excessive mucus which causes choking, and they frequently pass a stool at feeding time. They have irregular breathing patterns and they grimace and gurgle. They are not, by these behaviors, responding to their mothers, but to inner drives. The mother needs to be helped to delay social gratification which will not come until the infant smiles *at* her at a later time. The mother-infant relationship will be influenced by the type of baby the mother has and how nearly it meets her expectations. Unmet expectations may cause much anxiety and may result in a disturbed mother-infant adaptation. The nurse should study her patient's personality and explore with her what her expectations are. Together the mother and nurse should study the infant. Is it an active, passive, irritable, or somnolent baby? The nurse must help the mother to correctly perceive reality and help her to view the child in terms of realistic expectations.

The nurse needs to be observant of how her patient relates to the infant as each contact is made. How long does it take the mother to move from fingertip touching to use of the hands? Does she permit the infant's head to come in contact with her face when she holds him on her shoulder to bubble? Does she enfold the infant in her arms permitting torso to torso contact? If the nurse senses delay in the claiming process, she can act as a role model to the mother. It is possible, as the nurse handles the crying infant, to comfort the child by holding him close to her body and caressing the infant before she hands the infant to the mother. She can talk to the mother about the importance of skin to skin contact for early development. Rocking, patting, and auditory stimulation (chatting) constitute the infant's first contact with the world. The bodily contact provides the essential source of comfort, security, warmth, and increasing aptitude for new experiences.[31] The nurse should ask the mother what the infant's name is and should use it in the mother's presence. Indeed, the crib card should carry the infant's first name so that all nurses can use the name when assisting the mother. Thus, the nurse helps the mother to study her child, to find ways to relate to the child in a meaningful manner, and to receive pleasure from the relationship (Fig. 29-4).

The goal of nursing should be to help the mother to stay relaxed, to handle the child in a warm, sensitive manner, using cutaneous and auditory stimulation, to adapt to the rhythm of the infant, to protect the infant from potentially stressful experiences, and to develop an empathic interaction with her child. This is creative work of a professional character.

CRITERIA FOR ASSESSING ADEQUATE MOTHERHOOD IN THE EARLY WEEKS OF INFANT LIFE*

Mother-infant unity can be said to be satisfactory when a mother can:

1. Find pleasure in her infant and in tasks for and with him.
2. Understands his affective states and can comfort him by relieving his states of unbearable tension.
3. Can read his cues for new experience; can sense his fatigue level. Examples: Can receive his eye contact with pleasure. Promotes his new learnings with use of her face, hands, and objects. Does not overstimulate for her own pleasure.

---

* From Morris,[32] with permission.

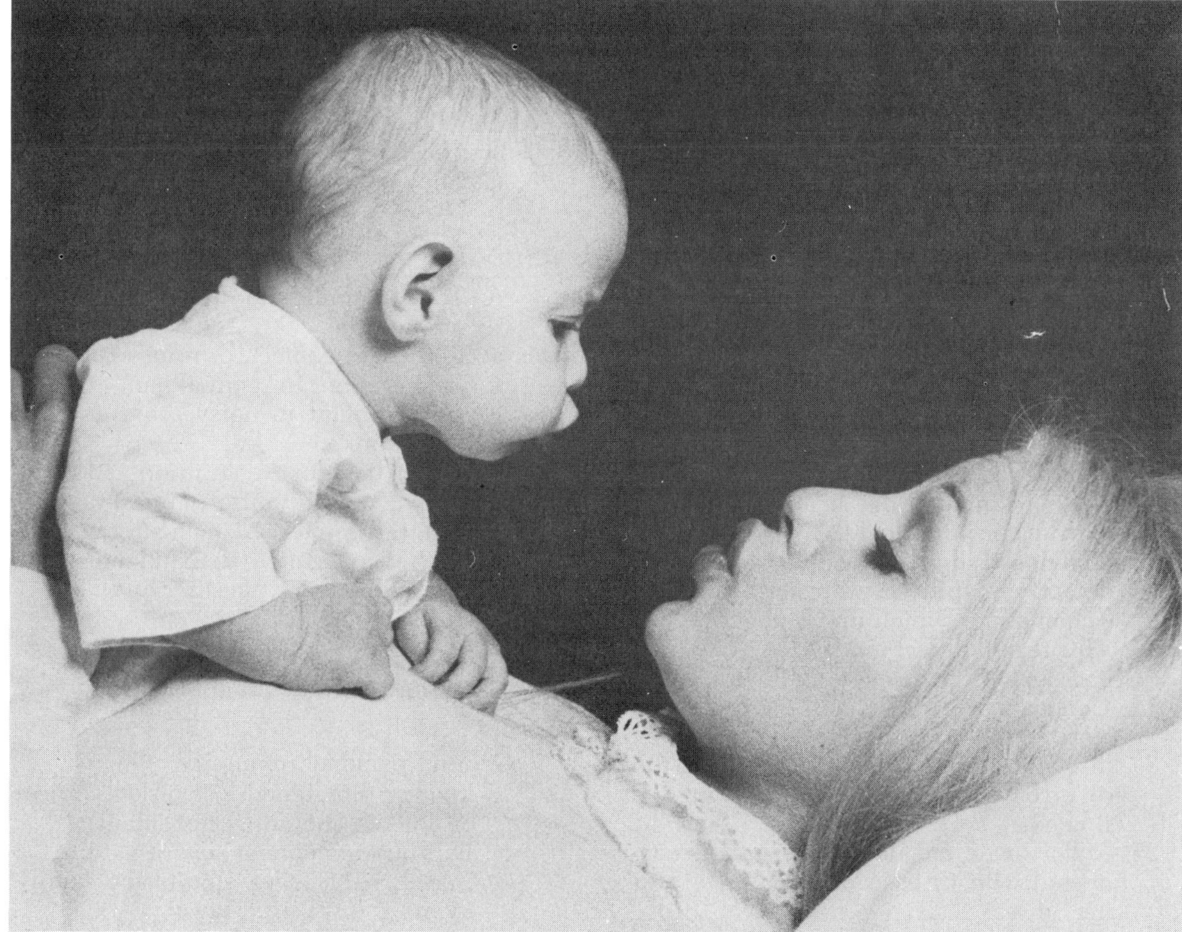

FIGURE 29-4. Mother and infant becoming acquainted with each other.

Signs Mothers Give When Not Adapting to Their Infants

1. See their infants as ugly or unattractive.
2. Perceive the odor of their infants as revolting.
3. Disgusted by drooling of infants.
4. Disgusted by sucking sounds of infants.
5. Upset by vomiting, but seem fascinated by it.
6. Revolted by any of infant's body fluids which touch them, or which they touch.
7. Annoyed at having to clean up infant's stools.
8. Preoccupied by odor, consistency, and number of stools.
9. Let infant's head dangle without support or concern.
10. Hold infants away from their own bodies.
11. Pick up infant without warning him by a touch or by speech.
12. Juggle and play with infant roughly after

feeding him even though he often vomits at this behavior.

13. Think infant's natural motor activity is unnatural.
14. Worry about infant's relaxation following feeding.
15. Avoid eye contact with infants, or stare fixedly into their eyes.
16. Do not coo or talk with their infants.
17. Think that their infants do not love them.
18. Consider that their infants expose them as unlovable, unloving parents.
19. Think of their infants as judging them and their efforts as an adult would.
20. Perceive their infant's natural dependent needs as dangerous.
21. Fears of infant's death appear at mild diarrhea or minor cold.
22. Convinced that their infant has some defect, in spite of repeated physical examinations which prove negative.
23. This feared defect tends to migrate from body system to disease, and back again.
24. Conceal the defect site or disease feared. If asked what they fear they disclaim knowing. They will reply to the reverse question of, "What do you hope it is not?"
25. Major maternal fears are often connected with disease perceived as "eating" diseases.
    Leukemia, or one of the other malignancies
    Diabetes
    Cystic fibrosis
26. Constantly demand reassurance that no defect or disease exists, cannot believe relieving facts when they are given.
27. Demand that feared defect be found and relieve.
28. Cannot find in their infants any physical or psychologic attribute which they value in themselves. (Probably the most diagnostic of these signs and readily elicited.)
29. Cannot discriminate between infant signs signaling hunger or fatigue, need for soothing or stimulating speech, comforting body contact, or for eye contact.
30. Develop inappropriate responses to infant needs:
    a. They over- or under-feed.
    b. Over- or under-hold.
    c. They tickle or bounce the baby when he is fatigued.
    d. Talk too much, too little, and at the wrong time.
    e. Force eye contact, or refuse it.
    f. Leave infant in room alone.
    g. Leave infant in noisy room and ignore him.
31. Develop paradoxical attitudes and behaviors. Example: Bitterly insist that infant cannot be pleased, no matter what is done, but continue to demand more and better methods for pleasing him.

Deterrents to Adequate Mothering

1. General personal immunity.
    a. Loss or threatened loss of love object or objects (including her infant).
    b. Disappointments of severe nature.
    c. Excessive fear of significant family member (own or in-laws).
    d. Father's criticism of mother or her infant.
    e. Rejection by her own mother or her in-laws of her or her infant.
    f. Financial worries.
    g. Husband's loss of job. This often provokes excessive fear of starvation on deep level, for self and infant.
    h. Father's punishing mother (openly or subtly) for own dependent needs.
    i. Serious illness of original parents or in-laws which constitutes the "first child" over the real infant, especially when mothers are directly involved in

care of their original parents or parents of her infant's father.
3. Current depersonalized and unrelated parturition and neonatal hospital practices.
4. Early discharge (from the second to fifth day) without sufficient help at home for maternal-infant adaptive tasks.
5. Failure in mother-doctor-family support system.

EXPANDING FAMILY ADAPTATIONS

Families with seemingly similar structures often respond differently when faced with a stress, since some families are more vulnerable to stress than are others. According to Hansen,[33] a family will better resist stress when two conditions exist:

1. Positional expectations are understood and accepted by all members.
2. Personal expectations are exceeded in voluntary actions intended to meet the perceived needs and desires of other members (these voluntary actions are recognized as such by the recipients).

In the organizational change when a new member is added to the family, nurses need to be sensitive to the manner in which *positional expectations* develop and whether they are understood and accepted by all members. As needs change for the new mother, the new father, and the children, the nurse also needs to assess if there are voluntary actions on the part of each dyad in the family (i.e., husband-wife, mother-child, father-child) to recognize and sensitively meet these *personal expectations.*

Children's Adaptation

The nurse can provide valuable assistance to multiparas in anticipating and understanding the behaviors manifested by children when a new infant is added to the family. This event may precipitate such behaviors as:

Changes in the mother-child relationship, particularly her relationship with the youngest child
Sibling competition and often sibling rivalry
Questions about pregnancy and birth.

Changes in Mother-Child Relationship

Many mothers experience separation anxiety and a sense of guilt in the changes brought about by the addition of a new baby. When they leave the child to go to the hospital, they miss the child and worry if their substitute is meeting the child's needs. Whereas they were content to remain in the hospital for their full postpartal stay after their first delivery, they now seem most anxious to return home as soon as their physician will permit them to do so. They often make frequent telephone calls and send little remembrances home to the child. They are anxious to know if the child misses them. They are concerned if his behavior indicates that he does. They worry about sleep problems, eating habits, and crying. They feel threatened if they are told "He is fine, doesn't seem any different—playful and happy" and they are devastated by "He hasn't asked about you, I don't think he misses you." If given the opportunity, they often talk to their nurse about their concern over needing to spend more time with the baby and that their older child may feel left out. They grieve over the necessary change in their relationship. Nursing assessment should include:

Age of the child and how dependent or independent he is
Who his present caretaker is and what their relationship is

- Whether the child is in his own home and own bed or in another home
- If in another home, whether he has previously visited there
- Mother's preparation of the child for this separation
- Reports the mother has had of the child's behavior since her hospitalization and her feelings about the reports
- Her knowledge of sibling competition and how she plans to handle any problems in this area.

Sibling Competition

Many mothers are threatened by the possibility that their child might be jealous, so it is better to avoid using this word when interviewing a mother. Many mothers will answer questions about the older child's possible adaptation with, "Oh, he'll love the baby." They can better handle less threatening questions. Universal statements and asking how she would act in a particular situation are useful techniques. For example:

- Most children get their noses a little out of joint when they have to share their mother with a new baby. How do you anticipate it will be in your home?
- What will you do if your son strikes the new baby?
- What will you do if your son demands the baby's bottle (or your breast)?
- What would you tell a mother who asked you what you would do about an older child who has begun to wet the bed again?

These types of interview questions will assist the nurse to understand the mother's ability to help her child handle his feelings and will also help the nurse to recognize areas where anticipatory guidance may be helpful.

Children sense that the relationship with their parents may not be the same. The child who asks, "When you come home, Mommy, can I sit on your lap?" wants to be assured that things will not change drastically.

Young children cannot understand why their all powerful mother had to leave them and go to the hospital. To punish her for such an act, the child may refuse to speak to her when she returns home. A question such as, "What will you do if your daughter shows anger toward you when you arrive home with the new baby?" will give the nurse insight into the mother's understanding of such a reaction and how she would handle the situation.

The postpartum unit of the hospital is an excellent place to institute group discussions of childrearing problems among multiparous mothers. Mothers can share their experience. The nurse, using a problem-solving approach, can help mothers to work through problems that concern them or that the nurse anticipates may concern them in the future. It is also an excellent place for nurses to learn much of practical value about childrearing from skilled mothers.

Sex Education

Children's questions about babies often begin when they learn that a new baby is to be added to the family. Additional questions are asked when the new brother or sister is brought home from the hospital. Parents need to be ready with answers that are factual and are based on the age of the child. If no questions arise by the age of four, the parents should find ways to stimulate the child's interest. Parents usually relate these facts to their children if:

- They feel the knowledge is appropriate for the child
- They themselves understand and have a vocabulary to explain the facts
- They are comfortable discussing the facts with their children.

Many parents have a vague understanding of the physiology of pregnancy and could not possibly explain the facts effectively to a young child. During the time the mother is in the hospital following delivery the nurse may make a valuable contribution toward helping parents be prepared to share the facts related to reproduction. Assessment should include:

Mother's attitude about relating these facts to her child
Mother's understanding of reproduction
Age of the child
Information, if any, the child has on the subject (questions that have been asked and information the parents have given).

The nurse must find ways to ascertain the mother's present knowledge in a nonthreatening way. She might begin by asking her what her own parents told her. If, as is often the case, she was not told at all or was told untruths and resents this, it may facilitate the nurse's further exploration. Peers, school, expectant parent classes, and other sources of information can be explored. If the mother needs further information, the nurse can furnish her with reading material to help her with the appropriate words to be used for a specific child or children. The nurse helps the mother understand that whether she answers her child's questions with facts, with fiction, or refuses to answer her child at all, she is teaching the child something about sex and sexuality.

The nurse should help the mother to focus on some specific ways to relate these facts. She can do this by asking such questions as:

What will you answer when he asks where the baby came from?
How will you answer if he asks how she got in there?
What will you say when he asks why she doesn't have a penis?

Many mothers are concerned about how much to tell the child about the relationship between the mother and father. The child does not need all of the facts, but what facts the parents do relate should include the love relationship of the two parents as well as honest facts about the anatomy and physiology of reproduction. Perhaps the best guideline for the very young child is to answer the questions he asks, but not go into further details. The parents should also expect the child to ask the same questions many times, distorting the facts until he gets it straight. For the older child, the parents might relate those facts with which they are comfortable and supply the child with a booklet or book which they then share.

Group discussions among multiparous mothers on a postpartal division with the leadership of a knowledgeable nurse would be an excellent way to structure one or two luncheons each week. The mothers could thereby receive support and learn from each other as they face this important task of parenthood.

The following books will make excellent references for your patients:

Baruch, D.: *New Ways in Sex Education*. Bantam, New York, 1962. (paperback) 60 cents.

The emphasis in this book is on the feelings and emotions associated with learning about sex. It covers the questions and concerns of preschoolers through adolescents with suggested methods of handling situations. As the author states, "you will need to adapt them to your own individuality and taste." It contains a special section of illustrations and stories for parents to use to help them discuss sex with their children.

Child Study Association of America: *What to Tell Your Child about Sex*. Permabooks,

New York, 1964. (paperback) 35 cents.

A handy paperback that helps parents handle sex education from the first questions of preschool children through the concerns of teenagers. It gives sample questions from both youths and parents for each of the developmental levels along with suggested answers. There are clear line drawings in a special section, "Facts of Life Illustrated," dealing with growing up, anatomy, reproduction, and birth.

Driver, H.: *Sex Guidance for Your Child*. Monona Publications, Madison, 1961. $4.50.

This book is written by a family life panel consisting of a child psychiatrist, minister, two teachers in physiology and biology, and a consultant in mental hygiene. It can be used not only by individual parents but as an outline for parent study groups. The emphasis is on healthy and respectful attitudes toward sex and it deals with children from infancy through adolescence.

Gruenberg, S. M.: *The Wonderful Story of How You Were Born*. Doubleday, New York, 1973. (paperback) 95 cents.

Although this book is written for young children, it may also be a useful reference for parents.

Father's Adaptation

Of all the people in the family unit, the father often receives the least attention when a new baby is added to the family structure. His needs are often subjugated to those of his wife, the newborn, and the other children. Yet he continues to have needs and must make considerable adjustments.

A father who as a child experienced feelings of displacement by a younger brother or sister may have those anxieties reactivated. When he observes his own child seemingly displacing him in his wife's life, he may react with resentment without recognizing the cause.[34] The hostility caused by feelings of rejection will make it difficult for him to respond to his wife with affection.

Sexual fulfillment, which likely has been delayed during the later part of pregnancy, is another area which may present problems. The obstetrician may suggest that the couple not become sexually active for up to six weeks after delivery. This puts considerable strain on the relationship at a time when the husband may need such fulfillment and when the wife may need reaffirmation of her femininity and her desirability as a sex partner. Most couples do not heed such advice. Nevertheless, they may feel guilty about not having done so, and worry about the consequences.

Family expansion is more orderly and less crisis-prone when each parent has concern for the other's needs. However, due to the extensive demands on the mother's time, the husband will have to assume major responsibility for seeing that his wife has some social relaxation. The mother needs a respite from the constant demands of a neonate and the husband should be encouraged to see that his wife obtains some relaxation. In the home, he should protect his wife from over-zealous friends and family whose visits and telephone calls may become a sensory overload.

The relationship between the new mother and father is reciprocal. Each will feel better able to parent, more comfortable with the role, and a greater sense of satisfaction and fulfillment when he or she feels the love and support of the other.

If there is a second child in the family, a new relationship may develop between the father and the older child. The father frequently assumes a more active role in providing physical care. He may also expand his role in the social life of the child. Since the child is now the older one, special privileges in keeping with his growth and development can be given and this enlarges the possible interaction with the father to the benefit of both.

Fathers vary greatly in their ability and willingness to take a part in the care of the infant. Many men are concerned about their ability and await some feedback from the infant before they participate. More often they are willing to help but it is the wife who, in her need to be all things to the infant, refuses to share the care with her husband or criticizes his inexpertness when he does try to assist. Occasionally, the husband assumes such a major role in caring for the infant or is so critical of his wife's care that she resents the "intrusion," feels jealous, and is happy when the husband returns to his job and leaves her with the care of the infant.

The nursing assessment should include:

Family constellation
Husband-wife relationship
Parent-children relationships
Close family and friends, their responses to the birth and their relationships with the family
Father's role, as he sees it in relation to the neonate, other children, and wife
Father's work and the hours available to the home and family
Family strengths

MOTHER-INFANT STUDY

The following patient study is presented to indicate a method of planning the nursing care of a new mother and her family, beginning with the first postpartal day and following through into the home.

Assessment (Chart) Labor and Delivery
Name: Mrs. Joan Simmons, a primipara
Age: 24
Occupation: "Housewife"
Religion: Protestant
Culture: Japanese-American
Residence: Apartment in residential part of the city
Husband: Age 26, Occupation: Clerical

Mrs. Simmons was admitted to the hospital at 11:02 AM on the day of delivery. Her membranes were leaking, but she was not in labor. Her pregnancy was then 41 weeks of gestation. She was accompanied by her husband who planned to support her in labor. They had both taken classes in Lamaze during the pregnancy.

She was given buccal Pitocin, followed by intravenous Pitocin which stimulated contractions of labor. She received Nisentil 40 mg. once during the transitional phase of labor and a pudendal block for the delivery. She was also given Deladumone OB, 2 cc. during the second stage of labor.

She delivered a girl child at 7:12 PM after 7 hours, 43 minutes of labor. The position: ROA (right occiput anterior). The type of delivery: NSD (normal spontaneous delivery). The infant was suctioned and given oxygen for one minute. The Apgar scores for the infant were 6-9-9.

The mother and child left the delivery suite in "good condition."

Assessment (Chart) D.D.
Fundus: Firm, I/U
Lochia: Rubra, moderate
B.P.: 110/80
Voided: 325 cc., 10:00 PM
Senokap $\dot{\overline{\text{T}}}$ H.S.
Slept at invervals during the night.

Assessment Data, P.P. Day 1
T.P.R.: 98.6-68-18
B.P.: 118/60
Fundus: Firm, U/U
Lochia: Rubra, moderate
Perineum: Slight edema. Complains of pain in the area.
Breasts: Soft
Voiding: Q.S.

Ordered Date	Ordered Hour	Checked R.N.	Routine Postpartum Orders
			1. Regular diet.
			2. On arrival from D.R., check for relaxation of fundus, excessive bleeding, and B.P. level.
			3. Ambulate with help as soon as patient desires.
			4. Darvon Compd. 65 mg. q2–3 hr. p.r.n. for discomfort. (Leave 6 caps. at bedside with instructions). Percodan tab. $\dot{\overline{\text{T}}}$ q4 hr. p.r.n., if no relief from Darvon.
			5. Catheterize, p.r.n., for bladder distention or distress. Notify physician if catheterization necessary more than 1X.
			6. Senokap 1–2, daily, H.S., X2 doses starting day of delivery and p.r.n. thereafter.
			7. If no B.M. by the 3rd postpartum day, insert one Dulcolax rectal suppository. May be repeated after 2 hr. if necessary.
			8. Hemoglobin, hematocrit, on 2nd postpartum day.
			9. Nupercainal Ointment at bedside if patient complains of hemorrhoids.
			10. Nembutal grs. 1½, H.S., p.r.n. May repeat one time after midnight, p.r.n.
			11. Instruct patient to use Dermoplast spray to episiotomy t.i.d. X2 days starting D.D. then t.i.d. as patient desires.
			12. ASA gr. x p.r.n. headache and temperature over 100° F.
			13. Rubella vaccine.

Environment: Mrs. Simmons shares a two bed rooming-in unit with another patient who also delivered yesterday. (This patient is a gravida 2, para 2.) The room has a number of floral bouquets. Mrs. Simmons is sitting up in bed having just finished her breakfast. (You note that she drank her orange juice, ate one piece of toast, and drank a cup of tea.)

8:00 AM—Patient: "I thought I'd be ravishing hungry, after all those months of being careful, but I'm not." (Said to no one in particular.)

You introduce yourself as her nurse and begin to add to your assessment while preparing her unit for morning care.

Nurse: Tell me about the baby's birth.

Patient: I was excited when I saw her. The first glance told me she was pretty normal. I saw she was a girl and I was happy. I said I wanted a boy for my husband, but secretly I wanted a girl. Isn't it funny—we had girls names picked out, but no boys—that's weird. She had that vernix over her, and quite a bit of hair. I was surprised. She looked like what I expected. I couldn't really distinguish anything that looked like us—except that hair—it looked like my husband's, stood straight up. She looked normal.

Nurse: How near did she meet your expectations?

Patient: It was all right then, but later when she got cleaned up I was disappointed. She looked like a boy, with that "pokey" hair.

Nurse: (as you begin the morning bath): Tell me about your labor.

Patient: Well, I woke up yesterday morning all wet, but no pains. I thought it might be my bag of waters. I called my doctor and he had me come to the clinic. They were ruptured, so they admitted me.

Nurse: Was your husband with you?

Patient: He stayed with me right through her birth. I didn't think he could do it, but he did. He was a big help.

Nurse: After you were admitted, what happened?

Patient: Well, they started my labor with something in my arm. It didn't take too long. I could follow Lamaze breathing pretty well until that other woman was admitted. She was screaming and carrying on. I began to worry that I'd act that way too. It didn't help when they told me it was her third baby either.

Nurse: And then?

Patient: I did okay until transition, then it began to get to me. I wanted to scream.

Nurse: What did you do? Would screaming have helped you to manage the pain?

Patient: Yes, I think it would have helped. I just twisted and turned and hid my face in the pillow. It was then they gave me something and it calmed me down. With my husband's help, I got control of things again. Then, in what seemed a short time, they took me to the delivery room, and I pushed and pushed. They gave me an injection in my bottom. I was so tired, I was afraid I couldn't do it. I wanted to see her born, but I had my eyes closed and was pushing so hard I missed most of it.

Nurse: What are your feelings about your performance?

Patient: Okay, I guess. My husband and the doctor said I did great.

Nurse: I'd say you did very well, too.

Patient: Oh, that back rub feels real good. My poor shoulder muscles ache this morning from all the pushing. They warned us about that during the classes.

Nurse: What happened after the delivery?

Patient: I came up here and my husband went home. Poor fellow, he must have been beat.

Nurse: And you?

Patient: Well, I was so excited I just couldn't sleep. I don't think I slept at all. I was just too excited with all that had gone on. And that's two nights without sleep. I was up the night before with a toothache. I've just finished having a root canal job done. That bath felt so good; I feel like a little girl again being taken care of that way. But, those stitches hurt. I've taken four of those Darvon already (in 18 hours).

10:00 AM—(rooming-in babies just brought from the nursery for the day) You note the mother has received Deladumone in the delivery room to inhibit lactation.

Nurse: How did you decide on the method to feed your baby?

Patient: In the beginning I wasn't sure how I wanted to do it. I didn't want my breasts large and out of shape. You hear all kinds of things. My friends who breast feed seem to have so many problems. One said to me that her baby wouldn't suck and she felt like such a failure. She cried over that. I thought bottle feeding might be easier. Another thing, they are laying people off in my husband's office. If he got layed off, I knew I'd have to go right back to work. (She paused.) Now, I'm sorry. I sorta wish I had tried.

The patient picked up the infant, smiled at her, held her in her left arm and offered it the formula. She did not use the infant's name. Most of her vocalization with the infant was imploring the infant to nurse. Twice she used a fingertip to caress the forehead. She handled the infant relatively skillfully. The infant was asleep most of the time and took less than ½ ounce of the formula. She kept prodding the infant and seemed anxious over the small amount.

Patient: She's getting cuter.

Nurse: Does she feel like she's really your baby?

Patient: I hadn't thought about it. I really don't know. I guess I'm not accepting it as a part of me. Then, I can't feel she's a part of the family. I never thought, "I'm your Mommy." I think in the hospital you feel uncomfortable. We'll feel more comfortable at home.

Nurse: Who is "we"?

Patient: Wow! I guess I really was talking about all three of us. (The telephone rings.)

Patient: Hello mother. Yes, I ate something. I skipped the eggs. I wasn't very hungry. She's cute, but she wouldn't eat this morning, only a few sucks. I guess I'll ask the pediatrician. Maybe she'll eat more later today.

Analysis:

Mrs. Simmons apparently needed to talk through her labor experience. In reviewing the labor record it seems she has the event clearly established in her mind. She felt the experience was painful and stressful but, largely due to feedback from husband and physician, she feels satisfied with her performance.

The infant is of the preferred sex (for her). It meets most of her expectations, except for its straight hair which she says looks like her husband's.

The mother-infant relationship shows claiming is beginning. The word "she" is used when talking about the infant. She is using fingertips to touch and caress the infant. She is beginning to relate the child to the family.

Mrs. Simmons is showing and accepting her dependency needs. The bath and back rub were gratefully accepted. She showed no objection to her mother inquiring about her food intake. She listened to instructions related to self-care and to the orientation instructions given by the nursery nurse.

This new mother shows some anxiety related to success as a mother. She chose to bottle feed because others told her of their failures with breast feeding. She seemed overanxious to have the infant take her feeding. She looks to the pediatrician for guidance.

She has sleep deprivation. Her perineal sutures are painful.

She seems to have some concern about body image—"I didn't want my breasts large and out of shape." More data is needed.

Nursing Care Plan—P.P. Day 1

Physiologic Needs

Sleep: Plan for uninterrupted nap late this morning. See that medication is given for sleep tonight.

Sutures: Use and teach use of Dermoplast spray. Sitz bath this PM

Vital Signs: Monitor uterus, lochia, breasts

Long Term Plans:

- Explore family planning
- Explore home assistance
- Check Hb. and Hct.

Psychosocial Needs

Infant Care: Support mother's efforts. Discuss sucking reflex, need for relaxed atmosphere. Help with questions. Be accessible during feeding period. Observe degree of anxiety. Class tomorrow.

Mother-Infant Relationship: Observe claiming process. Help mother study infant

Long Term Plans: Explore body image; begin exercises. Explore pregnancy, family relationships

---

Assessment Data, P.P. Day 2

- T.P.R.: 98-78-18
- B.P.: 100/60
- Fundus: U/I
- Lochia: Rubra, moderate
- Perineum: Still painful. Area less edematous.
- Breasts: Soft
- Voiding: Q.S.
- Hb.: 11.11
- Hct.: 33.5

Nurse: Good Morning. How's the appetite?

Patient: Oh, much improved. I enjoyed this breakfast. And I had a really good sleep last night. I really am beginning to feel like myself now.

Nurse: And the baby?

Patient: She's still pokey. She took an ounce yesterday evening, but only a few sips at the last feeding. I know you said she didn't need much for now, but I'd like to see her wake up and take notice somehow. I wish I had nursed her now. (looking at her abdomen)

I'm anxious to get back in shape. My mother came in last night and said, "Looks like there is another one in there." I guess lots of people expect me to be flat.

Nurse: That bothered you?

Patient: No. Well, I did find it necessary to explain things to them. I guess it did a bit.

Nurse: Tell me, what were your feelings during pregnancy when your body began to change?

Patient: I hated it in the beginning. My breasts enlarged first, even larger than my abdomen at first. I was sort of ashamed of that. Afterwards, I got used to it.

Nurse: And at the end of pregnancy?

Patient: I didn't mind that. But I was glad to get it over with. I got weighed early this morning.

Nurse: And?

Patient: It looks hopeful.

Nurse: What kind of goals do you and your husband have in terms of family size?

Patient: When we first got married we wanted three, but with the high cost of everything, two will be enough now.

Nurse: How soon?

Patient: Oh, not before 2½–3 years.

Nurse: How will you accomplish that?

Patient: I'm not sure. I haven't thought too much about it. I haven't given it serious thought. We sorta used rhythm before. Then we were married for four years and it didn't matter. We weren't trying not to get pregnant, but we weren't trying to get pregnant either. (seems reluctant to go on)

Nurse: You're going home tomorrow. How will you manage?

Patient: Well, my husband was to help, he's been on a week's vacation, but the baby was a week late and he has to go back to work. My Mom works, but she's offered to take a couple days off to help. My mother-in-law offered, so did some friends.

Nurse: What will your mother do?

Patient: Oh, she'll help any way I need. She and I are very close. My husband gets along well with her, too. And same on the other side of the family—get along well.

When the infant arrives for its morning feeding, you, the nurse, observe the mother-infant interaction and record it on the Observation Guide form as shown on the next page.

While the infant was feeding, the mother related to the nurse her fears concerning the baby.

Patient: I was exposed to German measles early in my pregnancy at about three months and I was real worried. I called up right away. They took antibody titer and I was assured all was okay, but I worried anyway. I knew some people with a deformed baby and I worked with a girl whose baby had a cleft palate and some abnormal fingers. That story worried me, too. My husband and I talked about the baby especially if it would be mentally retarded. I think I could handle that, but I'm not sure what his reaction would be.

Nurse: Did you have dreams about the baby?

Patient: Yes, but it was always normal.

Nurse: Are you saying you are concerned that this baby may not be normal?

Patient: Nooo, not really. But I do wish she would be more alert.

Analysis:

Mrs. Simmons has caught up on her sleep needs. Her perineal sutures are still painful.

She is concerned about her body image and wants assistance to get back to her former shape.

The mother-infant relationship is progressing at the anticipated rate. She is still concerned about her ability to feed the infant. Needs instruction on infant care. This mother continues to display anxious behavior about the infant's normalcy.

She plans to space her children, but has not decided on a method.

Patient needs iron rich food to improve her Hb. count.

Observation Guide: Maternal Touch

Tenderness	2	2	2	2	2	2	2	2	2	2	Total
Patting (comfort)	√				√					√	3
Caressing	√	√			√	√				√	5
Rocking	√	√	√	√	√	√	√	√	√	√	10
Cuddling	√	√	√	√	√	√	√	√	√	√	10
Expressing love	√										1
Chatting	√	√	√	√	√	√	√	√	√		9
Lulling											
Total											38

Description of behavior, words used, appropriateness.

Category
√ Solicitous
____ Casual
____ Unskilled
____ Anxious

Addressed the child as Kimberly and used the name twice. Most verbalization, which was constant, had to do with eating. Mother was concerned about the infant's lack of food intake, besides that said, "I got your eyes open." "What's over there?" (to sound in next bed). "Hey, your eyes are getting heavy, I shouldn't rock you, you go to sleep." "I think you had a bath this morning, that helped your appetite." "You have your father's hair."

Holding and Moving — Description of position of mother, relationship of infant's body to mother's, skill in handling the baby.

When baby arrived, reached into crib, lifted infant carefully, placed in left arm and rocked baby throughout most of feeding. Caressing was done only to face and one hand with one fingertip. Once placed infant on bed, unwrapped and looked at body, but did not touch body, rewrapped gently. Held infant well supported. When bubbled infant, held face close to baby's head.

Feeding
____ Breast
____ Glucose
✓ Formula

Description of maternal ability, infant's response, maternal frustration level, verbalization related to infant's feeding.

Handles child well. Feeding taken poorly (1 oz. in 20 min.). At times seemed frustrated, but generally accepted the behavior and didn't force the infant. "You don't like hospital food? Okay." "You look so contented, just want to be left alone?" "Okay, I won't nag."

Other Maternal Behavior (Cleaning, covering, scolding, telephoning, watching TV, chatting with roommate, etc.)

Spoke to observer, "Well, I can't believe it, this is the first time she's eaten. I'm afraid to take it out, for fear she won't start again." Spoke to roommate several times, but kept the focus on her child.

Nursing Care Plan—P.P. Day 2

Physiologic Needs

Sutures: Give sitz bath b.i.d. today.
Vital Signs: Monitor uterus, lochia, breasts.
Nutrition: Go over diet, be sure understands importance of iron in diet and how it can be assured.
Rest: Discuss need for rest after going home.
Family Planning: Give booklet to read.
Long Term Plans: Explore family planning.

Psychosocial Needs

Infant Care: Formula and bath class. Support mother's efforts.
Mother-Infant Relationship: Help mother study infant, using modified Brazelton assessment tool.
Self Concept: Discuss breast feeding vs. formula feeding. Mother's decision.
Body image: Begin exercises.

Assessment Data, P.P. Day Three
T.P.R.: 98.4-72-18
Fundus: U/3
Lochia: Rubra, scant
Perineum: Tender, but less painful
Voiding: Q.S.
Bowels: Movement yesterday

Nurse: Good morning. I see you are already packed.

Patient: Yes, this is the big day, and I really feel up to it. Kimberly opened her eyes last night and almost seemed to smile. She now has a good rooting reflex and took three ounces of milk this morning.

Nurse: You are encouraged?

Patient: Yes, but I am certainly glad you were here for me to turn to. I know now it was just a matter of time. She's okay and so is my decision to bottle feed this time. Incidentally, thank you for those booklets on birth control. The pill is out, I know that. I'm pretty sure I'll have an IUD put in when I come back for my checkup. I know I should wait until then, but if we don't, we'll use a condom in the meantime. I don't like the idea of taking pills every day, not even vitamins. And the side effects worry me. So that's what I'll do.

Nurse: I wanted to ask—you are Japanese-Caucasian, and your husband?

Patient: He's Korean, Hawaiian, Swedish.

Nurse: Are there cultural practices you follow in relation to raising children?

Patient: Not really. We live like many island people—enjoy lots of all the practices. My mother is Japanese, but even my grandparents spoke English. I don't even understand much about that culture—we love the food, though. You know, this is the first grandchild for both sets of parents. I think we can manage it though. Al and I will keep control of the important things.

The mother-infant relationship during the morning feeding was full of tenderness. The mother is responding to every throaty sound, cough, etc. She is holding the child in a close embrace and talking with her. The infant took 2½ oz. of formula and bubbled well. While the mother holds the infant over her shoulder to bubble, she nestles close to its face and presses her lips to the cheek.

The mother verbalizes awareness of the sleepless nights which may follow. The nurse has talked with her about her possible conflicts and the transient depression that could follow. She knows some things to help avoid the problem.

Assessment Data: Week 1 (by telephone)
Physical:

The suture area feels "heavy."

There is still a small amount of bright red lochia, mostly in the afternoon.

Sleep is broken. Got only four hours last night due to the infant's erratic schedule (sleep all day, up at night).

"First night home was terrible. Every little noise we were both up checking her. The second night I was so tired. My husband got up. He tries hard to help, but he gets nervous when he changes her, she keeps kicking. He's all broken out in a sweat when he finishes."

"Mother and mother-in-law were here during day over weekend. I'd rather do things myself. I get nervous with them taking care of my home. I'm right there doing it along with them. I feel guilty lying down with them working."

"Yesterday I mopped and vacuumed and my bottom hurt so I could hardly stand up."

"Baby's appetite has picked up. She's eating three ounces now. The only problem I have is with burping her. But she never throws up."

Nursing Care Plan—Week 1

Physiologic Needs

Household Help: Suggest try to get local teenager to help with heavy cleaning, and allow husband (who is willing) to help.
Fatigue: Suggest plan for rest period, reduce housekeeping standards for this period.
Lochia: Report lochial flow to M.D. if increases.
Infant Schedule: Suggest keep awake during day, will improve length of night periods.

Psychosocial Needs

Relaxation: Plan for some social activity within the week.
Self Concept: Congratulations on managing infant so well.

REFERENCES

1. Caplan, G.: *An Approach to Community Mental Health*. Grune and Stratton, New York, 1961.
2. LeMasters, E. E.: *Parenthood as a crisis*. In Parad, H. J. (ed.): *Crisis Interventions: Selected Readings*. Family Service Association of America, New York, 1965.
3. Kievet, M. B.: *Family roles*. In Clark A. L., et al. (eds.): *Parent-Child Relationships*. Rutgers University, New Brunswick, New Jersey, 1968.
4. Werner, H.: *Comparative Psychology of Mental Development*, rev. ed. International Universities Press, New York, 1964.
5. Clark, A. L.: *The generation gap and childrearing practices*. Nurs. Forum 11:177, 1972.
6. Ibid.: *The adaptation problems and patterns of an expanding family: the neonatal period*. Nurs. Forum 5:92, 1966.
7. Kievet: op. cit., p. 9.
8. Benedek, T.: *Motherhood and nurturing*. In Anthony E. J. and Benedek, T. (eds.): *Parenthood: Its Psychology and Psychopathology*. Little, Brown and Co., Boston, 1970, p. 154.
9. Ibid.: *The psychosomatic implications of the primary unit: mother-child*. Am. J. Orthopsychiatry 19:642, 1949.
10. McFarland, M. B. and Reinhardt, J. B.: *The development of motherliness*. Children 6:48, 1959.
11. Gail, S.: *The Housewife*. In Fraser, R. (ed.): *Work*. Penquin Books, London, 1968.
12. Rubin, R.: *Maternal touch*. Nurs. Outlook 11:828, 1963.
13. Benedek: *Motherhood and nurturing*, op. cit.
14. Pollack, G. H.: *Mourning and adaptation*. Internat. J. Psychoanal. 42:341, 1961.
15. Gordon, R. E., Kapostins, E. E. and Gordon, K. K.: *Factors in postpartum emotional adjustment*. Obstet. Gynecol. 25:158, 1965.
16. *Report of Phase No. 1 of a Study of Emotional Patterns of the New Mother*. Ross Laboratories Medical Department, Columbus, Ohio.
17. Colman, A. D. and Colman, L. L.: *Pregnancy: The Psychological Experience*. Herder and Herder, New York, 1971, p. 144.
18. Litz, T.: *The Person*. Basic Books, New York, 1968, p. 344.
19. Mead, G. H.: *Mind, Self and Society: From the Standpoint of a Social Behaviorist*. Charles W. Morris (ed.), University of Chicago Press, Chicago, 1934.
20. Shainess, N.: *The psychologic experience of labor*. N. Y. J. Med. 33:2923, 1963.
21. Rubin, R.: *Puerperal change*. Nurs. Outlook 9:753, 1967.
22. Ibid.: p. 775.
23. Anderson, E. H.: A *Study of Postpartum Depression: Implications for Nursing*. Convention Clinical Session, Design for Nursing Interaction, American Nurses' Association, 1964, p. 5.
24. Fieve, R. R.: *Depression in the 1970's*. In *Exerpta Medica*. The Hague, Zuidhollandsche Drukkerij, p. 7.
25. Rubin: *Maternal touch*. op. cit.
26. Morris, M. G.: *Maternal claiming-identification processes: their meaning for mother-infant mental health*. Am. J. Orthopsychiatry 35:302, 1965.
27. Robson, K. S., Howard, M. D. and Moss, A.: *Patterns of determinants of maternal attachment*. J. Pediatr. 77:978, 1970.
28. Cohler, B. J., Weiss, J. L. and Grunebaum, H. U.: *Child care attitudes and emotional disturbance among mothers of young children*. Genet. Psychol. Monogr. 82:5, 1970.
29. Parke, R. D.: *Mother-Father-Newborn Interaction: Effects of Maternal Medication, Labor, and Sex of Infant*. Proceedings, 80th Annual Convention, American Psychological Association, 1972.
30. Robson, K. and Moss, H.: *Patterns and determinants of maternal attachment*. J. Pediatr. 77:984, 1970.
31. Montagu, A.: *The Human Significance of the Skin*. Columbia University Press, New York, 1971, p. 80.
32. Morris, M. G.: *Maternal claiming-identification processes: their meaning for mother-infant mental health*. In Clark, A., et al.: *Parent-Child Relationship: Role of the Nurse*. Rutgers University, New Brunswick, New Jersey, 1968, p. 35–36.

33. Hansen, D. A.: *Personal and positional influence in formal groups: propositions and theory for research on family vulnerability to stress.* In King, R. (ed.): *Family Relations: Concepts and Theories.* Glendessary Press, Berkeley, California, 1969, p. 108.
34. Taylor, K. W.: *The opportunities of parenthood.* In Becker, H. and Hill, R. (eds.): *Family, Marriage and Parenthood.* Heath, Boston, 1948, p. 460.

BIBLIOGRAPHY

Adams, M. *Early concerns of primagravida mothers regarding infant care activities.* Nurs. Research 12:72, 1963.

Anthony, E. J. and T. Benedek (eds.): *Parenthood: It's Psychology and Psychopathology.* Little, Brown and Co., Boston, 1970.

Applebaum, R.: *The modern management of successful breastfeeding.* Child and Family 9:61, 1970.

Benedek, T.: *The psychosomatic implications of the primary unit: mother-child.* Am. J. Orthopsychiatry 19:642, 1949.

Ibid.: *Parenthood as a developmental phase.* J. Am. Psychoanal. Assoc. 7:389, 1959.

Benson, L.: *Fatherhood A Sociological Perspective.* Random House, New York, 1968.

Bernal, J.: *Crying during the first ten days of life, and maternal responses.* Dev. Med. Child Neurol. 14:362, 1972.

Bibring, G., et al.: *A study of psychological process in pregnancy and the earliest mother-child relationship.* Psychoanal. Study Child 26:9, 1961.

Blank, M.: *Some maternal influence on infants' rates of sensorimotor development.* J. Am. Acad. Child Psychiatry 3:668, 1964.

Bolin, R. H.: *Sensory deprivation: an overview.* Nurs. Forum 13:240, 1974.

Brody, S.: *Patterns of Mothering.* International Universities Press, New York, 1956.

Broussard, E. R. and Hartner, M. S.: *Maternal perception of the neonate as related to development.* Child Psychiatry Hum. Dev. 1:16, 1970.

Burstein, I., Kinch, R. A. H. and Stern, L.: *Anxiety, pregnancy, labor and the neonate.* Am. J. Obstet. Gynecol. 118:195, 1974.

Cantoni, K.: *The family: a conceptual framework.* Child and Family 9:37, 1970.

Carreras, F.: *Third day blues.* Briefs 30:106, 1966.

Clark, A. L.: *The beginning family.* Am. J. Nurs. 66:802, 1966.

Ibid.: *The adaptation problems and patterns of an expanding family.* Nurs. Forum 5:92, 1966.

Ibid.: *The generation gap and childrearing practices.* Nurs. Forum 11:177, 1972.

Clark, A. L. and Hale, R. W.: *Sex during and after pregnancy.* Am. J. Nurs. 74:1430, 1974.

Cohen, R. L.: *Some maladaptive syndromes of pregnancy and the puerperium.* Obstet. Gynecol. 27:562, 1966.

DeLissovoy, V.: *Child care by adolescent parents.* Child. Today 2:22, 1973.

Detrick, N.: *Sexuality in pregnancy and the puerperium.* Birth and Family Journal 1:5, 1974.

Eppink, H.: *Catheterizing the maternity patient.* Am. J. Nurs. 75:829, 1975.

Falicov, C. J.: *Sexual adjustment during first pregnancy and postpartum.* Am. J. Obstet. Gynecol. 117:999, 1973.

Greenberg, M. and Morris, N.: *Engrossment: the newborn's impact upon the father.* Am. J. Orthopsychiatry 44:520, 1974.

Gordon, R. E., Kapostins, E. E. and Gordon, K. K.: *Factors in postpartum emotional adjustment.* Obstet. Gynecol. 25:158, 1965.

Halstead, L.: *The use of crisis intervention in obstetric nursing.* Nurs. Clin. North Am. 9:69, 1974.

Hogenboon, P.: *Man in crisis: The father.* J. Psychiatr. Nurs. 5:457, 1967.

Howells, J. G. (ed.): *Modern Perspectives in Psycho-Obstetrics.* Brunner/Mazel, New York, 1972.

Josselyn, I. M.: *Cultural forces on motherliness and fatherliness.* Am. J. Orthopsychiatry 26:264, 1956.

Kennell, J., et al.: *Maternal behavior one year after early and extended postpartum contact.* Dev. Med. Child Neurol. 16:172, 1974.

Klaus, M. H., et al.: *Maternal attachment. Importance of the first postpartum days.* New Engl. J. Med. 286:460, 1972.

Ibid.: *Human maternal behaviors at the first contact with her young.* Pediatrics 46:187, 1970.

Korner, A. F.: *Individual differences at birth, implications for child care practices.* Birth Defects 10:51, 1974.

Korner, A. F. and Thoman, E. B.: *The relative efficiency of contact* and vestibular proprioceptive stimulation in soothing neonates. *Child Development,* 43:443, 1972.

Larson, V. L.: *Stresses of the childbearing year. American Journal of Public Health,* 56:32, 1966.

LeMasters, E. E.: Parenthood as a crisis. In Parad, H. J. (ed.) *Crisis Intervention: Selected Readings.* New York: Family Service Association of America, 1965.

Lewis, M.: *State as an infant environment interaction: an analysis of mother-infant interaction.* Merrill-Palmer Quarterly 18:95, 1972.

Lubic, R. W.: *The effect of cost on patterns of maternity care.* Nurs. Clin. North Am. 10:229, 1975.

McBride, A. B.: *The Growth and Development of Mothers.* Harper and Row, New York, 1973.

Meerloo, J. A. M.: *The psychological role of the father.* Child and Family 7:102, 1968.

Menaker, E.: *The social matrix: mother and child.* Psychoanal. Rev. 60:45, 1973.

Morrison, I.: *The elderly primigravida.* Am. J. Obstet. Gynecol. 121:465, 1975.

Murdaugh, A. and Miller, L. E.: *Helping the breastfeeding mother.* Am. J. Nurs. 72:1420, 1972.

Nelson, S. A.: *School age parents.* Child. Today 2:31, 1973.

Newton, N. *Maternal Emotions.* Hoeber, New York, 1955.

Ibid.: *Psychologic differences between breast and bottle feeding.* Am. J. Clin. Nutr. 24:993, 1971.

Nilsson, A., Uddenberg, N. and Almgren, P. E.: *Parental relations and identification in women with special regard to paranatal emotional adjustment.* Acta Psychiatr. Scand. 49:57, 1971.

Norris, A. S.: *The tired mother.* Child and Family 5:11, 1966.

Osofosky, H. J. and Osofosky, J. D.: *Adolescents as mothers.* Am. J. Orthopsychiatry 40:825, 1970.

Otte, M. J.: *Correcting inverted nipples–an aid to breastfeeding.* Am. J. Nurs. 75:454, 1975.

Parke, R. D., O'Leary, S. and West, S.: *Mother-father-newborn interaction: effects of maternal medication, labor and sex of the infant.* Proceedings of the 80th Convention of the American Psychiatric Convention, 1972.

Perez, A., et al.: *First ovulation after childbirth: the effect of breastfeeding.* Am. J. Obstet. Gynecol. 114:1041, 1972.

Porter, C.: *Maladaptive mothering patterns: nursing intervention.* In *A.N.A. Clinical Sessions.* Appleton-Century-Crofts, New York, 1972.

Prelude to Action. Maternity Center Association, New York, 1968.

Reeder, S.: *Becoming a mother: role transition.* In *A.N.A. Regional Clinical Conferences.* Appleton-Century-Crofts, New York, 1967.

Rich, O.: Hospital routines as rites of passage in developing *maternal identity.* Nurs. Clin. North Am. 4:101, 1969.

Richardson, S. A. and Guttmacher, A. F. (eds.): *Childbearing–Its Social and Psychological Aspects.* Williams & Wilkins, Baltimore, 1967.

Rising, S. S.: *The fourth stage of labor: family integration.* Am. J. Nurs. 74:870, 1974.

Robson, K. S. and Moss, H. A.: *Patterns and determinants of maternal attachment.* J. Pediatr. 77:976, 1970.

Ibid.: *The role of eye-to-eye contact in maternal-infant attachment.* J. Child Psychiatry, 8:13, 1967.

Rossi, A. S.: *Transition to parenthood.* Journal of Marriage and Family, 30:26, 1968.

Rubin, R.: *Basic maternal behavior.* Nurs. Outlook 9:683, 1961.

Outlook 9:753, 1961.

Ibid.: *Maternal touch.* Nurs. Outlook 11:828, 1963.

Ibid.: *The family-child relationship and nursing care.* Nurs. Outlook 12:36, 1964.

Ibid.: *Attainment of the maternal role. Part I.* Nurs. Research 16:237, 1967.

Ibid.: *Attainment of the maternal role. Part II, Model and referrants.* Nurs. Research 16:342, 1967.

Sexual Relations During Pregnancy and the Post Delivery Period. SIECUS Study Guide No. 6. Sex Information and Education Council of the United States, New York, 1967.

Shainess, N.: *Psychological Problems Associated with Motherhood.* In Arieti, S., et al. (eds.): *American Handbook of Psychiatry, vol. III.* Basic Books, New York, 1966.

Shaw, N. R.: *Teaching young mothers their role.* Nurs. Outlook 22:695, 1974.

Shulman, J. J.: *Contraceptive provisions in the immediate postpartum period.* Obstet. Gynecol. 40:403, 1972.

Spaulding, M. R.: *Adopting postpartum teaching to the mother's low income style.* In Gergersen, B., et al. (eds.): *Current Concepts in Clinical Nursing.* C. V. Mosby, St. Louis, 1969.

Tanner, L. M.: *Assessing the needs of new mothers in the postpartum.* In Duffey et al. (eds.): *Current Concepts in Clinical Nursing, vol. III.* C. V. Mosby, St. Louis, 1970.

Ibid.: *In-hospital care and post-hospital follow up.* Clin. Obstet. Gynecol. 14:1124, 1971.

Thompson, M.: *Establishment of lactation.* Nurs. Forum 10:292, 1971.

Warrick, L.: *Femininity, sexuality and mothering.* Nurs. Forum 8:224, 1969.

Womanly Art of Breast Feeding, The. La Leche League, Franklin Park, Illinois.

Wooden, H. E.: *Impact of the industrial revolution on hospital maternity care.* Nurs. Forum 1:91, 1961.

Wooden, H. E.: *Impact of the industrial revolution on hospital maternity care.* Nurs. Forum 1:91, 1961.

Ibid.: *The family-centered approach to maternity care.* Nurs. Forum 1:63, 1962.

UNIT 8

THE NEONATE

30 *Physiologic Perspectives*

DYANNE D. AFFONSO, R.N., M.N.

Birth plunges a new baby into an environment of obligatory changes. Survival is dependent upon the neonate's transition to extrauterine life. Some babies make the transition smoothly, while for others the process is complicated. It is essential to understand the process of transition to extrauterine life because such knowledge allows the nurse to facilitate the process. However, before discussing this transitional process, review of the infant's intrauterine environment is necessary to appreciate the impact of extrauterine transition.

SYNOPSIS OF INTRAUTERINE LIFE EXPERIENCES

Fetal growth varies in accordance with the functional capacity of the placenta; at first it is rapid, but then it decreases after about 38 weeks of gestation. (Growth then accelerates again immediately after birth and decreases again later in infancy.) The fetal-maternal exchange necessary for growth of the fetus takes place at the interface or contact point between maternal blood filling the intervillous spaces and the placental villi dipping down into those spaces and carrying the fetal capillaries. The intervillous spaces were formed when the chorionic villi from the embryo penetrated into the endometrium of the uterus and eroded out the spaces, leaving the bare tips of uterine arteries to spurt maternal blood into the intervillous spaces and uterine veins to carry it away after fetal-maternal exchange has taken place.[1]

The essential life activities, such as respiration and circulation, have unique features in the fetus. These are discussed in detail later in this chapter in the section on Perinatal Physiology. One needs to appreciate that the fetus lives under hypoxic conditions but, unlike the adult, he is able to survive because of unique adaptive mechanisms. Such mechanisms allow the fetus to use his limited available resources optimally to sustain life.

The world of the fetus is basically one of restrictions. He is restricted in space by his mother's uterine cavity; he is restricted in oxygen supply by the capability of the maternal-placental system; he is restricted in his ability to absorb nutrients and eliminate waste to keep his environment ecologically safe and his own system in balance. Therefore, the fetus is forced to institute an "energy conservation and waste disposal program." The manner in which this is done is truly a wonderment! Organs whose functions are limited during the intrauterine period are maintained primarily by the maternal-placental system, thus more nutrients can be diverted to organs essential for intrauterine functioning. For example, various structures such as the ductus arteriosus and ductus venosus divert blood flow away from the lungs and liver. Thus, available blood can be used for other organs which must sustain intrauterine growth and development. The fetus also discharges his waste at varying periods of gestation so as not to pollute his environment. He actively participates in this clean-up campaign. For example, the fetus is known to urinate into the amniotic fluid, but also swallows portions of it which is speculated to help regulate the quantity of the amniotic fluid.[2]

The world of the fetus has been compared to that of an astronaut in outer space (Fig. 30-1). In their book, *The Secret World of the Baby*,[3] Day and Liley delightfully provide an impression of the fetal world. Excerpts from their descriptions follow:

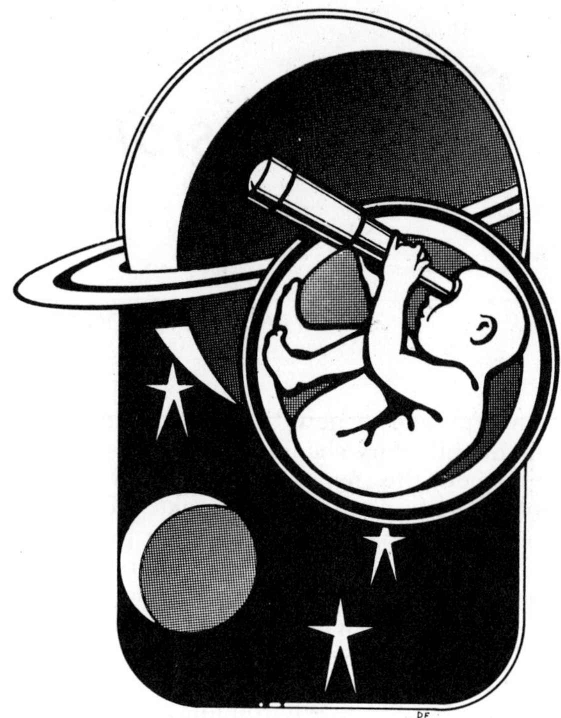

FIGURE 30-1. The fetus resembles an astronaut in outer space. (Drawn by Dave Fisher, Arizona Medical Center A-V Division, Tucson, Arizona.)

> Before he is born, the baby lives a very different life than he will live when he reaches the outside world. Inside his capsule he is like a submerged swimmer, existing in fluid rather than air. His balloon of fluid is something like the capsule that astronauts live in when they fly into outer space. Inside his capsule he does not feel the force of gravity, or "pull" from the earth. You and I cannot easily move away from the earth because gravity draws us toward ground level. It was quite a feat for each of us to learn to stand upright against gravity in the first place. The unborn baby has no such "pull" to earth. He is weightless, in much the same way as the astronauts are when they float free, so far up in space.
>
> When an astronaut floats in space, he is sometimes right side up, from our point of view on earth, and sometimes upside down. It is the same with the unborn baby. Since there is no pull of gravity, it does not bother the baby to be upside down. And, as long as his body is smaller than his space capsule, so that he moves about freely inside of it, he very often is upside down. Tethered to the placenta, his supply base, he swims, floats and circles inside his watery space capsule, as buoyant as you are when you swim in salt water.
>
> Because this inner world of his mother's womb is so different from the outside world where we all live, the baby needs some very special equipment to exist there—just as the spacemen need special suits and life lines to survive in space.
>
> Therefore, the body of the unborn baby is more complex than ours. Before he is born, the baby has several extra parts to his body, which he needs only so long as he lives inside his mother. He has his own space capsule, the amniotic sac. He has his own

life line, the umbilical cord. And he has his own "root system," the placenta. These all belong to the baby himself, not to his mother. They all developed from his original cell.

The amniotic sac—the baby's private space capsule—is surrounded by membranes of living tissue and contains fluid in which he floats.

The climate that the unborn baby lives in within his capsule is quite different from the outside world. Inside the womb, it is very warm—about ninety-nine degrees—and the temperature stays the same all the time. The fluid, which completely surrounds his body, also serves as a shock absorber. If his mother should accidentally fall, the jar would have little effect on the baby, since he is buoyant and is protected by the fluid around him. He is also unlikely to be sick, because there are no germs inside his sealed balloon.

Since the baby is so well protected, warmed and fed while he is in the womb, it is not surprising that people assumed that he was like a little plant. But the baby is not a plant, nor does he behave like one. If we want to compare him to another living creature, we could say he resembles, more than anything else, an aquatic animal. Like a playful baby seal, he is lively and active—swimming, diving, floating. Since his joints are more flexible than yours or mine and his spine is relatively elastic, the baby is as supple as an accomplished acrobat. He can get into all sorts of postures and positions that would be difficult or even impossible, for a child or adult.

THE STRESS OF BIRTH

The process of birth is a time of stress for the baby. If we consider the various stressful events (stressors) that occur during labor and delivery, we can rightfully use the term "birth stress."[4–6]

During labor, a major stressor to the fetus arises from the contractile activity of the uterus. Changes in pressure exerted in the amniotic cavity occur from the contracting uterus. Pressures range from 8 to 12 mm. Hg during periods of relaxation and from 20 to 60 mm. Hg at the height (peak) of uterine activity.[7] Too often there is not an appreciation of the impact of these changing intrauterine pressures on the fetus. The intrauterine pressure (usually measured in millimeters of mercury) can be translated into centimeters of water pressure: approximately 10 mm. Hg = 14 cm. of water.[8] Figure 30-2 provides an analogy of the amount of pressure the fetus experiences during a contraction as similar to pressures exerted during a deep water dive. Thus, the fetus resembles a swimmer during the relaxation phase of uterine contractions, and a diver as intrauterine pressure increases. One manifestation of these "swimming and diving procedures" by the fetus is slight changes in his blood pressure.[9]

Some of the fetal reactions to uterine contractions and how contractions create stress on the fetus are outlined in Table 30-1. In summation, a uterine contraction is a stressor to the fetus in three major ways:

1. Impedes placental blood exchange (exchange of blood in the intervillous space)
2. Applies pressure to the fetal body
3. Compresses the umbilical cord.[10]

Once the baby is born, he is bombarded by sensory stimuli, many of which are harsh as contrasted to the secure quiescence of the intrauterine environment. Examples of sensory stimuli contributing to birth stress are outlined in Table 30-2.

Stressors which act upon the fetus and neonate during the process of birth do not produce typical alarm reactions (such as shock) as they would in the adult. *Maturation pre-*

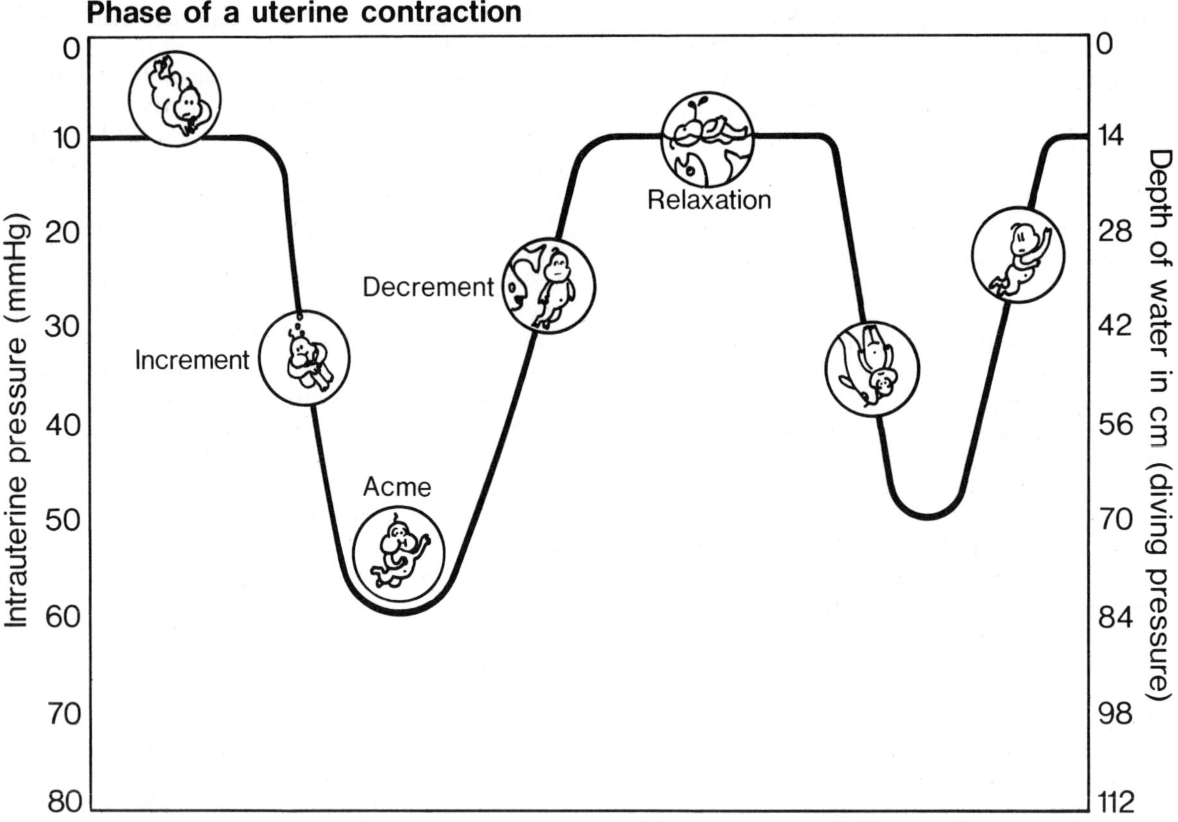

FIGURE 30-2. Graphic illustration of the analogy of intrauterine pressures as similar to pressures exerted during a deep water dive. (Drawn by Dave Fisher, Arizona Medical Center A-V Division, Tucson, Arizona.)

pares the organism of the newborn for the transition from intrauterine to extrauterine environment. *Postnatal adaptation assists* the developmental course by accelerating the maturation according to needs. *Neonatal tolerance protects* the organism from premature exhaustion of energy reserves. The rationale for this is related to developmental factors which protect the fetus by preparing him to cope with the stressors or by rendering stressors ineffective. Examples of these factors are the fetus' ability to maintain higher levels of amino acid and concentrations of hemoglobin, and available reserves for energy such as the ability to produce glucose to protect the baby from exhaustion in his confrontation with birth stress.[11]

It is important to note that a manifestation of birth stress can be seen in fluctuations in the fetal heart rate. A brief fall in rate can occur about 15 seconds after the rise of intrauterine pressure, with return to basal levels before the contraction ends.[12] However, any persistent fluctuation of heart rate, whether acceleration or deceleration, during or after a contraction should be immediately reported and measures instituted to rule out fetal distress.

TABLE 30-1. How Uterine Contractions Can Contribute to Birth Stress*

Stressor by Contraction	*Change Elicited*	*Effect on Fetal Welfare*
1. Compression of maternal abdominal aorta	Decreases blood flow through uterine arteries	Decreased blood flow to intervillous space reduces oxygen to fetus
2. Decrease in blood flow through intervillous space by constriction of arterial supply	Alters fetal acid-base balance	Produces hypoxia, hypercapnia, and acidosis
3. Increase in amniotic pressure	Alters fetal blood pressure and heart rate (usually recovers to basal levels before contraction ends)	Persistent deviation or prolonged recovery of blood pressure and heart rate indicates fetal distress
4. Mechanical pressure on presenting part		
a. Vertex	Molding of cranial bones; caput succedaneum	Little known about effects of temporary alteration in the shape of the cranium
b. Difficult breech	Sudden or prolonged pressure changes to fetal head	Neurologic abnormalities more frequent as compared to vertex presentations
5. Mechanical compression of umbilical cord by presenting part or other causes	Stops oxygenated blood flow to fetus	Predisposes to hypoxia and anoxia

* Data for table taken from Towell.[5]

TABLE 30-2. Sensory Stimuli Contributing to Birth Stress in the Newborn

Type of Sensory Stimuli	*Cause for Stress*
1. Thermal	Change from fluid to air medium Exposure to fluctuating environmental temperatures (e.g., coolness in air conditioned delivery rooms) Instability of temperature regulating system at birth
2. Tactile	Numerous manipulations by doctor to facilitate rotations for birth Measures to establish and maintain patent airway (slapping soles, suctioning) Positional changes to facilitate drainage of mucus by gravity Wrapping with blankets to ensure warmth; unlike warmth of amniotic sac Routines for identifications and provisions to ensure safety (administration of vitamin K, silver nitrate to eyes)
3. Chemical	Interruption of umbilical blood flow decreases oxygen and increases carbon dioxide; this results in changes in acid–base balance as reflected in blood gases taken at birth Hypoxia combined with hypercapnia predisposes to metabolic acidosis Acidosis will affect metabolic processes of the body Effects of medications given to the mother causing chemical imbalances in the fetus
4. Mechanical/Physical	Squeezing effect on fetal thorax by maternal vaginal walls (rather than causing stress it helps to expel fluid from respiratory tract and provides first portion for lung aeration) Compression of the umbilical cord or its twisting around the body (usually the neck) Manipulations to facilitate birth (e.g., use of forceps) or difficult presentations can result in trauma to body parts Other environmental stimuli such as bright lights, loud sounds

THE TRANSITIONAL PROCESS

Transition from intrauterine to extrauterine existence involves complex change processes. Obligatory change is demanded immediately after birth when the infant enters the atmospheric environment. Because the numerous change processes need time to become regulatory, the newborn experiences a period of instability. This period of instability may occur for the first six to eight hours or extend through the first 24 hours of life. This period has come to be known as the transitional period. Many progressive nurseries have come to value its importance by providing intensive observation of the neonate during this time. The physiologic importance of this transitional period is described by Pierog and Ferrara:[13]

> Once the infant is delivered he undergoes a radical change of environments. From an intrauterine existence (dark, warm, and watery; where there was minimal sensory stimulation and nutrition was performed by the maternal organism),he is expelled into an environment in which the medium is air, temperatures unstable, sensory stimuli are increased and constant, and the physiologic functions of respiration and nutrition must be performed by him.
>
> The cardiovascular hemodynamics change at birth.[14] As the cord is cut and the infant's lungs expand with his first breath, the pulmonary vascular bed opens, pulmonary vascular resistance is lowered, and aortic pressure becomes higher. Blood flow through the ductus arteriosus becomes unidirectional (left-to-right), eventually ceasing altogether. With the placental circulation removed, systemic venous return is now considerably diminished, so that pressure in the right atrium diminishes while that in the left atrium increases as the blood flow from the pulmonary area increases. The valve of the foramen ovale closes functionally because of the greater pressures within the left atrium.

The infant begins to breathe spontaneously within seconds after delivery; what actually occurs to cause the infant to draw his first breath is not clearly established, though it may be a number of stimuli that excite the respiratory center—a decrease in fetal oxygen tension and pH stimulating chemoreceptors, an increase in sensory stimuli (thermal, tactile, and so on), an increase in the infant's blood pressure after cord clamping (stimulating the baroreceptors), or elastic recoil of the compressed thorax as the infant emerges from the vaginal canal. Negative intrathoracic pressures from 20 to 70 cm. H_2O have been found as the infant draws the first few breaths;[15,16] as he cries, the lungs become completely and evenly expanded.

The infant is a true homeotherm and must adjust to the extrauterine environment to maintain a normal body temperature of 97 to 99° F. At delivery the infant's body temperature falls rapidly; he responds by vasoconstruction and an increased metabolic rate, which is evidenced by an increase in oxygen consumption.[17–22]

Desmond and co-workers,[23] in a study of the normal newborn immediately after birth, observed that the infant passes through a period of physiologic instability in the first 6 to 8 hours of life. This interval of adjustment they divide into two periods: the *first period of reactivity* lasts up to 30 minutes after delivery, and the *second period of reactivity* occurs at about the fourth to sixth hour of life. In the first 15 to 30 minutes of life the infant is alert and active, his body temperature falls, and he has tachycardia (with some fluctuation of the heart rate) and rapid and irregular respirations. Air begins to enter the gastrointestinal tract, and bowel sounds are noted. The infant's activity gradually diminishes, and he sleeps. In the second period of reactivity the infant again becomes alert, his respirations and heart rate become labile, and gagging may occur (Fig. 30-3). The sequence of clinical activity within

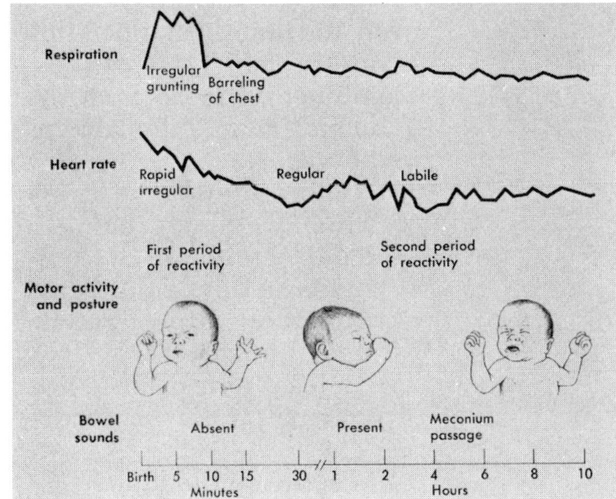

FIGURE 30-3. Some physiologic changes in the neonate in his adjustment to extrauterine life. (From Pierog and Ferrara,[4] with permission.)

these two periods occurs in all infants, regardless of the route of delivery or gestational age. However, the length of time these two periods last will vary, being affected by the length and difficulty of labor, the amount of stress to the fetus during labor, maternal medication and/or anesthesia, and other factors.

Arnold and associates[24] have outlined the extrauterine adaptive processes in six overlapping steps. Only after the successful completion of all steps can a neonate be said to have attained successful adaptation.

Step 1. Receives stimulation from pressure changes by uterine contractions and loss of uterine volume with ruptured membranes during labor.
Step 2. Encounters an avalanche of stimuli, e.g., cold, gravity, light, sounds during delivery.
Step 3. Must initiate air breathing.
Step 4. Must change the functions of its organ systems, e.g., lungs to maintain respirations, changes from fetal to neonatal circulation.
Step 5. Must reorganize metabolic processes, e.g., activitation of liver, renal, and gastrointestinal tract for passage of meconium.
Step 6. Must achieve a steady level or equilibrium in metabolic processes, e.g., production of enzymes, increase blood oxygen saturation, decrease acidosis associated with birth.

HIGHLIGHTS OF PERINATAL PHYSIOLOGY*

This is a theoretical discussion on selected physiologic functions in the fetus and neonate. A synthesis is presented on data relative to selected body functions. Because this is only an attempt to synthesize the multitude of data, the reader is encouraged to investigate the literature for more theoretical depth. Perinatal physiology is a dynamic field with new discoveries constantly emerging. Thus, the data presented here may change or be challenged by the time it reaches the reader.

1. The Respiratory System

Fetus: The primary respiratory organ is the placenta. Gas exchange occurs through diffusion at the intervillous space, which is governed by pressure gradients of oxygen and carbon dioxide. (Chapter 19 explains these gradients.) Certain factors help favor oxygen diffusion to the fetus from the mother. These are:

a. Uterine arterial blood flow favors the intervillous space; 25 per cent goes to uterine muscle, 75 per cent to placenta.
b. Fetal blood has greater affinity for oxygen than maternal blood.

---

*Data for this synthesized outline is taken primarily from Stave, U. (ed.): *Physiology of the Perinatal Period, vols. 1 and 2.* Appleton-Century-Crofts, New York, 1970, with permission. Page numbers refer to content location in the original text.

c. Hemoglobin concentration in the fetus is greater than in the mother.

d. Bohr effect: Blood with high acidity or high PCO_2 has less affinity for oxygen. Maternal blood increases in acidity as it gains carbon dioxide from the infant, while fetal blood decreases in acidity thereby increasing its affinity for oxygen (pp. 45–49).

Anatomic and Functional Development of the Lungs:

Lung buds appear	3.5 wks.
Lobar branching	6 wks.
Bronchi branching completed	10–16 wks.
Cilia in peripheral air passages	13 wks.
Primitive air sacs	20 wks.

By 28 weeks, two significant anatomic events occur: a) Blood vessels invade the mesenchyme to allow gas exchange, and b) Production of surfactant allows alveoli stability by altering surface tension during expansion and contraction, so these air sacs can fill with air. This alveolar development proceeds during the third trimester and is still incomplete at birth (p. 69).

In terms of functional development, the lungs are nonfunctional before 26 weeks of gestation primarily because of the lack of the two anatomic events mentioned above. Fetal respiratory movements do exist but are more like fine spasms than respirations as we know them.

Neonate: Entrance into an atmospheric environment demands immediate respiratory function. Some of the mechanisms involved in initiating the mandatory respirations after birth are:

a. Peripheral chemoreceptors are stimulated by low oxygen and high carbon dioxide resulting when the cord is severed and umbilical blood flow is interrupted.

b. Combined effects from the following may stimulate respirations:
   (1) Cold; altered heat loss from wet body being in contact with air
   (2) Release from a fluid environment alters gravitational forces
   (3) Release of resistance from vaginal walls on infant's chest
   (4) Tactile stimulation

c. Pulmonary reflexes help inflate the lung by initiating inspiratory gasps. These reflexes usually diminish within 48 hours of age (pp. 79–91).

Note that the *combined* effects of the above can help to stimulate respirations. However, they produce short passive respiratory movements (gasps) and cannot sustain respirations by themselves. Therefore, it is undesirable to utilize vigorous stimuli to aid respirations such as excessive slapping to soles or exposing to cold. These excessive stimulators become stressors which tend to inhibit rhythmic respirations.

Chapter 19 offers more details regarding the onset of respirations. What the nurse should appreciate about the neonate's first breath is that it was possible only after the infant overcame resistive forces from surface tension, viscosity of fluid in the airway, and tissue resistance.

There is a transitional period for respiratory patterns in the neonate. The rationale for this is related to the "hypoxic challenge" associated with birth from which the healthy infant recovers within 10 minutes. An important concept to note is:

Delivery is asphyxiating to the neonate, whether it is vaginal or abdominal. Thus, if an infant takes longer than ten minutes

TABLE 30-3. Serial Blood-Gas Tensions Reflecting Acid–Base Balance during the First Hour of Life

Determination	*Acid–Base Balance in Healthy Neonates 1–3 Days of Age**	*Normal Serum Values in Newborn†*	*Time Period in Minutes**				
			2–5	*6–10*	*11–20*	*21–40*	*41–64*
Pa_{O_2}, mm. Hg (oxygen tension in arterial blood)	70–90		19.5	48.7	56.3	56.7	61.7
P_{CO_2}, mm. Hg (CO_2 tension in the blood)	30.0–34.1		76.4	57.2	46.3	39.2	38.0
pH (H^+ concentration)	7.39–7.44	7.35–7.45	7.10	7.19	7.25	7.31	7.34
Na		135–145	139.0	136.0	135.0	135.0	134.0
K		4.0–4.5	9.1	8.4	8.0	8.5	8.0
Mg			2.0	2.1	2.5	1.8	0.5
Total protein			6.4	6.2	6.4	5.9	6.1

* Data from Oliver et al.[25]
† Data from McKilligin.[33]

to establish and maintain respirations, it should go to intensive care for assist in ventilation and/or correction of acid-base balance.[25]

This hypoxic challenge is documented in Table 30-3.

The neonate responds to the hypoxic challenge in two ways: a) Bi-phasic respiratory responses which are hyperventilation for two minutes and then reduction in ventilation, and b) Decrease in metabolism to minimize oxygen consumption (pp. 97, 98).

The maintenance of breathing in the neonate is influenced by acid-base balance, gas tensions, and the elastic properties of the lung and chest involved in the mechanics of inspiration and expiration.

2. The Circulatory System

Fetus: The cardiovascular system functions early; first heart beat occurs by three weeks of gestation and chemoreceptors respond to decrease blood flow by two months of gestation. Fetal circulation differs from that in the neonate in several ways:

a. High blood flow to placenta; approximately 50 percent of total cardiac output.
b. Anatomic structures which divert blood to organs performing priority life-sustaining functions.
   (1) Ductus venosus—arterialized blood from umbilical vein goes to inferior vena cava (on the way, it provides the liver with arterial blood).
   (2) Foramen ovale—permits major portion of oxygenated blood entering the heart to go directly to the left atrium, left ventricle, and out the ascending aorta so as to immediately

supply the heart and brain.

(3) Ductus arteriosus—blood from the right ventricle bypasses the lung through this structure into the descending aorta.

c. Oxygenated blood to the fetus travels via the umbilical *vein* and unoxygenated blood returns to the placenta via the umbilical *arteries* (pp. 148–151).

To ensure more oxygen *to* the fetus in his hypoxic environment, there are two arteries and one vein in the umbilical cord.

3. The Course of Fetal Circulation (Fig. 30-4)

"The classic concept of circulatory pathways in the fetus based on observations in animal fetuses has been that of two pumps circulating blood through a low resistance placental and a high resistance pulmonary vascular bed. Blood of relatively high oxygen saturation from the umbilical vein arrives at the ductus venosus to join a relatively small volume of desaturated blood from the lower extremities and, passing into the left atrium via the foramen ovale, reaches the left ventricle and ascending aorta. Desaturated venous blood from the upper extremities, head and neck passes through the superior vena cava, right atrium, right ventricle and pulmonary artery in turn. The major portion of blood reaching the main pulmonary artery then passes through the ductus arteriosus to the descending aorta. Blood from the descending aorta divides into a major portion which eventually reaches the placenta through umbilical arteries and a minor portion which passes into the inferior vena cava."[26]

Changes at Birth

Certain anatomic changes take place after birth which permit oxygenation of the blood by the lungs in place of the placenta:

Immediately after delivery, the baby begins to breathe and the pulmonary circulation changes. A much larger amount of blood is pumped into the *pulmonary arteries* by the *right ventricle* and a smaller amount passes through the *ductus arteriosus*. The *ductus arteriosus* begins to atrophy and eventually is known as the *ligamentum arteriosum*.

The pulmonary circulation increases and more blood is returned from the *lungs* to the *left atrium*. Since the pressure rises in the *left atrium* the *foramen ovale* closes. The placental circulation ceases to function when the cord is tied. The ends of the *hypogastric arteries* atrophy, and are then known as the *hypogastric ligaments*.

The *ductus venosus* becomes occluded and is known as the *ligamentum venosum*. The *umbilical vein* becomes obliterated and is known as the *ligamentum teres*.[27]

4. Neonatal Circulation

Normal blood volume ranges between 85 to 100 ml./kg. at birth, stabilizing to 85 ml./kg. by the second day (p. 224). Factors which influence blood volume in the neonate are:

a. Maternal blood volume which in turn is affected by mother's iron intake and maternal diseases.
b. Competency of the placenta such as any alteration by pathology in the surface area available for diffusion.
c. Uterine contractions increase blood volume by propelling blood under pressure to the fetus.
d. Amount of blood loss associated with delivery (e.g., placenta previa). Maternal losses above the range 500 ml. can leave the baby with a lower oxygen carrying capacity.
e. Placental transfusion at birth. In-

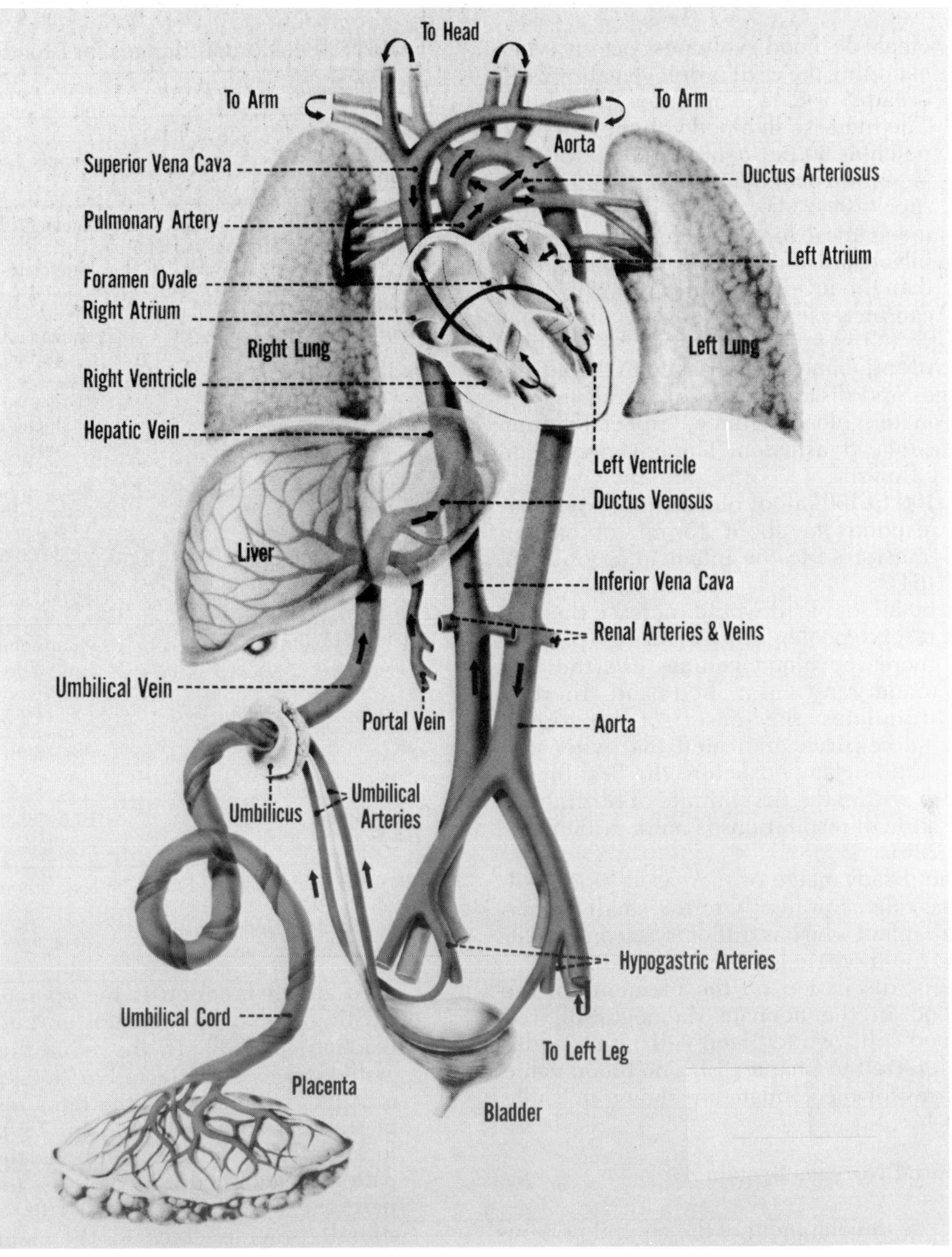

FIGURE 30-4. Diagram of fetal circulation. (Courtesy of Ross Laboratories.)

creased blood volumes occur when clamping the cord is delayed after 2 to 3 breaths or 2 to 3 minutes after birth. The increase in blood volume can be as much as 60 per cent or 100 to 150 ml., all within one to five minutes after birth (pp. 209–211). It is believed that mechanical forces such as milking an intact cord and holding the infant lower than the level of the uterus during birth can increase blood volume.

Attention must be directed to the advantages and disadvantages of increasing the neonate's blood volume, especially from placental transfusion. Thc advantages are as follows:

a. 100 to 150 ml. of blood transferred corresponds to about 15 ml. of oxygen transferred to the infant in seconds (p. 164).
b. 60 ml. of blood would increase the iron reserve pool by close to 32 mg. (p. 218).
c. Increased blood volume fills the pulmonary vascular bed and thereby stimulates the onset of breathing. Studies have indicated that when the cord is clamped before the first breath or within the first minute of birth, initiation of respirations is more difficult (p. 226).

The disadvantage of increased blood volume relates primarily to the small premature infant who has difficulty accommodating the increased volume (p. 218).

For discussion on the elements of the blood in the neonate (hemoglobin, red blood cells, white blood cells), the reader is referred to Chapter 19. The blood value norms for the neonate are shown in Table 30-4.

TABLE 30-4. Normal Ranges for Blood Values

Blood Elements	*Fetus*	*Full-Term Neonate*
Red blood cells (RBC), million/mm.	1.5–4.4*	mean: 4.638± range: 4.5–5.7
Hemoglobin, g./100 ml	12 wks.: 8–10 28 wks.: 14.5 34 wks.: 15	mean: 16.8 range: 16–18
Platelets, per mm.^{3}		mean: 200,000 range: 100,000–300,000
Leukocytes (white blood cells; greatest variation occurs in perinatal period), per mm.^{3}		(Great variation among references) range: 6,400–34,450 mean in first 10 days: 15,208 18,000 at birth to 23,000 in first 12 hours† 45,000 after birth‡
Differential WBC		Neutrophils make up 70% from birth to 4 days Lymphocytes dominant from first week to seventh week
Blood volume, ml./kg.		Birth: 85–100 mean: 85

* All values taken from Stave[6] unless otherwise indicated.
† Value stated by Hong (Chapter 19).
‡ Value taken from Guyton.[34]

5. Central Nervous System

The development of the central nervous system is an orderly, integrated process; each added function is incorporated into existing ones which creates an integrated reaction (p. 789). In the fetus this integrated process is reflected in "total pattern reflexes" which means the fetus responds to stimulation as a whole (p. 789). Later local reflexes will develop as the total pattern reaction diminishes. In the neonate these reflex responses to various stimuli provide clues to the neurologic functioning of the central nervous system (these reflexes are described later).

One important factor in the central nervous system is the blood–brain barrier or the hematoencephalic exchange system. This refers to the lack of myelin in the brains of young infants which allows increased penetration by certain substances in the blood. Myelin acts as a barrier to the entrance of substances into the brain but myelinization of the brain is not complete until about five years of age. This has implications for the effects of drugs. The hematoencephalic exchange makes it possible for drugs in the fetal and neonatal circulation to enter the brain. The neonate's response to a drug is more potent because of the interaction of the following factors: greater brain permeability due to the hematoencephalic exchange, larger surface area in proportion to weight which increases the response, and enzymatic activity for drug degradation and excretion is immature at birth.

6. Gastrointestinal Functions

Fetus: The gastrointestinal tract in utero is relatively inactive, although there is some activity as demonstrated by fetal ingestion and absorption of amniotic fluid, and production of meconium. It is speculated that there is insufficient peristalsis to expel a significant amount of meconium from the bowels. However, fetal asphyxia has been related to the release of meconium into the amniotic fluid primarily by increasing intestinal activity (peristalsis) and relaxing the anal sphincter.[28]

Neonate: The gastrointestinal tract shows development of secretory and absorption activities. There are adequate enzymes to digest and absorb simple carbohydrates and amino acids. Digestive functions develop adaptively; as the baby grows, gastrointestinal functions slowly increase.

There are many inabilities and limitations after birth which cannot be listed easily. The limitations primarily relate to anatomic structures and the neutrality of the gastric contents. According to Smith,[29] these limitations and their consequences are identified as:

a. Lesser supporting musculature due to deficient longitudinal fibers over the greater curvature of the stomach and deficient elastic fibers in the intestinal submucosa. This creates alterations in visceral relationships, especially the shape and size of the stomach; thus, the common distended appearance of the abdomen.
b. Unpredictability in relaxation of cardia and pyloric sphincters. The mild regurgitation or slight vomiting seen in newborns is due to the inability of the cardia sphincter to prevent reverse flow of stomach contents.
c. Tendency for "air pocketing" in upper curvature of the stomach, especially when infant is flat. Air easily enters the stomach during feedings and crying. This creates the need for frequent burping during feedings.
d. Irregularities in peristaltic motility occur along the gastrointestinal tract.

There is a delay in passage of ingested contents through the stomach and upper intestine. The consequence is a slow stomach emptying; begins 1½ to 2 hours after a feeding and is not complete until 3 to 4 hours later. This creates a need for interval feedings to allow stomach emptying.

Peristalsis increases in the lower ileum and is rapid with no delay in the colonic musculature. The result is stool frequency, averaging between one to six per day. Absence of stool within 48 hours after birth is indicative of intestinal obstruction.

e. Gastric contents are neutral at birth.

It becomes more acid each day after birth. However, this initial neutrality prevents growth of the normal bacterial flora of the stomach and bowels. This may lead to a deficiency in vitamin K, which is dependent upon the bacterial flora for its formation or upon ingested sources of vitamin K.

The above indicate the importance of the noenate receiving its nutritional requirements through interval feedings. The variations in stomach size (capacity), increased air into the stomach during feedings, and delayed emptying of stomach contents make it impossible for the infant to ingest the necessary quantity in three full meals a day as adults do.

7. Renal Functions

There is evidence of functional immaturity in the neonate's renal physiology as evidenced by tests such as urea clearances, renal plasma blood flow, and glomerular filtration rate. This is due primarily to the gradual development of renal functioning which does not meet adult performance levels until some time during the second year of life. The limitations in renal functioning in the neonate arise primarily from the diminished renal blood flow which is related to low arterial blood pressure at birth and increased renal vascular resistance (p. 698). Therefore, neonatal renal limitations are reflected in low glomerular filtration rate and immature tubular function. Volume and composition of body fluids can easily be disturbed.

The consequences of such limitations in renal functioning in the neonate are:

a. Decreased ability to concentrate urine due to the low tubular reabsorption rate and low levels of circulating antidiuretic hormone.
b. Hindered ability to maintain water balance by excretion of excess water or retaining water when needed. The newborn needs more water to excrete a certain amount of salt. Water loss accounts for the 5 to 6 per cent weight loss seen in the first few days of life. Obligatory losses occurs via the skin, pulmonary functions, and other metabolic activities which are elevated at this phase of life. Water loss also occurs as part of the physiologic process of maturation with accelerated tissue growth. Thus, the neonate is in a precarious position between rapid dehydration because of obligatory water losses and low water reserves due to limited kidney function.
c. Compromised ability to maintain acid–base compensatory mechanisms. Sluggish excretion of electrolytes, especially sodium and the hydrogen ions, results in accumulation of these

substances which predisposes the infant to disturbances such as dehydration, hyperkalemia, and mild acidosis (pp. 670, 693).

In spite of these limitations the healthy neonate can maintain an average pH and carbon dioxide value as efficiently as the adult.

The nurse needs to know that jeopardy to the neonate relative to its limited renal functioning occurs with the following:

a. Hypoxia and mild acidosis associated with prolonged delivery.
b. Pathologic losses with vomiting, diarrhea, excessive perspiration, excessive weight loss.
c. Prolonged restriction of oral intake, improper diet, excessive parenteral fluids high in electrolytes.
d. Retention of certain electrolytes and fluid when endocrine control of excretion does not develop properly.[30]

8. Hepatic Functions

The liver plays a primary role in metabolic processes through its high enzymatic activities. In the fetus some activities were handled by the maternal-placental unit. However, the neonate is forced to initiate these functions with birth. Liver function in the first week of life is hindered primarily from lack of gastrointestinal tract activity and limited blood supply due to the thick and narrow intrahepatic structure of the portal vein (p. 194). Major consequences of the limited liver function are:

a. Decreased ability to conjugate bilirubin (rationale for physiologic jaundice). Bilirubin is an end-product of hemoglobin degradation. It needs to be conjugated and is excreted in the bile and through the kidneys. Essential enzymes for conjugation (glucuronyl transferase) are insufficient in liver cells at birth. This results in hyperbilirubinemia due to the increased hemolysis of red blood cells in the first few days after birth. This creates the condition called icterus neonatorum or physiologic jaundice which occurs during the first week of life. The liver is overtaxed to handle the increased amounts of bilirubin for conjugation at a time when it is trying to establish its full enzymatic activity (p. 602).

Other factors which can influence the conjugation process of bilirubin need to be recognized because they help identify infants who are predisposed to icterus neonatorum (jaundice). These factors are:

(1) Prematurity which creates a situation of incompetent hepatic enzyme activities.
(2) Maternal-fetal blood factor incompatibility, which leads to hemolysis and simply overloads the system.
(3) Albumin is necessary for binding and transport of bilirubin and relative hypoalbuminemia occurs in the newborn due to rapid shifts of tissue compartments.
(4) Bilirubin dissociates completely from protein (albumin) binding at pH levels of 7.0 and below. Acidosis associated with birth leads to less binding and more free bilirubin.
(5) The step before the conjugation of bilirubin by glucuronyl transferase requires oxygen and glucose. Hypoxia and hypoglycemia associated with birth will hinder the process.
(6) Organic anions such as salicylates and sulfisoxazole may displace bilirubin from its albumin-binding sites thereby increasing unbound bilirubin which may then accumulate in the tissues. Mothers receiv-

ing large amounts of aspirin or sulpha drugs during pregnancy will predispose their infants to hyperbilirubinemia (pp. 602, 603).

b. Decreased ability to regulate blood sugar concentrations (rationale for neonatal hypoglycemia). Enzymatic activities which determine the uptake and release of glucose from storage (glycogen) and which facilitate the formation of glucose from amino acids (gluconeogenesis) are deficient. Thus, the process of birth results in a fall in blood sugar called neonatal hypoglycemia (p. 424). Blood sugar levels fall abnormally low when:
   (1) Glycogen stores in liver are low as with prematurity, a stressful birth process, asphyxiation at birth, cold, or intrauterine malnutrition.
   (2) The fetus of a diabetic mother produces extra amounts of insulin making the fetal tissues suffer from hyperinsulinemia (fat baby).
   (3) Carbohydrate regulating hormones (cortisol, epinephrine, glucagon) are insufficient as with genetic, metabolic disorders.[31]

c. Deficient production of prothrombin and other coagulation factors dependent upon vitamin K for synthesis such as PTC, proconvertin, Stuart Power Factor (rationale for neonate's predisposition to hemorrhage).

   Vitamin K is deficient at birth because its formation is dependent upon bacterial flora in the colon. This flora is absent at birth and is established in several days as gastric acidity increases. This vitamin K deficiency predisposes the newborn to hemorrhage during the first few days of life.

   Manifestations indicative of hemorrhage may be present in the second to third day. These are bloody or black stools, hematuria, bleeding from nose or circumcision site, oozing from umbilicus, and bleeding into the scalp and skin (ecchymosis).

   Administration of vitamin K is effective for prevention and treatment: vitamin K, 0.5 to 1 mg. intramuscularly for prevention and vitamin K, 1 to 2 mg. intravenously for treatment because the intramuscular route may cause large hematomas in a bleeding infant.

9. Endocrine Functions

"It appears that at birth, the endocrine glands are better organized for function than many other systems. The temporary unsteadiness of homeostatic control by the adrenals, parathyroids, pituitary is due largely to the impairment of target organs rather than hormone secretion."[32]

Adrenal cortical activity exists in utero and at birth. Such activity is speculated to play a role in favorable responses to the stresses at birth and the adaptive processes required. Interpretation of this activity can be obtained from concentrations of the hormones and allied substances in the blood and urine. Some consequences to the fetus and neonate as a result of living in a maternal-provided hormone environment are:

a. Vaginal discharge (and/or bleeding) in female infants.
b. Enlargement of mammary glands in both sexes. This is related to increased estrogen, luteal and pituitary prolactin activity.
c. Acne neonatorum.
d. Disturbances related to maternal endocrine pathology. For example:
   (1) Infants of diabetic mothers have hyperplasia of beta cells in the pancreas.
   (2) Infants whose mothers lack dietary iodine intake may have enlarged thyroids or congenital goiter at birth.

With birth, the infant must take over the endocrine functions formerly provided by the mother. His endocrine functioning must regulate the following:

a. Calcium-phosphorus balance. Parathyroid hormone regulates intestinal transport and stabilization of calcium and phosphorus. The neonate is functionally hypoparathyroid because of lack of its stimulation in utero. This results in higher serum phosphorus which lowers the serum calcium. Hypocalcemia increases susceptibility to tetany (signs are tremors, twitching, spasticity). Its treatment involves vitamin D and calcium intake either by oral or intravenous routes (pp. 704–708).
b. Regulation of blood glucose concentrations and effects on fat and protein synthesis. Glucose and fatty acids are the primary energy sources for tissue growth and metabolic processes. Glucose is the main source of energy for *neurons*. Insulin, the pancreatic hormone, stimulates peripheral utilization of glucose by:
   (1) Facilitating the entrance of glucose into muscle and fat cells.
   (2) Activating glycolysis and lipolysis.

   The role of insulin in the fetus is to promote and maintain growth and maturation. In the neonate there is a fall in blood glucose during the first hours of life, followed by a period of glucose instability. This is due to the cut in the placental glucose source and lack of supply from oral feedings. The neonate is now dependent upon the liver for its glycogen stores and enzymatic production to provide glucose for the brain. The enzymatic activity of the liver is dependent, among a number of things, upon the presence and amount of insulin (pp. 959–966).

   Consequences of too little or too much insulin are as follows:

   Lack of insulin results in muscle and fat cells excluding glucose and decreased enzymatic activity in the liver.

   Excessive insulin results in hypoglycemia due to increased glucose utilization. It is accompanied by hyperplasia and hypertrophy of beta cells in islets of Langerhans within the pancreas.

10. Thermogenesis and Regulation

Neonates are homeothermic; that is, they have mechanisms to maintain stable body temperatures. This is very important because at birth their body temperature falls 2 to 3° C. The fetal temperature is approximately 0.5° C above the mother's, even during labor and delivery (p. 197).

There are several factors which contribute to the heat loss associated with birth:

a. Termination of the heat exchange protection by the uterus.
b. Unfavorable big surface area relative to body volume.
c. Conduction heat loss which occurs when the neonate's body is in contact with a cooler solid object.
d. Convection heat loss occurs when temperature differences in the air (usually cooler) carry heat away from the body.
e. Radiation loss occurs when heat from the body radiates to cooler wall surroundings or objects. The amount of heat loss decreases with the square of the distance away from the cooler walls or objects.
f. Evaporation from the skin and respiratory tract accounts for 10 to 20 per cent of total heat loss. Major portion of heat loss at birth occurs through evaporation of amniotic fluid covering the baby (pp. 523–525).

The neonate quickly develops two important mechanisms to counterbalance heat loss. These are a) to retain the heat by vasoconstriction and insulation, and b) heat production. Let us examine these two compensatory mechanisms.

Retention of heat occurs primarily by vasoconstriction in response to decreased temperature. The blood is directed away from the skin surface, decreasing peripheral circulation. Heat transfer occurs via the deep blood vessels which do not influence skin color as do the smaller capillaries.

Therefore, one is cautioned not to assess skin temperature by color criteria alone because a baby may be flushed but cold. The temperature of the skin (axillary) versus the deep core temperature (rectal) is important because it provides an early clue of the neonate's ability to compensate for heat loss. Retention of heat also occurs via insulation from subcutaneous adipose tissue which stores and releases fatty acids. The neonate's limited amount of subcutaneous fat, especially in infants of low birth weight, limits successful heat conservation via insulation.

A very important compensatory mechanism is the ability to produce heat by so-called "non-shivering thermogenesis" (NST). It is elicited by the sympathetic nervous system's response to decreased temperature and is activated by adrenalin. Adipose tissue plays a vital role in the metabolic process of heat production. Recently, researchers have differentiated adipose tissue into "white" and "brown," the latter having unique contributions in the maintenance of body heat. However, in the human newborn it is not easily possible to distinguish between the two kinds of adipose tissue. The reader needs only to appreciate that adipose tissue in the human newborn is metabolically very active in heat production.

Thermoregulation is primarily controlled by thermoreceptors located in the skin, hypothalamus, and spinal cord which relay messages regarding when to produce and dissipate heat. The mechanism is outlined below:

> Cold → stimulates NST via receptors in skin and hypothalamus → increases temperature in adipose tissue → heat flow from interscapular adipose tissue to spinal cord → heat in spinal cord depresses shivering (pp. 532–533).

Shivering in the neonate is a late manifestation of prolonged exposure to cold. It occurs when the spinal cord temperature falls, indicating failure of the NST compensatory mechanism. (This is in contrast to the shivering seen in adults as a compensatory mechanism to generate heat.) Some signs indicative of jeopardy to life activities from exposure to cold are: decreased respirations, decreased heart rate, decreased blood sugar, edema of extremities, apathy, refusal of food, decreased rectal temperature.

Some principles relative to thermoregulation in the neonate are:

a. Higher thermal conductance occurs with smaller subjects (p. 523). This means greater heat loss can be expected in infants of low birth weight or preterm gestational age (due to the increased surface area exposed in proportion to the body size).
b. Instability of body temperature in the neonate is due to discrepancies between the efficiency of the effector system (thermal receptors) and body size (p. 539).

Fluctuation in body temperature can be seen in early infancy. Immature infants will have greater difficulty in maintaining stable temperatures because of less developed receptors to relay messages for response to heat loss.

c. Duration of quiet sleep activity provides a criterion to determine range of thermal neutral environment or thermal comfort (p. 542).

Thermal comfort is the temperature range in which the least amount of oxygen is consumed. This range varies with size of the baby and is narrower in smaller infants. Assessment of the neonate's duration and quality of sleep provides clues of his thermal comfort. Restlessness, agitation, or hyperactivity may be indicative of heat loss as it further increases oxygen consumption. Thus, lack of thermal comfort can predispose the infant to difficulties in maintaining essential life activities.

11. Immunoglobulin Synthesis

This refers to serumglobulins whose main function is antibody activity. They are synthesized in plasma cells located primarily in the spleen, lymph nodes, and intestinal mucosa (p. 323).

In the fetus, immunity is a passive process, that is, the uterus and placenta protect the fetus from immunologic stress. Passive immunity continues to be effective up to the first six months after birth. Table 30-5 lists types of antibodies the infant has from passive immunity. Knowledge of such data provides direction for the need for active immunization in infants because of decreasing immunity.

The production of immunoglobulin is limited in both the fetus and neonate. Thus, when placental protection fails and permits a fetal infection (such as prenatal syphilis), the fetal spleen produces more plasma cells and antibodies. Research is being conducted on synthesis of immunoglobulins by the fetus, placenta, and amniotic membrane. In the neonate, plasma cells are absent from the bone marrow until about 4 to 6 weeks of life when full synthesis begins. It is interesting to note that absorption of immunoglobulins from colostrum and breast milk occurs in very small, insignificant amounts. It therefore does *not* provide a rationale for immunologic transfer via breast feeding. Breast-fed babies appear better resistive to infections possibly due to local action of some suitable types of antibodies in the infant's intestinal tract since breast milk is superior in regard to enteric pathogens (pp. 359–361).

TABLE 30-5. Identification of Passive Immunity Levels in the Neonate*

A. *Good* protection from antibody transfer across the placenta occurs for:

1. Diphtheria
2. Scarlet fever
3. Tetanus
4. Purtussis
5. Measles
6. Herpes simplex
7. Poliomyelitis
8. Japanese B encephalitis
9. Vaccinia
10. Coxsaxie
11. Varicella zoster
12. Rubella
13. Influenza
14. Mumps

B. *Lower* (some) level of protection from antibody transfer across the placenta occurs for:

1. Influenza
2. Dysentery bacilli
3. Salmonella typhi (H antigen)

C. *No* Protection (no antibody transfer across the placenta) occurs for:

1. Rh antigen
2. Typhoid
3. Rheumatoid
4. Shigella dysenteriae
5. E. coli
6. Salmonella typhi (G antigen)

* From Stave.[6]

REFERENCES

1. Hughes, J.: *Synopsis of Pediatrics,* ed. 3. C. V. Mosby, St. Louis, 1971, p. 202.
2. Korones, S., Lancaster, J. and Roberts, F.: *High Risk Newborn Infants.* C. V. Mosby, St. Louis, 1972, pp. 7, 12, 180.
3. Day, B. and Liley, M.: *The Secret World of the Baby.* Random House, New York, 1966, pp. 13, 17, 18.
4. Pierog, S. and Ferrara, A.: *Approach to the Medical Care of the Sick Newborn.* C. V. Mosby, St. Louis, 1971, p. 49.
5. Towell, M.: *Influence of labor on the fetus and the newborn.* Pediatr. Clin. North Am. 13:575, 1966.
6. Stave, U. (ed.): *Physiology of the Perinatal Period, vol. 1.* Appleton-Century-Crofts, New York, 1970, pp. 29–43.
7. Towell: op. cit.
8. Eskes, T.: *Intrauterine pressure and the human foetus.* In Gevers, R. and Ruys, J. (eds.): *Physiology and Pathology in the Perinatal Period.* Springer-Verlag, New York, 1971, p. 33.
9. Ibid.
10. Turbeville, J.: *Nurse's role in intrapartum care.* Hosp. Top. 50:87, 1972.
11. Stave: op. cit.
12. Towell: op. cit.
13. Pierog and Ferrara: op. cit., pp. 50, 51.
14. Stahlman, M.: *Perinatal circulation.* Pediatr. Clin. North Am. 13:753, 1966.
15. James, L. S.: *Onset of breathing and resuscitation.* Pediatr. Clin. North Am. 13:621, 1966.
16. Karlberg, P., et al.: *Respiratory studies in newborn infants, II: Pulmonary ventilation and mechanics of breathing in first minutes of life, including onset of respiration.* Acta Paediatrica 51:121, 1962.
17. Adamson, K., Jr.: *The role of thermal factors in fetal and neonatal life.* Pediatr. Clin. and North Am. 13:599, 1966.
18. Adamson, K., Jr., Gandy, G. and James, L. S.: *The influence of thermal factors upon oxygen consumption of the newborn infant.* J. Pediatr. 66:495, 1965.
19. Adamson, K., Jr., and Towell, M. E.: *Thermal homeostasis of the fetus and newborn.* Anesthesiology 26:531, 1965.
20. Dawes, G. S.: *Foetal and Neonatal Physiology.* Year Book Medical Publishers, Chicago, 1968.
21. Moore, R. E. and Underwood, M. C.: *Possible role of noradrenaline in control of heat production in the newborn mammal.* Lancet 1:1277, 1960.
22. Scopes, J. W.: *Metabolic rates and temperature control in the human baby.* Brit. Med. Bull. 22:88, 1966.
23. Desmond, M. M., Rudolph, A. J. and Phitaksphraiwan, P.: *The transitional care nursery.* Pediatr. Clin. North Am. 13:651, 1966.
24. Arnold, H., et al.: *Transition to extra-uterine life.* Am. J. Nurs. 65:77, 1965.
25. Oliver, T. K., Demis, J. A. and Bates, G. D.: *Serial blood-gas tensions and acid-base balance during the first hour of life in human infants.* Acta Paediatrica 50:358, 1961.
26. Rowe, R. and Mehrizi, A.: *The Neonate with Congenital Heart Disease.* W. B. Saunders, Philadelphia, 1969, p. 18.
27. *Fetal Circulation.* Nursing Education Series No. 1, Ross Laboratories, Columbus, Ohio, 1957.
28. Korones: op. cit.
29. Smith, C.: *The Physiology of the Newborn Infant.* Charles C Thomas, Springfield, Ill., 1959, pp. 228–250, 363.
30. Ibid.
31. Korones: op. cit.
32. Smith: op. cit., p. 395.
33. McKilligin, H.: *The First Day of Life.* Springer, New York, 1970, p. 108.
34. Guyton, A.: *Textbook of Medical Physiology,* ed. 4. W. B. Saunders, Philadelphia, 1971, p. 996.

BIBLIOGRAPHY

Chamberlain G. and Banks, J.: *Assessment of the Apgar Score.* Lancet 2:1225, 1974.

Cozen, L.: *Orthopedic examination of the infant and child.* Am. Fam. Physician 4:60, 1971.

Crelin, E.: *Functional Anatomy of the Newborn.* Yale University Press, New Haven, 1973.

Dahm, L. and James, L.: *Newborn temperature and a calculated heat loss in the delivery room.* Pediatrics 49:504, 1972.

Davies, P., et al.: *Medical Care of Newborn Babies.* Spastics International Medical Publications, London, 1972.

Desmond, M., Arnold, R. and Phitaksphraiwan, P.: *Transitional care nursery.* Pediatr. Clin. North Am. 13:651, 1966.

Dubowitz, L., Dubowitz, V. and Goldberg, C.: *Clinical assessment of gestational age in the newborn infant.* J. Pediatr. 77:1, 1970.

Eoff, M., Meier, R. and Miller, C.: *Temperature measurements in infants.* Nurs. Res. 23:457, 1974.

Gevers, R. and Ruys, J.: *Physiology and Pathology in the Perinatal Period.* Springer-Verlag, New York, 1971.

Keay, A.: *Craig's Care of the Newly Born Infant.* Churchill, London, 1974.

Leeuwen, G.: *A Manual of Newborn Medicine.* Year Book Medical Publishers, Chicago, 1973.

Lockman, L.: *Neurological assessment in the first year of life.* Postgrad. Med. 50:80, 1971.

Long, G.: *Toweling newborn babies.* J. Pediatr. 75:157, 1969.

Lubchenco, L.: *Assessment of gestational age and development at birth.* Pediatr. Clin. North Am. 17:125, 1970.

McKilligan, H. R.: *The First Days of Life.* Springer, New York, 1970.

McLean, F. H.: *Significance of birth weight for gestational age in identifying infants at risk.* J. Obstet. Gynecol. Nurse 3:19, 1974.

Mingeot, R. and Herbaut, M.: *The functional status of the newborn infant. A study of 5,370 consecutive infants.* Am. J. Obstet. Gynecol. 115:1138, 1973.

Moore, M. L.: *The Newborn and the Nurse.* W. B. Saunders, Philadelphia, 1972.

Motil, K., Blackburn, M. and Pleasure, J.: *The effects of four different radiant warmer temperature set-points used for rewarming neonates.* J. Pediatr. 85:546, 1974.

O'Doherty, N. and Zinkin, P.: *A routine neurological examination for the full-term newborn infant.* Proc. R. Soc. Med. 64:476, 1971.

Papadatos, C., et al.: *Immunoglobulin levels and gestational age.* Biologia Neonatorum 14:365, 1969.

Prechtl, H. and Beintema, D.: *The Neurological Examination of the Full Term Newborn Infant.* W. S. Heinmann Medical Books, New York, 1964.

Reed, B.: *Management of the infant during labor, delivery, and the immediate neonatal period.* Nurs. Clin. North Am. 6:3, 1971.

Roberts, J.: *Suctioning the newborn.* Am. J. Nurs. 73:63, 1973.

Slumek, M.: *Screening newborns for hearing loss.* Nurs. Outlook 19:115, 1971.

Smith, C. A.: *The Physiology of the Newborn Infant.* Charles C Thomas, Springfield, Ill. 1975.

Smith, R.: *Temperature monitoring and regulation.* Pediatr. Clin. North Am. 16:643, 1969.

Stave, U. (ed.): *Physiology of the Perinatal Period, vols. I and II.* Appleton-Century-Crofts, New York, 1970.

Webb, C. H.: *Evaluation of the routine physical examination of infants in the first year of life.* Pediatrics 45:960, 1970.

Whitner, W. and Thompson, M.: *The influence of bathing on the newborn infant's body temperature.* Nurs. Res. 19:30, 1970.

31 Application of Physiologic Perspectives

DYANNE D. AFFONSO, R.N., M.N.

This chapter identifies nursing actions relative to the physiologic aspects of health care needed by the neonate. However, there is first a general discussion on the nursing role with all aspects of care, physiologic as well as psychosocial, integrated into the nursing care plan for the neonate. The rationale for this is to give the reader a perspective of the total nursing care plan. Attempting to include all aspects of nursing care in one chapter would result in an overwhelming amount of content for any reader to handle. Thus, the role of nursing is divided, with this chapter examining the physiologic aspects of neonatal care, and Chapter 33 examining the psychosocial aspects of neonatal care.

THE ROLE OF THE NURSE

WHY THE NURSE?

The significance of the nurse in the delivery of health care during the neonatal period arises from her continuing exposure to the newborn. The nurse is the only member of the health team who provides care through *continuous presence.* Nurses are present during every significant aspect in the maintenance of life during the first few days after birth. The nurse witnesses the infant's emergence from the birth canal and can immediately assess the infant's response to the beginning of extrauterine life. Frequently, it is the nurse who gives immediate assistance to the infant to facilitate respirations, provide warmth, and protect from stimuli which can be hazardous to life. While other members of the health team may be occupied with other tasks or not available, the nurse is there to give attention to the newborn. The nurse witnesses the extrauterine adaptation process and can facilitate it, or call attention for interventions when it is not occurring smoothly. The nurse's impact on the neonate's life continues into its daily basic needs. Provisions to ensure maintenance for ingestion, elimination, sleep, and stimulation are the responsibility of the primary care agent—the nurse.

NURSING PLAN FOR CARE

The components of nursing care to the neonate include:

1. *Assessment.* This involves the nurse's decision-making process to determine if the infant is or will be at risk in his adaptive process. The nurse proceeds to identify the needs of the baby which arise from possible difficulties encountered in extrauterine adaptation. Clinical

decisions (nursing diagnosis) are possible when the nurse collects necessary information and utilizes knowledge to identify infants at risk, possible causes for risk factors, and what the nurse can do about it. When the nurse promptly shares her assessment data with other members of the health team, medical management can be instituted and the nurse can support the therapy. Assessment does not relate only to physical findings. The psychosocial component of the assessment process focuses on determining the infant's ability to receive and react to stimuli, thereby developing his interaction potential.

2. Nursing actions to *protect* the neonate. These are actions which block stimuli which can impose additional stress to extrauterine adaptation.
3. Nursing actions to *nurture* the neonate. These are actions which help the neonate to maintain a continuing adaptive state after he has emerged successfully from the initial trauma and transition of birth.
4. Nursing actions to *stimulate* the neonate. These are actions which provide environmental and social input to enrich the neonate's behavioral development. These are discussed in detail in Chapter 33.

Thus, the uniqueness of the role of nursing during the neonatal life experience is in assessment for physical and behavioral status, and in implementing actions which will protect, nurture, and stimulate the neonate's physical growth and behavioral development. The nurse can also foster parent-infant relationships by teaching parents how to protect, nurture, and stimulate their infants. Through such sharing, the nurse transfers the performance of the actions to the parents so that such actions can be continued in the home environment.

GOALS OF NURSING

In the application of physiologic and psychosocial concepts for neonatal nursing care, the following major goals become evident:

1. Assessment of the neonate to
   a. Determine physical status immediately after birth
   b. Estimate and classify according to birth weight, gestational age, and intrauterine growth
   c. Determine physical status by a complete, detailed, physical examination after the initial transitional period
   d. Determine behavioral state to the reception of various stimuli which will enhance its interaction potential.
2. Protection of the neonate by
   a. Promoting establishment and maintenance of life-supporting activities such as respiration and circulation
   b. Minimizing the loss of body heat and the increased oxygen consumption which are usually associated with the birth process
   c. Instituting prophylactic treatments against infections and hemorrhagic disorders
   d. Providing proper identification of the infant.
3. Nurturance of the neonate's daily physical needs by
   a. Continuously assessing to identify risks which might become evident later
   b. Initiating and evaluating feeding
   c. Minimizing environmental dangers for infection
   d. Attending to general care for skin, healing of the umbilical stump, weight gain or loss, vital signs, activity, and sleep.
4. Stimulation of the neonate's behavioral development by
   a. Providing environmental input to

stimulate or arouse the capacity for interactive behaviors

b. Facilitating and promoting the acquaintance process between baby and parents (primarily the mother figure).

NURSING ACTIONS

This chapter is divided into two major parts: 1) Neonatal assessment for physiologic status, and 2) Actions which protect and nurture. The discussion begins by identifying the components in the nursing assessment process for the evaluation of the infant's physical status. Next, the nursing actions to protect and nurture are identified relevant to three periods in the neonate's early life: immediately after birth, during the transitional period, and during the remainder of the hospital stay. Actions to protect and nurture are presented in a listing format. The rationale is that such actions are straightforward and directive, and further explanations would not necessarily add to the content. The behavioral components of the assessment process and nursing actions to stimulate the neonate and his family will be presented in Chapter 33.

NEONATAL ASSESSMENT PROCESS

RATIONALE FOR NURSE'S INVOLVEMENT

Frequently, physical assessment of the neonate is done by the physician. However, nursing is emerging with new and dynamic roles reflecting ability for increased responsibilities. These new roles are long overdue. Often the nurse is the only person available to appraise the infant immediately after birth and during the entire transitional period. These emerging roles expand the nurse's impact from "merely watching the newborn closely" to doing an assessment which yields data to determine a clinical nursing diagnosis. There is a distinction in this process of assessment when done by the nurse as contrasted to that done by a physician, although the two should complement each other. The data obtained from the nurse and the doctor may be the same but the distinction occurs in how the data directs the plan for neonatal care. For example, the physician assesses to determine risk factors indicative of possible anomalies or complications, and to formulate a plan for their medical treatment or management. The nurse also assesses to determine risk factors, but for the purpose of planning actions which will assist the neonate to maintain daily activities, even if a risk or complication is present and the baby is being medically treated. Such daily activities include nutritional intake, elimination, conservation of energy, and maintenance of respiration. Both medical and nursing diagnoses should be directed toward the common goal of instituting plans for intervention early enough to facilitate and maintain extrauterine adaptation and optimal growth and development. It should be emphasized that the nurse and doctor should pool their assessment data so that plans for the neonate can incorporate all aspects of care: prevention, treatment, and support. In this way, assessment of the neonate will benefit the *neonate*, rather than the convenience of the nurse or doctor.

ASSESSMENT OF PHYSICAL STATUS

Goal: *Determine physical status immediately after birth.*

Assessment immediately after birth is done primarily through the Apgar scoring system and screening procedures to rule out congenital anomalies.

1. Apgar Score

   This is a tool to appraise the neonate's

SIGN	0	1	2
Heart Rate	Absent	Slow (below 100)	Over 100
Respiratory Effort	Absent	Slow Irregular	Good Crying
Muscle Tone	Flaccid, Limp	Some Flexion of Extremities	Active Motion
Reflex Irritability	No Response	Grimace	Cough, Sneeze or Cry
Color	Blue Pale	Body Pink Extremities Pale	Completely Pink

FIGURE 31-1. Apgar scoring system.

cardiopulmonary functions. It consists of five criteria with an optimum score of ten points (Fig. 31-1). An Apgar score should be given at least twice, at one minute and five minutes after birth. The five criteria in order of importance are:

a. *Heart Rate.* Provides an indication of the effects from asphyxia associated with the delivery process. It should be counted for a minimum of thirty seconds with a stethoscope for the most accurate count. Other means for checking are counting the pulsations of the umbilical artery, or feeling the epigastric area for pulsations of the aorta. When the heart rate is less than 100 beats per minute (score of 1), resuscitation measures should be instituted immediately.
b. *Respiratory Effort.* Assessment of inspiratory and expiratory efforts. This can be observed while the heart rate is checked. Respirations are good in vigorous crying (score of 2), slow, irregular (score of 1), or absent (score of 0).
c. *Muscle Tone.* Refers to the degree of flexion and resistance in the extremities when one attempts to straighten them. A score of 2 is given for well flexed extremities which resist attempts to extend. A score of 0 is given for limp, slack arms and legs. Anything in between is given a score of 1.
d. *Reflex Irritability.* Two ways to check for this are tickling the infant's nostril with a catheter or slapping the soles of the infant's feet. The response indicates the score.
e. *Color.* Attention is directed to the presence or absence of cyanosis. Most babies manifest acrocyanosis (extremities and mouth area bluish while the rest of the body is pink). Good places to assess color are the fingernails, palms, soles, tongue, and lips. Color is the least significant criterion.

At times, especially in acute emergencies when a baby is severely distressed, it may be helpful to remember that cues for each criteria in the descending order of the Apgar system are provided by the score given to the criteria above it. For example, a baby who has a good heart rate and respirations will most likely have adequate muscle tone, reflexes, and color. However, an infant who has a heart rate of less than 100 will have problems breathing and this lack of oxygen will make him limp, hyporeflexive, and cyanotic. This is important to note because when a heart rate is absent or below 100 and the infant is not breathing and is limp, the nurse should immediately act to aid the infant rather than continue the Apgar scoring. It should be noted that an Apgar score cannot be determined unless each criteria has been evaluated.

The value of the Apgar score is that it allows anticipatory preparation for the management of newborns. Apgar scoring has led to the following classification of infants for management:[1]

Apgar score of 7 and above: These infants usually do not need extra therapy beyond the routines to ensure patent airwav, heat, and continued observation.

Apgar score of 4 to 6 (moderately depressed infants): These infants may have problems establishing respirations and may need ventilation support. The larynx may need to be visualized and the trachea suctioned for blood clots, meconium, mucus, or vernix. An airway may be inserted and oxygen administered via mask and bag apparatus. The infant usually begins to breathe spontaneously after such efforts.

Apgar score of 0 to 3 (severely depressed infants): Time is of the essence in management of these infants and deliberate, planned actions are imperative. If the heart rate is below 100 and there is no response to stimulations to aid respiration, the nurse should stop the Apgar evaluation and provide resuscitation immediately. Endotracheal intubation, inflating the lungs with oxygen, external cardiac massage, use of cardiac stimulants, and correction of metabolic acidosis and hypoglycemia might all be part of the therapeutic management.

2. Screening Procedures

Procedures to rule out (r/o) congenital anomalies should be performed only after the newborn's condition stabilizes (approximately 5 to 10 minutes after birth). The American Academy of Pediatrics[2] recommends that the following be performed on all infants as soon as possible after delivery:

a. Breathing observed to see if infant can breathe with his mouth closed (r/o choanal atresia).
b. Soft tube passed through the mouth into the stomach (r/o esophageal atresia).
c. Gastric contents aspirated quantitatively at the same time (more than 15 to 20 ml. leads to suspicion of high intestinal obstruction).
d. Passing of soft catheter into rectum if no meconium seen (r/o anal atresia).

In addition to the above, many progressive hospitals and medical centers have expanded the screening procedures done by the nurse to include assessments such as:

e. Measurement of head circumference (r/o microcephaly).
f. Palpation of palate (r/o clefts).
g. Passage of #8 catheter through the mouth into the stomach to obtain gastric aspirate for quantity (as stated previously); culture specimen and smear for bacteria and polys (r/o infection).
h. Auscultation of lungs and heart (r/o diaphragmatic hernia, congenital heart disease, etc.).
i. Ortolani's maneuver (r/o congenital dislocation of hip). See Figure 31-2.

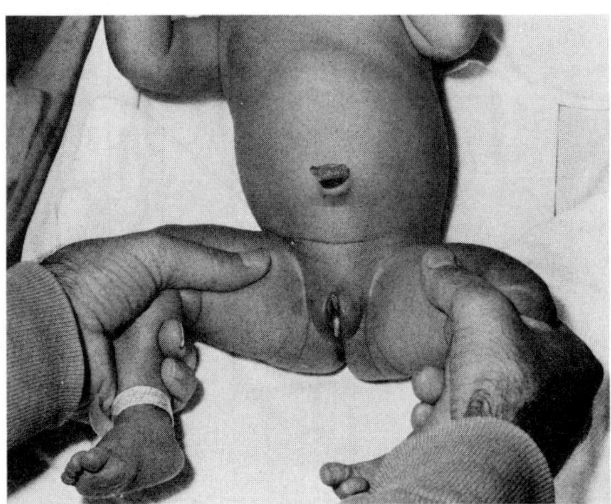

FIGURE 31-2. Ortolani's maneuver to check for congenital dislocation of the hips. The thighs are abducted (moved away from the midline) and a click is heard as the head of the femur is reduced back into the hip socket.

j. Count the number of vessels in the umbilical cord. There should be two arteries and one vein. Any discrepancies lead to anticipation of possible respiratory distress and/or congenital anomalies.

3. Estimation and Classification of Infants by Birth Weight, Gestational Age, and Intrauterine Growth

Examination First Hours

PHYSICAL FINDINGS		WEEKS GESTATION 20–48							
Vernix		Appears	Covers body, thick layer	On back, scalp, in creases	Scant, in creases	No vernix			
Breast tissue and areola		Areola and nipple barely visible no palpable breast tissue	Areola raised	1–2 mm nodule	3–5 mm	5–6 mm	7–10 mm	?12 mm	
Ear	Form	Flat, shapeless	Beginning incurving superior	Incurving upper 2/3 pinnae	Well-defined incurving to lobe				
	Cartilage	Pinna soft, stays folded	Cartilage scant, returns slowly from folding	Thin cartilage, springs back from folding	Pinna firm, remains erect from head				
Sole creases		Smooth soles without creases	1–2 anterior creases	2–3 anterior creases	Creases anterior 2/3 sole	Creases involving heel	Deeper creases over entire sole		
Skin	Thickness & appearance	Thin, translucent skin, plethoric, venules over abdomen, edema	Smooth, thicker, no edema	Pink	Few vessels	Some desquamation pale pink	Thick, pale, desquamation over entire body		
	Nail plates	Appear		Nails to finger tips	Nails extend well beyond finger tips				
Hair		Appears on head	Eye brows and lashes	Fine, woolly, bunches out from head	Silky, single strands, lays flat	?Receding hairline or loss of baby hair, short, fine underneath			
Lanugo		Appears	Covers entire body	Vanishes from face	Present on shoulders	No lanugo			
Genitalia	Testes		Testes palpable in inguinal canal	In upper scrotum	In lower scrotum				
	Scrotum		Few rugae	Rugae, anterior portion	Rugae cover	Pendulous			
	Labia & clitoris		Prominent clitoris, labia majora small, widely separated	Labia majora larger, nearly cover clitoris	Labia minora and clitoris covered				
Skull firmness		Bones are soft	Soft to 1" from anterior fontanelle	Spongy at edges of fontanelle, center firm	Bones hard, sutures easily displaced	Bones hard, cannot be displaced			
Posture	Resting	Hypotonic, lateral decubitus	Hypotonic	Beginning flexion, thigh	Stronger hip flexion	Frog-like	Flexion, all limbs	Hypertonic	Very hypertonic
	Recoil - leg	No recoil	Partial recoil	Prompt recoil					
	Arm	No recoil	Begin flexion, no recoil	Prompt recoil, may be inhibited	Prompt recoil after 30" inhibition				

20 21 22 23 24 25 26 27 28 29 30 31 32 33 34 35 36 37 38 39 40 41 42 43 44 45 46 47 48

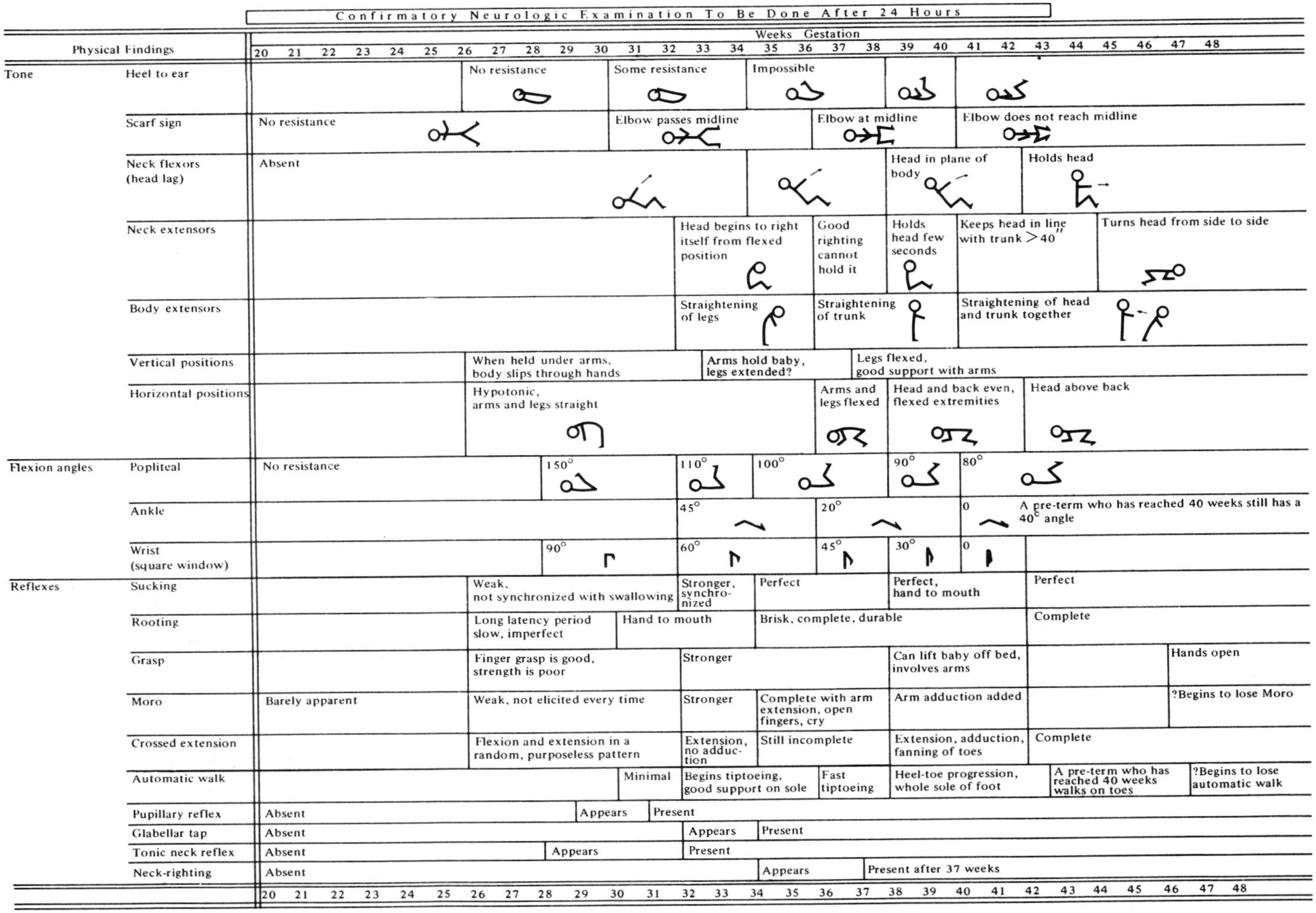

Confirmatory Neurologic Examination To Be Done After 24 Hours

Weeks Gestation: 20 21 22 23 24 25 26 27 28 29 30 31 32 33 34 35 36 37 38 39 40 41 42 43 44 45 46 47 48

	Physical Findings					
Tone	Heel to ear	No resistance	Some resistance	Impossible		
	Scarf sign	No resistance	Elbow passes midline	Elbow at midline	Elbow does not reach midline	
	Neck flexors (head lag)	Absent		Head in plane of body	Holds head	
	Neck extensors	Head begins to right itself from flexed position	Good righting cannot hold it	Holds head few seconds	Keeps head in line with trunk > 40″	Turns head from side to side
	Body extensors	Straightening of legs	Straightening of trunk	Straightening of head and trunk together		
	Vertical positions	When held under arms, body slips through hands	Arms hold baby, legs extended?	Legs flexed, good support with arms		
	Horizontal positions	Hypotonic, arms and legs straight	Arms and legs flexed	Head and back even, flexed extremities	Head above back	
Flexion angles	Popliteal	No resistance	150°	110°	100°	90° / 80°
	Ankle	45°	20°	0	A pre-term who has reached 40 weeks still has a 40° angle	
	Wrist (square window)	90°	60°	45°	30°	0
Reflexes	Sucking	Weak, not synchronized with swallowing	Stronger, synchronized	Perfect	Perfect, hand to mouth	Perfect
	Rooting	Long latency period slow, imperfect	Hand to mouth	Brisk, complete, durable	Complete	
	Grasp	Finger grasp is good, strength is poor	Stronger	Can lift baby off bed, involves arms		Hands open
	Moro	Barely apparent	Weak, not elicited every time	Stronger	Complete with arm extension, open fingers, cry	Arm adduction added; ?Begins to lose Moro
	Crossed extension	Flexion and extension in a random, purposeless pattern	Extension, no adduction	Still incomplete	Extension, adduction, fanning of toes	Complete
	Automatic walk	Minimal	Begins tiptoeing, good support on sole	Fast tiptoeing	Heel-toe progression, whole sole of foot	A pre-term who has reached 40 weeks walks on toes; ?Begins to lose automatic walk
	Pupillary reflex	Absent	Appears	Present		
	Glabellar tap	Absent	Appears	Present		
	Tonic neck reflex	Absent	Appears	Present		
	Neck-righting	Absent	Appears	Present after 37 weeks		

Weeks: 20 21 22 23 24 25 26 27 28 29 30 31 32 33 34 35 36 37 38 39 40 41 42 43 44 45 46 47 48

FIGURE 31-3. A tool for clinical estimation of gestational age. (From Kempe, C. H., Silver, H. K. and O'Brien, D.: *Current Pediatric Diagnosis and Treatment, ed. 3.* Lange, Los Altos, 1974, with permission.)

A

NEUROLOGIC SIGN	SCORE 0	1	2	3	4	5
POSTURE						
SQUARE WINDOW	90°	60°	45°	30°	0°	
ANKLE DORSIFLEXION	90°	75°	45°	20°	0°	
ARM RECOIL	180°	90-180°	<90°			
LEG RECOIL	180°	90-180°	<90°			
POPLITEAL ANGLE	180°	160°	130°	110°	90°	<90°
HEEL-TO-EAR MANEUVER						
SCARF SIGN						
HEAD LAG						
VENTRAL SUSPENSION						

B

External Sign		Score: 0	1	2	3	4
Edema		Obvious edema of hands and feet; pitting over tibia	No obvious edema of hands and feet; pitting over tibia	No edema		
Skin texture		Very thin, gelatinous	Thin and smooth	Smooth: medium thickness; rash or superficial peeling	Slight thickening; superficial cracking and peeling, especially of hands and feet	Thick and parchment-like; superficial or deep cracking
Skin color		Dark red	Uniformly pink	Pale pink; variable over body	Pale; only pink over ears, lips, palms, or soles	
Skin opacity (trunk)		Numerous veins and venules clearly seen, especially over abdomen	Veins and tributaries seen	A few large vessels clearly seen over abdomen	A few large vessels seen indistinctly over abdomen	No blood vessels seen
Lanugo (over back)		No lanugo	Abundant; long and thick over whole back	Hair thinning, especially over lower back	Small amount of lanugo and bald areas	At least half of back devoid of lanugo
Plantar creases		No skin creases	Faint red marks over anterior half of sole	Definite red marks over anterior half; indentations over anterior third	Indentations over anterior third	Definite deep indentations over anterior third
Nipple formation		Nipple barely visible; no areola	Nipple well defined; areola smooth and flat; diameter 0.75 cm.	Areola stippled, edge not raised; diameter 0.75 cm.	Areola stippled, edge raised; diameter 0.75 cm.	
Breast size		No breast tissue palpable	Breast tissue on one or both sides; diameter 0.5 cm.	Breast tissue on both sides; one or both 0.5-1.0 cm.	Breast tissue on both sides; one or both 1.0 cm.	
Ear form		Pinna flat and shapeless; little or no curving of edge	Incurving of part of edge of pinna	Partial incurving of whole of upper pinna	Well-defined incurving of whole of upper pinna	
Ear firmness		Pinna soft, easily folded; no recoil	Pinna soft, easily folded; slow recoil	Cartilage to edge of pinna but soft in places; ready recoil	Pinna firm, cartilage to edge; instant recoil	
Genitals	Male	Neither testis in scrotum	At least one testis high in scrotum	At least one testis right down		
	Female (with hips half abducted)	Labia majora widely separated, labia minora protruding	Labia majora almost cover labia minora	Labia majora completely cover labia minora		

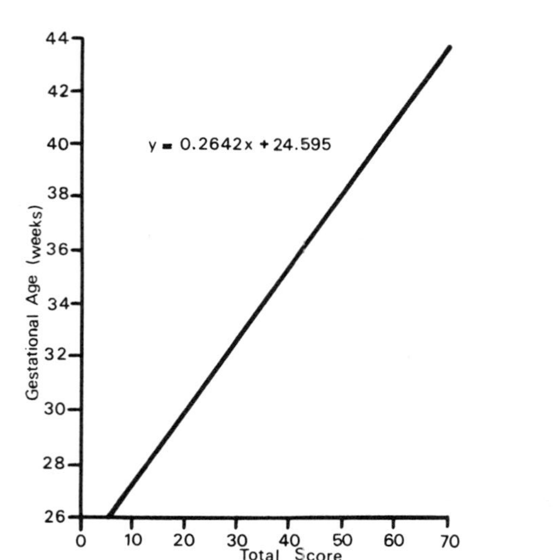

C

FIGURE 31-4. The Dubowitz tool for clinical assessment of gestational age. *A*, Scoring system for neurologic criteria. If the score differs on the two sides, take the mean. The following are notes on techniques of assessment:

Posture. Observed with infant quiet and in supine position. Score 0: arms and legs extended; 1: beginning of flexion of hips and knees, arms extended; 2: stronger flexion of legs, arms extended; 3: arms slightly flexed, legs flexed and abducted; 4: full flexion of arms and legs.

Square window. The hand is flexed on the forearm between the thumb and index finger of the examiner. Enough pressure is applied to get as full a flexion as possible, and the angle between the hypothenar eminence and the ventral aspect of the forearm is measured and graded according to diagram. (Care is taken not to rotate the infant's wrist while doing this maneuver.)

Ankle dorsiflexion. The foot is dorsiflexed onto the anterior aspect of the leg, with the examiner's thumb on the sole of the foot and other fingers behind the leg. Enough pressure is applied to get as full flexion as possible, and the angle between the dorsum of the foot and the anterior aspect of the leg is measured.

Arm recoil. With the infant in the supine position the forearms are first flexed for 5 seconds, then fully extended by pulling on the hands, and then released. The sign is fully positive if the arms return briskly to full flexion (score 2). If the arms return to incomplete flexion or the response is sluggish, it is graded as score 1. If they remain extended or are only followed by random movements the score is 0.

Leg recoil. With the infant supine, the hips and knees are fully flexed for 5 seconds, then extended by traction on the feet and released. A maximal response is one of full flexion of the hips and knees (score 2). A partial flexion scores 1, and minimal or no movement scores 0.

Popliteal angle. With the infant supine and his pelvis flat on the examining couch, the thigh is held in the knee-chest position by the examiner's left index finger and thumb supporting the knee. The leg is then extended by gentle pressure from the examiner's right index finger behind the ankle, and the popliteal angle is measured.

Heel-to-ear maneuver. With the baby supine, draw the baby's foot as near to the head as it will go without forcing it. Observe the distance between the foot and the head as well as the degree of extension at the knee. Grade according to diagram. Note that the knee is left free and may draw down alongside the abdomen.

Scarf sign. With the baby supine, take the infant's hand and try to put it around the neck and as far posteriorly as possible around the opposite shoulder. Assist this maneuver by lifting the elbow across the body. See how far the elbow will go across and grade according to illustrations. Score 0: elbow reaches opposite axillary line; 1: elbow between midline and opposite axillary line; 2: elbow reaches midline; 3: elbow will not reach midline.

Head lag. With the baby lying supine, grasp the hands (or the arms if a very small infant) and pull him slowly towards the sitting position. Observe the position of the head in relation to the trunk and grade accordingly. In a small infant the head may initially be supported by one hand. Score 0: complete lag; 1: partial head control; 2: able to maintain head in line with body; 3: brings head anterior to body.

Ventral suspension. The infant is suspended in the prone position, with examiner's hand under the infant's chest (one hand in a small infant, two in a large infant). Observe the degree of extension of the back and the amount of flexion of the arms and legs. Also note the relation of the head to the trunk. Grade according to diagram.

B, Scoring system for external characteristics.

C, Graph for conversion of total score for an estimated gestational age.

(From Dubowitz, L. M. S., Dubowitz, V. and Goldberg, C.: *Clinical assessment of gestational age in the newborn infant.* J. Pediatr. 77:1, 1970, with permission.)

Previously, newborns were classified as premature or term on the basis of birth weight alone:

A premature infant was one born weighing 2,500 g. (5 lb. 8 oz.) or less.

A term infant was one born weighing 2,501 g. (5 lb. 9 oz.) or more.

It is now accepted that the degree of a baby's maturity (and ability to adjust to extrauterine life) is more closely related to gestational age than to birth weight. Therefore, the following classification is preferred:

A term infant is one born between 38 to 41 weeks of gestation.

A preterm infant is one born before 38 weeks of gestation.

A post-term infant is one born after 42 weeks of gestation.

Furthermore, clinical studies have brought into focus infants who are born weighing less than their gestational age would suggest (small for date infants). These infants were found to be at risk in their neonatal adaptation and it is speculated that certain factors interfered with their intrauterine growth. Therefore, the current recommendation is that each neonate be appraised as to rate of intrauterine growth, or amount of weight gained per unit of gestational age. This is done by determining both birth weight and gestational age, and comparing the individual baby's rate of growth with normal standards obtained from a large number of babies. Assessment tools for these purposes include the following:

a. Guides for clinical assessment of gestational age on the basis of neurologic and physical-external findings or criteria.

   Figure 31-3 is a chart by which the nurse examines the newborn for the criteria listed and makes a conclusion on the estimated gestational age based on the patterns of the findings. The criteria identify the changes which can be manifested when intrauterine growth is altered, such as breast tissue, sole creases, etc. It is recommended that the chart be used only as a guide.

   The Dubowitz tool (Fig. 31-4) is a guide based on a series of neurologic responses dependent mainly on muscle tone and primitive reflexes as well as external features. The total score for the combined neurologic and external findings is a maximum of 70. The graph is used to correlate the total score with the estimated gestational age. For example, a total score of 60 corresponds to 40 weeks of gestation.

b. Classification of newborns in terms of being large, appropriate, or small for gestational age (Fig. 31-5).

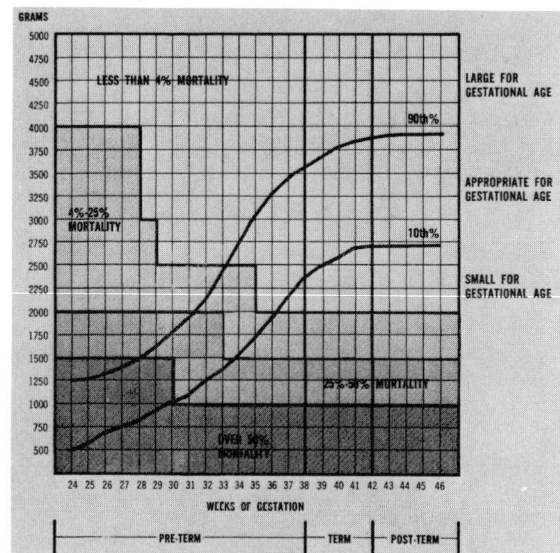

FIGURE 31-5. Classification of newborn infants by birthweight, gestational age and intrauterine growth to determine appropriateness, and large or small for gestational age. (From Battaglia, F. C. and Lubchenco, L. O.: *A practical classification of newborn infants by weight and gestational age.* J. Pediatr. 71:159, 1967, with permission.)

The recognition of infants small or large for date allows anticipatory preparation to treat complications which may arise.

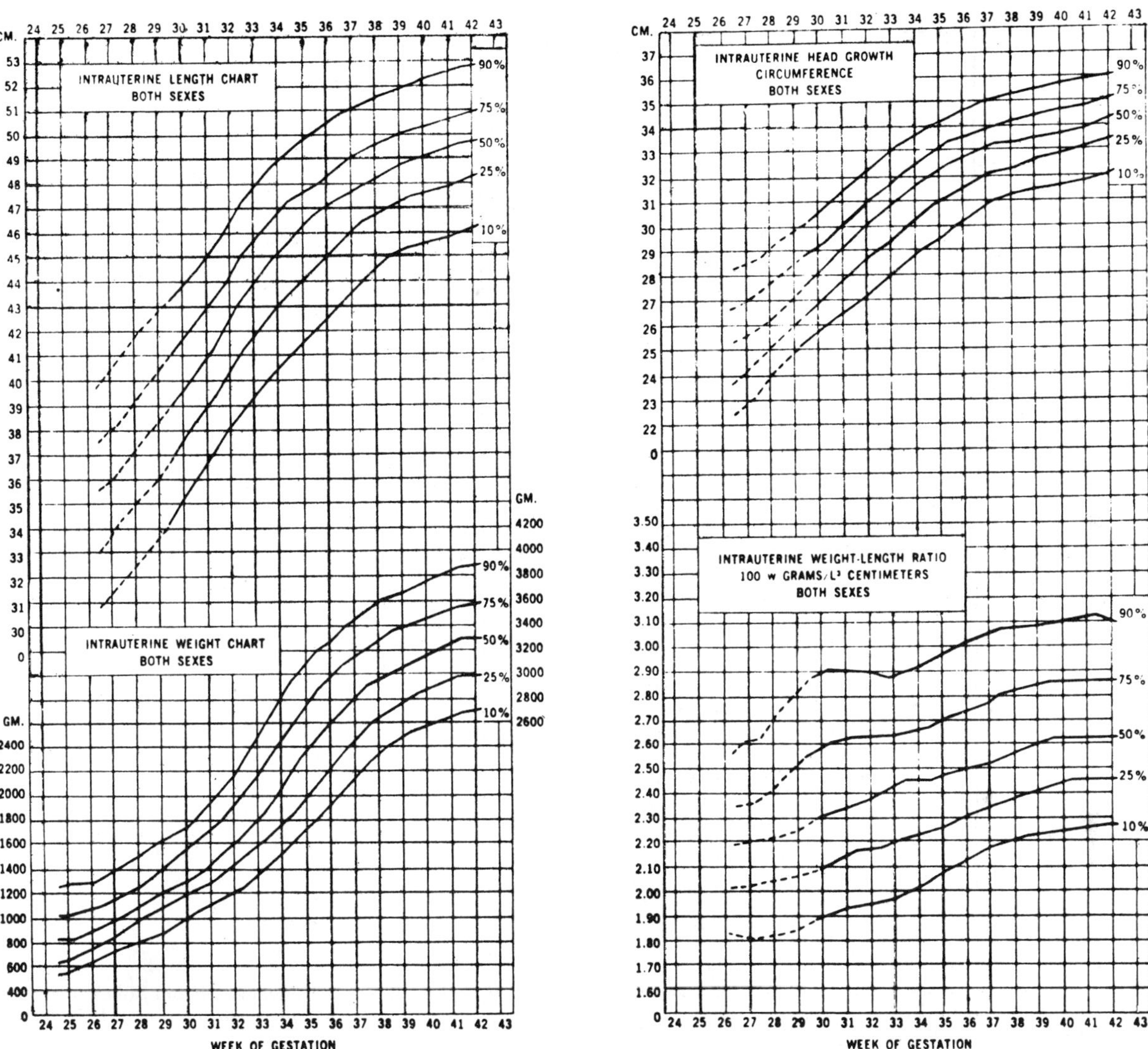

FIGURE 31-6. Colorado intrauterine growth charts. Percentiles of intrauterine growth in weight, length, head circumference, and weight-length ratio. (From Lubchenco, L. O.: *Intrauterine growth in length and head circumference as estimated from live births at gestational ages from 26 to 42 weeks.* Pediatrics 37:404, 1966, with permission.)

c. Intrauterine growth charts (Fig. 31-6).

These serve as standards of references for percentiles of intrauterine growth in weight, length, head circumference, and weight/length ratio. These are important because discrepancies in intrauterine growth will be reflected first in the infant's weight, then the length, and eventually (in severe cases) the head circumference.

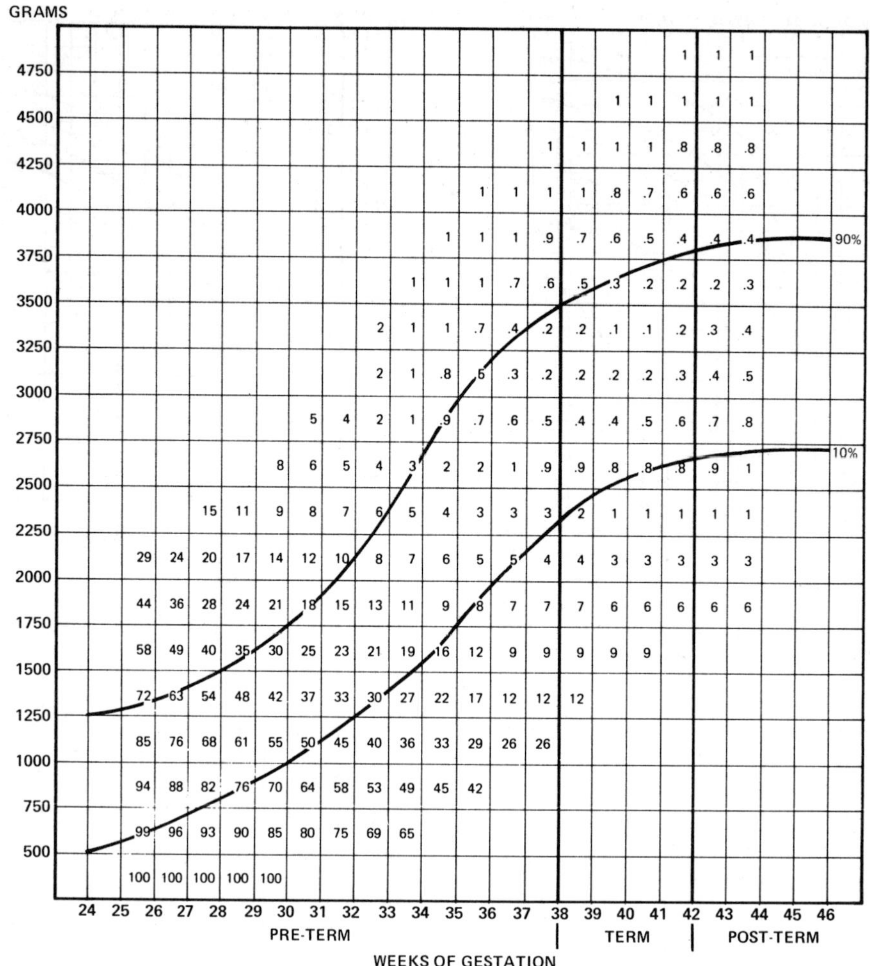

FIGURE 31-7. Newborn classification and neonatal mortality risk, by birth weight and gestational age. (From Lubchenco, L. O., Searls, D. T. and Brazie, J. V.: *Neonatal mortality rate: Relationship to birth weight and gestational age.* J. Pediatr. 81:814, 1972, with permission.)

The value of such classifications is identification of the neonate at risk and early management to curtail risk factors and enhance extrauterine adaptation. Clinical evaluation tools are invaluable in helping the nurse assess for the high-risk neonate. Figure 31-7 is one tool developed specifically for identifying neonates who are at risk. This allows the nurse to prepare the expected therapeutic plan without losing precious time.

4. Determining of Physical Status by Complete Examination

After initial examination at birth, every infant should have a thorough physical examination. The purpose is to:

a. Reassess the infant's continuing adaptive responses to extrauterine life.

b. Casefind abnormalities which may have been missed in the initial exam when priorities focused on the establishment of respiratory and circulatory adaptation.
c. Casefind complications which are manifested later rather than in the initial hours after birth.
d. Share findings with parents to reassert infant's well-being or possible risk factors at a time when parents can receive supportive help from hospital staff.

The physical examination should involve an orderly, systematic process to ensure completion of all segments of the examination. The sequence is usually cephalocaudal (from head to toe). However, instead of establishing a rigid sequential order, the system should be flexible enough for accommodation to the particular situation presented by the baby and environment. The nurse is in a unique position to perform the physical examination due to the constant care she provides to the neonate. Therefore, it is imperative for nurses to recognize and utilize all available opportunities for data collection. For example, certain physical findings are best elicited during baths, feeding, sleep, and so forth.

The physical examination described in this book involves the nurse in an expansion of traditional roles in neonatal assessment. Four dimensions of the physical examination process are highlighted:

1. *Inspection:* looking closely at the body parts to assess variables such as symmetry, size, color, contour, and position. Certain instruments are used to increase visualization with additional light sources, e.g., opthalmoscope for eyes, otoscope for ears, flashlight for pharynx.
2. *Palpation:* touching to assess variables such as vibrations, consistency, degree of tenderness, presence of masses. Also aids in localization of an organ and determination of its size. Usually performed with the flat surface of the finger or fingertips.
3. *Percussion:* tapping to assess sounds influenced by the presence of gas, fluid, or masses which can contribute to distention. Performed by placing the fingers of one hand firmly against the body part and using the index or middle finger of the other to tap, as with a hammer.
4. *Auscultation:* listening to body sounds with a stethoscope. Usually reveals significant findings in assessment of a neonate. The stethoscope should have a diaphragm and bell and fit the ears properly to decrease the introduction and misinterpretation of extraneous sounds.

NEONATAL ASSESSMENT GUIDE

The following is a guide for evaluation of the full-term neonate through physical examination. Norms and common variations are outlined as well as significant factors to consider as one is performing the physical examination. Table 31-1 presents the normal values for vital signs in the neonate.

Guidelines for Evaluation of the Normal Full-Term Neonate through Physical Examination

Checklist of Manifestations and Norms	*Significant Considerations*
I. General Appearance Inspection: A. Weight ranges: 2500–4300 g. (5½–9½ lb.) average weight: 3400 g. (7½ lb.) B. Length ranges: 19–21″	

Guidelines—*Continued*

Checklist of Manifestations and Norms	*Significant Considerations*
C. Head circumference: 33–35 cm. (13–14 inches) D. Chest circumference: 30–33 cm. (12–13 inches)	Head should exceed chest; if much smaller indicative of microcephaly; if larger (4 cm. greater than chest) may indicate hydrocephaly, increased intracranial pressure.
E. Neck short, as if head fits on shoulders	
F. Assumes posture similar to that in utero; proverbial fetal position: head flexed to chin, arms close to trunk, extremities flexed, back bent, flexion at knees with dorsiflexion onto anterior aspects of the legs[3]	Known as position of comfort for neonate; he can be made to stop crying when gently curled up into this position. Proverbial fetal position dependent upon normal muscle tone. If no attempt is made to assume the position of flexion, there is diminished muscle tone from trauma, hypoxia, or criteria reflecting preterm in gestation.
G. Head ¼ of total length, torso appears longer than extremities, arms appear longer than legs	
H. Symmetry of body parts	Asymmetry may indicate congenital defects, birth trauma.
I. Good time to note vital signs (see Table 31-1 for norms)	
II. Manifestations of the Skin Inspection and Palpation:	Observe generally first and then inspect closely as each area of the body is examined.
A. Any coatings 1. Vernix caseosa: cheesy, whitish substance left over from intrauterine life; protective to skin while in utero	Differing philosophies of its value and whether to make deliberate efforts to remove it. May be excessive in skin folds around genitals, neck, elbows. Usually dries and flakes off within 24 hours. Excess indicates preterm; absence may indicate post-term.
2. Lanugo: fine, downy hair prevalent over back, shoulder, facial areas; prominent in younger gestational age	One criterion used to estimate gestational age. Explanation to mother helps to alleviate anxiety.
B. Texture 1. Epidermis is thin, soft to touch, smooth and delicate 2. 2nd–3rd day it becomes dry, flaky or peeling 3. Subcutaneous tissue (adipose pads) can be felt in the cheeks, buttock	Skin that feels firm is usually associated with distress such as extreme cold, shock, infections. Hard skin is called sclerema. Excessive desquamation (scaling) at birth is related to post-term gestational age. Check the cheeks for adipose tissue. Significant lack of adipose tissue may relate to retarded intrauterine growth, or indicate that fat deposition did not occur in the last trimester, or reflect a preterm gestational age. Lack of adipose tissue will predispose the infant to difficulty with thermogenesis.
C. Hydration Neonates have turgor, due to increased intercellular hydration of subcutaneous tissues.[4] Edema of subcutaneous tissue may occur from pressure exerted during birth process.	Technique to assess: grasp skin with finger and thumb; skin should spring back to original shape without an indentation, fold or wrinkled appearance (indicates lack of turgor). Edema most noted around eyes and dorsal aspects of extremities.
D. Color Normal skin usually has blush, reddened appearance due to the thin epidermis increasing visualization of the skin's capillaries.	Technique to assess: Blanching of the skin: put both index fingers next to each other, apply steady pressure and simultaneously separate the fingers to allow visualization of the skin area. Blanching is necessary to differentiate manifestations such as jaundice and ecchymosis which may be masked by the reddened skin color.

Guidelines—*Continued*

Checklist of Manifestations and Norms	*Significant Considerations*
1. Acrocyanosis: localized cyanosis in peripheral locales such as nose, hands, feet. Possibly related to hypoxia associated with birth which increases peripheral resistance and results in sluggish peripheral circulation.	Newborns at birth are seldom completely pink. However, cyanosis which is generalized (not localized) to the body is indicative of distress. Localized cyanosis may occur with difficult presentations due to pressure against the cervix. *Example:* cyanosis of buttock and legs with breech and cyanosis of scalp with marked caput succedaneum.
2. Harlequin color change: curious phenomenon in which the color on the dependent half in a side-lying position turns pink, while the upper half is pale. The colors reverse when baby is turned.[5] Its significance is unknown.	In the supine or prone positions, color distribution should be even. Explanations to mother will alleviate anxiety.
3. Telangiectatic nevi ("stork bites"): capillary dilatation creates these flat, localized reddened areas.	Common on upper eyelids, back of neck, occiput. May appear during crying periods. Explanations to the mother are important because it may recur throughout the first year. Disappears with blanching because blood is drained from the engorged capillaries.
4. Jaundice (icterus; yellowish skin color): may manifest between 2nd–3rd day of life due to icterus neonatorum (see discussion of Hepatic Functions in Chapter 30).	Blanching technique necessary for assessment of its presence which can be masked by reddened hues. Typical erythema associated with the newborn and moderate icterus together produces a ripe peach color. Jaundice before the 2nd day indicative of hemolytic disease and demands immediate attention.
E. Vesicles or Rash	
1. Erythema toxicum: pink papular rash which may have purulent vesicles on it, having no apparent significance.	Common on trunk and diapered area; usually transient. Appears at 1–2 days of life and usually disappears spontaneously within 1st week.
2. Milia: small, white papules representing distended sebaceous glands whose functions are limited at birth.	Prevalent on chin, cheeks, nose, forehead; usually disappears spontaneously within a few weeks. Instruct mother not to prick the pimple-like spots.
F. Hemorrhagic Sites	
1. Ecchymoses: appear as bruises, black and blue contained areas usually from trauma associated with labor and delivery or rough handling by personnel.	Should be reported because they can be indicative of serious infection or bleeding disorders. The size should be noted because the extravasated blood in it when broken down can elevate serum bilirubin to dangerous levels.[6]
2. Petechiae: minute hemorrhagic areas due to fragility of capillaries easily ruptured with increased pressure from labor and delivery.	Usually prevalent over the face and upper trunk as a result of pressure during descent and rotations during labor and birth. Ecchymoses and petechiae do not disappear with blanching because the blood is contained in the tissues. Usually disappear in 1–2 days; if not, may indicate infection or thrombocytopenia (low platelet count).
G. Pigmentation	
Mongolian spots: bluish, or purple irregular bruise-like spots over parts of the body. Bluish color caused by the presence of large, branching chromatophore-like cells in the corium.[7] Prevalent among Negro, Asian, and some European ethnicities.	Prevalent over the buttock and sacrum but may extend over the back and shoulders. Explanations to mother that they are harmless are important since spots may remain through the preschool years of life.

Guidelines—*Continued*

Checklist of Manifestations and Norms	*Significant Considerations*
Note: Pigmentation begins at *birth* in basal layer of epidermis.[8]	Human beings are undifferentiated in utero. Different skin pigmentations of various races begin in the postnatal period of life.
III. Significance of the Skin	
A. Infant's skin is a growth index: Skin thickness and subcutaneous tissue serve as an index of nutritional status. Well-nourished infants have well-defined layers of subcutaneous fat over their bodies.[9]	Prominent bony landmarks (clavicle, ribs) upon inspection may indicate prematurity and/or malnourishment.
B. It participates in disturbances of other organ systems through alterations of its own metabolism.[10]	The relationship between the skin and systemic diseases is demonstrated in examples such as increased sodium in the skin with cystic fibrosis and hyperpigmentation in disturbed protein metabolism, as PKU. Therefore manifestations of the skin can provide clues to the presence of pathologic processes in the body.
IV. Body Parts	
A. Head	
Inspection and Palpation:	
Common variations in shape occur with vaginal delivery, cephalic presentation. Primarily a result of pressure exerted during labor and delivery.	More commonly seen in firstborn and with prolonged labors. Head of a firstborn faces the tighter resistance offered by maternal birth canal and structures while prolonged labor forces the head to sustain more pressure.
1. Moulding: overlapping of the calvarium bones and narrowing of the sutures caused by normal compression during delivery to accommodate passage through birth canal.	Measurement of the head is done by placing the tape above the eyebrow and around the most prominent aspect of the occiput. Some degree of molding expected in all vertex, vaginal deliveries. Disappears in a few days. Palpitation reveals overriding of bones or overlap of what feel like ridges (sutures). Cesarean sections or breech presentations may result in an undisturbed head shape.
2. Caput succedaneum: diffuse swelling of the soft tissues of the scalp due to pressure. Swelling is not confined and may extend across suture lines.	Palpate the head, edema is detected by softness to touch. Ecchymotic coloration may be seen. Explanations to mother imperative as it resembles a bruise-like injury which can generate feelings of guilt and anxiety in parents. Disappears within a few days.
3. Cephalhematoma: subperiosteal hemorrhage in which blood collects beneath the periosteum and the bone. Swelling confined to an individual bone and thus the swollen area does not cross suture lines.	Inspection may reveal swelling several hours later because the trauma is deep. Parents need to know that resolution of the process takes time, average of 6 weeks or longer. Such visible signs of a difficult birth arouse anxiety and/or guilt feelings.
4. Fontanelles: soft membraneous areas where each suture meets. They allow the variations in shape by which the head is accommodated through the birth canal. Two significant fontanelles:	

Guidelines—*Continued*

Checklist of Manifestations and Norms	*Significant Considerations*
a. Anterior: between sagittal and coronal sutures; diamond shaped, up to approximately 5 cm.; enlarges as molding resolves; closes approximately 18 months of age.	Feel and measure fontanelles: bulging—indicative of increased intracranial pressure larger but flat and soft—indicative of malnourishment, hydrocephaly, retarded bone age (hypothyroidism).
b. Posterior: between sagittal and lambdoid sutures; triangular; smaller than anterior; closes approximately 2 months of age.	depressed, sunken—indicative of dehydration.
5. Inspection and palpation of the scalp and hair	Report unusual lesions, bleeding, coarse, brittle hair.
6. Inspection for Facial Symmetry	
a. Facial symmetry between parts: lopsided appearance may be seen when the shoulder is pressed into the neck, usually attributed to an intrauterine position of latero flexio of the head.	Asymmetry disappears within a few weeks or months. Facial asymmetry may also result from injury to the nerves from birth trauma (facial nerve palsy).
b. Symmetry between left and right sides: asymmetry can also occur from sustained pelvic pressure on the fetal head during the birth process.	Asymmetry may persist into adult life, frequently masked by hair growth. Some infants have a tendency to turn their heads more to one side than the other, giving an asymmetrical appearance.
B. Eyes Inspection may reveal the following normal variations:[11]	
1. Reflections of Anatomic Immaturity:	
a. Scleral color: bluish tint because they are thin.	Icterus (jaundice) may first be evident in the sclerae where it is not masked by the ruddy color of the skin.
b. Eye color: iris usually grayish-blue in Caucasian infants, grayish-brown in infants of other races.	Final eye color achieved by deposition of pigment by 6–12 months of age.
Brushfield spots (speckles on the iris) may be seen.	Often associated with Down's syndrome but may occur in normal infants.
c. Tears: lacrimal glands not fully functional until 1–3 months.	Explain to parents to avoid concern about baby's tearless crying.
d. Pseudostrabismus: irises do not appear to be centered but more toward the bridge of the nose. This is due primarily to facial structures which create an illusion of internal strabismus: the bridge of the nose is wide and flat, and the epicanthal folds of the upper eyelid obscure the inner canthus.	Explanations to parents are essential as this is a frequent source of questions. Be sure to inspect for true deviation to right or left.
e. Eyelids: closed most of the time but when open may appear asymmetrical and to operate independently of one another, producing pseudoptosis.	Stimuli which promptly cause closing are: bright lights, loud noises, touching the eyelashes or cornea. Attempts to forcefully open the eyelids are met with resistance and such attempts cause blepharospasms. Opening of the eye can be accomplished by manipulating the above stimuli and/or gently rotating the head when held upright.
2. Reflections of Neuromuscular Immaturity: Lack of muscular function, incomplete myelinization of the cerebral neural pathways, and visual cortex can result in:	Explanations to parents essential as these are frequently a stressor.

Guidelines—*Continued*

Checklist of Manifestations and Norms	*Significant Considerations*
a. Incoordinate eye movements due to incomplete neuromuscular control of orbital muscles and lack of muscular development. Random, jerky, uneven eye movements producing transient strabismus.	
b. Setting sun sign: the irises deviate downward and appear to sink beneath the lower eyelid due to lid lag.	Observed as transitory in normal infants but may be indicative of pathology (hydrocephalus). Report its manifestation.
c. Doll's eye phenomenon: when an infant is in the supine position and has his head turned from one side to the other or up and down, his eyes may lag behind without adjusting to the new head position.	Almost always seen from birth to 10 days; disappears by 2–3 months. Demonstrates lack of integration of head-eye coordination.
3. Reflections of Trauma:	
a. Subconjunctival hemorrhage: bright red crescentic band located on the side or near the iris. Due to rupture of small conjunctival vessels from increased pressure during the birth process.	Blood absorbs within 10 days.
b. Chemical conjunctivitis: eyelids become edematous and a purulent discharge may appear. Results from irritation from silver nitrate treatment.	Subsides within 2–7 days.
4. Determine the presence of the following:	
a. Red reflex: small red-orange circular spot seen with the ophthalmoscope light at the pupils. Red reflex caused by light falling on the retina.	Absence indicates opacity of the lens or obstruction to light passing through it (such as cataracts).
b. Blink reflex: elicited by shining a bright light at the eyes, results in quick closure of eyelids.	Absence may indicate impaired light perception.
c. Corneal reflex: touching the cornea lightly will result in eye closure.	Inspect the appearance of the cornea; should be bright and shiny (not hazy and dull) when illuminated by light.
d. Reactions of pupils to light: easily done by shading one eye for a moment or two and then exposing it to the light source.	Note its presence or absence; asymmetry or poor response to light may indicate neurologic dysfunction.
Sphincter muscle gives pupil movement in response to light but dilator muscles not functional until six months of life.	Also note shape (round, oval, etc.) and size (constriction or not) of pupils.
C. Ears	
External Inspection:	
1. Position: top of ear should be at the same level as the eye (if you draw an imaginary line from the eye to the ear).	Low-set ears may indicate chromosomal abnormalities and/or congenital renal disorders.
2. Cartilage formation: some cartilage should be felt on palpation.	Lack of cartilage indicative of preterm gestation.
Internal Inspection (with otoscope)	It is recommended that nurses do not probe the ears internally as a routine procedure. During the neonatal period the ear canal is short and can easily be damaged by the otoscope in the hands of an inexperienced nurse.

Guidelines—*Continued*

Checklist of Manifestations and Norms	*Significant Considerations*
D. Neck Inspection:	
1. Position and movement: should have flexible movements in rotation from side to side and from flexion to extension.	Examination in prone position allows appropriate data collection on neck position and movements.
2. Length: an appropriate neck length is visible without being hidden by folds or hyperextension.	Excessive folds (webbing) and hyperextension (opisthotonus) may be associated with pathologic conditions.
3. Demonstrates some degree of head control by flexion of neck muscles and contraction of shoulder and arm muscles (Fig. 31-8).	When lifting the full-term neonate by the wrists to a sitting position, head control is manifested by the head not falling onto the chest; if the head should fall forward, it prompts correcting to an erect position. Failure of the head to correct its position may be indicative of hypotonia due to early gestational age or pathology such as Down's syndrome or previous hypoxia.

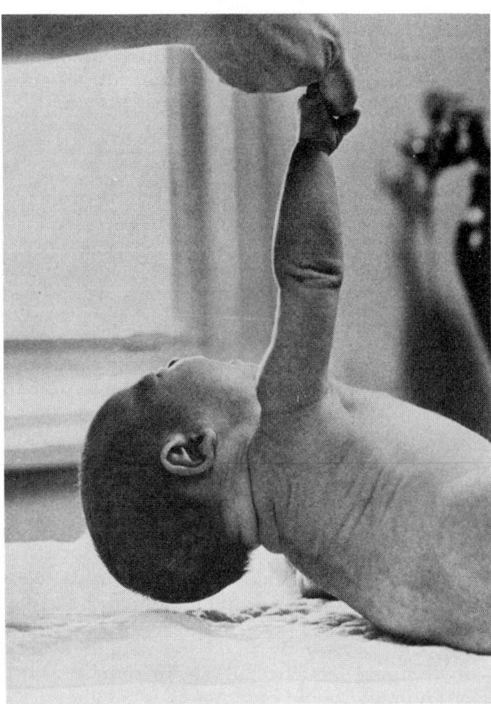

FIGURE 31-8. The full-term neonate demonstrates some degree of head control when lifted by the hands.

Checklist of Manifestations and Norms	*Significant Considerations*
Palpation: Feel for swellings, edema, masses, presence of lymph nodes or enlarged thyroid.	
E. Thorax Inspection:	
1. Shape and size: ribs should be flexible and the xiphoid cartilage at the lower end of the sternum may be prominent beneath the skin.	Pectus excavatum (funnel breast) is often seen in prematures with respiratory distress. An increased A-P diameter of the chest often indicates air trapping after aspiration.

Guidelines—*Continued*

Checklist of Manifestations and Norms	*Significant Considerations*
2. Breathing movements: respiratory movements are predominantly diaphragmatic. Thoracic cage rarely moves, while the abdomen rises and falls with inspiration and expiration. (See Table 31-1 for norms in assessment of respirations.)	
3. Breast area: assess size and position of breasts Supernumerary nipples may be found in line with regular nipples.	Breast enlargement and secretion may be seen due to maternal hormonal influences. In many congenital syndromes, such as Turner's syndrome, the breasts may be positioned farther apart than normal. Extra nipples rarely contain glandular tissue and are harmless.
Palpation: Feel for tenderness in the clavicle area; prominent bony masses; presence or absence of breast tissue.	Screening to rule out clavicle fractures. Amount of breast tissue is a criterion for estimation for gestational age.
F. Lungs Percussion: Reveals less valuable data in the newborn than in any other age period because the chest is so small that localization of vibrations is difficult.	
Auscultation: Detect breath sounds with stethoscope.	Reduced breath sounds indicate poor air exchange. Asymmetrical breath sounds may indicate penumothorax.
G. Heart Inspection: Location of pulsations: should be visible in midclavicular line toward the lateral half of the left thorax, near the 5th intercostal space.	Indicates heart size; if found in epigastrum, suspect heart enlargement.
Palpation: Apical pulse should be found at the 5th intercostal space.	Detection of other positions can lead to suspicion of conditions such as pneumothorax, diaphragmatic hernia, etc.
Auscultation: The first and second heart sounds should be clearly audible and are discernible from each other.	The area listened to should include the entire precardium, extending to the left scapula through the axilla region.
Closure of the mitral and tricuspid valves elicits the first sound, while closure of the aortic and pulmonic valves gives the second sound.	Heart sounds may be rapid but should be regular in rhythm and rate. Irregularity in sounds, rate of beats or murmurs should be reported immediately. Cardiac valve sounds are best heard in the following: 1. Apex (mitral valve) 2. Second interspace at the left sternum (pulmonic valve) 3. Second interspace at the right sternum (aortic valve) 4. Junction of xiphoid and sternum (tricuspid valve).[13]

Guidelines—*Continued*

Checklist of Manifestations and Norms	*Significant Considerations*
H. Abdomen Inspection: 1. Contour may be cylindrical with slight protrusion. 2. Umbilical stump is normally bluish-white, moist, and shiny; by 24 hours it becomes yellowish-brown, dull and dry; eventually becomes blackish-brown and shrivels (process due to loss of Wharton's jelly and exposure to air).	Make special notations of: 1. Distention (tight skin making subcutaneous vessels visible)—suspicion of bowel obstruction or weakened abdominal muscles 2. Localized bulging at flanks—suspicion of enlarged kidneys, ascites, or absent abdominal muscles 3. Signs of impending infection (redness, wetness, odor) in umbilical area.
Palpation: Usually light or gentle palpation precedes deep palpation. Feel for:	
1. Edge of liver: found in right lower to upper quadrant (right costal margin). 2. Tip of spleen: feels like a slight mass in the lateral aspects of the left upper quadrant.	These organs may not be easily palpated until the nurse gains experience in doing so.
3. Kidney: in posterior flank (place a finger there with upward pressure while the other hand presses downward toward that finger; oval-like structure is felt).	Feel for any masses (tumors, cysts, structural defects).
4. Femoral area: feel for pulsation as well as for lumps and masses.	Femoral pulse gives clues about peripheral circulation and inguinal hernias may be detected (more common in the male infant).
5. Bladder distention: firm globular mass felt in suprapubic area.	Persistence of distention even after voiding may indicate obstruction.
Percussion: May indicate presence of gas and demarcation of organs.	
Auscultation: Intermittent tinkling sounds indicative of peristalsis.	It is suggested that the nurse auscultate the abdomen prior to palpating it to decrease external stimulations causing bowel sounds.
I. Genitals Inspection: 1. Structure Females: may be edematous, engorged due to maternal hormonal influences; presence of labis majora, labia minor, clitoris, vaginal opening. Hymenal tag may protrude from vagina.	Meatus difficult to visualize so voidings should be noted.
Males: position of external meatus should be at the end of the glans penis; scrotum checked for symmetry and size; prepuce (piece of skin) covers the glans penis and is not retractable in neonates. This is usually removed by circumcision.	Meatal openings on the underneath portion of the glans penis indicative of hypospadias. Look for lack of urine flow or signs of infection resulting from interference by the prepuce.

Guidelines—*Continued*

Checklist of Manifestations and Norms	*Significant Considerations*
2. Discharge In females a milky white discharge, at times blood-tinged, is seen.	Due to hormonal influence of mother; disappears within weeks.
Palpation: 1. Two testes, about 1 cm. in diameter, should be felt in the scrotum of the male.	Any masses, tenderness or bulging indicative of pathology.
2. Anus: inspection for patency and location.	Note character of stools.
J. Extremities Inspect the following: 1. Digits: polydactyly is extra fingers or toes; syndactyly is fusion of digits or webbing.	Most extra digits can be eliminated by tying them off, allowing necrosis and eventual falling off. (This procedure depends on the degree of involvement of polydactyly.)
2. Position at rest (resting posture): some degree of flexion should be noted in arms, hands, and legs. Legs may have a mild degree of medial rotation (bowing) and be in slight abduction at the hips.	Lack of flexion indicates hypotonia possibly from hypoxia, motor depression, anomalies, or underdeveloped gestation. Pathologic deviations are: 1. Limbs lying flat on surface (frog posture) 2. Opisthotonic posture—head retroflexed and lower limbs extended 3. Head turned constantly towards one side 4. Any asymmetrical posture 5. Strong rigid flexion of upper and lower limbs 6. Both hands constantly held in front of mouth
3. Spontaneous motor activity: a. Athetoid postures and movements may be seen: some fingers flex while others extend; simultaneous extension or flexion of the elbow with rotation of wrist and upper limbs.	Note condition of extremities with movements. Marked reactions such as tonicity, clonicity, twitching of face, prolonged tremors to whole body, are indicative of pathology.
b. Slight tremors may be seen in the arms.	Note frequency, magnitude and area of involvement with the tremors.
Palpate for: 1. Movements: range of motion (ROM). Normal ranges for the different joints are as follows:[14] a. Neck: 1) bending forward and backward = 110° 2) turning face side to side = 150° 3) bending head to side with nose pointing forward at all times = 90°	It is not necessary to assess the exact number of degrees but whether the range of movement is less than normal or significantly beyond. Never use extra force to assess ROM or to the point of making the infant cry.
b. Shoulder: 1) abduction of arm from trunk = 120° 2) rotation of arm = 260–270° c. Elbow: 1) forearm flexes through = 170° d. Wrist: 1) flexion = 110° 2) extension = 80° e. Hips: 1) flexion and extension = 160–170° f. Knee: 1) full range of 170° 2) knees should not hyperextend and legs should flex onto thigh	Asymmetry in range of motions may indicate weakness, paralysis, fractures. Failure to move an extremity may indicate spinal cord injury. Marked resistance to putting an extremity through ROM may indicate muscular disorders. Instability in the hip when attempting to flex and abduct, as well as excessive skin folds in the anterior and posterior aspects leads to suspicion of congenital hip dislocation.

Guidelines—*Continued*

Checklist of Manifestations and Norms	*Significant Considerations*
g. Ankle: 1) maximum flexion and extension of the foot = 130°	
2. Determine resistance to passive movements: arms and legs should promptly return to degree of flexion after attempts to extend them.	Prolonged extension may indicate hypotonia.
3. Examine creases: a. Palm of hand: simian crease may lead to suspicion of Down's syndrome	
b. Soles of feet: gives clues for estimated gestational age	Decrease of creases indicates less gestational age (Fig. 31-9).

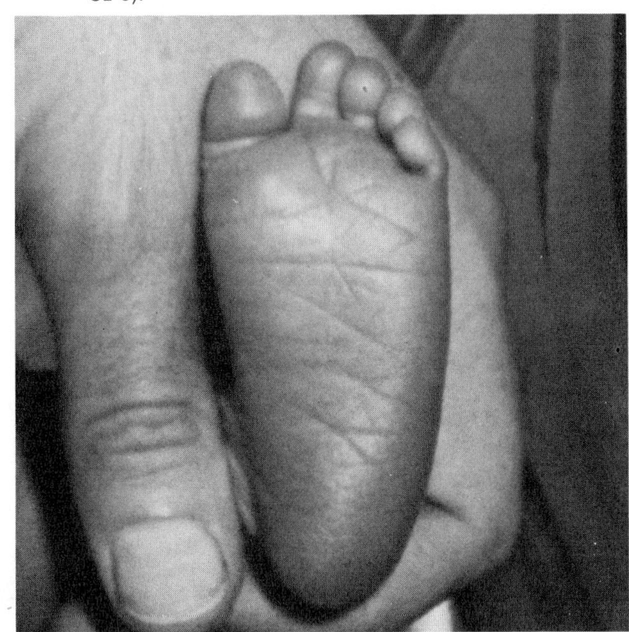

FIGURE 31-9. The foot of a full-term neonate shows a complex series of creases over the entire sole.

Checklist of Manifestations and Norms	*Significant Considerations*
4. Assess alignment and proportion: arms usually longer than the legs; feet usually in varus or valgus position.	Note any unusually long extremity.
5. Assess color and temperature.	Check nailbeds for color (or cyanosis); note temperature differences between extremities and any excessive coldness or warmness to touch.
6. Elicit reflex responses (see Part V. Presence or Absence of Basic Responses).	Check for symmetry and completeness in reflex responses.
K. Spinal Column Inspect and palpate the dorsal spine with infant in prone position.	Note any abnormal curvatures or masses. Examine skin for any tufts of hair over the spine; suspicion of spina bifida. Examine for any pilonidal dimple in coccygeal area; look closely for any pilonidal cysts or sinus and any signs of infection at this site.

Guidelines—*Continued*

Checklist of Manifestations and Norms	*Significant Considerations*
V. Presence or Absence of Basic Reflexes Assessment of basic reflexes contributes to neurologic evaluation of the newborn. Other components in the neurologic exam have previously been discussed, such as muscle tone reflected by movement and resistance of extremities, head lag or control, eye movements and pupil reactions, and general posture. Assessment for certain reflexes should be a mandatory part of every physical examination. These are categorized below. Assessment of all other reflexes present at birth should be part of a neurologic evaluation. The following reflexes are described according to Prechtl and Beintema.[16] Essential reflexes to assess in routine physical exam: A. Oral Responses 1. Rooting: stroking corners of the mouth, upper or lower lip results in head turning toward the stimulated side. The mouth usually opens with stimulation to lips (Fig. 31-10). 2. Sucking: placing object in mouth elicits rhythmic sucking.	The rationale for checking reflex responses in the neonate is that it elicits significant data on the status of neurologic functioning. Neurologic examination of the newborn is of special value because abnormal signs present in the first days or weeks of life may disappear to be followed months or years later by the appearance of abnormal findings.[15] Absence, weakness, or asymmetry of responses may be indicative of central nervous depression from drugs or anoxia; central nervous system or spinal cord defects or lesions; presence of immaturity as seen in preterm infants.

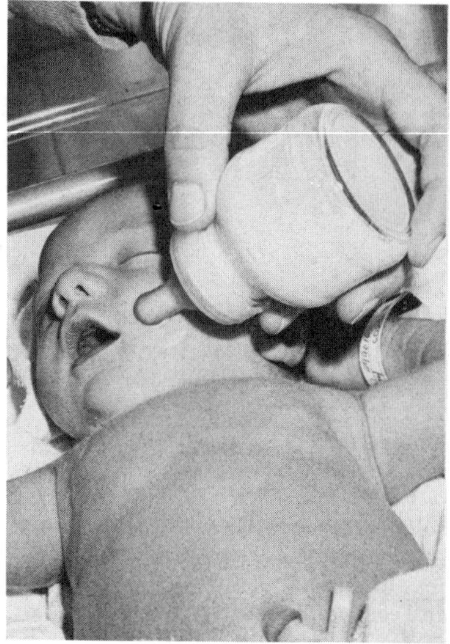

A

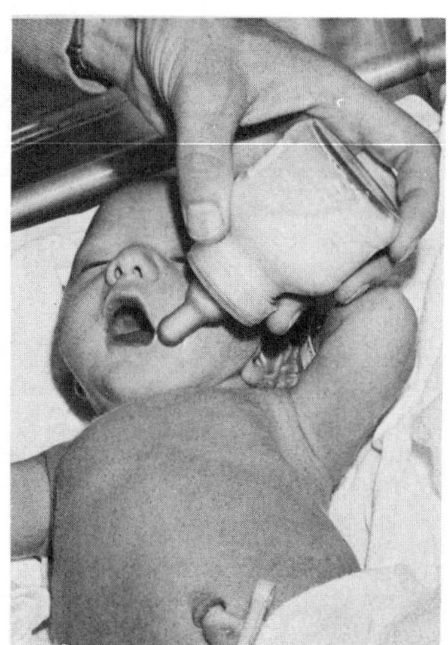

B

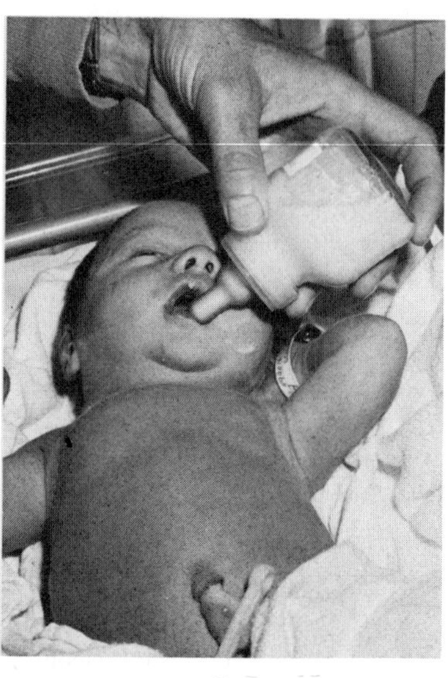

C

FIGURE 31-10. The rooting reflex. *A*, Stimulus applied to the cheek. *B*, Head turning toward to the stimulus. *C*, Sucking response elicited.

Guidelines—*Continued*

Checklist of Manifestations and Norms	*Significant Considerations*
B. Grasping Responses 1. Palmar: press palmar surface of hands and flexion of fingers (grasp) around examiner's fingers results. 2. Plantar: press thumbs against ball of feet and flexion of all toes results.	
C. Traction Responses Grasp infant's hands at the wrist and pull slowly to sitting position. Response should be extension of the arms at the elbows with some degree of head control.	Head control is a joint function of the strength of the neck muscles and activity of the labyrinth (structures regulating equilibrium).[17] Provides cues on equilibrium-regulating mechanism.
D. Moro Response (Startle Response) Elicit by sudden, rapid movement of the head by dropping it a little while infant is held; if head lowering is contraindicated, suspend baby horizontally and lower hands rapidly coming to abrupt halt. A complete response consists of two phases (Fig. 31-11):	Most significant singular reflex indicative of CNS status. Also elicited by sudden tap on surface which baby is lying. Movement must be sudden, rapid, and abrupt to elicit response. Note threshold for elicitation (easily or needing many stimuli), asymmetry of responses, completeness of response.

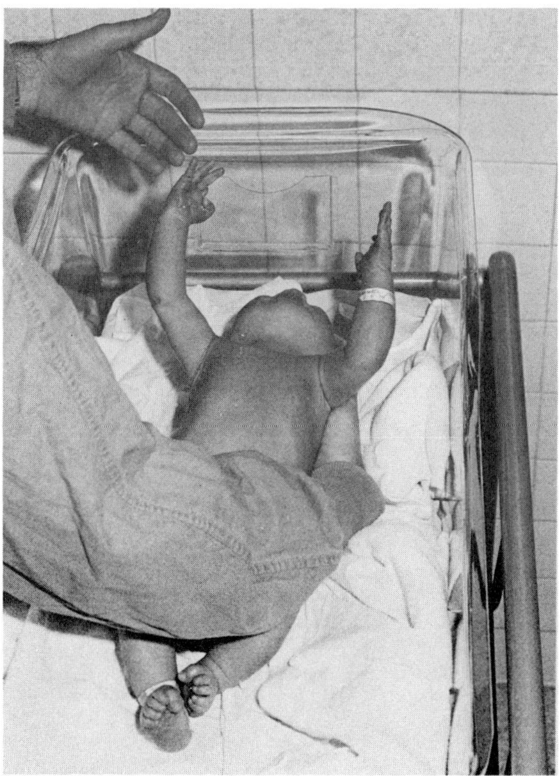

FIGURE 31-11. The Moro reflex.

Guidelines—*Continued*

Checklist of Manifestations and Norms	*Significant Considerations*
Phase 1: Quick flexion of forearm at the elbow followed by abduction of the upper limb at the shoulder, extension of the forearm at the elbow, extension of fingers. Phase 2: Subsequent adduction of arm at the shoulders.	
Additional reflexes to assess in neurologic exam: E. Those demonstrated spontaneously by infant: yawning, stretching, swallowing, sneezing, hiccups.	These have been related to increasing oxygen intake, clearing nasal passage, and elimination of gas. Increased yawning, sneezing, and hiccupping are frequently seen in drug withdrawal syndrome in infants of addicted mothers.
F. Response while prone 1. Bauer's response (spontaneous crawling): Pressing hands gently on soles of the feet elicits spontaneous crawling efforts. 2. Incurvature of the trunk: Scratching the side of the vertebral column slowly results in the trunk curving to the stimulated side.	
G. Responses while Upright 1. Placing: Lifting the baby so the dorsal part of the foot lightly touches an edge results in spontaneous lifting of the feet onto the surface by flexion of the knees and hips. 2. Stepping: Lifting the baby, allowing the soles of the feet to touch the surface of a table results in alternating stepping movements with both legs (Fig. 31-12).	

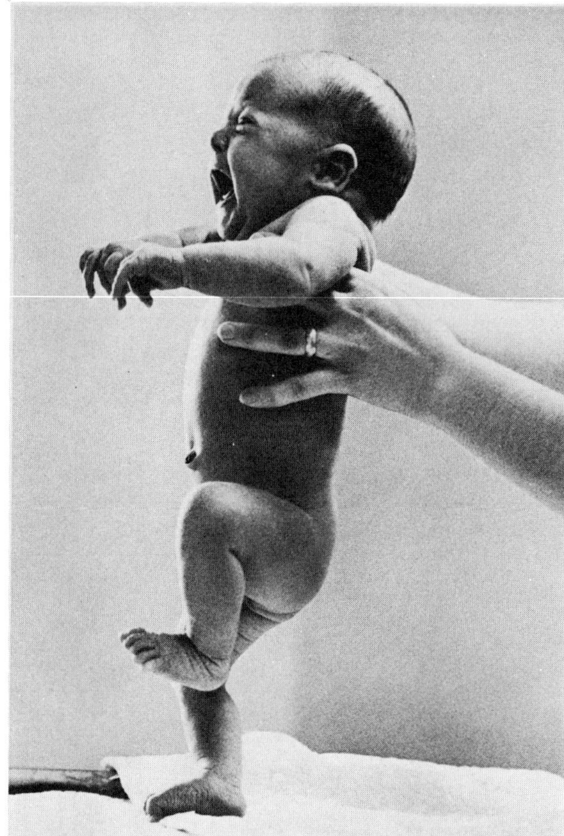

FIGURE 31-12. The stepping response. (Courtesy of Mead Johnson Laboratories, Evansville, Indiana.)

Guidelines—*Continued*

Checklist of Manifestations and Norms	*Significant Considerations*
H. Response while Supine	
1. Tonic Neck Reflex: Turning the head to the side results in extension of the arm on the side which the head is turned, and flexion of the opposite arm.	
I. Responses in Extremities	These are less pronounced in the newborn, becoming more distinct with age.
1. Biceps Reflex: tapping of the biceps muscle in the elbow area results in short contraction felt in the biceps muscle and in the infant's wrist.	Assessment for numerous other reflexes can be included in a neurological exam. The few having relevance to the nursing role in assessment have been highlighted here.
2. Babinski Reflex: light stroking of the sole of foot from heel to toes results in dorsiflexion of big toe and spreading of smaller toes.	
3. Patella Deep Tendon Reflex: relax both legs, then tap the tendon below the patella; the knee jerks from extension of the knee by contraction of quadriceps muscles.	
4. Achilles Deep Tendon Reflex: dorsiflex the foot and tap the back of the heel; ankle jerk occurs.	
5. Ankle Clonus: press both thumbs against the distal part of the soles of the feet; a quick dorsiflexion of the feet occurs.	
6. Withdrawal Reflex: prick soles of foot with a pin and withdrawal occurs with simultaneous flexion of hip, knee, and foot.	
VI. Sensory Modalities	An extensive application of sensory capacities on behavioral development is presented in Chapter 32. This section merely presents the physiologic data.
A. Visual Visual behavior is active at birth as evidenced by the following:[18]	Nurses need to appreciate the neonate's visual capacity, relate information about it to parents, and help parents provide visual enrichment to their babies.
1. Visual acuity is about 20/200; improves rapidly; refractive error usually hyperopic.	Neonate is far-sighted, vision beyond 20 feet is normal while near vision unclear.
2. Fixation present immediately at birth; preferential fixation for vertical edges versus horizontal.	Newborn has more fixations with vertical angles; parents should present themselves and objects in vertical rather than horizontal plane.
3. Retinal development complete except for refinement of macula.	Eyes are light-sensitive; the macula contributes to keen vision which develops later.
4. Pupils reactive to light.	Newborn will blink, squint, or even sneeze in response to light. Bright lights such as flash bulbs do not harm vision but produce discomfort.
5. Presence of well developed visual cone system.	This system contributes to discriminative vision. Newborn has ability to see fine details of form, contrast and color.
6. Myelination of optic pathways not completed until 4 months of age.	The limiting link in the newborn's visual system is the nervous system's participation in voluntary object-elicited eye movements.
7. Eyes move well in response to vestibular stimuli and moving objects.	Newborn can follow object when it is in the center of the field; his eyes move with body rotations such as head movements.

Guidelines—*Continued*

Checklist of Manifestations and Norms	*Significant Considerations*
B. Auditory Hearing hindered at birth due to amniotic fluid in middle ear. Once it is absorbed and replaced by air, auditory system is active.	Initially the newborn appears oblivious to sound. Presence of hearing manifests in responses to noise such as eye movements (blinking, staring), startle reaction, crying. (Can be tested with a bell or other sounds.) Differentiation of sounds and location of its direction does not occur until weeks later.
C. Taste Differentiation between bitter and sweet flavors is present; more neutral flavors are not discernible.	Newborn responds to displeasurable flavors by turning away or protruding the tongue as if to rid the flavor; pleasurable flavors accepted by active sucking.
D. Smell Appears to be present but its development at birth is questionable.	Speculations that the infant can smell breast milk by turning his head toward the breast. Part of the neonate's learning environment involves the smell of his mother/parents.
E. Tactile/Touch Appears to be keen at birth as evidenced by responses to touch (rooting, sucking).	Tactile is primary mode by which the infant learns about his environment. Sensitivity to touch appears to have a systematic process of development. It is speculated to begin through the mouth with sucking; then to the face where contact of the cheek initiates rooting and stimuli to the lips initiate sucking; to face where contact with breasts or mother's body brings feelings of comfort; to fingers where contact elicits the grasp.
Sensitivity to painful stimuli and extreme temperatures appears to be present but not distinct. Therefore, pain threshold is high.	Newborn quickly associates warmth, gentleness, and firm, secure handling with pleasure; while cold and rough, unstable handling makes him uncomfortable. Newborn appears to withdraw from painful stimuli (pressure, cold, etc.). His reactions are sluggish and delayed initially, becoming more violent and rapid with age.

TABLE 31-1. Vital Signs in the Neonate

Vital Sign	*Rate*	*Comments*
I. Respirations		
A. First period of reactivity (up to 30 minutes of life)	50-60/min.*	Great fluctuations in rate and pattern: gasps are seen initially; periodic breathing (short periods of nonbreathing without drop in heart rate) can occur; apnea (nonbreathing with fall in heart rate) frequently associated with birth asphyxia.
B. Second period of reactivity (4-6 hours)	50-70/min.†	Biphasic responses frequent. Apneic spells more likely to occur now. If associated with drop in heart rate, neonate needs to be stimulated to begin breathing again. Close observation imperative.
C. Stabilization period (1-2 days)	30-40/min.‡ upper range of 50 occasionally seen	Respirations now regular in rhythm. Normal respiratory movements are mainly diaphragmatic (abdomen rises and falls with inspiration and expiration while thoracic cage remains immobile). The neonate is also an obligatory nose breather. Abnormal manifestations indicative of distress are: intercostal retractions; retractions of the xyphoid; grunting on expiration; flaring nostrils; persistent elevated rates.

TABLE 31-1. *Continued*

	Vital Sign	*Rate*	*Comments*
			Take respirations for full minute. If above 60 or below 25/min., notify the physician.
II.	Heart Rate	Range of 100–180 beats/min.; at birth peak of 180/min.; within 30 min. drops to 120–140/min.§	Heart sounds resemble "toc-tic." The first heart sound is not as high in pitch or as sharp as the second. The two heart sounds should be clearly audible and well defined.
III.	Temperature	36.5–37° C (97.7–98.6° F)** normal range	Deviation from this range deserves consideration. Abdominal skin temperature is an indicator for internal thermal state. Therefore, best monitor is through the axillary method which reflects skin temperatures. Rectal temperature is misleading because it is often normal even with cold stress, becoming subnormal only after metabolic activity can no longer maintain a normal core temperature. When the rectal temperature does fall, it indicates failure in the compensatory mechanism of the body to maintain its core temperature.††

* Stave, U.: *Physiology of Perinatal Period, vol. 1.* Appleton-Century-Crofts, 1970, p. 223.

† McKilligan, H.: *The First Day of Life.* Springer, New York, 1970, p. 43.

‡ Avery, M. and Normand, C.: *Respiratory physiology in the newborn infant.* Anesthesiology 26:511, 1965.

§ Moore, M.: *The Newborn and the Nurse.* W. B. Saunders, Phildelphia, 1972, p. 81.

** *Standards and Recommendations for Hospital Care of Newborn Infants, ed. 5.* American Academy of Pediatrics, Evanston, Illinois, 1971, p. 89.

†† Korones, S.: *High Risk Newborn Infants: The Basis for Intensive Nursing Care.* C. V. Mosby, St. Louis, 1972, p. 63.

NURSING ACTIONS TO PROTECT AND NURTURE

The physical care given to the neonate focuses on actions to protect and nurture the newborn. Protective acts are those which *block* stimuli which can impose additional stress to extrauterine adaptation. Protective nursing acts are numerous immediately after birth and in the initial transition period. Nurturing acts are those which *help* the neonate to continue his adaptive state optimally. Nurturing nursing acts are numerous after the baby has achieved some degree of stabilization from birth. Protective and nurturing acts are not necessarily separate from each other. They interrelate in their effects to promote infant well-being. For example, the nursing plan for infant feeding serves to protect the infant from increased hypoglycemia as well as to nurture his daily caloric needs.

TRANSITIONAL CARE CONCEPT

Why should nurses protect and nurture the neonate? Recently, the *transitional care concept* emerged, fostering the attitude that newborns are analogous to postsurgical patients because delivery is accompanied by physiologic stresses, as with surgery.[19] Arnold and associates[20] strongly support the transitional care concept stating that routine care exposes the neonate to "limbo" or lost periods of attention during his first natal day when he is at highest risk. Remember, the neonate begins life with a period of intense activity, the first period of reactivity which lasts about 30 minutes after birth. This period is characterized by outbursts of purposeless movements, instability of respirations such as hyperventilation, transient flaring of the alae nasi, chest retractions, some grunting, and tachycardia as high as 180 beats per minute in the first three minutes.[21] After all this activity the neonate becomes quiet, unresponsive, and settles into a sleep which begins about two hours after birth and lasts from minutes to between two to four hours. This is almost an attempt by the neonate to "charge up his batteries" for a second period of reactivity which begins between four to six hours of life. Again the neonate is active and responsive to stimuli. His heart rate increases as he attempts to reorganize his various metabolic processes and organ functions for extrauterine survival. During this second period of reactivity there is a tendency for the infant to have periodic breathing (spells in which respiration ceases for seconds) and also an increase of mucus in his oral cavity.[22,23] Therefore, there is a need to protect the baby from prolonged apneic spells and from choking on the mucus he cannot rid by himself.

The transitional care concept promotes the attitude that newborns should be monitored as intensely as postsurgical patients. It suggests that newborns leave the delivery room and make a progression to various areas in the nursery which are prepared to best meet the needs presented by the baby. Progressive hospitals have created a transitional care area in their nurseries where newborns are admitted for close observation, similar to the recovery room for surgical patients. The purposes of such transitional care areas are to monitor the

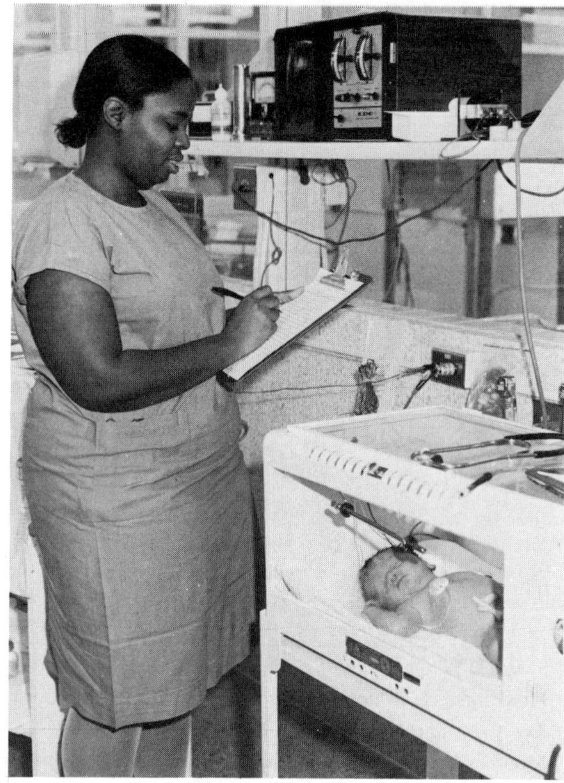

FIGURE 31-13. Nurse monitoring a neonate in the transitional nursery.

neonate's physiologic adjustments in extrauterine transition and to plan care in anticipation of any risks which might complicate the transitional process (Fig. 31-13). Thus, neonates can be closely watched and protected. The nurse is constantly ready to implement life-saving measures such as suctioning for mucus or stimulation to break transient periodic breathing.

When infants are stabilized and doing well, they are eventually transferred to rooming-in to be with mothers or to the central nursery. Other infants, depending upon the degree of stabilization, may be transferred to the intensive care area or remain for further observations to have their needs met.

Nurses working with neonates all begin their care with one priority action—hand washing. Before any contact with the neonate, proper hand washing must be done as a primary act to protect the baby. Too often the proper technique for hand washing is taken for granted or sacrificed. Because of its significance in protecting the neonate, a brief explanation of the technique as recommended by the Academy of Pediatrics[24] is presented.

Before washing, remove all jewelry and roll up sleeves above the elbows. A small amount of antiseptic preparation should be placed in the palm of the hands, and the hands, wrists, and forearms washed thoroughly up to the elbow. All areas should be lathered, including between fingers and lateral aspects. The initial wash upon entering the nursery should be a *minimum* of two minutes. A fifteen-second wash is required between handling of infants. A soft brush, which does not irritate the skin, should be used with the initial hand wash. Fingernails should be cleaned with a plastic or orange wood stick at this time. Hands should be thoroughly rinsed and dried. *Always remember to wash hands between babies.*

NURSING ACTIONS

The following is an outline of suggested nursing actions to protect and nurture the neonate. Actions are identified relevant to goals for specified periods in the extrauterine adaptation process. These actions are appropriate for the normal full-term neonate. Actions for infants at risk will be discussed in Chapter 38.

Period: Immediately after birth
Nature of Acts: Protective

Goal: Promote establishment and maintenance of respirations

Actions	*Rationale/Considerations*
1. Position infant briefly with head slightly lower than chest or in side-lying position.	Gravity facilitates drainage of mucus and amniotic fluid from naso-oral cavity
2. Suction nostrils and oropharynx with bulb syringe, De Lee trap.	Removes mucus to ensure patent airway. Gentle, brief suction preferred to long, vigorous activity which leaves the baby "airless." Hand devices preferred over machines which may have too much power for the infant's air volume.
3. Slap soles of the feet or rub the infant's back, without undue force.	Provides additional stimuli to aid institution of ventilation by promoting baby's crying.

Goal: Minimize loss of body heat associated with birth

Actions	*Rationale/Considerations*
1. Immediately wipe off amniotic fluid from entire body as quickly as possible with warm towel.	Immediate heat loss occurs through *evaporation* of amniotic fluid.
2. Place baby on padded warm surface instead of cold one without padding.	Reduces *conductive* loss which occurs via skin contact with cooler solid object.
3. Supply warmth from overhead heat-radiating device	Reduces *convective* loss by decreasing flow of cool surrounding air.
4. Locale of baby should not be up against delivery room walls.	Amount of heat lost by *radiation* varies inversely with the square distance between the infant and a cold object.[25]

Actions	*Rationale/Considerations*
5. Help baby to maintain a semi-flexed position.	Flexion of the extremities reduces heat loss by decreasing surface area exposed to the environment.
6. Transport baby rapidly and with warm covering (blankets). Position should be one of least exposure to the environment. Ideally infant should be in a covered conveyance.	Reduces heat lost by having infant covered and held snugly or in a conveyance which decreases exposure to cool surrounding air.

Goal: Collect pertinent data for initial assessment

Actions	*Rationale/Considerations*
1. Apgar scoring at one and five minutes. 2. Classify for birth weight, gestational age, intrauterine growth. 3. Do screening procedures to rule out anomalies (see text).	Procedures should be done only after the infant has established respirations successfully.

Goal: Institute prophylactic treatments against gonorrhea ophthalmia and hemorrhagic disorder

Actions	*Rationale/Considerations*
1. Give prophylactic treatment with 1% silver nitrate. The silver nitrate is the method recommended by law in most states. Instill one drop of silver nitrate into each conjunctival sac; it should remain in contact with the area for a minimum of 15 seconds.	Drug is effective against the gonorrhea bacillus which may have been present in maternal tissues. Antibiotic ointments are not recommended by the American Academy of Pediatrics as a method for prophylaxis because of the possibility of resistance to the antibiotic by certain strains of the gonococci.[26]
Saline rinses should not be used; use distilled water.	Saline may cause silver chloride precipitate which increases the tendency toward chemical conjunctivitis.[27]
2. Administer vitamin K, 0.5 to 1 mg. IM (Fig. 31-14).	Prevents hemorrhagic tendencies which result from lack of liver's production of clotting factors, dependent upon vitamin K for synthesis. Vitamin K is deficient because of lack of normal bacterial flora in intestines (due to gastric neutrality).

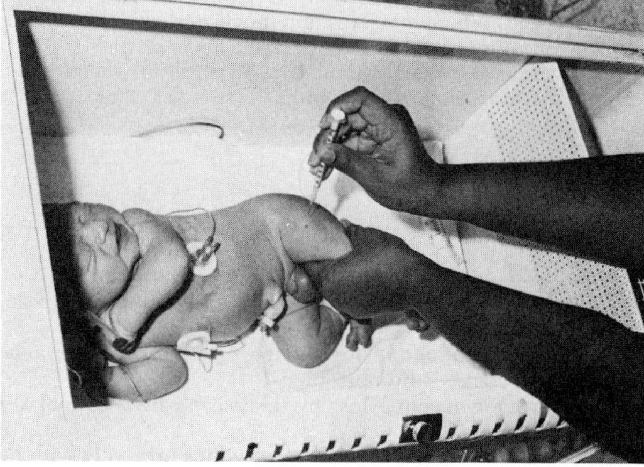

FIGURE 31-14. Nurse administering vitamin K, IM, in the lateral aspect of the thigh. Note how the leg is held securely.

Goal: Proper identification of the infant

Actions	*Rationale/Considerations*
1. Apply ID bands to wrist, ankles.	Besides insuring proper maternal-infant interaction, there are legal implications.
2. Take prints of infant's foot, palms, and fingers; also of mother's palms and fingers (if recommended by hospital policies).	Check ID's on baby and mother before leaving delivery room.
3. Prints are useless unless completely legible without smudges.	Easy removal of ink from infant's and mother's hands or feet can be done with petroleum jelly.
4. Always compare identification of mother and infant to ensure accuracy.	Unnecessary anxiety and stress can be generated when the wrong baby is brought to a mother.

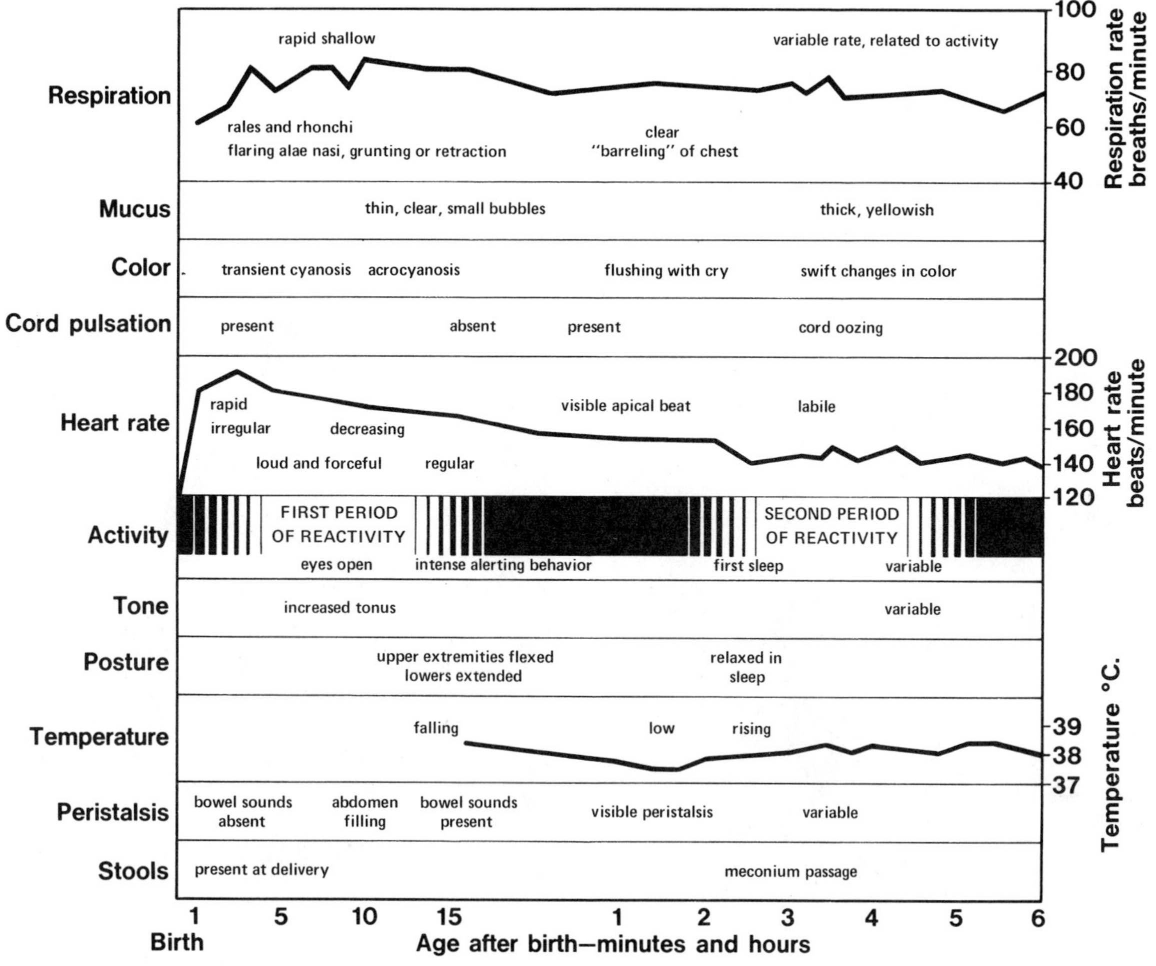

FIGURE 31-15. Graph illustrating fluctuations of activity and vital signs during the transitional period in the neonate.

Period: Transitional period
Minimum period of 6–8 hours with upper limits of 24 hours until condition stabilizes. After that time infant is transferred to appropriate area to meet his needs.
Nature of Acts: Protective and Nurturing

Goal: Primary goal is provision for continuous assessment through observations and routine screening procedures

Actions	*Rationale/Considerations*
1. Assess the neonate's physiologic and behavioral patterns during the transition period (Fig. 31-15). Check heart rate, respiratory rate and character, color, behavior, at intervals of 15–30 minutes the first hour, then every 1–2 hours until stable. (See Table 31-1 for norms of vital signs.)	Vital signs should be recorded and easily accessible for rapid general evaluation of physiologic adjustments.
2. Obtain other assessment data, if not previously done: classifications for gestational age, birth weight, length, chest-head circumference (Fig. 31-16).	Provides baseline norms for anticipation of risk.
3. All infants should be examined within the first 6–8 hours of life and before first feeding.[28]	

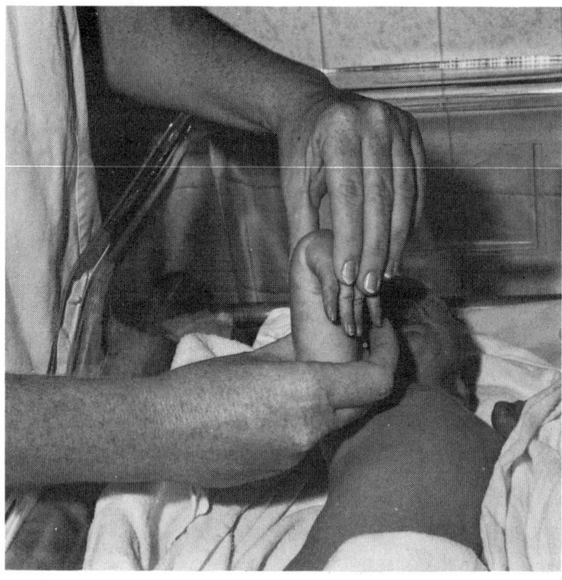

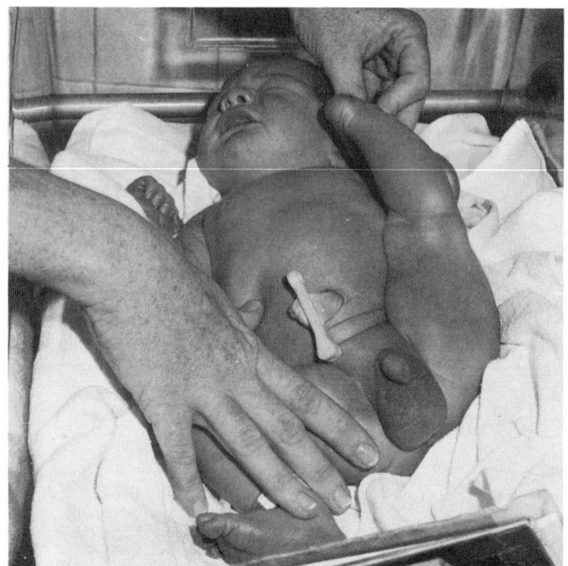

FIGURE 31-16. Nurse using the Dubowitz tool to estimate gestational age. *Left,* Square window sign. *Right,* Heel to ear maneuver.

Goal: Continue assessment for thermoregulation status

Actions	*Rationale/Considerations*
1. Immediate attention to body temperature a. Take initial temperature rectally. b. Provide warmth through mechanical devices or snuggling with warm blankets. c. Continue considerations of factors increasing heat loss through evaporation, conduction, convection, radiation.	Unessential procedures which expose the infant should be held until later with priority for providing body warmth. This decreases oxygen consumption which may be already taxed by trauma of birth.
2. Continued temperature regulation a. Axillary temperatures should be taken (after initial rectal temperature to assure anal patency). b. Use separate thermometer for each infant.	Routine rectal temperatures are not recommended as they predispose to rectal mucosa irritation. Axillary temperatures provide valuable data in terms of the body's compensatory mechanism to maintain thermoneutrality. Rectal temperature is a core temperature while axillary is a skin temperature. Heat is transferred from the core of the body to the skin in the body's heat regulatory system. Therefore, a decrease in axillary temperature allows time for successful management without undue harm while a fall in core temperature indicates failure in the body's compensatory heat regulation.[29]
c. Procedure: place thermometer in axilla by pressing the infant's arm gently, but tightly, against it and the side of the body for 3 minutes.	Taken properly, axillary temperatures are dependable.
d. Routine: minimum of every hour for the first 4 hours and every 4 hours in the first 24 hours.[30]	
e. Attention to deviations from 36.5–37° C (97.7–98.6° F).	Investigate for considerations relative to fever, cold stress, general deterioration, or thermal conditions in the environment.

Goal: Promote safeguards against infection

Actions	*Rationale/Considerations*
1. Constant attention to individual techniques a. Wash hands before and after infant and equipment handling (technique described previously). b. Care given in infant's own environmental area. 2. Limit contacts by various personnel in nursery area. 3. Organize nursing assignments to limit traffic and exposure of infant. 4. Respect institution's regimen for infection control through dress standards and screening of personnel.	Each infant should be handled as a potential source of infection and each infant's equipment should be considered an individual isolation unit.[31]

Goal: Initiate and evaluate feeding ability

Actions	*Rationale/Considerations*
1. Determine readiness for feeding by behaviors such as rooting and sucking, swallowing reflexes, hand to mouth activity, alertness.	Vital signs should be stable before feeding is attempted.
2. Give clear sterile water or dextrose water approximately 15–30 cc. from 4–6 hours after birth when found to be stable.	Water is usually given first before milk to check sucking reflex and loosen any mucus so it can be regurgitated. Sterile water, if aspirated, is least irritating to the lungs.
3. First milk intake should be approximately three to four minutes suckling time at the breast or between 30–50 cc. of formula.	The newborn's stomach capacity is approximately 30–60 cc.[32] and capable of much dilatation. Infants who are stable should not have feedings withheld for long periods simply because of routines since it predisposes to further hypoglycemia.

Period: Continued care after transition period (first three days of life)
Nature of Acts: Primarily to Nurture

Goal: Daily attention for general care

Actions	*Rationale/Considerations*
1. Continued observation for activity, appearance, color.	Specific attention for signs of jaundice; other significant signs indicative of risk are dyspnea, cyanosis, vomiting, hemorrhage, twitching, lethargy.
2. Care of the umbilical stump. Use of agents to promote drying such as alcohol, hexachlorophene, merthiolate. Simply swab the umbilical stump several times a day. Expose area to the air to enhance drying by positioning diaper below umbilicus.	When the cord is severed, it will necrose and dry primarily because of the lack of blood supply and the loss of Wharton's jelly which previously lubricated the vessels. The goal is to promote drying and prevent infection. The cord usually detaches or falls off between 5–8 days of life (or up until the second week of life).
Check area for any bleeding, excessive oozing, foul odor.	These signs are indicative of an unhealed stump promoting the possibility of infection. Oozing is most likely to occur within the first six hours of life, especially when the infant cries or passes meconium. Tub baths are not recommended until after the cord drops. Dressings over the cord are also undesirable as they prevent drying from exposure to the air.
3. Circumcision care a. Keep area clean, and observe for bleeding. b. Sterile gauze with petrolatum is applied over the raw surface during the first 24 hours. c. Keep infant off of abdomen for a few hours after the procedure.	Goal is to promote healing by keeping area clean and dry thereby eliminating a medium for bacterial growth. The petrolatum gauze should be changed after each voiding during the first day unless the physician has applied a gauze firmly and wishes it to remain on the site for 24 hours. Observe penis for bleeding frequently (hourly) and do not cover the area thickly with diapers. Position off the area to eliminate discomforts and pressure or friction from contact with bed clothing. Report bleeding promptly for treatment, frequently by controlled pressure or medicinal application such as adrenalin solution (1:1,000). Mothers need to be taught how to care for the circumcision after discharge; ideal to send the petrolatum gauze home with the baby if it is still being used.

Actions	*Rationale/Considerations*
4. Skin care	The skin is a protective covering, offering a line of defense to the body. In the newborn the skin is thin, delicate, tender, and easily irritated. Care must be taken to prevent breaks in its surface, leading to invasion by bacterial agents (infection).
5. Neonate's bath a. Use clean soft washcloth or cotton balls, and gentle wiping. Forcibly removing old blood or vernix caseosa by rubbing leads to irritation and possible skin breakdown.	Techniques may vary but basic principles must be valued. Examples are: prepare all necessary equipment before the procedure, ensure safety factors such as temperature of the environment and bath water, never leave infant alone, prevent undue exposure of the infant, start from cleanest areas using motions which will prevent re-entry of substances into cleaned areas.
b. Check pH of the soap, preferably use one that is neutral. Use of concentrated hexachlorophene is undesirable because of its tendency to cause skin irritation and brain damage if absorbed through the skin in significant quantity.	The average pH of the skin is below 5 between 2–24 weeks of age. Washing with substances with a higher pH, such as a value of 10, increases the pH of the skin; taking about 60 minutes for it to return to normal. The pH of the washing substance can therefore compromise the skin's acid-base balance.
c. Shampoo: use firm but gentle circular motions. A moderately firm scrub brush is ideal to prevent build-up of the scaling scalp which can predispose to cradle cap.	Attention to fontanels where scaly build-up is likely to occur. Should cradle cap occur, it can be treated by rubbing oil on the scalp to help loosen the scales and then brushing. Allow the oil to soak the scalp before brushing.
d. Face, eyes, and ears: wipe eyes and face with water only. Start with eyes wiping from inner area outward. Wipe nose and mouth area clean. Wipe outer ear and its entrance to the canal (not inside).	Eyes are wiped from inside outward to prevent dislodged mucus from re-entering the eye. A rule to remember is never place any object smaller than your elbow into orifices such as nostrils and ears. They have their own cleaning and protective systems such as the hair in the nares and the wax in the ears.
e. Neck: may be difficult to clean because of the many folds. Gently hyperextend the neck by positioning jaw forward or use object so infant can hyperextend voluntarily by fixation on the object.	Neck folds are good places for collection of substances. During warm weather such folds may predispose to heat rash (also folds in elbow and under the knee). Prickly heat rash usually starts around the neck and shoulders and spreads to other areas. It can be effectively controlled by dusting with cornstarch or making a paste with water and bicarbonate of soda to apply to the area. Prickly heat consists of minute pink pimples (tiny blisters may form on them) and is not harmful but may be uncomfortable for the infant and distressing to parents.
f. Torso and extremities: quick, efficient way to clean is use of your hands to soap and rinse.	Use of hands provides infant with stimulation directly from the human touch.
g. Genitals *Male babies*—clean the penis and substances which have accumulated. The foreskin can be gently retracted for cleaning.	Smegma (a secretion) may be formed and collected under the prepuce behind the glans penis. The foreskin of uncircumcised babies should be gently retracted and replaced immediately to prevent edema to the area.
Female babies—principles for adult hygiene should be used; wipe vaginal areas using one stroke, one cotton ball, in a front to back direction. The folds of the labia should be gently spread to remove accumulations of secretions.	Front to back strokes prevents reentry of substances into cleaned areas. Vaginal discharge, slight bleeding, and smegma must be cleansed.

Actions	Rationale/Considerations
h. Buttocks: keep clean and dry as possible. Do not rub area vigorously, rather use patting motions. Excessive use of powder is not recommended as it may lead to aspiration of powder and causes drying of the skin which predisposes to cracking and eventual skin breakdown.	Buttock area is susceptible to redness and skin breakdown because of contact with urine and feces. The ammonia in the urine and the nitrogen by-products in the stools cause acid reactions which predispose to diaper rash or skin breakdown.
If diaper rash occurs, use of protective ointments such as A and D ointment, petroleum jelly, or cornstarch may promote drying. If skin breakdown occurs, the use of zinc oxide, exposing the area to air, warm daylight or lamp treatments can promote healing.	Cornstarch sprinkled onto the area with a salt shaker is very effective in treating ordinary diaper rash. Do not use plastic pants when diaper rash occurs. If lamp treatments are used, be sure the screened bulb is no stronger than 40 watts and no closer than 12–16 inches from the exposed buttock. Such treatments should average 20 minutes and no longer than 30 minutes. Mothers need to be told that care in washing diapers can reduce bacteria causing ammonia dermatitis (diaper rash). Simple facts are to use *hot* (boiling) water, thorough rinses, use antibacterial agents such as vinegar or Borateem, and dry in *hot* dryers or direct sunshine. Sunshine is very effective in destroying bacteria.
6. Attention to weight curve: weights taken every day to determine gain or loss should be done in a systematic manner. a. Prepare scale with fresh cover for each infant. b. Balance scale properly. c. Avoid chilling caused by undue exposure of the infant. d. Protect infant from injury by keeping one hand over the infant while on the scales.	There is a 5–6% weight loss in the first few days of life, primarily due to water loss associated with the high metabolic rates, obligatory losses via the skin and pulmonary activities, and the larger surface area of the newborn which increases water loss through evaporation. Weight loss above 10% predisposes the infant to dehydration leading to water-electrolyte imbalances.[15]
7. Attention to stool patterns:	Stool patterns involve changes in consistency, color, odor, frequency, depending upon food intake.
First stools are *meconium*—dark greenish to black, sticky, odorless. Persists for 3 days.	Meconium consists of secretions which have accumulated in gastrointestinal tract in utero: epithelial and epidermal cells, lanugo, and bile pigments are the components.
Transitional Stools: changes to greenish-brown eventually becoming greenish yellow about the third to fourth day.	Ingestion of milk changes the color.
Subsequent stool pattern is dependent upon the type of food ingested: *Breast-Fed:* Color: bright, golden yellow; at times, light greenish Consistency: unformed but not watery; soft (mushy) Frequency: initially less than formula-fed babies; one or two a day, but increases to more than four a day by second week Odor: aromatic, sweet smelling *Formula-Fed:* Color: pale yellow or yellowish-white Consistency: more formed, firmer Frequency: initially more frequent and regular than breast-fed babies, but declines to about three a day in the second week Odor: foul smelling	Abnormal stool patterns are: no stools within 48 hours—indicative of intestinal obstruction. Meconium passed but no other stools—indicative of obstruction in the ileum. Thick, putty-like meconium—indicative of meconium ileus, an early symptom of cystic fibrosis. Diarrhea—indicative of gastroenteritis or overfeeding. Bloody stools—bright red or tarry (old blood) stools are indicative of intestinal bleeding. Flecks of blood may be due to an anal fissure.

Actions	*Rationale/Considerations*
Changes in color are also related to treatments: a. Receiving iron—stools darker and firmer b. Under bililight—stools bright green c. Receiving gentian violet for thrush—stools faintly purple	
8. Maintain adequate nutritional intake: promote feeding method of choice by considering the following:	
a. Breast-fed neonate—see Chapter 28 for nursing actions to help the mother. Consider flexible feeding schedules so infant may eat when ready (demand feeding).	The principle of "supply and demand" states that maximum milk production increases with frequent and/or complete emptying of the breast. This provides the rationale for demand feeding so the infant can maximally empty the breast, thereby increasing production and maintaining adequate supply for intake.
b. Formula-fed neonate—consider the following with use of ready-to-eat formulas: (1) Store in cool place, at room temperature; does not need prewarming. (2) Use within four hours after bottle opened. (3) Do not reuse disposable equipment.	Most hospitals currently use prepared formula because it is less expensive than maintaining a formula division.
Considerations regarding the technique for bottle-feeding:	
(1) Baby in semi-upright position. Neck of bottle filled with milk.	Facilitates entry of contents into the stomach by gravity. Decreases the amount of air entering the stomach during feeding.
(2) Be sure tongue is down when inserting nipple into mouth.	To allow sucking and swallowing reflex to participate in feeding.
(3) Burp during feeding and after by holding infant upright, over the shoulders or sitting with back and neck supported straightforward.	This position allows air to reach a free passage out of stomach.
(4) Quality and amount of feeding should meet the minimum requirements for the neonate. (See Chapter 17 for discussion.)	

REFERENCES

1. Korones, S., Lancaster, J. and Roberts, F.: *High Risk Newborn Infants.* C. V. Mosby, St. Louis, 1972, pp. 50–53, 62, 92–94.
2. *Standards and Recommendations for Hospital Care of Newborn Infants.* American Academy of Pediatrics, Evanston, Illinois, 1971.
3. Korones: op. cit.
4. Gleiss, J. and Stuttgen, G.: *Morphologic and functional development of the skin.* In Stave, U. (ed.): *Physiology of Perinatal Period, vol. 2.* Appleton-Century-Crofts, New York, 1970, pp. 892–900.
5. Korones: op. cit.
6. Ibid.
7. Finnerud, C. W. and Webster, J. R.: In *Brenneman's Practice of Pediatrics, vol. IV.* W. F. Prior Co., Hagerstown, Maryland, pp. 10–15.
8. Gleiss: op. cit.
9. *The Skin, number one of a series on variations and minor departures in normal infants.* Produced by Mead Johnson Laboratories, Evansville, Indiana, 1968.
10. Gleiss: op. cit.
11. *The Eyes, number three of a series on variations and minor departures in normal infants.* Produced by Mead Johnson Laboratories, Evansville, Indiana, 1968.
12. Walton, D.: *The visual system.* In Stave, U. (ed.): *Physiology of the Perinatal Period, vol. 2.* Appleton-Century-Crofts, New York, 1970, pp. 875–886.
13. Clausen, J., et al.: *Maternity Nursing Today.* McGraw-Hill, New York, 1973, p. 694.
14. Prechtl, H. and Beintema, D.: *The Neurological Examination of the Full Term Newborn Infant.* The Spastics Society Medical Education, London, 1964, p. 25.
15. Ibid.
16. Ibid.

17. Arnold, H., et al.: *Transition to extra-uterine life.* Am. J. Nurs. 65:77, 1965.
18. Walton: op. cit.
19. Korones: op. cit.
20. Arnold et al.: op. cit.
21. Ibid.
22. Ibid.
23. McKilligan, H.: *The First Days of Life.* Springer, New York, 1970, p. 43.
24. *Standards and Recommendations for Hospital Care of Newborn Infants.* op. cit.
25. Korones: op. cit.
26. *Standards and Recommendations for the Hospital Care of Newborn Infants,* op. cit.
27. Pierog, S. and Ferrara, A.: *Approach to the Medical Care of the Sick Newborn.* C. V. Mosby, St. Louis, 1971, pp. 68, 73.
28. Ibid.
29. Korones: op. cit.
30. *Standards and Recommendations for the Hospital Care of Newborn Infants,* op. cit.
31. Ibid.
32. Smith, D.: *The Physiology of the Newborn Infant.* Charles C Thomas, Springfield, Illinois, 1975, p. 363.
33. Gleiss: op. cit.

BIBLIOGRAPHY

Chamberlain G., and Banks, J.: *Assessment of the Apgar Score.* Lancet 2:1225, 1974.

Cozen, L.: *Orthopedic examination of the infant and child.* American Family Physician 4:60, 1971.

Crelin, E.: *Functional Anatomy of the Newborn.* Yale University Press, New Haven, 1973.

Dahm, L. and James, L.: *Newborn temperature and a calculated heat loss in the delivery room.* Pediatrics 49:504, 1972.

Davies, P., et al.: *Medical Care of Newborn Babies.* Spastics International Medical Publications, London, 1972.

Desmond, M., Arnold, R. and Phitaksphraiwan, P.: *Transitional Care Nursery.* Pediatr. Clin. North Am. 13:651, 1966.

Dubowitz, L., Dubowitz, V. and Goldberg, C.: *Clinical assessment of gestational age in the newborn infant.* J. Pediatr. 77:1, 1970.

Eoff, M., Meier, R. and Miller, C.: *Temperature measurements in infants.* Nurs. Res. 23:457, 1974.

Gevers, R. and Ruys, J.: *Physiology and Pathology in the Perinatal Period.* Springer-Verlag, New York, 1971.

Keay, A.: *Craig's Care of the Newly Born Infant.* Churchill, London, 1974.

Leeuwen, G.: *A Manual of Newborn Medicine.* Year Book Medical Publishers, Chicago, 1973.

Lockman, L.: *Neurological assessment in the first year of life.* Postgrad. Med. 50:80, 1971.

Long, G.: *Toweling newborn babies.* J. Pediatr. 75:157, 1969.

Lubchenco, L.: *Assessment of gestational age and development at birth.* Pediatr. Clin. North Am. 17:125, 1970.

McKilligan, H. R.: *The First Days of Life.* Springer, New York, 1970.

McLean, F. H.: *Significance of birth weight for gestational age in identifying infants at risk.* J. Obstet. Gynecol. Nurse 3:19, 1974.

Mingeot, R. and Herbaut, M.: *The functional status of the newborn infant. A study of 5,370 consecutive infants.* Am. J. Obstet. Gynecol. 115:1138, 1973.

Moorc, M. L.: *The Newborn and the Nurse.* W. B. Saunders, Philadelphia, 1972.

Motil, K., Blackburn, M. and Pleasure, J.: *The effects of four different radiant warmer temperature set-points used for rewarming neonates.* J. Pediatr. 85:546, 1974.

O'Doherty, N. and Zinkin, P.: *A routine neurological examination for the full-term newborn infant.* Proc. R. Soc. Med. 64:476, 1971.

Papadatos, C., et al.: *Immunoglobulin levels and gestational age.* Biologia Neonatorum 14:365, 1969.

Prechtl, H. and Beintema, D.: *The Neurological Examination of the Full Term Newborn Infant.* W. S. Heinmann Medical Books, New York, 1964.

Reed, B.: *Management of the infant during labor, delivery, and the immediate neonatal period.* Nurs. Clin. North Am. 6:3, 1971.

Roberts, J.: *Suctioning the newborn.* Am. J. Nurs. 73:63, 1973.

Slumek, M.: *Screening newborns for hearing loss.* Nursing Outlook 19:115, 1971.

Smith, C. A.: *The Physiology of the Newborn Infant.* Charles C Thomas, Springfield, Illinois, 1959.

Smith, R.: *Temperature monitoring and regulation.* Pediatr. Clin. North Am. 16:643, 1969.

Stave, U. (ed.): *Physiology of the Perinatal Period, vols. I & II.* Appleton-Century-Crofts, New York, 1970.

Webb, C. H.: *Evaluation of the routine physical examination of infants in the first year of life.* Pediatrics 45:960, 1970.

Whitner, W. and Thompson, M.: *The influence of bathing on the newborn infant's body temperature.* Nurs. Res. 19:30, 1970.

32 *Psychosocial Concepts*

DYANNE D. AFFONSO, R.N., M.N.

This chapter discusses psychosocial influences in the development of the newborn into a distinct individual. This is an exciting area to explore as it is relatively new in its development and many interesting conclusions are emerging from numerous research findings. The following content reflects a synthesis of the available literature beginning with the impact of prenatal influences and continuing on to an investigation of the neonate's interactional adaptation with its environment.

PRENATAL INFLUENCES

What determines what a baby will be like? It was once commonly accepted that human life began with birth. The nine-month interval between conception and delivery was largely neglected as being significant in human development. However, Montagu emphasizes the importance of intrauterine events and their influences on postnatal development:

> From the moment of conception until delivery nine months later, the human being is more susceptible to his environment than he ever will be again.[1]

> The human gestational period . . . of the earliest experience is truly fundamental, foundational, since it is during this time that we are made into the organism which makes its appearance at birth and develops afterward.[2]

The reader is referred to Montagu's book for a discussion on the effects of various stimuli (e.g., nutrition, maternal age, drugs, smoking, etc.) on prenatal and postnatal life. For the purpose of relating psychosocial concepts, this section highlights two variables, maternal age and maternal emotions.

MATERNAL AGE

The chronologic age of a woman is not as significant to prenatal and postnatal life as her biologic age. This refers to the woman's reproductive capacity reflected in the prerequisites for reproduction, i.e., ovulation and maintenance of a fertilized egg within the uterus. The following is a generalized classification by Montagu[3] on maternal age effects:

1. Ages 23± to 29: This is viewed as the optimum developmental period for reproduction. The largest proportion of healthy outcome from pregnancy occurs at this time.
2. Ages below 23: This is the period between the establishment of menstruation and optimum reproductive capacity. It is characterized by physiologic efforts to

regulate ovulation and the uterine environment through hormonal secretions. It is viewed as a time of reproductive inefficiency and thus, any fetus developing in such a climate is at a disadvantage.

3. Ages above 28, especially above 35: Risk factors increase due primarily to deterioration of the hormonal regulation to provide an optimum environment to nurture the development of the egg and endometrial growth.

What about effects from the father's age? Paternal age does not significantly affect fetal and neonatal development, primarily because the reproductive capacity of the male continues (even beyond 70 years), as contrasted to reproductive capacity terminating in the mid-forties for females.

MATERNAL EMOTIONS

Throughout history, folklore has implied that the pregnant woman's emotional state can affect her unborn baby. Studies to determine if such a relationship does exist have revealed interesting findings which appear to indicate the following:

1. Maternal emotions can modify fetal and neonatal behaviors.
2. Maternal emotions can affect the uterus, sometimes jeopardizing the pregnancy.
3. Maternal emotions can contribute to malformations.

It is worthwhile to explore the contributing factors to the above effects.

Relationship to Fetal and Neonatal Behaviors

It is speculated from numerous studies that a possible relationship exists between maternal emotional disturbance (e.g., anxiety, tension) and hyperirritability in the fetus and newborn.

Whitehead, as early as 1867, wrote the following in a description of a case of convulsions in the fetus of a mother experiencing stress.

> Severe physical shocks such as falling from a height may leave the fetus unperturbed and unharmed. But it seems otherwise . . . when the mental system of the mother becomes unbalanced by violent and sudden shocks of anguish or by prolonged and severe anxiety. . . .[4]

Sontag, who has made extensive contributions to the study of maternal-fetal emotional interactions, states:

> Deeply disturbed maternal emotions produce a marked increase in the activity of the fetus, probably as a result of increased adrenalin level in the maternal and therefore, fetal blood.[5]

> After birth these infants remain irritable and hyperactive for weeks or months. They cried a great deal, slept for short periods only. There appeared also to be an autonomic or psychosomatic component of such behaviors as expressed in gastro-intestinal functions. Most infants exhibited a food intolerance, cardiospasm and frequent loose stools. They failed to gain weight for a long period. They burn more of their food supply for energy and store less as fat and possibly even as muscle.[6]

Sontag, from his research, makes two interesting speculations. First, infants from emotionally-stressed pregnancies do not have adequate response patterns to negotiate successfully with their environment and thus are more susceptible to neurosis.[7] Second, such infants become children who exhibit unstable behaviors and manifest functional disturbances (especially of the gastrointestinal system).[8] Sontag's views are supported by other studies which demonstrated signs of restlessness, excessive crying, irritability, vomiting, and loose stools in infants whose mothers were emotionally stressed during pregnancy[9] and demonstrated attitudes of rejection toward their pregnancy.[10]

What is the mode through which maternal emotions exert behavioral changes in the infant? The primary mechanism is the neurohumoral system. There are reciprocal secretions from both maternal and fetal endocrine functioning which come into contact with each other through the placental circulation system. This results in a "common endocrine pool," the neurohumoral bond.[11] Emotional states such as stress and tension are accompanied by the release of hormones and chemical substances, primarily cortisone compounds and adrenalin. An excess of these acts upon the body to elicit physical manifestations such as dilation or constriction of muscles and blood vessels. Bodily patterns can also be disturbed as seen in increased respiratory rates in the fetus. The neurohumoral bond is responsible for the physical manifestations observed in the baby.

Relationship to Uterus

There appears to be a relationship between stress and hyperirritability of the uterus, causing it to abort its contents. The uteri of habitual aborters have been found to be hypersensitive to emotional stimuli, causing contractions to be easily initiated.[12] One study made an interesting correlation between emotional stress and an antigen-antibody reaction in tissue cell metabolism which caused an interference with the maintenance of gestation.[13]

Relationship to Congenital Malformations

In a study examining the relationship between stress and the incidence of cleft palate in human infants, Strean and Peer concluded:

> It is possible and perhaps probable, that two factors operate in the production of this congenital abnormality—genic activity and stress. One operating without the other may be unable to produce cleft palate. . . . Severe emotional stress, particularly when associated with hyperemesis, appears to have been the most important single factor. Stressor agents are known to influence adrenal cortical activity. . . . Excess of this hormone (hydrocortisone) inhibits fibroblastic proliferation and produces histochemical changes in collagen fibers.[14]

Fibroblastic and collagen activities are essential components in the formation of bone (palate).

In summation, there appears to be strong support from research findings that the pregnant woman's emotional state can influence the maintenance of gestation, affect a newborn's activity level, and predispose the fetus to anomalies.

PSYCHOANALYTIC MEANING OF BIRTH

Psychoanalytic theories view birth as a traumatic life experience, the impact of which affects the newborn's later development. This viewpoint focuses on the interrelationship among the concepts of sensory alteration, loss, and anxiety. Psychoanalytic theories propose the following theme: the events associated with birth involve a state of sensory overcharge or bombardment of stimuli to the fetus (Fig. 32-1). The emergence from the maternal uterus creates feelings of loss for the security and tranquility of intrauterine life. Such sensory overload and suffering from intrauterine loss create feelings of helplessness which lead to the first cause for anxiety in human existence. Here is a closer examination of each component in this theme.

Sensory overload to the fetus and neonate at birth arises from two major factors: 1) preparation for birth through descent into the pelvic cavity and passage through the birth canal, and 2) mandatory physiologic adjustments to be

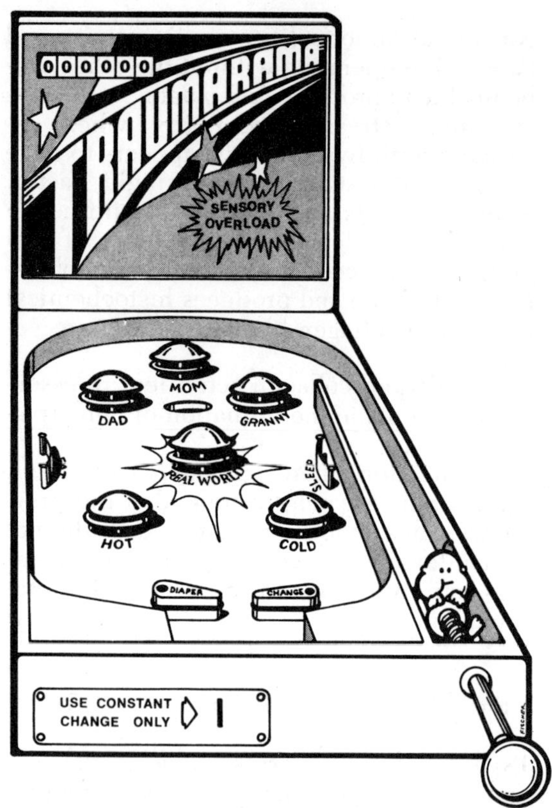

FIGURE 32-1. Psychoanalytic theories view birth as a life experience thrusting the individual into a state of sensory bombardment. (Cartoon by Dave Fisher, Arizona Medical Center A-V Division, Tucson, Arizona.)

made by the neonate at birth to sustain life activities previously performed by the maternal-placental system. A feeling of loss is predicted to occur with birth and is related to the fetus' severance from the maternal womb. Intrauterine existence is characterized by stability; temperature, pressures, and movements are all within a constant, predictable range. In contrast, birth thrusts the baby into an environment in which the only constant is change. According to Rank, this experience of loss associated with birth results in a tremendous psychic shock:

> The whole of later existence becomes a reaction to extrauterine suffering and loneliness and every pleasure has as its final aim the re-establishment of intrauterine primal bliss.[15]

The separation from the mother through birth is speculated to precipitate feelings of apprehension and helplessness, giving rise to the first anxiety experienced in life.[16,17]

To some readers this discussion on the psychoanalytic meaning of birth may appear too extreme. Such theories are presented to stimulate thought about the differing impact on human development which can emerge from an experience common to all men—birth. It should be stated that psychoanalytic theories do not always predict an outcome of despair for the future development of the individual. Some infants emerge successfully from the trauma of birth through adaptive behaviors acquired through interactions with their environment (primarily the parents). Those who are unsuccessful in adaptation usually manifest some degree of neurosis as adults.

THE PROCESS OF INTERACTIONAL ADAPTATION

It was once theorized that the newborn emerged into the world as an "empty slate" with limited or no capacity to exert any influence on its environment. The infant was viewed as a passive recipient of stimuli with total dependence on its environment. However, this theory has been greatly challenged. Studies have demonstrated the significance of the prenatal environment[18,19] as well as the presence of perceptual capacities in the infant from the moment of birth.[20–22] The newborn was observed to respond to and discriminate stimuli, thus influencing which stimuli will be reinforced or extinguished.[23] The newborn was also observed to have the capacity to manifest social responses (smiling) very early in life.[24] Thus emerged the significance of obtaining knowledge about the process by which the newborn will interact and thereby adapt to its environment. The process of *interactional adaptation* is defined as *the active participation by the newborn to orient and acquaint itself with the environment, working to establish a social relationship with others and eventually distinguish itself as a separate entity.* Thus, the process contributes to the early formation of the ego.

The process is also supported by a feedback mechanism necessary for its maintenance. The infant's responses to environmental stimuli must be reinforced or such behavioral reactions will diminish. Such infant responses also become feedback for the continuity or termination of input from the environment (such as from the mother).

It is beyond the scope of this book to present all aspects of interactional behaviors seen in infants. Because the focus of this chapter is the neonatal period, the discussion will be limited to the exploration of interactional patterns during the first four to five weeks of life. Specifically, the following areas will be explored because of their relevance to the role of nursing:

1. How the neonate derives and processes information from its environment.
2. Contributing factors which stimulate the neonate to interact with the environment.
3. Factors influencing the neonate's participation in the acquaintance process (primarily with its mother).

How the Neonate Derives and Processes Information from the Environment

The neonate can see, hear, smell, and feel from the moment it arrives in the world. Thus, the baby is not passive but is a sensory-active human being.

Through its senses, the neonate processes information or stimuli. This involves both the perceptual capacity to receive stimuli, or input, and the capacity to elicit behavioral reactions to the stimuli, known as output. The neonate must be able to recognize, attend, and discriminate stimuli. Then there must be an ability to manifest behavioral responses. Here is a brief overview of the behavioral capacities in the neonate revealing the ability to perceive stimuli and react to them.

Visual alertness has been demonstrated through such abilities as to fixate on an object, track it briefly (follow it), and distinguish preference for patterns and contour.[25,26] It should be noted that in the early weeks of life an infant is able to focus clearly on objects that are eight or nine inches from the eyes.[27] Visual alertness is very important in neonatal behavioral development for two reasons. First, it enables the neonate to explore its environment, and second, it is an important prerequisite for eliciting social responses in the very early phases of life. Eye-to-eye contact is important in the development of social interchange between parent and offspring, as it is in adult communications.[28]

Other sensory capacities are active in the neonate. Definite responses were observed to various auditory stimuli (bell, bird whistle, human voices) within the first week of life.[29] The neonate was also observed to respond to an odor as well as to discriminate it from other odors as early as the first few days of life.[30] Infants were shown to be sensitive to tactile stimulation within the four-day lying-in period (hospital stay).[31]

Sensory capacities in the newborn are not limited to reception of stimuli but extend to discrimination (preference) for various stimuli. Preferences in visual stimuli were observed as early as 48 hours after birth.[32] The neonate clearly preferred stimuli containing patterns or contour, color, and solid objects (as opposed to flat ones). The favor for patterns was especially marked for that of a human face. A crucial factor in visual preference up to about two months of age was movement.[33] Preference in auditory stimuli was also observed, notably for a "high-pitched human voice."[34] Discriminating responses to olfactory stimuli also occurred within the first four days of life when the baby was able to distinguish disguised mixtures of odors, making similar responses to odors with common ingredients.

These discriminating abilities in the neonate are very important in behavioral development. Such capacity allows the baby to exert an influence on its environment. The infant has a say as to the type of stimuli it wants to receive. The infant's reactions to a stimulus (indicating pleasure or displeasure) will affect the environment in terms of providing feedback, either reinforcement or not for the stimulus. Such feedback affects the neonate's (and others') *choice* for subsequent behaviors. Note the word choice for it implies that behavioral responses can determine whether the stimuli will be continued, changed, or terminated. Bowlby describes this further:

> Thus, owing to the selective sensitivity with which a baby is born, different sorts of behaviors are elicited by different sorts of stimuli and much more attention is paid to some parts of the environment than to other parts . . . some sorts of behavioral sequence are rapidly augmented (reinforced) whilst other sequences are rapidly diminished (habituated).[36]

Factors Which Stimulate the Neonate to Interact with the Environment

This section explores the factors which can stimulate the neonate's potential for interactive behaviors. The literature appears to identify three main theories suggesting how the newborn can be stimulated to interact with the environment. These are: 1) exploratory behaviors, 2) infant-state, and 3) basic drives or needs.

Exploratory Behaviors

The capacity for searching the environment by looking is viewed as the most prominent activity of the newborn during its waking hours; "the newborn looks as a response to most stimuli such as sounds, movement or positional changes."[37] Gesell described the infant as "picking up the environment with his eyes alone at a time of its development when exploration was not possible by motor ability."[38] Fantz adds support to the importance of visual exploration by stating that the newborn's capacity to resolve, organize, and discriminate visual stimuli directs its motivation (desire or initiative) to explore its surroundings.[39] Schaffer states that curiosity, arousal seeking, exploratory drives (call it what you like) is one of the most important attributes with which a child comes into the world.[40]

Attentive behaviors in the neonate are accompanied by decreased heart rate, respiratory rate, and motor activity.[41] It is generally agreed that the most stimulating input to arouse attentive behaviors comes from the human subject, especially the human face.[42–44] The human face is attended to for significantly longer periods than any other visual stimulus.[45] The rationale for this is expressed by Rheingold:

> If one analyzes the social object, the human being . . . one is struck by its extraordinarily high stimulating qualities. Visually, the human face is bright, parts of it shine, it has contour and complexity. It moves almost constantly, bringing stimulus change with every movement. It produces sound. The human body offers tactile stimulation. Above all, the social object moves in response to the infant's own movements. The human being is but another complex of stimuli, but because he is living, he is more interesting, and because he is human, he is more responsive.[46]

One additional note: as with adults, the newborn will become bored with the repetition of the same stimulus. The stimulus will come to lose its effectiveness to elicit a response, a process called habituation. However, if the stimulus is withheld for an interval, it again will have eliciting powers when reintroduced. This is regarded as a very important aspect of the learning process in early life.

Infant-State

This is also referred to as the infant's state of behavior. It pertains to the various levels of tension or perceptual arousal in the neonate's behavior, reflecting both his need and availability for contact with the external environment.[47] Infant-state is viewed as a variable which determines the effectiveness and range of interactions the infant will have with his environment.[48] The significance of infant-state on the neonate's interactional patterns is expressed by Brazelton:

> His use of state to maintain control of his reactions to environmental and internal stimuli is an important mechanism and reflects his potential for organization.[49]

Various authors have defined and described infant-states into such categories as differential sleep patterns (irregular, disturbed, deep), alert levels (alert, focused, reactive, non-alert), and differential crying behaviors.[50,51]

The infant's response to a stimulus will differ depending upon the state of the infant when the stimulus is received. For example, the presence or absence of visual and auditory pursuit movements is greatly affected by whether the infant is crying, sleeping, or alert. Also, responses to auditory stimuli during sleep will resemble startle movements as contrasted to eyes widened (as if to listen) when the stimulus is received during an alert state. It is important to note that variations in infant-state can occur from environmental input. An infant's state of behavior can be manipulated to make him more susceptible to interact with the environment. Studies have demonstrated that the infant's state of behavior to explore his environment can be activated by the attentiveness of his mother, as well as specific aspects in maternal care involving physical contact between the mother and infant.[52,53] One study revealed an interesting finding that vestibular stimulation, such as changing an infant's position to being held upright, greatly increased visual attention in the neonate.[54]

Another interesting factor in infant-state concerns consolability, described as the degree to which an infant in an upset (crying) state could quiet himself or be quieted by some external stimulus.[55] Consolability has relevance to interactive behaviors because a crying infant cannot attend to a stimulus and prepare itself for interaction with the environment. Studies have investigated how the following stimuli can elicit soothing effects on the neonate: oral pacification,[56] visual attention to a stimulus,[57] and rhythmic tactile stimulation such as tapping, rubbing, and rocking.[58]

The importance of infant-state is emphasized by Rosenthal:

> The importance of infant-state in the process of interaction is far from being trivial and more research is needed on the role it plays in infant-environmental interaction.[59]

Basic Drives or Needs

The main theme here is that biologic needs evoke stimuli and in the process of receiving gratification for such needs, the infant also receives stimuli to arouse his interactive behaviors. The most frequent illustration relates to the instinctual drive of hunger. All babies must eat and the ingestion of food gratifies the hunger need. However, in the process of sucking the breast or bottle, more than hunger satisfaction occurs. The baby can be exposed to a multitude of stimuli at the same time (depending upon the feeding technique, baby's position, and mother's behaviors). Stimuli arise mainly from direct contact. Tactile contact can come from the baby touching mother as well as the mother touching the baby. Visual contact can occur with the mother looking at the baby and the baby looking back. Auditory contact occurs when the mother talks to the baby during the feeding time. Thus, the feeding situation is a good opportunity by which the infant's perceptual and exploratory behaviors can be activated. The best stimuli are present: the human face, voice, and touch. The infant should be positioned in such a manner that contact through visual, auditory, and tactile means is possible. Mothers need to be aware that feeding times are also opportunities by which the infant can gain more than just hunger satisfaction.

There is another important development which occurs during the feeding situation. It is called *anticipatory orientation* and is the anticipation by the infant of coming into contact with a stimulus (mouth to breast or bottle), observable as early as the fourth feeding.[60] At first, a baby's anticipatory movements are elicited not by the sight of the bottle or breast, but by the tactile and/or proprioceptive (kinesthetic) stimuli received when placed in the nursing position.[61] Proprioceptive or kinesthetic stimuli refer to stimulation of the muscles, joints, and ligaments when in the nursing position. This anticipation orientation is viewed as an important precursor to the concept of the ability to wait. The ability to wait is regarded as significant in ego development, whereby the infant will distinguish itself from the environment and gain confidence that his needs will be satisfied.[62]

The need for stimulation of the sense modalities has been viewed as part of the infant's repertoire of instinctual drives. Satisfaction of such drives always requires some kind of interaction with the environment. Its significance on later ego development is described below:

> The satisfactions of a number of needs are often experienced together and hence become linked. In the course of associating outside processes with need satisfaction there begins to develop in the baby the possibility of identifying or recognizing that there is something outside him as compared to something just inside.[63]

The above discussion has shown the critical role of stimuli from the environment to evoke or arouse the neonate's behavioral potential to interact with his environment. Evoking-type stimuli are noted to raise the infant's level of general responsiveness and it is reasonable to assume that the highly responsive infant is in active interaction with his environment.[64] Such a highly responsive infant is able to exhibit a variety of behaviors and thereby maximize his amount of stimuli input. Thus, the evoking or arousal quality of a stimulus makes a very important contribution to infant learning. When an infant is aroused and responsive, he is in a position to receive potent reinforcing stimuli provided by the environment's responses to him. One word of caution is necessary. Effects from excessive, continuous, and repetitive stimulations must be considered. Research findings indicate that overstimulating can lead to regression;[65] repetitive stimulations lead to habituation thereby inhibiting the learning process;[66] and continuous stimulation has no significant impact in arousing an infant's interactive behaviors.[67] Thus, in the provision of stimuli for the purpose of arousing the infant's behaviors, consideration must be given to the preferential status of the stimulus, its frequency, variety, and pattern in the input scheme.

How the Neonate Participates in the Acquaintance Process

In Chapter 29 the mother-infant interaction was discussed primarily from the viewpoint of the mother's role in the process. Interaction implies a two-way interchange, involving changing patterns of mutual stimuli-input and responses-output by both mother and baby. The responses of each to the behaviors of the other provides the feedback necessary to maintain or terminate future interactions. Thus, an examination of what each party brings to an interaction is necessary, and this section is the counterpart to the discussion in Chapter 29. For too long the emphasis has been on the mother because the infant was viewed as a passive recipient of maternal care. What the infant brings to the mother-infant relationship, what he represents from the very start, is frequently overlooked.[68]

That the infant indeed participates in the interaction process toward developing a social relationship was observed by Ainsworth:

> I was struck by the active part the baby himself plays in the development of attachment. All of (his) behaviors show initiative. . . . The striking part played by the infant's own activity in attachment lead me to the hypothesis that it is largely through his own activity that the child becomes attached, rather than through stimulation, or through passive satisfaction of creature comfort needs.[69]

The process by which an infant develops a relationship or attachment first to his mother and then to others is complex, consisting of various phases and extending beyond the neonatal period. Interaction in the early phases of life is a result of exploration of both infant and mother, as each orients to the other. Since this chapter focuses on the neonatal period of life, the following discussion highlights how interaction is facilitated by exploratory behaviors.

The Acquaintance Phase

Before any interchange can occur between two individuals, they must acquaint themselves with each other. Acquaint means to gain knowledge about or to familiarize oneself with the characteristics of an object or person. The neonate possesses various behaviors which help him to orient and respond to others. Exploratory behavior by the infant is viewed as important an activity as eating,[70] and provides the foundation for social responsiveness in human life.[71]

Let us examine the infant's exploratory behaviors. Bowlby[72] states that the behavioral equipment which helps the baby to acquaint to its mother, takes three main forms:

1. Perceptual equipment: Activation of the sense organs so the infant can sample and familiarize itself with the stimulus (such as mother).
2. Effector equipment: Helps the infant to establish and maintain contact to obtain more information about the stimulus.
3. Signalling equipment: A form of early communication the infant employs to bring his mother to him. This has profound effects upon the mother's subsequent reactions to the baby.

Perceptual equipment (Fig. 32-2)

It has already been shown that the infant processes environmental stimuli through keen selective sensitivity. How does this sensitivity promote acquaintance of baby with mother?

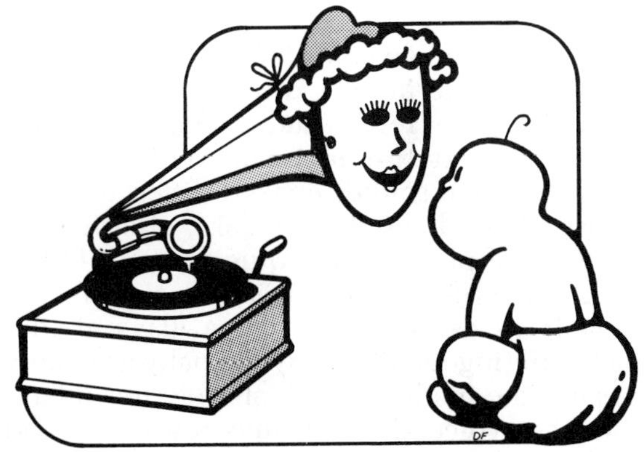

FIGURE 32-2. The infant's perceptual equipment of preference for a human face and voice contributes to the acquaintance process with his mother. (Cartoon by Dave Fisher, Arizona Medical Center A-V Division, Tucson, Arizona.)

One factor is the baby's visual preference for the human face, in combination with its ability to fixate on it, follow it, and thereby explore its features. During infant-care tasks the mother can ideally be in a position which provides face-to-face orientation between her and baby. Through such frequent exposures, the infant familiarizes himself with his mother's face and eventually distinguishes it from others. Such visual experiences are usually reinforced by the mother's behaviors. For example, when a mother notices her baby is visually attending to her, it is likely that the mother will increase her contacts with the baby by such actions as talking, singing, or touching her baby. The mother thereby becomes not only a rewarding subject to watch but interesting too, because of her varied responses. The significance of visual contact in promoting attachment between baby and mother is illustrated by Ainsworth:

> The baby, when apart from his mother but able to see her, keeps his eyes more or less continuously oriented towards her. When held by someone else, he can be sensed to be maintaining a motor orientation toward the mother; he is neither ready to interact with the adult holding him, nor to relax in her arms.[73]

The second main contribution to exploratory behaviors is the infant's discrimination of auditory stimuli. Hetzer and Tudor-Hart demonstrated that the maternal voice (high-pitched human sound) evoked differential responses as early as three weeks, eliciting expressions of pleasure and quiescence.[74] Other investigators feel this discrimination is observable as early as one to two days of life. Such quieting responses by the baby are likely to cause the mother to talk more to her infant. Thus, her voice also becomes rewarding and the infant is provided with more input of her voice. The opportunities to attend to the mother's voice, and eventually distinguish it from others, are thus increased.

Effector equipment

Bowlby describes this as the use of organs to make physical contact with another human being, primarily with head and mouth, and hands and feet. There have been interesting speculations that the baby's stimulation for orienting behaviors is associated with its reflex responses. Many of the reflex responses result in the infant facing or coming into contact with a stimulus (such as his mother). Here are some illustrations.

Behavioral responses related to head movements and sucking. The rooting reflex, whereby the baby turns its head in the direction of tactile stimulation to the cheeks, appears to have some orienting function. One study suggested that rooting behaviors served as the "reflex response of the neonate toward orientation" because the result is that it brings the infant to face the stimulus[75] (the eyes are in a better position to explore the stimulus). For example:

> A baby is held upright, head resting on mother's shoulder. The baby turns his medial ventral line (body) towards the mother's face in response to her touch to his left cheek. The mother in turn faces the baby and makes contact with his right cheek, as her shoulder supports the left side of his head. Stimulated on both sides, the infant will come to rest his head against her neck.[76]

Thus, in the above study, the researchers suggest that the infant's repetitive responses to stimulation-eliciting and rooting, and the mother's continuing reactions to the baby's rooting response, form the basis for early interaction. Behavioral responses related to the sucking reflex were described as having an orientation function because the baby is in contact with his environment during sucking activities, mainly with the subjects or objects delivering food.[77] Thus, it is speculated that in addition to meeting ingestive needs, head movements and sucking behaviors have the effect of orienting the baby to its mother.

Behavioral responses related to grasping, clinging, and reaching. Grasping, clinging, and reaching are means by which animals attach themselves to their mothers, mainly to prevent separation when mothers are moving. In the human infant such behaviors have been correlated to responses seen in the Moro, grasp, and traction reflexes. Interestingly, one study revealed that "palmar grasp reflex and strengthened clinging were noted when the Moro reflex was elicited with traction of the infant's hands and arms."[78] Reflexes have been viewed as providing primitive responses by which the neonate can grope or seek physical contact, and once it is made, maintain the contact such as by tight grasping (Fig. 32-3).

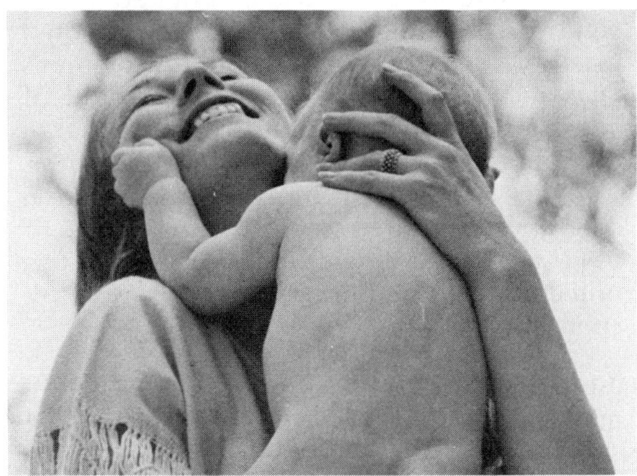

FIGURE 32-3. The grasp reflex allows the infant to maintain physical contact with a human being.

Signalling equipment

This involves the neonate's mode of communication through gestures and vocalizations (mainly smiling, babbling, and crying). The significance of such signals is the social response it evokes from others. Here is the beginning of social interaction in human existence. Smiling and babbling act as social releasers, that is, they elicit a predictable outcome of social interaction between baby and companion.[79] This occurs because the behaviors are pleasurable and attempts are made to encourage them. Also, social stimulus (such as the presence of a human being) is the primary elicitor and reinforcer for smiling and babbling behaviors. In contrast, crying is not viewed as a desired behavior and it evokes responses to discourage the behavior. Usually the best stimulus to terminate crying comes from the human voice, face, or touch. Thus, such signalling behaviors bring human stimuli to the baby and interaction can occur. A brief examination of these signalling behaviors reveal interesting findings.

Smiling. A baby's smile is one of the most important contributions it can make to initiate and maintain social exchange. It is the foundation by which social responses are developed in the early experiences of life. Old beliefs and folklore led mothers to believe that smiling arose from "gas in the baby" or would not occur until several weeks or months after birth. Mothers and fathers therefore anxiously awaited the "first smile" which was to come as the baby grew older. However, observations by Wolff revealed new perspectives about smiling behaviors in the neonate:

> A baby was observed to grimace as early as 2 to 12 hours after birth. Note the word grimace, for movements involved only the mouth, suggestive of a smile. Smiling behaviors tend to occur with high frequency at the moment when a neonate would close its eyes. Grimacing was elicited by a variety of sounds during irregular sleep without preference to an auditory stimuli. During this first week of life, such smiling behaviors did not evoke significant social responses because the observer frequently was uncertain that behavior was a smile.
>
> During the second week the smile was more distinct, "mouth stretched open, cheek muscles contracted, and eyes wrinkling,

giving the impression that the entire face was smiling." Two significant advances occurred. First, the infant's smiles were elicited more frequently by a human high-pitched (maternal) voice, and second, smiles were more frequent immediately after a meal and with the eyes open. During the third week, the human voice elicited a smile more often than any other stimulus. The crucial change is that the infant now smiles when alert, eyes open and attending to a stimulus. This greatly contributes to the communication value of the smile in promoting social interaction.

The fourth week is critical in the development of the infant's smiling repertoire. Increased efficiency in visual abilities makes a major impact on smiling behaviors. The infant, through coordinated eye-head movements now has a tendency to focus on the observer's eyes, providing eye-to-eye contact for the first time. First the baby searched the face, looking at the hairline, mouth, and other facial features. When the baby made eye-to-eye contact, he was then noted to smile. During this time proprioceptive and tactile stimuli can also elicit smiling. Playing a game of pat-a-cake elicited smiling, even when the infant could not hear or see his companion. Thus, visual stimuli become the primary elicitors for smiling as auditory stimuli lose their eliciting powers.[80]

The infant's ability to focus efficiently on the human face and to maintain eye contact with it is regarded as a landmark in the social interactive process between mother and baby. Such abilities increased mother-infant interactions. Wolff noted that mothers commented, "Now he can see me" or "Now he is fun to play with" and spent more time playing with their babies. After the neonatal period, the infant learns to associate social responses with smiling (such as greeting a person with a smile).

Babbling. The developmental process for babbling is similar to that of smiling. Again, it was Wolff who described the babbling process:

> At birth, the baby makes a variety of sounds such as grunting with stools, sighs with yawns, crying, and other noises. Eventually these are replaced with gurgles and coos. This occurs about the same time the baby smiles in response to auditory and visual stimuli (approximately 3 to 4 weeks of age). By the fifth week the infant frequently gurgles or coos with an open mouth and becomes so excited that its vocalizations resemble a chortling laughter. At this time the human voice (especially mother's) can elicit more babbling than smiling, and it is possible to carry on conversations in excess of ten to fifteen vocalizations by imitating the baby's sounds. Babbling can also be elicited by the sight of a moving face. The baby was noted to babble the most when it both saw mother's face and heard her voice. The amount of vocalizations by the infant is proportional to the reinforcement received for the behavior. For instance, babbling increased when mothers responded with conversations or other sounds, and babbling decreased or terminated when mothers made no verbal response to it.[81]

Babbling is a social releaser because it promotes mutual social interchange between mother and baby by keeping mother in close proximity to her infant.

Crying. This behavior usually conveys distress (such as hunger or discomfort from a wet diaper) to parents. The responses it evokes are directed toward termination or prevention of the behavior.

Wolff explored the behavior in depth and found that:

> There are four distinct types of crying, of which the most common are hunger cries and cries indicating pain. There is a distinction between these cries which mothers quickly learn, thereby manifesting different re-

sponses to the two cries. To the pain cry, mothers are apt to respond immediately while to hunger cry they will respond more calmly. Hunger cries are rhythmic, starting with a low intensity which builds up in time. It is usually followed by a brief silence, and a short inspiratory whistle. Pain cries are sudden in onset, high intensity from the beginning, and arrhythmic. They consist of a long inspiratory whistle immediately followed by a long expiratory cry. There are various elicitors for crying dependent upon the various differences in newborns. During the second week of life, the infant was observed to cry when naked, and quickly stopped when a blanket or something of thickness was placed over its ventral body surface or when redressed. During the third week of life, crying is significantly related to the infant's state; a fussy baby cried when presented with a silent, nodding head, or a quiet baby cried when disturbed.

Many interventions were noted to arrest crying which was not due to hunger. For example:

- pacifier sucking
- continuous non-painful stimulation such as a white light (had a sustained hypnagogic effect)
- rhythmic tapping to various parts of the body repeatedly
- swaddling which immobilizes the baby and generated a constant background of tactile stimulation
- picking up the baby to give rise to a complexity of visual, olfactory, and kinesthetic stimulations
- pressure on the abdomen with the flat of the hand or pressing the infant's hands on his own chest
- presenting a human face within the baby's visual field.[82]

Bowlby also demonstrated that crying behaviors could cease when the baby heard a sound (preferably a human voice), and was rocked (preferably at a rate of at least sixty cycles per minute for effective vestibular simulation).[83]

The significant consideration for neonatal crying behaviors is that whatever measure is used to arrest the behavior, it should be predicted to offer the infant visual, auditory, tactile, kinesthetic, and vestibular stimulation. Such stimulations are most effective in terminating crying when offered by a human being. Thus, crying is one way a baby can bring himself human interaction.

There appears to be a reciprocal interchange in the interaction between the baby and his companion when elicited by crying behaviors. This relates to the duration of infant crying. Some nurses have noted that when mothers (or nurses) respond quickly to an infant's cry, the behavior can be terminated easily by the actions previously described. However, when the infant has been crying for a long time and his cries have not elicited any human stimulus, then it takes longer and more comforting actions to stop the crying.

The preceding information on crying behaviors has significant value for both parents and health professionals. First, there should be an appreciation of crying as a signal behavior for the infant to maintain interaction with the environment. Second, there are many ways to terminate crying behaviors besides infant feeding. These other means involve some type of contact with human stimuli, thus giving rise for interaction.

The above discussion emphasized the neonate's contribution to the acquaintance process. If one takes the time to closely observe an interaction between two parties, it becomes evident that each is eliciting many behaviors which will affect the other's responses. The mother-child interaction is a two-way street, representing a true reciprocal exchange.[84] The initial approach toward interaction can come from either party. The mother may take the initiative by merely looking at her baby or by talking to the infant. The baby may take the initiative by spontaneous crying, smiling, or fixation on the mother's face. For interaction to occur there must be a reciprocal response to a stimulus which will facilitate the exploration of each party by the other. Stimuli which are of critical importance during the first four to five weeks of life are auditory, visual, tactile, vestibular, and kinesthetic. These arouse exploratory behaviors in both mother and baby. It is by hearing, seeing, touching, being touched, and having freedom for positional changes and spontaneity in movements that both baby and mother get to know each other better and eventually distinguish each other as different from other stimuli. Important considerations for stimuli in the interaction process are:

1. The infant's perceptual capacities are stimulated more effectively from input provided by a human subject.
2. The mother's interactive responses to her baby increase significantly when she perceives that the baby is capable of responding to her.
3. The development of social responsiveness early in life is directly related to the infant's ability to fixate, both visually and aurally, to a human stimulus. The reinforcers for such social responses also come from social input, such as continued looking, talking, or touching contact provided by mother.

After the acquaintance phase, the next step in the establishment of a mother-child relationship (or attachment) is the infant's discrimination of the mother as separate from the self and others. This phase is inhibited when the infant is hindered in acquainting himself with his mother by lack of stimuli input from her. It has also been noted that infants who fail or have difficulty discriminating the primary social figure (mother), will be retarded in their ability to establish interaction and relationships with others in their environment, such as the father, siblings, grandparents, and so forth. In the later phase of the first year of life, the infant's attachment to his mother is greatly enhanced by his developing locomotive skills.

Thus, the precursor in the formation of any relationship is the exploration of each party by the other. Interaction between baby and mother during the early phases of life is more likely to be strengthened when mutually positive reinforcements are given for behavioral responses to auditory, visual, and tactile stimuli, especially when provided by a human subject.

SIGNIFICANCE OF EARLY LIFE EXPERIENCES

The importance of the earliest life experiences is vividly expressed by Frank:

> The infant arrives as a young mammalian cub with all the capacities needed for biological existence. But since he must grow up to live in a symbolic cultural world and to participate in the social order of his group, he must be humanized and transformed into a personality for this uniquely human way of living. The first stage of being enculturated occurs in infancy. . . . What the infant experiences during the first year of life establishes many of his basic patterns which persist and largely govern what he will learn and what he will do and feel in his ensuing years.[85]

The infant's early experiences and their subsequent effect on later development are related to individual behavioral differences present at birth.[86] Such differences arise from the wide range of sensory-perceptual capacities. Korner[87] states, ". . . the most enduring characteristic of an individual derives from his capacity to take in and synthesize sensory stimuli." Such perceptual differences in early life affect how the infant will cope and respond to events in the world as he develops into an adult. Personality appears to depend on one's own spontaneous reaction to the conditions of his life; the most critical of all conditions are those affecting the ability to act (behavioral responses).[88] Differences will manifest in the perception of the self (self concept), and perception of the world (as evoking pleasure or stress), and thus determine the achievement of successful adaptation in the environment.

PERCEPTION OF THE SELF: EGO DEVELOPMENT

Early interactional experiences provide the structure or foundation by which the infant eventually discriminates the self as a separate entity from the environment. The beginnings of ego formation are laid during the neonatal period by two possible modes: 1) the neonate's scanning and exploration of the environment, and 2) the eventual discrimination for preferential social responses (such as smiling). Frank lends support to the first mode:

> Central to the task of living in a shared world with others and utilizing what it offers . . . is learning to distinguish "me" from "not me"—a task which involves selective awareness and discriminating perceptions. This involves a cumulative and progressive orientation which he gains by scanning the environment, locating and perceiving what he selects therefrom, which then becomes labeled with names that he gradually learns to recognize and use.[89]

Engel supports the second mode:

> The smile in response to specific individuals (such as mother) and not to others, is an early point at which an observer can recognize that the adult is acquiring for the infant some sort of identity separate from the self.[90]

Neonatal life experiences provide a beginning in the creation of one's own *life space.* Life space refers to the individual's unique imprint left upon the many events and people encountered in his daily life activities; it becomes observable as the person makes choices, decisions, accepts, ignores, rejects, and responds differentially to whatever he encounters.[91] While in early life the opportunity for the selection of forming one's life space may be limited (by the input from the environment and the neonate's limited ability to make choices), it is nonetheless demonstrative of how early patterns provide a directive for the infant's continued behavioral development in his child-rearing processes (Fig. 32-4).

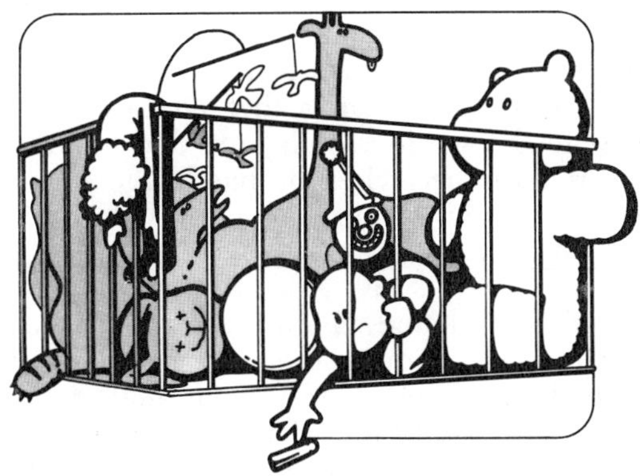

FIGURE 32-4. The infant's life space is created by the many events and people he encounters in his daily life activities. (Cartoon by Dave Fisher, Arizona Medical Center A-V Division, Tucson, Arizona.)

PERCEPTION OF THE WORLD

Early life experiences influence the neonate's perception of the world and its subsequent childhood events.[92] This perception is very important because it forms the foundation on which the child's future interpersonal relationships will be built. The degree to which the world is regarded as eliciting pleasure or frustrations will influence the neonate's future initiative to interact with the environment. The neonate's perception of the world comes from two major modes of input: 1) the type of stimuli received to arouse its sensory capacities, and 2) the phenomenon of human imprinting.

First, a look at the type of stimuli input. Although the sensory capacities are present at birth, their developmental efficiency is dependent upon stimuli which will arouse them. Thus, "the more a child has heard and seen, the more he wants to see and hear."[93] The impact of stimuli input on the infant's perception of the world can be vividly illustrated with a discussion on the significance of touch.

> Tactile contacts with humans, the kind of tactile comforting received in cuddling and mothering, may be one of the largest components in the infant's initial orientation to the world, developing that confidence or trust in the world which provided comforts and reassurance when he has little capacity for sustained disturbances and for self-stability.[94]

There is evidence which indicates that lack of tactile stimulation in the early phase of life can lead to physical and emotional disturbances. The inhibition of tactile perceptions was shown to profoundly retard behavioral development as well as hinder the ability to establish relationships with others.[95]

Now for a look at the phenomenon of *human imprinting*. Several authors have indicated there is a sensitive period (or periods) for the development of social responses in early life.[96,97] There are discrepancies as to when this critical period begins. Some say it occurs between six weeks to six months.[98] Others state there are two phases in this sensitive period. The first period begins with the infant's visual fixation and pursuit of the human face (as early as two weeks), and the second period begins with the eventual discrimination of mother from others (4 to 5 months of age).[99] Human imprinting is speculated to occur in these sensitive time periods in an infant's early development. Imprinting in animals is the phenomenon by which the animal learns how to respond and behave in the environment by following maternal behaviors. In humans, some investigators regard imprinting as an inborn desire to learn the parent.[100] Others believe imprinting is not innate but a learned ability to integrate features of the environment from input provided by maternal behaviors.[101] The imprinting phenomenon is significant because of its contribution to the infant's perception of the human species. Ambrose describes this:

> The infant is gradually piecing together and building his picture of what a human being is like. He learns this from the first member of the human species he interacts with, namely his mother. When he learns the characteristics of the species via her, one of the things he learns is what the human face and clothed body are like, also the voice, touch, smell, of the human being.
>
> Furthermore, all the variety of behaviors she carries out have effects in satisfying his physiologic needs. . . . That is, the infant also learns from the nature of the mother's responsiveness what sort of behavior he can expect from a human being. [102]

ADAPTATION OR MALADAPTATION TO THE ENVIRONMENT

Studies have indicated how early life experiences can predispose an infant to anxiety.[103,104] Neurosis is the common manifestation of this predisposition to anxiety. Freud stated, "Each individual ego is endowed from the beginning with its own peculiar disposition and tendencies (to anxiety)."[105] This unique predisposition may also occur from many other factors such as imprinting of undesirable maternal behaviors. For example:

> Depending on what his mother is like, his picture of a human being may turn out to be anything between two extremes. At one ex-

> treme, it may be a loving, or need-satisfying, anxiety-reducing person . . . at the other it may be a hating, rejecting, poor need-satisfier, who frequently elicits anxiety. . . . In other words, some infant's picture of a human being will be one which elicits in them more anxiety than from others.[106]

There is speculation that variations in the primary ego apparatus (arising from early life experiences) may influence the choice of defense mechanisms seen in later life.[107]

THE LEARNING PROCESS

There is the belief that learning processes in human life result from the individual's behavioral interaction with his environment during everyday life activities.[108] The various contacts or interactions in life provide the basis for important behavioral skills to be learned. Such skills, called the basic behavioral repertoires, are acquired as the result of responses to environmental situations which occur consistently (repeatedly) and for which the infant's responses are appropriately reinforced.[109] Intellectual development or learning is viewed as the cumulative acquisition of various basic behavioral repertoires which have evolved from a behavioral-environmental interaction. Some of the basic behavioral repertoires acquired in early life and constituents in the development of learning are:

1. Availability of stimuli to activate the neonate's sensory capabilities.
2. Development of sensory-muscular coordinations for responses to stimuli.
3. Discrimination for selective stimuli.
4. Attending to a stimuli.
5. Pairing of the response with rewarding conditions or positive reinforcement for the desired response.[110]

Does this sound familiar? It's like outlining sections previously presented. It becomes obvious that early life experiences involving environmental interaction do contribute to the learning process. Piaget lends support to this by emphasizing the significance of "exercising or stimulating" the infant's sensory capacities. In his discussion of the first stage of primitive intelligence (birth to one month) he states:

> By repetitive and successful action of the thing in the environment (behavioral responses), this schema (patterns of behavior) is not only crystallized as mental experiences but is also used in furthering adjustment to and learning about the environment.[111]

Brazelton also emphasizes the importance of stimulation on learning:

> Each stimulus adds to the new baby's experiences . . . many repetitions of this go into the "learning" or "conditioning" that will eventually result in his ability to react. . . .
>
> With each stimulus reaction an infant's brain has the opportunity to store up experiences for future learning.[112]

Stimuli input in early life is important to arouse the neonate's behavioral potential so that appropriate behaviors can be reinforced. In this process the infant will build up his basic behavioral repertoires which are the foundation for learning. When environmental stimuli are absent, the development of the basic repertoires will be deficient, abnormal, or absent.

REFERENCES

1. Montagu, A.: *Life Before Birth.* Signet books, New York, 1964, introductory page.
2. Ibid.: *Prenatal Influences.* Charles C Thomas Publishers, Springfield, Illinois, 1962, p. 4.
3. Ibid., 117–123, 192.

4. Whitehead, J.: *Convulsions in utero.* Brit. Med. J. 2:59, 1867.
5. Sontag, L.: *The significance of fetal environmental differences.* Am. J. Obstet. Gynecol. 42:1000, 1941.
6. Ibid.: *Differences in modifiability of fetal behavior and physiology.* Psychosom. Med. 6:154, 1944.
7. Ibid.: *War and fetal-maternal relationship.* Marriage and Family Living 6:5, 1944.
8. Ibid.: *Some psychosomatic aspects of childhood.* The Nervous Child 4:296, 1946.
9. Turner, E.: *The syndrome in the infant resulting from maternal emotional tension during pregnancy.* Med. J. Aust. 1:221, 1956.
10. Ferreira, A.: *The pregnant woman's emotional attitude and its reflection on the newborn.* Am. J. Orthopsychiat. 30:550, 1960.
11. Montagu, A.: *Prenatal Influences,* op. cit.
12. Dunbar, F.: *A psychosomatic approach to abortion and the abortion habit.* In Rosen, H. (ed.): *Therapeutic Abortion.* Julian Press, New York, 1954.
13. Weil, R. J. and Tupper, C.: *Personality, life situation and communication: a study of habitual abortion.* Psychosom. Med. 22:448, 1960.
14. Strean, L. P. and Peer, L. A.: *Stress as an etiologic factor in the development of cleft palate.* Plast. Reconstr. Surg. 18:5, 1956.
15. Rank, O.: *Trauma of Birth.* Brunner Books, New York, 1952.
16. Freud, S.: *Introductory Lectures on Psycho-Analysis.* Allen and Unwin Company, London, 1922, pp. 331–332.
17. Brody, S. and Axelrad, S.: *Anxiety and Ego Formation in Infancy.* International Universities Press, New York, 1970.
18. Norris, A. S.: *Prenatal factors in infant and emotional development.* J. A. M. A. 172:413, 1960.
19. Abramson, J. H., Singh, A. R. and Mbambo, V.: *Antenatal stress and the baby's development.* Arch. Dis. Child. 36:42, 1961.
20. Fantz, R. and Nevis, S.: *Pattern preferences and perceptual cognitive development in early infancy.* Merrill-Palmer Quarterly 13:77, 1967.
21. Gough, D.: *The visual evidence of infants during the first few weeks of life.* Proceedings of Research in Social Medicine 55:308, 1962.
22. Lipsitt, L., Engen, T. and Kaye, H.: *Developmental changes in the olfactory threshold of the neonate.* Child Dev. 34:371, 1963.
23. Kagan, J. and Lewis, M. *Studies of attention in the human infant.* Merrill-Palmer Quarterly 11:95, 1965.
24. Ambrose, J. A.: *The development of the smiling response in early infancy.* In Foss, B. M. (ed.): *Determinants of Infant Behavior, vol. 1.* John Wiley and Sons, New York, 196, pp. 179–196.
25. Fantz, R. L.: *Pattern discrimination and selective attention as determinants of perceptual development from birth.* In Kidd, A. J. and Rivoire, J. L. (eds.): *Perceptual Development in Children. International Universities Press,* New York, 1966.
26. Watson, J.: *Perception of object orientation.* Merrill-Palmer Quarterly 12:73, 1966.
27. Fantz: op. cit.
28. Wolff, P.: *Observations on the early development of smiling.* In Foss, B. M. (ed.): *Determinants of Infant Behavior, vol. 2.* John Wiley and Sons, New York, 1963, pp. 117–130.
29. Ibid.
30. Lipsitt, Egen and Kaye: op. cit.
31. Lipsitt, L. and Levy, N.: *Electro-tactual threshold in the neonate.* Child Dev. 30:547, 1959.
32. Fantz: op. cit.
33. Wolff, P.: *Observations on newborn infants.* Psychosom. Med. 21:110, 1959.
34. Wolff: *Observations on the early development of smiling,* op. cit.
35. Lipsitt, L.: *Learning processes of human newborns.* Merrill-Palmer Quarterly 12:45, 1966.
36. Bowlby, J.: *Attachment and Loss, vol. I: Attachment.* Basic Books, New York, 1969, pp. 265–298.
37. Rheingold, H.: *The effect of environmental stimulation upon social and exploratory behavior in the human infant.* In Foss, B. M. (ed.): *Determinants of Human Behavior, vol. 1.* John Wiley and Sons, New York, 1961, pp. 166–168.
38. Gesell, A.: *The First Five Years of Life.* Harper and Row, New York, 1941.
39. Fantz: op cit.
40. Schaffer, H. R.: *Some issues for research in the study of attachment behavior.* In Foss, B. M. (ed.): *Determinants of Infant Behavior, vol. 2.* John Wiley and Sons, New York, 1963, p. 194.
41. Kagan and Lewis: op. cit.
42. Ambrose: op. cit.
43. Rheingold: op. cit.
44. Schaffer: op. cit.
45. Kagan and Lewis: op. cit.
46. Rheingold: op. cit.
47. Brown, J.: *States in newborn infants.* Merrill-Palmer Quarterly 10:313, 1964.
48. Rosenthal, M.: *The study of infant-environment interaction: some comments on trends and methodologies.* J. Child Psychol. Psychiat. 14:308, 1973.
49. Brazelton, T. B.: *Assessment of the infant at risk.* Clin. Obstet. Gynecol. 16:370, 1973.
50. Brown: op. cit.
51. Brazelton, T. B.: *Observations of the neonate.* J. Am. Acad. Child Psychiat. 1:38, 1962.
52. Rubenstein, J.: *Maternal attentiveness and subsequent exploratory behavior in the infant.* Child Dev. 38:1009, 1967.
53. Korner, A. and Thoman, E.: *Visual alertness in*

neonates as evoked by maternal care. J. Exp. Child Psychol. 10:67, 1970.
54. Ibid.
55. Brazelton, T. B.: *Neonatal Behavioral Assessment Scale.* J. B. Lippincott, Philadelphia, 1974.
56. Rovee, C. and Levin, G. *Oral pacification and arousal in the human newborn.* J. Exp. Child Psychol. 3:1, 1966.
57. Korner, A. and Grobstein, R.: *Visual alertness and related to soothing in the neonates: implications for maternal stimulation and early deprivation.* Child Dev. 37:867, 1966.
58. Wolff, P.: *The natural history of crying and other vocalizations in early infancy.* In Foss, B. M. (ed.): *Determinants of Human Behaviors,* vol. 4. John Wiley and Sons, New York, 1969, pp. 81–111.
59. Rosenthal: op. cit.
60. Call, J.: *Newborn approach behavior and early ego development.* Int. J. Psycho-Analysis 45:286, 1964.
61. Bowlby: op. cit.
62. Engel, G.: *Psychological Development in Health and Disease.* W. B. Saunders, Philadelphia, 1964, pp. 41, 49, 59.
63. Ibid.
64. Gewirtz, J.: *A learning analysis of the effects of normal stimulation, privation, and deprivation on the acquisition of social motivation and attachment.* In Foss, B. M. (ed.): *Determinants of Infant Behavior, vol. 1.* John Wiley and Sons, New York, 1961, pp. 213–290.
65. Kahn, J.: *Human Growth and the Development of Personality,* ed. 2. Pergamon Press, London, 1971, p. 46.
66. Lipsitt: op. cit.
67. Rosenthal: op. cit.
68. Korner, A.: *Individual differences at birth: implications for early experience and later development.* Am. J. Orthopsychiat. 41:608, 1971.
69. Ainsworth, M.: *Patterns of attachment.* Merrill-Palmer Quarterly 10:57, 1964.
70. Piaget, J.: *The Psychology of Intelligence.* Harcourt, Brace, New York, 1950.
71. Ambrose: op. cit.
72. Bowlby: op. cit.
73. Ainsworth, M.: *The development of infant-mother interaction among the Ganda* In Foss, B. M. (ed.): *Determinants of Infant Behavior, vol. 2.* John Wiley and Sons, New York, 1963, p. 77.
74. Hetzer, H. and Tudor-Hart, B. *Die fruhesten reaktionen auf die menschliche stimme,* as interpreted by Bowlby, J.: *Attachment and Loss, vol. I: Attachment.* Basic Books, New York, 1969, p. 270.
75. Blauvelt, H. and McKenna, J.: *Mother-neonate interaction: Capacity of the human newborn for orientation.* In Foss, B. M. (ed.): *Determinants of Infant Behavior, vol. 1.* John Wiley and Sons, New York, 1961, pp. 4, 5.
76. Ibid.
77. Prechtl, H.: *The directed head turning response and allied movements of the human baby.* Behavior 13:212, 1958.
78. Prechtl, H.: *Problems of behavioral studies in the newborn infant.* In Lehrman, D. S., Hinde, R. A. and Shaw, E. (eds.): *Advances in the Study of Behavior, vol. 1.* Academic Press, New York, 1965.
79. Bowlby: op. cit.
80. Wolff: *Observations on the early development of smiling,* op. cit.
81. Ibid.
82. Wolf, P. *The natural history of crying and other vocalizations in early infancy,* op. cit.
83. Bowlby: op. cit.
84. Korner, A.: *Mother-child interaction: one- or two-way street?* Social Work 10:47, 1965.
85. Frank, L.: *On the Importance of Infancy.* Random House, New York, 1966, p. 6, 99–103.
86. Korner: *Individual differences at birth,* op. cit.
87. Ibid.
88. Bettelheim, B.: *Where self begins.* Child and Family 7:5, 1968.
89. Frank: op. cit.
90. Engel: op. cit.
91. Frank: op. cit.
92. Korner: *Mother-child interaction,* op. cit.
93. Hunt, J.: *The psychological basis for using preschool education as an antidote for cultural deprivation.* Merrill-Palmer Quarterly 10:209, 1964.
94. Frank: op. cit.
95. Spitz, R. A.: *Hospitalism.* In Freud, A., et al. (eds.): *The Psychoanalytic Study of the Child, vol. 1.* International Universities Press, New York, 1945.
96. Ambrose, J. A.: *Concept of a critical period for the development of social responsiveness in early human infancy.* In Foss, B. M. (ed.): *Determinants of Human Behavior, vol. 1.* John Wiley and Sons, New York, 1961, pp. 201–225.
97. Hinde, R. A.: *Nature of imprinting,* In Foss, B. M. (ed.): *Determinants of Human Behavior, vol. 1.* John Wiley and Sons, New York, 1961, pp. 227–233.
98. Gray, P. H.: *Theory and evidence of imprinting in human infants.* J. Psychol. 46:155, 1958.
99. Brody and Axelrad: op. cit.
100. Gray: op. cit.
101. Gewirtz: op. cit.
102. Ambrose: *Concept of a critical period,* op. cit.
103. Brody and Axelrad: op. cit.
104. Benjamin, J.: *The innate and the experiential in development.* In Brosin, H. (ed.): *Lectures on Experimental Psychiatry.* University of Pittsburg, Pittsburg, 1961.
105. Freud, S.: *Analysis terminable and interminable.* In *Collected Papers, vol. 5.* Hogarth Press, London,

1950.
106. Ambrose: Concept of a critical period, op. cit.
107. Hartmann, H.: *Ego Psychology and the Problem of Adaptation.* International Universities Press, New York, 1958.
108. Staats, A.: *Child Learning, Intelligence, and Personality.* Harper and Row, New York, 1971.
109. Ibid.
110. Ibid.
111 Piaget: op. cit.
112. Brazelton, T. B.: *Infants and Mothers: Differences in Development.* Delacorte Press, New York, 1969, p. 25.

BIBLIOGRAPHY

Barnett, K.: *A theoretical construct of the concepts of touch as they relate to nursing.* Nurs. Res. 21:102, 1972.

Bernal, J.: *Crying during the first 10 days of life and maternal responses.* Dev. Med. Child Neurol. 14:362, 1972.

Blaesing, S. and Brockhaus, J.: *The development of body image in the child.* Nurs. Clin. North Am. 7:597, 1972.

Bowlby, J.: *Attachment and Loss, vol. I: Attachment.* Basic Books, New York, 1969.

Brazelton, T. B.: *Does the neonate shape his environment?* Birth Defects 10:131, 1974.

Ibid.: *Infants and Mothers: Differences in Development.* Delacorte Press, New York, 1969.

Ibid.: *Neonatal Behavioral Assessment Scale.* Spastics International Medical Publications, London, 1973.

Buss, A.: *A conceptual framework for learning effecting the development of ability factors.* Hum. Dev. 16:273, 1973.

Campbell, D.: *Sucking as an index of mother-child interaction.* Symp. Oral Sensory Perception 4:152, 1973.

Clark, L.: *Care of the well child: Introducing mother and baby.* Am. J. Nurs. 74:1483, 1974.

Day, B. and Liley, M.: *The Secret World of the Baby.* Random House, New York, 1966.

Emde, R. and Koenig, K.: *Neonatal smiling and rapid eye movement states.* J. Am. Acad. Child Psychiat. 8:57, 1969.

Foss, B. M. (ed.): *Determinants of Infant Behavior, vols. 1–4.* Wiley and Sons, New York, 1961, 1963, 1965, 1969.

Fouts, G.: *Elimination of an infant's crying through response prevention.* Percept. Mot. Skills 38:225, 1974.

Freud, W.: *The Baby Profile, II.* Psychoanal. Stud. Child 26:172, 1971.

Friedman, S.: *Habituation and recovery of visual response in the alert human newborn.* J. Exp. Child Psychol. 13:339, 1972.

Greenberg, M. and Morris, N.: *Engrossment: the newborn's impact upon the father.* Am. J. Orthopsychiat. 44:520, 1974.

Hiernaux, J.: *Environmental and genetic influences upon growth.* J. Anat. 107:181, 1970.

Hirschman, R. and Katkin, E.: *Psychophysiological functioning, arousal, attention, and learning during the first year of life.* Adv. Child. Dev. Behav. 9:115, 1974.

Honig, A.: *The role of the nurse in stimulating early learning.* J. Nurs. Educ. 9:11, 1970.

Hulsebus, R.: *Operant conditioning of infant behaviors: a review.* Adv. Child. Dev. Behav. 8:111, 1973.

Hutt, C., et al.: *Habituation in relation to state in the human neonate.* Nature 220:618, 1968.

Jeffrey, W. and Cohen, L.: *Habituation in the human infant.* Adv. Child. Dev. Behav. 6:63, 1971.

Junker, K.: *Selective attention in infants and consecutive communicative behavior.* Acta Paediatr. Scand. (Suppl.) 231:1, 1972.

Kaplan, L.: *The concept of the family romance.* Psychoanal. Rev. 61:169, 1974.

Katz, S., Rivinus, H. and Barker, W.: *Physical anthropology and the biobehavioral approach to child growth and development.* Am. J. Phys. Anthropol. 38:105, 1973.

Kobre, K. and Lipsitt, L.: *A negative contrast effect in newborns.* J. Exp. Child Psychol. 14:81, 1972.

Kulka, A., Fry, C. and Goldstein, F.: *Kinesthetic needs in infancy.* Am. J. Orthopsychiat. 30:562, 1960.

Lenard, H., von Bernuth, H. and Prechtl, H.: *Reflexes and their relationship to behavioral state in the newborn.* Acta Paediatr. Scand. 57:177, 1968.

Levy, D.: *Behavioral Analysis: Analysis of Clinical Observations of Behavior as Applied to Mother-Newborn Relationships.* Charles C Thomas, Springfield, Illinois, 1958.

Mahler, M. S.: *Symbiosis and individuation: the psychological birth of the human infant.* Psychoanal. Study Child 29:89, 1974.

Michaelis, R., et al.: *Activity states in premature and term infants.* Develop. Psychobiol. 6:209, 1973.

Mills, M. and Melhuish, E.: *Recognition of mother's voice in early infancy.* Nature 252:123, 1974.

Montagu, A.: *Prenatal Influences.* Charles C Thomas, Springfield, Illinois, 1962.

Rebelsky, R. and Hanks, C.: *Fathers' verbal interaction with infants in the first three months of life.* Child Dev. 42:63, 1971.

Rose, S., Katz, P. and Samsky, J.: *Influence of visual enrichment on infants' visual preferences.* Percept. Mot. Skills 35:960, 1972.

Rosenthal, M.: *The study of infant-environment interaction: some comments on trends and methodologies.* J. Child Psychol. Psychiat. 14:301, 1973.

Rubin, J., Provenzano, F. and Luria, A.: *The eye of the beholder: parents' view on sex of newborns.* Am. J. Orthopsychiat. 44:512, 1974.

Salk, L.: *The critical nature of the post-partum period in the human for the establishment of the mother-infant bond: a controlled study.* Dis. Nerv. Syst. 31(Suppl.):110, 1970.

Southwood, H.: *The origin of self-awareness and ego behavior.* Int. J. Psychoanal. 54:235, 1973.

Stark, R. E., and Nathanson, S.: *Spontaneous cry in the newborn infant; sounds and facial gestures.* Symp. Oral Sensory Perception 4:323, 1973.

Stevenson, R.: *The Fetus and Newly Born Infant: Influences of the Prenatal Environment.* C. V. Mosby, St. Louis, 1973.

Stone, L., Smith, H. and Murphy, L.: *The Competent Infant.* Basic Books, New York, 1973.

Tautermannova, M.: *Smiling in infants.* Child Dev. 44:701, 1973.

Tempesta, L.: *The importance of touch in the care of newborns.* J. Obstet. Gynecol. Nurse 1:17, 1972.

Thomas, A. and Autgaerden, S.: *Locomotion from Pre- to Post-Natal Life; How the Newborn Begins to Acquire Psycho-Sensory Functions.* W. S. Heinemann, New York, 1966.

Wolff, P.: *The Causes, Control and Organization of Behavior in the Neonate.* International Universities Press, New York, 1966.

Zern, D.: *The relationship between mother-infant contact and later differentiation of the social environment.* J. Genet. Psychol. 121:107, 1972.

33 Application of Psychosocial Concepts

DYANNE D. AFFONSO, R.N., M.N.

Including *Behavioral Assessment of the Neonate*
by T. Berry Brazelton, M.D.

This chapter focuses on the application of the content presented in the previous chapter to the nursing purposes in working with the neonate and his family. The behavioral aspects in neonatal assessment are highlighted as well as identification of nursing actions which stimulate. Nursing actions to stimulate the neonate are those actions which provide environmental and social input to maximize the neonate's potential for behavioral development.

PSYCHOSOCIAL ASSESSMENT

The psychosocial component in neonatal assessment consists of evaluation in two areas:

1. Daily behavioral patterns
2. Determination of the infant's behavioral state for interaction with the environment

DAILY BEHAVIORAL PATTERNS

This refers to the neonate's patterns of daily life activities, primarily feeding, elimination, and sleep-activity. There have been many studies investigating such behavioral patterns.[1-4] The most relevant contribution to nursing's purpose in assessing daily patterned activities was done by Craig.[5] As a nurse-midwife, Craig recorded the neonate's behavioral patterns for feeding, elimination, and sleep-wakefulness. Her purpose was to enhance nursing knowledge of the newborn so that the best care could be given to the infants by nurses, and so that nurses could help parents to understand these behaviors. Craig's major findings are summarized below to serve as a baseline for norms in neonatal assessment of daily behavioral patterns.

1. Feeding Patterns

   Breast-fed babies: they increased the time spent at the breast from 6 minutes in the first few days to 18 minutes by the last three days in the first week. A plateau was reached by the fifth to seventh day of approximately 110 minutes of feeding per day. Babies of multiparous mothers had greater intake than those of primiparous mothers. By the end of the first week, breast-fed babies ate approximately every 3¾ hours or close to 7 times a day.

   Formula-fed babies: on the first day they drank an average of 45 cc. at each feeding. By the third day they averaged 60 cc. per feeding and between the fourth to sixth day the intake was approximately 70 cc. The average intake per feeding in the second week of life was about 90 cc. By the end of the first week they ate, on the average, every 4½ hours or close to 5 times a day. Infants of multiparous mothers ate 40 to 150 cc. more formula daily than those of primiparous mothers.

2. Elimination Patterns

   During the first four days of life an infant averaged 2 to 4 bowel movements per day. The frequency of bowel movements appeared related to the frequency and amount of food intake. During the first half of the first week of life, formula-fed infants had more bowel movements, about 4 per day, than breast-fed infants. However, after the fourth day the breast-fed infants had more bowel movements, possibly related to the establishment of lactation. Infants averaged a daily frequency of urination beginning from 3 to four times in the first few days of life to between 5 to 6 times per day in the latter half of the first week.

3. Sleep-Wakefulness Patterns

   Newborns slept approximately 16¼ hours each day. The longest interval of sleep was an average of 5½ hours in the first few days, which decreased to a little over 4 hours by the latter part of the first week. In general, breast-fed newborns of multiparous mothers slept the most, while breast-fed babies of primiparous mothers and formula-fed babies of multiparous mothers slept the least.

   Newborns fussed 20 to 25 percent of their waking time, or a daily average of 1¾ hours during the first week of life. The fussing pattern was minimum during the first 2 days and increased to a maximum on the third to fourth day of life. Generally, breast-fed babies and those of primiparous mothers fussed more than their counterparts.

The preceding is a very brief outline of Craig's findings and the reader is encouraged to read her study for more details. What significance is there in having such knowledge about the neonate's daily behavioral patterns? This knowledge demonstrates the need for nurses to assess the newborn's unique needs and then plan nursing care to meet these needs instead of performing routines which are created for the convenience of the staff. Also, such knowledge allows the nurse to help parents recognize expected behavioral patterns so they, too, can modify their approaches to meet such needs. When parents feel that their parenting skills are satisfying their infants, their self-confidence increases and they will interact more with their infants. This builds the foundation for healthy parent-child relationships.

Nurses are encouraged to explore the daily behavioral patterns in the neonates they care for. Differences in what are considered normal patterns may become evident and be related to the uniqueness of the specific locale and its population's life style. Clinical assessment is important because it provides the means by which nursing care can optimally meet the unique needs of a specific newborn and his parents.

BEHAVIORAL POTENTIAL FOR INTERACTION

Currently, the most respected and published tool to achieve this type of assessment is a behavioral rating scale developed by Brazelton.[6] The scale scores a newborn's interactive behaviors, that is, the infant's available responses to his environment, and in turn, how he affects the environment. The scale also contributes to an evaluation of the infant's neurologic functioning, but its main focus is behavioral. The scale has made a major contribution toward identifying the sensory capacities in a newborn infant as well as demonstrating the baby's potential for interactive behaviors. The scale also contributes to identifying infants who are at risk in terms of not being able to achieve optimal interaction with their environment. The authors are honored to have Dr. Brazelton contribute to this section of the book with the following description of his behavioral tool.

BEHAVIORAL ASSESSMENT OF THE NEONATE*

Physicians and nurses, and, in particular, those who see children and their new parents, are at the most influential front I know of. We have an opportunity to participate in the ongoing development of an immature organism at a time when our support and guidance may have real potential value for infuencing the outcome of this development. Although we do not know what outcome may be optimal in all cases, we must be ready to team with the parents in an effort to produce it for each child. In order to do this, we must 1) be willing to listen to and work with parents as individuals, and 2) we must avail ourselves of every opportunity to see the developing child's individual assets and his particular needs from his environment. In this effort, I see our role as starting before birth with the parents, and at birth with the child himself. I feel that the kind of infant he is becomes the most powerful influence in shaping his future. If we as professionals can help the parents credit and understand his individuality, his future will be assured in all likelihood. I have developed the Neonatal Behavorial Assessment to alert professionals to the potential individual strengths of the neonate, and hope that they will use their information to support the parents of the neonate in understanding him as an individual.

BEHAVIORAL EXAM

Having noted the inadequacy of Apgar scores and standard neurologic exams in predicting later outcome, I began to try to develop an assessment scale which measured the responses which pediatricians and neonatal nurses take into account as they assess newborns in the first few days.[7] The scale has developed over many years, and with the assistance of many of my colleagues in psychology, we have been able to develop a manual to score the 26 behavioral items on a 9-point system and the 20 reflex items on a high-medium-low scale. After two days of training, we have been successful in bringing observers from the disciplines of medicine, nursing, and psychology to .85 agreement and reliability among observers which must be obtained to make the data collected on different samples of neonates of comparable value. Newborn and four-week retest measurements of reliability across observers and subjects has been achieved successfully. This has also been borne out more recently in studies with low birth weight infants.[8]

Determination of State

The behavioral evaluation tests and documents the infant's use of state behavior (state of consciousness) and his response to various kinds of stimulation administered by a caretaker. Since his reactions to all stimuli are dependent on his ongoing "state," any interpretation of them must be made with this in mind. His use of state to maintain control of his reactions to environmental and internal stimuli is an important mechanism and reflects his potential for organization. State no longer need be treated as an error variable but serves to set a dynamic pattern to allow for the full behavioral repertoire of the infant. Specifically, our examination tracks state changes over the course of the exam, its lability and direction. The variability of state points to the infant's capacities for self-organization. His ability to quiet himself as well as his need for stimulation also measure this adequacy.

An important consideration throughout the tests is the state of consciousness or "state" of the infant. Reactions to stimuli must be interpreted within the context of the presenting

*This section was written by T. Berry Brazelton, M.D.

state of consciousness, as reactions may vary markedly as the infant passes from one state to another. State depends on physiologic variables such as hunger, nutrition, degree of hydration, and the time within the wake-sleep cycle of the infant. The pattern of states as well as the movement from one state to another appear to be important characteristics of infants in the neonatal period, and this kind of evaluation may be the best predictor of the infant's receptivity and ability to respond to stimuli in a cognitive sense. Our criteria for determining state are based on our own experiences and on those of others, and are comparable with the descriptions of Prechtl and Beintema.[9]

Sleep States

1. Deep sleep with regular breathing, eyes closed, no spontaneous activity except startles or jerky movements at quite regular intervals; external stimuli produce startles with some delay; suppression of startles is rapid, and state changes are less likely than from other states. No eye movements.
2. Light sleep with eyes closed; rapid eye movements can be observed under closed lids; low activity level, with random movements and startles or startle equivalents; movements are likely to be smoother and more monitored than in deep-sleep state; responds to internal and external stimuli with startle equivalents, often with a resulting change of state. Respirations are jagged or irregular, sucking movements off and on.

Awake States

3. Drowsy or semi-dozing; eyes may be open or closed, eyelids fluttering; activity level variable, with interspersed, mild startles from time to time; reactive to sensory stimuli, but response often delayed; state change after stimulation frequently noted. Movements are usually smooth.
4. Alert, with bright look; seems to focus attention on source of stimulation, such as an object to be sucked, or a visual or auditory stimulus; impinging stimuli may break through, but with some delay in response. Motor activity is at a minimum.
5. Eyes open; considerable motor activity, with thrusting movements of the extremities, and even a few spontaneous startles; reactive to external stimulation with increase in startles or motor activity, but discrete reactions difficult to distinguish because of general high activity level.
6. Crying; characterized by intense crying which is difficult to break through with stimulation.

Components of Exam

The behavior exam tests for neurologic adequacy with 20 reflex measures and for 26 behavioral responses to environmental stimuli, including the kind of interpersonal stimuli which mothers use in their handling of the infant as they attempt to help him adapt to the new world. In the exam, there is a graded series of procedures—talking, hand on belly, restraint, holding and rocking—designed to soothe and alert the infant. His responsiveness to animate stimulation—voice and face, etc.—and to inanimate stimulation—rattle, bell, red ball, white light, temperature change, etc.—is assessed. Estimates of vigor and attentional excitement are measured as well as assessment of motor activity and tone, and autonomic responsiveness as he changes state. With this examination given on successive days we have been able to outline:

1. The initial period of alertness immediately after delivery—presumably

the result of stimulation of labor and the new environmental stimuli after delivery.

2. The period of depression and disorganization which follows and lasts for 24 to 48 hours in infants with uncomplicated deliveries and no medication effects, but for longer periods of 3 to 4 days if they have been comprised from medication given their mothers during labor.
3. The curve of recovery to "optimal" function after several days. This third period may be the best single predictor of individual potential function and it seems to correlate well with the neonate's retest ability at 30 days.[10] The shape of the curve made by several examinations may be the most important assessment of the basic CNS intactness of the neonate, his ability to integrate CNS and other physiologic recovery mechanisms, and the strength of his compensatory capacities when there have been compromising insults to him during labor and delivery.

Neurologic Items

The exam should be accompanied by a complete neurologic evaluation if there is any reason to question the neurologic intactness of the infant. Short of that, the neurologic items in the scale will act as an initial screening for central nervous system damage. The neurologic items are used to elicit the neonate's behavioral responses as well as to register his neurologic adequacy. They are:

Ankle clonus
Plantar grasp
Palmar grasp
Babinski responses
Standing reflex
Stepping reflex
Placing reflex
Incurvation (spinal reflexes)
Crawling response in prone
Glabella reflex
Vestibular responses (tonic deviation head and eyes)
Ocular nystagmus
Tonic neck reflex
Moro reflex
Rooting
Sucking
Responses of extremities and spinal musculature to passive movement

Behavioral Items

1. *Response decrement to light* (scored in sleep states)—One of the most impressive mechanisms in the neonate is his capacity to decrease responses to repeated disturbing stimuli. In this test, an attempt is made to measure the decrement which occurs in a quiet state (1 or 2), after the infant has responded with an aversive reaction to a flashlight shone briefly in his eyes (closed or open). The response decrement over time is assessed on the basis of the neonate's ability to control the fol-

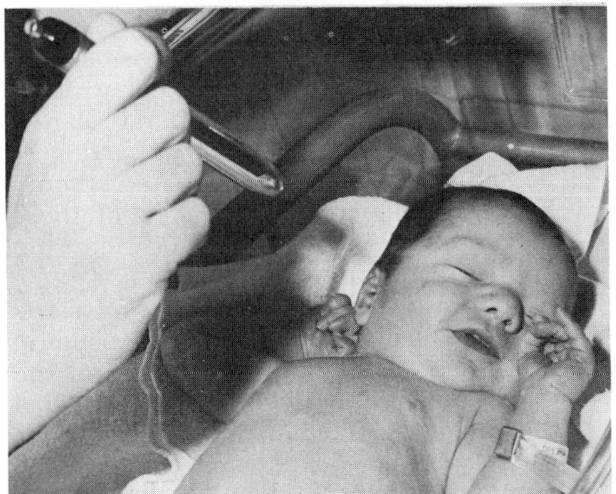

FIGURE 33-1. The neonate's response to light is assessed using a flashlight.

lowing reactions: a) all or none startles of the entire body, b) delayed and graded localized startle, c) respiratory changes, and d) blinks of the eyelids. The delaying and finally the suppression of any reactions are degrees of the same kind of habituation. The infant's performance is evaluated after 10 flashes, unless he has successfully shut down his response before that (Fig. 33-1).

2. *Response decrement to rattle* (scored in sleep states)—Using a rattle to break through his sleep state to produce an initial startle, the neonate's response decrement is measured and scored over 10 stimuli, in the same way as to the light.
3. *Response decrement to a bell* (scored in sleep states)—This item and Item 2 above are designed to measure the neonate's ability to shut out a disturbing auditory stimulus. Hence, as in Item 1, the stimulus must be able to break through the ambient conditions and create a startle response. The bell may be more successful in doing this, especially in a noisy nursery. Often, the rattle may bring the baby out of his generally shut-down state, in which case testing should be continued with the bell. The bell should be similar to the one used in a standard Gesell Test.

   The infant is scored (as above) according to his ability to delay and shut down his aversive reactions (general startle, tight blinking, and respiratory changes) as he habituates himself to repeated stimuli. Even a temporary suppression of these reactions is evidence of his ability to shut out the disturbing stimuli.
4. *Response decrement to pinprick* (scored in sleep states)—As a test of response decrement to tactile stimulation, the diaper pin may be used to prick the heel of the infant's foot when he is quiet. This may be repeated several times. The examiner watches for how totally and how rapidly the whole body responds to this pinprick. In an immature or CNS-damaged infant, the opposite foot withdraws and the whole body responds as quickly as the stimulated foot (a demonstration of the all-or-none aspect of an immature organism). The degree, rapidity, and repetition of this "spread" of stimulus to the rest of the body is measured here. The other aspect is the infant's capacity to shut down this spread of a generalized response. When he continues to respond in an obligatory, repetitive way, he rates a low score. As he demonstrates a suppression of responses to the stimulus and changes his state to a more alert, receptive one, he deserves a high score. Many infants demonstrate some but not all of this behavior, and it may be evidence of excellent CNS function. Middle scores are saved for infants who demonstrate some habituation but not an accompanying state change of alertness.
5. *Orientation response–inanimate visual* (scored in alert state 4)—Since most neonates will demonstrate some ability to fix on a visual object (a contrasting bright or shiny object, e.g., a bell, red ball, white mask) and follow it horizontally for brief excursions, this is a measure of that ability. It is highly state-related, and may not be demonstrated in any one exam, but, under optimal conditions (a quiet, semi-dark room), it is repeatable; following with the eyes is also accompanied by head-turning to follow. Vertical following seems of an even higher order, and many babies will stretch their necks to follow up and down.

   The infant may respond with a) alerting (decrease in random activity, focus on examiner's face when it is in his line of vision, slow regular respirations, and follows face when it moves in arcs), and b) brightening (change in facial expression, widening of eyes and brighter look, jagged respiration, with an associated decrease in random activity).

6. *Orientation response–inanimate auditory* (scored in alert state 4)—This is a measure of his response to a rattle or soft bell when he is in an alert state. One can observe brightening of his face, shifting of his eyes to the sound, and finally head turning to the sound. He may then be seen to search for the stimulus with his eyes.
7. *Orientation—animate visual* (alert state 4)—The next three items score the attention which is called up be the examiner's social cues—voice, face, cuddling, holding, rocking, and so forth. The infant may respond with alerting, brightening, and settling into the arms. He may turn his head to seek the voice or face. Having caught the examiner he may rivet his attention, and "lock" on for long periods. No interest is unusual. How he is held may strongly influence this, and the examiner should attempt to reproduce two maneuvers commonly used by mothers: a) hold the infant in a cuddled position in the arms up against the chest, and b) upright on the shoulder in a bubbling position.

   For the "visual only" item the examiner places his face in the infant's line of vision then moves it slowly in lateral and vertical arcs until the infant stops following.

   The infant will follow with 30 to 60° arcs with eyes and often with his head, showing real alert interest as he does so.
8. *Orientation—animate auditory* (alert states)—The examiner removes his face from infant's line of vision and talks to him from one side (6 to 12 inches from ear). Continuous, soft, and high-pitched speech is the best stimulus, e.g., infant's own name. The infant will quiet, become alert, and turn repeatedly toward the examiner's voice, searching for the source of his voice as he alerts.
9. *Orientation animate—visual and auditory stimuli* (alert state)—The same criteria for scoring are used as in Items 5 and 7. The same conditions pertain except that the examiner's voice is used to reinforce face, both on the bed and when infant is held. Voice is continuous while face is moving.
10. *Alertness* (in most alert state)—This assesses the frequency of the best periods of alertness as shown by his responsivity to the examiner within these best periods. These periods can occur at any time during the exam period. Often this is elicited while the examiner holds the infant. Since newborns are so variable, and are alert for such a short period, one must assume that any period of alertness in a 30-minute exam may be taken as an index of the infant's "capacity for responsiveness." In a less randomly selected time sample than this, or when one can wait for a spontaneous period of alertness, this measure might be a better index of his availability, but I have found that most infants show small periods of alert behavior during an exam. These should be assessed. Alerting is defined as brightening and widening of eyes, while orienting is used for the response of turning toward the direction of stimulation.
11. *General tone—predominant tone* (in alert states)—This scores the motor tone of the baby in his most characteristic state of responsiveness. Since this is a summary assessment, it should include the overall use of tone as he responds to being handled. This should be assessed in state 4, unless there is no opportunity to produce such an assessment. This should then be assessed in state 6.

    Tone becomes a summary assessment of motor responses as evaluated when he is at rest and is confirmed by handling assessed in such maneuvers as spontaneous activity, pull to sit, holding him over hand horizontally, prone placement, etc., and should be an overall assessment of his body tone as he reacts to all of these.
12. *Motor maturity* (alert states)—Motor

maturity is demonstrated by smooth movements of the extremities and a free, wide range of movement. This is a measure of motor responses, spontaneous and elicited, assessed throughout the exam in the alert states. The arm movements become the easiest to score. The assessment is of a) smoothness versus jerkiness which reflects the balanced flexors and extensors versus the unbalanced cogwheel movement of the premature of CNS irritation with flexors and extensors competing, and b) freedom of arcs of movement (90°) (arms on bed) versus restricted arcs (45° etc.) (arms and legs in flexion). The premature has unlimited freedom of movement (floppy) in lateral, sagittal, and cephalad areas, but the movements are jerky and cog-like, overshooting their marks. The very mature infant has both freedom of movement in all directions associated with a smooth, balanced performance (not floppy). The average newborn is somewhat limited in arcs of movement, especially those above the head, and somewhat in the lateral plane.

13. *Pulled to sit* (in awake states)—The examiner places a forefinger in each of the infant's palms. With the arms extended, the infant's automatic grasp is used to pull him to sit. The shoulder girdle muscles should respond with tone, and muscular resistance to stretching his neck and lower musculature as he is pulled into a sitting position. Usually he will also attempt to right his head into a position which is in the midline of his trunk and parallel to his body. Since his head is heavy and out of proportion to the rest of his body mass, this is not usually possible and his head falls backward as he comes up. In a seated position, he attempts to right his head, and it may fall forward. Several attempts to right it can be felt via the shoulder muscles as the examiner maintains his grasp on the infant's arms. A few infants make no attempt at all.
14. *Cuddliness* (in awake states)—This is a measure of the infant's response to being held. There are several components which are scored in summary of his responses to being held in a cuddled position against the examiner's chest, and up on his shoulder. The responses are a measure of his negative or positive responses, as well as none at all. The baby can mold to the examiner's body and against his shoulder, turning to nuzzle and nestle his head into the crook of neck.
15. *Defensive movements* (in awake states)—A small cloth is placed with examiner's fingers asserting light pressure over the upper part of the face which would partially occlude the nose, and is kept in place for two minutes, or until the infant responds with a series of responses: a) general quieting, b) mouthing, c) head turning and rooting from side to side, d) head turning lateral as well as neck stretching up and down, e) general undirected increase in activity, f) directed swipes in general area of cloth, g) directed swipes in specific area of cloth which removes the cloth.
16. *Consolability with intervention* (tested in crying state)—This measures the number of activities on the part of examiner which are necessary to interfere with this fussing state and allow the baby to move to a quieter state. Some infants will quiet only when they are dressed and left alone. Any stimulus from the environment disturbs them. Others will quiet when they are held and actively rocked. A steady hand held on a crying baby's belly will act as a soothing stimulus. Others need one or both arms held in addition to the hand on the belly. Holding the arm or arms interferes with the disturbing startle activity which is triggered by crying or fussing. A few babies will even quiet to the examiner's voice or face and are easily consoled by any maneuver.
17. *Peak of excitement* (upset state)—This is a

measure of how much motor and crying activity the infant gives off to the observer at his peaks of excitement, and responsiveness pulls him toward the mean. The kind of intense reactions which some infants demonstrate when they reach their peak of excitement shows an unavailability to the outside world, and must be scored high. Others are hardly able to be jogged to respond at all, and their peak is very low. An average and optimal response would fall in the moderate, reachable range, in which the infant could be brought to respond to stimuli in spite of a high degree of upset or excitement, but then return to more moderate states. This is scored to differentiate motor excitement as opposed to alertness (Item 10) which scores sensory excitement.

18. *Rapidity of buildup* (from sleep to crying)—This is a measure of use of states from a quiet state to an agitated state. It measures the timing and the number of stimuli which are used before he changes from his initially quiet state to a more agitated one. Since this implies that we start with an initially quiet baby, it measures the period of "control" which he can maintain in the face of increasingly aversive stimuli as well as the additive effect of these stimuli in changing his initially quiet state. The first preference is when one can observe the infant as he changes from a sleep state or a quiet awake one (state 5) to an agitated crying one (state 6).
19. *Irritability* (in alert states)—This measures the number of times he gets upset as well as the kind of stimuli which make him cry.
20. *Activity* (in alert states)—This is a summary of the activity seen during the entire observation, especially during the alert states. The activity consists of two kinds: a) spontaneous, and b) in response to the stimulation of handling and the stimuli used by the observer.
21. *Tremulousness* (in all states)—Since in its severe form this may be a measure of CNS irritation or depression, or may occur for metabolic reasons, or may be a sign of immaturity, it becomes one more way of indicating all of these. If it is severe, the baby should become suspect and a neurologic evaluation is indiated. Milder forms of tremulousness are demonstrated at the end of a startle, and as a baby comes from sleeping to awake states. There is some tremor of the chin and extremities which can be expected in the neonate's first week. As the infant is dehydrated normally in the second and third day, metabolic imbalances cause some tremulousness. In light sleep or as he startles in deep sleep, tremors of the extremities are noted. As he becomes alert and active, the tremulousness should be overcome with smooth, voluntary behavior of the limbs. Aversive stimuli set off a startle which is followed by a return of tremulousness of the chin and extremities. Mildly aversive stimuli should not cause observable tremors in their reactions. Quivering and tremors are synonymous. Shivering may occur after the infant has been undressed for a period, and would need to be differentiated from tremulousness.
22 *Amount of startles* (during entire exam)—Both spontaneous startles and those which have been elicited in the course of stimulation are included in this. Some infants never startle during an exam, except when a Moro reflex is elicited. Abnormally sensitive infants overreact to any disturbing stimulus with a startle, and have observable startles for no reason. Hence they must be considered "spontaneous" or due to internal stimuli.
23. *Lability of skin color* (as he wakes up and is handled during exam)—This measures the changes of color and vascularity which take place in a period of exam, e.g., the acrocyanosis of peripheral mild cyanosis when the extremity is left uncovered, the change from pink to pale or purple when

the baby is undressed—mottling and a web-like appearance may occur in an effort to maintain body heat. A normal newborn is likely to demonstrate mild color changes several times in an exam during which he has been undressed, disturbed, and upset.

24. *Lability of states* (all states)—This measures the infant's state performance over the exam period. Frequency of state changes over a recognizable wide swing are counted (alert to awake, crying to alert, sleep to crying, crying to sleep).
25. *Self-quieting activity* (when upset)—This is a measure of activity which the baby initiates in a fussing state in an observable effort to quiet himself. The number of activities which can be observed is counted. Their success is measured by an observable state change which persists for at least 5 seconds. The activities which can be seen are: a) hand to mouth efforts, b) sucking on fist or tongue, and c) using visual or auditory stimuli from the environment to quiet himself (more than a simple response is necessary to determine this).
26. *Hand to mouth facility* (in all states)—This is measured in all states. A hand to mouth reflex is inborn, and seems to be a response to stroking the cheek or the palm of the infant's hand. It can be triggered by mucus and gagging in the neonate, by discomfort, and by placing him in a prone position. It is seen spontaneously as the neonate attempts to control himself or comfort himself when upset. This is a measure of his ability to bring his hands to his mouth in a supine position as well as his success in insertion. Some infants bring their hands to their mouths repeatedly, insert a part of the fist or fingers, and suck actively on the inserted part.
27. *Smiles* (all states)—Smiles are seen in the neonate. They surely can be of reflexive grimacing in nature, and they also occur "appropriately," i.e., in response to soft auditory and/or visual cues. Occasionally, when the baby is handled and restrained in a cuddling position, a smile comes across his face as he relaxes. I have seen close replicas of "social smiles" in the newborn period—when an examiner leans over his crib and talks softly to him. They are difficult to be sure of, may consist primarily of a softening and brightening of the infant's face with a reflex grimace thrown in, and they may certainly be difficult to reproduce. Hence, one hesitates to call these social "smiles," but they surely are the facial precursors of such smiling behavior. A mother reinforces them as such.

We feel that the behavioral items are tapping in on more important evidences of cortical control and responsiveness, even in the neonatal period. The neonate's capacity to manage and overcome the physiologic demands of this adjustment period in order to attend to, to differentiate, and to habituate to the complex stimuli of an examiner's maneuvers may be an important predictor of his future central nervous system organization. Certainly, the curve of recovery of these responses over the first neonatal week must be of more significance than the midbrain responses detectable in routine neurologic exams. Repeated behavioral exams on any two or three days in the first 10 days after delivery might be expected to be sensitive predictors of future cortical function.

In predicting future risk for the baby, it may be as important to estimate the effect of his neonatal responses on the environment around him.

Bowlby[11] has stressed the importance of observing the earliest interactions between mother and infant as predictive of the kind of attachment a mother may form for the infant. He suggests that there is a kind of "imprinting" of responses from her which may be triggered by the neonate's behavior. Moss[12] and Goldberg[13] point to the trigger-like value of the newborn's small size, helpless appearance, and distress cries in setting off mothering activities. Klaus and Kennell[14] have described the kinds of initial contacts which mothers make with their newborn infants and the distortions in this behavior when the mother is depressed by abnormalities in the baby, such as prematurity, illness in the neonatal period, and so forth. Eye-to-eye contact, touching, handling, and nursing behavior on the part of the mother may be assessed and judged for predicting her ability to relate to the new baby. Changes in these behaviors over time are stressed as indicators of recovery or non-recovery of maternal capacity to attach to the baby by mothers who have been depressed and unable to function optimally by having produced an infant at risk.[15]

The ability of the baby to precipitate and encourage her attachment and care-taking behavior must be taken into account. With an unresponsive neonate, the feedback mechanisms necessary to fuel mothering behavior are severely impaired. In a series of medicated newborns of normal mother-infant pairs, the effect on neonatal sucking coupled with the physiologic effect of the medication on her milk production delayed recovery of weight gain by 36 to 48 hours in a normal group.[16] Since this is an observation of rather gross level, interference in the interaction dyssynchrony of more subtle "lack of fit" in the earliest mother-infant attachment interaction should be carefully watched for and observed over time. The possibility of creating or compounding the problems of infants at risk by a distortion of the environment's reactions to him is too important, and our tools for predicting this in the lying-in period should be sharpened. The opportunity for observing the pair together is never again as available, and surely we are missing valuable predictive information when we do not make regular, repeated observations of interactive situations, such as feeding periods, "play" periods after feeding, and bathing—documenting the maternal behavior and the infant's responses to it, as well as the changes in each which occur over time in a supportive, protective situation such as the lying-in hospital. In the case of infants at risk, it is vital to fostering their capacity for recovery and integration of any intact mechanisms for development that we provide them with the best possible environment. Without an early assessment of this environment as it reacts to the baby, we may miss an invaluable opportunity to support the parents and improve the environment for an infant at risk.

The Neonatal Behavioral Assessment has been developed as a research tool, and its value as such will depend on investigators' reliability in order to compare groups of neonates. This reliability demands that all who wish to use it for gathering data in the neonatal period reach interscorer reliability of .85 on all items.

However, it can also be used as part of a nurse's or physician's clinical assessment. The items lend themselves to being added to the usual pediatric examination, and attention to these remarkable capacities on the part of the neonate will add considerably to the predictive skill and the pleasure of a nurse clinician as he or she examines the neonate.

NURSING ACTIONS TO STIMULATE

The purpose of these actions is to stimulate the neonate's interaction potential and thereby enhance his growth and development. The nurse is ready to implement nursing actions which stimulate after completion of a behavioral assessment (such as described by Brazelton). Behavioral assessment is a prerequisite to action because it provides information on the neonate's sensory-perceptual capacities which indicate the infant's readi-

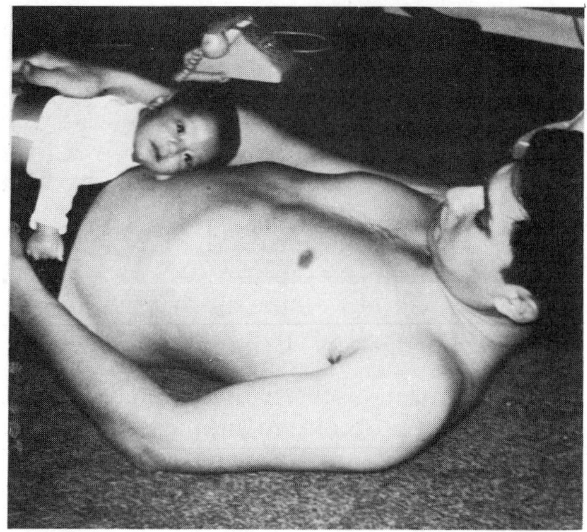

FIGURE 33-2. This father has developed a unique style to arouse alert behaviors in his 2-week-old son by providing a most potent stimulus—father's bodily touch and voice.

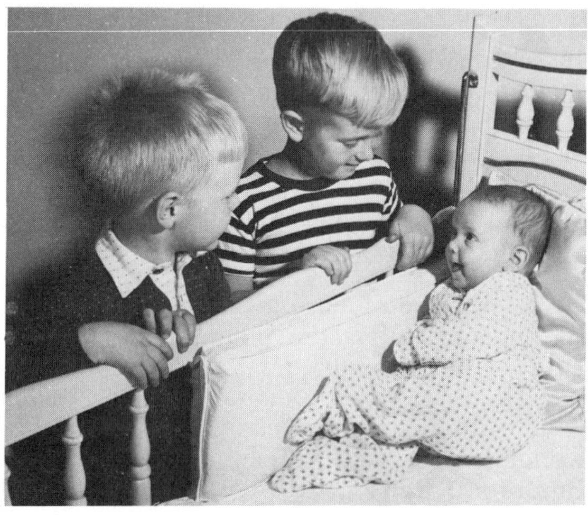

FIGURE 33-3. Infant receiving visual and auditory stimulation from older siblings.

ness and potential for interactive behaviors. It is not feasible to identify every possible action by which the nurse can stimulate the neonate and his family. Many actions are presently unknown and will emerge through creative endeavors by nurses who value the importance of infant stimulation. Thus, the following are examples of possible nursing actions. Nursing actions are identified relative to major goals in the nursing care plan for stimulating the neonate and his family.

Goal: *Provision of environmental input to stimulate the neonate's interaction potential.*

Inherent to attaining this goal is that the nurse share with parents the approaches effectively used for infant stimulation. This is crucial because the hospital is a pseudoenvironment for the infant to establish interaction patterns. It is the family environment with its unique family members and life style that will be the natural habitat where interaction must be established (Figs. 33-2 and 33-3). Therefore, parents need to know how to best present themselves and their home environment to build the foundation for interaction patterns which will be mutually satisfying to the infant and all in the family. Here are some suggested approaches and considerations to stimulate the newborn's interaction potential.

Proper Position of Both Infant and Stimulus

Are the infant's sense organs (eyes, ears, nose, hands, and feet) able to receive stimuli as well as elicit responses to them? Sometimes the infant's visual field is obstructed with too many stimuli, such as equipment or harsh lights, or the infant cannot attempt to locate a stimulus because he is restricted in movements. For example, too tight bundling will prevent the infant from turning his head to follow a stimulus and also prevent receiving touch or touching others. Another example is a beautiful mobile hanging in the center of the nursery, too high or out of visual range for infants whose bassinettes are not close by.

The position of the human stimulus is also important. Can the baby see, hear, and feel the mother or nurses as they come in contact with him? It is important to remember that the most ideal position to promote behavioral development is when both the baby and the parent or nurse have face-to-face orientation with each other. The stimulation potential is strengthened when the face-to-face contact is accompanied by the human voice and touch. Some questions a nurse or parent should ask themselves regarding position are:

> Am I within the baby's visual field, or too close or too far away for him to fixate on me?
>
> How do I position the baby during feedings? Are his hands free to make contact with the bottle, breast, or other parts of my body? Can he turn his head freely when he desires to take a break during his feeding, to explore his surroundings? Or am I holding him too snugly so that he is restrained in movements?
>
> Do I take the time to change the infant's position in his bassinette so he can absorb all aspects of his environment?
>
> How do I carry the baby? Are his eyes, ears, and hands free for exploration, or are they obstructed by parts of my body? Or am I holding him too tightly or so insecurely that his infant state of behavior is tense, precluding his availability of energy for attending to stimuli?

One last factor concerns an interesting hypothesis by Dr. Lee Salk who proposes that carrying an infant on the left side, close to the heart, serves an important psychobiologic process.[17] This position apparently has a soothing effect on the baby which is speculated to result from an association between the rhythmic maternal heart beat and a tension-free state which developed during gestation.

Consider Quality and Amount of Stimuli Input

Remember that neonates have selective preferences (discrimination) as to which stimuli will arouse their interaction potential. Therefore, parents and nurses should evaluate stimuli for their ability to activate the infant's attending processes. Unfortunately, many times stimuli are chosen because of influences from advertisements or relating quality with monetary cost. It has already been stated that the best arousal-evoking stimulus is the human one, which doesn't have a price tag. Parents and nurses should choose inanimate objects which are bright, shiny, moving, and have pattern or contour. Auditory input should be soft and rhythmic, rather than harsh and loud. Tactile stimulation should be gentle, warm, and smooth, rather than rough, jerky, and cold. Consider the type of auditory and tactile input provided by nurses. How often have you entered a nursery and heard nurses talking loudly to each other across the room? The nursery can sometimes provide auditory bombardment with a multitude of sounds from equipment, voices, traffic, water, and so forth. In such an environment, the baby will have difficulty attending to a specific sound. The infant will usually block reception of the stimulus because it has difficulty organizing the multitude. Another factor for consideration is how often do nurses bother to assess whether their hands are warm or cold before proceeding to handle a baby when giving care?

The maximum benefits of human stimuli can also decrease when the human face, voice, and touch are not presented long enough for the neonate to attend. For example, a quick glance at the baby or uttering two sounds is not adequate to arouse the infant. Unfortunately, in the nursing world such fleeting contacts are a common occurrence because the nurse is so task-oriented. This was validated by the findings in a study which explored nurse-infant interaction:

> In routine care, from first observations, it seems that the child is not looked at much, or smiled at or spoken to; neither is he tickled much, fondled nor moved around. . . .
>
> The concern of the nurse is over food intake, digestive process, production of stools, burps, and cleanliness. When speaking occurs, it is often when something goes wrong with one of these things. The good child is the one who drinks fast, burps promptly, has a stool before a clean diaper is put on. . . . (Such good behavior by the infant) does not bring much more stimulation or attention from the nurse. In general, nurses have a low tolerance for crying or suffering. These are met by indifference and not infrequently with impatience and resentment; the child is blamed for being naughty. . . .
>
> All this shows that communication between the nurse and infant is rare.[18]

There is also another danger inherent in nurses who demonstrate behaviors indicative of lack of involvement or communication with the infants. At times parents observing the nurses may begin to perceive that such task-orientation is the ideal or expectation for the "parenting role." The danger lies in parents "imprinting" the nurses' behaviors of trying to achieve a task in the least time, regardless of effects on the infant.

The solution is that nurses must take more time in their routine care to give attention by looking, talking, and touching the baby, and trying to elicit behavioral responses. Cues indicative of the attending process in the neonate are: decrease in motor activity; quieting, settling down behaviors; visual fixation by glassy-eyed staring; auditory fixation as if listening; head turning toward a stimulus; subtle responses such as decreased heart and respiratory rate. Parents and nurses need to recognize these behaviors as significant interaction responses. When parents and nurses take more time in giving themselves to the baby, they will come to find that the baby can be fun to talk to, touch, and look at. Here is the genesis for interaction. When parents look at, talk to, and touch the baby, and perceive that the baby has received their input, then they will continue to interact. Likewise, the baby who is given more to look at, to listen to, and to touch, will be better able to see, hear, and feel. Thus, the baby will take the initiative to bring stimuli input into his world.

Recognition of Opportunities for Infant Stimulation

Our present life style is one perceived as having too much to do in too little time. Nurses, and also mothers (especially multiparas), are easily caught in the "too busy syndrome." This refers to the attitude that one is too busy to do anything extra or beyond the usual or routine. Nurses and mothers easily agree that their role is to feed and diaper the baby but may not be too receptive if given a mandate to talk to the baby for a minimum period of 10 to 15 minutes. Who has ten minutes to spare? The solution may be simple. In the process of meeting the newborn's essential needs for maintaining respirations, ingestion, warmth, and diaper changes the nurse and parents are exposing the infant to social contact. These everyday, routine times of contact can significantly influence behavioral development. The frequency and repetition of stimuli input provide the patterning of behavioral responses. Infant care tasks bring the best stimuli input to the baby—the human being. Thus, nurses and parents must learn to slow down their pace and maintain facial, voice, and touch contacts long enough for the infant to explore the stimulus and react to it.

Another important consideration is recognition of the interaction potential in the neonate's reflexes. Nurses and parents need to appreciate that reflex responses also have an orientation function. For example, when the rooting reflex is elicited by touching the infant's cheek, he turns his head toward the stimulus to face it. Parents and nurses should meet the infant half way by also turning toward the baby to allow a face-to-face orientation. Likewise, the palmar grasp is elicited by touching the palm. Many parents recognize the interaction potential in the infant's grasp because they show genuine excitement that their infant is "holding on to me." However, what is the impact of the grasp on the busy nurse? Is excitement also felt or does the nurse become perturbed that her task is interrupted and time must be taken to pry the little fingers loose?

Nurses and parents must ask themselves, "When am I providing human contact to the baby?" Human contact should be provided during the infant's optimum behavioral state for reception and reaction to human stimuli, the alert states. It is obvious that a crying, fussy, hungry, or drowsy baby will not be able to attend efficiently to human stimuli in attempts to activate its interaction potential. Thus, a baby should be played with and talked to when he is also awake and quiet. Too often, babies are given human input primarily when they are crying. The danger is that the infant will associate crying as eliciting human stimuli and quieting behaviors as not bringing the pleasurable human stimuli. Parents and nurses also need to know how they can manipulate the infant's state of behavior to make him more receptive to activate his interaction potential. Attempts by the baby to quiet himself through random motions to get the hands near the mouth should not be abruptly stopped. Also, nurses and parents need to know how to console crying and irritable behaviors by means other than feedings. Again the human input of face, voice, and touch is very effective to terminate crying. Other measures to elicit soothing effects are: rocking, rhythmic tapping, stroking, or patting parts of the body, such as the chest and abdomen; maintaining constant tactile contact by carrying and cuddling the baby, preferably on the left side so additional input can occur from the heart beat; placing the baby into a flexed position resembling the comfort of the in utero position; non-nutritive (pacifier) sucking. Parents should experiment with various techniques to console their infant. The uniqueness of the interaction between parent and child may be expressed when a method for consolability elicits soothing behaviors only when performed by the distinct voice, touch, or face of the parent.

Mutual Reinforcement for Behavioral Input and Reactions

Feedback is the mechanism by which interaction is maintained. The mutuality of the feedback is important because interaction implies mutual input and output. Parents will not continue to provide stimulation to their infants unless they feel their actions are meaningful. Meaning is found when they can perceive that the baby received their input and likes it. Likewise, the baby will not continue to attend to a stimuli unless it finds pleasure in doing so. The rewards are different for the infant as compared with adults. The most rewarding stimulus for the infant is the continued input of the human being looking, talking, touching, and playing with him. However, adults expect more, primarily because of their expectations of social rewards they have acquired in their years of interacting with the world. Thus, parents and nurses are looking for higher levels of social responses such as smiling and babbling from the infant. Although the potentials for these higher level responses are present at birth, they must be developed through stimulation. Therefore, adults must be reoriented to recognize the unique expression of the neonate to convey that he is pleased with the parents' attempts to convey love and care. Parents need help to appreciate that the infant's attending processes, their ability to console the infant, and the unrecognizable grimaces and uncoordinated vocalizations resembling groans or grunts can indeed be rewards from the infant. The simple responses of the neonate become meaningful when the adult perceives such behaviors as communicating, "Mommy and Daddy, I like you." Positive feedback is highly enriching to the ego of both parents and the infant. The infant will come to perceive the world as eliciting pleasure and satisfactions in him, and parents and nurses will feel good that they can instill pleasure in others.

Goal: *Promote acquaintance process between parents and infant (primarily between mother and infant).*

The nurse's involvement in facilitating parent-child interaction should have begun in the prenatal period, continued through the intrapartal experience, and reach peak involvement during the postpartal phase. Now with the baby's presence in the world, he also contributes to the acquaintance process with his parents. The nurse must integrate these infant contributions in the nursing plan to facilitate parent-child interaction. Whereas other chapters have focused primarily on the parent (mother), the aim here is to focus on the child's involvement. This discussion complements those found in other chapters (especially Chapter 29). This discussion offers some important suggestions to promote parent-child interaction, primarily from the infant's viewpoint.

First, both mothers and babies must be allowed to explore each other. Environmental arrangements which allow the infant to be with the mother according to the mother's desires seem to facilitate exploration behaviors. Rooming-in with the assistance of a knowledgeable nurse can help the mother and infant to familiarize themselves with each other. Remember, exploratory behaviors are influenced by physical and emotional stability of both mother and baby. Thus, the nurse must give consideration to the mother's state of comfort as well as her perception of her own readiness and desire to have contact with her infant. Some mothers may be very eager to interact with their infants immediately in the delivery room and should not be denied this interaction. Other mothers may not be so eager and may need more time to work through their feelings about the child they produced. Such mothers should not have their newborns forced upon them but rather the nurse should focus on the mother and her concerns. The nurse must also consider the baby's state of behavior. An infant having difficulty establishing physiologic adaptation should not be taxed with environmental stimulation. The baby's energies may be needed for his physiologic functioning and he should not have his behavioral potential aroused until he is physiologically stable.

Nurses should permit parents to explore their infants in privacy. Parents may be reluctant to initiate exploratory behaviors if they feel they are being observed or that others can overhear their comments to the baby. Thus, the nurse should ask the parents if they would like to be alone with their new infant. If the room is shared with other patients, the curtain can be drawn to ensure some privacy.

A second important nursing action is assisting parents to identify the unique behaviors in their newborn infants. One way to accomplish this is by sharing Brazelton's behavioral assessment tool with parents. Nurses should demonstrate the assessment as well as involve parents in its participation. The rationale for this is that it allows the parents to recognize the infant's perceptual abilities and teaches parents how to activate their infant's exploratory behaviors. The nurse can tell the mother that she is the best elicitor to activate the baby's sensory arousal. Nurses can demonstrate this by talking, touching, and looking at the infant during his alert state and pointing out to the mother the behavioral responses she might not recognize as having interaction potential. Nurses should also tell parents that they are the best elicitors for the development of social responses which are highly rewarding. Smiles and babbling manifest earlier when infants are provided with their mothers' voice, face, and touch repeatedly during contacts in daily living. Mothers should elicit the rooting reflex and grasp reflex to allow the baby to see them better and to maintain contact with the fingers. The value of the nurse doing a behavioral assessment with the mother present is that the infant can clearly demonstrate to the mother that he is capable of seeing her, hearing her voice, and touching her, and eventually will prefer her stimulations to those from inanimate objects or strangers.

The following assessment tool is an example of how a group of concerned nurses have modified Brazelton's tool to share with parents (mothers especially), with the nurse assisting the mother to assess her infant's behavioral responses.

NEWBORN ASSESSMENT TOOL*

(Application of Brazelton Assessment Tool to the Nursing Assessment of the Newborn)

This tool can have four uses:

Initial and ongoing assessment of neurologic and behavioral responses	1. It can be used as an initial assessment instrument of the newborn's behavior and of his neurologic responses. It can be used as an assessment of the important beginnings of emotional and cognitive development of the infant. It can be used as a day-to-day assessment of the subtle changes of the neonate as he recovers from the birth shock and from the effect of medication.
Predictor of initial parent/child relationships	2. It can be used as a predictor of the manner in which the infant, because of his behavorial responses, affects his environment. It further can be used as a predictor of parental reactions and the resulting parent-infant patterns that are likely to develop.
Parental assessment and attachment	3. When shared with the mother and father, it can help them to focus on the infant's individuality and to assess his needs more adequately. It can be a potent instrument to help them understand their child and develop a deeper attachment to him.
Instrument to establish a preventive relationship with parents	4. Establishing your interest as a caregiver of the individual assets and strengths of the newborn, the parents can identify with your approach to the "total" child, and feel a different kind of support from you.

* Developed by Ann Clark in association with a group of selected nurses at Kaiser Medical Center, Honolulu, Hawaii, 1974.

Parental Adaptation to Infant's Behavior

TO:

FROM: Your Nurses

Today is the first day of your child's life and the first day of your lives together.

I am sure you are aware of how important this day is. You are facing quite a responsibility. Life with the baby won't always be happy, but in understanding his behavior and his responses you can not only learn to live with him but can find much joy and happiness in doing so. Your new baby is not totally helpless. As you well know, he can already do many things. As erratic as his behavior may seem to us at times, it does not occur by accident. It has purpose. One of your tasks will be to discover his early developmental responses to you and to his environment for they will effect the relationship that will develop between you. In focusing on his behavior you can help him to become organized, to grow physically and emotionally, and to reach his learning potential. What more creative work can there be in all this world?

You and your baby are important to your nurses and your doctor. We would like to help you discover your infant's responses and his adaptation to his new world as he struggles to gain some mastery over himself. By doing so, one can begin to predict the kind of interaction he is likely to set up with his environment (sights, sounds, smells, touch, etc.) and what environment will be most enriching to his enfolding personality.

His day of birth was likely a trying time for him. Hopefully, he'll never have another birthday as stressful as his first one. From a warm, secure, quiet, dark aquatic environment, he was pushed and squeezed into a world full of sounds, lights, chilled dry air, and rough textures. He likely was a bit shocked (physically). It will take him several days to completely recover from the experience and we must be patient with him.

1. RESPONSE TO SIGHT AND TO SOUND

Before the baby wakes up, let us see what are his responses while asleep. Sleep is of two types. In deep sleep he seems oblivious to all around him. Generally he is quiet, but occasionally he startles, making auditory sounds and thrusting his arms and legs out. In a less deep sleep, but a sleep nevertheless, there is eye movement under closed lids. He is more active and it may seem to you he is not really asleep. It is true he can be more easily awakened.

Now, before he awakens, we will check to see how he responds to a light flashed over his closed eyes a number of times. We will then follow this with a bell, and finally a rattle.

Babies vary greatly in how, or if, they respond to this kind of stimulation. Some babies respond very little, others are disturbed at first but slow down the responses, finally ignoring the light or the sound.

2. ALERTNESS

VISUAL RESPONSE

Your baby can see. As soon as the edema has disappeared around his eyelids he can open them. His interest in looking at and following a bright shiny object will be tried first. Then we will follow that stimulation with a face. Hold him upright facing you. Can he be alerted to look at your face, will he follow your face if you move it to the right or left?

AUDITORY RESPONSE

Move your face from his line of vision and talk to him from one side. A soft, high-pitched voice is the best stimulus. Repeat his name and encourage him to turn his face toward your voice, over and over again. Don't despair if he doesn't respond at first. He is learning, it may take time.

Note how alert he is when you try to get a visual or auditory response from him.

3. CUDDLINESS

What is your child's response to being held?
How does that response meet your expectation or what you hoped your baby would be like?

Some babies nestle in your arms in a very relaxed manner. Other babies tend to be stiff and seem to be trying to escape from the person holding them. They seem to respond better to activity such as rocking, bouncing, etc., than to being held quietly.

4. CONSOLABILITY

The baby's cry is his main mode of communication. Some of his crying you will learn to understand, others may confuse you. When your baby is upset, how long does he cry? What seems to precipitate the crying?

Some infants seem to be easily disturbed by any stimuli in their environment. Being undressed, picked up, etc. may set off the crying.

Does your baby have an ability to quiet himself without intervention? This would demonstrate a high degree of consolability. Without picking him up, will placing your hand on his abdomen be enough to quiet him? Try holding his arms on his abdomen (this will keep the startle reflex from frightening him when he cries). This may be all that is needed to quiet him. Some babies are quieted by a face or by a voice. Some babies find their fist and suck on that to console themselves.

Picking up, caressing, rocking, and cuddling, all necessary experiences for any child, may be what it takes to quiet him. (Incidentally, offer these experiences to your child often, not just in response to his cries). Many mothers are concerned about "spoiling" their baby by picking him up. Your baby's cry should be responded to. He should not be left to cry for long periods of time. It is all right to try to comfort your crying child. However, in spite of your best effort, he may continue to cry.

Note when your infant is presented with an interfering stimuli how much does it take to upset him? How upset does he become? How long is he upset? What quiets him? All of these observations give you some measure of the control he can maintain in the face of an irritating stimuli. Babies vary greatly and you need to know what you can expect from your child.

5. PROTECTIVE REFLEXES

Your child has a number of reflexes. One of these (the sucking reflex) helps him to search for food. Some serve him as protective reflexes and it will make life more secure for you to know about them.

We will place a cloth over the baby's face and exert light pressure over the upper part of his face. Note his response to this intrusion as he moves his head to facilitate adequate breathing. Unless he were to get tangled in some loose garment or get his head wedged into a small place, he can be depended on to struggle to keep his head clear of external obstruction and to breathe.

He has other reflexes to protect him also. He yawns to get more oxygen, coughs and sneezes to clear his nasal passages, and blinks to protect his eyes from bright lights and from objects coming in contact with his eyes.

6. OTHER REFLEXES

The MORO (startle) reflex is your baby's response to something that frightens him. Loud sounds, a sudden jolt, or a loss of balance will precipitate this behavior. It even occurs sometimes during his sleep. He responds by throwing out both arms in an embrace, drawing up his legs and then crying. It is a normal reflex which will disappear in a few months.

ROOTING, SUCKING, SWALLOWING. Your baby learns much about his world through his sensitive lips and his mouth. He roots for an object whenever his cheek or lips are touched. Once the object is within his grasp he mouths it and tries to swallow it. It is a reflex with which you will cooperate as he learns to suck and later to eat. There is one exception, your baby does have taste discrimination. He will refuse some bitter and very salty tastes.

GRASP REFLEX. Anything placed in the palm of your infants hand will be grasped and held tightly for a short period of time. His feet, too, have a grasp reflex. Stimulate the soles of his feet by stroking from heel to toe and you will see the toes turn downward in a grasplike motion.

DANCING reflex may be demonstrated by your baby. Hold him upright with your hands under his armpits and allow his feet to touch the crib mattress. In this manner he may be assisted in taking little stepping motions.

7. MUSCLE TONE

Your baby's motor activity is demonstrated by how smooth or how jerky he moves his arms and legs. Note how far he swings his arms and legs and how close he pulls them to his body. Is he a "floppy" baby (like a rag doll)? A stiff, tense, jittery baby? How much does he stretch his arms and legs?

SITTING UP. Place him in a sitting position, but do not support his head as you usually do. He may, momentarily, bring his head up, only to drop it backwards or forward due to the weight of the head and the undeveloped neck muscles. Some babies make no such effort.

8. OTHER OBSERVATIONS

HICCOUGHING. We do not know what precipitates a hiccough, but we do know that it will disappear within ten minutes, even if we do nothing. It is caused by spasms of the chest muscles your child uses in breathing, going into spasm. The baby seems less disturbed by the phenomena than do the adults about him.

SMILING. Yes, your baby can smile. Some of these smiles seem to be precipitated by the internal working of his body, others seem to be a social response. They are hard to elicit. You will be excited with what seems to be a positive feedback.

BREATHING PATTERN. Now uncover your infant's chest and note his breathing pattern. It is unusually rhythmic, but at times he seems to be holding his breath momentarily and then speeds up his breathing as if to catch up.

SKIN COLORING. Observe the color of your child's skin and how it changes when he is active, cries or is asleep. For the first few days you may note some cyanosis (bluish color) around his lips or of his hands or feet.

TREMULOUSNESS. Babies may have brief episodes of trembling. Usually it is the arms that are involved, but greater areas of the body, including the chin, may tremble. Some tremulousness is to be expected during the first week of life.

Do ask your nurse if you note other responses or if you have further questions. We enjoy studying your infant, too.

A third nursing consideration is to help parents find meaning in the acquaintance process, meaning in their infant's behavioral responses and to make their own responses to their infants more meaningful. There is a reciprocity to "meaningfulness" in the acquaintance process. Too often parents do not understand their infant's behaviors and these behaviors elicit feelings of anxiety or guilt in the parent instead of pleasure. Likewise, for the infant, some parents may constantly talk, touch, or stimulate their infants with a barrage of input so that the infant is easily fatigued instead of being aroused for interaction. The nurse's role is twofold: provide parents with information about normal neonatal behavioral responses (as described previously with the use of behavioral assessments), and help parents to coordinate their exploratory behaviors with those of the infant. The significance of the correlation among the sequence of behaviors to enhance the acquaintance process is beautifully illustrated in the following description of a mother trying to elicit smiling in her infant.

> The mother smiles and vocalizes to the infant and moves her head rhythmically towards and away from his face. The infant first responds by rapt attention, with a widening of his eyes and a stilling of his body movements. Then his excitement increases, body movements begin again, he may vocalize and eventually a smile spreads over his face. At this point he turns away from his mother before beginning the whole cycle once again. Throughout this sequence the mother's actions are carefully phased with those of the infant. During the infant's attention phase the mother's behaviour is restrained but as his excitement increases she vocalizes more rapidly and the pitch of her voice rises. At the point when he is about to smile her movements are suddenly reduced, as if she was allowing him time to reply. However, not all mothers behave in this way. Some subject their infants to a constant and unphased barrage of stimulation. The infant is given no pauses in which to reply and he seems to be totally overwhelmed by his mother. Instead of playing this game for long periods, he is quickly reduced to fussing and crying and shows sustained and prolonged turning away from the mother's face.[19]

Some examples of nursing actions to provide meaning in the mother-infant acquaintance process are:

1. Help parents to recognize the infant's behavioral clues indicating readiness for interaction. Examples of behaviors indicative of a neonate's attending abilities are: decrease in movements in an active baby or increase in movements in a quiet baby;[20,21] visual fixation by glassy-eyed staring or eyes widening;[22] auditory atten-

tion by head turning to a stimulus, eyes blinking or staring;[23,24] decreased respiratory rate.[25]

2. Help parents to understand that infant behaviors indicative of negative responses (such as crying or turning away) may reflect the infant's reactions to his internal physiologic state rather than a response to the mother's care (such as feeding, bathing, diapering). Nurses need to have a general appreciation that parents (especially the mother) may perceive the baby's behaviors as indicative of his general attitude or feeding toward the parent. This is illustrated below:

    Mothers tend to believe that their newborn likes them and appreciates their ministrations when the infant's behavior is characterized by nursing eagerly, cuddling, smiling after feeding, focusing in the direction of the mother's face, listening to her voice, quieting when touched, and sleeping for relatively long periods after feeding. Behavior that leads mothers to believe their infants have a critical, rejecting attitude toward them includes refusal to suck, vomiting, crying during or after a feeding, angry crying, turning away from the mother's touch, resisting being held closely, or closing the mouth firmly.[26]

3. Help parents to feel that their input to their infant is meaningful by providing positive reinforcement for their behaviors. During the initial phases in the acquaintance process the parents' egos may be fragile in terms of their perception of being "good parents" to their new child.

The nurse can demonstrate that parental input does not have to be in a set or correct way. There is no right and wrong to the infant in his early life experiences. All that is needed to "turn him on" to his parents is to see their faces, hear their voices, and feel their touches long enough to explore and familiarize himself with the input. Soon the infant will want more of the simple pleasures that his parents bring him. Too often, mothers are seen to be very anxious about their abilities to perform infant care tasks. To these mothers the nurse can explain that her input of talking, playing, and conveying love and attention during the tasks will outweigh any advantage from her performing the task efficiently (Fig. 33-4).

Another important nursing consideration is to help parents identify the infant be-

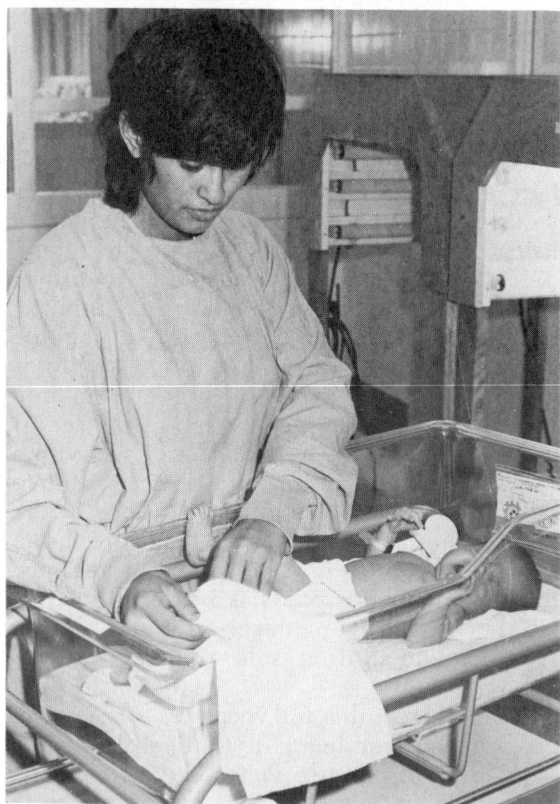

FIGURE 33-4. This mother is encouraged to care for her baby while he is still in the nursery receiving phototherapy for jaundice. This will increase her confidence in caring for her baby when he is ready to be discharged.

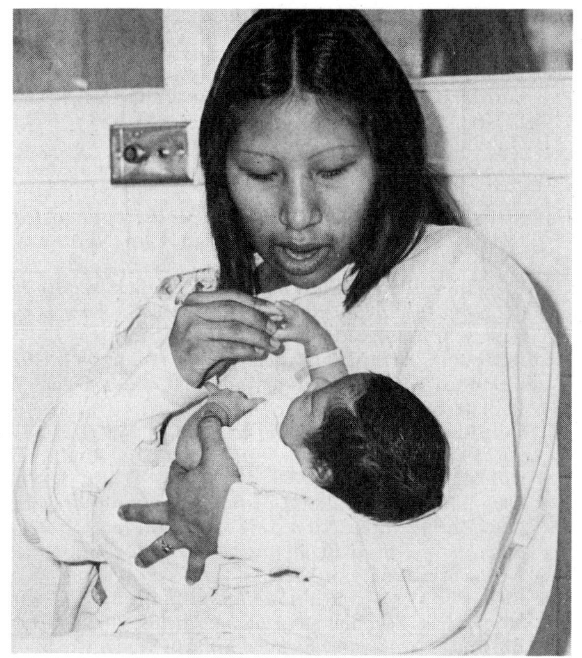

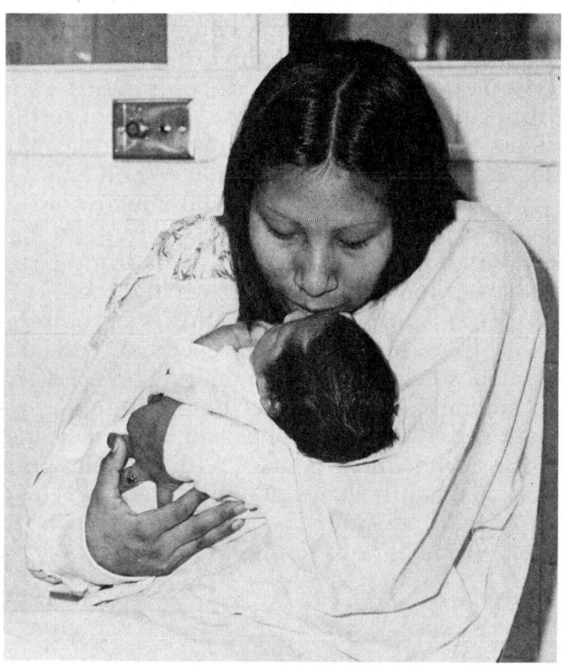

FIGURE 33-5. *Left,* This mother is providing her baby with opportunities to differentiate her from others. *Right,* She rewards the baby for his efforts to visually fixate on her face.

haviors which are most pleasurable to them. Then the nurse can help parents to elicit these behaviors as the necessary feedback to continue interaction between the parent and child. For example, smiling and babbling are social releasers by continuing parental attention. Mothers only need to know that her voice and face contact encourage the development of such behaviors with more vocalizations.

The nurse must also help mothers to appreciate the significance of their infants being able to discriminate them from others. This ability is the antecedent toward the infant establishing relationships with others (such as father, sibling, relatives). It has been shown that an infant is retarded in ability to relate to others if it has difficulty discriminating the mother from others. The most obvious way a baby will learn to discriminate the mother is when she makes her face, voice, and touch readily available to him during daily life activities. Thus he can explore her features and come to recognize her as different from others (Fig. 33-5).

The preceding discussions represented a beginning in the identification of the multitude of approaches nurses can use to stimulate the infant and to help parents have mutually satisfying interactions with their infants. During the neonatal period of life the infant's behavioral responses may be awkward or unrecognizable to parents. Thus, the nurse calls attention to the behavioral cues the infant offers indicating readiness for interaction. Apparently, the best stimulation to enhance behavioral development stems from the concept of love. Love means to care for someone, to show respect, to make oneself readily available to the other. Thus, when this concept of love is integrated into the daily life activities such as feeding, bathing, sleeping, the infant is also being stimulated toward his optimum potential in behavioral development. It is important to note that the specific action done to the infant is not as crucial as the manner in which it is done. When stimuli are presented via mechanical means or by humans whose nonverbal behaviors do not convey love and interest, the long term effects of the stimuli are greatly reduced.

We all must value that the type of relationship an individual will establish with the human world is built upon the foundations of interaction laid in its beginning life experiences—the neonatal period. Thus, parents, nurses, and all in contact with the newborn and his family have an unlimited gift (use of oneself) to offer the baby in attempts to attain optimal behavioral development.

REFERENCES

1. Parmelee, A.: *Infant sleep patterns: from birth to sixteen weeks of age.* J. Pediatr. 65:576, 1964.
2. Laupus, W.: *The feeding of infants* in *Nelson's Textbook of Pediatrics.* W. B. Saunders, Philadelphia, 1964, p. 140.
3. Brazelton, T. B.: *Crying in infancy.* Pediatrics 29:582, 1962.
4. Arnold, H., et al.: *Transition to extra-uterine life.* Am. J. Nurs. 65:77, 1965.
5. Craig, M.: *Normal neonatal behavior patterns: the first week of extrauterine life.* Child and Family 9:303, 1970.
6. Brazelton, T. B.: *Neonatal Behavioral Assessment Scale.* National Spastics Society Monograph No. 50. Heinemann and Son, London, 1973.
7. Ibid.
8. Scarr, S. and Williams, M.: *The assessment of neonatal and later status in low birth weight infants.* Child Dev. 44:94, 1973.
9. Prechtl, H. and Beintema, O.: *The Neurological Examination of the Full Term Newborn Infant.* William Heinemann, London, 1964.
10. Horowitz, F. D., et al.: *Newborn and four week retest on a normative population using the Brazelton Newborn Assessment procedure.* Paper presented at the Annual Meeting of the Society for Research in Child Development, Minneapolis, 1971.
11. Bowlby, J. *Attachment and loss, vol I: Attachment.* Basic Books, New York, 1969.
12. Moss, H. A.: *Methodological issues in studying mother-infant interaction.* Am. J. Orthopsych., 35:482, 1965.
13. Goldberg, S.: *Competence reconsidered: A model of parent-infant interaction.* Personal communication, 1975.
14. Klaus, M. H. and Kennell, J. H.: *Mothers separated from their newborn infants.* Pediatr. Clin. North Am. 17:1015, 1970.
15. Brazelton, T. B., Koslowski, B. and Tronick, E.: *Study of neonatal behavior in Zambian and American babies.* J. Am. Acad. Child Psychiatry, in press.
16. Brazelton, T. B.: *Psychophysiologic reactions in the neonate: No. 2, Effect of maternal medication,* J. Pediatr. 58:513, 1961.
17. Salk, L.: *The role of the heart beat in the relations between mother and infant.* Scientific American 228:24, 1973.
18. David, M. and Appell, G.: *A study of nursing care and nurse-infant interaction.* In Foss, B. M. (ed.): *Determinants of Infant Behavior, vol. 1.* Wiley and Sons, New York, 1961, pp. 132-133.
19. Richards, M.: *Social interaction in the first weeks of human life.* Psychiat. Neurol. Neurochir. 74:38, 1971.
20. Brown, J.: *States in newborn infants.* Merrill-Palmer Quarterly 10:313, 1964.
21. Wolff, P.: *Observations of newborn infants.* Psychosom. Med. 21:110, 1959.
22. Fantz, R.: *Pattern discrimination and selective attention as determinants of perceptual development from birth.* In Kidd, A. J. and Rivoire, J. (eds.): *Perceptual Development in Children.* International Universities Press, New York, 1966.
23. Wolff: op. cit.
24. Brazelton, T. B.: *Observations of the neonate.* J. Am. Acad. Child Psychiat. 1:38, 1962.
25. Kagan, J. and Lewis, M.: *Studies of attention in the human infant.* Merrill-Palmer Quarterly 11:95, 1965.
26. Kennedy, J.: *The high risk maternal-infant acquaintance process.* Nurs. Clin. North Am. 8:551, 1973.

BIBLIOGRAPHY

Barnett, K.: *A theoretical construct of the concepts of touch as they relate to nursing.* Nurs. Res. 21:102, 1972.

Bernal, J.: *Crying during the first 10 days of life and maternal responses.* Dev. Med. Child Neurol. 14:362, 1972.

Blaesing, S. and Brockhaus, J.: *The development of body image in the child.* Nurs. Clin. North Am. 7:597, 1972.

Bowlby, J.: *Attachment and Loss, vol. I: Attachment.* Basic Books, New York, 1969.

Brazelton, T. B.: *Does the neonate shape his environment?* Birth Defects 10:131, 1974.

Ibid.: *Infants and Mothers: Differences in Development.* Delacorte Press, New York, 1969.

Ibid.: *Neonatal Behavioral Assessment Scale.* Spastics International Medical Publications, London, 1973.

Buss, A.: *A conceptual framework for learning effecting the development of ability factors.* Hum. Dev. 16:273, 1973.

Campbell, D.: *Sucking as an index of mother-child interaction.* Symp. Oral Sensory Perception 4:152, 1973.

Clark, L.: *Care of the well child: introducing mother and baby.* Am. J. Nurs. 74:1483, 1974.

Day, B. and Liley, M.: *The Secret World of the Baby.* Random House, New York, 1966.

Emde, R. and Koenig, K.: *Neonatal smiling and rapid eye movement states.* J. Am. Acad. Child Psychiat. 8:57, 1969.

Foss, B. M. (ed.): *Determinants of Infant Behavior, Vols. 1-4.* Wiley and Sons, New York, 1961, 1963, 1965, 1969.

Fouts, G.: *Elimination of an infant's crying through response prevention.* Percept. Mot. Skills 38:225, 1974.

Freud, W.: *The Baby Profile, II.* Psychoanal. Study Child 26:172, 1971.

Friedman, S.: *Habituation and recovery of visual response in the alert human newborn.* J. Exp. Child Psychol. 13:339, 1972.

Greenberg, M. and Morris, N.: *Engrossment: the newborn's impact upon the father.* Am. J. Orthopsychiat. 44:520, 1974.

Hiernaux, J.: *Environmental and genetic influences upon growth.* J. Anat. 107:181, 1970.

Hirschman, R. and Katkin, E.: *Psychophysiological functioning, arousal, attention, and learning during the first year of life.* Adv. Child. Dev. Behav. 9:115, 1974.

Honig, A.: *The role of the nurse in stimulating early learning.* J. Nurs. Educ. 9:11, 1970.

Hulsebus, R.: *Operant conditioning of infant behaviors: a review.* Adv. Child. Dev. Behav. 8:111, 1973.

Hutt, C., et al.: *Habituation in relation to state in the human neonate.* Nature 220:618, 1968.

Jeffrey, W. and Cohen, L.: *Habituation in the human infant.* Adv. Child. Dev. Behav. 6:63, 1971.

Junker, K.: *Selective attention in infants and consecutive communicative behavior.* Acta Paediatr. Scand. [Suppl.] 231:1, 1972.

Kaplan, L.: *The concept of the family romance.* Psychoanal. Rev. 61:169, 1974.

Katz, S., Rivinus, H. and Barker, W.: *Physical anthropology and the biobehavioral approach to child growth and development.* Am. J. Phys. Anthropol. 38:105, 1973.

Kobre, K. and Lipsitt, L.: *A negative contrast effect in newborns.* J. Exp. Child Psychol. 14:81, 1972.

Kulka, A., Fry, C. and Goldstein, F.: *Kinesthetic needs in infancy.* Am. J. Orthopsychiat. 30:562, 1960.

Lenard, H., von Bernuth, H. and Prechtl, H.: *Reflexes and their relationship to behavioral state in the newborn.* Acta Paediatr. Scand. 57:177, 1968.

Levy, D.: *Behavioral Analysis: Analysis of Clinical Observations of Behavior as Applied to Mother-Newborn Relationships.* Charles C Thomas, Springfield, Ill., 1958.

Mahler, M. S.: *Symbiosis and individuation: the psychological birth of the human infant.* Psychoanal. Study Child 29:89, 1974.

Michaelis, R., et al.: *Activity states in premature and term infants.* Dev. Psychobiol. 6:209, 1973.

Mills, M. and Melhuish, E.: *Recognition of mother's voice in early infancy.* Nature 252:123, 1974.

Montagu, A.: *Prenatal Influences.* Charles C Thomas, Springfield, Ill., 1962.

Rebelsky, R. and Hanks, C.: *Fathers' verbal interaction with infants in the first three months of life.* Child Dev. 42:63, 1971.

Rose, S., Katz, P. and Samsky, J.: *Influence of visual enrichment on infants' visual preferences.* Percept. Motor Skills 35:960, 1972.

Rosenthal, M.: *The study of infant-environment interaction: some comments on trends and methodologies.* J. Child Psychol. Psychiat. 14:301, 1973.

Rubin, J., Provenzano, F. and Luria, A.: *The eye of the beholder: parents' view on sex of newborns.* Am. J. Orthopsychiat. 44:512, 1974.

Salk, L.: *The critical nature of the post-partum period in the human for the establishment of the mother-infant bond:* a controlled study. Dis. Nerv. Syst. 31(Suppl.): 110, 1970.

Southwood, H.: *The origin of self-awareness and ego behavior.* Int. J. Psychoanal. 54:235, 1973.

Stark, R. E. and Nathanson, S.: *Spontaneous cry in the newborn infant; sounds and facial gestures.* Symp. Oral Sensory Perception 4:323, 1973.

Stevenson, R.: *The Fetus and Newly Born Infant: Influences of the Prenatal Environment.* C. V. Mosby, St. Louis, 1973.

Stone, L., Smith, H. and Murphy, L.: *The Competent Infant.* Basic Books, New York, 1973.

Tautermannov's, M.: *Smiling in infants.* Child Dev. 44:701, 1973.

Tempesta, L.: *The importance of touch in the care of newborns.* J. Obstet. Gynecol. Nurse 1:17, 1972.

Thomas, A. and Autgaerden, S.: *Locomotion from Pre- To Post-Natal Life; How the Newborn Begins to Acquire Psycho-Sensory Functions.* W. S. Heinemann, New York, 1966.

Wolff, P.: *The Causes, Control and Organization of Behavior in the Neonate.* International Universities Press, New York, 1966.

Zern, D.: *The relationship between mother-infant contact and later differentiation of the social environment.* J. Genet. Psychol. 121:107, 1972.

UNIT 9

PATHOPHYSIOLOGIC RISKS DURING CHILDBEARING

34 Health Problems Complicating Pregnancy

DYANNE D. AFFONSO, R.N., M.N.
HARLAN R. GILES, M.D.

A number of medical disorders antedating or arising during a gestation may profoundly affect the outcome of pregnancy. Reciprocally, pregnancy itself may significantly modify the natural course of certain diseases. This chapter deals with the relationships between certain common medical conditions, the gestational process, and the unborn child.

Over the past few years advances in obstetric facilities and techniques have succeeded in decreasing perinatal mortality (stillbirths plus neonatal deaths) to the present rate of approximately 15 per 1,000 live births. Recent evidence confirms that the significant majority of such perinatal deaths can be ascribed to a minority of pregnant patients who are identified as high risk. Medical complications such as diabetes mellitus, hypertension, and cardiorespiratory disorders in the mother may increase her chances of a fetal loss by three- to fivefold. The thrust of perinatal care today lies in the identification and intensive management of such high-risk patients in order to achieve a further reduction in perinatal mortality. Application of the highest standards of nursing care is essential for the high-risk parturient and her unborn fetus if obstetric tragedy is to be prevented.

DIABETES

Diabetes mellitus, perhaps to a greater extent than any other single disorder, exerts a profound effect on pregnancy outcome. Conversely, pregnancy itself may dramatically alter the severity of the diabetes. An appreciation of this interrelationship is essential if one is to render expert prenatal care to the diabetic.

Before the nurse can appreciate the impact diabetes and pregnancy have upon each other, there must be an understanding of the diabetic disease process. "Diabetes mellitus is a chronic systemic disease characterized by disorders in 1) metabolism of insulin, and of carbohydrate, fat and protein, and 2) the structure and function of blood vessels."[1] Diabetes is sometimes classified as an endocrine disease because it arises from delayed release, deficiency, or absolute lack of insulin. Insulin is a highly specialized protein with powerful hormonal action and is secreted by the beta cells in the islands of Langerhans of the pancreas.[2] Insulin greatly affects metabolism, as is evident by its three significant functions:

1. Facilitates conversion of glucose to fat (lipogenesis) in adipose tissue and liver.
2. Speeds conversion of glucose to glycogen, especially in muscles, and oxidation of glucose in insulin-sensitive tissues.
3. Affects rates at which amino acids enter the cells and rate of protein synthesis.[3]

When there is insufficient insulin, there is a depression of these functions. The following is an outline of the course of events arising from insulin lack:*

- I. General effects of insulin lack
  - A. Depression of insulin functions results in "Adaptation of Cells to Starvation Syndrome" (Hunger)
    1. Decrease in utilization of glucose by peripheral tissues
    2. Increased mobilization of fatty acids
    3. Increased breakdown of amino acids
    4. Results in some ketonemia (elevation of ketone bodies in the blood)
    5. Some ketonuria (excretion of ketone bodies in the urine)
- II. Specific consequences of insulin lack on metabolic activities
  - A. Carbohydrate metabolism
    1. Conversion of glycogen in liver to glucose (glycogenolysis)
    2. Blood glucose rises (hyperglycemia)
    3. Elevation of blood sugar limited by renal threshold (normal threshold 160–180 glucose/100 ml. blood)
       - a. Results in glycosuria (loss of glucose in urine)
    4. Effects of glycosuria
       - a. Dehydration—especially if nausea and vomiting prevent food intake
       - b. Osmotic diuresis manifests through polyuria
         - (1) Water and electrolyte (K + Na) lost
       - c. Progressive dehydration leads to
         - (1) Hemo concentration
         - (2) ↓ blood volume, blood pressure, circulation to tissues
         - (3) Generalized tissue anoxia causes anaerobic metabolism
         - (4) Anaerobic processes increase lactic acid in blood which decreases oxygen supply and results eventually in cardiac failure
  - B. Fat metabolism
    1. Fat stores mobilized in form of fatty acids in blood (ketogenesis)
    2. Accumulation of fatty acids in the blood (ketonemia) leads to metabolic acidosis
    3. Elevated ketoacids exceed kidney capacity—results in ketouria
    4. Effects of ketouria
       - a. Loss of sodium and potassium ions
       - b. Water-holding power of extracellular fluid decreases = dehydration
       - c. Same results ensue as above (A-c)
  - C. Protein metabolism
    1. Protein catabolism exceeds anabolism especially in the muscles
    2. Amino acids in blood rise
    3. Acids excreted—nitrogen bound (NH_2) in the urine
    4. Catabolism results in loss of nitrogen and potassium creates hypovolemia (cellular dehydration)
    5. Same results ensue as above (A-c)
- III. Manifestations of disturbed metabolic activities—described in Table 34-1.

The most widely accepted classification of diabetes in pregnancy is that proposed by White (Table 34-2). Class A, or chemical diabetes, refers to patients who have a positive glucose tolerance test during a pregnancy, but exhibit no symptoms or outward manifesta-

*Data for this outline were taken from Beland, I.: *Clinical Nursing: Pathophysiological and Psychosocial Approaches,* ed. 2. Macmillan, New York, 1970, pp. 852–857.

TABLE 34-1. Consequences and Manifestations of Insulin Lack*

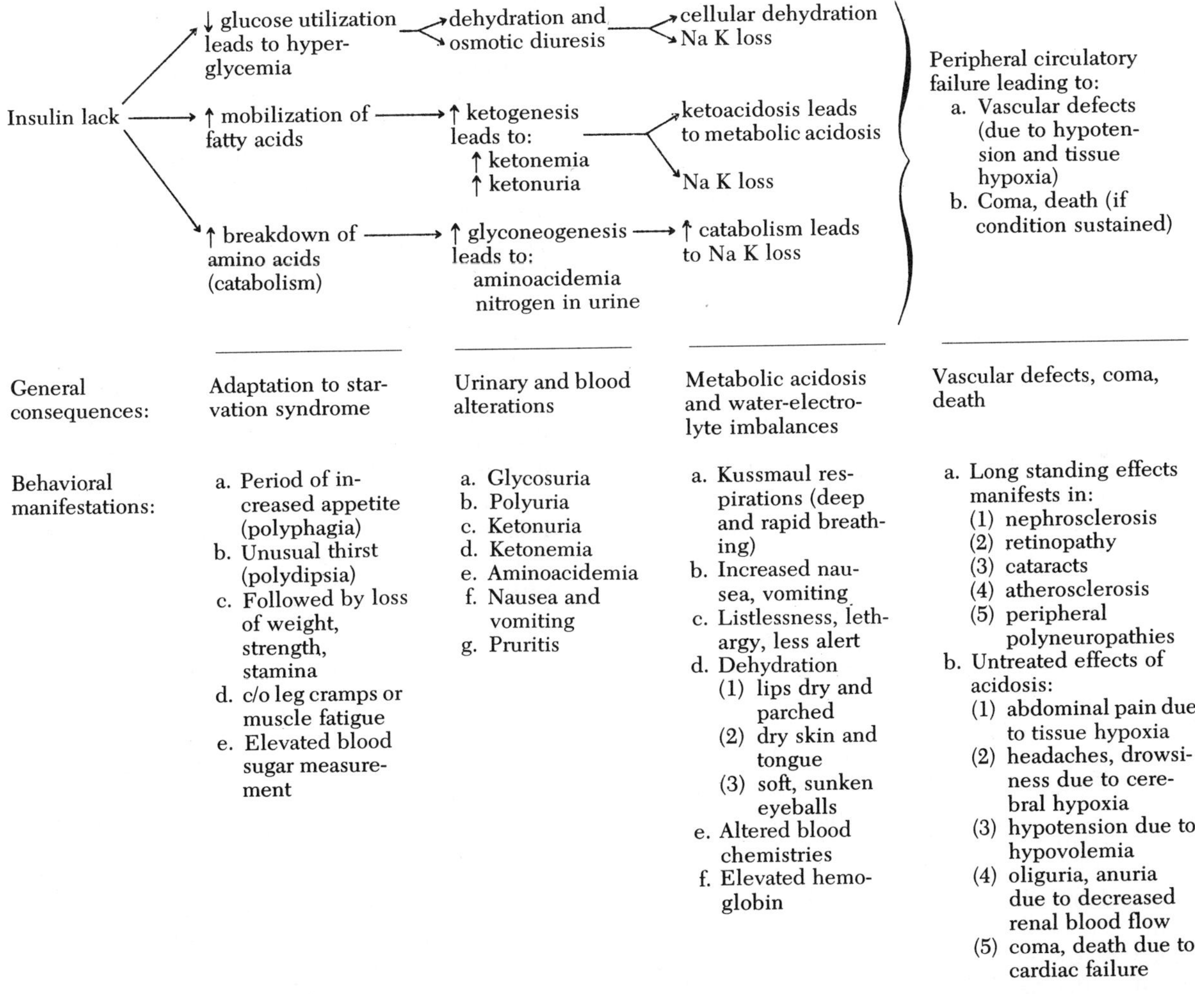

General consequences:	Adaptation to starvation syndrome	Urinary and blood alterations	Metabolic acidosis and water-electrolyte imbalances	Vascular defects, coma, death
Behavioral manifestations:	a. Period of increased appetite (polyphagia) b. Unusual thirst (polydipsia) c. Followed by loss of weight, strength, stamina d. c/o leg cramps or muscle fatigue e. Elevated blood sugar measurement	a. Glycosuria b. Polyuria c. Ketonuria d. Ketonemia e. Aminoacidemia f. Nausea and vomiting g. Pruritis	a. Kussmaul respirations (deep and rapid breathing) b. Increased nausea, vomiting c. Listlessness, lethargy, less alert d. Dehydration (1) lips dry and parched (2) dry skin and tongue (3) soft, sunken eyeballs e. Altered blood chemistries f. Elevated hemoglobin	a. Long standing effects manifests in: (1) nephrosclerosis (2) retinopathy (3) cataracts (4) atherosclerosis (5) peripheral polyneuropathies b. Untreated effects of acidosis: (1) abdominal pain due to tissue hypoxia (2) headaches, drowsiness due to cerebral hypoxia (3) hypotension due to hypovolemia (4) oliguria, anuria due to decreased renal blood flow (5) coma, death due to cardiac failure

* Based on data obtained from Beland, I.: *Clinical Nursing: Pathophysiologic and Psychosocial Approaches,* ed. 2. Macmillan, New York, 1970; and Tepperman, J.: *Metabolic and Endocrine Physiology*, ed. 3. Year Book Medical Publishers, Chicago, 1973.

tions of the diabetic state. Classes B through F include overt diabetics with varying age of onset and progression of disease.

In general, increasing severity or duration of diabetes is correlated with a less favorable prognosis for both mother and fetus. However, even Class A diabetics have a higher incidence of early miscarriages, stillbirths, and congenital anomalies, and should therefore receive equal obstetric attention.

TABLE 34-2. White's Classification of Diabetes*

Class A —	Glucose tolerance test diabetes
Class B —	Onset over age 20 Duration 0–9 years No vascular disease
Class C —	Onset age 10–19 Duration 10–19 years No vascular disease
Class D —	Onset under age 10 Duration 20-plus years Vascular disease Calcification in legs Retinitis
Class E —	Calcified pelvic vessels
Class F —	Patients with diabetic renal impairment

* From Nelson, B., Gillespie, L. and White, P.: *Pregnancy complicated by diabetes mellitus.* Obstet. Gynecol. 1:219, 1953, with permission.

The diagnosis of diabetes in pregnancy, especially Class A diabetes, depends upon a high index of suspicion. Patients with a prior history of fetal wastage, including early miscarriages, congenital anomalies, and stillbirths should recieve a 5-hour glucose tolerance test. Other factors suggestive of diabetes include excessive birth weight infants (greater than 4,000 grams) or a family history of diabetes or recurrent toxemia. Physical signs, such as marked obesity, excessive weight gain in pregnancy, or polyhydramnios may indicate underlying diabetes. Although glucosuria may be seen in pregnancy from physiologic causes, it is essential that diabetes be excluded in each case by testing the blood sugar. Class A diabetes will never be diagnosed unless the disorder is frequently suspected. Glucose tolerance tests are most sensitive when performed in the second or third trimester. The intravenous route may be chosen, but most investigators prefer the 5-hour oral test because it is more physiologic.

HOW PREGNANCY AFFECTS DIABETES

There is an increasing appreciation that pregnancy exerts a *diabetogenic action*, that is, that pregnancy itself creates a "diabetic" condition. This concept is discussed by Gerbie:*

> Most problems associated with the management of the diabetic pregnancy patient are related to changes in glucose tolerance, alterations in insulin utilization, and an increased tendency to ketosis. Difficulties are especially likely to arise in conjunction with hyperemesis gravidarum, dietary indiscretion, and pregnancy-related nutritional imbalance. Such complications of pregnancy as pyelonephritis and toxemia further increase the difficulties involved in control of the diabetes. Drastic alterations in the internal secretions accompany the pregnant state, including changes in the secretion of estrogen, progesterone, corticosteroids, and growth hormone, and all play some part in the mechanism of the diabetogenic effect of pregnancy.
>
> The concept that pregnancy is itself diabetogenic has arisen from data indicating that there is a loss of reactivity to insulin usually beginning in late pregnancy, followed by a decrease in the peripheral utilization of carbohydrate. The pertinent evidence includes a measurable decrease in the production of lactate, a drop in inorganic phosphate, and lessening hypoglycemia. These changes appear to result from a hormonal antagonism to insulin, from placental degradation of insulin, or from a combination of both mechanisms. It is well established that the utilization of carbohydrates may be influenced by certain extra-pancreatic endocrine secretions, notably cortico-

*From Gerbie, A.: *Endocrine diseases complicated by pregnancy.* In Haynes, D. (ed.): *Medical Complications during Pregnancy.* McGraw-Hill, New York, 1969, pp. 336, 337, with permission.

steroids and substances released from the hyperactive pituitary gland. Elevations of the blood sugar can be the result of a number of endocrine changes characteristic of pregnancy, including increased excretion of glucocorticoids and an increase in the production of growth hormone, possibly potentiated by placental lactogen.

Overproduction of growth hormone has the effect of decreasing insulin sensitivity while stimulating insulin production and lessening insulin's hypoglycemic effect. It can be shown that there is a marked increase in the growth-promoting activity of the plasma of pregnant rats, and that this activity persists after hypophysectomy, an observation which suggests that the placenta is the source of the phenomenon. Data from the human being indicate that hypophysectomized pregnant women show impairment of glucose tolerance and increased insulin resistance during pregnancy, with reversion to normal glucose tolerance after delivery. Glucocorticoids also produce hyperglycemia, and there is a marked increase in plasma cortisol levels during pregnancy, particularly in the third trimester. The placenta has also been credited with producing adrenal cortical hormones.

Freinkel and Goodner[4] propose that placental degradation of insulin may play a part in the mechanism of the diabetogenic effect of pregnancy. This degradation has been demonstrated by incubating insulin tagged with I^{131} with placental extracts and by the finding in pregnant rats of a markedly accelerated turnover of I^{131} insulin, which reverts to normal following delivery. Several independent workers (Spellacy and Goetz,[5] Bleicher and coworkers,[6] and Burt[7]) have shown that the plasma insulin level is consistently elevated during pregnancy. Although some have postulated that carbohydrate metabolism in the liver contributes to the diabetogenic effect of pregnancy, glycogen synthesis, storage, and breakdown do not alter significantly during gestation.

The clinical demonstration of the diabetogenic effect of pregnancy is provided by the fact that insulin requirements in any given patient usually increase during gestation, only to decrease markedly following delivery. Also, the incidence of clinical diabetes mellitus increases precipitously with parity. Thus, a para 5 is three times more likely to develop diabetes than is a nullipara, while Murphy[8] has shown that one-half of all women with 10 or more children are diabetic.

HOW DIABETES AFFECTS PREGNANCY

It is necessary to preface this discussion with the comment that optimal maternal-fetal-neonatal outcomes can be achieved through constant monitoring and control of the diabetes during gestation and with skillful obstetric and pediatric interventions. However, a diabetic pregnancy is not without hazards. The effects of diabetes are best exemplified by the complications to which a diabetic pregnancy is most vulnerable.

1. *Hydramnios.* Approximately 10 per cent of diabetic pregnancies manifest polyhydramnios.[9] It is believed that diabetic pregnancies do have more accumulated amniotic fluid than do those of nondiabetics.[10] Although the exact reason for this is unknown, "increased osmotic pressure, hypersecretion of amniotic fluid, and a diuresis resulting from fetal hyperglycemia are suspected theories."[11] The significance of hydramnios is debatable. White[12] states there is a threat from premature rupture of membranes leading to premature delivery prior to viability, while Driscoll and Gillepsie[13] do not consider this a significant complication. In excessive hydramnios, aminocentesis may be indicated, making

the pregnancy vulnerable to the hazards associated with the procedure.

2. *Acidosis.* Acidosis accounts for the greatest fetal risk in a diabetic pregnancy. Driscoll and Gillepsie state "it constitutes an emergency of major proportions and actual or impending acidosis requires immediate hospitalization."[14] White states "the degree of ketoacidosis develops rapidly in midpregnancy and intrauterine death in the second trimester is caused most commonly by ketoacidosis."[15] (The effects of diabetes on the neonate are discussed later in Chapters 37 and 38)
3. *Effects of vascular complications.* When vascular disease is present, the pregnancy is vulnerable to the risk of toxemia. In the diabetic with renal disease, increased proteinuria and hypotension are serious complications requiring hospitalization.[16]
4. *Other complications.* The diabetic pregnant woman who develops hyperemesis gravidarum is at risk to severe metabolic disturbances if the condition does not subside with frequent small feedings and/or pharmacologic agents. Early hospitalization may be mandatory. Anemia may develop into a serious problem in the diabetic with vascular disease. Its early detection (hemoglobin and hematocrit measurements) and correction is essential. Vaginal infections such as monilial vaginitis are also more prevalent in pregnant diabetic women. Driscoll and Gillepsie describe a complication known as the "pregnant headache" which can be manifested in as many as 10 per cent of pregnant diabetic women.[17] They describe it as beginning in the second or third trimester, progressing to a severe encephalalgia. Hospitalization is usually required with narcotic, intraveneous, and bed rest treatments bringing relief within a few days. Driscoll and Gillepsie believe such headaches predispose to the development of acidosis if untreated.

NURSING MANAGEMENT

Nursing management of the Class A diabetic differs little from the care afforded a normal uncomplicated pregnancy. Although some dietary restrictions may become necessary as outlined below, most patients do quite well on a normal diet, avoiding only marked excesses of carbohydrate intake. The urine should be tested for sugar at each prenatal visit. Positive results should be corroborated with a blood sugar determination. Since peak blood sugar values are most often obtained 2 hours after a meal, this is an ideal time for testing. It is also important to check fasting blood sugars, especially if the patient has symptoms suggestive of hypoglycemia.

Although most patients with Class A diabetes require no pharmacologic intervention, an occasional patient will manifest fasting blood sugar levels above 120 mg. % and 2 hour postprandial values above 180 mg. %. When this occurs, insulin therapy may be necessary. This is generally instituted on a sliding scale until a daily or twice daily dosage schedule can be established. The urinary threshold must be identified, as this serves as the main index of control when the patient leaves the hospital. Oral hypoglycemics are mentioned only to be condemned. Such agents may cause fetal abnormalities and rarely provide sufficient control of the diabetes. They are today considered contraindicated in pregnancy.

The risk of intrauterine fetal death dictates that patients with Class A diabetes should not be allowed to go past term. In addition to the usual hazards, induction of labor in such patients may be difficult due to the excessive fetal weight. Consequently, the incidence of cesarean delivery rises somewhat. Postpartum, the infant must be watched closely for signs of hypoglycemia. (This is discussed in detail in Chapters 37 and 38.)

For the overt diabetic, nursing management is more complex. The patient should be seen as early as possible in the pregnancy and re-evaluated at frequent intervals (at least every two weeks during the first two trimesters and weekly thereafter.) Complications must be recognized promptly and managed aggressively. The central role of nursing lies in patient education. The nurse must understand the diabetic illness and appreciate in detail the effect of pregnancy on the diabetes. More importantly, she must effectively communicate this to the patient. It is only through patient instruction and cooperation that optimal pregnancy outcome will be realized.

Rigid control of the diabetes is mandatory to prevent the grave complications of ketosis and coma. Changes in sugar tolerance during pregnancy are neither constant nor predictable. Moreover, the diabetes may become quite brittle, requiring meticulous attention to dietary as well as insulin requirements. Most experts advise the following diet content:

30–40 calories per kilogram
150–250 grams of carbohydrate
60–80 grams of protein
80–90 grams of fat.

It should be emphasized that no single dietary plan is ideal for all patients, and modifications are often necessary to maximize diabetic control. The trend today is toward higher caloric intake with administration of sufficient insulin to drive the sugar inside the cells.

Liberal use of hospitalization is essential to good diabetic management. Most overt diabetics should be hospitalized relatively early in pregnancy to reassess the patient's physical status and to regulate the diabetes. Blood and urine sugar levels must be correlated to establish a threshold. There are many methods of determining insulin requirements, most of which are quite satisfactory. Each physician-nurse team must select the approach that works best for them. The general principles involved in any scheme of regulation include:

1. Determination of dietary requirements.
2. Frequent sampling of blood and urine sugars.
3. Calculation of daily insulin requirements.
4. Condensation of multiple insulin doses into one or two daily injections.
5. Re-evaluation of diabetic control.

The blood sugar ideally should be maintained between 120 to 150 mg. % fasting and 150 to 180 mg. % 2 hours after meals. Such control can be shown to markedly enhance fetal salvage and decrease the obstetric problems related to excessive birth weight. The nurse should know which urine sugar values correspond to the above ranges of blood sugar, and continually reassess control in the light of these values as well as patient symptoms. Hypoglycemic episodes must be avoided meticulously, as fetal blood sugar levels usually run 20 to 30 mg. % below maternal levels, and fetal growth and development may be impaired. On the other hand, maternal ketoacidosis presents an even more serious challenge to the fetus, whose system tolerates acidosis quite poorly. Fetal death will almost certainly result if the mother's condition is not corrected rapidly. Rehospitalization may be necessary from time to time to maintain rigid control. During these admissions, fetal growth and well-being must be assessed. Careful clinical measurements of fundal height and use of diagnostic ultrasound provide documentation of satisfactory growth and detection of complications such as polyhydramnios and excessive birth weight infant. Chemical tests such as blood or urinary estriol levels may provide some index of fetal well-being.

Overt diabetics are usually admitted one or two weeks prior to anticipated delivery for final regulation. Because of the risk of fetal death, delivery is usually accomplished between 36 and 38 weeks of gestation. Fetal maturity is generally confirmed by amniocentesis prior to delivery, If the pelvis is adequate, the cervix ripe, and the infant of reasonable size, induction of labor is initiated with oxytocin. The fetus should be continuously monitored for signs of distress. If the cervix fails to progress, or if fetal distress occurs, cesarean section is performed without delay. In either case, pediatric assistance should be present in the delivery room to guard against the neonatal complications of hypoxia and/or hypoglycemia.

Postpartum, maternal insulin requirements may fall precipitously, and it is not uncommon for mothers to require no insulin at all for the first 24 to 48 hours after delivery. As in early pregnancy, regulation of the diabetes is necessary in the puerperium and may require extension of the usual hospital stay.

The diabetic pregnancy generates enormous psychologic, social, and economic impact upon the family. The nurse must continually and enthusiastically support the medical intervention plan, and seek to alleviate the patient's anxiety concerning her pregnancy. The nurse must often serve as coordinator between obstetrician, internist, social worker, hospital personnel, the patient, and her family in maximizing the effectiveness of patient care. She should encourage the patient to receive continued medical care and counseling regarding the prognosis for subsequent pregnancies.

CARDIAC DISEASE

The majority (90 to 95 per cent) of heart diseases during pregnancy is attributed to lesions of rheumatic origin, while a smaller percentage occurs from congenital defects, and from coronary, atherosclerotic, and thyroid origins. Heart disease is considered a major risk factor during pregnancy because it is the fourth leading cause for maternal mortality. Suggested goals in the nursing management of a pregnant woman with heart disease are:

1. Assess the impact pregnancy can impose upon the heart's functional capacity.
2. Protect the maternal heart by maintaining a balance between cardiac load and cardiac reserve.
3. Nurture the woman to cope and adapt to the many restrictions imposed upon her during pregnancy.

NURSING MANAGEMENT

Prenatal Period

The woman must be continuously evaluated to estimate the heart's capacity in tolerating the stresses imposed by pregnancy. Prenatal supervision and care is mandatory for successful outcomes. The woman may be seen twice a week or more often by the health team, consisting of the obstetrician, cardiac specialists, dietitian, nurse, and social worker. During the prenatal period, assessment and reassessment of the cardiac functional capacity (also known as cardiac functional reserve) are done by numerous tests. The New York Heart Association has developed a classification for cardiac disease which helps to clue the health team on the anticipated course and outcome of the pregnancy (Table 34-3).

The nurse must always be alert for early signs of cardiac decompensation. Congestive heart failure is the main cause for maternal death, demonstrating the heart can no longer meet the demands of pregnancy. Abrupt or gradual appearance of any of the following should be reported immediately.

1. Rales heard with a stethoscope at the base of the lungs.
2. Progressive generalized edema.
3. Progression of dyspnea upon exertion.
4. Frequent coughs (with or without hemoptysis).
5. Episodes of palpitation.

TABLE 34-3. Classification for the Severity of Cardiac Disease*

Classification	*Criteria—Patient Behaviors*
Class I	No limitation on physical activities Normal physical activity causes no discomforts. No symptoms of cardiac insufficiency or anginal pain.
Class II	Slight limitation on physical activities Normal physical activity causes fatigue, dyspnea, or anginal pain.
Class III	Moderate to marked limitation of physical activity Less than ordinary activity creates excessive fatigue, palpitation, dyspnea, or angina pain.
Class IV	Unable to carry out physical activity without experiencing discomforts symptoms of cardiac insufficiency or angina pain even at rest.

Women in Classes I and II usually emerge with a normal childbearing experience while those in Classes III & IV are more vulnerable to complications.

* From *Nomenclature and Criteria for Diagnosis of Diseases of the Heart and Blood Vessels*, ed. 5. The New York Heart Association., New York, 1955, with permission.

6. Any difficulty breathing or sense of smothering.

The above signs are indicative of cardiac decompensation, demanding priority medical actions to correct the cardiac status. Until the cardiac condition improves, obstetric manipulations should be withheld because any procedure, no matter how slight, may be enough of a stimulus to stress the heart into cardiac failure.

Pregnancy is a stressor to the heart because it creates an increase in the cardiac workload, forcing the heart to work harder. There is no problem if there is a balance between the cardiac reserve (the heart's functional work capacity) and the cardiac load (the demands made by the body). However a heart afflicted with disease may not have adequate reserves to keep pace with the increased demands during pregnancy. Therefore, the diseased heart of a pregnant woman must be protected from overwork (leading to possible cardiac failure) by ensuring equilibrium between the heart's workload and its functional capacity.

The following are nursing actions which help to protect the afflicted maternal heart during pregnancy:

1. Promotion of rest
   Rest prevents fatigue in cardiac functioning and is a vital part in management of heart disease. The pregnant woman needs to value sleep patterns which include a minimum of 8 to 10 hours daily, with frequent rest periods. Rest is so vital that if a woman is unable to rest adequately at home, hospitalization may be necessary.
2. Restriction of physical activities
   The woman must be protected from physical exertion which leads to fatigue. This is not to propose that all physical activity be omitted. It is encouraged as long as it does not lead to shortness of breath or fatigue.
3. Assessment and alleviation of anxiety
   An anxious woman has an elevated basal metabolism rate. Therefore, anxiety must be kept at a minimum so as not to overwork the afflicted heart. Understanding her cardiac condition and its impact upon the pregnancy can greatly reduce maternal concern.
4. Adequate nutrition
   A diet high in iron, protein, and other essential nutrients is especially important for the pregnant woman with cardiac disease to meet the increased needs for oxygen and blood-plasma volume.
5. Protection from infection

Any additional insult to the body (such as a common cold, sore throat, etc.) predisposes the woman to possible cardiac failure. The additional energy needed to combat the infection may not be met by the already overworked heart.

6. Constant monitoring of the pregnancy

   Every effort is made to protect the woman from factors predisposing to complications such as excessive weight gain, edema, and anemia. This is possible only through frequent, regular, prenatal care.

Ideally, all the above measures can be implimented with the woman at home. However, if this is impractical, hospitalization may be required in order to maintain a balance between the cardiac reserve and workload. The patient should receive special attention during 28 to 32 weeks of gestation as this is the period of maximum cardiac output. During this time cardiac decompensation is most likely to occur.

Labor and Delivery

The normal process of childbirth is a potentially hazardous period for the woman with cardiac disease because of the increased cardiac output and the mandatory muscular exertion which predisposes to fatigue. Necessary nursing actions are discussed below:

1. In addition to the normal routines for monitoring the labor process, the pulse and respiratory rates should be checked at least every 15 minutes and more frequently as labor progresses. Any rise in rates such as a pulse of over 100 and respirations above 25 per minute needs immediate attention and may demand therapeutic intervention.
2. The chest should be auscultated frequently to detect any rales.
3. The ideal position in bed is semirecumbent with head and shoulders elevated and supported. This allows maximum expansion of the thoracic cavity for optimum ventilation.
4. Support medical therapy which may include:
   a. Administration of broad-spectrum antibiotics as prophylaxis against valvular damage. Patients with valvular defects require antibiotic prophylaxis, preferably broad-spectrum, during labor and delivery to prevent further valvular destruction from infection of the valves themselves.
   b. Administration of oxygen for ventilatory support.
   c. Digitalization if early signs of cardiac decompensation exist.
   d. Drugs for sedation to ensure proper rest.
   e. Diuretics if fluid retention (edema) is pronounced.
   f. Analgesics, usually combined with a tranquilizer, to offer adequate pain relief.
5. Every effort is made to decrease the length of the second stage and minimize bearing down efforts. Optimal mode for delivery is via low forceps under a local or regional anesthesia, to allow a controlled delivery with minimal trauma and hemorrhage. Regional and/or local anesthesia permits the least interference with oxygenation of the mother and fetus.

Postpartal Period

After delivery, intensive nursing care to the mother must continue because risks of cardiac failure and death are great. The early puerperal phase is a danger time because there is a remobilization of extravascular fluid into the blood stream and a significant rise in cardiac output. This increased blood volume creates a burden on the heart. Actions to protect the mother during the postpartal period are:

1. Hospitalization and bed rest are extended, often for as much as a week after delivery, because decompensation has been known to occur as late as the fifth to sixth day after delivery.
2. Continue to position the woman in ways that enhance respiratory and cardiac function.
3. Ambulation and other physical activities are initiated gradually to assess the heart's tolerance to activity.
4. Although the woman should not be separated from her baby just because she has a heart condition, the nursing staff must understand that contacts with the baby should not include demands for the mother to care for the baby. Infant care tasks put additonal strain on already overworked heart.
5. Help the mother prepare for discharge to the home. Explore with the woman and her family the availability of help needed to manage the new baby, other family members, and the household. Ideally a nurse will visit the home to assess the woman in her own unique environment. Assessment of the woman's sleep and rest patterns usually elicts valuable information on the woman's physiologic and psychologic adaptation.

INFECTIONS

Infections occurring during pregnancy may impose a significant threat to mother and fetus. Prompt recognition and treatment and sound nursing support are essential. Therapeutic regimens must be predicated on fetal as well as maternal welfare.

Bacterial Infections

The principal site for bacterial infections in pregnancy is the urinary tract. Studies of pregnant women reflect an incidence of asymptomatic bacteriuria between 5 and 10 per cent. It is not surprising, therefore, that cystitis is a frequent problem in pregnancy. More importantly, the compression of the ureters by the uterus and ovarian blood vessels causes stasis and obstruction to flow of urine from the kidneys. Bacterial organisms ascend from the bladder, and renal infection, or pyelonephritis, follows. Pyelonephritis is a serious infection which is characterized by high fever, chills, and flank pain.

Nursing management begins with prompt recognition of the symptoms of urinary tract infection. Dysuria, pyuria, hematuria, and increasing urinary frequency should suggest a bladder infection, while the additional symptoms of flank pain, fever, and chills should alert one to the possibility of pyelonephritis. In the former, attention to adequate fluid intake and the antibiotics prescribed by the physician are usually sufficient. When pyelonephritis is suspected, bed rest with elevation of the feet is mandatory to allow proper urinary drainage. Antibiotics are generally administered parenterally.

Although other bacterial infections, such as streptococcal pharyngitis, otitis, and pneumonia are encountered in pregnancy, their incidence is no higher than in the nonpregnant population. Regardless of the site of infection, nursing care should focus on the principles of adequate hydration and rest, and close adherence to the antibiotic regimen outlined by the physician. Of special importance in any infection is control of the maternal temperature. Because the fetal "core" temperature is always somewhat higher than that of the mother, high fever in pregnancy creates a significant hazard to the fetus. Consequently, aspirin, sponge baths, or a cooling blanket are often necessary to keep the maternal and fetal temperatures within reasonable range.

Viral Infections

Due to their small size, viruses are capable of crossing the placenta and infecting the fetus. Exposure to viral infections within the first 12 weeks of gestation may cause developmental anomalies. Perhaps the best known example of this is the congenital rubella syndrome, which results in congenital cataracts, deafness, and cardiac malformations when exposure occurs between the fifth and tenth weeks of intrauterine life. Other viruses have been associated with different teratogenic effects. Exposure to viral illness in the second or third trimester may lead to intrauterine growth retardation or to a serious neonatal viral syndrome.

Pregnant women should be screened routinely for susceptibility to rubella. Negative titers show no prior exposure and thus no immunity to rubella. Patients in this category should be cautioned to report any possible exposures promptly. Rubella vaccine can be safely administered to such patients postpartum, but another pregnancy should not be undertaken for three to four months after injection.

Viral Hepatitis. Perhaps the most serious viral infection for both mother and fetus is viral hepatitis. This disease is associated with a high incidence of fetal wastage, including first trimester miscarriage, intrauterine fetal death, and stillbirth. If the disease becomes progressive, it can lead to hepatic failure and maternal death. Pregnant patients exposed to viral hepatitis should receive an injection of immune globulin.

Nursing care for the pregnant patient who has contracted hepatitis should be carried out under strict isolation techniques, and nurses who are pregnant should not care for such patients unless absolutely mandatory. Patients uniformly require bed rest and careful attention to diet including an adequate but not excessive protein intake. Satisfactory fetal growth should be carefully documented.

Alterations in the patient's general status or specific clinical laboratory findings should be promptly discussed with the physician.

Fungal Infections

Due to hormonal influence during gestation, pregnant women have an increased incidence of monilial vulvovaginitis. Details of this disorder and its treatment have been discussed previously in Chapter 21. It should be noted however, that vaginal suppositories such as nystatin or candicidin should be inserted manually to avoid applicator trauma to the cervix or uterus. Recurrent infection is not uncommon.

THYROID DYSFUNCTION

Thyroid dysfunction in pregnancy is not a common complication. This may be attributed to the fact that the patients with either hypothyroidism or hyperthyroidism usually ovulate irregularly and thus have difficulty becoming pregnant. Those who become pregnant suffer a high incidence of fetal wastage.

The major risk for the hyperthyroid patient is that of thyroid storm. This frightening development consists of severe tachycardia, hypertension, sweating, and possible congestive heart failure. In addition, mental function is erratic and the patient may even become acutely psychotic. Hospitalization and prompt pharmacologic intervention are mandatory to prevent maternal death.

The threat of thyroid storm demands careful surveillance of the hyperthryoid pregnant patient. It should be remembered that pregnancy itself has a pronounced effect on thyroid function tests, often making them difficult to interpret. Thus the nurse should be alert to the clinical symptoms of increasing thyroid function such as tachycardia, sweating, heat intolerance, nervousness, diarrhea, and insomnia.

A variety of drugs are used in the hyperthyroid patient to either block the uptake of iodine by the thyroid gland or interfere with the production of thyroid hormone. It should be noted that such drugs may cross the placenta and interfere with the thyroid function in the fetus. Most patients with mild hyperthyroidism can be managed effectively with mild sedation alone, such as phenobarbital. Medications prescribed by the physician must be administered precisely and promptly. Occasionally, patients fail to respond to pharmacologic management and surgical intervention to resect all or part of the thyroid gland becomes necessary. When feasible, this is best carried out in the second trimester to decrease untoward fetal effects.

Rh SENSITIZATION

Blood grouping for type and Rh factor is an essential facet of the obstetric work-up. Any patient who is Rh negative should receive special attention because of the possibility of Rh sensitization. Sensitization commonly occurs when an Rh negative mother carries an Rh positive fetus. Red blood cells from the fetus may enter the maternal circulation and provoke antibody formation against the Rh factor. Because this generally occurs following delivery, the first baby is usually unaffected. However, during a subsequent gestation, these maternal antibodies may cross the placenta and cause severe hemolysis in the fetus. This causes anemia which is proportionate in severity to the degree of sensitization in the mother. If allowed to progress unchecked, the anemia may cause marked fetal edema and congestive heart failure, a symptom complex known as erythroblastosis fetalis.

Although management of the erythroblastotic infant is discussed in Chapter 37, intensive prenatal care for the Rh sensitized mother can exert a salutary effect upon fetal outcome. When a patient is found to have a positive antibody titer, she is followed quite closely to determine the severity of the disease. Although serial determinations of the titer or strength of the antibody can be obtained, the best appraisal of fetal status is gained by sampling the amniotic fluid. Bilirubin, a breakdown product of the hemolyzed blood, can be measured in the amniotic fluid and provides the best correlation with the degree of Rh sensitization. This testing may begin as early as 26 weeks of gestation and is repeated at intervals until the fetus is ready to be delivered. When amniotic fluid bilirubin levels reach a severe-risk level, the baby is delivered prematurely. If the chances for survival outside the uterus are poor, additional time may be gained by intrauterine transfusion. In this technique, a needle is advanced under fluroscopic control into the uterus and then into the fetal abdomen. Rh negative red blood cells can then be administered to the fetus to correct the anemia. Such cells are either obtained from the mother or cross-matched to her blood. Intrauterine transfusion may be repeated several times until fetal maturity is attained. Early delivery and prompt, intensive neonatal care are essential elements in fetal survival.

The number of Rh sensitized patients is dwindling rapidly thanks to the development of an immune globulin (RhoGAM) which prevents antibody formation. Administered intramuscularly within 72 hours postpartum, this globulin attacks fetal red cells which have gained access into the maternal blood stream at the time of delivery. Antibody formation, therefore, cannot occur. Unfortunately, immune globulin is of no benefit to patients who are already sensitized, but in unsensitized individuals it is 99 per cent effective.

NURSING CARE DURING HIGH-RISK PREGNANCY

When working with a woman whose pregnancy is at risk, the nurse must value the following:

1. Protect the woman and fetus from physiologic dangers which can arise as a result of medical disorders in pregnancy.

The nurse must have an understanding of the disease and it's impact on pregnancy as well as how pregnancy can influence the medical disorder. The nurse must be able to assess and implement skills that will support medical therapy. Close monitoring of the woman during the entire childbirth experience is essential.

2. Nurture and support the woman and her family to cope and adapt to the stresses associated with the pregnancy. The pregnancy may be plagued by many situations which are not always pleasant, such as restrictions on daily activities, imposed by frequent prenatal visits as well as from the disease itself. Thus the woman may begin to feel that pregnancy is a burden rather than a satisfying experience. Some women may continue to fear for their own safety and that of the baby and such concerns are often legitimate. The nurse assists the woman toward optimal adaptation by simple actions such as:
   a. Encouraging expression of feelings and concerns at every nurse-patient encounter.
   b. Generously providing positive reinforcement for the woman's cooperation in adhering to medical therapy and the imposed restrictions.
   c. Nurturing the family members also for their lives are greatly affected by the woman's physical and emotional condition.
3. Appreciate that there may be a delay in the initiation and development of maternal-infant interaction. Frequently, the risks associated with pregnancy may inhibit or prevent the mother from witnessing the delivery and seeing or touching her infant immediately after birth. At times, the mother's condition necessitates physical separation from the baby. It is essential that such mothers be allowed time to express their feelings about the baby and to at least see the infant whenever possible. The nurse must ensure that contacts between mother and baby are as pleasurable as possible. The mother may also have increased feelings of inadequacy regarding the care of the new baby because she was delayed in the initiation of such tasks. The nurse should help to promote maternal success in attempts at infant care. Success helps to build the reservoir for maternal self-confidence.

REFERENCES

1. *Diabetes Mellitus,* ed. 7. Eli Lilly and Company, Indianapolis, 1973, p. 1.
2. Ibid., p. 29.
3. Beland, I.: *Clinical Nursing: Pathophysiological and Psychosocial Approaches,* ed. 2. Macmillan, New York, 1970, p. 852.
4. Freinkel, N. and Goodner, C: *Insulin metabolism and pregnancy.* Arch. Intern. Med. 109:235, 1962.
5. Spellacy, W. and Goetz, F.: *Plasma insulin in normal late pregnancy.* N. Engl. J. Med. 268:988, 1963.
6. Bleicher, S., O'Sullivan, J. and Freinkel, N.: *Carbohydrate metabolism in pregnancy,* N. Engl. J. Med. 271:886, 1964.
7. Burt, R.: *Insulin resistance in pregnancy.* Obstet. Gynecol. 25:43, 1965.
8. Murphy, R.: *The hidden diabetic.* Conn. Med. 2:306, 1957.
9. Gerbie, A.: *Endocrine diseases complicated by pregnancy.* In Haynes, D. (ed.): *Medical Complications during pregnancy.* McGraw-Hill, New York, 1969, p. 339,
10. Driscoll, J. and Gillepsie, L.: *Obstetrical considerations in diabetes in pregnancy.* Med. Clin. North Am. 49:1031, 1965.
11. Gerbie: op. cit., p. 339.
12. White, P.: *Pregnancy and diabetes, medical aspects.* Med. Clin. North Am. 49:1016, 1965.
13. Driscoll and Gillepsie: op. cit., p. 1032.
14. Ibid.
15. White: *op. cit.,* p. 1017.
16. Driscoll and Gillepsie: op. cit., p. 1032.
17. Ibid., p. 1033.

BIBLIOGRAPHY

Bates, G. W.: *Management of gestational diabetes.* Postgrad. Med. 55:55, 1974.

Bonica, J.: *Obstetric Complications.* F. A. Davis, Philadelphia, 1965.

Ibid.: *Maternal respiratory changes during pregnancy and parturition.* Clin. Anesth. 10:1, 1974.

Brewer, D., et al: *The physiology of pregnancy. Clinical pathologic corrections.* Postgrad. Med., Part I, 52:110, 1972; Part II, 53:221, 1973.

Burstein, I., et. al.: *Anxiety, pregnancy, labor, and the neonate.* Am. Obstet. Gynecol. 118:195, 1974.

Caleel, G. T.: *Thyroid disease in pregnancy.* J. Am. Osteopath. Assoc. 72:635, 1973.

Carrington, E.: *Diabetes in pregnancy.* Clin. Obstet. Gynecol. 16:28, 1973.

Cianfrani, T. and Conway, M.: *Ectopic pregnancy.* Am. J. Nurs. 63:93, 1963.

Cranley, M. and Frazien, S.: *Preventive intensive care of the diabetic mother and her fetus.* Nurs. Clin. N. Am. 8:489, 1973.

Danforth, D.: *Textbook of Obstetrics and Gynecology*, ed. 2. Harper and Row, New York, 1971.

DeAlvarez, R: *Hypertensive disorders in pregnancy.* Clin. Gynecol. 16:47, 1973.

Delaney, J. J., et al.: *Management of the pregnant diabetic.* Acta Diabetol. Lat. 8:1, 1971.

Desforges, J.: *Anemia complicating pregnancy.* J. Reprod. Med. 10:111, 1973.

Donald, I.: *Practical Obstetrical Problems.* J. B. Lippincott, Philadelphia, 1969.

Dudgeon, J.: *Intrauterine infections.* Ciba Found. Symp. 10:1, 1972.

Essex, N., et al.: *Diabetic pregnancy.* Br. Med. J. 4:89, 1973.

Feitelson, P. J., et al.: *Management of hypertensive gravidas.* J. Reprod. Med. 8:111, 1972.

Fields, H.: *Induction of Labor.* Macmillan, New York, 1965.

Friedman, E.: *Labor: Clinical Evaluation and Management.* Appleton-Century-Crofts, New York, 1967.

Garnet, J.: *Pregnancy in women with diabetes.* Am. J. Nurs. 69:1900, 1969.

Gonzalez, L. F.: *Heart disease in pregnancy.* Md. State Med. J. 19:137, 1970.

Gottesman, R., et al.: *Diagnosis and management of thyroid diseases in pregnancy.* J. Reprod. Med. 11:19, 1973.

Greene, J. W., et al.: *The use of urinary estriol excretion in the management of preganacies complicated by diabetes mellitus.* Am. J. Obstet. Gynecol. 91:684, 1965.

Greenhill, J.: *Biological Principles and Modern Practice of Obstetrics.* W. B. Saunders, Philadelphia, 1974.

Gusdon, J., et al.: *Amniotic fluid antibody titers and other prognostic parameters in erythroblastosis.* Am. J. Obstet. Gynecol. 108:85, 1970.

Hardy, J.: *Answers to questions on infections in the pregnant patient.* Hosp. Med. 6:44, 1970.

Hasen, J. M., et al.: *Maternal cardiovascular dynamics during pregnancy and parturition.* Clin. Anesth. 10:21, 1974.

Haynes, D.: *Medical Complications during Pregnancy.* McGraw-Hill, New York, 1969.

Hellman, L. and Pritchard, J.: *Williams Obstetrics,* ed. 14. Appleton-Century Crofts, New York, 1971.

Hendricks, C. H., et al.: *Toxemia of pregnancy: relationship between fetal weight, fetal survival, and the maternal state.* Am. J. Obstet. Gynecol. 109:225, 1971.

Jacobson, H. and Reid, D.: *High-risk pregnancy. II. Maternal and child care.* N. Engl. J. Med. 271:302, 1964.

Kahn, C. B., et al.: *Laboratory assessment of diabetic pregnancy.* Diabetes 21:31, 1972.

Laugharne, E., et al.: *Gestational diabetes—when teaching is important.* Can. Nurse 69:34, 1973.

Leeman, C. P.: *Dependency, anger, and denial in pregnant diabetic women.* Psychiatr. Q. 44:1, 1970.

Leon, J.: *High-risk pregnancy: graphic representation of the maternal and fetal risks.* Am. J. Obstet. Gynecol. 117: 497, 1973.

Light, H., et. al.: *Maternal concerns during pregnancy.* Am. J. Obstet. Gynecol. 118:223, 1974.

MacLeod, S. C.: *Relationship between elevated blood pressure and urinary estriols during pregnancy.* Am. J. Obstet. Gynecol. 109:375, 1971.

McCarry, J., et al.: *Time of onset and duration of labor in women with cardiac disease.* Lancet 1:483, 1973.

McFee, J.: *Anemia: A high-risk complication of pregnancy.* Clin. Obstet. Gynecol. 16:153, 1973.

Naeye, R., Dellinger, W. and Blanc, W.: *Fetal and maternal features of antenatal bacterial infections.* J. Pediatr. 9:733, 1971.

Naeye, R. and Blanc, W.: *Relation of poverty and race to antenatal infection.* N. Engl. J. Med. 283:555, 1970.

Nesbitt, R.: *Coincidental Medical Disorders Complicating Pregnancy.* In Danforth, D. (ed.): *Textbook of Obstetrics and Gynecology,* ed. 2, Harper and Row, New York, 1971.

Nesbitt, R. and Aubry, R.: *Recognition and care of high-risk obstetrical patients. Part I.* Hosp. Med. 3:43; *Part II* 3:41, 1967.

Neuberg, R.: *Drug addiction in pregnancy. Review of the problem.* Proc. R. Soc. Med. 65:867, 1972.

Oparil, S., et al.: *Heart disease in pregnancy.* J. Reprod. Med. 11:2, 1973.

O'Sullivan, J. B., et al.: *Medical treatment of the gestational diabetic.* Obstet. Gynecol. 43:817, 1974.

Perlmutter, J. F.: *Drug addiction in pregnant women.* Am. J. Obstet. Gynecol. 79:569, 1967.

Philipp, E., Barnes, J. and Newton, M.: *Scientific Foundations of Obstetrics and Gynaecology.* F. A. Davis, Philadelphia, 1970.

Ray, M., et al.: *Clinical experience with the oxytocin challenge test.* Am. J. Obstet. Gynecol. 114:1, 1972.

Reid, D.: *Principles and Management of Human Reproduction.* W. B. Saunders, Philadelphia, 1972.

Report of working group on the relation of nutrition to fetal growth and development. In *Maternal Nutrition and the Course of Pregnancy.* Committee on Maternal Nutrition, National Research Council, 1970.

Report of working group on nutrition and the toxemias of pregnancy. In *Maternal Nutrition and the Course of Pregnancy.* Committee on Maternal Nutrition, National Research Council, 1970.

Rose, P. A.: *The high risk mother-infant dyad–A challenge for nursing?* Nurs. Forum 6:94, 1967.

Rovinsky, J. and Guttmacher, A.: *Medical, Surgical and Gynecologic Complications of Pregnancy,* ed. 2. Williams & Wilkins, Baltimore, 1965.

Schneider, J.: *The high risk pregnancy.* Hosp. Prac. 6:133, 1971.

Selenkozo, H.: *Thyroid function and dysfunction during pregnancy.* Clin. Obstet. Gynecol. 16:66, 1973.

Sise, H.: *Hypofibrinogenemic states in obstetrics.* J. Reprod. Med. 10:115, 1973.

Spellacy, W.: *Diabetes and pregnancy.* Am. J. Obstet. Gynecol. 113:855, 1972.

Speroff, L.: *Toxemia of pregnancy. Mechanism and therapeutic management.* Am. J. Cardiol. 32:582, 1973.

Sullivan, J.: *Blood Pressure elevation in pregnancy.* Prog. Cardiovasc. Dis. 16:375, 1974.

Tyson, J. E.: *Medical aspects of diabetes in pregnancy and the diabetogenic effects of oral contraceptives.* Med. Clin. North Am. 55:947, 1971.

Ibid.: *Obstetrical management of the pregnant diabetic.* Med. Clin. North Am. 55:961, 1971.

Ueland, K., et al.: *Hemodynamic response of patients with heart disease to pregnancy and exercise.* Am. J. Obstet. Gynecol. 113:47, 1972.

Weir, J. G.: *Pregnant narcotic addict, a psychiatrist's impression.* Proc. R. Soc. Med. 65:869, 1972.

White, P.: *Pregnancy Complicating Diabetes.* Am. J. Med. 7:609, 1949.

Waters, W.: *Management of renal disease in pregnancy.* J. Reprod. Med. 8:48, 1972.

Worley, R. J., et al.: *Hyperthyroidism during pregnancy.* Am. J. Obstet. Gynecol. 119:150, 1974.

35 Complications Arising during Pregnancy

DYANNE D. AFFONSO, R.N., M.N.
DAVID DANFORTH, M.D.

This chapter focuses on problems resulting from pregnancy which can threaten the well-being of both mother and fetus. Although there are many such problems, two major complications will be explored in depth: toxemia and third trimester bleeding. The latter part of this chapter briefly highlights other complications that result specifically from pregnancy.

TOXEMIA OF PREGNANCY

Toxemia of pregnancy is a disease that occurs only in pregnancy. In almost all reports of maternal mortality, toxemia ranks either as the second or third leading cause of death. The purpose of this discussion is to outline the essential features of this complication. Toxemia is typically characterized by hypertension above any prepregnant level, proteinuria above any prepregnant level, and edema. Toxemia usually occurs in the last three months of pregnancy, but may be manifest earlier, especially in the presence of a hydatidiform mole. Women in their first pregnancy are particularly vulnerable, but the disease can appear during subsequent gestations. The disease occurs in 2 to 10 per cent of pregnant women, varying with their socioeconomic stratum. The higher figure is characteristic for those who are medically deprived, whose prenatal care is inadequate, who cannot or will not follow the balanced diet and the program that are necessary for normal pregnancy, and for those among whom the incidence of predisposing factors is very high. The lower figure is typical for those of higher socioeconomic status.

Toxemia has been classified in many ways. For the purposes of this discussion the following categories are used:

Incipient toxemia
Moderate toxemia
Severe toxemia
Eclampsia

Since any case of toxemia can presumably progress to eclampsia during pregnancy, some prefer to classify toxemia using the terms "mild preeclampsia," "moderate preeclampsia," and "eclampsia."

The final stage of toxemia is characterized by generalized tonic and clonic convulsions, loss of consciousness, and coma. The number of convulsions may vary from one or two to more than 100. The higher the number of convulsions, the greater the likelihood of death, which usually results from cerebrovascular accident, pulmonary edema, or extreme acidosis. Death may not always occur immediately, it may occur after a few days as the result of renal failure, aspiration pneumonia, or hepatic failure.

CAUSES

The *predisposing causes* for toxemia of pregnancy are hypertensive vascular disease, chronic renal disease, diabetes mellitus, polyhydramnios, multiple pregnancy, and hydatidiform mole. The incidence of toxemia is high among those who have these diseases. Pure toxemia is almost limited to women in their first pregnancy; if it occurs in later pregnancies, it is almost always superimposed upon one of the aforementioned predisposing factors.

The *exact cause* of toxemia is not known. At present, it appears that overstretching of the uterus (as occurs in multiple pregnancy, hydramnios, hydatidiform mole, and in certain first pregnancies) may be an important factor. This, as well as hypertensive vascular disease, can result in impairment of the uterine blood supply which in turn may cause ischemic damage to the placenta, with consequent elaboration into the maternal circulation of some unidentified substance which produces vasospasm and the other manifestations of toxemia.

SIGNS AND SYMPTOMS

Edema. Some edema of the ankles and fingers occurs in 60 per cent of women whose pregnancies are wholly normal. In toxemia the accumulation of water is much greater. In severe cases there may be pitting edema of the lower legs over the tibia, presacral edema, puffiness of the face and eyelids, swelling of the backs of the hands and, rarely, massive edema of the vulva. The bell of the stethoscope may leave a ring on the abdominal wall after listening for the fetal heart tones. The presence of swelling beyond that which is normally expected in pregnancy should alert the attendent to the possibility of toxemia. Also, weight gain in excess of one half pound per week may suggest excessive accumulation of water even in the absence of manifest edema.

Hypertension. No fast rules can be set regarding the blood pressure levels that are characteristic of incipient, moderate, and severe toxemia. Indeed, fatal eclampsia has occurred in women whose blood pressures were only slightly elevated. If generalizations can be made, an elevation of 30 mm. Hg systolic or 15 mm. Hg diastolic over the levels found in the first six months is considered abnormal and characteristic of toxemia of pregnancy. As a rule, in severe toxemia the blood pressure is of the order of 160/90 or higher, and in moderate toxemia it is 140/90 or above.

Proteinuria. Traces of proteinuria may result from contamination by a vaginal discharge. If it is present in a midstream specimen in the last trimester of pregnancy, it must be regarded as significant. Proteinuria is a late and usually ominous sign of toxemia. If the blood pressure is also elevated, the appearance of protein in the urine may suggest that the toxemia is severe.

Hyperreflexia. In severe toxemia, but rarely in mild or incipient cases, the deep tendon reflexes are significantly increased. The presence of transient or sustained ankle clonus and hyperactive biceps jerks suggests that eclampsia may be imminent. With the arm partially flexed, the biceps jerk, if it is hyperactive, can be readily elicted by sharply striking the middle finger of one hand against the thumb of the other which is placed against the biceps tendon in the antecubital fossa. The ankle jerk is elicted by bending the knee outward to one side, and sharply flexing the foot forward.

NURSING MANAGEMENT

Nursing Goals

Suggested nursing goals are:

1. Protect the mother and fetus from detrimental effects of toxemia.

2. Support the medical plan to control the condition and prevent eclampsia (convulsive stage).
2. Nurture the woman and family so they can cope as best as possible and have healthy outcomes in spite of this complication.

The nurse must be able to identify women who are vulnerable to toxemia of pregnancy. Predisposing factors, as previously described, are:

1. Hypertensive vascular disease
2. Chronic renal disease
3. Diabetes mellitus
4. Polyhydramnios
5. Multiple pregnancy
6. Hydatidiform mole.

In addition to the above, other risk factors for nursing assessment are:

7. *Age*. Women less than 20 years old or over 30 years old, especially over 35, are most vulnerable.
8. *Parity*. Although the primigravida is most vulnerable, multigravidas with over 5 gestations can be at risk due to age and socioeconomic factors.
9. *Race*. It is observed than nonwhites have an increased incidence of preeclampsia.
10. *Life style*. Socioeconomic status will determine whether a life style will nurture or stress the gestation. Socioeconomic conditions influence maternal diet, whether prenatal care is sought, valued, and maintained, and the degree of stresses and anxieties that plague the pregnant woman. In our modern society, financial stressors can be a major deterrent to healthy gestation.

The nurse should gather information about the above variables at the initial prenatal contact to immediately identify women who are likely to develop toxemia of pregnancy. In addition, assessment includes monitoring of blood pressure, weight, urine testing for protein, and alertness to other signs as listed in Table 35-1. Sometimes subtle clues indicative of toxemia are not remarkable, as illustrated in the following incident:

A 24-year-old primigravida, 32 weeks pregnant, was seen in a general hospital emergency room with vague complaints of headache, pains in the abdomen, and some vomiting. Her husband brought her to the hospital because she seemed "very excited, irritable, and uncomfortable." The intern taking a history found that she had been plagued by headaches for several weeks. She had seen her physician for routine prenatal visits twice during this time and was told such complaints were not uncommon but "normal for this stage of pregnancy." The intern suspected premature labor but felt no contractions and recommended that his medical superior check her. Meanwhile, a nursing student entered the room and began interacting with the woman. The student noticed that the woman's hands were slightly edematous and when she inquired about it, the woman revealed that she had not been able to twirl her wedding ring around her finger in weeks. Upon taking a blood pressure reading, the student found the systolic and diastolic only 8 to 10 cm. above what she remembered as the normal limits. However, she was concerned because both systolic and diastolic were elevated. She asked the woman to void, checked the urine, and found it to be positive for protein. At that point she told the woman not to move from her seat until she returned. She sought the intern to share her assessment data and asked, "Do you think the woman is preeclamptic?" The woman was diagnosed to be preeclamptic and treated properly. Later the intern revealed that he never suspected preeclampsia because he was looking at each symptom individually instead of interrelating the complaints and seeking more data.

TABLE 35-1. Symptomatology for Toxemia of Pregnancy*

Symptoms	*Theory*	*Comments*
Preeclampsia is characterized by a triad of symptoms:		Prenatal care is crucial in the prevention of preeclampsia because the woman may not be aware of this triad of early symptoms and may feel perfectly healthy in spite of the symptoms.
1. Edema reflected in sudden excessive weight gain. + minimal edema of the pedal and predtibial areas. ++ marked edema of lower extremities. +++ edema of the face, hands, lower abdominal wall and sacrum. ++++ anasarca with ascites.	Retention of water and impairment in sodium excrecretion possibly due to arteriolar thickening reflecting impairment of renal function. Sudden excess weight gain reflects water retention in the tissues.	Weight gain in excess of 1 lb. per week in the first 32 weeks of gestation or excess of 2½ lb. per week after the 34th week may suggest preeclampsia.
2. Hypertension (↑BP)	Arteriolar vasoconstriction manifests in an elevated systolic and diastolic pressure. Peripheral vascular spasms are best reflected in an elevated diastolic.	A rise of 30 mm. Hg systolic and 15 mm. Hg diastolic *above baseline norms* must be considered a risk factor suggestive of preeclampsia in a pregnant woman.
3. Proteinuria	Vasoconstriction of the afferent glomerular arterioles alters the permeability of the glomerular membrane allowing escape of protein.	The normal pregnant woman should not exceed 300 mg. daily excretion of protein, at maximum. Levels above this may be suggestive of preeclampsia.
The following are danger signs indicating progression oj the disease:		
1. Visual disturbances a. Blurred vision b. Scotoma (spots before the eyes) c. Double vision	Vasoconstriction creating edema and spasms in the retinal area leading to possible detachment of the retina.	Complaints of visual disturbances warrant assessment of the fundi with an opthalmoscope to detect any edema or vasospasms in the retinal area.
2. Headaches, vertigo (dizziness), nervousness, excitability, apprehension, nausea, vomiting	Vasoconstriction can create cerebral edema and hypoxia leading to hyperirritability of the cerebral cortex.	Complaints of headaches and these vague symptoms should not be dismissed or treated with routine remedies (aspirins) until further assessment is done to rule out toxemia.
3. Hemoconcentration (↑ Hematocrit)	Fluid accumulation in the tissue results in shift of fluid from the intravascular to the extravascular compartment.	Adequate fluid replacement becomes essential to maintain intravascular volume and adequate urinary output.

TABLE 35-1. *Continued*

Symptoms	*Theory*	*Comments*
Progression of the following symptoms indicates eclampsia is imminent:		
1. Epigastric pain	Indicates possible ischemia (reduced blood flow) in areas served by major abdominal vessels, such as bowel or liver.	Possible infarction of these areas should be considered, and liver function should be evaluated.
2. Oliguria (less than 30 cc./hour) leading to possible anuria	Indicates renal impairment due to decreased circulation.	Urine output will show an increase in protein as well as the presence of casts and red blood cells.
3. Hyperactive reflexes (sustained ankle clonus)	Indicates possible increased cerebrovascular resistance.	Increasing reflexes may forecast an impending seizure, and additional medication may be warranted.
4. Convulsions (occurrence indicates eclampsia)	Massive electrical discharge from central nervous irritability and/or ischemia.	Warning signs that a convulsion is imminent are severe epigastric pains, headaches, tightness around the chest, increased restlessness, decreased pulse and respirations.
5. Drowsiness—loss of consciousness	Progression into coma	Assess the level of consciousness to determine the patient's orientation to "person, place and time." Decreased responsiveness is suggestive of ensuing coma.

* Based on data obtained from: Dennis, E. and Hester, L.: *Toxemia of pregnancy.* In Danforth, D. (ed.): *Textbook of Obstetrics and Gynecology*, ed. 2. Harper and Row, New York, 1971; and Greenhill, J. and Friedman, E.: *Biological Principles and Modern Practice of Obstetrics.* W. B. Saunders, Philadelphia, 1974.

Nursing Actions Which Protect

Protective acts aim to minimize or prevent detrimental effects of toxemia on mother and fetus. Detrimental effects arise because toxemia is associated with peripheral arteriolar vasconstriction and vasospasms. Vasoconstriction decreases blood flow thereby diminishing nutrients and oxygen to the cells. Consequently maternal and fetal organ functions are altered. Thus, every attempt must be made to minimize vasoconstriction. Suggested nursing actions, protective in nature, are:

1. Conservation of Energy
   Energy conservation is important in decreasing the metabolic rate to minimize the demand for oxygen at a time when oxygen supply is compromised. In mild toxemia the woman is encouraged to take rest periods in the morning and afternoon and to sleep at

least 8 hours for a minimum total of 12 hours rest within a 24-hour period. The nurse is challenged to make specific suggestions as to how a busy wife and mother might organize her daily routines to ensure essential rest periods. If toxemia is moderate to severe, hospitalization is necessary to maintain bed rest and restrict physical activities. Bathroom privileges are allowed accordingly. Bed rest has the additional benefit of enhancing diuresis to combat edema. The hospital is not the best environment for peace and quiet. Thus, the nurse may need to manipulate the environment by turning off bright lights, drawing curtains to curtail sunlight, controlling traffic in and out the woman's room, and minimizing unnecessary conversations and sounds near the woman. This control of the environment is crucial when toxemia is severe because any sudden sensory stimulation can precipitate a convulsion.

2. Assessment for Anxieties and Concerns

   Anxiety stimulates the sympathetic-adrenal system in the body thereby causing a physiologic response of vasoconstriction. Fear and undue concerns intensify the toxemic condition. Therefore, the nurse must recognize clues indicative of anxiety and allow opportunities for the woman to express her concerns for herself, baby, and family. The nurse can help the woman to initiate problem-solving approaches.

3. Promotion of Comfort

   Provisions for personal hygiene such as bed baths, clean linens and clothes, oral care, and grooming can make the hospitalized woman who is confined to bed feel fresh and revitalized. The nurse must also consider the woman's position in bed. Frequently, women are in a semi-upright position, but hunched or sliding down in the bed, making them vulnerable to backaches. Check to see if the woman is in a position which prevents undue pressure from body parts. The simple act of giving a backrub has multiple benefits of releasing muscle tension, enhancing relaxation, and providing time for the woman to share her feelings.

4. Support Medicinal Therapy

   The toxemic patient is usually on a drug regimen to control the condition. At one time, toxemic women were frequently given diuretics to assist mobilization of retained water. However, studies have shown that diuretics can create adverse effects in human pregnancy.[1] Thus, while the current medical regimen is to encourage diuresis by such measures as rest and sleep, a toxemic woman may also be managed with diuretics at the discretion of her physician. At times, additional warmth (such as use of blankets, etc.) may be used to increase perspiration, thus aiding loss of retained fluid. Some women may be given sedatives to ensure adequate rest and sleep. The hospitalized patient may need additional drugs such as anticonvulsants (magnesium sulfate), narcotics (morphine sulfate), sometimes antihypertensives, and rarely, vasodilators. Magnesium sulfate is frequently the drug of choice because of its multiple effects of causing central nervous system depression to prevent convulsions, promoting vasodilation, and enhancing diuresis to aid in mobilization of retained water. It is preferably given intravenously for immediate onset of action, but may be given intramuscularly. There are certain factors the nurse must consider in the administration of magnesium sulfate, remembering that 1 g. of magnesium sulfate is equivalent to 2 cc. of a 50 per cent solution:

   a. Use intravenous equipment that will allow careful regulation for the prescribed flow rate.

b. When the drug is to be given intramuscularly, consider the following:
   (1) Administer the drug deep into the gluteal muscle for best absorption and minimal irritation to the subcutaneous tissues.
   (2) It is good technique to change the needle after withdrawing the solution to prevent leakage of the solution from the needle during the injection.
   (3) Inject the dosage equally into each buttock if the amount to be given is large.
   (4) Disperse the solution in as wide an area as possible by slightly moving the needle during the injection to prevent accumulation of the drug in one area.
   (5) Massage the area after injection to enhance absorption.
   (6) Administration of magnesium sulfate is painful. Sometimes a local anesthetic is administered or added to the solution to minimize discomfort. If not, the woman should be forewarned to anticipate discomfort since the elicitation of pain may be enough of a stimulus to provoke a convulsion. Warm compresses may be used to minimize discomfort and also aid absorption.

c. Recognize toxic effects. Because magnesium sulfate is largely excreted via the kidneys and the patient's kidney function may be comprised by toxemia, the nurse must be alert to overdosage from accumulation of the drug. Toxicity is characterized by loss of the deep tendon reflex (knee-jerk), quickly followed by depression of respirations (below 12 to 14 per minute) and lowered pulse. Nursing precautions involve checking the deep tendon reflex, respirations, and pulse, before and after administration of the drug. The drug should be withheld if there is no reflex, respirations are below 14 per minute, heart rate is markedly decreased, or urine output is less than 30 cc. per hour.

d. Prepare the antidote for toxicity. Calcium gluconate should always be readily available as an antidote via intravenous administration. The nurse must know the precautions associated with any drug before giving it. Patients should be continuously monitored for side effects and bed rails should be used to prevent accidents such as falling out of bed during heavy sedation.

5. Safety and Protection of Mother and Fetus

Monitoring of the toxemic patient is mandatory to protect her from entering eclampsia. Respiratory rate, pulse, and blood pressure should be checked at least every four hours, or more frequently as the situation warrants. Weight should be checked daily to assess whether fluids are being retained or excreted. Weights should be taken on the same scale, at the same time each day to ensure consistency in results. Weights are best taken upon waking, prior to routine daily activities such as food intake. The intake and output record is a valuable data source. If toxemia is severe, a Foley catheter is inserted to ensure precise measurement of urinary output. Oral intake may be withheld and intravenous therapy maintained. The degree of output will help regulate the amount of intravenous intake to prevent fluid overload in the body. Intravenous fluids are also given to overcome hemoconcentration. Twenty-four hour urine specimens are collected for protein analysis to assess effects of the disease on renal function. Specific tests such as creatinine clearance may be necessary and often show substantial reduction in renal flow. The fetal heart rate should also be monitored. Should the heart rate decrease or become irregular, the physician should be notified immediately. If the fetal distress does not respond to conservative management (change in normal position, oxygen by mask, etc.), cesarean delivery may be warranted.

Protecting the Eclamptic Patient

The nurse must constantly be alert to symptoms warning that eclampia is imminent (see Table 35-1). Eclampsia is a dangerous complication distinguished by convulsions leading to possible coma. Maternal mortality increases dramatically, and convulsions frequently result in intrauterine death through premature separation of the placenta. Preeclampsia may cause premature labor with all the attendant physiologic risks, or the fetus may be stressed by poor uteroplacental circulation. Convulsions also predispose the mother to pneumonia from aspiration of mucus. In severe cases, congestive heart failure and pulmonary edema are encountered. Other dangers include central nervous system hemorrhage, hepatic or renal damage, and self-injury during convulsions.

The definitive cure for toxemia is delivery. The baby is often safer, even if premature, in an intensive care nursery than in the hostile intrauterine environment. Sometimes eclampsia will precipitate spontaneous labor and delivery, or if eclampsia occurs during labor, it augments uterine contractions making labor rapid. However, an assisted delivery is not possible until convulsions are controlled. The eclamptic woman must never be left alone, but constantly watched for a possible convulsion. Sensory stimuli should be minimized because any sudden stimulus is likely to evoke a convulsion. A quiet, dark room, absolute bed rest, and sedation of the patient are usually ordered. The nurse must remember that she is a source of sensory stimulation and should speak softly, walk quietly, and perform nursing assessments gently. Other safety measures include using bedrails and assuring availability of padded tongue blades or other devices to prevent biting of the tongue during a convulsion. (Use of a bandage roll, a rolled wash cloth, or rubber tubings will also suffice.)

Convulsions

The patient may not be able to communicate that a convulsion is imminent. However, there may be nonverbal clues such as epigastric pain, tightness around the chest, decreased pulse and respirations, irritability, restlessness, staring, or "aura" appearance. A convulsing person, expecially a pregnant one, presents a frightening scene. However, the nurse must control her anxiety in order to make important observations and protect the woman during the convulsive attack. The nurse must observe when the convulsion begins, the parts of the body involved, and its duration. Convulsions usually last 10 to 15 seconds but may last as long as a couple of minutes. Ziegel and Van Blarom[2] describe a convulsive attack:

> Convulsions both tonic and clonic, occur in eclampsia. At first all muscles go into a state of tonic contraction; then they alternately contract and relax. The convulsions are sometimes preceded by an aura, but often are so entirely unheralded that they occur while the patient is asleep. They ordinarily begin with a twitching of the eyelids or facial muscles. The eyes are wide open and staring, and the pupils are usually dilated. Next the whole body becomes rigid, and then alternate contraction and relaxation of muscles begin. The twitchings proceed from the muscles about the nose and mouth to those of the neck and arms, and so on until

the entire body is in spasm. The patient's face is usually cyanotic and badly distorted, with the mouth being drawn to one side. She clenches her fists, rolls her head from side to side, and tosses violently about the bed. She is totally unconscious and insensible to light, and during the seizure respirations cease. Her head is frequently bent backward. Her neck forms a continuous curve with her stiffened, arched back. Another distressing feature is the protruding tongue and the frothy saliva, which is blood stained if the patient is not prevented from biting her tongue by use of a mouth gag between her teeth. Finally, muscular movements become milder, and then the patient lies motionless. After a long, deep breath respiratory movements are resumed.

During the acute stage the respirations are, as a rule, labored and noisy, and cyanosis may be present. The temperature is often normal, or may rise to 38.3° C (101° F). It may go as high as 40° C (104° F) in severe cases and this is a serious prognostic sign.

Significant nursing actions for the patient who convulses are:

1. Insert the padded tongue blade to protect the tongue.
2. Release or loosen restraints to prevent injury from fracture to bones.
3. Protect the woman from cuts and bruises if she is hitting herself against the bedrails by placing a pad or pillow between her and the object.
4. After the convulsion an oral airway may be inserted to maintain patency of the airway. The woman should be positioned on the side or with head slightly down to facilitate drainage of secretions and prevent aspiration.
5. Suction appropriately to remove accumulated secretions.
6. Restrict oral intake and maintain intravenous intake until the condition improves.
7. Monitor maternal and fetal status frequently (urinary output, blood pressure, fetal heart tones, pulse, respirations, temperature). Also, assess for labor because a convulsion can initiate spontaneous contractions but the woman may not be aware of such sensations.

After the convulsion, several nursing actions should be provided as the woman enters into a coma. During the comatose period the nurse must act appropriately to sustain life activities through such measures as ensuring a patent airway, maintaining proper position, promoting circulation, monitoring vital signs, and preventing skin breakdown. This is a period when active communication with the woman is neither desired nor possible. (After the coma period, the woman may not remember what has happened and the nurse will need to orient her back to reality in terms of time, person, and place.)

The nurse should also check for any vaginal bleeding and/or abdominal rigidity which might indicate a premature separation of the placenta (abruptio placentae). The nurse also needs to assess for impending labor which can be initiated by the stress of convulsions. Cervical dilatation can occur rapidly and delivery may be imminent. If labor does not occur spontaneously, it can be initiated as a plan for medical management. Thus the nurse must anticipate nurturing the woman through labor and delivery.

As soon as is feasible, labor may be induced with oxytocics. If unsuccessful, a cesarean section is performed. The nurse should monitor uterine contractions and fetal heart rate, be alert to impending convulsions, and anticipate care for a high-risk neonate. Emergency equipment should be readily available for both mother and baby.

Intensive nursing care to the eclamptic patient must continue even after delivery. Danger of convulsion does not end with delivery and the woman needs to be closely monitored in the early postpartal period. After delivery there is usually rapid improvement from the toxemia. The most favorable response is that of increased urinary output which usually occurs within 48 hours after delivery. As diuresis ensues, edema usually diminishes and the weight and blood pressure return to normal.

Nursing Actions Which Nurture and Stimulate

The woman at risk from toxemia needs input to nurture her in coping with the condition and to stimulate toward optimal maintenance of daily living patterns. The nurse nurtures by keeping the woman and family informed of the situation, thereby lessening anxieties (which can activate the sympathetic-adrenal system and augment vasoconstriction). Nurturance also includes positive reinforcement for efforts to help one's self by adhering to therapy (taking medications and rest periods). The nurse also nurtures by communicating understanding that pregnancy is difficult and more of a hardship because of the limitations imposed by toxemia. The nurse needs to help the family understand what toxemia is and how it is a hazard to pregnancy so that limitations and therapy can be better accepted.

To stimulate optimal health during gestation, the nurse must continuously reinforce the value of prenatal care to the toxemic woman. Special efforts should be made to make the woman feel that the time, money and energy invested in a prenatal visit yield valuable and rewarding results. Sometimes a woman may feel guilty and blame herself for causing toxemia because she has not sought prenatal care or did not follow recommended therapy for diet, rest, and medications. The nurse needs to explore why the woman may not have been able to seek prenatal care or to maintain prescribed therapeutic plans. Rather than being punitive, the nurse must convey to the woman that her past behaviors are not as important as what she does now. Hopefully, such acceptance and understanding by the nurse will stimulate the woman to value and adhere to therapy.

The woman may need help to modify daily living patterns, especially if her life style fosters stress and augments toxemia. This endeavor may prove a nursing challenge because suggestions for modifying daily routines of sleep, diet, and activity must be relevant to the woman's home environment. Suggestions must be feasible or the woman can easily say "yes" in the clinic but return to her normal routines when she is at home. The dietary regimen is always a hard pattern to modify. Women often need help preparing foods that are not excessive in sodium. Unfortunately, women of lower socioeconomic status usually prepare meals by using ingredients high in sodium or use additional salt to flavor meals. This may be a hard meal pattern to break because foods not rich in salt may be less palatable. Regarding diet therapy, it was once believed that strict salt restriction was necessary for the toxemic woman. However, current research has challenged this because there is an increased need for sodium during pregnancy to maintain fluid and electrolyte balance. Thus, women are currently advised not to eliminate their normal intake of sodium but rather to avoid excessive intake of sodium through salty foods (such as potato chips, salted crackers, and canned foods packed in sodium) and in the preparation of their meals as previously mentioned.

The hospitalized patient with severe toxemia may find her diet restricted in sodium and calories as a therapeutic plan to manage the symptoms. For these women, meals may appear less appetizing and the nurse may need to make meal times pleasant and rewarding by providing additional attention and positive reinforcement for efforts to adhere to the therapy. Also, whenever feasible, every attempt should be made to include the woman's preferences in the diet. The nurse must also stimulate the woman who is losing protein in her urine to increase her dietary intake of protein to compensate the loss. Again the nurse must make specific suggestions of foods rich in protein but within the family's budget.

The nurse needs to value what is occurring in the home environment during and after hospitalization for toxemia. This is an important aspect for assessment because stressors related to family living will be deterrents to the mother's recovery. For example, a mother who is not receiving help with child care may be preoccupied with the welfare of her children. Likewise, her children may feel neglected because of the mother's decreased ability to carry on the routines which have become a source of security to the children. The nurse may need to refer the family to community resources (such as through social services) and/or mobilize the extended family to support the woman through her recovery period.

The nurse should stimulate the toxemic woman and her family to actively participate in monitoring the condition. The family should be taught danger signs and told to seek medical attention immeditely if such signs are present. When the nurse effectively nurtures and stimlates the family, then every day of the pregnancy can be meaningful in spite of the limitations and risks posed by toxemia. Hopefully, such nursing actions will result in a successful outcome for mother and baby.

THIRD TRIMESTER BLEEDING

Late pregnancy bleeding can result from several causes. Although some are trivial, *any* bleeding must be regarded as potentially fatal until the serious causes are ruled out. The possible causes include:

1. Placenta previa
2. Premature separation of the placenta (abruptio placentae)
3. Rupture of the uterus
4. Vasa previa
5. Circumvallate placenta or placenta membranacea
6. Lesions of the cervix (e.g., polyp, carcinoma)
7. Lesions of the vagina (e.g., laceration due to trauma, hemangioma)
8. "Bloody show" may precede labor by hours or days. It is usually scanty, mixed with mucus, pink in color, and stops rather promptly.

In all cases of vaginal bleeding after the twentieth week (except those clearly due to bloody show) the following are to be done at the time of admission to the hospital:

1. Bed rest
2. Gentle examination of the abdomen, but *no pelvic or rectal examination*
3. Hemoglobin and hematocrit
4. Urine for protein and sugar
5. Cross-match at least two units of blood (more if history of heavy bleeding or if double set-up examination [see below] is contemplated).

The two classic causes of bleeding after the twentieth week of pregnancy are placenta previa and premature separation of the placenta.

PLACENTA PREVIA

In placenta previa, the placenta is implanted low in the uterus, either on the lower uterine segment or over the internal os. As the lower uterine segment develops, retracts, and dilates to an extent in the last weeks of pregnancy, the anchoring villi are torn and uterine sinuses at the placental site are opened, thus permitting the escape of variable amounts of blood depending on the number and size of the sinuses that are opened. The amount of bleeding may be scanty at first, or it may be very profuse.

Causes

The exact cause is unknown. Placenta previa occurs in about one of every 200 deliveries, and is more common in multiparas. It is also more common in women who have had a prior low cervical cesarean section, since implantation tends to occur at the site of the uterine scar.

Classification

1. *Total placenta previa* is the condition in which the placenta completely covers the internal os.
2. *Partial placenta previa* is the condition in which a part of the internal os is covered by the placenta. (For purposes of definition one considers the cervix to be 2 cm. dilated.)
3. *Marginal placenta previa* is the condition in which the placental edge can be felt inside the internal os, but does not cover any part of it.

Types of placenta previa are shown in Figure 35-1.

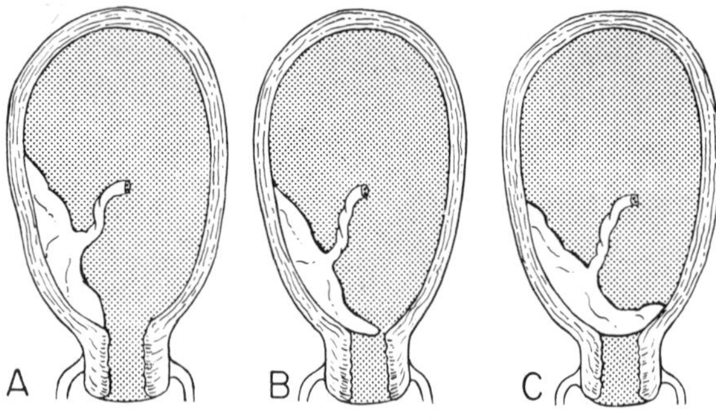

FIGURE 35-1. Types of placenta previa. *A*, Low implantation of placenta. *B*, Partial placenta previa. *C*, Total placenta previa. (From Bonica, J.: *Principles and Practice of Obstetric Analgesia and Anesthesia.* F. A. Davis, Philadelphia, 1972, with permission.)

Symptoms and Signs

Painless vaginal bleeding is the cardinal sign of placenta previa. Whenever this occurs in the last three months of pregnancy, regardless of whether it is scanty or copious, placenta previa should be considered to be present until it is ruled out. The blood is bright red in color.

The first hemorrhage is usually, but not always, scanty, and *if no rectal or vaginal examinations are made,* it usually stops spontaneously, to recur again within hours or days. Each subsequent hemorrhage is usually more profuse than the last one.

The uterus remains soft, and if labor is beginning, it relaxes completely between contractions.

The fetal heart is unaffected unless there is major placental detachment or maternal shock due to blood loss.

Since the presence of the placenta deep in the pelvis may prevent the head or buttocks from engaging, the presenting part may be entirely unengaged; transverse and oblique lies are frequent.

Diagnosis

The *direct diagnosis* of placenta previa is made by feeling the placenta through the cervix. However, this examination can provoke the most violent bleeding, and it is to be undertaken *only* in two specific circumstances: 1) When pregnancy has advanced beyond 37 weeks and nothing is to be gained in the interest of the baby by delaying delivery, and 2) When repeated hemorrhages or unremitting bleeding of such magnitude have occurred that postponing delivery would endanger the mother's life. This examination is referred to as "the double set-up examination," and it is never to be made unless everything is in instant readiness to perform cesarean section at once if heavy bleeding should be provoked.

The *indirect diagnosis* of placenta previa is

made by tests which are designed to localize the placenta without the need for a digital examination. If, by such tests, the placenta is found to be implanted high in the uterus, then placenta previa can be ruled out. The methods available for making this indirect appraisal are:

1. X-ray soft tissue placentography, with or without dye in the bladder can sometimes demonstrate the position of the placenta. However, this method is so often misleading that it is no longer recommended.
2. Placental localization using *radioisotopes* is relatively simple, highly accurate, and not harmful to mother or baby. Chromium 51-tagged erythrocytes, technetium 99-tagged albuminate, and radio-iodinated serum albumin (RISA) are used most commonly. RISA requires that the mother receive Lugol solution before the test is performed to saturate the fetal thyroid and block fetal uptake; this is not necessary for either of the other techniques.
3. *Ultrasound scan* is highly accurate and simple to use. In institutions where it is available, it is used almost to the exclusion of all other indirect techniques.
4. *Femoral arteriography* with retrograde catheterization and dye injection above the level of the hypogastric artery is accurate, technically difficult, moderately hazardous, and rarely indicated or needed.

Management

The management of a patient with painless late pregnancy bleeding is based upon 1) the amount of bleeding and 2) the duration of pregnancy at the time of the first hemorrhage.

A. *If the duration of pregnancy is less than 37 weeks and bleeding is either scanty or is stopped after a prior hemorrhage:*

1. Take *indirect* steps to localize the placenta.

   If placenta previa is ruled out, digital and speculum examinations are made to determine vaginal or cervical sources of the bleeding.

   If placenta previa is confirmed by the indirect tests, *expectant management* is appropriate. The purpose of expectant management is to permit the baby to grow a little larger and, hopefully, to delay the need for delivery until 37 weeks of gestation. It has no purpose after 37 weeks and indeed is not without risk because of the increasing likelihood of violent bleeding as term is approached. In conducting expectant management the following are to be scrupulously observed:

   a. Continued bed rest with bathroom privileges only.
   b. No rectal or vaginal examinations.
   c. *Matched blood* (2 units) available at all times for immediate transfusion if it should be needed.
   d. Cesarean section should be done, regardless of pregnancy duration, if bleeding is frequently recurrent, persistent, or profuse.

At 37 weeks, steps are taken to deliver the baby, and the decision must now be made whether vaginal delivery is feasible and appropriate, or whether cesarean section is preferable. This decision is based on exact knowledge of 1) the degree of placenta previa, that is, whether it is central, or is only marginal, and 2) the feasibility of induction of labor and delivery without jeopardizing either mother or baby. These determinations are made by what is termed *double set-up examination,* which means a sterile vaginal examination in the operating room where all is in readiness to perform cesarean section or vaginal delivery.

It is emphasized that vaginal or rectal examination in the presence of placenta previa may be followed by instant hemorrhage that can be fatal unless cesarean section can be performed within minutes. The double set-up therefore requires that the examination be made on the operating table; that all personnel for cesarean section be present (circulating nurse, anesthetist, and someone to provide immediate care for the baby); that the scrub nurse and at least one physician assistant be scrubbed; that all instruments, sutures, and ligatures be open and set up for immediate use for either abdominal or vaginal delivery; that an infusion be running through a large bore needle that can be used for the rapid transfusion of blood if it should be needed; and that at least two units of matched blood be immediately available.

It was noted before that after expectant management of placenta previa, the double set-up examination is made at 37 weeks with the intention of proceeding to delivery. Accordingly, at the time of the examination one either ruptures the membranes to induce labor if it is appropriate, or proceeds at once to cesarean section. The principles upon which this decision is based are as follows:

a. *Rupture the membranes* if the placenta does not cover the internal os and none of the following indications for cesarean section is present.
b. *Perform cesarean section:*
   (1) If the placenta covers the internal os.
   (2) If profuse bleeding results from examination regardless of the degree to which the placenta covers the internal os.
   (3) If an oblique or transverse lie is found, such that no presenting part is in the pelvis.
   (4) If the cervix is uneffaced and rupture of the membranes is technically not feasible.
   (5) If, after rupture of membranes, heavy bleeding or any evidence of fetal embarrassment ensues, or if labor does not follow in normal fashion.
   (6) If there are any other circumstances (e.g., previous cesarean section, prior vaginal plastic operation) for which delivery by cesarean section would be preferable to vaginal delivery.

B. *If the duration of pregnancy is 37 weeks or more at the time of the first admission,* proceed at once to double set-up examination, as outlined above. If placenta previa is confirmed, either the membranes are ruptured or cesarean section is performed as outlined above. If placenta previa is ruled out, other possible sources of bleeding are sought.

C. *If the patient is admitted with heavy, unremitting, painless, red vaginal bleeding of shock-producing proportions and the clinical picture is of placenta previa,* transfuse at once as needed and perform cesarean section without prior double set-up examination. If placenta previa is not confirmed at operation, a meticulous search is made after operation for vaginal or cervical sources of bleeding.

Prognosis

In the present day, and under satisfactory circumstances, the likelihood of death or even serious hemorrhage from placenta previa should be approximately nil. The prognosis for the baby is less favorable, the perinatal mortality being approximately 15 per cent; most of the infant deaths are due to prematurity.

PREMATURE SEPARATION OF THE PLACENTA

Premature separation of the placenta (abruptio placentae) is the circumstance in which the normally situated and normally implanted placenta suddenly separates from the uterine wall before the baby is delivered. Bleeding occurs from the uterine surface from which the placenta has detached. The source of the blood, just as in placenta previa, is from the maternal circulation, and it is released under considerable pressure. The concomitant presence of hypertension may compound the problem and the uterus, being still distended by the baby and amniotic fluid, cannot contract sufficiently to close off the bleeding uterine vessels. In some of the cases the blood may be entirely trapped behind the placenta, causing further separation of the placenta from the uterus. This is referred to as the *concealed hemorrhage.* In some cases the blood may find its way to the vagina by seeping between the fetal membranes and the uterine wall. This is known as *external or revealed hemorrhage.* In the remaining cases a portion of the blood may find its way to the outside, and part of it may remain either beneath the placenta or between the membranes and the uterine wall. This is known as *partially concealed hemorrhage,* and it occurs with sufficient frequency that the amount of external bleeding gives no indication of the amount of blood that is lost from the maternal circulation or of the seriousness of the problem. When external bleeding occurs, the blood is usually dark in color, rather than red as it is in placenta previa. Types of abruptio placentae are shown in Figure 35-2.

If there is no easy egress for the blood, its force may cause it to burst through the fetal membranes into the amniotic sac. In almost all of the cases the blood is under sufficient pressure that some of it extravasates into the uterine wall between the muscle fibers, thus accounting for the uterine irritability that is a cardinal sign of premature separation of the placenta. If this should be extreme, bluish ecchymotic areas are present on the serosal surface of the uterus. In some cases this is sufficient to cause the uterus to be almost entirely blue in color and to prevent it from contracting properly after the baby has been delivered. This is the so-called *Couvelaire uterus,* named after the obstetrician who first described it.

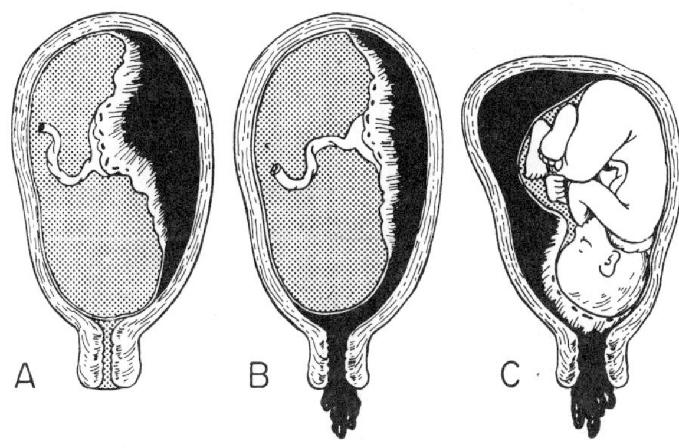

FIGURE 35-2. Abruptio placentae. *A*, Internal or concealed hemorrhage. *B*, External hemorrhage. *C*, Prolapse of the placenta. (From Bonica, J.: *Principles and Practice of Obstetric Analgesia and Anesthesia.* F. A. Davis, Philadelphia, 1972, with permission.)

As the result of damage to the uterine wall and retroplacental clotting, large quantities of thromboplastin are released into the maternal circulation. This in turn can result in the formation of myriad tiny clots, the so-called *disseminated intravascular coagulation.* Because of this, renal perfusion is seriously impaired, with resulting acute tubular necrosis (which may be reversible) or acute cortical necrosis (which can be fatal). Oliguria and proteinuria are therefore extremely ominous signs in premature separation of the placenta.

In addition to the aforementioned problems, huge quantities of fibrin may be laid down both within the blood vessels and, especially, in the retroplacental clot. This can be sufficient to deplete the liver fibrinogen more rapidly than it can be restored. The result is *hypofibrinogenemia*, with increased bleeding not only from the uterus, but in other organs as well.

Premature separation of the placenta, in greater or lesser degree, occurs in about 2 per cent of pregnancies that reach the last trimester and accounts for more than half of the instances of late pregnancy bleeding.

Causes

The cause of premature separation of the placenta is not known. It is much more common in multiparous than primiparous women, and in women over the age of 35. Toxemia of pregnancy clearly predisposes to this complication, especially in women who have underlying hypertensive vascular disease. Folic acid deficiency was once thought to be an etiologic factor, but this is no longer accepted.

Trauma is concerned in some cases. A direct blow to the abdomen, or amniocentesis if the needle traverses the placenta, can produce premature separation, but they are extremely rare causes.

Signs and Symptoms

The clinical signs usually vary according to the degree of detachment of the placenta. In the marginal type they are usually trivial, whereas complete detachment may be quickly fatal unless it is dealt with at once. Hence, the clinical designations of mild, moderate, and severe separation.

Premature separation of the placenta is to be suspected if the uterus is excessively irritable and fails to relax well. *The amount of external bleeding bears little relation to the severity of the process:* there may be none in precipitous massive abruption; in lesser degrees of separation the bleeding may be scant, moderate, or heavy depending on the proportion of blood that escapes to the vagina. Uterine discomfort and tenderness may be early signs of marginal sinus or *mild separation* (less than one fourth of the placental surface). Scant to moderate bleeding may or may not be present. Signs of *moderate separation* (more than one fourth and less than two thirds of the placental surface) include continuous uterine pain and tenderness, sustained firm or partial contraction of the uterus, and, usually, signs of fetal embarrassment (excessive fetal movements, irregular fetal heartbeat). *Severe separation* (more than two thirds of the placental surface) is usually characterized by knife-like pain, shock, a board-like uterus, and fetal death. *Clotting defects* are common in moderate and severe abruption. *Predisposing conditions* (toxemia, trauma, multiparity) may be present.

Management

In general, the management of abruptio placentae depends on the degree of separation and to a lesser extent on the duration of pregnancy. The customary orders in the various situations are summarized as follows:

Mild Abruptio Placentae

1. *Pregnancy less than 36 weeks, not in labor.* (In the presence of bleeding, the differential diagnosis is from placenta previa.)
   a. No vaginal or rectal examination.
   b. Indirect tests for placental localization.
   c. If placenta previa is ruled out: 1) make speculum examination for vaginal or cervical sources of bleeding, and 2)

observe for 48 hours. If no bleeding and no labor after ambulation, and if uterus relaxes well, discharge home with instructions to return instantly if any pain or bleeding.

2. *Pregnancy less than 36 weeks, early or active labor.*
   a. Double set-up examination.
   b. If no placenta previa, *rupture membranes.* (This *permits* the uterus to contract to an extent around its contents which are not reduced in bulk, and may diminish the bleeding.)
   c. Oxytocin infusion if labor is desultory. Start at 2 mu/min. and increase by 2 mu/min. every 5 minutes until contractions of good quality. (The oxytocin "drip" for stimulation of labor is an obsolete device that probably accounts for many of the disasters that result from oxytocin infusions. Each maternity unit should have as part of its standard equipment at least one infusion pump to deliver exact amounts of oxytocin at preselected rates.)
3. *Pregnancy more than 36 weeks.*
   a. Double set-up examination.
   b. If no placenta previa, *rupture membranes.*
   c. Meticulous fetal monitoring, preferably by fetal ECG.
   d. Oxytocin infusion if labor is desultory.
   e. *Cesarean section* if there is fetal distress, continued bleeding, or failure of uterus to relax well between contractions.

Moderate Abruptio Placentae

1. Cross-match at least 3 units of blood.
2. Set up tubes for evaluation of clotting defect. Administer fibrinogen *only* as clearly indicated by demonstration of hypofibrinogenemia *and* continued bleeding. Repeat clotting test every 15 minutes.
3. *Rupture membranes* regardless of whether abdominal or vaginal delivery is anticipated.
4. If no immediate labor, oxytocin infusion.
5. *Cesarean section:* a) If baby is viable and there is fetal distress, b) if there is not effective labor within 2 hours, or c) if delivery cannot be anticipated within 6 hours of membrane rupture.
6. *If shock is present or imminent:*
   a. Monitor CVP and Foley catheter output.
   b. Human serum albumin (250–500 ml. 5%) while awaiting cross-match.
   c. If urgent need for blood, transfuse unmatched Rh negative type O with added Witebsky substance.
   d. Nasal oxygen, elevate legs 20° Trendelenburg.

Severe Abruptio Placentae

Management is the same as for moderate separation except that much more blood is needed and the clotting defect is apt to be far more profound. The baby usually needs no serious consideration since it is probably either dead or doomed, and the priority is to institute measures for the preservation of the mother's life.

1. *Rupture membranes at once regardless of shock* and regardless of proposed method of delivery.
2. Replace blood quickly (4 to 8 units usually needed), with care to avoid circulatory overload. Calcium gluconate (10 ml. 10%) IV after every 6 units of banked blood.
3. Correct clotting defect as indicated by clotting tests.
4. *Cesarean section:* a) If there is any chance the baby may still be alive, b) if

rupture of the membranes is not followed promptly by effective labor, or c) if at the time the membranes are ruptured, the cervix is such that delivery cannot be anticipated within two hours. (The longer the patient is undelivered the more likely irreversible maternal complications.)

Prognosis

In the severe cases, where most of the placental surface is detached, the infant mortality is almost 100 per cent regardless of treatment, and the outlook for the mother is ominous unless the problem is dealt with promptly and skillfully. In the lesser degrees of separation the outlook for the baby depends in large measure upon its maturity, and the degree and duration of anoxia or hypoxia.

For the mother, the prognosis depends on the combined insult of several factors, including the amount of blood lost from the maternal circulation, the severity of a coagulation defect (that is, hypofibrinogenemia or disseminated intravascular coagulation), and the number of hours that ensue between the placental accident and delivery. The mother's prognosis is also greatly influenced by certain complications to which women with premature separation of the placenta are predisposed; they include postpartum hemorrhage, renal failure, and pituitary necrosis (Sheehan's syndrome).

ROLE OF NURSING

Nursing responsibilities in the management of a woman bleeding during pregnancy are primarily to:

1. Collect information on the extent of bleeding and protect the woman until medical intervention begins.
2. Initiate diagnostic work-up for continued assessment.
3. Prepare for possible emergency labor and delivery or cesarean section.
4. Assess for shock and implement protective acts should it occur.

During the initial contact between the woman and nurse, information should be collected on the nature of the bleeding—its onset, amount, color, and frequency. Nurses must be cautioned against use of such terms as mild, moderate, or plentiful. Blood loss must be accurately assessed in measurable terms (e.g., "cupful," "completely saturated two vaginal pads"). Experiment with various measures to estimate the amount of bleeding. For example, one nursing student used blood left from a routine delivery to measure how many cc.'s it took to saturate parts and all of a vaginal pad. Ask the woman how frequently she changes her pads or how many pads she has used to gain some insight into the degree of bleeding. Remember that the amount of vaginal bleeding is not an accurate indication of the severity of the condition because bleeding may be concealed behind the placenta. Other important data to collect are whether pain is present and does the uterus feel hard, firm, and tender to touch (indicative of abruptio placentae). To protect the woman from dangers associated with hemorrhage, the nurse should immediately place the woman on bed rest and keep her quiet. Activity and sensory stimulation can aggravate the bleeding as well as elevate the basal metabolic rate thereby increasing oxygen consumption. The woman should be transferred from the room via a stretcher. An intravenous system should be started to provide fluids to increase the lowered blood volume. Lactated Ringer's solution acts as a better volume expander than dextrose in water. The IV also allows administration of blood when necessary. The nurse should also monitor pulse, respirations, blood pressure, and fetal heart tones at appropriate intervals, depending on the situation.

The nurse may be needed to institute measures for laboratory diagnosis. All women who are bleeding should have blood drawn for hemoglobin, hematocrit, type and cross-match for units of blood, and analysis for clotting defects such as hypofibrinogenemia. Other diagnostic tests will be ordered by the physician as necessary, such as radiologic and isotope studies to localize the placenta. The nurse should protect the woman by assuring that no vaginal or rectal examination be performed unless it is done under the physician's direction.

The nurse must anticipate an emergency delivery, either vaginally or abdominally, as part of the care plan. Thus, the abdomen as well as the perineum should be shaved. A Foley catheter may need to be quickly inserted if a cesarean section is done. During a double set-up examination the nurse must always be ready for a delivery and will function to position and prepare the woman, as well as to circulate necessary equipment and medications as a member of the health team. Preparation for an emergency delivery must also include the woman and family. Imagine the stress and anxiety if a woman enters a room expecting only to be examined and suddenly is bombarded with the hurried arrangements for a delivery! The climate during an emergency delivery is anxiety-provoking for all involved —patient, doctor, nurse. Therefore, extra efforts must be made to support the woman, keep her informed of her status and her baby's, and to positively reinforce her attempts to cope with the situation.

The bleeding woman is vulnerable to vascular collapse and must be protected from shock, usually by transfusion of blood and intravenous fluids to increase circulatory volume. Other necessary nursing actions include elevating the legs to a 20° Trendelenburg position, administering oxygen, and monitoring respirations, pulse, blood pressure, and the central venous pressure. A discussion of nursing actions relative to shock is presented in Chapter 36.

The woman at risk from bleeding during pregnancy requires much nurturance to minimize anxieties about her own welfare and her baby's. A valuable and appreciated nurturing action is the physical presence of the nurse. When the nurse is with the patient, anxieties can be expressed, information given to allay fears or misconceptions, and a feeling of trust and self-worth is gained. The nurse must also realize that these women will need assistance in performing their daily routines when they return home (as discussed in the section on toxemia). The nurse needs to communicate to the woman the significance of returning for follow-up laboratory studies (such as for hemoglobin, hematocrit). In addition, any woman who experiences blood loss will need information regarding the importance of iron intake, both in diet and in supplements through iron tablets.

OTHER CONDITIONS

HYDRAMNIOS

Excessive accumulation of amniotic fluid results in a condition known as hydramnios. The incidence of this condition is 1 in 1,000 deliveries. Although the volume of amniotic fluid in a normal term pregnancy ranges from 800 to 1200 ml., the volume in hydramnios may reach 5 liters or more. The etiology of hydramnios is unclear, but there is speculation that disturbances in the fetal ability to swallow during gestation contribute to the excessive accumulation of fluid.

Possible Consequences

1. Premature rupture of the membranes may occur due to distention by the excessive fluid.
2. Premature labor and delivery of the infant may result.
3. Prolapse of the umbilical cord may occur

when there is a sudden loss of the large amount of fluid during spontaneous or artificial rupture of the membranes.

4. Premature separation of the placenta may occur when the uterus contracts to adapt to the reduced volume of its contents.
5. There is substantial perinatal mortality associated with hydramnios. Major congenital anomalies may also be present, most often involving the central nervous system (e.g., anecephaly, spina bifida, myelomeningiocele).

Clinical Signs

Clinical signs suggestive of hydramnios include:

1. Unusually large uterine size (distended uterus).
2. Distant or inaudible fetal heart tones.
3. Indistinct fetal parts.

The diagnosis may be confirmed by ultrasound or by conventional roentgenography. Using these techniques, multiple pregnancies or significant fetal anomalies can be excluded and the excessive fluid visualized.

The nurse needs to appreciate that hydramnios commonly is associated with multiple pregnancies, especially in single-ovum twins, maternal diabetes, erythroblastosis fetalis, and toxemia.

Treatment

Treatment depends upon the symptoms. If the large uterus causes abdominal discomfort, edema of the lower extremities, and/or edema of the abdominal walls, the woman is hospitalized. She is placed on bed rest and moderate sodium intake. Diuretics may be ordered, but are of uncertain value. Such conservative management is usually continued until labor spontaneously ensues. However, if symptoms pose a maternal threat, such as dyspnea, orthopnea, and vomiting, some of the amniotic fluid may be removed by amniocentesis, withdrawing only sufficient volume to bring maternal symptomatic relief.

EXTRAUTERINE PREGNANCY

The zygote may sometimes implant in sites other than the normal uterine corpus. This is usually referred to as an *ectopic pregnancy* (nidation of the zygote is usually outside the uterus or in an abnormal location within the uterus). Figure 35-3 illustrates the various locations of ectopic pregnancies. There is an increased incidence of ectopic pregnancy in the nonwhite (1 in 120 pregnancies) contrasted with the white population (1 in 200 pregnancies).[3]

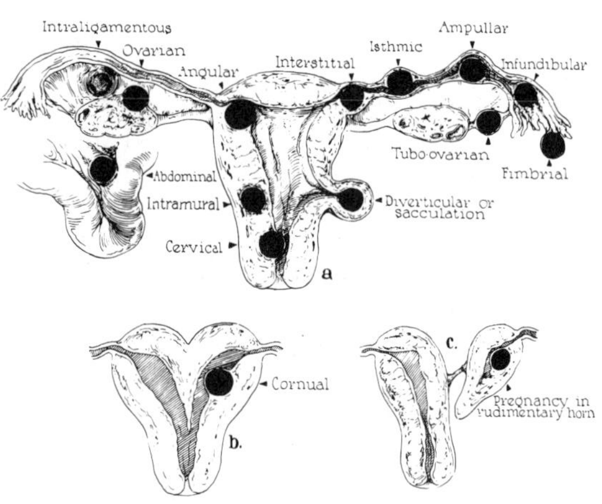

FIGURE 35-3. Various types of ectopic pregnancies. (From Danforth, D. (ed.): *Textbook of Obstetrics and Gynecology*, ed. 2. Harper and Row, New York, 1971, with permission.)

Clinical Signs

1. Pelvic pain which may be sharp or dull, constant or intermittent. The pain may be felt throughout the lower abdomen and is usually associated with vaginal bleeding.
2. Menstrual delay with or without vaginal bleeding.
3. Changes in vital signs. Rise in pulse and fall in blood pressure is suggestive of impending shock. The temperature may be elevated or normal.
4. Urinary frequency may be observed.

Although difficult to diagnose, ectopic pregnancy is strongly suggested by findings of a minimally enlarged uterus and a tender adnexal mass. Laboratory confirmation is made by a falling hematocrit or hemoglobin, and possible leukocytosis. Pregnancy tests may be helpful when positive, but a negative pregnancy test does not exclude an ectopic pregnancy.

Treatment

The most frequent type of extrauterine pregnancy is a *tubal gestation*. Conditions may exist that prevent or retard the passage of the fertilized egg through the fallopian tubes, e.g., gonorrheal infection, or tubal adhesions. A tubal pregnancy usually terminates by the rupture of the fallopian tube with resulting intraperitoneal hemorrhage. This results in increased pain, and the patient may present in shock. A large gauge intravenous line should be immediately established and vital signs monitored continuously until stable. Blood should be made available for immediate transfusion. The treatment is surgical. The affected tube and ovary are generally excised intact, and every effort is made to preserve reproductive functions. If extensive infection is encountered, complete removal of the uterus, tubes, and ovaries may be indicated. If a normal tube and ovary can be spared with the uterus, then future childbearing can be anticipated.

Other less common types of extrauterine pregnancies include cervical and abdominal gestations. Such experiences usually create a painful gestation and may result in a threat to the woman's life because of excessive blood loss. Although treatment is surgical, it is interesting to note that abdominal pregnancies have been known to produce near term infants.

HYPEREMESIS GRAVIDARUM

Nausea and vomiting (morning sickness) are frequent discomforts in the first trimester of pregnancy. However, when nausea and vomiting persist, leading to difficulty in retaining oral intake, the condition is known as hyperemesis gravidarum. Although the exact cause of this condition is not clear, numerous theories are proposed, such as:

1. High levels of chorionic gonadotrophin creating endocrinologic imbalances.
2. Disturbances in the metabolic changes which are mandatory during pregnancy.
3. Decreased gastric motility during pregnancy.
4. Disturbances related to pyschologic adjustments to pregnancy and the role of mothering.

It is generally accepted that hyperemesis is a result of the interplay between physiologic and psychologic forces during pregnancy. Psychologic forces have become an increasing important area for exploration in research related to hyperemesis. It was once speculated that vomiting represented a symbolic rejection,[4] an oral attempt toward abortion, in terms of the child or of motherhood.[5] However, experimental studies failed to validate such a relationship.[6,7] Later, Chertok and coworkers[8,9] did numerous studies that supported the hypothesis that indeed there is a relationship between vomiting during pregnancy and the woman's feelings about the fetus. In one study there was support that a strong relationship existed between hyperemesis and maternal attitudes of ambivalence toward the child. He states his main findings as:

1. A positive correlation between vomiting and the mother's ambivalent attitudes towards the prospective child.
2. A positive correlation between vomiting and the mother's negative experience of the first foetal movements (quickening).
3. A negative correlation between vomiting and the husband's "positive contribution" to the marital partnership.[10]

Nursing Actions

Physiologic needs. One nursing goal is to protect the woman from dehydration and starvation. The woman is usually hospitalized if vomiting persists. Oral intake is restricted and parenteral therapy instituted with glucose and saline solutions supplemented with minerals and vitamins (especially vitamin B complex). Parenteral therapy allows the gastrointestinal tract a period of rest after being overstimulated by vomiting actions. As during any intravenous therapy, the nurse should monitor the woman for intake and output (fluid intake, urinary output, amount vomited). As the woman responds favorably by decreased vomiting, small, frequent feedings are instituted. This usually consists of alternate fluid feedings (tea, juices, ice chips) and bland solid feedings (toast, crackers, dry cereal). These feedings are usually at intervals of 2 to 3 hours to assess the woman's tolerance. The diet is gradually increased according to the woman's tolerance until a regular diet is achieved.

Another nursing goal is to provide physiologic comfort during this time. Nursing actions to achieve this are:

1. Oral hygiene after vomiting.
2. Removal of vomitus promptly.
3. Change of clothing and/or linens as necessary.
4. Considerations given to the temperature (not too hot or cold) and the appearance of foods so that meal times can be a pleasurable experience.
5. Manipulation of the environment to provide rest and sleep as excessive vomiting can result in fatigue and exhaustion.

Psychologic needs. The nurse must be able to penetrate the unpleasant physical manifestations of the vomiting. The woman who has hyperemesis usually needs a tremendous amount of support in terms of being understood and accepted. She needs reassurance that she is someone worthy of attention. The nurse needs to actively apply many of the concepts in Unit 2 of this book to achieve nursing goals such as:

1. Help the woman to feel she is important and her feelings are legitimate. The nurse needs to be a good listener and remain nonjudgmental. Remember that a woman with ambivalent or negative feelings about the pregnancy or baby may be reluctant to expose herself for fear of rejection. A prerequisite to encouraging ventilation of feelings is the development of a nurse-patient interaction that is characterized by trust and mutual respect.
2. Help the woman to identify her own feelings. This is an important step in problem solving. Until the woman can recognize and accept her feelings she may continue to reject reality and resort to fantasies and misconceptions. The nurse should encourage the woman to identify the problem as the woman perceives it. It is beneficial to have the woman state her problem or situation in her own words.

3. Finally the nurse helps the woman initiate problem-solving approaches. This usually involves collaboration with other disciplines and family members if success is to be achieved. Women with ambivalent feelings toward the pregnancy, baby, husband, themselves, or others, will need help expressing and handling such feelings. The woman may need help in exploring what alternatives are available to her in her unique life style. The nurse needs to assess the woman's situational supports and the stressors confronting her.

The area of hyperemesis during pregnancy is largely unexplored in the nursing literature. Therefore, the reader is encouraged to investigate clinical situations of hyperemesis and to share approaches in the care of such women through the nursing literature.

REFERENCES

1. Brewer, T. H.: *Human maternal-fetal nutrition.* Obstet. Gynecol. 40:868, 1972.
2. Ziegel, E. and VanBlarcom, D.: *Obstetric Nursing*, ed. 6. Macmillan, New York, 1972, p. 210.
3. McElin, T.: *Ectopic pregnancy.* In Danforth, D. (ed.): *Textbook of Obstetrics and Gynecology*, ed. 2. Harper and Row, New York, 1971, p. 357.
4. Freud, S. and Breuer, J.: *Studies on hysteria.* In Freud, S.: *Complete Psychological Works: Standard Edition, vol. 2.* Hogarth Press, London, 1955.
5. Chertok, L.: *The psychopathology of vomiting in pregnancy.* In Howells, J. (ed.): *Psycho-Obstetrics.* Brunner/Mazel, New York, 1972.
6. Coppen, A.: *Vomiting in early pregnancy: psychological factors and body build.* Lancet i:172, 1959.
7. Bernstein, I.: *An investigation into the etiology of nausea and vomiting of pregnancy.* Minnesota Med. 5:34, 1952.
8. Chertok L., Mondzain, M. and Bonnaud, M.: *Psychological, social and cultural aspects of sickness during pregnancy.* Act. Nerv. Super. 4:394, 1962.
9. Ibid.: *Vomiting and the wish to have a child.* Psychosom. Med. 25:13, 1963.
10. Chertok, op. cit., p. 280.

BIBLIOGRAPHY

Bonica, J.: *Obstetric Complications.* F. A. Davis. Philadelphia, 1965.

Ibid.: *Maternal respiratory changes during pregnancy and parturition.* Clin. Anesth. 10:1, 1974.

Brewer, D., et al: *The physiology of pregnancy. Clinical pathologic corrections.* Postgrad. Med. Part I 52:110, 1972. Part II 53:221, 1973.

Burstein, I., et al.: *Anxiety, pregnancy, labor, and the neonate.* Am. J. Obstet. Gynecol. 118:195, 1974.

Cianfrani, T. and Conway, M.: *Ectopic pregnancy.* Am. J. Nurs. 63:93, 1963.

Dansforth, D.: *Textbook of Obstetrics and Gynecology,* ed. 2. Harper and Row, New York, 1971.

DeAlvarez, R.: *Hypertensive disorders in pregnancy.* Clin. Obstet. Gynecol. 16:47, 1973.

Desforges, J.: *Anemia complicating pregnancy.* J. Reprod. Med. 10:111, 1973.

Donald, I.: *Practical Obstetrical Problems.* J. B. Lippincott, Philadlephia, 1969.

Feitelson, P. J., et al.: *Management of hypertensive gravidas.* J. Reprod. Med. 8:111, 1972.

Fields, H.: *Induction of Labor.* Macmillan, New York, 1965.

Friedman, E.: *Labor: clinical evaluation and management.* Appleton-Century-Crofts, New York. 1967.

Greenhill, J.: *Biological Principles and Modern Practice of Obstetrics.* W. B. Saunders, Philadelphia. 1974.

Haynes, D.: *Medical Complications during Pregnancy.* McGraw-Hill, New York, 1969.

Hellman, L. and Pritchard, J.: *Williams Obstetrics,* ed. 14, Appleton-Century Crofts, New York, 1971.

Hendricks, C. H., et al.: *Toxemia of pregnancy: relationship between fetal weight, fetal survival, and the maternal state.* Am. J. Obstet. Gynecol. 109:225, 1971.

Jacobson, H. and Reid, D.: *High-risk pregnancy II. Maternal and child care.* N. Engl. J. Med. 271:302, 1964.

Jones, W.: *Ectopic pregnancy.* Ala. J. Med. Sci. 9:310, 1972.

Leon, J.: *High-risk pregnancy: graphic representation of the maternal and fetal risks.* Am. J. Obstet. Gynecol. 117:497, 1973.

Light, H., et al.: *Maternal concerns during pregnancy.* Am. J. Obstet. Gynecol. 118:223, 1974.

MacLeod, S. C.: *Relationship between elevated blood pressure and urinary estriols during pregnancy.* Am. J. Obstet. Gynecol. 109:375, 1971.

McFee, J.: *Anemia: a high-risk complication of pregnancy.* Clin. Obstet. Gynecol. 16:153, 1973.

Nesbitt, R.: *Coincidental medical disorders complicating pregnancy.* In Danforth, D. (ed.): *Textbook of Obstetrics and Gynecology,* Harper & Row, New York, 1971.

Nesbitt, R. and Aubry, R.: *Recognition and care of high-risk obstetrical patients. Part I.* Hosp. Med. 3: 43, 1967. *Part II* Hosp. Med. 3:41, 1967.

Page, E.: *On the pathogenesis of pre-eclampsia and eclampsia.* J. Obstet. Gynaecol. Br. Commonw. 79:883, 1972.

Palmer, R. L.: *A psychosomatic study of vomiting of early pregnancy.* J. Psychosom. Res. 17:303, 1973.

Patten, B. M.: *Neurological signs in preeclampsia.* Bull Los Angeles Neurol. Soc. 36:61, 1971.

Philipp, E., Barnes, J. and Newton, M.: *Scientific foundations of obstetrics and gynaecology.* F. A. Davis, Philadelphia. 1970.

Pilowsky, I., et al.: *Psychological aspects of preeclamptic toxemia.* J. Psychosom. Res. 15:193, 1971.

Ray, M., et al.: *Clinical experience with the oxytocin challenge test.* Am. J. Obstet. Gynecol. 114:1, 1972.

Reid, D.: *Principles and management of human reproduction.* W. B. Saunders, Philadelphia, 1972.

Rose, P. A.: *The high risk mother-infant dyad–A challenge for nursing?* Nurs. Forum 6:94, 1967.

Rovinsky, J. and Guttmacher, A.: *Medical, Surgical and Gynecologic Complications of Pregnancy,* ed. 2. Williams & Wilkins, Baltimore, 1965.

Schneider, J.: *The high risk pregnancy.* Hosp. Prac. 6:133, 1971.

Sise, H.: *Hypofibrinogenemic states in obstetrics.* J. Reprod. Med. 10:115, 1973.

Speroff, L.: *Toxemia of pregnancy. Mechanism and therapeutic management.* Am. J. Cardiol. 32:582, 1973.

Sullivan, J.: *Blood Pressure elevation in pregnancy.* Prog. Cardiovasc. Dis. 16:375, 1974.

Report of working group on the relation of nutrition to fetal growth and development. In *Maternal Nutrition and the Course of Pregnancy.* Committee on Maternal Nutrition, National Research Council, 1970.

Report of working group on nutrition and the toxemias of pregnancy. In *Maternal Nutrition and the Course of Pregnancy.* Committee on Maternal Nutrition, National Research Council, 1970.

36 Complications of Labor and Delivery

DYANNE D. AFFONSO, R.N., M.N.

The term *dystocia* is used to describe any interference in the normal processes of labor. The causative factors may be maternal, fetal, or a combination of both. The three major causes are abnormalities of uterine contractions, abnormalities of position and presentation, and abnormalities of the pelvis (Table 36-1). The consequences of difficult childbirth include:

1. Labor is prolonged. Progress may be slow, minimal, or absent.
2. The woman and fetus are vulnerable to physiologic dangers. Examples of such hazards are rupture of the uterus, increased infection and hemorrhage, lacerations from difficult obstetric manipulations, dehydration, fatigue, and fetal-neonatal distress.
3. Spontaneous vaginal delivery may not be probable or possible. Delivery may need to be assisted through use of forceps, abdominal delivery (cesarean section), or other obstetric manipulations.
4. The woman is vulnerable to crisis due to the psychologic impact of the stressors associated with the risk factors.

An appreciation of these consequences is necessary in order to achieve the following nursing goals:

1. Assessment of the labor pattern to detect or predict any deviation from normal.
2. Support medical intervention to increase the effectiveness and successful outcome of labor.
3. Protect the woman and fetus from physiologic dangers to which they are vulnerable.
4. Prepare and nurture the woman to optimally cope with the events in the situation.
5. Implement crisis intervention to protect the woman and her family from detrimental psychologic consequences which can arise as a result of the complications.

Goal: Nursing Assessment of Labor Patterns

Assessment of uterine contractile patterns is important because early detection of deviations may be initially identified by the nurse during her frequent encounters with the laboring woman. The nurse should be familiar with normal labor (as discussed in Chapter 24) and also be able to identify signs suggestive of complications as identified in Table 36-2. The nurse should be able to assess uterine contractile patterns to detect dytocia due to abnormal or inadequate uterine activity. The three types of uterine contractile patterns and their consequences on the labor process are presented in Table 36-3. There are several clinical tools

TABLE 36-1. Three Major Causes of Dystocia*

I. Abnormalities Due to Uterine Contractions
   A. Significant prolongation of any phase of labor, called uterine dysfunction. Two major types of uterine dysfunction:
      1. Subnormal or hypotonic patterns
         a. Infrequent
         b. Poor intensity
         c. Contributes to minimal or lack of labor progress
      2. Abnormal or hypertonic patterns
         a. No relaxation between contractions

II. Abnormalities of Position and Presentation
   A. Faulty presentations
      1. Persistent occiput posterior
      2. Breech (sacrum)
      3. Face (mentum)
      4. Brow (frontum)
      5. Shoulder
      6. Compound presentation
   B. Abnormalities in fetal development
      1. Excessive fetal size
      2. Malformations
      3. Hydrocephalus

III. Abnormalities of the Pelvis
   A. Contractions of the pelvis whereby the diameters are decreased and thus also the capacity of the pelvis
      1. Contraction of the pelvic inlet—the antero-posterior diameter is 10.0 cm. or less and the transverse diameter is 12 cm. or less
      2. Contraction of the midpelvis—suspected if the ischial spinous diameter is below 9.5 cm.
      3. Contraction of the pelvic outlet—the inter-ischial tuberous diameter is 8.0 cm. or less
   B. Pelvic deformities
      1. Dwarf pelvis
      2. Asymmetry due to childhood injuries or other diseases

*Based on data obtained from Pearse, W. and Danforth, D.: *Dystocia due to abnormal fetopelvic relations.* In Danforth, D. (ed.): *Textbook of Obstetrics and Gynecology*, ed. 2. Harper and Row, New York, 1971, pp. 629–649; Hendrick, C.: *Dystocia due to abnormal uterine action.* In Danforth, D. (ed.): *Textbook of Obstetrics and Gynecology*, ed. 2. Harper and Row, New York, 1971, pp. 650–661; and Hellman, L. and Pritchard, J.: *William's Obstetrics*, ed. 14. Appleton-Century-Crofts, New York, 1971, pp. 894–918.

TABLE 36-2. Summary of Danger Signs in Labor*

Observation or Finding	*Possible Significance*
Rapid, slow, or irregular fetal heart tones	Fetal hypoxia (fetal distress)
Greenish-brown amniotic fluid (vertex presentation)	Fetal distress
Port-wine colored amniotic fluid	Ruptured vasa previa; premature separation of placenta
Unengaged presenting part	Disproportion or malpresentation
Failure of progress in dilatation	Prolonged labor with increasing danger of perinatal loss
Failure of presenting part to descend after full dilatation	Disproportion or error in estimate of dilatation
Bleeding (liquid or clots)	Separation of placenta; torn maternal tissue
Rising blood pressure	Preeclampsia
Low blood pressure	Shock; postural hypotension; reaction to drug
Fever	Amnionitis; extrauterine infection
Maternal tachycardia	Impending shock
Foul or purulent vaginal discharge	Amnionitis (eventual fetal pneumonia or sepsis)
Abnormal abdominal pain and tenderness	Separation of placenta; rupture of uterus; abdominal condition necessitating surgery
Uterine tetany (failure of uterus to relax between contractions)	Intrauterine bleeding due to premature separation of placenta
Excessive complaint of pain	Hysteria; undetected abnormality; reaction to medication
Prolapsed cord	Without instant action by attendant, perinatal death
Contractions getting farther apart, weaker, and more irregular	Uterine inertia; too much medication
Unconsciousness	Eclampsia; shock; hysteria; heavy sedation; epilepsy
Pallor; cool damp skin; air hunger	Bleeding; shock
Cyanosis	Aspiration of vomitus; cardiac failure

* From Danforth, D. (ed.): *Textbook of Obstetrics and Gynecology*, ed. 2. Harper and Row, New York, 1971, p. 568, with permission.

TABLE 36-3. Patterns of Uterine Contractions and Their Consequences

Pattern	*Characteristics*	*Clinical Effects*	*Occurrence*	*Cause*	*Dangers*	*Clinical Management and Consequences*
Normal	Fundal dominance Good intensity at peak Good relaxation between contractions (frequency) Good duration (averages over 35 seconds)	Effacement of the cervix Dilatation of the cervix Descent of presenting part Discomforts during contractions	Normal labor and delivery	Term gestation	—	Spontaneous vaginal delivery
Hypotonic or Subnormal	Fundal dominance Weak intensity (mild) Long periods of relaxation (long intervals between contractions) Less than 30 seconds duration	Resembles beginning phase of labor Slow or no progress from latent to active phase Effacement may occur Dilatation minimal or absent	Frequently seen in active phase Can appear in both first and second stage of labor	Inadequacy of myometrial function to overcome resistance from the lower uterine segment and cervix Too early or too heavy administration of medications, especially during latent phase	Fatigue, exhaustion Fetal distress due to prolonged labor	Promote better relationship between presenting part and cervix by: rupture of membranes walking sitting or upright position Augmentation of labor with oxytocics
Hypertonic or Abnormal	No fundal dominance (may be midsegment) Irregular intensity No relaxation Irregular duration No pattern established	Labor progress is hindered	Frequently appears in latent phase Patients who are highly anxious are most vulnerable Abrupt appearance usually in first stage	Etiology unclear	Fetal distress acute Danger of ruptured uterus	Sedation to stop abnormal patterns Regional block to anesthesize nerves supplying the fundus where contractions originate Oxytocics are contraindicated as they will enhance abnormal patterns

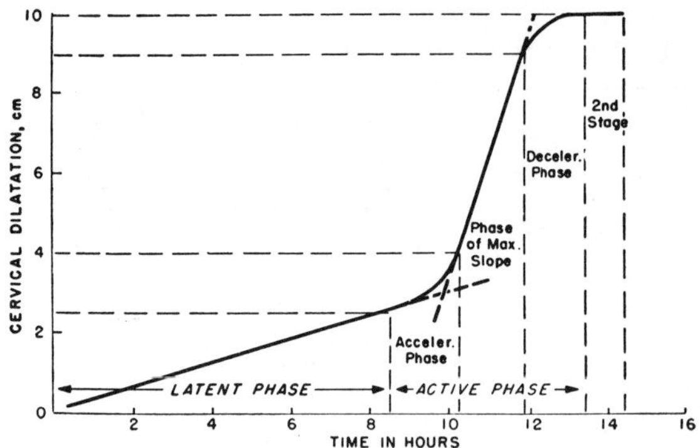

FIGURE 36-1. Labor patterns in nulliparas. (From Friedman, E.: *Primigravid labor: A graphicostatistical analysis.* Obstet. Gynecol. 6:569, 1955, with permission.)

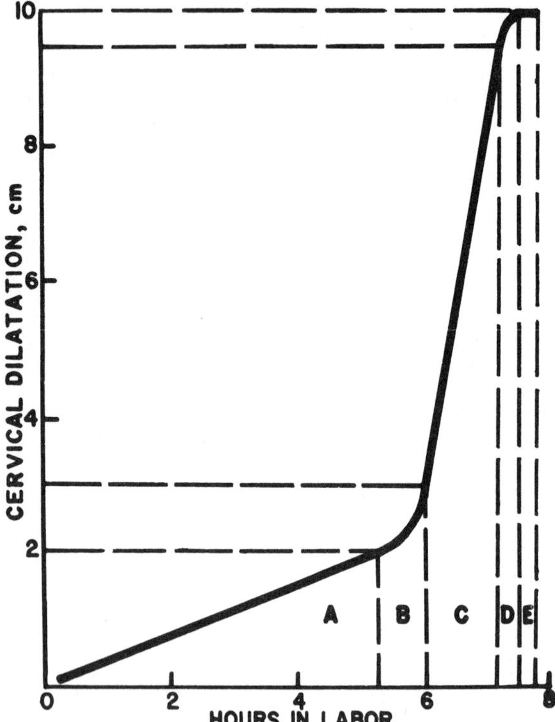

FIGURE 36-2. Labor pattern in multiparas. *A*, Latent phase. *B-D*, Active phase: *B*, Acceleration phase; *C*, Phase of maximum slope; *D*, Deceleration phase. *E*, Second stage. (From Friedman, E.: *Labor in multiparas: A graphicostatistical analysis.* Obstet. Gynecol. 8:692, 1956, with permission.)

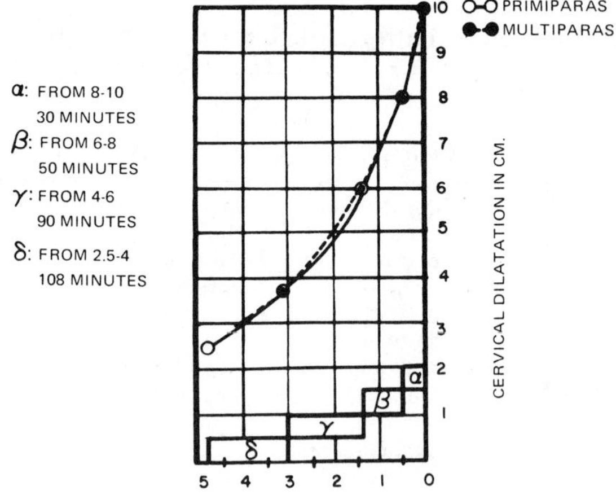

FIGURE 36-3. Normal curve of cervical dilatation. (From Hendrick, C. H., Brenner, W. and Kraus, G.: *Normal cervical dilatation in late pregnancy and labor.* Am. J. Obstet. Gynecol. 106:1065, 1970, with permission.)

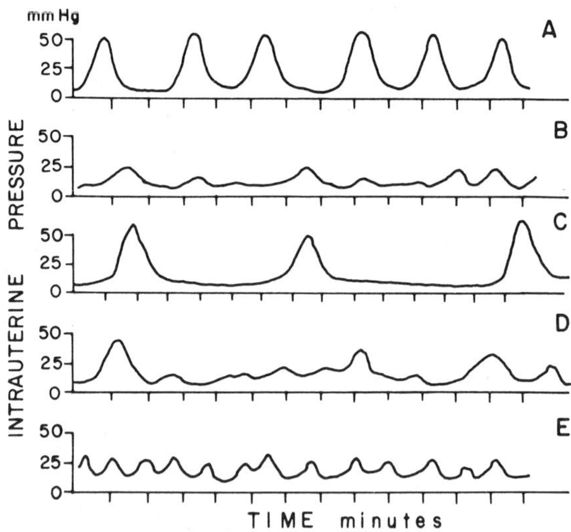

FIGURE 36-4. Uterine contractility patterns in labor. *A*, Typical normal labor. *B*, Subnormal intensity with frequency greater than needed for optimal performance. *C*, Normal contractions but too infrequent for effective labor. *D*, Incoordinate activity. *E*, Hypercontractility. (From Hendrick, C.: *Dystocia due to abnormal uterine action.* In Danforth, D. (ed.): *Textbook of Obstetrics and Gynecology*, ed. 2. Harper and Row, New York, 1971, with permission.)

available which help to predict whether a woman's cervical dilatation course is comparable to a normal pattern. Figures 36-1 to 36-3 illustrate normal curves of cervical dilatation in nulliparas and multiparas. When electrical monitoring is available, the nurse can recognize deviations from the printout recording of the intraterine pressures (Fig. 36-4). Any deviation should be reported immediately to the physician to allow early confirmation of dystocia and to plan therapy.

Goal: Support Medical Intervention to Increase the Effectiveness and Successful Outcome of Labor

The plan for medical intervention depends upon the type of complication which presents. The optimal goal of the obstetrician is to ensure a healthy delivery by the least traumatic means to both mother and baby. The nurse should have a general understanding of the type of medical therapy that may need nursing monitoring and support. This section focuses on the nurse's role when the following situations exist:

1. Simple techniques are needed as a stimulus to enhance labor.
2. Dytocia due to decreased or subnormal contractile patterns.
3. Dystocia due to hypercontractile patterns.
4. Dystocia due to abnormal fetopelvic relationships.
5. Prolapse of the unbilical cord.

Stimuli to Enhance Labor

When the doctor has ascertained that lack of labor progress is not due to any type of dystocia, he may order various procedures as attempts to increase the effectiveness of labor. Examples are:

1. Empty a distended bladder which can impede descent of the presenting part and cervical dilatation. Throughout labor the nurse should check for signs of impending bladder distention and encourage voiding at intervals to prevent unnecessary bladder catheterizations.
2. Give an enema to enhance uterine contractions and also to prevent mechanical obstruction to the presenting part due to distended maternal bowels. Optimal effects are best achieved when the enema is given early in labor. Enemas may be contraindicated when the cervix is more than three-fourths dilated and/or the presenting part is at a low (plus) station.
3. Change the woman's position. In general, contractions are better coordinated and more intense, although less frequent, when the woman is in the side-lying position rather than the supine position.[1] The nurse should always remember that the best position during labor is one which makes the woman most comfortable. Never force the woman to assume a certain position. However, the nurse should suggest a change in position, especially if the woman has not moved for a period of time.
4. Sometimes the promotion of a better relationship between the presenting part and the cervix can enhance labor. This can be done in several ways. Better relationships can be achieved with the help of gravity. Unless contraindicated, the woman may be encouraged to walk in the hall, sit in a chair, or assume an upright position. However, when the amniotic membranes have ruptured and the fetal head is not engaged, the woman should not be permitted out of bed in order to prevent possible prolapse of the cord. Another technique to promote better relationship between the cervix and presenting part is *amniotomy* (artificial rupture of the amniotic membranes) by the

physician. There are several nursing implications when an amniotomy is to be done:

a. Prepare the woman for what the procedure entails and the expected consequences.
b. Observe the color of the fluid; discoloration may indicate fetal distress.
c. Assess the fetal heart rate to ascertain the fetus' tolerance to the procedure.
d. Keep the woman in bed until assessment reveals there is no danger from prolapse of the cord.
e. Record the time and results of the procedure in the chart.

Dystocia Due to Decreased or Subnormal Contractile Patterns

The primary interventive measure to correct this type of dystocia is stimulation of uterine activity by a pharmacologic agent. Oxytocin is the drug most widely used because it is believed to be the safest and most effective agent. Current research investigations are exploring the possible use of prostaglandins to enhance uterine contractile activity. Augmentation of labor with oxytocics is primarily a medical responsibility. The physician makes the decision for its use, determines the route of administration, regulates and reassesses for the therapeutically safe dosage, and evaluates its effects. What, then, is the nurse's role?

Nursing role during oxytocin therapy

Because the physician and nurse collaborate in providing optimal care to the woman during labor, the nurse assists with medical intervention by participating in the monitoring of the mother and fetus to ensure a healthy outcome. Specifically, the nurse-physician team collaborate to achieve the following:

1. Safe Preparation and Administration of Oxytocin

The nurse should know that the ideal way to administer oxytocin is dilution in an intravenous infusion, with the use of an intravenous infusion pump to maintain an exact flow rate. Oxytocin comes in ampules labeled *IU* (international units) which means there is an international standard for the dispensing of the drug. Because oxytocin must be diluted, the nurse must have an understanding of the equivalent of an international unit of the drug when mixed in milliliters of an intravenous solution. This is described below:

1 IU = 1,000 milliunits (mU)

When 1 IU of oxytocin is added to 1,000 ml. of IV fluid, each milliliter of the solution contains 1 mU of oxytocin. (Likewise, 5 IU to 1,000 ml. [IV fluid] = 5 mU of oxytocin/milliliter of the solution.) The dosage of oxytocin used in therapy refers to the number of mU in the intravenous solution to be given per minute. When standard intravenous equipment is used, which delivers 15 drops per milliliter, each drop contains 0.33 mU of oxytocin; thus to administer oxytocin at 2 mU/min.—begin infusion at 6 drops/min; at 5 mU/min.—begin infusion at 15 drops/min.[2]

Calculated formula: (A) $\frac{.33\text{ mU}}{1\text{ drop}} = \frac{2\text{ mU}}{X\text{ drops}}$

$$X = 6$$

(B) $\frac{.33\text{ mU}}{1\text{ drop}} = \frac{5\text{ mU}}{X\text{ drops}}$

$$X = 15$$

Although the above discussion seems directed to the physician because he orders the dosage, the nurse should have an understanding of how dosages are calculated to ascertain whether a physician's desired dosage for oxytocin is congruent with his specific flow rate for the intravenous infusion. The nurse should also ensure that a two-bottle intravenous system is used. This permits prompt discontinuation of the oxytocin solution while the other bottle with unmedicated fluid can be used to keep the vein open. It is a safe nursing measure to keep a hemostat near the intravenous setup in case emergency clamping of the tubing is needed to terminate oxytocin infusion.

Sometimes oxytocin is administered through the nasal or oral cavity. Intranasal administration involves placement of a nasal pack saturated with a dosage of oxytocin or spraying oxytocin into the nostril. Transbuccal administration of oxytocin involves placement of oxytocin tablets in the mouth (usually under the tongue). Intranasal or transbuccal oxytocin is administered at specified intervals (30 minutes to an hour). The nurse should be aware that administration of oxytocin other than by the intravenous route carries additional hazards primarily because the rate of absorption of the drug is unpredictable.

The nursing role when oxytocin is administered other than intravenously is to recognize the potential hazards and let the physician take full responsibility for the administration of the drug. After administration of buccal oxytocin the woman should be offered oral hygiene.

2. Protect the Woman from Being Alone and Unsupervised during Oxytocin Therapy

   The single most important action is to prevent a situation whereby the woman receiving oxytocin is not constantly monitored. Optimum management of the woman includes close monitoring by a physician and/or nurse with use of electrical monitoring equipment when possible. An infusion pump is also desirable to ensure prescribed flow rate of the solution. It is unrealistic to expect the physician to be physically present every minute and he may need to be relieved for short intervals. The nurse can be a capable substitute in his absence but should make certain the physician returns to assume his primary responsibility of monotoring and regulating the situation.

3. Monitor Maternal-Fetal Responses during Oxytocin Administration

   The physician and nurse collaborate to evaluate the following:

   a. Uterine contractions—subnormal contractile patterns show favorable response to therapy when they increase in frequency, intensity, and duration. However, if contractions are of prolonged duration (over 70 seconds), are constant with no interval or relaxation phase, or are violently intense, the oxytocin should be stopped immediately to prevent consequences from increased intrauterine pressure such as rupture of the uterus, separation of the placenta, and hypoxia to the fetus.
   b. Blood pressure and fetal heart rate—should be checked at least every 15 minutes or more often to assess maternal-fetal tolerance to the augmentation effects of oxytocin.
   c. Patency of the equipment—the intravenous system should be checked periodically to ascertain whether the desired dosage of oxytocin is being infused. The flow rate may have been altered by a change in the woman's position or obstruction in the tubings.

4. Knowledge of the Pharmacologic Actions of Oxytocin

   The physician-nurse team should be

knowledgeable of the action, effects, and the potential lethality of the drug that is being infused. This is useful in informing personnel of the desirable and undesirable consequences of oxytocin therapy. Any standard pharmacologic text provides in-depth information on oxytocic drugs.

Dystocia Due to Hypercontractile Patterns

Uterine hypertonicity leading to abnormal contractions can be suspected when there is no complete relaxation between contractions and the woman complains of severe pain during contraction. Usually, complaints of pain are out of proportion to the clinical effects of the contraction. The nurse also notes that complaints of pain or tenderness are expressed between contractions. Any of these findings should be reported to the physician immediately. Electrical monitoring of the intrauterine pressure helps to confirm the presence of hypercontractile patterns. The nurse should be aware that primigravidas who are highly anxious are most vulnerable to this type of dystocia. The abnormal contractions usually appear abruptly in the latent phase of labor, before active labor progress is established. Medical intervention usually consists of sedation or regional anesthesia in an attempt to stop the hypercontractile patterns. After the woman has rested, contractions may begin spontaneously or be augmented with oxytocin therapy.

The nurse can make a significant contribution to the total management of the patient by working to promote rest and decrease the anxiety level. Initially, the nurse's priority is to promote rest because both mother and fetus are fatigued. Also, the fetus is exposed to a reduction in oxygen due to decreased blood flow through the placenta. Suggested nursing actions are:

1. Manipulation of the environment to decrease noise, lights, traffic.
2. Administration of sedatives as ordered.
3. Observing for any reactions to the drug.
4. Using the siderails to prevent injury.
5. Promoting comfort by facial sponges, back rubs, fresh bed clothes, change of position, or whatever else brings comfort.

In performing these actions, the nurse also meets the greatest need of a highly anxious individual—the need to be sustained by another human being. The nurse continuously appraises the situation and without overloading the woman, slowly begins to intervene to lower anxiety by implementing the actions described by Peplau in Chapter 9. The nurse is in an excellent position to achieve this because of her continuous contact with the patient. The nurse utilizes all her own resources and collaborates with other disciplines to help institute problem-solving approaches to meet the unique needs of the woman.

Dytocia Due to Abnormal Feto-Pelvic Relationships

This type of dystocia usually requires the obstetrician's assistance in delivering the infant through use of forceps, surgery, or other obstetric manipulations. Nursing responsibilities arise from an appreciation of the impact fetopelvic disproportions can have on the woman and how best to nurture (support) her through the experience. This discussion will briefly outline implications for care which should be considered as part of the nurse's role. (Nursing care relative to postoperative care of the cesarean section patient will be discussed later.)

Occiput Posterior Fetal Position. The nurse needs to realize that labor will be prolonged, with increased discomforts in the lower back. The woman may be required to push actively during a maximum second stage of 2 hours to help the fetal head rotate spontaneously. The physician may assist rotation of the head manually or by forceps. Consider nursing actions to combat fatigue, ensure hydration, promote

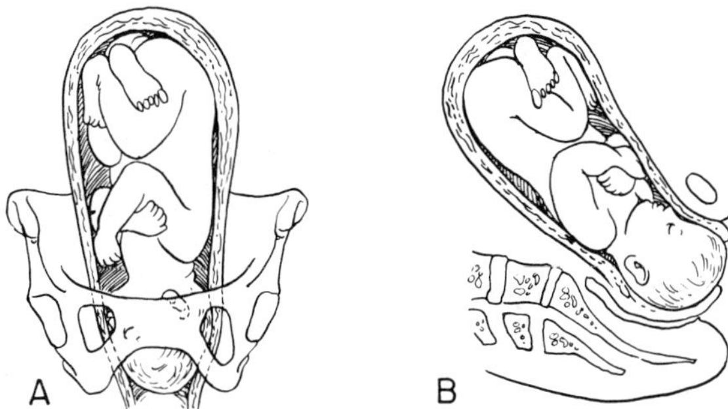

FIGURE 36-5. Brow presentation. *A*, Anterior view. *B*, Sagittal view. (From Bonica, J.: *Principles and Practice of Obstetrical Analgesia and Anesthesia.* F. A. Davis, Philadelphia, 1972, with permission.)

comfort, and prevent discouragement, frustration, and fears. Prepare parents to anticipate molding of the baby's head due to the prolonged second stage.

Brow Presentation (Fig. 36-5). When the occipitomental diameter (13.5 cm.) of the fetal head presents, a cesarean section is usually planned because vaginal delivery is not probable. However, if the brow converts into a face presentation (head eventually flexes), a vaginal delivery can be anticipated when accommodation between the fetus and pelvis is adequate.

Face Presentation (Fig. 36-6). The woman in labor needs to know that chances for a vaginal delivery are good if the chin presents anteriorly. If the chin remains posterior, it is best managed by a cesarean section because attempts to rotate it are very hazardous and frequently unsuccessful. When a baby is born with a face presentation, parents need to be prepared for the infant's appearance. The face may appear bruised, eyelids and lips swollen, and the occipital area flattened and elongated. With time, such manifestations resolve themselves. If a cesarean section is planned, the woman should be prepared in ample time to allow expression of feelings which hopefully will lead to better acceptance of such a decision. The nurse needs to convey to the woman that the events precipitating the need for a cesarean section do not reflect a failure on the part of the woman herself.

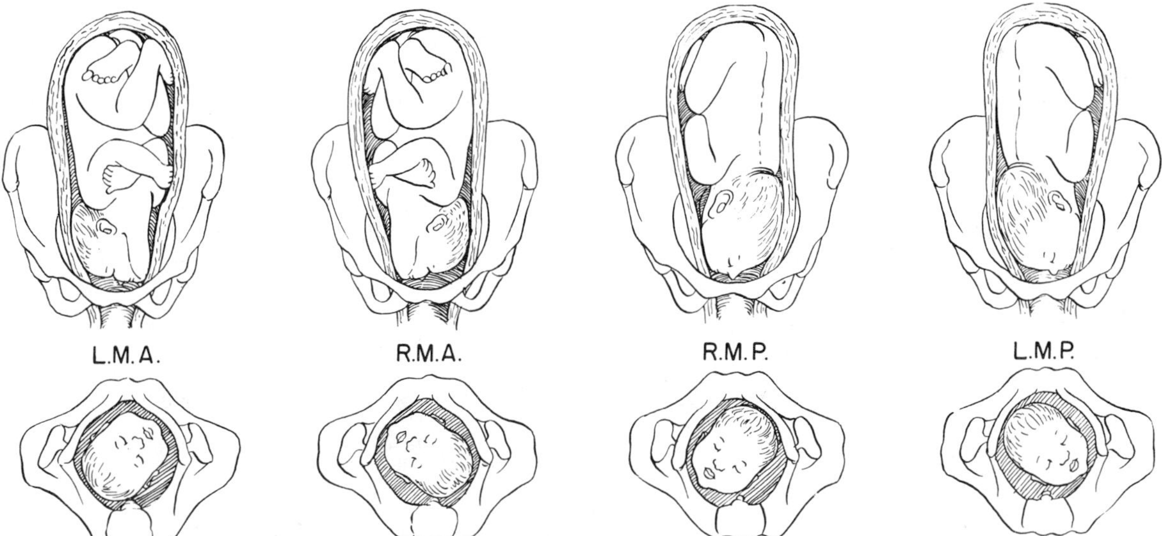

FIGURE 36-6. Face presentations. Left mentoanterior (LMA); Right mentoanterior (RMA); Right mentoposterior (RMP); Left mentoposterior (LMP). (From Bonica, J.: *Principles and Practice of Obstetric Analgesia and Anesthesia.* F. A. Davis, Philadelphia, 1972, with permission.)

Transverse Arrest. When arrest of the fetal head in the transverse position occurs and there is no labor progress for over 30 minutes, the nurse needs to prepare the woman as to what to expect. The labor will be prolonged, oxytocin therapy may be instituted, a maximum 2-hour second stage with demands on the woman to push, and use of forceps to advance the fetal head are events that can be anticipated. The nurse will need to work intensely to protect and nurture the woman so she will not experience great anxiety.

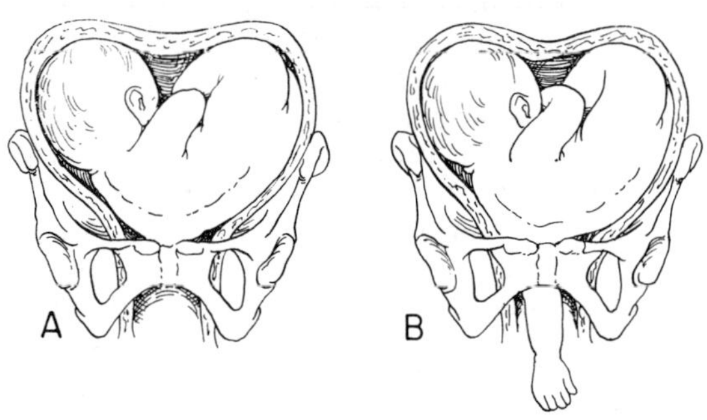

FIGURE 36-7. Transverse presentation. *A*, Right scapuloanterior. *B*, Prolapse of an arm in transverse lie. (From Bonica, J.: *Principles and Practice of Obstetric Analgesia and Anesthesia*. F. A. Davis, Philadelphia, 1972, with permission.)

Transverse Lies and/or Compound Presentations (Fig. 36-7). If labor begins when the fetus is in a transverse lie, cesarean section is believed to be the best management. For compound presentations, the woman needs to be prepared for obstetric manipulations and/or cesarean section. The nurse prepares the woman and her husband appropriately.

Breech Presentation (Fig. 36-8). When the fetus presents with the sacrum or buttocks (breech) the obstetrician makes an assessment of the feasibility for vaginal delivery. When the size of the infant is compatible with the pelvic diameters, the obstetrician assesses the position of the fetal legs because it greatly influences the course and outcome of labor. Labor usually terminates in a successful vaginal delivery with a frank breech and complete breech. In such instances the sacrum allows satisfactory cervical dilatation, although the frank breech is a more effective dilating wedge against the cervix. However, in an incomplete or footling breech, labor is prolonged because of the lack of an effective dilating wedge and there is great danger of prolapse of the cord due to the available space between the cervix and presenting part through which the cord can slip. Thus, an incomplete or footling breech may be best managed by cesarean section, depending upon the situation.

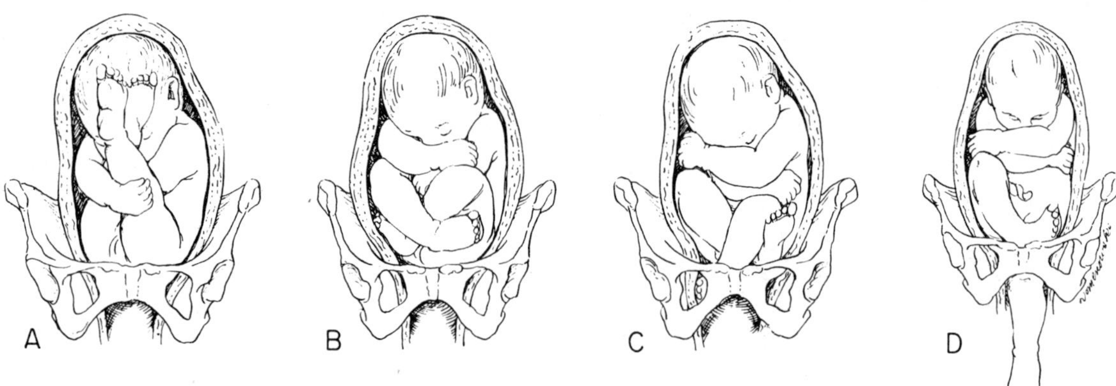

FIGURE 36-8. Types of breech presentations. *A*, Frank. *B*, Complete. *C*, Incomplete. *D*, Footling. (From Bonića, J.: *Principles and Practice of Obstetric Analgesia and Anesthesia*. F. A. Davis, Phildelphia, 1972, with permission.)

The nurse needs to prepare and support the woman for the following consequences relating to a breech presentation:

1. Labor may be prolonged, depending upon the degree of effectiveness of cervical dilation by the presenting part.
2. A period of trial labor may be expected during which the progress of labor is evaluated. If progress is poor, cesarean section is the alternative.
3. The ideal mode for delivery is an *assisted breech delivery*. The mother needs to know she is to be an active part in an assisted breech delivery. This process involves delivery of the baby by the woman's own contractile powers to the level of the umbilicus, with assistance at this point by the obstetrician for the delivery of the head.[3] The mother's active participation involves voluntary abdominal powers demonstrated through bearing down efforts until the baby is delivered to the level of the umbilicus.
4. Because the woman's participation is critical, she can anticipate anesthesia in the form of regional or local blocks such as a pudendal. These interfere least with the voluntary abdominal powers.
5. At times, breech extraction delivery is necessary when the presenting part is not able to reach the level of the pelvic floor without assistance by the obstetrician. Breech extraction is also performed when the cervix contracts around the neck or obstructs delivery of the head.
6. To decrease perinatal mortality and morbidity, progressive obstetric departments require that two qualified physicians be present during a breech delivery. The second physician serves as a consultant or assistant as necessary. The mother needs to anticipate such a medical team during the delivery to decrease anxiety which may arise over the unexpected appearance of a second physician.
7. The nurse must appropriately give positive feedback to a woman who had a breech vaginal delivery to reinforce that the successful outcome was attributable in a large part to a woman's participation in the labor process.
8. Parents also need to be prepared for the appearance of the infant. The buttock, scrotal, and perineal areas may be edematous and bruised while the legs may assume the intrauterine position of extension. Such manifestations resolve spontaneously with time.

Prolapse of the Umbilical Cord

Prolapse of the umbilical cord represents an acute obstetric emergency because of hazards to the fetus from compression of the cord leading to anoxia and possible death (Fig. 36-9). Priority interventions consist of decreasing pressure on the cord followed by prompt delivery of the baby. Nursing responsibilities in dealing with the risks of cord prolapse focus on three nursing goals.

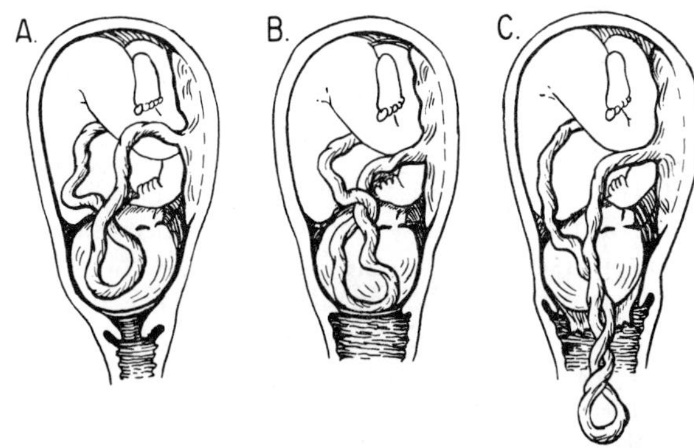

FIGURE 36-9. Prolapse of the umbilical cord. *A*, Occult prolapse with intact membranes—there is little risk of pressure on the cord. *B*, Forelying cord—increasing risk of compression. *C*, Frank prolapse—risk of compression is high. (From Bonica, J.: *Principles and Practice of Obstetric Analgesia and Anesthesia.* F. A. Davis, Philadelphia, 1972, with permission.)

The first nursing goal is to casefind women who are vulnerable to cord prolapse. The risk of cord prolapse increases when there is space between the presenting part and the cervix in which the cord can be compressed or slip out. Factors which lend themselves to this situation are:

1. Prematurity
2. Transverse lie
3. Breech presentations (frequency of incidence in descending order are: single footling, double footling, complete breech, and frank breech)
4. Multiple pregnancy
5. Polyhydramnios
6. Premature rupture of the membranes (especially if the head is unengaged).

The second nursing goal is to recognize clinical signs suggestive of cord prolapse. A diagnosis of prolapsed cord means that the cord is at or below the level of the presenting part. The most obvious confirmation of the diagosis is sight of the cord protruding from the introitus. However, the cord is prolapsed even when it is lying next to the presenting part, as felt upon vaginal examination. Therefore, the nurse must be able to recognize signs indicating possible cord prolapse. Signs of fetal distress may suggest cord prolapse. Early clues may be alteration in the fetal heart rate, meconium-stained amniotic fluid, or passage of meconium in a presentation that is not breech. The nurse should carefully assess the fetus after rupture of the membranes as the cord is most likely to descend at that time. It is good nursing practice to frequently check the perineum to ascertain that nothing unusual is emitting from the vagina. Also take heed of the patient's comments. One woman in labor who had a prolapsed cord made the following comment: "I feel something down there. It almost feels like a string or something hanging low."

The third nursing goal is to protect the fetus by actions which decrease compression of the cord. Time is of the essence when the cord prolapses. The fetus will not be able to tolerate anoxia without damaging consequences. Priority action is to relieve pressure on the cord. A position whereby the mother's head is below the level of the hips helps to displace the presenting part away from the cord. Elevation of the hips with pillows, lowering the patient's head, or the knee-chest position help to decrease pressure. These positions are especially important during contractions when pressure exerted on the cord is greatest. It is difficult to completely relieve pressure during a contraction unless the physician places his hand into the vagina to keep the presenting part away from the cord. The nurse should never leave the woman unattended. Help should be summoned by other personnel or use of emergency call signals. While awaiting the arrival of the physician, maintain the woman in the position that exerts the least pressure on the perineal area. *Never elevate the knee-gatch of the bed* as this only adds pressure by gravity to the perineal area. Oxygen by mask or catheter can be administered to the mother to minimize anoxia to the fetus. The nurse should continuously assess the fetal heart rate or if the cord is visible, check and count the pulsations. The environment will be tense and anxiety-provoking. The nurse must remember to reassure the mother about what has happened and that measures are being taken to protect the fetus. Simple, short sentences, in a calm, reassuring tone of voice can frequently convey confidence and prevent panic in the woman. Every effort must be made not to increase the woman's anxiety level because her cooperation is necessary in terms of maintaining the proper position, breathing the oxygen, and remaining still. As soon as feasible the nurse should institute measures regarding priority preparations for prompt delivery. Delivery is usually by cesarean section. If the cord has prolapsed out of the vagina, it should be protected with sterile towels moistened with saline to prevent drying and further contamination. The nurse shold not make attempts to reinsert the cord into the vagina as this increases perinatal morbidity.

It is important to discuss the nurse's role when the cord prolapses and immediate delivery is not possible. An example is when the nurse receives a telephone call describing what appears to be a prolapsed cord. The priority is to get the woman to a hospital immediately; use an ambulance or helicopter if private transport is not available or feasible. During transport, stress the importance of keeping the woman in a position whereby her head is lower than her hips. If the cord is visible, it should be protected with a clean, moist towel. Oxygen should be used if available during transport. The nurse needs to calmly stress the urgency of time as a determinant for a successful outcome.

Goal: Protection of the Mother and Fetus from Physiologic Hazards to Which They Are Vulnerable

When labor is prolonged and/or delivery is difficult, the incidence of perinatal morbidity and mortality increases. The mother is in danger from uterine rupture and is vulnerable to infection, postpartum hemorrhage, dehydration, and increased lacerations from difficult obstetric manipulations. The fetus is jeopardized due to prolonged exposure to the stress from uterine contractions. The nurse needs an understanding of what prolonged labor means in order to protect the mother and baby from its effects. The nurse should frequently call the physician's attention to the length of a woman's labor, especially when the physician is distracted by other priorities regarding decisions for therapy and plans for the mode of delivery.

At one time prolonged labor meant a labor of more than 24 hours. However, this is not a feasible criterion because no woman or fetus should be subjected to the forces of labor for as long as 24 hours. A labor is currently viewed as prolonged if any phase deviates from the established normal labor curve (Fig. 36-10).

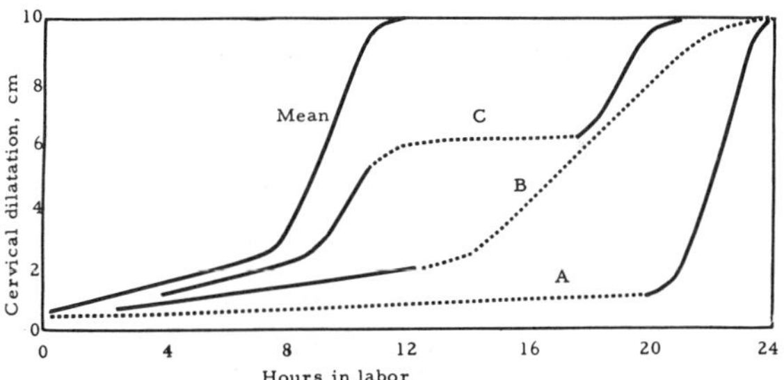

FIGURE 36-10. Major labor aberrations shown in comparison with the mean cervical dilatation time curve for nulliparas. *A*, Prolonged latent phase. *B*, Protracted active phase dilatation (primary dysfunctional labor). *C*, Secondary arrest of dilatation. (From Friedman, E.: *Dysfunctional labor.* In Greenhill J. P. (ed.): *Obstetrics*, ed. 13. W. B. Saunders, Philadelphia, 1965, with permission.)

Hendrick states that the upper time limit for the performance of normal labor should be 18 hours; that is, the physician should be suspicious of dysfunctional labor during the first six hours of labor, institute therapy before the twelfth hour of labor, and complete delivery within 18 hours after the onset of labor.[4] Dangers to the fetus increase significantly after 15 hours in the first stage labor, while hazards to the mother and fetus increase significantly when the second stage is longer than two hours. Detrimental consequences to the mother arise primarily from prolongation of the second stage of labor, of which the greatest danger is rupture of the uterus.

Let us examine the consequences of prolonged labor and what the nurse can do to protect the mother and fetus.

One outcome is maternal fatigue and exhaustion. Labor means work, and after hours of muscle activity the cells become fatigued and need rest to replenish their energy supply. The danger in prolonged labor is that the uterus may no longer be able to tolerate any more pressure and may suddenly break (rupture of the uterus) or the muscle cells may become so fatigued that they are no longer able to contract, creating uterine atony and predisposing to postpartal hemorrhage. The ultimate effect from complete maternal exhaustion is inability of all cells to function, resulting in maternal death. The nurse can prevent detrimental effects from maternal fatigue by making special efforts to promote rest, comfort, and tranquility of both body and mind when labor is predicted to be prolonged. The woman needs help to learn to relax between contractions and demands on her should be reduced to a minimum. The nurse must continuously assess the woman's anxiety level and manipulate to keep anxiety at low levels. Anxiety stimulates the sympathetic-adrenal system which increases the metabolic rate thereby increasing energy expenditure. Thus, anxiety is an additional burden when labor is prolonged because the existing energy supply is already low.

Intensive nursing care must continue even after delivery because fatigue makes the woman vulnerable to postpartal hemorrhage. The woman should be regarded as high risk and observed closely in the early postpartal period. She should not be left unattended until the uterus is firmly contracted, lochia flow is within normal limits, and vital signs and blood pressure have stabilized. Any woman who is exposed to prolonged labor should be typed and cross-matched for blood in anticipation of hemorrhage. The woman may be supported in the immediate postpartal period with intravenous oxytocin and intravenous fluids to augment the blood volume (lactated Ringer's solution is preferred over routine dextrose in water). The nurse should be prepared to implement measures to combat shock and make certain that a physician is readily available should hemorrhage occur.

Another danger is the predisposition to infection. Due to the many obstetric manipulations necessary to manage the difficult labor and delivery, the woman is a good candidate for pathogenic growth. The nurse can protect the woman by preventing exposure to pathogens carried by people, places, and things. When labor is complicated, the woman is usually supported with antibiotic therapy and the nurse should ensure that the proper drug and dosage are maintained. An especially important nursing action is hygiene to the perineal area because the moisture from the lochia flow provides a good environment for pathogenic growth. Initially, the nurse must perform the perineal care because the woman should not be forced to expend additional energy. Fatigue lowers the woman's resistance, thereby increasing her vulnerability to infection.

Dehydration may also occur in prolonged labor. Restriction of oral intake of solids and fluids is typical during childbirth in the United States. Therefore, with each additional hour of labor the woman's fluid and nutrient supply is lowered and needs to be replenished. The nurse should make certain that the woman has intravenous fluids which meet her minimum requirements. Assessment for the state of hydration includes checking the skin for turgor and noting whether the eyes appear sunken. Later, blood chemistries should be done to assess the fluid and electrolyte status. As soon as possible, the woman should be allowed oral fluid intake.

Prolonged labor endangers the fetus due to the prolonged stress from uterine contractions. The nurse must participate in the close monitoring of the status of the fetus either by electrical equipment or frequent checking of the heart rate by intermittent auscultation. The nurse should also recognize signs of fetal distress and report them immediately. When labor is prolonged, a pediatrician should be on call to manage the infant at birth due to the anticipated fetal distress. Specific nursing actions to protect the fetus during labor and birth were discussed in Chapter 26. Care of the distressed neonate at birth was discussed in Chapter 31.

Goal: Prepare and Support the Woman for the Type of Delivery That Is Indicated

A normal delivery is often approached with some degree of apprehension and anxiety. When delivery is expected to be difficult, anxiety increases proportionately. When anxiety rises, it narrows the individual's perceptual field, making the person preoccupied with his own perceived needs. The woman may become preoccupied with her own safety and the survival of her baby. Family members may also share this concern, in addition to being plagued by feelings of helplessness. The physician may be bombarded by decisions as to how the situation can best be managed. The nurse can make a significant contribution in the anxiety-provoking situation of a complicated labor and delivery. The nurse is in a unique position to manipulate the anxiety level in the environment because she is not burdened by obstetric priorities and can therefore be patient-focused. The nurse can assess the anxiety level of the individuals, implement measures to decrease an elevated level, and thereby maximize coping efforts of the woman, family, and even the physician. Because anxiety is highly contagious, decreasing its level in one individual makes an impact in decreasing the anxiety levels of others. Implementation of measures to control anxiety and maximize coping efforts represents a significant aspect of the care the nurse provides to nurture the individual. This nurturance care can be viewed as nursing's unique contribution in the total management of the patient when labor and delivery are complicated.

Regardless of the mode of delivery, every woman facing childbirth, and particularly when childbirth deviates from normal, needs nursing nurturance in terms of the following:

1. Preparation as to what to expect in terms of events and stimuli to be felt, heard, and seen. To prepare the woman appropriately, the nurse must be aware of the impact anxiety has on the learning process. Explanations to an anxious person should be simple, direct, using short phrases or sentences. The nurse is cautioned not to overload the woman with technical, detailed knowledge which can be an additional source of anxiety. Until the anxiety level decreases, the woman is primarily concerned with the "here and now" and needs to know what is happening to her and her baby. Later, when anxiety decreases, the nurse can prepare the woman for events to come. Audiovisual aids can be used to enhance verbal explanations.
2. Protection from being exposed to sudden changes without being notified. This is a nursing challenge because when labor and delivery are complicated, emergency situations may dictate immediate changes in terms of procedures, medications, and monitoring equipment. A classic example is the woman in prolonged labor who has become accustomed to the routine events in her room. Suddenly a change in the labor process dictates that she must rapidly be moved into another room for vaginal or abdominal delivery. Amidst the priorities in preparation for delivery, the woman does not receive notification of the change but is wisked off into the new environment. During transport she becomes restless, agitated, and begins to shout. Her actions should not be labeled as an exhibition of bizarre behavior but rather a manifestion of increased anxiety (panic). The nurse can prevent this by telling the woman the change about to occur, even if short explanations must be given while the change is being implemented. Never underestimate the woman's ability to tolerate change. Most women who have an understanding that their labor is complicated anticipate sudden changes in the plan to ensure a healthy outcome. It is simply

respect for the patient's rights that a word of explanation be given.[5]

3. The need to be sustained by another human being increases proportionately with anxiety and thus a priority nursing action is to remain with the woman as much as possible during the delivery. When labor is complicated, the need for increased obstetric manipulations may give the appearance that the area most worthy of attention is the perineum. After the nurse ascertains that the physician does not need any priority help, she should position herself near the woman's head. In this way eye-to-eye contact can be provided, a feature that has been demonstrated to be very important in human interaction. Close to the woman's head, the nurse can hear the woman's comments, observe for nonverbal gestures, and provide a sense of human closeness through touch and physical presence even if no words are spoken. When feasible, the husband should be permitted to support his wife. However, the reality is that during complications an additional person in the delivery room may not be feasible or permitted. If so, the woman may have no one else for support but the nurse.
4. Accept the woman's comments and concerns as legitimate. Anxiety frequently leads to a distorted perception of reality and it is not unusual for women with complicated labors to maximize their fears or exaggerate their concerns. The woman does indeed perceive her situation as she expresses it. Her comments should not be ridiculed, minimized, or ignored because the long-term effects from such actions can be devastating to the ego. The nurse needs to provide opportunities for expression of feelings, acknowledge that what the patient says is important, and offer explanations to correct any misconceptions.
5. The nurse must remember to keep the woman and her family informed of the status of both mother and baby. This prevents the woman and family from having to resort to fantasies or imagining increased dangers perceived in the situation. Simple information such as sharing results from checking vital signs and fetal heart tones may be most appreciated.
6. When labor is prolonged, progress is slow which easily breeds disappointment and frustration. The nurse must consciously plan to provide positive reinforcement at frequent intervals to prevent the woman from feeling that her situation is hopeless. The nurse uses her own unique personality and style of communication to convey that the mother is coping as well as can be expected and that her efforts are appreciated and will be meaningful for the future outcome.
7. When labor and delivery are complicated, the immediate maternal-infant claiming process may be delayed. The impact of the childbirth experience on the woman may prevent her from being able to spontaneously initiate contact with the new baby. A multitude of factors contribute to this, such as fatigue, discomfort, unmet expectations, and feelings of disappointment. Immediately after delivery the woman may have a need to focus on herself, as if to assimilate the many events that have happened to her. Nursing assessment is critical during this phase. The nurse takes her clues from the mother as to whether a woman desires and is able to initiate interaction with her baby. When interaction is desired, it should not be prohibited. When a woman shows no interest in the baby, the infant should not be forced upon her until she is ready. Health professionals should be cautioned not to make hasty judgmental comments when a woman shows no interest or desires not to see her baby.

They should realize the woman is giving a clue that her priority need is to receive attention herself rather than give attention to the baby.

Nursing Care during Obstetric Operations

Operative obstetrics refer to the special manipulative procedures the obstetrician must perform to ensure a successful delivery, either vaginally or abdominally. While the obstetrician's primary focus is to perform the procedure efficiently, the nurse participates in the total care of the patient by helping to prepare the woman so she can accept the procedure to be performed. This discussion examines the role of the nurse during forceps delivery and cesarean section.

Forceps delivery

When a forceps delivery is indicated (Table 36-4), the woman needs to know the function of the forceps and the consequences and risks to the baby and herself. Forceps are used principally to assist the baby through the vaginal canal and/or rotate or manipulate the head so it can present itself more favorably to accommodate the pelvic passageway. The woman needs to know that skillful use of forceps means the obstetrician will attempt to enhance the normal mechanisms of labor by providing additional force to maneuver the fetal head through the birth canal. When forceps are applied skillfully, the dangers are minimal. In fact, in America, the use of outlet or prophylactic forceps has become a part of the plan for many normal deliveries.

Outlet forceps delivery means the application of forceps when the fetal head has reached the pelvic floor and is crowning. The physician may elect to deliver via outlet forceps because of various benefits:

1. There is more control of the delivery by the obstetrician instead of relying on the unpredictable voluntary efforts of the patient.
2. The head is not exposed to undue pressure against the perineum because the obstetrician lifts it up over the perineum with the forceps.
3. Trauma to maternal soft tissues is minimized when forceps are used in conjunction with an episiotomy.[6]

TABLE 36-4. Indications and Prerequisites for the Use of Forceps for Delivery*

I. INDICATIONS
   A. Any condition threatening the life of the mother or infant which can be relieved by delivery.

Examples of Maternal Indications	*Examples of Fetal Indications*
eclampsia	prolapsed cord
heart disease	premature separation of the placenta
acute pulmonary edema	excessive pressure exerted upon fetal head from prolonged perineal arrest
intrapartal infection	decreased fetal heart rate
uterine dysfunction	meconium in vertex presentation

   B. Forceps delivery may be elective (elective low forceps or outlet forceps delivery). This occurs when the physician elects to bring forth delivery knowing that a spontaneous vaginal delivery can eventually occur. The rationale is to prevent prolonged pressure of the fetal head against a rigid perineum, thus protecting the infant from possible cerebral injury.

II. PREREQUISITES
   A. Head must be engaged.
   B. Fetus must be either in a vertex or face presentation.
   C. Position of the head must be known (to effect rotation as necessary).
   D. Cervix must be completely dilated.
   E. Membranes must be ruptured.
   F. There should be no disproportion between the size of the head and that of the pelvis.

* Based on data obtained from Hellman, L. and Pritchard, J.: *Williams Obstetrics*, ed. 14. Appleton-Century Crofts, New York, pp. 1121–1123.

The other type of forceps delivery involves some manipulation (usually rotation of the fetal head) for extraction of the infant. This is referred to as *midforceps delivery*. The dangers associated with forceps delivery depend upon the position and level of the presenting part and the ability of the obstetrician to apply and use the forceps. The higher the presenting part, the more the dangers. Application of forceps at any time prior to full engagement of the head is not justified in modern obstetric practice. Because forceps are capable of exerting great force, a successful outcome also depends on the obstetrician's ability to guide the presenting part out of the vagina.

TABLE 36-5. Indications for Primary Cesarean Section*

Condition	*Occurrence, %*
I. Dystocia	51.4
A. Contracted pelvis	23.8
B. Malpresentation	11.2
C. Large fetus	10.1
D. Uterine dysfunction	6.3
II. Hemorrhage	11.8
A. Placenta previa	6.9
B. Abruptio placentae	4.9
III. Toxemia	3.3
A. Preeclampsia	2.0
B. Chronic hypertension	1.3
IV. Other High-Risk Factors	23.6
A. Fetal distress	8.7
B. Concurrent disease	4.5
C. Prolapse of cord	3.6
D. Prolonged rupture of membranes	2.3
E. Intrapartal infection	1.9
F. Elderly primigravida	1.7
G. Rh incompatibility	1.0
V. Previous Surgery	3.1
VI. Miscellaneous	6.7

* Data obtained from Hellman, L. and Pritchard, J.: *Williams Obstetrics*. ed. 14. Appleton-Century-Crofts, New York, 1971, p. 1166.

Cesarean section

A cesarean section is delivery of the infant through incisions in the abdominal and uterine cavities. The indications for a cesarean section are listed in Table 36-5.

Preoperative Nursing Care. The nurse participates in the preparation of the woman who is to have a cesarean section by performing such actions as:

1. Obtain proper consent forms signed by the woman or, in case of emergency, signed by a family member.
2. Assure that proper lab tests have been done such as roentgenograms, blood counts, and blood typing and cross-match for units of blood should it be needed.
3. Prepare the abdominal area by shaving. The area from below the breasts to the pubic region is usually shaved.
4. Assure that the bladder is emptied so as not to obstruct the delivery. Sometimes a Foley catheter is ordered to ensure that the bladder will not become distended.
5. Assure that an intravenous system is inserted to keep an open route for administration of medications, fluids, and blood. The needle should be of adequate size to allow the administration of blood if necessary.
6. Assess vital signs and fetal heart rate prior to the procedure. Alterations in the fetal heart rate may be an indication for an emergency cesarean section.
7. Assure that the mother is properly identified and that the baby will be properly identified after delivery. Some nurses prepare the infant's identification card with only the infant's last name and attach it to the chart so it can be properly completed after the baby is born.
8. Provide adequate explanations about what to expect regarding the delivery and allow expression of feelings. Answer any questions and clarify any misconceptions.

9. Assess whether the mother plans to breast or bottle feed because some medications to inhibit lactation (such as Deladumone) should be given as soon as possible after the delivery. If cesarean section is to be done in a surgical unit, the obstetric staff may need to prepare the medication and send it with the woman so that it can be given at the proper time.

In an emergency, some of the above actions may not be feasible. The nurse needs to constantly assess and make proper judgments so that nursing actions are in accord with the priorities presented in the unique situation.

Postoperative Nursing Care. Nursing care after cesarean section is very similar to that given to any surgical patient. Nursing consideration must be given to the following:

1. Assurance of a patent airway and immediate protection from respiratory obstruction by actions such as suctioning and positioning which facilitates drainage of mucus to prevent possible aspiration.
2. Close monitoring of vital signs and blood pressure for clues of impending complications.
3. Promote comfort through proper positioning, use of medications as ordered, and assistance with personal hygiene such as oral care and bed baths.
4. Assessment of the incision area for proper healing. Any bleeding, swelling, redness, or odor should be reported immediately. The area should be protected by keeping it clean and dry. Undue pressure on the area should be prevented by assuring that the woman's position in bed is not creating pressure on the incision area.
5. Assess that the woman's intake and output are adequate. Some woman have difficulty voiding immediately after the delivery and may need to be catheterized until they are able to urinate without difficulty.
6. One of the best measures to prevent cardiovascular and pulmonary complications after surgery is early ambulation. The woman may initially be reluctant to attempt such a venture for fear of pain. The nurse can help significantly by first explaining the rationale for the action, then what is to be involved in the first attempt to ambulate, and finally assisting the woman to actually ambulate. When the nurse can explain the steps which lead to successful ambulation, then the woman will not be overwhelmed when asked to perform the task. The nurse should always offer positive reinforcement for efforts made during ambulation to increase the woman's confidence in her ability to ambulate again.
7. Anticipate management of a pain experience from the surgery, such as discomforts at the operative site or from gas pains. In addition, some women, especially multiparas, may experience "after-birth pains" as the uterus contracts to maintain its tone. The nurse should plan to minimize the perception of pain through the use of ordered medications and other measures to provide comfort and decrease anxiety.
8. Assessment of the body's adjustment to the delivery is important because a cesarean section is indeed a delivery process. Monitoring of the fundus and lochia flow should not be forgotten. Assessing the firmness and level of the fundus may be difficult because of the tenderness at the incision area. Thus, checking for the amount of bleeding becomes increasingly important.

The psychologic impact of having a cesarean section is discussed in the next section.

Goal: Implement Crisis Intervention to Prevent Detrimental Psychologic Consequences

The nurse must have an appreciation of the possible impact a complicated labor and delivery can have on the woman and her family. Building upon the concepts presented in Unit 2, let us briefly examine their application when physiologic risks are associated with the childbirth experience.

One major impact will be increased anxiety due to the additional stressors to which the woman is exposed. Examples of these stressors are:

1. Increased obstetric manipulations needed to assess and manage the situation.
2. The unknown is ever present in terms of not knowing exactly what the outcome will be, not knowing when an emergency will arise because of acute dangers to mother or baby, and not knowing exactly how long one must endure the processes of labor.
3. The expectation for an uneventful labor experience will not be met. Peplau in Chapter 9 discussed how anxiety increases when expectations are not met.

Increased anxiety can be a deterrent to labor progress. Physiologically, highly anxious women have been found to be more vulnerable to abnormal contractile patterns leading to prolonged labor. Psychologically, the highly anxious woman is more apt to have a distorted perception of events, thereby increasing perceived dangers in the situation. Increased anxiety can create fears not only during the present childbirth experience but can be projected for future childbearing experiences. Increased anxiety also leads to decreased ability to comprehend the situation. There is also decreased active participation in enhancing the labor process. Therefore, the woman may be less able to understand explanations or to follow through with commands when her active participation is needed. This latter point is important because frequently the woman's cooperation in terms of voluntary efforts, such as to push or remain still, is necessary for successful management of the situation.

Another impact concerns the concept of loss. When labor is complicated, the woman is more apt to experience feelings of loss for a valued aspect of herself or for a valued person, such as the baby. The woman will have legitimate reasons for grieving. For example, she may grieve for the anticipated loss of the baby if she is told the baby is endangered. She may grieve the loss of expectations in terms of what she expected labor and delivery to be like, her concept of her ability to participate and maintain control of the situation, and any other feelings of loss directed to the self in terms of body image, ability to communicate, and trust and confidence in the self. The husband also has legitimate reasons for grieving. He may begin to grieve for the anticipated loss of both the mother and baby when he realizes the dangers associated with the situation. Grief regarding loss of an aspect of the self may be directed to the self concept in terms of one's perceived ability to help or participate in the experience.

During the childbirth experience, the health professionals may become so preoccupied with priorities in the physical management of the situation that they fail to recognize the manifestations of grief. Benoliel in Chapter 10 described that the normal grieving process consists of emotional responses such as:

1. Period of numbness and shock.
2. Feelings of anger and fear.
3. Sense of helplessness and a wish to be helped.
4. Feelings of despair and emptiness, sometimes coupled with guilt and shame.
5. A renewal of hope and reorganization of behaviors to cope with the reality of the consequences associated with loss.

TABLE 36-6. Behavioral Reactions to Grief during the Childbirth Experience

Normal Stages of Grief	*Expected Behaviors*	*Nursing Considerations*
Period of numbness and shock	Decreased responsiveness to the environment; appears disinterested in events occurring. Appears withdrawn. Manifests immobile behaviors such as staring at the walls, rigid positioning, lack of movements.	Do not have unrealistic expectations of the woman such as demanding she be able to communicate effectively. Do not respond by also withdrawing because the woman acts like she's not interested in nursing actions. Demonstrate acceptance of this grief stage by actions such as physical presence, gentle touch.
Feelings of anger and fear	Aggressive behaviors may be directed to others such as use of vulgar language, physical aggression, or finding faults. Fears may be expressed verbally or by nonverbal clues through the sympathetic-adrenal responses. Lack of sleep and irritability are also other clues indicative of this phase.	Accept aggressive behaviors without retaliating with punitive comments or actions. Provide a listening ear to communicate that the woman's concerns and behaviors are important. Try to communicate an understanding of the woman's difficulties that must be coped with.
Sense of helplessness	Increased dependency needs may manifest through behaviors such as: a. Frequent commands in asking for things to be done b. Regressive behaviors such as resorting to childish mannerisms may be seen c. Mourning behaviors (crying) are increased d. Sense of helplessness may be expressed directly by verbal comments.	The physical presence of the nurse is necessary to combat feelings of helplessness and a sense of abandonment. Accept mourning behaviors without ridiculing or minimizing the behaviors.
Sense of despair	May begin to share morbid comments about the outcome of childbirth. May demonstrate withdrawal behaviors and act as if nothing matters. May express feelings of guilt and attach blame for the situation on the self.	The nurse must work diligently to instill trust and confidence in the woman and her family about the medical management of the situation. Because labor may be prolonged, fatigue leads to discouragement and loss of hope. Measures to promote rest and comfort may help to forestall excessive fatigue, and thereby curb a sense of total despair.
Reorganization of behaviors to enhance coping	This phase is marked by a renewal of interest and energy in the woman. She may at last be able to talk about the experience spontaneously, ask many questions, seek to reestablish previous communication patterns with others.	The nurse's key role is to listen, clarify, and provide missing facts to help the woman integrate the reality of the loss that occurred. Remember, psychologic recovery from the pain of loss takes time. Therefore, nursing intervention may need to be continued in the home through visiting nurse agencies and/or referral to other disciplines.

The goal of nursing is to assist the woman and her husband through the above phases so that a healthy resolution of the loss occurs. However, in the clinical situation this may not be so simple because there will be priorities directed to the physical management of the labor process. Often the woman's behavioral responses of grief are misinterpreted, resulting in negative or punitive reactions by the health team. Table 36-6 explores nursing implications regarding the behavioral reactions of grief.

The concept of sensory alteration is also applicable when labor and delivery are at risk. Sensory overload can occur from the use of many electrical devices to monitor the baby and the labor process. A feeling of overload also arises because the pace of events is usually more rapid, especially during an emergency. Amidst all this environmental bombardment, the woman may experience a sense of sensory deprivation. Presence of the husband may be limited by frequent interruptions to assess and perform procedures to enhance labor. The staff may be so preoccupied with the management of the labor process that priority attention is given to the status of equipment, and the woman is easily forgotten.

The self concept can be threatened if the woman and her family feel a sense of failure or cannot find meaning in the childbirth experience. This leads to detrimental effects on the individual's future behavioral development. If the individual cannot accept the consequences of a childbearing experience that is complicated, then mental health can be jeopardized.

It may be necessary for the nurse to institute crisis intervention to prevent detrimental psychologic consequences when the childbirth experience is complicated. The nurse needs to work to help the woman and her family in:

1. Gaining a realistic perception of the event.
2. Facilitating the presence of situational supports.
3. Working to help the woman to utilize adequate coping mechanisms.
4. Doing whatever else is necessary to aid in problem-solving for healthy resolution of crisis.

Psychologic Impact of Cesarean Section

A classic example of a woman vulnerable to crisis is when a cesarean section must be performed because there is no progress after a trial labor. During informal interviews conducted by the author, women who had to have a cesarean section after a trial labor expressed the following:

1. Although most women were relieved that their labor was terminated, there was a sense of failure or defeat because the woman felt she was unable to complete the normal, expected process of bringing forth a baby. When the trial labor failed, women felt they were personally responsible. They conveyed a feeling that somehow they should have been better able to manipulate the forces of labor. The process of labor was seen as an extended part of the self, rather than under involuntary control.
2. Many women were observed to be in a grieving process. The grief varied. Some grieved for the loss of a vaginal delivery. Others grieved because they did not feel an active part of the delivery as they had desired. The grief seemed to focus primarily on the loss of a desired aspect of the self, especially regarding the woman's perception of her own performance.
3. Women had increased anxieties about their own welfare and that of their babies.
4. Major stressors after a cesarean section were fatigue and pain. Women were noted to be exhausted and had difficulty resting or sleeping. Pain in the postpartal period, especially intestinal discomforts

(gas pains), appeared to be a stressor. Most women expressed that is wasn't fair that after suffering during labor and delivery they should still be plagued by pain now that it was over. Some women expressed feelings of envy on seeing vaginally delivered women "pop in and out of bed with ease," while they had to make special maneuvers and efforts to perform such simple acts.

5. Most women expressed initial concerns about their babies. However, after being reassured that the infant was well (especially after seeing the baby themselves), most women were not anxious for facts about infant care. Rather there was an initial need to be given attention and to be ministered to in attempts to meet dependency needs. Women appeared to respond favorably when they received nurturing care which did not have to be shared with anyone, especially the baby.
6. It was noted that women who had support by visits from spouses or other family members made a faster recovery than those who were forced to recuperate without significant situational support. Husbands and family members were helpful in encouraging and aiding the women toward early ambulation and self-care. Women who were forced to face the recovery period alone were noted to be slower in finding meaning in the childbirth experience and in initiating interaction with the infant.
7. Most women were not favorable toward future childbearing experiences as compared with their vaginally delivered counterparts. Women who had cesarean sections were anxious to receive knowledge on contraceptives and a few of the younger patients said they wanted no more children.

The above are not necessarily the predicted or normal responses for every woman who has a cesarean section. Rather, they are shared as a stimulus for the nurse to collect data about women's responses to a cesarean section. Some women may have very different reactions from those described. However, we cannot add to nursing knowledge unless each nurse in the clinical setting takes the initiative to assess the impact an experience has on the woman. In the area of the psychologic impact from a cesarean section, nursing has a responsibility to add more knowledge by clinical assessment of a woman's reactions.

Postpartal Hemorrhage

The process of delivery involves a certain amount of blood loss. However, any blood loss above 500 cc. is considered postpartal hemorrhage. Factors which predispose to this complication are listed in Table 36-7. The nurse should have two goals in mind when postpartal hemorrhage presents:

1. Protect the woman by measures which include monitoring the amount of bleeding and preventing additional blood loss.
2. Support medical intervention to prevent hemorrhage or to manage the situation when it exists.

Nursing actions to prevent excessive bleeding after delivery were described in Chapter 28. One of the most important nursing actions is massage of the uterus. The nurse should be able to perform massage as described in Chapter 28. She should also attempt to express any clots, reporting the amount, color, and size of clots expelled. Helping to keep the uterus firm by manual compression through massage is so important that when hemorrhage occurs, the nurse may need to do it constantly until the physician arrives to manage the situation. Thus, any woman who is vulnerable to or is hemorrhaging should never be left unattended. At such times, the uterus may need to be monitored constantly to be sure it is con-

TABLE 36-7. Major Factors Predisposing to Postpartal Hemorrhage

Cause	*Predisposing Factors*
A. Uterine atony or uterine inertia Inability or failure of the myometrical cells to contract and constrict the blood vessels within the muscle fibers. This results in open sinuses at the sites of placental separation. Largely due to muscle fatigue, exhaustion, or bleeding into the muscle, such as during premature or incomplete separation of the placenta.	1. Overdistention of the uterus due to a large baby, multiple gestation, or hydramnios. Amount of blood loss is directly proportional to the size of the intrauterine mass. 2. Prolong labor leading to muscle fatigue. 3. Maternal exhaustion. 4. Excessive medications or deep ether anesthesia whereby the muscle fibers are too relaxed and unable to maintain muscle tone. 5. Difficult obstetric operations resulting in trauma to the muscle cells. 6. Grand multiparity resulting in diminished muscle tone with each pregnancy. 7. Abnormalities in the third stage in which the placenta fails to separate, separation is incomplete, or obstetric manipulations force separation too early.
B. Retained placenta fragments Any piece of the placenta (regardless of size) remaining in the uterus interferes with the complete constriction of the blood vessels. It is recommended that after delivery the placenta be inspected for any tears or missing areas. Evidence of torn blood vessels is highly suggestive of retained placenta.	1. Defects in the decidua causing incomplete or difficult separation of the placenta. 2. Too early a manipulation to force the placenta out of the uterus during the third stage of labor. 3. Uterine inertia in the third stage of labor.
C. Laceration of the perineum, vagina, cervix, or lower uterine segment. Unrepaired tears, especially when deep in the vagina, cervix, or uterus, can result in profuse bleeding. Hematoma (bleeding into the tissues) can occur from trauma to blood vessels in the area. Bleeding is slow, frequently involving the vulva and under the vaginal mucosa. A hematoma can occur without a distinct laceration.	1. Difficult deliveries dictating aggressive operative manipulations. 2. May be seen in spontaneous vaginal deliveries.
D. Blood-coagulation defects Reduction in fibrinogen levels (hypofibrinogenemia) leading to interference with blood-clotting mechanisms. Usual techniques to control bleeding are unsuccessful until the low fibrinogen level is corrected (frequently by intravenous administration of fibrinogen)	1. Severe premature separation of the placenta, missed labor, multiple prior transfusions, and known hemorrhagic disorders all contribute to a reduction in blood fibrinogen level.

tracting. The nurse also assists with other actions such as maintaining the oxytocin infusion.

During hemorrhage, oxytocin may be given via rapid intravenous infusion as a stimulus for the myometrium to contract. This is the one instance when the nurse does not need to be concerned about the drip rate relating to an exact dosage of the drug. Rather, the goal is to assure rapid infusion of the oxytocin. Another nursing activity involves getting laboratory tests for typing and cross-matching for blood and other tests to rule out coagulation defects. Valuable time can be saved when the nurse anticipates and orders such tests instead of merely waiting for the physician's orders.

Shock

Hemorrhage is an insult to the body and can lead to shock. Shock constitutes an emergency because it decreases blood flow to vital organs, thereby threatening life. The nurse must be able to assess and implement life-saving measures because excessive loss of blood can occur rapidly should the uterus not contract properly after delivery. To implement appropriate actions, the nurse must understand the physiologic mechanisms involved in shock and the symptoms which reflect the consequences. Such theoretic knowledge is described by Royce[7] in a reference the reader is encouraged to read. An excerpt from the reference is presented below:

> After a major insult such as cardiac arrest or hemorrhage, physiologic compensatory mechanisms are set into immediate motion. Catecholamines are released by the adrenal cortex to constrict the arterioles and venules in the skin, the lungs, the liver, the kidneys and the bowel, allowing more blood to flow to the heart and brain (Figure 36-11). This selective ischemia interferes with normal oxidative metabolism and becomes detrimental if shock is prolonged. Cells in the peripheral circulation metabolize glucose anaerobically, resulting in an increase of lactic acid and uncompensated cellular acidosis. Catecholamines which initially caused vasoconstriction of the arterioles and venules and increased peripheral resistance are no longer effective in maintaining cardiac output. A decreasing serum pH causes vasodilation of the arterioles while the venules continue to constrict (Figure 36-12).

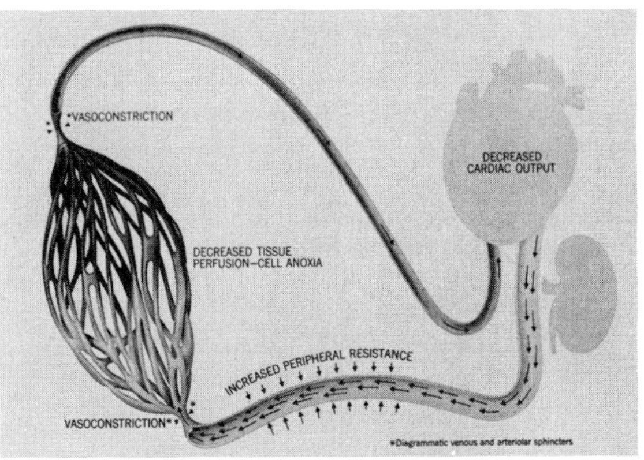

FIGURE 36-11. Hemodynamic alterations in ischemic shock. (Courtesy of The Upjohn Company.)

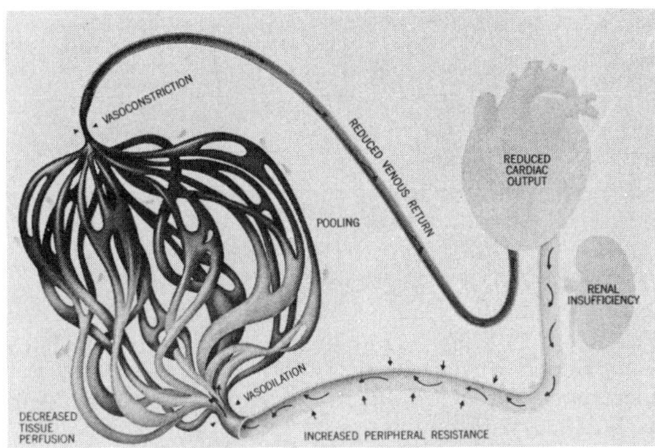

FIGURE 36-12. Hemodynamic alterations in stagnant shock. (Courtesy of The Upjohn Company.)

> This results in a further decrease of perfusion with resulting tissue anoxia, acidosis, edema, and pooling of blood. The cell membranes and mitochondria are destroyed by the accumulation of lactic acids and altered enzymes. Although increased potassium levels would be expected due to the loss of cell membrane integrities, hyperkalemia is rare in shock.

When the nurse understands that shock primarily involves decreased perfusion of the cells, then the symptoms become meaningful.

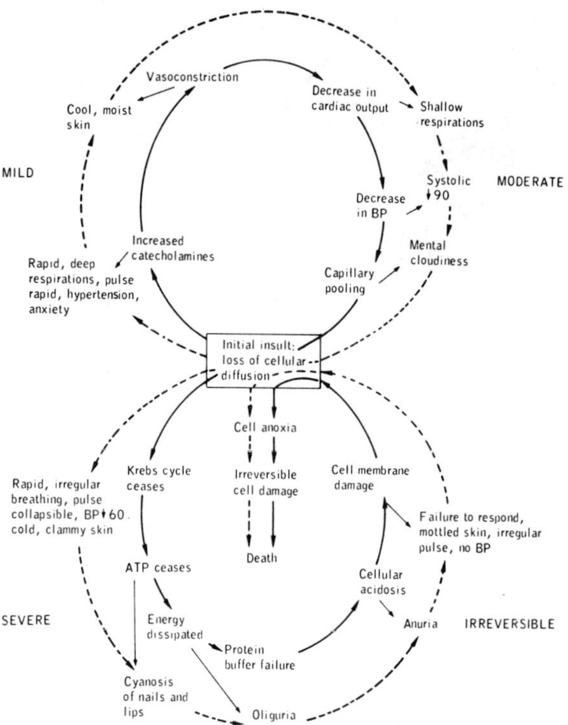

FIGURE 36-13. Diagram of physiologic alterations in shock in relation to symptoms. (From Royce, J.: *Shock—Emergency nursing implications.* Nurs. Clin. North Am. 8:377, 1973, with permission.)

The physiologic alterations in shock in relation to symptoms are shown in Figure 36-13. Because the nurse should also recognize signs of impending shock, the symptoms presented in Table 36-8 help to identify signs relative to the degree of shock.

In the care of the patient in shock, Royce[8] recommends the following nursing considerations:

1. Insert an airway and start an intravenous solution of 50 per cent dextrose in water while awaiting the physician. These actions provide a patent airway and help prevent venous peripheral collapse.
2. Never leave the patient. Rather, ask other staff members to gather priority equipment needed, such as blood sample tubes, suction apparatus, Foley catheter with urinometer, central venous pressure apparatus, stethoscope and blood pressure equipment, and the emergency cart with a defibrillator.
3. Constantly monitor the respiratory and cardiac status and institute measures to increase blood flow to the tissues. This is achieved through the following activities:
   a. Be sure intravenous solutions are flowing adequately. Whole blood, plasma, and albumin may be given to increase blood volume. Dextrose in water and lactated Ringer's solution may also be given to reduce hemoconcentration to improve blood flow by decreasing viscosity of the circulation. The nurse must take caution not to run fluids too rapidly leading to fluid overload. Any moist-sounding respirations or abnormal muscular action during breathing may be suggestive of pulmonary edema.
   b. Central venous pressure is important because it indicates the pumping ability of the heart in relation to blood volume. Thus, it indicates whether blood volume is adequate, deficient, or excessive. CVP readings below 6 cm. H_2O may indicate blood volume deficits, while readings above 12 cm. H_2O indicate increased blood volume from too rapid IV infusion or impending cardiac or peripheral vascular failure. Each nurse should be able to operate the CVP apparatus.
   c. Urinary output should be assessed. Output below the normal rate of 30 to 50 cc. per hour is suggestive of deterioration in the patient's status. Increased urinary output is an indication of improvement.
   d. Monitor respirations and blood pres-

TABLE 36-8. Symptoms of Shock*

	Mild	*Moderate*	*Severe*	*Irreversible*
Respirations	Rapid, deep	Rapid, becoming shallow	Rapid, shallow, may be irregular	Irregular, or barely perceptible
Pulse	Rapid, tone normal	Rapid, tone may be normal but is becoming weaker	Very rapid, easily collapsible, may be irregular	Irregular apical pulse
Blood pressure	Normal or hypertensive	60–90 mm. Hg systolic	Below 60 mm. Hg systolic	None palpable
Skin	Cool and pale	Cool, pale, moist, knees cyanotic	Cold, clammy, cyanosis of lips and fingernails	Cold, clammy, cyanotic
Urine output	No change	Decreasing to 10–22 cc./hr. adult	Oliguric (less than 10 cc.) to anuria	Anuric
Level of consciousness	Alert, oriented, diffuse anxiety	Oriented, mental cloudiness or increasing restlessness	Lethargy, reacts to noxious stimuli, comatose	Does not respond to noxious stimuli
CVP	May be normal	3 cm. H_2O	0–3 cm. H_2O	

* Developed by M. M. Wagner as appeared in Royce, J.: *Shock: emergency nursing implications.* Nurs. Clin. North Am. 8:380, 1973.

sure. Rapid respirations are a way for the body to get rid of accumulated acids during shock. Hyperventilation usually indicates deficiency in gas exchange and a need for ventilatory assistance. Oxygen and/or respirator therapy may be needed. Blood gases should always be done to prevent oxygen toxicity during oxygen therapy. The nurse is cautioned not to rely solely on blood pressure readings. Decrease in systolic pressure is a manifestation of shock in its later phases at which time detrimental effects of circulatory pooling and stagnation may exist. Thus, a significant drop in blood pressure is usually indicative of severe shock, which may be irreversible and fatal.

e. Assessment of the skin is a good indicator of the degree of shock because compensatory mechanisms will sacrifice blood flow to maintain skin temperature and color. Thus, ischemia of the skin, in which it is cool and pale, may exhibit in early, mild shock. As shock increases, the skin becomes cooler, cyanotic, and moist to touch. In severe shock petechiae indicate damage to the cells, while mottling indicates cell anoxia and death. Therefore the nurse must value the skin as providing early clues of impending shock. Areas to assess for ischemia are the eyelids, buccal mucosa, gums, tongue, and nailbeds. Improvement of skin color indicates an increase in peripheral circulation.

f. Assessment of the level of consciousness gives an indication of the degree of cerebral blood flow. Early signs of decreased perfusion to the brain are increased anxiety or restlessness, dim vision, vertigo, and orthopnea, Increasing cerebral hypoxia is suspected with progression of mental confusion, lethargy, and decreased ability to react to stimuli.

Thus, the role of the nurse during postpartal hemorrhage is to protect the mother from impending death or complications from the therapy such as pulmonary edema, and any damage to the lungs should oxygen and respirator therapy be necessary. One word of caution—it was once accepted that placing the woman in a Trendelenburg position helped to increase blood flow to the brain during shock and so this action was often used injudiciously. However, research has indicated that this position can impair cardiac filling and may be more detrimental than beneficial.[9] Therefore, the nurse is now cautioned not to use the position unless specifically ordered by the physician. The factor to value in preventing postpartal hemorrhage is close monitoring of the state of contractility of the fundus after delivery. In nursing the woman in shock the nurse must work quickly to implement measures because brain death can occur within five minutes after perfusion ceases.[10]

Puerperal Infection

Infection of the maternal reproductive system during or after childbirth is a grave complication with a high mortality rate. A maternal temperature of above 100.4° F (38° C) after the first 24 hours after delivery which remains elevated for over 24 hours with no other defined cause for the fever is an indication for the diagnosis of puerperal sepsis. The various types of infection, their symptoms, and nursing implications are listed in Table 36-9.

TABLE 36-9. Common Types of Puerperal Infection

I. Reproductive Tract (genital) Infections

May originate from two primary sources:
- endogenous—bacteria in the normal vaginal flora become virulent when tissues are traumatized
- exogenous—introduction of pathogens via transmission from personnel, break in aseptic technique, or contamination from sources such as feces

Common causative organisms: streptococci, Escherichia coli, Staphylococcus albus or hemolytic Staphylococcus aureus, Clostridium perfrigens, Neisseria gonorrhoeae

A. Infections may be localized in the vulva or vagina (called vulvitis and vaginitis), and to the episiotomy site

Signs/Symptoms
- localized perineal pain, redness, edema to the area
- persistent low grade fever
- cloudy, white exudate and/or purulent discharge from the episiotomy site or lacerations
- complaints of dysuria (pain upon urination)

Treatment
- analgesics
- sitz baths
- perineal heat lamp
- drainage at the abscess
- administration of antibiotics

TABLE 36-9—*Continued*

B. Infection of the cervix (cervicitis) and/or endometrium (endometritis). Majority of puerperal sepsis is attributed to endometritis.

Signs/Symptoms
elevated temperatures. During first 48 hours may be only low grade but by the third postpartal day, it is above 38° C and remains elevated.
uterine tenderness
malaise
foul smelling, copious lochia

Treatment
culture and sensitivity done and appropriate antibiotics given.

C. Infection extended beyond the endometrium into surrounding pelvic structures (pelvic cellulitis and venous thrombosis)

Signs/Symptoms
high temperature such as 104° F
chills
thrombosis in the uterine or ovarian veins is suspected with danger of pulmonary embolism
elevated leukocytes (above 20,000)
positive blood and uterine cultures

Treatment
bed rest
administration of appropriate antibiotics according to culture and sensitivity test results
administration of oxytocics to promote the uterus to expel any accumulated matter
maintain hydration with intravenous fluids
isolation techniques imperative
transfusions of whole blood if hemoglobin decreases

II. Urinary Tract Infections

Three predisposing factors—dilatation, stasis, and bacteriuria, all of which usually result from trauma to the bladder and/or ureters from the impact of labor and delivery

Common causative organism: Escherichia coli

Signs/Symptoms
frequent, small voidings or inability to urinate
pain upon urination
hematuria
bacteria and pus cells found in laboratory diagnosis of the urine
(The above would indicate lower urinary tract infection, e.g., cystitis.)
chills
tenderness over one or both kidneys (kidney and flank tenderness)
malaise
elevated temperature
GI—nausea, vomiting
(The above are associated with upper urinary tract infection; acute pyelonephritis.)

Treatment
bed rest
force fluids
antibiotic therapy

TABLE 36-9. *Continued*

III. Mastitis (acute infection of the breast)

May be a result of organisms entering through a fissure in the nipple or acquired from infant through breast feeding

Common causative organism: Staphylococcus aureus

Signs/Symptoms
- minimal signs if breasts are adequately drained during nursing
- occlusion of the ducts results in
  - engorged, tender, red breasts
  - chills
  - fever
  - headache
  - malaise
  - tender mass palpated in the breast

Treatment
- discontinue breast feeding
- antibiotic therapy
- analgesics for discomfort
- surgical drainage of the abscess may be indicated
- support breasts with a binder or well-fitted brassiere

REFERENCES

1. Hendrick, C.: *Dystocia due to abnormal uterine action.* In Danforth, D. (ed.): *Textbook of Obstetrics and Gynecology*, ed. 2. Harper and Row, New York, 1971, p. 653.
2. Reynolds, S. and Hendrick, C.: *Physiology of uterine contractions and onset of labor.* In Danforth, D. (ed.): *Textbook of Obstetrics and Gynecology*, ed. 2. Harper and Row, New York, 1971, p. 515.
3. Pearse, W. and Danforth, D.: *Dystocia due to abnormal fetopelvic relations.* In Danforth, D. (ed.): *Textbook of Obstetrics and Gynecology*, ed. 2. Harper and Row, New York, 1971, p. 644.
4. Hendrick, C.: op. cit., p. 657.
5. Quinn, N. and Somers, A.: *The patient's bill of rights.* Nurs. Outlook, 22:240, 1974.
6. Russell, K.: *Clotting defects, transfusions, and shock.* in Danforth, D. (ed.): *Textbook of Obstetrics and Gynecology*, ed. 2. Harper and Row, New York, 1971, p. 677.
7. Royce, J.: *Shock—Emergency nursing implications.* Nurs. Clin. North Am. 8:377, 1973.
8. Ibid.
9. Ibid.
10. Ibid.

BIBLIOGRAPHY

Bonica, J.: *Obstetric Complications.* F. A. Davis, Philadelphia, 1965.

Ibid.: *Maternal respiratory changes during pregnancy and parturition.* Clin. Anesth. 10:1, 1974.

Burstein, I., et al.: *Anxiety, pregnancy, labor, and the neonate.* Am. J. Obstet. Gynecol. 118:195, 1974.

Danforth, D. (ed.): *Textbook of Obstetrics and Gynecology*, ed. 2. Harper and Row, New York, 1971.

Donald, I.: *Practical Obstetrical Problems.* J. B. Lippincott, Philadelphia, 1969.

Dudgeon, J.: *Intrauterine infections.* Ciba Found. Symp. 10:1, 1972.

Fields, H.: *Induction of Labor.* Macmillan, New York, 1965.

Friedman, E.: *Labor: Clinical Evaluation and Management.* Appleton-Century-Crofts, New York, 1967.

Greenhill, J.: *Biological Principles and Modern Practice of Obstetrics.* W. B. Saunders, Philadelphia, 1974.

Hasen, J. M., et al.: *Maternal cardiovascular dynamics during pregnancy and parturition.* Clin. Anesth. 10:21, 1974.

Hellman, L. and Pritchard, J.: *Williams Obstetrics*, ed. 14. Appleton-Century Crofts, New York, 1971.

Jacobson, H. and Reid, D.: *High-risk pregnancy II. Maternal and child care.* N. Engl. J. Med. 271:302, 1964.

Leon, J.: *High-risk pregnancy: graphic representation of the maternal and fetal risks.* Am. J. Obstet. Gynecol. 117:497, 1973.

Nesbitt, R. and Aubry, R.: *Recognition and care of high-risk obstetrical patients. Part I.* Hosp. Med. 3(9):43, 1967; *Part II* Hosp. Med. 3(10):41, 1967.

Philipp, E., Barnes, J. and Newton, M.: *Scientific Foundations of Obstetrics and Gynaecology.* F. A. Davis, Philadelphia, 1970.

Ray, M., et al.: *Clinical experience with the oxytocin challenge test.* Am. J. Obstet. Gynecol. 114:1, 1972.

Reid, D.: *Principles and management of human reproduction.* W. B. Saunders, Philadelphia, 1972.

Rose, P. A.: *The high risk mother-infant dyad–A challenge for nursing?* Nurs. Forum 6:94, 1967.

Rovinsky, J. and Guttmacher, A.: *Medical, Surgical and Gynecologic Complications of Pregnancy*, ed. 2. Williams & Wilkins, Baltimore, 1965.

Schneider, J.: *The high risk pregnancy.* Hosp. Prac. 6:133, 1971.

37 *Major Risks to the Neonate*

THOMAS R. HARRIS, M.D.

Before discussing a number of important diseases encountered in the newborn period, their causes and effects on function (etiology and pathophysiology) and recommended modes of nursing management, we need to ask ourselves three fundamental questions:

1. Are neonatal diseases basically different from those of adulthood?
2. Are we dealing with a patient who responds differently to disease than would an adult?
3. Will we encounter diffuculties with the newborn that will necessitate a different approach to his disease as regards our assessment and plan of supportive management and treatment (protect, nurture, and stimulate)?

The answer to the first question is "yes" in a number of cases. Certain lethal congenital conditions do not permit survival beyond the newborn period or infancy, so are not seen in adult medicine. Examples are hypoplastic left heart syndrome and asphyxiating thoracic dystrophy. Such conditions represent potential frontiers of ultra-aggressive neonatal intensive care, challenging us to develop new surgical approaches and even better postoperative supportive teams and techniques. Their discussion is beyond the scope of this book.

A second group of syndromes and diseases exclusive to the newborn can often now be detected early and either avoided completely or quite well managed thanks to recently acquired knowledge of pathophysiology and development of better supportive techniques. Examples discussed in some detail are asphyxia neonatorum, meconium aspiration, and Rh and ABO erythroblastosis.

Then there is a host of problems peculiar to the newborn period and especially accentuated in the premature infant that can best be characterized as "diseases of development or immaturity." These are the results of poor synthesizing ability, low enzymatic activity, underdeveloped regulatory function, persistance of a fetal condition, or incompletely developed structures that limit function at less-than-adult levels. Examples discussed in this area include idiopathic respiratory distress syndrome or hyaline membrane disease, hyperbilirubinemia, hypoglycemia and hypocalcemia, and late metabolic acidosis of the premature.

Lastly, there are certain iatrogenic (caused by the doctor) diseases or complications of treatment that we only see in the newborn. They are in part dependent on the degree of immaturity of the patient or represent accentuated responses of developing tissues to toxic effects. Examples are retrolental fibroplasia and bronchopulmonary dysplasia.

We must answer the second fundamental

question in the affirmative also. We are dealing with a patient who responds differently to disease than does the adult precisely because of his immature structures and functions. This is the real heart of neonatal medicine and nursing. One must know the various structural and functional limitations of the newborn and premature infant in order to best protect him from excesses and compensate for his weaknesses. One must know what compensatory mechanisms are already functioning so these may be further supported or duplicated in kind and effect. One must know the quite different "normal" values or acceptable limits of variation in the newborn so as not to demand too much of him or overshoot in our treatment. Chapter 30 discussed the functional status, norms, and limitations of the newborn. The present chapter reiterates many of these, tracing the effects of the physiologic limitations upon specific disease processes. Special attention is focused on the premature and small-for-date (intrauterine growth retarded) newborn.

Our third fundamental question is likewise answered "yes." There are a number of difficulties encountered in dealing with the newborn that necessitate a quite different nursing approach than when working with the usual adult. Assessment of problems in a patient who cannot talk or who can hardly express subjective symptoms forces one to rely heavily on historical data provided by the mother and obstetrician. Prenatal and intrapartal risk factors assume utmost importance as early clues or warning signs in place of subtle symptoms recalled by the patient. The diagnostic work-up of the newborn is further hampered by the very limited sample supply (blood volume is only 80 cc. per kg. body weight), the need for miniaturization and microtechniques, and the problem of a patient who is unable to cooperate. Moreover, symptoms of organ dysfunction or failure may be late in onset since up until the time of birth the mother and placenta may well have provided the entire function. There may also be quite different expression or presentation of symptoms in the newborn as compared with the adult. Seizure activity, for instance, may be expressed as apneic episodes or sudden atonic (limp) spells rather than frank convulsions. This chapter points out some of these unusual forms of symptom presentation.

Regarding supportive management and treatment, screening tests and monitoring are of particular importance in neonatology. Given the newborn's inherent structural and functional immaturity and his subsequent regulatory instability, it becomes of great importance to detect deviant trends as early as possible before they get out of hand and require major intervention with all of its further risk. If detection must await the appearance of really obvious symptoms, we may already be faced with an irreversible situation or one in which permanent damage to the individual has already occurred. Neonatal nurses play as crucial a role in determining final patient outcome as anywhere else in medicine. Likewise, sophisticated equipment that both provides a stable environment for the fragile neonate and detects the slightest deviation of a vital sign from normal has become an integral part of newborn nursing care (Fig. 37-1). The modern neonatal nurse must familiarize herself with this equipment and understand its basic mode of operation.

This chapter attempts to provide the reader with the means to *assess* the severity of a number of common neonatal conditions, as well as point out whenever possible any clues that may lead to anticipation of the initial or subsequent problems and thus possibly protect the baby from further difficulty. By emphasizing the pathophysiologic mechanisms (explanations for disordered function) involved in these representative diseases, it is hoped that the reader may gain a deeper understanding of the basic problems and may fashion a more rational plan of medical and nursing management to *nurture* and *stimulate*

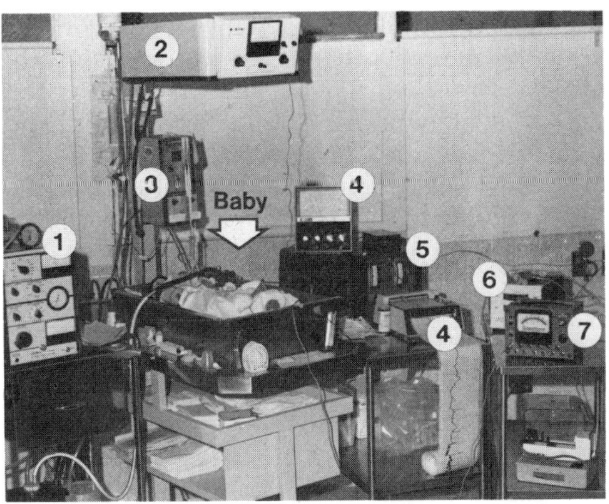

FIGURE 37-1. Supportive equipment for the critically ill neonate. 1) Bourns infant ventilator to assist ventilation. 2) KDC radiant heat warmer to provide servo-control of infant's body temperature. 3) IVAC infusion pump to deliver exact fluid amount through IV or umbilical catheter. 4) IBC oxygen analyzer with strip chart recorder to continuously monitor O_2 concentration of gas being delivered to patient and oxygen tension of arterial blood. 5) KDC EKG and respiration monitor with limit alarms to warn of apnea or arrhythmias and display EKG and respiration patterns. 6) Hewlett-Packard blood pressure module with transducer to directly measure arterial blood pressure. 7) Yellow Springs telethermometer to provide accurate reading of patient or air temperature.

the high-risk neonate. Chapter 38 discusses in considerable detail the specifics involved in the major nursing procedures performed on newborn infants. When machines are involved in these procedures, the theory of their mode of operation is briefly described.

DISORDERS OF TRANSITION

With the transition from fetal to extrauterine life at birth, a number of momentous physiologic changes and adjustments take place, the likes of which are never again duplicated in an entire lifetime. As described in detail in Chapter 19, respiration (the exchange of oxygen [O_2] for carbon dioxide [CO_2]) that previously was accomplished by the placenta, must now be taken over by the lungs of the newborn. This means that O_2-containing air must be brought into the alveoli (terminal air sacs) in close proximity with CO_2-laden blood flowing through the pulmonary (lung) capillaries. Fluid that previously filled the lungs has to be replaced with air, the lungs expanded further, and the alveoli stablized (kept from fully collapsing at the end of expiration). Blood flow that previously in large part bypassed the lungs now has to be redirected through the lungs to pick up the O_2 and excrete the CO_2. This involves shutting off the fetal shunts (short-cuts between heart chambers or big vessels) that allowed circumvention of the lungs. That is to say, the foramen ovale and ductus arteriosus must be closed. Rhythmic respirations have to be instituted, maintained, and constantly adjusted to meet the metabolic needs of the newborn, i.e., provide him with adequate O_2 for energy-producing processes while eliminating sufficient CO_2 to keep the blood pH (acid level) within normal range.

Many metabolic functions, such as temperature regulation and maintenance of glucose (sugar) level, which were previously taken care of by the mother must now be taken over by the infant. Foodstuffs (carbohydrates, protein, and fat), electrolytes (sodium, potassium, chloride, calcium, magnesium, and so forth), and water must be absorbed through the intestines instead of the placenta. Likewise, waste products such as urea, bilirubin, and nonvolatile acids (those acids other than CO_2 that cannot be eliminated through the lungs) must now be excreted through the liver, intestines, and kidneys. It is astounding that such a large percentage of newborn infants are able to handle all this with a minimum of support . . . that the majority of newborn babies can be considered "normal."

But what about the 10 to 20 per cent of all neonates that do encounter difficulties in making this transition from fetal to extrauterine life?

Perhaps their embryologic development was abnormal and they were born with congenital anomalies (malformations) making certain key functions, e.g., lung ventilation or perfusion, difficult or impossible.

Perhaps they suffered hypoxia (lack of oxygen) or birth trauma during delivery and were asphyxiated (depressed in vital functions) at birth.

Perhaps they had an untimely birth, born either too early (prematurely) and thus not fully equipped to make all the necessary changes, or too late (postmaturely) and thus handicapped in other ways.

Perhaps they were malnourished in utero and suffered growth retardation, resulting in inadequate energy stores to make the transition smoothly.

Perhaps they were handicapped by the effects of maternal complications of pregnancy such as Rh sensitization or an endocrine disorder such as diabetes.

If one looks closely, all processes (normal and abnormal) occurring in the immediate newborn period are influenced by the stresses imposed in making the transition from fetal to extrauterine life. This section deals with a number of conditions that make the transition very difficult or nearly impossible. Basically, these conditions present mechanical or regulatory problems that, if not quickly overcome, will lead to overwhelming metabolic disturbances disruptive of further life functions. The stage may be set already by prior fetal distress due to maternal metabolic problems or placental dysfunction but at the actual time of birth, the focus is on mechanical and regulatory problems involving the lungs, heart, and circulation. Secondarily, metabolic disturbances may arise that influence all other major organ systems including the central nervous system, liver, blood, and kidneys.

MECHANICAL PROBLEMS INVOLVING THE AIRWAYS AND LUNGS

Mechanical problems involved with breathing include anything that obstructs or restricts air movement into the lungs. The principle *obstructive defects* encountered in the immediate newborn period, starting with the upper airway and moving downward to the alveoli (terminal air sacs) are illustrated in Figure 37-2 and the disorders of function they bring with them are outlined below.

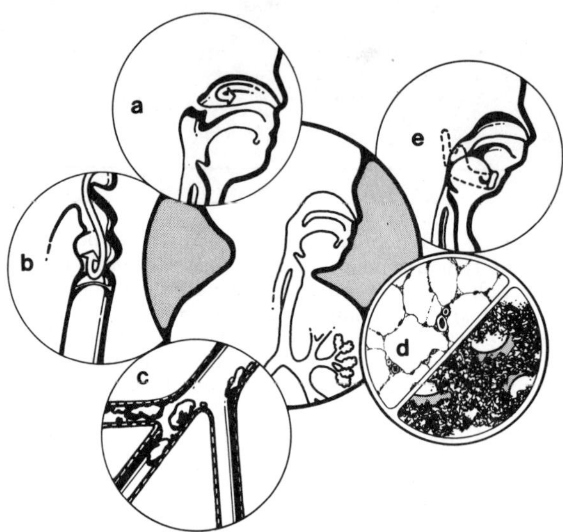

FIGURE 37-2. Obstructive defects of the respiratory tract. *a*, Choanal atresia. *b*, Laryngeal web. *c*, Meconium aspiration. *d*, Hyaline membrane disease. *e*, Micrognathia and glossoptosis.

Choanal atresia, or congenital obstruction of the posterior nares (nasal passages) (Fig. 37-2*a*). Since most newborns are obligatory nose breathers, respiratory distress and even asphyxia can occur quickly if the child is not made to cry (forcing him to breathe through his mouth), or if his mouth is not kept open (by use of an oral airway or nipple with cut-off tip).

Laryngeal (voice box) *web* (Fig. 37-2*b*) above, at, below the true vocal cords may partially or completely obstruct the airway. The newborn makes respiratory efforts but to no avail if the obstruction is complete, and will die of asphyxia if one is unable to "punch through" the web with the endotracheal tube used for intubation or if the obstruction cannot quickly be bypassed by a tracheostomy (most difficult to perform in a newborn).

Meconium aspiration syndrome (Fig. 37-2*c*) (see below under Problems of Postmaturity). Depending upon the amount and consistency of the material aspirated (breathed into the lungs by mistake) either the trachea itself or more distal airways (mainstem, segmental, or terminal bronchi) can be partially or completely blocked off, making adequate ventilation impossible. Here again the airway must be cleared, either by direct suctioning or by lavage (rinsing out) followed by suctioning if the baby is to avoid immediate suffocation or subsequent respiratory failure due to inflammation and swelling, closing off the lower airways.

Alveolar atelectasis (collapse of the alveoli) (Fig. 37-2*d*). Atelectasis can result from total obstruction of proximal airways or deficient surfactant (a substance produced in the alveolar lining cells to reduce wall tension and overcome the tendency of the small air sacs to collapse). The most common condition involving alveolar atelectasis in the newborn is hyaline membrane disease, to be discussed under Problems of Prematurity. The two principle methods of support in this situation are to provide enriched oxygen concentration to breathe to overcome the associated hypoxia, and to apply a constant positive distending pressure to the airways to forcefully keep the alveoli from collapsing.

Micrognathia (small lower jaw) and *glossoptosis* (posterior positioning of falling back of the tongue) (Fig. 37-2*e*). Micrognathia associated with a cleft palate, as in the Pierre Robin syndrome, not only leads to upper airway obstruction when the tongue falls back to the posterior wall of the pharynx blocking off the lower pharynx, but also if the tip of the tongue goes through the cleft and fills the midportion of the nasal passages. Emergency treatment is needed to establish an oral or nasal airway around and behind the tongue.

Restrictive defects interfering with lung expansion may originate from within (intrinsic) or from without the lung (extrinsic), or both. Important *intrinsic* pulmonary restrictive defects are illustrated in Figure 37-3 and outlined below.

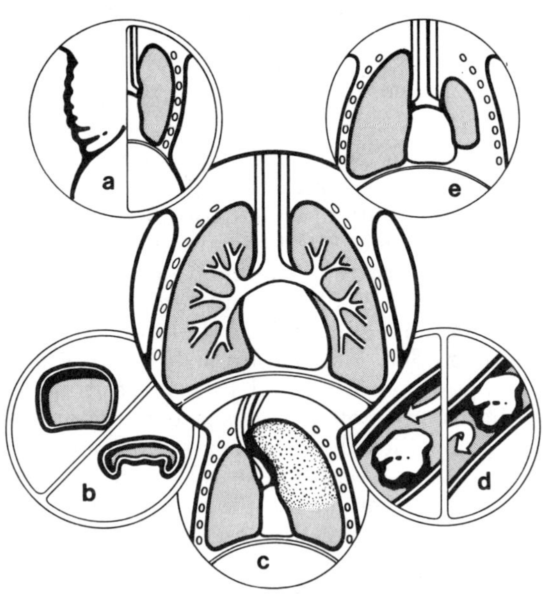

FIGURE 37-3. Intrinsic restrictive defects of the respiratory system. *a*, Thoracic dystrophy (small chest cage). *b*, Tracheal collapse as mechanisms for development of lobar emphysema. *c*, Lobar emphysema. *d*, Air trapping behind partial occlusion of bronchus as mechanism for development of lobar emphysema. *e*, Hypoplastic.

Hypoplastic (underdeveloped) *lungs* (Fig. 37-3*e*). A lung or both lungs may fail to develop fully due to an inherent growth disturbance or because of some early restriction of the space in which the fetal lungs develop. The latter situation is seen in *congenital diaphragmatic hernia* (see below) in which abdominal contents in the chest from early gestation restrict the space needed for lung development, or in *thoracic dystrophy* (Fig. 37-3*a*) in which an inherently small chest cage prevents full lung expansion and development. Treatment involves careful support of ventilation until the lungs have developed to the point where they can provide the necessary gas exchange themselves.

Lobar emphysema (overdistention of one or more lobes of the lung) (Fig. 37-3*c*). The selective trapping of air in one portion of the lung may result from a number of causes. Bronchi tend to expand on inspiration and contract on expiration due to the negative and then positive pressure exerted upon them during the respiratory cycle. If a *foreign body* (Fig. 37-3*d*) is partially occluding the lumen of the main airway leading to that lobe, air will be allowed in on inspiration when the air tube widens, but will not be able to escape on expiration as it narrows around the occluding object. If the cartilage framework of a major airway is deficient, as in *tracheal malacia* (Fig. 37-3*b*), it will tend to collapse on expiration and trap air behind it. If the overdistended lobe is seriously compressing other portions of normal lung or shifting the mediastinum (soft tissue space between the lungs, and including the heart and major vessels) so as to compromise return of blood to the heart by way of the great veins, then that lobe must be surgically resected if no intraluminal obstructing object can be found on bronchoscopy (viewing of the lumen of the bronchi with an optical instrument called a bronchoscope).

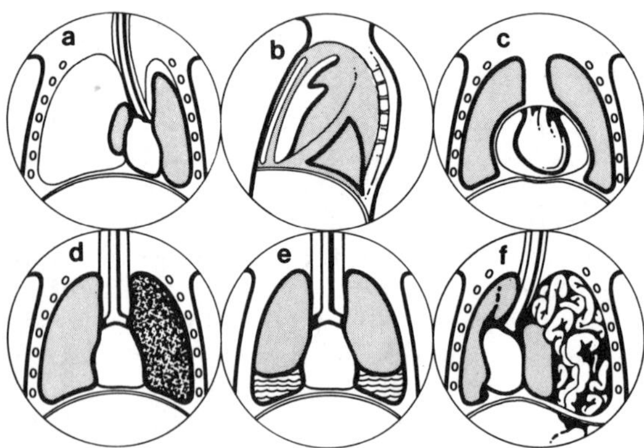

FIGURE 37-4. Extrinsic restrictive defects of respiratory system. *a*, Tension pneumothorax. *b*, Pneumomediastinum. *c*, Pneumopericardium. *d*, Pulmonary interstitial emphysema. *e*, Pleural effusion. *f*, Congenital diaphragmatic hernia.

Extrinsic causes of lung restriction are much more common and tend to present a more acute situation. Important extrinsic restrictive defects are illustrated in Figure 37-4 and outlined below.

Pulmonary air leak, or accumulation of air leaked out of ruptured alveoli into spaces where air is not normally found, such as the intrathoracic space (*pneumothorax*) (Fig. 37-4*a*), mediastinum (*pneumomediastinum*) (Fig. 37-4*b*), pericardial sac (*pneumopericardium*) (Fig. 37-4*c*), or interstitual space of the lung tissue (*pulmonary interstitial emphysema*) (Fig. 37-4*d*). When pressure builds up in these spaces, surrounding lung tissue or vital organs (great vessels, mediastinum, heart) can be restricted and their function impeded. Ventilation, venous blood return to the heart, or diastolic filling of the heart chambers, and therefore, cardiac output (amount of blood advanced by the heart per minute) are diminished as a result. Treatment when possible is achieved by placing a tube into the space and attaching it to a one-way valve, allowing the trapped air under pressure to escape but not allowing outside air to enter the space when a negative pressure is produced by the patient during deep inspiration.

Pleural effusion, or collection of fluid in the intrathoracic space (Fig. 37-4*e*). Most commonly, pleural effusions are associated with generalized edema or hydrops as seen in severe Rh erythoblastosis (see below), severe maternal anemia, or hypoproteinemia and congenital nephrosis. The effusion generally resolves as the resulting anemia or hypoproteinemia in the newborn is corrected. If respirations are restricted to the point of respiratory failure (severe hypoxia and/or CO_2 retention), then the fluid must be tapped off (thorocentesis), or the baby provided with mechanical support of ventilation and enriched oxygen to breathe until the effusion is reabsorbed.

Abdominal distention restricting downward movement of the diaphragm. Since newborns, and especially prematures, predominantly breathe with their diaphragms, restrictive abdominal distention of any cause poses a serious threat and demands immediate decompression of the stomach (by way of a nasogastric tube) and correction of the underlying cause of distention once it is identified.

Congenital diaphragmatic hernia (Fig. 37-4*f*) involves an early developmental defect most often in the posterolateral (to the back and side) portion of the left hemidiaphragm. Abdominal contents find their way through the defect and compress the lung on that side, shift the mediastinum to the opposite side, and thereby compress the right lung as well. Hypoplasia of the rapidly developing lungs results, worse on the left side than on the right. If one attempts to rapidly expand such underdeveloped lungs they are likely to rupture, which results in pneumothorax and a rapid worsening of the condition. This is still true after surgery when the abdominal contents are back in the abdomen. Extreme care must be exercised in supporting ventilation in this situation, and frequently all efforts are to no avail since the lungs are just too small to provide adequate gas exchange.

MECHANICAL PROBLEMS INVOLVING THE PULMONARY CIRCULATION

Mechanical problems of transition involving the pulmonary circulation include those situations which result in continued bypassing of the lungs by blood through right-to-left (R→ L) shunts at the atrial and ductal level (as in the fetal circulation), and congenital heart defects involving obstruction of blood flow into or out of the lungs.

Persistent Pulmonary Vascular Obstruction. This is the term now used to describe persistence of the fetal-type circulation beyond the usual time after birth. This condition is not uncommon, yet has just recently been appreciated. Resistance to flow of blood through the pulmonary circulation remains high, so that the blood continues to take the easier routes across the foramen ovale or through the ductus arteriosus instead of to the lungs. The reasons why pulmonary vascular resistance does not drop quickly after birth in the usual fashion to let the blood flow through are not yet fully understood. We do know, however, that chronic fetal hypoxia with thickening of the pulmonary arterioles, and polycythemia (excessive number of red blood cells) may have this effect, as can any condition that limits lung expansion (see above) or delays the rise in oxygen tension in the blood after birth (see below under Asphyxia Neonatorum). Since these babies are often severely cyanotic and have a relatively normal chest roentgenogram, they mistakenly may be thought to have some form of congenital heart disease and are then subjected to cardiac catheterization. Instead, conservative treatment is indicated which involves maximum expansion of the lungs, oxygen therapy, and acidosis correction until such time as the pulmonary resistance subsides and blood flow through the lungs increases. A number of these infants cannot be helped and die of increasing hypoxia.

Patent Ductus Arteriosus. One might think that a patent (still open) ductus alone could lead to continued shunting of blood past the lungs going right-to-left from the pulmonary artery directly to the aorta. This undoubtedly is the case to a large degree in persistent pulmonary vascular obstruction described above, and to a lesser degree in the early stages of hyaline membrane disease where the ductal R→ L shunt may amount to as much as 5 to 8 per cent. However, the much more common situation is for the blood to flow left-to-right (L → R) through the ductus because the pressure in the aorta is generally higher than that in the pulmonary artery. This also turns out to be the case in the baby with hyaline membrane disease who has passed the peak of his disease and is now getting better. As the lungs open up and pulmonary vascular resistance drops, blood starts shunting L → R though the ductus which floods the pulmonary circulation with blood and puts a great strain on the left side of the heart which has to pump the blood out again when it returns to the left heart from the lungs. As the left heart begins to fail and blood backs up behind it into the lungs, the baby's respiratory status worsens—his oxygen requirements go back up and the work of breathing with a stiffer lung also increases. If heart action cannot be adequately strengthened by digitalis, or the water in the lungs eliminated by diuretics, then surgical correction by ligating (tying off) the ductus must be carried out, no matter how small the baby is at the time.

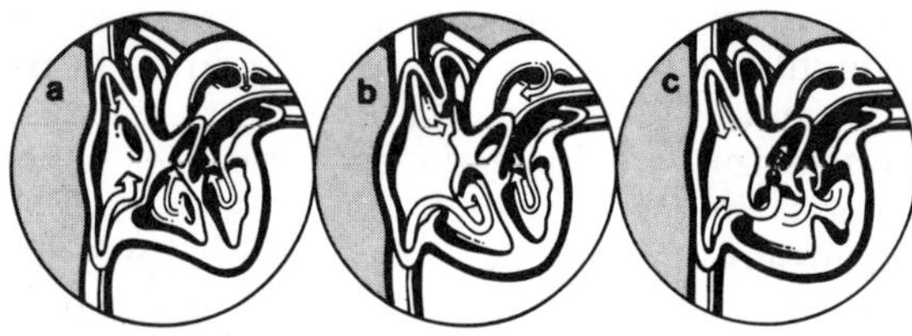

FIGURE 37-5. Congenital heart defects obstructing blood flow to the lungs. *a*, Tricuspid atresia. *b*, Pulmonary valvular atresia. *c*, Tetralogy of Fallot.

There are a number of *congenital heart defects* that involve *obstruction to right outflow*, or blockage of the movement of blood from the right side of the heart to the lungs (Fig. 37-5). Two of the more common forms of this, tricuspid atresia and pulmonary atresia, are often associated with a very small (hypoplastic) right ventricle. Clinically they are characterized by marked cyanosis that does not respond to oxygen, chest roentgenograms that show a small heart and underperfused lungs, initial lack of respiratory distress, and good pulses and blood pressure since left-sided cardiac output is normal or even increased.

Tricuspid Atresia (Fig. 37-5*a*). In cases where there is complete aplasia (total lack of development) of the tricuspid valve (between the right atrium and right ventricle), all blood returning to the heart must go across the foramen ovale to get to the left side. From there it must take one of two devious routes to get to the lungs: either it can go out the aorta from the left ventricle and double back L → R through the ductus to the pulmonary artery and lungs, or it can go across a high ventricular septum defect to the small right ventricle and out the pulmonary artery to the lungs. Real difficulties may arise when the ductus closes and/or the ventricular septum defect gets smaller. Tricuspid atresia may be associated with other heart anomalies such as pulmonary valve hypoplasia, or with transposition of the great vessels (see below). Incomplete blockage of the tricuspid valve (tricuspid stenosis) with or without other heart defects is also known to occur.

Pulmonary Atresia (Fig. 37-5*b*). If there is total blockage of blood flow through the pulmonary valve (between right ventricle and the pulmonary artery) and there is no associated ventricular septum defect, the only way blood can get to the lungs is through the ductus L → R after it has gone across the foramen ovale and down and out the left ventricle and aorta. When the ductus closes in this situation, the baby dies unless the pulmonary valve can be sprung open in surgery, or another connection between the aorta and (right) pulmonary artery (Waterston shunt) can be made. To increase the flow of blood from the right to the left side and thus circumvent the right outflow obstruction, a bigger hole is also made in the atrial septum (between right and left atrium) by balloon septostomy (Rashkin procedure). This involves passing a catheter across the foramen ovale into the left atrium, blowing up a small balloon on the tip of the catheter, and then pulling it back to the right side smartly, thus opening up a bigger hole in the septum for blood to flow through R → L.

Pulmonary atresia with an open ventricular septum (*pseudotruncus arteriosus*) also occurs, but offers no advantage to the newborn since right outflow is still completely obstructed and there is almost complete dependence on the ductus.

Pulmonary Stenosis (narrowing of a lumen). This occurs rarely below the pulmonary valve (infundibular stenosis), most commonly at the valve (pulmonic valvular stenosis) or very rarely out in the pulmonary arteries (peripheral pulmonary arterial stenoses). The main mechanical problem in all these cases is an obstruction to blood flow out the right side of the heart to the lungs and difficulty achieving a higher pressure beyond the obstruction than is present in the left atrium so that blood can flow through the lungs in sufficient quantity. These conditions rarely give the newborn clinically evident difficulty unless the stenosis is very tight or there are associated heart defects.

Pulmonic stenosis in conjunction with a high ventricular septum defect and an aorta that rides over that defect receiving blood from both the right and left ventricles constitutes the *tetralogy of Fallot* (Fig. 37-5*c*). The hemodynamic (blood flow mechanical) problem here is that the resistance to flow out the pulmonary artery due to the stenosis is greater than it is out the aorta. Thus, blood preferentially shunts R → L across the ventricular septum defect and out the aorta or straight up into the overriding aorta. Since a considerable portion of the blood being pumped by the heart thus gets over to the left side without having to go through the lungs, the baby is left cyanotic to a greater or lesser degree. Few newborns with tetralogy get into serious difficulty, because neither heart chamber is pumping blood against a high pressure, and so heart failure is very unlikely to occur. Complete surgical correction can be accomplished at a later date by closing the ventricular septum defect and opening up the stenotic pulmonary valve.

Other congenital heart defects that affect pulmonary circulation and leave the baby cyanotic include *t*otal anomalous venous return, *t*runcus arteriosus, and *t*ransposition of the great arteries (Fig. 37-6). All three of these can be diagnosed in the newborn period and when combined with the other two defects described above that also begin with a "t" (*t*ricuspid atresia and *t*etralogy of Fallot) they constitute well over half of all congenital cyanotic heart disease.

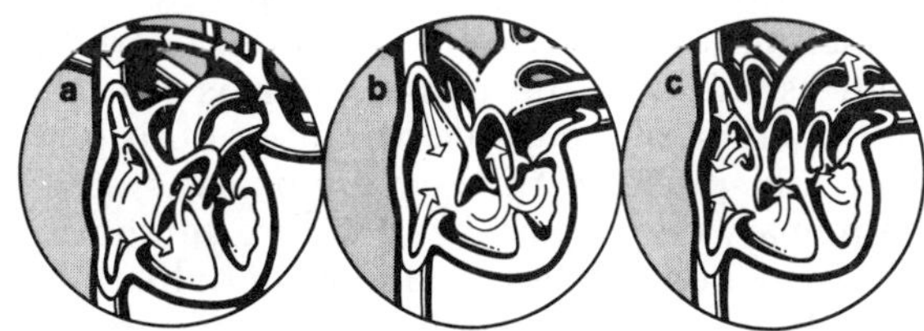

FIGURE 37-6. Cyanotic congenital heart defects. *a*, Total anomalous pulmonary venous return. *b*, Truncus arteriosus. *c*, Transposition of the great arteries.

Total Anomalous Pulmonary Venous Drainage, or transposition (reversal) of the pulmonary veins (Fig. 37-6*a*). This condition involves an aberrant system of blood return from the lungs. Rather than returning the oxygenated blood to the left atrium, it is dumped back into the right side of the circulation to go around again. Drainage from the lungs may be either above the diaphragm into the superior vena cava, azygous vein, or sinus venosus, or below the diaphragm into the portal vein or ductus venosus. Frequently, pulmonary venous obstruction is involved with backing up of blood into the lungs (pulmonary venous congestion) and subsequently increased pressure in the pulmonary arteries, against which the right heart has to pump. Pulmonary edema (leakage of fluid out of the lung veins into the lung tissues and alveoli) and right ventricular hypertrophy (compensatory enlargement) with later dilation and failure can all occur. In these cases, surgery must be performed quickly if the baby is to survive, yet it is often very difficult or impossible to hook up the pulmonary vein(s) back to the left atrium.

Truncus Arteriosus (Fig. 37-6*b*). Signs include a large heart (cardiomegaly), increased pulmonary blood flow, and high pressures in the pulmonary circulation. In this defect, only one great artery comes out of the heart on top of one valve that spans the outflow tracts of the right and left ventricles. Invariably there is a large ventricular septum defect between the two pumping chambers. The pressure and blood flow in the pulmonary arteries that branch off this main trunk are often nearly as high as those in the aorta which is just the continuation of the trunk. Because of this high flow and pressure in the pulmonary system, pulmonary edema and heart failure can occur. This may be palliated (temporarily helped) by "banding" (constricting) the pulmonary arteries. A string is tied around the vessels narrowing their lumen so that the pressure and blood flow beyond the point of banding is reduced to a tolerable range. Later, when the child gets bigger, complicated corrective surgery may be performed.

Transposition of the Great Arteries (Fig. 37-6*c*). This may also lead to pulmonary venous congestion and respiratory distress due to pulmonary edema (in cases where there is an intact ventricular septum). However, the main problem is one of hypoxemia (low oxygen level) in the blood going out to the body. Unless there is some other means of mixing blood between the right and left sides of the circulation through a ventricular or atrial septum defect or open foramen ovale or ductus arteriosus, the baby will quickly die of hypoxia. This is because the oxygenated blood returning from the lungs gets pumped right back out to the lungs, since the pulmonary artery comes off the left ventricle and the aorta comes off the right. Balloon septostomy (described above) then becomes an emergency procedure before the ductus (the one remaining point of mixing) closes spontaneously.

There are many more forms of congenital heart disease that are not discussed here. Defects such as atrial septum defect (ASD), ventricular septum defect (VSD) and coarctation (tightening or narrowing) of the aorta are all relatively common, and are frequently associated with other malformations. Coarctation of the aorta, large VSD's, hypoplastic left heart syndrome (underdeveloped left ventricle, aortic valve, and ascending aorta), and patent ductus arteriosus with L → R shunting are the most common causes of left heart failure in the newborn period. Prior to going into failure, these patients are not cyanotic. Excepting left heart hypoplasia, these defects can frequently be managed conservatively (using digitalis to strengthen the contractility of the heart, diuretics to remove excess water from the lungs, and enriched oxygen to breathe). With newer surgical and supportive techniques (discussed in the next chapter) some of these otherwise lethal conditions can be palliated or totally corrected even in the newborn period.

ASPHYXIA NEONATORUM

Asphyxia neonatorum is the broad term used to indicate delayed onset of breathing at the time of birth. Literally, the word asphyxia means "no pulse," which implies depression of heart action and collapse of the circulation. Certainly serious cardiac and circulatory malfunction does occur in any prolonged delay in the onset of breathing, as will be described in more detail below. However, of more immediate importance is the reduced availability of oxygen (hypoxia) or total lack of O_2 (anoxia) and the inability to eliminate CO_2 (hypercarbia) which accompany the asphyxia.

Causes of newborn asphyxia or hypoxia can originate in the mother, the placenta, the delivery process, or the baby himself. A number of the more common causes are listed in Table 37-1. Basically, we are dealing with problems of transport, exchange, or regulation, as is made clear in the following examples:

1. Prenatally, the total amount of maternal

TABLE 37-1. Causes of Asphyxia Neonatorum

I. Maternal Causes
  A. Reduced blood flow to the placenta
    1. Maternal heart disease affecting the pumping of blood
    2. Maternal vascular disease affecting the flow of blood
      a. Preeclampsia or toxemia
      b. Arteritis due to advance diabetes, lupus, etc.
    3. Compression of the abdominal arteries and veins by the uterus
    4. Maternal hypotension or acute shock
    5. Prolonged uterine contractions
  B. Reduced oxygen content of the blood flowing to the placenta
    1. Maternal hypoxia due to cyanotic heart disease or severe lung disease
    2. Maternal anemia
    3. Abnormal hemoglobin or oxygen binding to hemoglobin
II. Placental and Cord Causes
  A. Placental insufficiency due to vascular disease, infarcts, edema (hydrops placenta), infection, fibrinosis, etc.
  B. Placental separation or placenta praevia
  C. True knot in cord, nuchal cord, or prolapsed cord.
III. Neonatal Causes
  A. Mechanical problems involving the airways and lungs
    1. Obstructive defects without or within, such as choanal atresia, glossoptosis, laryngeal web, aspiration syndrome, etc.
    2. Restrictive problems within or without the lungs such as lobar or interstitial emphysema, hyaline membrane disease, pneumothorax, pneumomediastinum, diaphragmatic hernia, eventration, pleural effusion, etc.
  B. Mechanical problems involving the flow of blood to or from the lungs
    1. Obstruction of right outflow, such as tricuspid atresia, Ebstein's anomaly, pulmonary stenosis or atresia
    2. Obstruction or abnormal return of blood back from the lungs, such as total anomalous venous return and transposition
  C. Depressed respiratory center
    1. Due to previous fetal distress and hypoxemia and acidosis
    2. Due to passage of depressant drugs or toxins from the mother to the fetus
    3. Due to increased intracranial pressure secondary to hemorrhage, infection, or congenital CNS anomaly.

blood flowing to the placenta was reduced (due to maternal cardiac or vascular problems, or excessive contraction of the uterus), or the oxygen content of that blood was reduced (due to maternal lung problems leading to low levels of oxygen dissolved in the blood, or to anemia resulting in low levels of hemoglobin to bind and carry the oxygen to the tissues).

2. There was a reduction in the amount of exchange of gases, foodstuffs, and waste products between the maternal and fetal sides of the placenta (due to placental insufficiency or abnormalities).
3. The flow of blood to and from the baby and the placenta was interrupted or diminished (due to umbilical cord anomalies or occlusion).
4. There was previous passage across the placenta of products of abnormal maternal metabolism, drugs, or bacteria or their toxins that depress the respiratory center or adversely influence cardiovascular and pulmonary function of the newborn.
5. There existed in the newborn certain anomalies that mechanically restricted or obstructed ventilation of the lungs, reduced pulmonary blood flow, or interfered with the regulation of respiration and heartbeat. The more important mechanical problems of transition in the newborn were discussed in detail above.

If one knows which maternal diseases are likely to reduce the quantity and O_2 content of blood flowing to the placenta, or if one utilizes the tests to evaluate placental function, or if one knows the drug history of the mother before and during labor, or if one knows the forewarning signs of congenital anomalies in the fetus, then one can anticipate impending neonatal asphyxia in the majority of cases and be ready for it. We also know that asphyxia neonatorum is seen more frequently in babies born postmaturely (delivery overdue by more than two weeks) or in babies who are small-for-dates (having suffered fetal growth retarda-

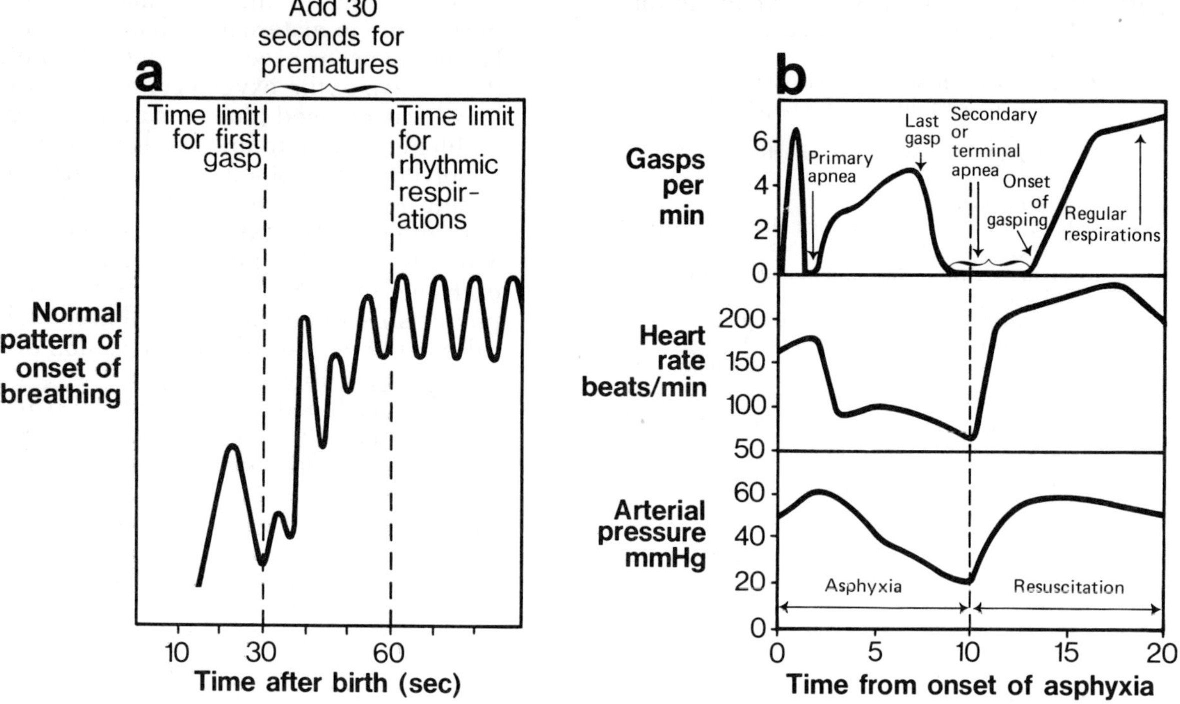

FIGURE 37-7. Clinical assessment of asphyxia. Normal (*A*) and abnormal (*B*) patterns of breathing and other vital signs.

tion). Other intrapartal signs suggestive of impending birth asphyxia include meconium staining of the amniotic fluid (hypoxia activates bowel movement) and certain patterns of fetal heart rate change monitored during labor. These patterns were discussed in detail in Chapter 26.

The degree of asphyxia or depression of a newborn at the time of birth can be assessed by clinical and laboratory means. The Apgar scoring system (see Chapter 31) allows quick clinical assessment by assigning 0 to 2 points for each of five objective signs: Color (*A*ppearance), heart rate (*P*ulse), reflex activity (*G*rimace), muscle tone (*A*ctivity level), and respiratory effort (*R*espirations). Any total score of less than 7 is considered to indicate asphyxia. "Mildly depressed" infants have scores between 4 and 6, while "severely depressed" infants have scores between 0 and 3 points. Thus, high-risk newborns can be assessed quickly and accurately for the presence and degree of asphyxia. The one-minute Apgar score identifies babies requiring immediate resuscitation, whereas the five-minute score better indicates the severity of the asphyxia and the possible outcome (prognosis). Convincing correlations have been demonstrated between these scores and actual blood chemistry changes known to occur during various degrees of asphyxia (see discussion below on blood gas changes in asphyxia).

Another means of clinically assessing the severity of asphyxia at birth is through accurate timing of the onset of breathing and close observation of the pattern of ensuing respirations. *Normal* term infants take their first breath around 15 seconds and never later than 30 seconds of life. After 3 to 5 gasp-like efforts, sustained rhythmic respirations should be established no later than 60 seconds after birth. Prematures may take 15 to 30 seconds longer to achieve these goals (Fig. 37-7*a*).

Intrapartum asphyxia delays the onset and alters the pattern of respiration, as do most analgesics and anesthetics administered to the mother just prior to delivery. From experiments on newborn Rhesus monkeys, which most closely resemble the human situation, we know that acute total asphyxia produced by clamping the cord and not allowing the animal to breathe air results in a definite time sequence of respiratory efforts (Fig. 37-7*b*):

1. After approximately one minute of struggling and rapid gasping, *primary apnea* (period of nonbreathing) sets in. During primary apnea, the heartbeat falls to about one half its normal rate and levels off, blood pressure actually increases as a means of compensation for the low pulse, and muscle tone persists. Primary apnea is followed by renewed gasping which then gradually decreases in strength and frequency over the next 4 to 5 minutes.
2. The "last gasp" comes after about 6 to 7 minutes of total acute asphyxia, and *secondary asphyxia* sets in. Now heart rate and blood pressure fall rapidly and all muscle tone is lost. If resuscitation is not begun immediately, permanent brain damage will occur. The longer the delay in providing assisted ventilation after secondary apnea begins, the greater the time elapses before spontaneous gasps and rhythmic respirations will be reestablished.

Since brain damage is associated with the early stages of secondary apnea even if subsequent resuscitation is successful, it is most important to distinguish between primary and secondary apnea. If the infant breathed or cried before becoming apneic, this is primary apnea. Likewise, if gasping returns before color improves or if spontaneous respirations can be induced by pain or cold stimulus, one is still dealing with primary apnea. Oxygen reserves are quickly depleted when the newborn stops breathing and he becomes cyanotic (*blue asphyxia*). However, circulation is maintained in this earlier stage of asphyxia since blood pressure rises in response to peripheral vasoconstriction and less vital areas of the body are excluded from the central circulation. On the other hand, secondary apnea is present if spontaneous respirations can no longer be induced by sensory stimuli, or if color improves before gasping returns in response to assisted ventilation. Since both heart rate and blood pressure have now fallen below tolerable levels, and muscle and vasomotor tone are no longer present, the newborn is in shock and appears more pale than cyanotic (*pallid asphyxia*).

As mentioned above, the degree of asphyxia as judged by Apgar scores correlates well with the extent of blood gas changes. The latter therefore represents another means of assessing the degree of asphyxia the infant suffered, with two important qualifications. First, one must know that every normal delivery involves a certain amount of "physiologic" asphyxia. The mean arterial oxygen tension (Pa_{O_2} or partial pressure of oxygen physically dissolved in arterial blood) is less than 20 mm. Hg (normal adult level is between 80 and 95), whereas the mean Pa_{CO_2} (partial pressure of carbon dioxide in arterial blood) in normal newborns at birth is about 50 mm. Hg (normal adult value is 40). The mean pH value is 7.26 (instead of the normal of 7.40), and the mean bicarbonate level in normal newborns is 19 mEq. per liter (normal adult value is 24). With the onset of respiration in normal newborns, these values quickly approach acceptable adult levels: Pa_{O_2} is up to 50 in less than

10 minutes and over 60 by one hour; $PaCO_2$ is down to 40 within 20 minutes, and compensates for more persistent metabolic acidosis (low bicarbonate) by going even below 40 mm. Hg by 30 minutes of age; pH consequently rises to about 7.30 by 30 minutes and 7.34 by one hour of age. These not-so-normal normal values of regular newborns must be appreciated before proper comparisons can be made with those of asphyxiated infants.

The speed at which blood gas values change for the worse during total acute asphyxia has been precisely determined for newborn monkeys: PaO_2 falls to near zero in less than 5 minutes; $PaCO_2$ rises at a rate of about 8 mm. Hg per minute; pH falls about 0.04 pH units per minute; and bicarbonate drops nearly 2 mEq. per liter per minute. However, and this is a second important qualification, asphyxia in the usual human situation is not one of pure acute total asphyxia starting at the time of birth. Rather, acute asphyxia is superimposed upon previous chronic asphyxia in utero. Thus, one would need to know how bad the blood gas values were at the time of birth plus how much time had elapsed before resuscitation was begun to be able to predict how much hypoxia, hypercarbia, and acidosis the baby suffered in the process.

The metabolic changes that occur with asphyxia and hypoxia eventually affect all bodily functions, but some more rapidly and severely than others. As available oxygen is quickly depleted, the organism is forced to switch from aerobic (utilizing oxygen) metabolism of glucose, which produces high quantities of energy plus CO_2 and water, to anaerobic (without O_2) breakdown of glucose (glycolysis), which yields lactate (a nonvolatile acid) and much less energy. Glucose is mobilized from glycogen stores in the liver (already reduced in prematures and newborns with prior fetal distress) in response to the excretion of adrenalin and steroids from the adrenal glands in answer to the stress of hypoxia. Lipolysis (breakdown of the triglyceride fats to glycerol and free fatty acids [FFA]) also is stimulated by the secretion of adrenalin, and some energy is thereby produced. This comes from the further oxidation of FFA and resulting ketone bodies, but is limited by the lack of oxygen and tends to produce more nonvolatile acids which further contribute to the metabolic acidosis.

The pathophysiologic effects of *hypoxemia* (low oxygen tension in arterial blood) in the newborn include:

1. Persistence of the fetal-type circulation with high pulmonary vascular resistance, poor blood flow through the lungs, continued patency of the foramen ovale and ductus arteriosus with right-to-left shunting of blood at the atrial and ductal level. The explanation for this is that high oxygen tension in the blood is essential for opening up the pulmonary circulation and closing the ductus.
2. Loss of ability to maintain body temperature during cold stress, since heat production involves oxygen-consuming metabolic processes, and cannot proceed without O_2.
3. Reduction in responsiveness of the respiratory center so that it becomes increasingly difficult to start respirations. Note: A little hypoxia stimulates respiration, whereas severe hypoxia paralyzes the respiratory center.

The extreme *hypercarbia* resulting from asphyxia also adversely affects the respiratory center. Note: A little CO_2 retention acts as a stimulus to respiration, whereas severe CO_2 retention "anesthetizes" the patient.

The pathophysiologic effects of the *acidosis* accompanying asphyxia are innumerable and include the following:

1. Many *metabolic processes* producing energy and new substances are pH-dependent, and are depressed under

conditions of acidosis. For example, the process of breaking down glycogen (the storage form of glucose) to lactate in order to produce energy when oxygen is scarce or lacking (as is the case during asphyxia) is itself depressed when the pH falls much below normal.

2. Likewise, the formation of certain *clotting factors* and other crucial proteins is inhibited during periods of metabolic acidosis.
3. *Cell membrane potentials* (necessary to regulate the movement of ions such as K^+ and Na^+ in and out of the cell), as well as *active transport systems* (energy-requiring processes that move other substances in and out of cells and organs) are strongly influenced by pH, and break down altogether in extreme acidosis.
4. *Myocardial* (heart muscle) *responsiveness* to sympathetic amines (such as adrenalin) is reduced by acidosis, and heart rate and cardiac output (amount of blood pumped per minute) are thus depressed.

Knowing the rapid course of events and pathophysiologic mechanisms involved in neonatal asphyxia aids us now in fashioning a rational plan of therapy.

1. The airway must be cleared (Fig. 37-8*A*) and the infant stimulated to cry. If this cannot be achieved by simple tactile (touch) or cold stimuli, then assisted ventilation (mouth-to-mouth, bag and mask [Fig. 37-8*B*], or mechanical ventilation with a respirator) must be instituted. Volume expansion of the lungs does much to lower pulmonary vascular resistance and increase the amount of cardiac output going to the lungs to pick up oxygen. Ventilation eliminates the respiratory component to the acidosis (see above).
2. Oxygen is to be administered in a concentration sufficient to raise the PaO_2

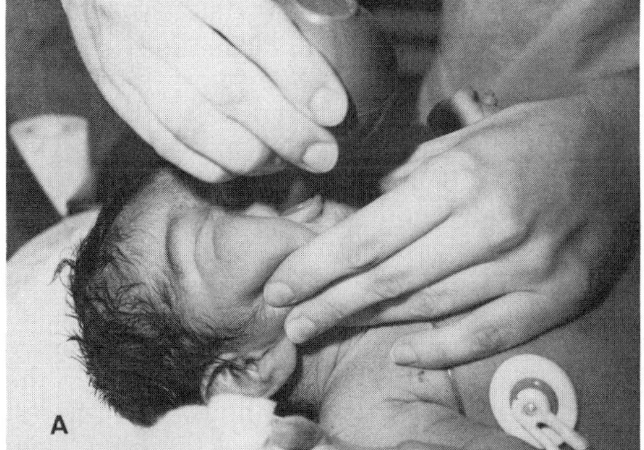

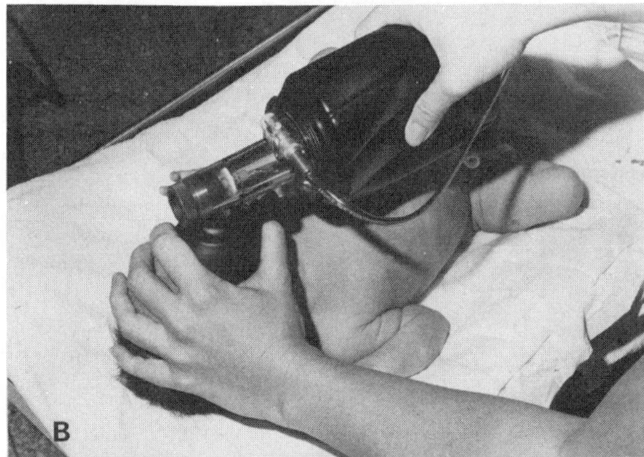

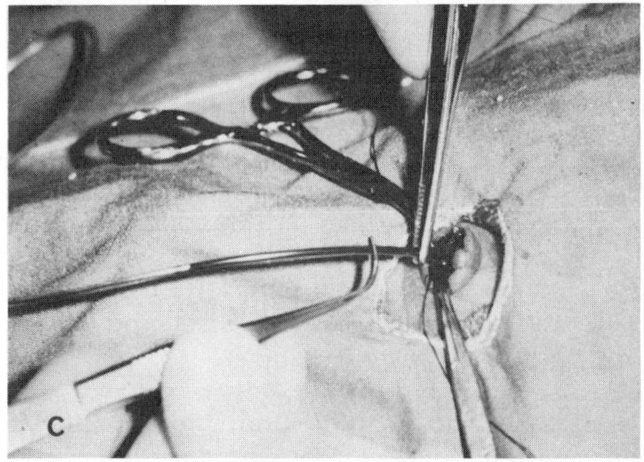

FIGURE 37-8. Plan of therapy for resuscitation of the newborn. *A*, Clearing the upper airway. *B*, Expanding the lungs and administering oxygen with a bag and mask set-up. *C*, Placement of umbilical catheter for administration of sodium bicarbonate and to measure blood pressure.

above 60 mm. Hg and thus largely saturate the hemoglobin of the body's blood. Depending on his hematocrit (portion of blood made up of red cells), the infant will lose his cyanosis and appear pink when about 80 to 85 per cent of his arterial blood is saturated with oxygen (see discussion on cyanosis below under Polycythemia). The rise in amount of oxygen in the lungs and blood further lowers pulmonary vascular resistance and increases blood flow through the lungs. This in turn reduces right-to-left shunting of blood around the lungs, and helps in closing the foramen ovale and ductus arteriosus. Oxygen is now available to tissues for energy production by the more efficient aerobic pathways.

3. Dilute sodium bicarbonate is administered intravenously (Fig. 37-8C) to correct the metabolic component of the acidosis. This restores responsiveness of the respiratory center and the myocardium, and reactivates a host of enzymatic processes. Pulmonary vascular resistance is also reduced, although this may be due more to the volume expansion of the circulation accompanying the bicarbonate infusion than to correcting the pH itself.
4. Blood pressure is kept above a systolic value of 45 mm. Hg by administering volume expanders (transfusing blood, plasma, or albumin) so as to maintain adequate cardiac output. This in turn assures adequate pulmonary perfusion, pick-up of O_2 in the lungs, transport of O_2 and substances to the tissues, and the removal of waste products.

Hypoxic damage to the brain, heart, kidneys, and liver of newborns who have suffered birth asphyxia has been studied extensively. It is important to know what this damage involves, so that one can anticipate funtional defects and problems that are likely to arise in newborns who have suffered asphyxia. Also, the ultimate prognosis for the infant can in large part be determined by observing the degrees of functional disability arising in the immediate postasphyxic period.

The amount and pattern of damage resulting from hypoxia is dependent upon the type, intensity, and duration of the hypoxia, and upon the degree of maturation of the organism. Which tissues are most damaged by hypoxia is dependent upon their O_2 and energy requirements (metabolic level) and the proportion of aerobic to anaerobic metabolism they are equipped to perform. All this has application to the newborn, but many specifics are yet to be worked out and the details are very complicated. Therefore, only a brief outline of the major points will be presented here.

Stagnant hypoxia (lack of oxgyen delivery to the tissues due to circulatory insufficiency or shock) is generally more damaging than *hypoxic hypoxia* (low Pa_{O_2} but intact circulation), because the tissues are also deprived of nutrients as well as oxygen and there is an accumulation of toxic waste products. The fetal heart and brain are best protected from stagnant hypoxia because they receive the majority of the blood returning from the placenta by way of direct line through the ductus venosus, foramen ovale, and ascending aorta. Under conditions of hypoxia, a greater proportion of the blood returning to the heart from the superior vena cava is shunted across the foramen ovale to maintain the amount of blood perfusing the heart and brain at a time when cardiac output is falling (see above).

Acute total asphyxia at the time of birth in a previously normal fetus results in major destruction to brainstem nuclei with postasphyxic difficulty in sucking and swallowing, as well as sensory loss over the extremities. In contrast, acute asphyxia at birth superimposed upon prolonged fetal hypoxia results in brain swelling and scarring in areas of the basal ganglia and paracentral cerebral cortex. The latter pattern of damage most closely resembles that seen in the majority of cerebral palsy cases. As regards the liver, the right half is likely to suffer more damage than the left in cases of fetal hypoxia because a greater portion of the blood returning from the placenta through the umbilical vein goes to the left side. After birth and the clamping of the cord, the left side of the liver is more apt to suffer stagnant hypoxic damage because it was relatively more dependent on the umbilical vein for its blood supply.

Newborns, and even more so prematures, are somewhat protected from hypoxic brain damage because of their immaturity and reduced cerebral metabolism rate as compared with adults. The less mature a brain is, the lower its energy requirements and the longer it can tolerate periods of hypoxia without irreversible damage. Generally speaking, it is also true that the ratio of anaerobic to aerobic metabolism is greater the more immature and undifferentiated (lacking in complex function) the central nervous system (CNS) is. This makes the more immature brain better able to carry on energy-consuming processes when oxygen is scarce. On the other hand, the more premature a newborn is, the more likely he is to suffer intracranial hemorrhage (subependymal, intraventricular, subarachnoid, and brainstem bleeding) secondary to hypoxic insult, and thus also suffer brain damage and/or death.

Specific problems that may be anticipated in the newborn who has suffered severe asphyxia and hypoxia involve malfunction of the CNS, lungs, heart, liver, adrenals, and kidneys. Apneic episodes, poor vasomotor (vessel diameter) and body temperature control, reduced or absent reflex responses, and seizures are early signs of postasphyxic brain damage. Some of these symptoms may be the result of temporary cerebral edema (brain swelling). Fluid intake therefore must be restricted to less than maintenance requirements (75 cc. per kg., first day) until this possibility has passed. Persistent seizures, lack of muscle tone, and poor swallow and suck are bad signs for the future.

There is no question that the premature who suffered fetal distress and/or asphyxia neonatorum will have an increased likelihood of developing hyaline membrane disease (see below) and will run a more severe course. In my own experience during a 32-month period (August 1971 to May 1974), only 5 out of 20, or 25 per cent, of prematures survived who were born with Apgar scores of less than 7 and required assisted ventilation for respiratory failure due to severe hyaline membrane disease. This is contrasted with a survival rate of 84 per cent (86 out of 102) for those prematures born with an Apgar score of 7 or greater who required assisted ventilation for respiratory failure due to severe hyaline membrane disease.

Cardiac function may also be affected after severe asphyxia. This is seen as heart enlargement on roentgenography, elevation of central venous pressure (reflecting back-up of blood behind the right side of the heart which is not keeping up with its pumping job) and pulmonary edema (reflecting back-up of blood behind the left side of the heart into the lungs). It may be necessary to digitalize (administer Digoxin to) postasphyxic patients to increase heart muscle contractility (strength of contraction) and avoid cardiac insufficiency and failure.

Postasphyxic hypoglycemia, abnormal clotting function, and hyperbilirubinemia may all reflect liver damage resulting from severe asphyxia neonatorum. Glucose IV, infusion of fresh blood or frozen plasma to supplement clotting factors, and close monitoring of bilirubin levels may be necessary in these babies. Phototherapy used to control hyperbilirubinemia is known to result in "bronzing" of the baby's skin if liver damage is present. Adrenal hemorrhage is a common finding at autopsy in babies who died of asphyxia at birth.

Renal tubular necrosis, which actually involves damage to both the glomeruli and tubules of the kidney, also is a common sequela (consequence) of severe asphyxia. It is characterized by an initial reduction in urinary output or anuria (complete lack of urine) followed by a diuretic phase (if the baby survives) in which increasing amounts of rather dilute urine are excreted with spillage of blood, protein, and other substances that normally are reabsorbed by the renal tubules. Fluid intake must be sharply reduced during the anuric phase since additional water (above insensible losses, or approximately 40 cc. per kg. per day) cannot be excreted and will further lead to cerebral edema and heart failure.

Thus, one can appreciate that the final outcome of an asphyxiated newborn rests not only on the degree and duration of the hypoxia suffered but also upon the severity of the resulting complications and just how these are anticipated and managed.

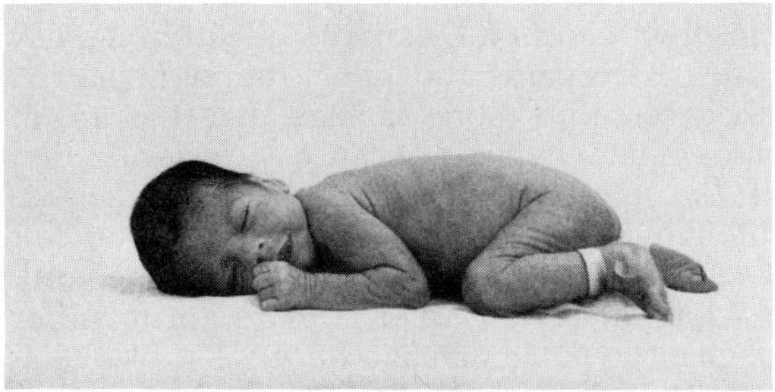

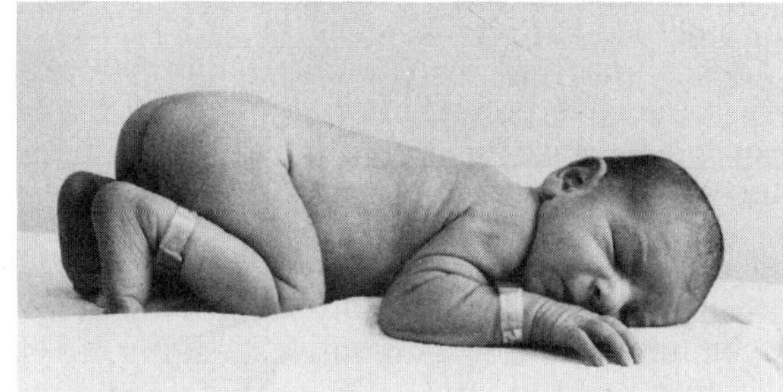

FIGURE 37-9. *Top*, premature infant. *Bottom*, full-term infant.

DISEASES OF THE PREMATURE INFANT

Prematurity implies being *born too early* or after a *short gestation*. Officially, a premature infant is any infant born at 37 weeks or less, calculated from the first day of the mother's last menstrual period (Fig. 37-9).

Prematurity is *not* synonymous with *low birth weight* (less than 2,500 grams or 5½ pounds) as was previously accepted to be the case. Approximately 20 per cent of all babies weighing less than 2,500 grams at birth are more than 37 weeks gestation. Conversely, about 4 per cent of babies weighing more than 2,500 grams at birth have gestational ages of 37 weeks or less. It is most difficult to separate factors associated with prematurity from those with low birth weight since the two overlap in both directions. The low-birth-weight infant may be premature or simply small for gestational age (small-for-date), or both (see section on SGA babies below).

Generally speaking, the etiologic factors leading to prematurity involve anything that expels the fetus prematurely, such as anomalies of the uterus and its cervix, abnormal implantation, premature separation of the placenta, or premature onset of labor. On the other hand, the etiologic factors leading to birth of a small-for-date baby generally involve alteration in the placental passage or fetal reception of nutrients (foodstuffs and oxygen). These include conditions that interfere with the general health and nutrition of the mother, the circulation and efficiency of the placenta, or the development and growth of the fetus. The problems frequently encountered by the two groups of newborns often overlap, yet distinct differences do exist.

Prematurity *is* synonymous with *immaturity* or functional limitation due to incomplete development. Anatomic, physiologic, and biochemical functions are all involved, each in its own degree. Deficiency of function in these various areas will affect the newborn's ability to meet all those demands not previously required of him in the protective environment of the uterus. Generally speaking, the more prematurely a baby is born, the less able he will be to meet the demands of extrauterine life. Duration of gestation is more closely related to functional maturity of a newborn than is birth weight.

In discussing the pathophysiologic mechanisms of diseases of prematurity, one is dealing largely with problems of immaturity. We will focus on five conditions: 1) hyaline membrane disease or idiopathic respiratory distress syndrome (IRDS), 2) periodic breathing and apnea, 3) hyperbilirubinemia, 4) hypolcalcemia, and 5) late metabolic acidosis of the premature. Table 37-2 presents a brief resume of the functional status of the premature infant. The list is not complete but does alert one to the major problems to be anticipated in the premature infant.

TABLE 37-2. Brief Outline of the Physiologic Status of the Premature Infant

Function and Status	*Problems to Be Anticipated*
Regulatory Functions:	
1. *Temperature regulation*	
Increased conductive and radiant heat losses due to increased total body water but reduced insulating fat; poor vasomotor control of blood flow to skin capillaries; and relatively large surface area to body mass ratio.	Hypothermia
Restricted metabolic rate and heat production due to reduced muscle and fat deposits, low enzyme activities, and reduced muscle activity.	
Poor sweat production due to sweat gland immaturity.	Overheating
2. *Respiratory regulation*	
Near-normal chemoreceptor response to changes in blood O_2, CO_2 and H^+ (pH), but accentuated dependancy on baroreceptor, lung stretch receptor, and cold stimulus input to maintain threshold activity level of respiratory center neurons.	Periodic breathing and apnea
Respiratory Function:	
Tendency toward CO_2 retention due to irregular breathing, weaker respiratory muscle activity and less rigid thoracic cage.	Hypoventilation (CO_2 retention)
Tendency toward alveolar collapse due to reduced surfactant production and sparse pulmonary elastic tissue; made evident by reduced compliance and low functional residual capacity.	Hypoxemia (low blood PO_2)
Weak gag and cough reflexes.	Aspiration
Cardiovascular Function:	
Tendency toward persistence of fetal circulation due to delayed closure of the ductus arteriosus and relatively higher pulmonary artery pressure.	Pulmonary hypoperfusion Venous admixture (R→ L shunting) and hypoxemia Patent ductus arteriosus
Reduced capillary density, so less gas exchange, foodstuff delivery, and waste product removal.	Tissue hypoxia and acidosis
Increased capillary fragility.	Petechiae, eccymoses, hemorrhage
Digestive Function:	
Weak suck and swallow, delayed stomach emptying, reduced intestinal mobility.	Slow weight gain, abdominal distention and necrotizing enterocolitis

TABLE 37-2. *Continued*

Function and Status	*Problems to Be Anticipated*
Low secretion of gastric acid and digestive enzymes.	Fat, protein and carbohydrate loss in stools
Delayed bacterial colonization of the gut and poor fat absorption.	Vitamin K deficiency bleeding
Liver and Metabolic Functions:	
Reduced glycogen, fat, vitamin and mineral storage (especially calcium) at birth.	Hypoglycemia Hypocalcemia
Reduced enzyme activites for intermediary protein metbolism.	Transient phenylketonuria, tyrosinemia, etc.
Reduced synthesis of proteins such as albumin, fibrinogen, and liver-dependent clotting factors.	Hypoalbuminemia and edema Hemorrhage
Poor clearance of bilirubin.	Hyperbilirubinemia
Renal Function:	
Reduced glomerular filtration rate.	Water retention, edema, and poor drug clearance
Reduced ability to concentrate urine or conserve water.	Dehydration
Reduced tubular reabsorption of glucose, amino acids, and bicarbonate.	Protein and glucose spillage; proximal renal tubular acidosis of prematurity
Reduced tubular secretion of fixed acid, phosphate, and drugs.	Metabolic acidosis, hyperphosphatemia and drug accumulation
Immune Function:	
Low levels of alpha and beta globulins or opsonization factors important for leucocyte phagocytosis.	Susceptability to viral and fungal infections
Low specific antibody (IgG) levels received passively from the mother.	Susceptibility to gram negative bacterial infections
Reduced WBC bacteria-killing ability due to perioxidase and other intracellular enzyme inactivity.	Sepsis

HYALINE MEMBRANE DISEASE OR IDIOPATHIC RESPIRATORY DISTRESS SYNDROME

Hyaline membrane disease (HMD) or idiopathic (of unknown cause) respiratory distress syndrome (IRDS) is essentially a disorder of prematurity with increasing incidence and mortality correlating directly with the degree of prematurity (Fig. 37-10). In babies born between 29 and 30 weeks of gestation, the incidence is nearly two thirds (66 per cent), between 31 and 32 weeks it is slightly over one third, between 33 and 34 weeks it is one fifth, and between 35 and 36 weeks it is one twentieth. The incidence is further increased in babies born by cesarean section before 37 weeks of gestation and without a prior trial labor. HMD is still the number one killer of prematures, accounting for nearly 40 per cent of all their deaths, or about 20,000 babies a year in this country.

Predisposing factors for HMD besides prematurity and birth by cesarean section include:

1. Acute complications of pregnancy, such as maternal bleeding, hypotensive episodes, or hypoxia, that lead to intrauterine anoxia before or during labor.
2. Birth asphyxia (may be related to the above-mentioned acute complications of pregnancy, or due to other causes as outlined in Table 37-1 above) reflected in low Apgar scores.
3. Maternal diabetes, insofar as it leads to premature delivery or birth by cesarean section.
4. Hypothermia and/or metabolic acidosis and hypotension in the immediate postpartal period.

In contrast, a number of other factors seem to protect the premature from developing HMD, or at least reduce its incidence in any comparable group of prematures. These factors involve chronic, less acute stresses on the

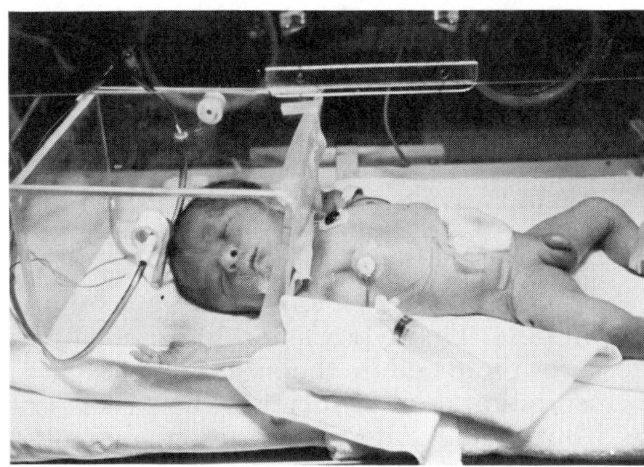

FIGURE 37-10. Infant with idiopathic respiratory distress syndrome. Note severe retractions.

fetus such as toxemia or hypertension in the mother, premature rupture of membranes, low-grade intrauterine infection, and heroin addiction of the mother. Theories as to why some factors should predispose to HMD and others protect against it are considered below.

Clinical symptoms of HMD include all of the classical signs of respiratory distress such as tachypnea, expiratory grunting, nasal flaring, sternal and intercostal retractions, and increasing cyanosis unless progressively higher concentrations of oxygen are administered. Ausculation of the lungs reveals very soft breath sounds (poor air movement) in spite of the baby's extremely labored respiratory efforts. Peripheral circulation is poor, as exemplified by acrocyanosis (coldness and blueness of the hands and feet) and slow return of color to an area blanched by pressure (delayed capillary filling).

The chest roentgenogram shows a diffuse haziness (fine reticulogranular or ground-glass appearance) in all lung fields, air bronchograms (clearly outlined bronchi appearing darker than the surrounding lung tissue) and hypoaeration (poor expansion).

The course of the disease is quite typical and any deviation from this usual course should raise one's suspicion that a major complication has developed (see below) or that there is some underlying anomaly or superimposed disease process also present. After a short symptom-free interval following birth, respiratory distress develops that either peaks, plateaus, and then improves within the space of 24 to 72 hours (mild to moderately severe cases), or that relentlessly progresses until the infant fades or crashes into respiratory failure (severe cases) and dies of cardiopulmonary arrest unless afforded assisted ventilation. Respiratory failure is best defined as intractable apneic episodes (see below) or severe hypoxia (arterial PO_2 of less than 50 mm. Hg while breathing 100 per cent oxygen) or severe CO_2 retention (PCO_2 of greater than 80 mm. Hg while breathing spontaneously).

If the infant dies, one finds that the lungs appear very much like liver . . . wet, solid, and heavy (sink in water). Under the microscope one sees scattered air spaces representing a few remaining partially-open alveoli lined with a hyaline (glassy-like) membrane which is composed of fibrin and alveolar cell debris. The lymphatics and capillaries appear dilated, but the pulmonary arterioles (small arteries) are constricted.

Prior lung function studies would have shown greatly diminished lung volumes (due to the atelectasis or air sac collapse), reduced compliance (increased stiffness of the lungs due to their wetness and resistance to expansion), and greatly restricted blood flow through the lungs (pulmonary hypoperfusion due to arteriolar constriction).

The main pathophysiologic mechanism at work here centers around reduced stability of the alveoli (increased tendency for them to collapse at the end of expiration) due to surfactant (a fatty substance) deficiency. Any time there is a meeting point or interface between air and a fluid film (such as that made up by a bubble, or the inside of an air sac in the lung), there is a strong force (surface tension) working to collapse the bubble or reduce the size of the interface. If however, a thin layer of a fatty substance such as soap or surfactant is spread over the air-fluid interface, the surface tension is greatly reduced and the bubble is less likely to shrink or the air sac less likely to collapse.

Surfactant (mainly represented by a surface-active substance called lecithin) is produced in the lining cells of the alveoli and secreted onto their surface to stabilize the air sacs from collapsing. However, if a baby is born prematurely, before his lungs are developed enough to produce or secrete this substance in sufficient quantity to do the job of reducing the surface tension of the alveoli, his air sacs will tend to collapse at the end of expiration when the inside air pressure drops to its lowest point. Also, if a fairly mature fetus suffers some acute distress due to a maternal complication that leads to hypoxia or compromised circulation, his alveolar cells (along with many other metabolically-active cells) may be damaged and the surfactant production temporarily turned off just at the time of delivery. In contrast, certain less acute stresses, such as placental insufficiency or vaginal delivery itself, actually stimulate the production of surfactant and prepare the baby for extrauterine life. It is now thought that this stimulating effect (or induction) is controlled by steroids, produced by the body in greater quantities at the time labor begins or in response to many forms of stress. In cases of premature labor, it may even be possible to support this induction process by administering additional steroid medicines to the mother.

A lack of surfactant in the lungs brings with it a number of ill effects associated with air sac collapse (atelectasis). Air cannot get into the air sacs to deliver its oxygen to the blood in the surrounding capillaries or to pick up the carbon dioxide brought in from the body. The scant amount of blood flowing through the lungs (see below) returns to the left heart to go back out to the body with only small amounts of oxygen so that the tissues become hypoxic. The combination of poor lung expansion and low oxygen levels in the blood keeps the pulmonary vascular resistance high (see above under Disorders of Transition) so that little blood flows through the lungs, as well as slows the process of closing the ductus arteriosus and foramen ovale so that much of the blood pumped by the right heart continues to bypass the lungs.

A number of other vicious circles are set into motion here. The hypoxia and high (negative) pressures produced (in the intrathoracic space) on inspiration tend to increase the leakage of fluid out of the lung capillaries, making the lungs stiffer and even harder to expand. Tissue hypoxia forces the body to revert to anaerobic (without oxygen) pathways to produce energy, which are much less efficient than aerobic (with oxygen) metabolism and result in the formation of fixed acids such as lactate and pyruvate. The resulting metabolic acidosis in turn adversely affects heart function (further compromising circulation to lungs and body), liver function (further reducing energy production and synthesis of important proteins such as clotting factors), and CNS function (leading to respiratory irregularities). If these vicious circles cannot be interrupted, serious complications and death may quickly ensue.

The most common complications occurring in idiopathic respiratory distress syndrome are apneic episodes, pulmonary air leak (pneumothorax, and so forth), and hemorrhage into the lungs or brain. All of these may themselves lead to respiratory failure and represent lethal complications. If significant bleeding does occur in the lungs or brain, it usually means death to the baby.

Treatment of IRDS or hyaline membrane disease should focus on overcoming the atelectasis and correcting the metabolic disturbances that result from it. Intermittent reexpansion of the lungs by periodically applying continuous positive airway pressure (CPAP) by mask and enriching the oxygen the baby breathes to overcome hypoxia is often all that is needed in mild cases. Correction of the metabolic acidosis by infusion of sodium bicarbonate, maintaining blood pressure and hemoglobin levels by albumin, plasma, or packed cell infusions, replacement of clotting factors with fresh plasma or whole blood transfusions, and assisting ventilation with CPAP by mask or by nasal prongs or intermittent positive pressure ventilation (IPPV) with positive end expiratory pressure (PEEP) may be necessary in the more severe cases. Temperature control and cautious gavage feedings or peripheral hyperalimentation are important supportive therapeutic measures. Surgical procedures such as placement of chest tubes to decompress a complicating pneumothorax or pneuropericardium, or ligation of a patent ductus arteriosus (see above) may also be necessary to save some babies. Utilizing all of these modes of therapy, we are now able to achieve an overall survival rate approaching 90 per cent for premature babies with hyaline membrane disease treated in our regional newborn intensive care centers.

PERIODIC BREATHING AND APNEIC EPISODES

Periodic breathing is a common occurrence in premature infants whereby they simply stop breathing for short periods of time. When these periods of "nonbreathing" are extended and/or are accompanied by bradycardia and cyanosis or require stimulation or actual bagging to reinstitute spontaneous breathing, they are called *apneic episodes*. The smaller and more immature the baby, the shorter period of time he can go without breathing before exhibiting bradycardia and cyanosis. For this reason apnea should not be defined by some arbitrary time period of nonbreathing. Some babies cannot even tolerate 5 seconds of nonbreathing without getting bradycardia and requiring stimulation to restart breathing. In contrast, bigger, more mature babies can often go up to 30 seconds without taking a breath or showing any ill effects, and can still start up again spontaneously.

The overall incidence of periodic breathing and apnea is directly proportional to the gestational age (and to a lesser degree, the birth weight) of the infant. It is encountered in nearly all true prematures with birth weights of less than 4 pounds. It usually begins around 16 to 48 hours of life, becomes increasingly frequent to reach a peak in about one third of the time it takes the baby to attain a weight of 4 pounds, and then gradually subsides to become almost nonexistent at about the time he achieves the usual 5-pound weight for discharge. Any deviation from this usual pattern should raise one's suspicion that something else besides just "immaturity of the respiratory center" is causing the irregularity.

A number of factors besides gestational age and maturity have been shown to influence the frequency and duration of periodic breathing in healthy premature infants. For instance, periodic breathing occurs almost exclusively during active or REM (rapid eye movement) sleep, and occurs more frequently when the surrounding temperature is increasing or the baby is being warmed. Conversely, it can be stopped altogether if the infant is given a critical concentration of CO_2 (usually around 2 to 4 per cent) or O_2 (anywhere between 25 and 90 per cent) to breathe. The critical concentration or turning point for O_2 that stops further periodic breathing depends on the baby's size and maturity at the time, and becomes less and less at a rate that is very similar for all babies. That is to say, the process of maturation of the respiratory center that eventually makes it capable of sustaining uninterrupted regular respirations proceeds at approximately the same rate in all healthy premature infants.

Apneic episodes leading to bradycardia, cyanosis, or mottled skin color are very dangerous for the premature infant since they can quickly lead to severe hypoxia and circulatory collapse, and thus lasting brain damage. The faster the heart rate drops, the more severe the spell is likely to be and the greater difficulty one will have getting the baby going again. Also, the longer one waits to intervene, the more rigorous and extended the resuscitative measures will have to be to overcome the apnea and restabilize the infant. A number of pathologic conditions lead to more frequent and severe apneic episodes:

1. *Hypoxia.* As mentioned above in the discussion on asphyxia, hypoxia reduces energy production and eventually interferes with cell function, including that of the respiratory neurons (nerve cells) that are responsible for rhythmic breathing.
2. *Extremely low or extremely high blood volume.* Shock due to blood loss, or heart failure due to fluid overload can produce apnea in a newborn infant and especially in a premature.
3. *Acidosis.* Extreme respiratory acidosis (CO_2 retention) or less marked metabolic acidosis (accumulation of fixed acid) can cause apnea by directly paralyzing the respiratory center or indirectly interfering with energy production by its effects on circulation and enzyme activities (see previous discussion of asphyxia).
4. *Infections.* Circulating toxins present during sepsis can adversely affect the respiratory center, as can local inflammation due to direct infection in the brain (meningitis and/or encephalitis). Increased apnea may be the first sign of infection.
5. *Hypoglycemia.* Here the energy source for brain cell function is directly taken away. Hypoglycemia must always be ruled out in a baby exhibiting more frequent apneic spells.
6. *Hypocalcemia.* Nerve potentials as well as cardiac muscular contractility and capillary permeability all seem to be dependent upon a normal level of ionized calcium in the circulating blood. There is thus a correlation between hypocalcemia and increased occurrence of apnea.
7. *Seizures.* Certain types of seizures in the newborn are actually capable of extinguishing all muscle tone and respiratory activity, and thus present as apnea.
8. *Increased intracranial pressure.* This may be due to hemorrhage in the brain, inflammation, or congenital malformations that obstruct flow of cerebral spinal fluid and eventually compress the cells of the respiratory center to cause apnea.

Because of frequent association between periodic breathing and apneic episodes, it is important to monitor all babies weighing less than 4 pounds as well as any newborn known to have one of the above conditions or a previous apneic spell. The methodology and instrumentation used for monitoring apnea and the steps to be taken when resuscitating an infant having a severe apneic spell are discussed in the next chapter. Precautionary measures that may be taken to keep periodic breathing and apneic episodes to a minimum, besides correcting any of the identified pathologic conditions listed above, include the following:

1. Servo-control body temperature to the lower end of the thermoneutral zone, i.e., between 35.8 and 36.5° C (96.6 and 97.8° F). The mild cold stress acts as a stimulus to respirations without causing increased oxygen consumption (still within the thermoneutral zone).
2. Avoid marked fluctuations in ambient (surrounding) temperature, or rapidly heating up a baby. The new proportional type convective or radiant heat incubators and warmers are preferable to the older all-or-nothing systems, since heat is emitted in proportion to what the baby needs (in accordance to how far away he is from the desired value) rather than just turning full-tilt on or off and

fluctuating between the extremes of too hot or too cold.

3. Perodically expand the baby's lungs by making him cry, bagging him, or applying continuous positive airway pressure by face mask intermittently. In cases of intractable apnea, especially in infants weighing less than 1,000 grams (2⅓ lb.), we have been most successful in controlling apnea by applying nasal-CPAP for extended periods of time. These procedures re-expand atelectatic (collapsed) areas of the lung and increase functional residual capacity, thereby affording more reserve oxygen in the lungs to tide the baby over during periods of nonbreathing.

PHYSIOLOGIC JAUNDICE AND HYPERBILIRUBINEMIA

As many as 80 per cent of all premature infants will exhibit jaundice (yellow discoloration of the skin and sclera, representing a serum bilirubin level of greater than 5 mg.%) in the first week of life. Bilirubin levels in cord blood are normally between 1.8 and 2.8 mg.%, for prematures as well as term infants. The rate of rise during the first two days is also about the same for the two groups, i.e., 1 to 2 mg.% per 24 hours. Thereafter, however, the level in the premature infant continues to rise rather than level off, and peaks on the average at about 8 to 10 mg.% (upper range 15 mg.%) on the fourth to fifth day before starting down. By the tenth day of life it should be below 2 mg.%.

Within these limits we are generally justified in speaking of *physiologic jaundice*, or that which can be expected in the normal premature infant. The reasons why the bilirubin level continues to rise after the second day in the premature as contrasted with the term infant and why it peaks at a higher level are discussed in detail below. Outside the limits outlined above, we can no longer consider it physiologic, but rather *pathologic jaundice*, falling into one of five major groups that demand a diagnostic work-up:

1. Early onset jaundice (appearing before 24 hours of age).
2. Rapidly rising bilirubin (greater than 5 mg.% rise in 24 hours).
3. Hyperbilirubinemia (bilirubin greater than 12 mg.% in term infants and 15 mg.% in prematures).
4. Elevated "direct" fraction of bilirubin (greater than 1.5 mg.%).
5. Prolonged jaundice (visible jaundice beyond 7 days in the term infant and 10 days in the premature).

The actual level of bilirubin in the blood is the sum of all that is produced, minus the amount excreted, divided by the space in which it is distributed over any set period of time. What this means is that to really understand why premature infants are inclined to have high bilirubin levels in their blood, we must know what factors influence the production, distribution, and excretion of bilirubin in prematures, and just how important each of these factors is from a quantitative standpoint.

Bilirubin is formed by the breakdown of heme pigments found in cell elements (nonerythrocyte bilirubin) as well as in hemoglobin of red blood cells. The newborn infant has a proportionally larger amount of nonerythrocyte bilirubin being formed, as well as a shorter erythrocyte (RBC) life span (about 88 instead of 120 days), so that the total production (or breakdown) of bilirubin is 2 to 3 times greater than in the adult on a per kilogram body weight basis. This is increased even further in the premature infant, and that increase is directly proportional to the degree of prematurity. Furthermore, this high rate of production comes just at a time when the baby's ability to clear bilirubin from his system is at its lowest point.

Because bilirubin is almost completely insoluble in water at normal pH ranges, it cannot be excreted directly in the urine. Rather, it must be excreted in the bile after being processed in the liver. To get to the liver it is bound to albumin, making it water-soluble, and thereby transportable in the plasma. However, the large albumin molecule to which it is bound prevents it from being filtered by the kidneys and excreted in the urine even though it is now water-soluble. Albumin-bound bilirubin also cannot penetrate the blood-brain barrier, so it causes no brain damage in this form. The amount of bilirubin that can be bound to albumin is dependent upon the amount of albumin available in the serum, as well as the concentration of other substances that compete with bilirubin for albumin binding sites. It also depends on the blood pH, since the affinity of albumin for bilirubin is reduced when a state of acidemia (low blood pH) is present. Prematures are at risk for having low albumin binding capacity for all three of these reasons: they tend to have low serum albumin levels (hypoalbuminemia), they have relatively large amounts of free heme (due to hemolysis) and free fatty acids (due to hypoglycemia) in the circulation that compete with bilirubin for albumin binding sites, and they tend toward acidosis with resulting low albumin-bilirubin binding affinity.

Once it is brought to the liver, the bilirubin is transported into the hepatocyte (liver cell) by mechanisms that are still poorly understood. The amount of bilirubin that can be held in the liver cells for processing, and consequently the total uptake of bilirubin into the liver, is in turn dependent upon two intracellular proteins labeled Y and Z. Here again the newborn, and particularly the premature, is disadvantaged in having a relatively low amount of Y protein. This deficiency may well represent the single most important factor contributing to the premature's poor ability to clear bilirubin through the liver. Added to this is the theoretical possibility that continued patency of the ductus venosus (the fetal circulatory short-cut between the portal sinus and inferior vena cava) may result in some bypassing of blood around the liver and subsequent reduction of hepatic bilirubin uptake.

The conjugation (coupling) process taking place in the liver cells and resulting in the attachment of bilirubin to glucuronic acid (made out of liver glycogen) so as to enable its secretion into the bile is dependent upon an enzyme system called glucuronyl transferase. The degree to which the activity of this enzyme system is reduced in the premature infant is open to considerable debate at present, but some degree of immaturity of the conjugating system is certainly present. In states of hypoglycemia and glycogen depletion, the basic substrate (building block) for glucuronic acid is reduced, and this, too, must limit conjugation of bilirubin in the premature.

From the liver cell, conjugated bilirubin is excreted into the tiny bile ducts and on into the common duct and duodenum. Further down in the intestines it is transformed (reduced) to urobilinogen by bacteria and excreted in the stool as a yellow-brown pigment. However there exists in the intestines an enzyme system called beta-glucuronidase that acts to split off (or deconjugate) the bilirubin from glucuronic acid if it is not first reduced by the bacteria. Once it is again detached from the glucuronic acid, the free bilirubin is reabsorbed through the intestinal wall (penetrating easily because it is again fat-soluble in the free state) and brought back to the liver by the portal vein to start the process all over again. This recycling of bilirubin is called the *enterohepatic circulation* and delays the ultimate clearance of bilirubin from the body. For the fetus, this system has obvious advantages since it brings the bilirubin back into the circulation where it can be cleared by the placenta. For the newborn, and especially the premature who has a very high beta-glucuronidase activity level as well as delayed bacterial colonization of his gut, the enterohepatic circulation may well play a major role in his reduced ability to clear bilirubin from his system.

Excessively high levels of bilirubin pose a grave danger to the newborn and especially to the premature, since it may leak out of the blood stream and find its way into crucial cells such as the neurons of the basal ganglion of the brain. Bilirubin is thought to damage these cells by interfering with their oxygen uptake and utilization. The final result is a condition called kernicterus, which is described in detail later under Erythroblastosis Fetalis.

The level at which bilirubin is no longer completely bound to albumin and is free to leak out of the blood stream into tissues and eventually through the blood-brain barrier into the brain to cause damage is dependent upon a number of factors, several of which have already been listed above. It follows then that infants at risk for developing kernicterus are those with bilirubin levels so high as to exceed even normal albumin binding capacity and those with factors that depress albumin binding of bilirubin or make brain cells more vulnerable to damage from bilirubin. These include:

1. Infants who were or are anoxic, hypoxic, or acidotic.
2. Babies with low serum albumin concentrations associated with prematurity, hyaline membrane disease, hydrops, liver disease, and so forth.
3. Infants exposed to cold who have an increased free fatty acid level due to fat breakdown for heat productin. The free fatty acids compete with albumin for binding sites.
4. Infants whose mothers received large dosages of sulfa drugs (which also compete with bilirubin for conjugation), or heparin, aspirin, and parenteral drugs containing sodium benzoate, all of which compete with bilirubin for albumin binding.

There are three principle modes of treating physiologic jaundice when it threatens to reach or has actually reached pathologic levels. The first two of these, early feedings and phototherapy, are discussed in this section, whereas exchange transfusions are discussed later under Erythroblastosis Fetalis. The nursing responsibilities involved with these modes of therapy will be discussed in Chapter 38.

The rationale for instituting *early feedings* in all infants at risk for developing hyperbilirubinemia touches on every aspect of bilirubin clearance discussed above. The calories or energy supplied by the food represents substrate or fuel to perform the work of synthesizing the necessary proteins, providing the glucuronic acid for conjugation and carrying on active transport and secretion processes. Early feeding also stimulates gut motility leading to early elimination of meconium (which contains bilirubin that may be reabsorbed) and more rapid bacterial colonization of the gut to aid the process of reducing the conjugated bilirubin before it can be deconjugated by beta-glucuronidase in the intestines and recycled through the enterohepatic circulation. Many clinical neonatologists consider early feedings to be the single most important routine to be instituted in newborn nurseries to minimize the incidence of hyperbilirubinemia and lower the number of exchange transfusions that need be performed.

Phototherapy is a widely used method of managing rising or high bilirubin levels, especially in premature infants. Its application is so simple that it tends to be used uncritically. In reality, phototherapy is still largely in the experimental stage since a limited amount is known about its mode of action, potential complications, and long-term effects. These topics will be reviewed briefly here.

In the test tube (in vitro), bilirubin carried in plasma is broken down to biliverdin and other photo-oxidation products when it is exposed to sunlight or artificial light of the right wavelength (particularly in the blue light range). This process is dependent upon the presence of oxygen and actually goes faster at lower pH levels (more acid environment). When these photo-oxidation products are then injected into the circulation of rats, they do not seem to get into the spinal fluid or brain cells to cause damage, but rather are excreted in the bile. In vivo (in the live animal situation), photo-oxidation of bilirubin occurs in the skin and not in the plasma. The photodecomposition (light breakdown) products are largely water-soluble dipyrrols (fragments of the heme molecule) which can then be excreted in the bile and urine and need not be bound to albumin for transport. Thus, bilirubin clearance is aided considerably under phototherapy, and bilirubin levels in the blood drop on the average from between 2 to 4 mg.% after 12 or more hours "under the lights."

Phototherapy has a number of other effects, some of which can lead to complications. It causes dilation of the capillaries of the skin which can result in temperature regulation problems, redistribution of the circulation, and increased insensible water losses. It activates the pigment-producing melanocytes in the skin causing "sun tanning." In babies with liver damage, the brown photo-oxidation products are not adequately excreted but are left in the skin to a large degree and result in the so-called "bronze baby" syndrome. There is also considerable experimental evidence that prolonged exposure to bright light may effect a number of biologic body rhythms such as normal temperature fluctuations, food consumption patterns, level of physical activity, and the secretion of a large number of hormones in the body. The end results may be an acceleration of glycogen breakdown (glycolysis), reduction in protein synthesis, and uncoupling of heat-producing metabolic processes. With all this evidence of known and potential effects of light exposure, one should definitely approach the use of phototherapy with some caution. A good rule of thumb should be to use phototherapy only when its risks are judged to be less than those of the hyperbilirubinemia itself or the risks that come from having to do an exchange transfusion. There is no justification for placing every premature baby "prophylactically" under the "bili-lights," since only 15 to 25 per cent will exceed a bilirubin level of 15 mg.% if left untreated, and less than 5 per cent will exceed that level if phototherapy is first begun when the baby's bilirubin is 10 mg.%.

HYPOCALCEMIA

Mean serum calcium levels in normal prematures are directly proportional to gestational age: the average calcium level for infants of 30 weeks gestation is about 7.0 mg.%, for 35 weeks 8.0 mg.% and for 40 weeks 9.0 mg.%. This is due to progressively increasing transplacental active transport of calcium from the mother to the fetus with increasing gestational age. If the baby is born prematurely, he is deprived of a comparable portion of the calcium that would have crossed over to be stored in bone and tissue.

There are a number of other factors besides gestational age that affect the calcium level in newborns, and all of these may apply to individual prematures at one time or another:

1. *Hyperphosphatemia* (high phosphate level in the blood) depresses serum calcium levels by fostering calcium deposition in the bones and by decreasing bone responsiveness to parathyroid hormone (which works to mobilize calcium from the bone). Phosphate is released into the blood in large quantities when tissue is broken down (as in birth trauma) or when the baby is forced to fall back on his own energy stores (by breaking down glycogen, fat, and protein) if unable to feed adequately. Some milk formulas have a relatively high phosphate content compared with breast milk.

2. *Asphyxia and acidosis* lead to hypocalcemia by a number of mechanisms. With the asphyxia comes tissue breakdown (hyperphosphatemia), poor calcium intake and reduced effectiveness of parathyroid hormone. Acidosis results in the mobilization of calcium from the bone to buffer (neutralize) the acid in the blood. Then when the acidosis is corrected (e.g., by the administration of sodium bicarbonate), the calcium returns to the bone leaving the blood depleted.
3. *Low serum protein levels* (as seen in prematures and especially those with hyaline membrane disease) result in less calcium being carried in the blood in bound form; total calcium level is proportionally reduced.

There is now strong evidence that the premature infant is relatively or functionally hypoparathyroid. That is to say, his parathyroid glands do not respond to the naturally low levels of calcium to the degree that they should be secreting enough parathyroid hormone (parathormone) to meet the need. Thus, serum calcium levels tend to remain relatively low in spite of the presence of hypocalcemia due to hyperphosphatemia, asphyxia, acidosis, hypoproteinemia, or whatever other cause.

The signs and symptoms of hypocalcemia in the newborn include the following:

1. Twitching of one or more extremities.
2. Convulsions (late sign).
3. High-pitched or squeaky cry.
4. Hypotonicity (floppiness).
5. Increased apneic episodes (see above) or cyanotic spells in prematures.
6. Edema (due to increased leaking of fluid from the capillaries).

As one can see, these are all nonspecific signs frequently associated with many other neonatal problems. However, it is quite helpful to always consider hypocalcemia as a possible cause if the premature was born asphyxic, suffered birth trauma, was acidotic and received bicarbonate, has respiratory distress, or has had inadequate milk intake.

The treatment of hypocalcemia varies from prophylactic early feedings or maintenance calcium in an IV for the groups listed above, to IV push of calcium gluconate (5 to 10 cc. of a 10 per cent solution diluted 50:50 with sterile water and given slowly while monitoring heart rate) in cases of severe twitching or convulsions. Calcium supplement to oral feedings may also be given (1 to 3 g. of a calcium salt per day), or one may use a commercial formula such as PM 60/40 which has a more favorable calcium to phosphorus ratio. The relatively high percentage of phosphorus in many prepared formulas (and especially diluted cows' milk with sugar added) loads the premature with phosphorus which he has difficulty excreting due to his immature kidneys. PM 60/40 has a calcium:phosphorus ratio of 2.0:1 which more closely resembles that of human milk (2.25:1) than does that of standard formulas with their 1.3:1 ratios.

When calcium is being given by IV push, one must be particularly careful to assure that it is given slowly and that the heart rate is being monitored to avoid bradycardia. Caution should also be used if the infant is receiving Digoxin for a cardiac problem or is hypokalemic (low potassium level), since calcium potentiates (amplifies) the effects of these.

LATE METABOLIC ACIDOSIS

All premature infants tend to become metabolically acidotic during the first few weeks of life even if they have had no major respiratory or cardiovascular problems. Their pH drops as does their bicarbonate or base excess (amount of bicarbonate and other base still available to neutralize the nonvolatile or fixed acid in the blood). They try to make up for this by blowing off extra volatile acid (CO_2) by hyperventilating. If they are fed a standard formula rather than breast milk, the acidosis may become quite marked and eventually interfere with their growth. Although these infants may remain vigorous and continue to ingest quantities that should be adequate in terms of fluid and caloric intake, they fail to gain weight or they "fail to thrive."

The reasons for this late metabolic acidosis of the premature rest with problems associated with their immature kidneys as well as with the inadequacies of the formulas we presently use to feed them. The frequency with which late metabolic acidosis severe enough to cause failure to thrive is encountered depends upon the population of prematures one is dealing with—how immature they are, what other problems they have had that might predispose to acidosis (e.g., asphyxia, hypoxia) or affect oral intake, and what type of formula they are being fed. One of the functional limitations of the premature kidney involved in acidosis is called proximal renal tubular acidosis of prematurity.

The proximal kidney tubules are responsible for reabsorbing a number of important substances that have been filtered through the glomeruli and would be lost to the urine if not reabsorbed into the blood. These substances include glucose, amino acids (protein), phosphate, and sodium bicarbonate. The renal threshold for these substances is the highest blood level at which they can still be completely reabsorbed by the kidney and not spilled in the urine. When these thresholds are exceeded, valuable substances needed for energy supply and growth are lost from the body, and they take equally valuable water with them through a process called osmotic diuresis.

The threshold for bicarbonate in the premature may be as low as 17 to 19 mmol. per liter, rather than the adult level of 26 to 28 mmol.; the more immature the baby, the lower the threshold. This means that any time the blood level exceeds that threshold, it will be spilled into the urine and lost to the body. The resulting blood bicarbonate level of only 17 to 19 mEq. per liter represents a rather severe metabolic acidosis, with a pH in the range of 7.25 to 7.30 (normal is 7.40) if no respiratory compensation has taken place. With the acidemia (acid blood) comes loss of sodium, potassium, and calcium in the urine, depleting bone and muscle stores of these electrolytes. The blood chloride level, on the other hand, goes up (hyperchloremic acidosis). Since bicarbonate continues to be spilled as long as one is still above the threshold, the urine is alkaline even though the baby is becoming acidotic. Once the blood bicarbonate level is equal to or lower than the threshold, the urine becomes acidic as it normally should be, in contrast to distal renal tubular acidosis where the urine can never be acidified below a pH of 6.0, no matter how acidotic the patient becomes.

The treatment of proximal renal tubular acidosis of the premature is relatively simple. One keeps replacing the bicarbonate faster than it is being spilled. This may require as much as 10 mEq. bicarbonate per kilogram body weight per 24 hours. We usually add 0.5 to 1 cc. of full strength sodium bicarbonate (1 mEq. per cc.) to each or every other feeding, and gradually decrease this according to the laboratory results as the baby matures. Bicarbonate supplement may be required for one week to one month.

The other problem involved with late metabolic acidosis of the premature is the composition of the formula used to feed him. More fixed acid is being released in the process of metabolism than the kidneys can deal with even though the net acid excretion of the premature with late metabolic acidosis is above normal. This acid comes from either the incomplete utilization of the protein in the formula itself or from the breakdown of the infant's own protein (catabolism) in the face of an inadequate offering of certain amino acids in the formula. The total amount of protein in the formula may be adequate or even more than enough, but the proportion of the various protein components (amino acids) may be out of line with the infant's real needs and thus lead to imbalance and acidosis. The premature infant's needs, in turn, are dependent upon the degree of maturation of the various enzyme systems he possesses to catabolize (breakdown) or anabolize (build up) protein and other foods. A formula that best matches his particular metabolism may be quite different from one best suited for older infants. It is interesting that prematures who are fed only breast milk never develop late metabolic acidosis.

This condition may also be successfully treated in some instances by discontinuing all protein intake for 24 to 48 hours and then starting over again with oral feedings. Premature diets that offer more than 4 mg. of protein per kilogram of body weight per day should be avoided from the beginning. High calorie diets instituted too abruptly in feeding premature infants have recently been cited as a possible cause of necrotizing enterocolitis which can lead to abdominal distention, bloody-mucous stools, air collection in the bowel wall and portal venous system, ruptured bowel, peritonitis, and frequent death in premature infnts. Our natural desire to "fatten up" and "put weight on" the small premature infant must be tempered by the realization that his immature digestive system can tolerate only so much formula of a limited degree of complexity and concentration; to exceed those limits may very well cause more harm than good.

PROBLEMS OF THE SMALL-FOR-DATE INFANT

With the realization that small babies (less that 2,500 grams or 5½ pounds) are not necessarily premature (37 weeks or less gestation), a new dimension is added to our thinking. We are now talking about rate of growth (change in weight, length, or size per unit time) while in the mother. This is a dynamic rather than static concept, focusing on rate of change rather than some arbitrary cut-off number.

Growth (increase in mass with time) is due to either an increase in the total number of cells in the body or increase in the size of the individual cells, or both. Likewise, intrauterine growth retardation might be due to a reduction in cell number or cell size. This distinction has been used to separate a *hypoplastic* group from a *malnourished* group of small-for-date babies. Hypoplasia, or incomplete development, implies something inherently or internally wrong with the individual that is restricting his growth and will continue to do so even after birth unless the *internal* defect or malformation affecting growth can be surgically corrected. The malnourished group, on the other hand, supposedly comes equipped with all the normal cells and growth potential, but has been deprived of adequate nourishment due to unfavorable external conditions. Once these are removed at the time of birth, one would expect "catch-up" growth to occur and the individual to eventually reach normal size and full potential. However, in reality, these distinctions do not always hold up, and we will be forced to modify our thinking as our understanding deepens.

Small-for-date babies having congenital anomalies with or without chromosomal defects, or babies who suffered certain types of intrauterine infection best fit the hypoplastic category. Congenital anomalies that are often associated with intrauterine growth retardation include:

1. Those that involve regulatory and endocrine function, such as severe CNS anomalies (e.g., anencephaly).
2. Those that affect the circulation in a manner that reduces blood flow to key

areas of the body, such as coarctation of the aorta or hypoplastic left heart syndrome.

3. Those that block or affect reabsorption of fluid through the fetal gut, such as esophageal atresia with or without tracheoesophageal fistula, and ruptured omphalocele or gastroschisis (intestines outside the abdominal cavity).

Nearly all of the easily recognizable chromosomal syndromes are associated with a high incidence of growth retardation. Newborns with Down's syndrome weigh 10 to 15 per cent less than the normal baby of same gestational age at birth, and are 2 to 3 cm. shorter. Trisomy 13 and 18 babies, as well as those with cri-du-chat (crying cat) syndrome are generally even more retarded in their growth. Possible reasons for the disorganized and restricted growth in chromosomal syndromes include: 1) disorderly cell division, 2) deletion or inactivation of genes that determine protein synthesis and body stature, and 3) imbalance of genetic material that distorts embryologic (developmental) processes.

Two common intrauterine viral infections frequently result in the birth of small-for-date babies, namely rubella and cytomegalic inclusion disease (CID). The mean birth weight of rubella babies is nearly two pounds under the average for normal newborns and more than half of them fall below the tenth percentile on the Colorado intrauterine growth charts. About 35 per cent of neonates infected with CID are small for gestational age (SGA). Careful morphologic (structural) studies of rubella babies have demonstrated the presence of true hypoplasia or actual decrease in the total number of cells in such organs as the heart, liver, kidneys, and brain.

By far the largest group of small-for-date infants comes from pregnancies that involve maternal disease or unnatural conditions that effect the supply of oxygen and/or nutrients to the fetus either directly or through insufficient function of the placenta. Such conditions include:

1. Preeclampsia, toxemia, or any other condition leading to maternal hypertensive vascular disease.
2. Maternal lung or heart disease, bleeding, or severe anemia.
3. Excessive maternal smoking, alcoholism, or heroin addiction (these frequently also involve some degree of maternal malnutrition),
4. Placental abnormalities such as anomalies of cord insertion (velamentous insertion in which cord vessels branch out on the membranes before entering the placental disc surface, and battledore insertion of cord vessels onto the edge of the placental disc), diffuse fibrinosis and hemangioma (vascular tumors) of the placenta.

The more long-standing and severe the fetal malnutrition is, regardless of the cause, the more severe the fetal growth retardation will be. This can involve body length and head size as well as birth weight. If, on the other hand, the fetal malnutrition comes late in the pregnancy or is less severe, the head is likely to be relatively unaffected, the body length somewhat reduced, and the body weight the most obviously affected of all. Plotting all three parameters on the Colorado intrauterine growth charts and comparing relative percentiles for head circumference, body length, and body weight thus allows one to establish a pattern of growth retardation that semiquantitatively reflects the severity and duration of the fetal malnutrition, and provides some prognostic value as to neonatal complications and future postnatal growth and development.

Other clinical findings besides reduced body weight and length in the small-for-date baby include wasted musculature, loose thin skin (Fig. 37-11) with the ribs showing through, sparse hair, wide-spread sutures and

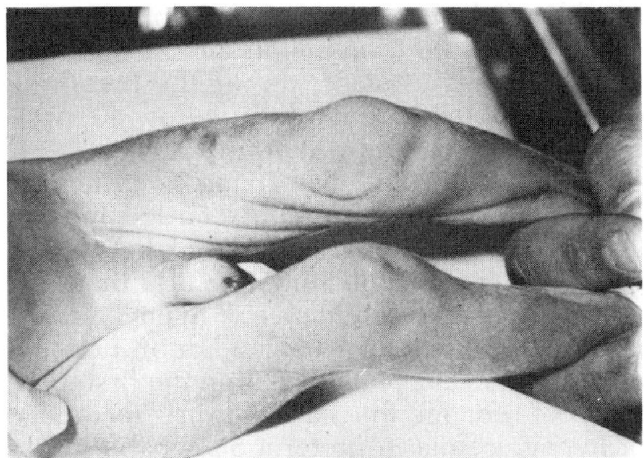

FIGURE 37-11. SGA baby with loose skin and wasted musculature.

large fontanels, and thin, brown-discolored umbilical cord. The face often has the expression of a "worried little old man" (Fig. 37-12).

The problems encountered by small-for-date neonates are often quite predictable and many can be managed satisfactorily if identified and treated early. It is very important, however, to sort out those problems associated with congenital or chromosomal anomalies or intrauterine infection from those that arise from fetal malnutrition, since the former groups have an infinitely poorer prognosis.

Gross (obvious or severe) congenital anomalies can be identified immediately by inspection, passage of feeding tubes or suction catheters, and auscultation of all SGA babies, as is done routinely in the transitional nursery by the nurse herself:

1. Inspect upper lip, gum, and palate to rule out clefts.
2. Pass a feeding tube or suction catheter down each nostril to rule out choanal atresia and on down into the stomach to rule out esophageal atresia or trachioesophageal fistula. Aspirate stomach contents; if more than 15–20 cc. of fluid are obtained, suspect upper intestinal obstruction.

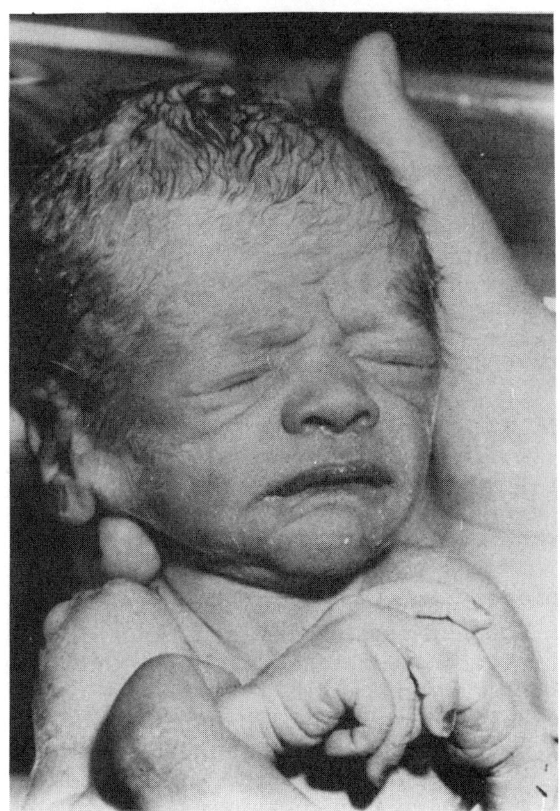

FIGURE 37-12. Worried expression of SGA baby. Note large, wrinkled hands with long nails.

3. Auscultate the heart for murmurs.
4. Inspect along the dorsal spine, neck, and head to rule out meningomyeloceles and encephaloceles.
5. Inspect anus and place rectal thermometer to rule out imperforate anus.

Less obvious congenital anomalies may be suspected in babies who show one or more of the following signs:

1. Low-set ears (a line extending laterally from the eyelid slit falls above the level of the ear lobe).

2. Single transverse palmar crease (simian line).
3. Incurved fifth finger.
4. Wide-spread nipples.
5. Single umbilical artery.
6. Joints that do not fully extend or can be hyperextended.
7. Abdominal distention with bilious gastric aspirate.
8. Failure to urinate within the first 24 hours or pass stool within the first 48 hours.

Signs of intrauterine infection that may have led to fetal growth retardation include:

1. Petechiae (small punctate red flecks that don't blanch when pressed), ecchymoses (patches of blood in the skin that look like small bruises), and skin rashes.
2. Hepatomegaly (enlarged liver) and/or splenomegaly (enlarged spleen) with early onset of jaundice (high direct fraction of bilirubin).
3. Chorioretinitis (inflammation of the choroid and retina of the eye, seen as dark or red spots on the eye grounds).
4. Lethargy when not aroused, and irritability when stimulated.

The four major problems encountered in neonates born small-for-gestational age due to placental insufficiency or fetal malnutrition are asphyxia neonatorum, hypoglycemia, polycythemia, and hypothermia. Asphyxia has been discussed previously. Its incidence in SGA babies is between 15 to 30 per cent. Polycythemia, which occurs in 15 to 50 per cent of SGA babies, will be discussed later in this chapter. Hypoglycemia and thermodysregulation associated with the small-for-date infant will now be discussed in more detail.

HYPOGLYCEMIA

Neonatal hypoglycemia is generally defined as a blood glucose level below 30 mg. per 100 cc. (30 gm.%) for term infants and 20 mg.% for low-birth-weight infants during the first three days of life; thereafter, a level below 40 mg.% is considered to represent hypoglycemia. If one applies the "less than 20 mg.%" criteria to SGA or intrauterine growth retarded infants, and measures their glucose level before the first feeding, one will find a greater than one third (33 per cent) incidence of hypoglycemia. Using the "less than 30 mg.%" definition and applying it to SGA infants within the first three hours of life, one finds a two-thirds incidence of hypoglycemia in preterm SGA babies (less than 38 weeks of gestation), one-fourth incidence for term (between 38 and 42 weeks of gestation) SGA infants, and about one-sixth incidence for post-term SGA babies (greater than 42 weeks of gestation).

These are very high odds indeed, and reflect the precarious position of the small-for-date infant as regards his glucose level and state of energy balance in the first few hours after birth. The reasons for this precarious state are now partially understood. First of all, the SGA baby has reduced carbohydrate stores to fall back on once he is cut off from the supply he received from the placenta. Glycogen reserves (glycogen is the storage form of glucose found in the liver and muscle) are used up almost immediately instead of after 2 or 3 hours of life as is the case in the normal newborn. Gluconeogenesis (the process of converting fat and protein to glucose) then takes over, but here again the SGA infant is at a grave disadvantage. Not only does he again have reduced reserves in the form of muscle protein and adipose (fat) tissue for the conversion to glucose (and ketone bodies which can also be used for energy), but he also has a reduced hyperglycemiac (blood sugar elevating) response to norepinephrine (from the adrenal glands) and glucagon (from the alpha cells of the pancreatic islets) which instigate the gluconeogenic process. The reason for the poor response to norepinephrine and glucagon even though they apparently are excreted at a higher than normal rate in SGA babies may be that the enzyme systems in the liver responsible for the production of glucose and ketone bodies from glycerol and free fatty acids (the basic components of fat), and glucose from amino acids (the basic components of protein) are delayed in their maturation. That is to say, the enzyme systems in the liver responsible for gluconeogenesis and ketogenesis (production of ketone bodies) in the SGA baby are functioning at a lower than normal level of activity, either because their development has been delayed for some reason or their activity level is being suppressed by some unknown factor or factors.

Symptoms of hypoglycemia in the newborn may be discrete (not obvious) and nonspecific (invariably have many other causes besides hypoglycemia). Clinical manifestations of hypoglycemia can include:

1. *Jitteriness or tremulousness* (repetitive shaking of the extremities). It may occur spontaneously or be brought on by stimulation (in contrast to seizures which cannot be elicited by stimulation).
2. *Cyanosis or dusky spells.* The cyanosis is usually peripheral rather than central, indicting reduced peripheral circulation, unless associated with apneic episodes which may lead to generalized cyanosis.
3. *Apneic episodes or irregular respirations* (see discussion of periodic breathing and apnea in the section on prematurity).
4. *Hypotonia or limpness and lethargy.* The child may be listless when left alone but jittery when stimulated. Poor feeding or refusal to feed is generally a problem also.
5. *Weak or high-pitched cry.* The high-pitched cry also characterizes heroin-addicted infants who frequently are SGA but usually quite vigorous and lusty in their cry.
6. *Seizures.* They occur in the more extreme cases and carry a poor prognosis. The same infant may be both jittery and have true seizures.

Every SGA infant should be screened for hypoglycemia, beginning shortly after birth. This is usually accomplished by performing Dextrostix determinations at 30 to 60 minute intervals, and obtaining a true blood glucose determination from the laboratory whenever the Dextrostix reads less than 45 mg.% or the child is symptomatic.

It is our practice to begin treatment whenever the true blood glucose is confirmed to be below 45 mg.%. The simplest form of treatment is institution of early feedings, either by nipple (after a trial of swallowing sterile water in case of aspiration) or by gavage. Ten per cent dextrose in water may be used, but will quickly lead to loose stools if continued for any length of time. Regular formula that also provides fat and protein should follow as soon as tolerated.

Undoubtedly the safest and most physiologic method of treating early hypoglycemia in SGA babies is to infuse glucose solution by peripheral IV. This provides a steady input of sugar (and a line for administering electrolytes and medications if necessary) until such time as adequate oral intake is established. By starting early, one can usually manage things with 5 per cent dextrose in water, but in more severe cases it may prove necessary to advance to 7½ or 10 per cent dextrose. Beyond that it becomes necessary to administer higher concentrations (12½ or 15 per cent dextrose) by way of a central line such as through an umbilical venous or arterial catheter.

The frequently recommended practice of injecting a bolus of 50 per cent dextrose in hypoglycemia in the newborn is both dangerous and unnecessary. If given through a peripheral IV, this hypertonic solution invariably scleroses the vessel and can cause local tissue damage if it infiltrates. Similar damage to the vessel can occur if given through an umbilical artery catheter, or to liver tissue if the umbilical venous catheter tip is in a hepatic vein rather than through the ductus venosus and in the inferior vena cava or heart. The point to be made is that all of these potential complications can be avoided if one realizes that the same total quantity of glucose can be delivered by reducing the concentration but increasing the amount given, instead of giving smaller amounts of dangerously-high concentrated solution.

THERMOREGULATION

The problems of temperature maintenance in the SGA infant are unique in many ways and teach us much about thermoregulation in newborns in general. Although rather severe limitations are placed upon the SGA baby by his relatively small body size and lack of energy stores and insulation, his homeothermic (temperature stabilizing) responses are comparatively well-developed, at least to the degree of his advanced gestational age.

Thermoregulation is a matter of balancing heat loss with heat production. One loses heat to (or gains heat from) the environment by radiation, convection, evaporation, and conduction. The amount of heat lost is dependent upon the difference between skin and air (or surrounding object) temperature, or the so-called external gradient, as well as the difference in temperature between the interior of the body (core temperature) and skin temperature, or the so-called internal gradient. If one is faced with an unfavorable external temperature gradient, one can attempt to minimize heat loss to the environment by reducing the portion of total body surface exposed to the outside, and by reducing the internal gradient through a process of restricting the flow of warm blood from the interior of the body to the skin where heat may be lost to the environment by one or more of the four mechanisms listed above.

The small-for-date infant has two advantages over the normal premature of equal size when it comes to minimizing heat loss to the environment. In the first place, he is better able to flex his extremities and thereby reduce the total amount of surface area exposed to the outside. Secondly, his ability to shut down his peripheral circulation through vasomotor control (reducing the inner size of the vessels by active constriction of muscle fibers in the walls of the vessels) is more advanced. However, the SGA infant shares the same unfavorably large surface area per unit of body mass as does the normal premature, and he also lacks tissue thickness and subcutaneous fat insulation to slow down the exchange of heat from the body to the environment.

As for heat production to offset excessive heat losses, the SGA infant is again slightly better off than is the normal premature infant of comparable size. As long as his energy supplies hold out, he is able to consume more oxygen to produce more heat than is his premature counterpart. The fuel to be burned with oxygen to produce heat is primarily glucose and fat. The latter is mobilized by the action of norepinephrine, and it has been shown that the SGA baby can increase norepinephrine excretion during cold stress to a greater degree than can premature babies of similar size. Again, however, the SGA baby faces the same (if not worse) lack of substrate (glucose and fat) to burn for heat as does the premature, and further heat production comes to a halt if he becomes hypoglycemic or hypoxemic. Likewise, if cold stress is allowed to continue for extended periods, lipid (fat) stores may become exhausted, and profound hypothermia (low body temperature) will then quickly result.

The therapeutic consequences of this knowledge of thermoregulatory mechanisms are obvious. One must reduce the external temperature gradient between skin and air by warming the surrounding air (as in the incubator), or one must constantly replenish the heat the baby is losing to the environment by an accessory heat source focusing on his body (as is done with a radiant heat warmer). Furthermore, one must provide the infant with substrate faster than he is able to burn it for heat production and growth so that he will not become hypoglycemic, hypoxemic, or run out of lipid stores. Supplemental modes of feeding (see section on parenteral alimentation) may thus prove necessary in the early days of life of these infants until their oral caloric intake becomes adequate.

Table 37-3 summarizes some of the major differences between the two major groups of low-birth-weight babies, the premature and the small-for-date infant.

TABLE 37-3. Comparison of the Two Major Groups of Low-Birth-Weight Infants

Premature	*Small-for-Date*
Higher neonatal mortality	Higher incidence of congenital anomalies
Major regulatory problems: Frequent apneic spells Cardiac arrhythmias common Accentuated temperature fluctuations High incidence of hypoglycemia and hypocalcemia	Problems due to low energy reserves: High incidence of fetal distress and asphyxia neonatorum Hypothermia when energy stores are exhausted Higher incidence of hypoglycemia Hypocalcemia occurs postasphyxia
Marked initial weight loss	Initial weight loss less severe or prolonged
Major respiratory problem is hyaline membrane disease	Most frequent respiratory problem is meconium aspiration pneumonia
High incidence of intracranial hemorrhage	High incidence of pulmonary hemorrhage
Accentuated physiologic anemia	Polycythemia
Accentuated physiologic jaundice	Less frequent nonhemolytic jaundice
Low resistance to neonatal bacterial infections	Intrauterine infections frequent cause of growth retardation

PROBLEMS OF THE POSTMATURE INFANT

Postmaturity is perhaps the most underrated high-risk condition in perinatology. One still encounters those who even question the existence of the "so-called postmaturity syndrome." Others simply have little appreciation of its significance.

Conservatively defined, an infant is postmature if gestation was 43 weeks (300 days) or more duration. The incidence of postmaturity using this definition is about 6 per cent. Yet postmaturity and its complications account for approximately 16 per cent of all perinatal deaths! This is because there is at least a twofold higher perinatal mortality (sum of fetal and neonatal deaths) in postmature versus term pregnancies. The high death rate is particularly pronounced (one in ten) in postmature babies born of primagravida mothers. This is due to related problems occurring more frequently in first pregnancies such as toxemia, hypertension, and prolonged labor (lasting longer than 24 hours). Half of the deaths are fetal deaths and the other half are the result of birth injuries, neonatal asphyxia, meconium aspiration with respiratory failure (see below), or severe congenital anomalies especially involving the CNS. This last point may have etiologic (causal) significance since we know that endocrine function of the fetus is important for the onset of labor, and central structures such as the thalamus, hypothalamus, and pituitary play key roles in endocrine regulation. Anencephalics (born with no brain) lack these structures, and they have an eightfold greater incidence of postmaturity than normally-formed infants.

Postmaturity occurs most frequently among primagravida and high parity mothers within any given age group. Furthermore, a positive history of prolonged gestation in the preceeding pregnancy is associated with a twofold increased incidence of repeat postmaturity. In addition to these predictive factors, there are a number of obstetric signs that may alert one to the possibility of postmaturity:

1. *Excessive* (greater than 5 pounds) *weight loss during the last weeks of pregnancy.*
2. *Oligohydramnios* or decreased amount (less than 300 cc.) of amniotic fluid. This finding may correlate with a decrease in uterine size during prolonged gestation.
3. Palpation during labor of a *hard fetal head*, or a *lack of cephalic molding.* The prolonged gestation allows for a more advanced degree of bone development, including the skull. Molding (conforming of the head to the shape of the birth canal) is resisted, and this may lead to high arrest of the fetal head, prolongation of labor, uterine inertia, and so forth.
4. *Meconium staining of the amniotic fluid.* As mentioned before, this is a reliable indication of fetal distress and may reflect reduced functioning of the postmature placenta and/or hypoxia associated with prolonged labor.
5. *Asphyxia at birth* not accounted for by abnormal labor or delivery. With current fetal monitoring techniques in wide use, such cases of "unexpected" newborn asphyxia are much less frequently encountered.

The postmature newborn has a number of characteristic physical findings. Some of these are not exclusive to the postmature infant. However, the more of the following signs that are present, the more likely is the clinical diagnosis of postmaturity:

1. *Wrinkled or macerated skin.* This is best seen on the hands and feet which have a "soaked in water" appearance. The skin is boggy, wrinkled, and elevated in large folds.
2. *Cracked, parchment-like skin.* This becomes pronounced once the skin dries. It may then desquamate or flake off, or peel off in sheets (Fig. 37-13).

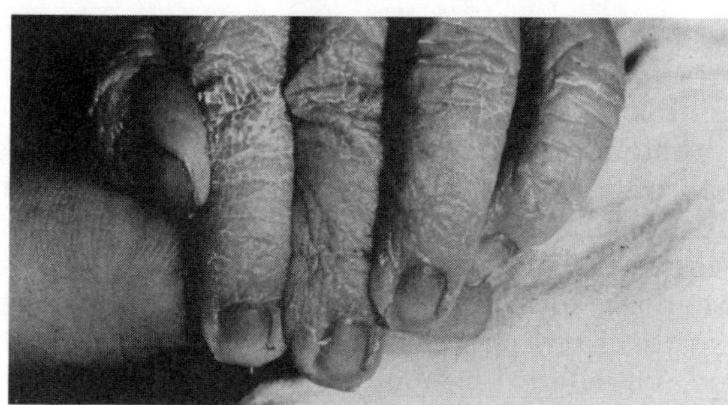

FIGURE 37-13. Cracked, parchment-like skin of the postmature infant. Note also the long, curved fingernails.

3. The above two skin changes are associated with an *absence of vernix caseosa* (cheesy skin coating normally covering the fetus). This lack of protective vernix exposes the epidermis (outer layers of skin) to the amniotic fluid and undoubtedly contributes to its maceration and desquamation.
4. *Reduced subcutaneous tissue and loose, pale skin.* These changes occur secondary to the acute weight loss late in gestation, and the ongoing cornification (stratifying) of the outer layers of the skin. The loose skin is especially evident over the thighs and buttocks. The increased cornification of the skin tends to obscure the underlying capillaries giving the skin its pale appearance.
5. *Long, curved fingernails and toenails.* The nails of the postmature continue to grow in utero past term and curve owing to their increased length (see Fig. 37-13).
6. *Green-yellow staining* of skin, nails and cord. The staining is caused by the presence of meconium in the amniotic fluid. Yellow staining implies that the meconium has been present for a sufficient time (six or more hours) to have become oxidized from green to yellow, and points to prolonged fetal distress.

Problems encountered in postmature infants may include all of the metabolic disturbances seen in small-for-date infants (see above), as well as complications arising from birth asphyxia (see section on asphyxia neonatorum above). Of special concern to neonatologists is the frequent association between postmaturity and the problems of massive meconium aspiration and polycythemia.

MECONIUM ASPIRATION

A large percentage of infants born with meconium staining of the amniotic fluid will have aspirated or inhaled some of this irritating substance into their lungs before or during birth. Although all fetuses make small rapid respiratory movements in utero, these are not sufficient to draw in amniotic fluid into their lungs. In fact, the lungs are constantly secreting fluid of their own which is periodically discharged into the surrounding amniotic fluid. Only when the fetus is stimulated prematurely to begin gasping respirations can amniotic fluid and its contents be brought into the lungs. The same stimulus that led to the premature passage of meconium, namely hypoxia or fetal distress, can also provoke premature onset of gasping respirations and subsequent meconium aspiration.

Since 5 to 10 per cent of all deliveries reveal meconium staining of the amniotic fluid, and nearly 60 per cent of these will be found to have meconium-containing material in their trachias, the problem of meconium aspiration represents a major cause of respiratory distress in the newborn. This is particularly the case in large infants or more mature (especially postmature) infants who have the muscle strength to suck in the thick material all the way down into their lungs. However, only about 25 per cent of all those with meconium staining will show roentgenographic changes suggestive of aspiration, and only half of these (or 10 to 15 per cent of the total) will exhibit respiratory symptoms of major concern.

The roentgenographic signs suggesting meconium aspiration in the newborn include:

1. Coarse, patchy areas of decreased aeration, collapse, or infiltration asymmetrically distributed throughout both lungs.
2. Fluid in the intralobar fissures (horizontal spaces between the lobes) and in the costophrenic angles (where the lateral diaphragm meets the chest wall).
3. Hyperaeration (air-trapping) or overexpansion of those areas not collapsed, with depression of the diaphragm.
4. Evidence of pulmonary air leak (interstitial emphysema, pneumomediastinum and pneumothroax).

Clinical symptoms in the infant with significant meconium aspiration include tachypnea (fast breathing) and tachycardia (fast pulse), inspiraory nasal flaring and retractions (sucking in above, between, and below the ribs), expiratory grunting, increased AP (anterior-posterior or front to back) diameter of the chest, palpable liver (brought down with the diaphragm) and noisy respirations with rales (rattles) and ronchi (snoring sounds) heard on auscultation of the lungs (listening with a stethoscope). The tachypnea may persist for many days, and in severe cases, the infant may show increasing cyanosis and difficulty breathing until he requires assisted ventilation to survive. In the most severe cases, the material is so thick that it blocks the trachea, and must be immediately removed at birth by suctioning or the infant will die quickly from asphyxia. These babies will be struggling frantically for air with deep retractions upon each gasp, or they already may be in secondary apnea (see above section on asphyxia) and are beyond the stage where they can struggle for breath.

Meconium may not only partially or completely block bronchi, but it is also very irritating and represents a good media (source of nutrients) for bacteria to grow. The inflammatory reaction (swelling due to increased blood flow and edema in the area) slowly worsens, eventually blocking off distal airways, just as the clumps of meconium did initially. That is to say, if the trachea is suctioned but the smaller or thinner meconium is driven down further into the lungs, the resulting delayed inflammatory reaction may later result in severe respiratory distress and eventual respiratory failure. So often one sees meconium-stained babies who are resuscitated at birth and subsequently do well for a period of hours. However, they then develop increasing respiratory distress, or they suddenly deteriorate upon developing a pulmonary air leak, just when things were thought to be going well.

The ball-valve mechanism that leads to air trapping and eventual pulmonary air leak with extrinsic restriction of alveolar expansion has been described previously in the discussion of mechanical problems involving the airways and lungs. The alveolus that finally ruptures need not be at the surface of the lung so that the leaking air immediately forms a pneumothorax. More often it is somewhere in the middle of the lung, so that the leaking air now must track along the loose connective tissue around the vessels and bronchi (interstitial emphysema), and either go out to the edge of the lung to break through the visceral pleura (single-layered membrane on the outer surface of the lung) or more likely go inward to the mediastinum. Here it fills a number of small chambers bordered by connective tissue around the large vessels and heart. It may push up the thymus so that its tip floats free like a sail (see Fig. 37-4B), or it may (as seen on roentgenogram) form a halo around the heart on the AP film. The leaking air may also tract down under the parietal pleura (membrane lining the inner chest cavity) of the mediastinum and along the diaphragm forming a halo over its upper border. Eventually it may break through the parietal pleura and again form a pneumothorax. It is extremely important to comprehend this possible chain of events if one is to correctly interpret newborn chest films and be able to anticipate impending life-threatening tension pneumothorax in a baby who has been identified as already having interstitial emphysema or a pneumomediastinum.

A new and effective but very aggressive form of treatment for babies suffering from massive meconium aspiration is gradually gaining acceptance and will undoubtedly save many lives in the future. Because it is impossible to avoid pushing further into the lungs some of the meconium remaining after quick suctioning of the trachia at birth and applying positive pressure ventilation to the infant (see section on assisted ventilation and resuscitation) to initially expand the lungs, it is necessary to find some method of later removing that meconium before it can cause the serious inflammatory reaction described above. This can in fact be achieved by lavaging (washing out) the airways with a nonirritating solution such as normal saline. This is done by passing a suction tube down into the mainstem bronchi, one at a time, and briskly squirting 3 to 5 cc. of normal saline into the distal airway. This is immediately suctioned out, removing large amounts of green meconium. The child is bagged with high oxygen concentration in between and then the process is repeated on alternate sides until the aspirate is completely clear of meconium. This may take 5 or 6 washings on a side, and if oxygen is used in abundance between lavages, the baby tolerates the procedure amazingly well. If performed within the first thirty minutes of life, there should be no significant subsequent inflammatory reaction. In my own experience over the past two years, there has not been a single case of massive meconium aspiration that went on to respiratory failure if the child was inborn and received early lavage treatment. However, it has been necessary to mechanically ventilate a large percentage of those infants transported from distant hospitals where lavage was not previously performed, and 5 out of 7 of these respirator babies were lost during the same two year period.

POLYCYTHEMIA

Polycythemia, or increased red blood cell volume (recognized by a high hematocrit or hemoglobin), is frequently seen in postmature infants. It is also common in SGA infants whose growth retardation is due to placental insufficiency, infants of diabetic mothers, and the larger of discordant twins (differing in appearance but originating from the same egg [monovular]). Of particular concern is the infant who is both postmature and small for gestational age since the degree of polycythemia is likely to be greater from the beginning and will become even worse over the first half-day of life, as the infant excretes a portion of his known excess extracellular water (see section on SGA infants).

A hematocrit taken from heel-stick blood is invariably higher than that measured from blood taken out of a vein or umbilical catheter because of sludging (packing together) of blood cells in the distal capillaries when peripheral circulation is slowed down for one reason or another. It is therefore preferable to define polycythemia in the newborn as any *venous (or central) hematocrit* (Hct.) over 60 per cent, and severe polycythemia as a hematocrit over 70 per cent. It is somewhere between these two levels of Hct. that blood viscosity (internal friction due to the sliding of one layer of fluid over another) increases radically. The resultant "hyperviscosity" may cause a decrease in blood flow and increased workload on the heart, as well as an increased blood clotting and bleeding tendency. Every postmature infant should have his hematocrit checked during the transitional period (first six hours of life), and if the peripheral Hct. is greater than 60 per cent, a repeat Hct. should be done on venous blood.

Some infants with polycythemia show no initial symptoms other than a ruddy appearance (plethora), or they may appear cyanotic when they cry. Cyanosis is determined by the absolute concentration of reduced hemoglobin (that which is not bound with oxygen) in the blood, and is present whenever there are 4 or more grams per 100 cc. of blood (g.%). The more hemoglobin (or higher hematocrit) an infant has, the more likely he is to have a total of 4 g.% hemoglobin in the reduced state and thereby appear cyanotic since this level can be attained now at near-normal percentages of oxygen saturation of the blood (percentage of hemoglobin bound or "saturated" with oxygen). For example, a normal infant with a hemoglobin of 18 g.% and a Hct. of 3 times that or 54 per cent) would have to have less than 78 per cent of his hemoglobin bound with oxygen to appear cyanotic, because it takes 22 per cent (100 − 78 = 22) of 18 g.% to equal the needed 4 g.% of reduced hemoglobin to make him appear cyanotic. However, an infant who is polycythemic and has a hemoglobin of 24 g.% (Hct. of 72 per cent), will appear cyanotic when his oxygen saturation is nearly within the normal range at 83 per cent (normal is greater than 85 per cent) since 17 per cent (100 − 83 = 17) of 24 g.% is also 4 g.%. Oxygen saturation is likely to be reduced (and therefore cause cyanosis) in the newborn who cries, because he ventilates less well when he holds his breath, and he shunts more blood R→L (bypassing the lungs) through his still-open ductus arteriosus and foramen ovale when he increases his intrathoracic (inside the chest cage) pressure during crying.

Other symptoms sometimes associated with polycythemia include the usual signs of respiratory distress (may also be the result of aspiration in the same baby), central nervous system abnormalities such as seizures (may also be secondary to asphyxia or metabolic disturbances in the same baby), signs of heart failure, and jaundice or hyperbilirubinemia.

The pulmonary, CNS, and cardiac symptoms seen in certain babies with polycythemia are best ascribed to the circulatory difficulties brought on by the increased blood viscosity, although the exact mechanisms are not yet completely understood. The hyperbilirubinemia and jaundice so frequently seen in babies that are polycythemic are best understood by knowing the usual processes involved with hemoglobin degradation (breakdown). One gram of degradated hemoglobin produces approximately 34 mg. of bilirubin that has to be cleared from the blood by the liver (see discussion of jaundice above). If the infant has 25 per cent more hemoglobin than normal (e.g., 24 g.% rather than 18 g.%, or Hct. of 72 per cent rather than 54 per cent), it means he must clear that much more bilirubin just in the process of keeping up with what is broken down daily. Assuming the normal life span of a newborn's red blood cells to be somewhere between 50 and 100 days, this means he is forced to clear the bilirubin produced by the degradation of 1 to 2 per cent of his hemoglobin every day. A polycythemic baby weighing 3 kilograms and having a blood volume of about 250 cc. (80 to 85 cc. per kilogram) and a total hemoglobin content of 60 grams (24 grams per 100 cc.) will have to clear 0.6 to 1.2 grams of degradated hemoglobin or 20 to 40 mg. of bilirubin (0.6 to 1.2 × 34) daily instead of 15 to 30 mg. if he had a hemoglobin of 18 g.%.

Polycythemia should be treated whenever a baby is symptomatic or if the central hematocrit is greater than 70 per cent. Treatment is accomplished by performing a partial exchange transfusion, using fresh frozen plasma rather than whole blood for the exchange. By using the following formula which allows calculation of the amount of plasma to be used (exchanging 10 cc. increments at a time), the baby's hematocrit can be lowered to the desired level of around 60 per cent:

$$\text{cc.'s of plasma for the exchange} = \frac{\text{blood volume} \times (\text{original Hct.} - \text{desired Hct.})}{\text{original Hct.}}$$

NEONATAL PROBLEMS DUE TO PREGNANCY COMPLICATIONS OR MATERNAL DISEASE

The following discussion is concerned with neonatal pathophysiologic processes that originate in the pregnancy itself or can be traced to maternal disorders or disease. As mentioned previously, prenatal and maternal history takes on great importance in neonatology since it provides the earliest clues or signals of potential problems which are more easily handled if detected early. Furthermore, everything that happens later in the newborn period has its roots in the prenatal, intrapartal, and transitional periods to some degree. A really close look at all pathophysiologic processes occurring in the immediate newborn period show some effects of prior maternal problems of pregnancy, labor or delivery, or the influence of events occurring during labor and delivery, or stresses imposed in making the transition from fetal to extrauterine life. However, there are a number of pathologic conditions encountered in the newborn period that stem directly from problems arising from the pregnancy itself or from prior maternal disease. Two such conditions to be described in detail here are erythroblastosis fetalis (due to Rh or ABO incompatability) and the problems encountered in the infant of a diabetic mother.

Rh AND ABO ERYTHROBLASTOSIS FETALIS

Erythroblastosis fetalis (hemolytic disease of the fetus) results from maternal sensitization or immunization against a fetal blood antigen (foreign substance that stimulates specific antibody formation) that she herself does not possess. The resultant antibodies produced by the mother cross the placenta and cause immediate or delayed destruction (hemolysis) of the fetal red blood cells. The fetus, or later the newborn, responds by increasing production (poiesis) of young erythrocytes (erythroblasts) in the bone marrow or other sites such as the liver and spleen (extramedullary erythropoiesis). If the rate of destruction exceeds the rate of new cell production, the fetus or newborn becomes anemic. If the amount of bilirubin produced from the hemoglobin released from the destroyed red cells exceeds the baby's ability to clear it, hyperbilirubinemia and jaundice result. If the level of bilirubin exceeds the capacity of the blood to bind it to protein, the free bilirubin may pass the blood-brain barrier and enter the nuclei of the brain causing damage or a condition called kernicterus.

The mechanisms by which the mother becomes sensitized or immunized against blood antigens possessed by the fetus but not by herself are well understood in the case of Rh erythroblastosis but poorly understood in the case of ABO erythroblastosis. In the Rh situation, it is most commonly a matter of fetal blood cells containing the antigen crossing the placenta and getting into the maternal circulation during the pregnancy, or at the time of delivery of a previous pregnancy or abortion. In the ABO situation, the immunizing process most likely has nothing to do with the pregnancy, but rather results from some other exposure to the A or B antigen known to occur in certain bacteria and foodstuffs. In both cases, a *critical amount* of exposure to the antigen is required to trigger the maternal antibody-producing mechanism. For Rh erythroblastosis, this amount has been estimated at approximately 1 cc. of Rh-positive cells entering the maternal circulation, or ½ cc. as a primary stimulus followed by $^1/_{10}$ or $^1/_5$ cc. as a booster stimulus during a subsequent pregnancy.

Approximately 15 per cent of all Caucasians have Rh-negative blood. About 80 per cent of Rh-negative females mate with Rh-positive males, accounting for nearly 12 per cent of all infants born. Since 65 per cent of the babies from such matings of Rh-negative females with Rh-positive males will have Rh-positive blood, one would expect that 1 out of 10 babies born would have Rh erythroblastosis if all such mothers were sensitized. Fortunately, even in the days before RhoGAM only about 1 in 20 Rh-incompatible matings resulted in fetal Rh hemolytic disease, for an overall incidence of 1 in 200 to 250 deliveries. Obstetric factors known to increase the likelihood of maternal Rh-sensitization include toxemia of pregnancy, amniocentesis, version procedures, cesarean section, breech delivery, manual removal of the placenta, and abortion. An important factor that reduced the incidence of Rh-sensitization in pregnancy was the presence of a double incompatibility, or ABO as well as Rh differences between mother and child. This was because the fetal cells that reached the mother were destroyed by the naturally-occurring anti-A or anti-B antibodies in her circulation before sensitization to the Rh antigen could take place. It was this realization that led to the use of anti-D gamma globulin (RhoGAM) to prevent Rh sensitization in Rh-negative mothers delivering Rh-positive babies. Such injection of the human immune globulin after delivery works to destroy the fetal cells that have reached the mother and to block maternal antibody production.

Approximately 20 per cent of all pregnancies involve ABO incompatibility, and half of these consist of an O-group mother with an A- or B-group baby. However, hemolytic disease is only seen in about 10 per cent of all ABO incompatible set-ups instead of 10 per cent of all deliveries because anti-A and anti-B immune antibodies do not pass as easily into the fetus as do anti-Rh antibodies. Also, the fetus has A or B antigen in other tissues besides the red cells so that the immune antibodies that do get across are absorbed in part by these other tissues and are less likely to affect the red blood cells.

In severe cases of Rh erythroblastosis fetalis, the production of new red blood cells by the fetus fails to keep up with the continuing hemolysis, and anemia becomes extreme. In a further attempt to compensate for reduced oxygen transport to the tissues, the fetus expands his blood volume by drawing in more fluid and by increasing his cardiac output. However, due to the need to maintain such a high cardiac output, and because of the tissue hypoxia that results from reduced oxygen-carrying capacity of the blood, the heart may fail and tissue edema may become increasingly severe. Fluid collects in the larger spaces too, such as in the pleural and peritoneal cavities, resulting in the overall picture of anasarca (hydrops fetalis).

Hydropic hemolytic disease is further characterized by abnormalities of the endocrine glands, namely hyperplasia (excessive enlargement) of the fetal zone of the adrenal cortex and of the pancreatic islets. This latter change results in an overproduction of insulin and the tendency of these infants to suffer from neonatal hypoglycemia similar to infants of diabetic mothers. Another problem frequently seen in these babies is their tendency to bleed. With the anemia there is associated thrombocytopenia (low platelet count). This fact, along with the hypoxic damage to the capillaries, may explain the bleeding tendency in these already-compromised erythroblastotic babies.

Emergency resuscitation and treatment is usually necessary at the time of birth in the more severely anemic (hemoglobin less than 8 to 10 g.%) or hydropic infants if they are to survive. O, Rh-negative "universal donor" packed cells should be on hand at the time of delivery in babies thought or known (by successive amniotic fluid analyses) to be severely affected. After respirations have been established, an umbilical venous catheter is placed and central venous pressure (CVP) is measured. Nearly half of the infants are already in shock (low CVP), whereas the other half are in high output cardic failure (high CVP). In the former group, rapid transfusion of 15 to 20 cc. per kg. of packed cells expands their blood volume and gets them out of shock as well as raises their hemoglobin level to improve oxygen-carrying capacity. In the latter group, one must first reduce the intravascular volume by drawing off sufficient blood to lower their CVP to the 10 to 15 cm. H_2O pressure range, and then raise their hemoglobin and hematocrit level by carrying out a modified exchange transfusion with the packed cells. Once their cardiovascular status is stabilized, the other problems one must anticipate include the hypoglycemia that can be controlled with IV glucose infusion, hyaline membrane disease if they are born prematurely as is so frequently the case, bleeding tendency, and early-onset jaundice that can rapidly lead to kernicterus if not controlled.

TABLE 37-4. Clinical Phases of Kernicterus*

Phase	*Time of Onset*	*Symptoms*
One	2nd–3rd day of life	Hypotonia, lethargy, and a poor sucking reflex.
Two	3rd–4th day of life	Spasticity and opisthotonus and fever.
Three	Second month of life	Gradual appearance of extrapyramidal signs (athetoid cerebral palsy).

*Adapted from Van Praagh, R.: Diagnosis of Kernicterus in the Neonatal Period. Pediatrics, 28:870, 1961.

Kernicterus presents in three rather clearly defined clinical phases as outlined in Table 37-4. Key factors in determining the level of bilirubin at which kernicterus will occur include the degree of maturity of the baby, his level of unbound albumin, and his acid-base status. The ideal measure to decide when an exchange transfusion is indicated in a particular baby would be his "free bilirubin level" throughout the course of his jaundice, since it is the free bilirubin that has access to the brain. Considerable effort is presently being devoted to develop such a laboratory test to determine free bilirubin level. In the meantime, one generally begins with the "absolute-maximal bilirubin level allowed" (widely accepted to be 20 mg.%) and lowers

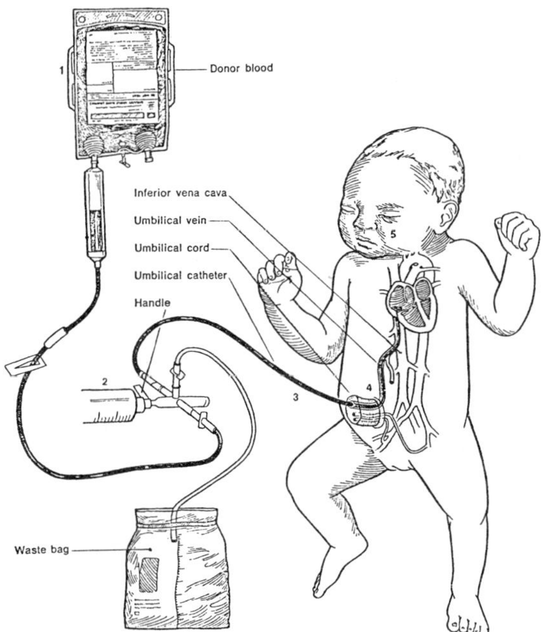

FIGURE 37-14. Five principal danger points in performing exchange transfusion. 1) Donor blood: transfusion reaction due to mismatched blood, blood too cold, blood too old, blood too acidic. 2) Syringing technique: too-rapid hemodynamic changes, overloading of circulation due to errors in syringing. 3) Umbilical catheter (external): air embolism, infection. 4) Umbilical catheter (internal): perforation of umbilical vessels, cardiac arrhthmias due to catheter irritation, rupture of spleen, subsequent portal hypertension. 5) Airway: asphyxia, aspiration pneumonitis. (From Pochedly, C.: *Minimizing risk exchange transfusion.* Am. Fam. Physician 2:75, 1970, with permission.)

the "exchange level" below this in accordance with the baby's degree of prematurity, hypoalbuminemia, and acidosis. Some babies need to be exchanged at bilirubin levels as low as 10 to 12 mg.%.

The technique of *exchange transfusion* is quite straightforward but fraught with risks to the baby. Figure 37-14 illustrates the principle points of danger in actually performing an exchange. One could add to this the danger of cardiac arrhythmias if the catheter is in the heart, or bradycardia if the calcium (to replenish that removed from blood anticoagulated with citrate) is injected too rapidly. Also there is the danger of subsequent development of necrotizing enterocolitis due to compromised bowel circulation from a misplaced catheter or thromboembolic processes. These potential complications necessitate that fresh blood be used, that the blood be warmed on its way to the baby, that the location of the catheter be verified by roentgenogram, that heart rate and body temperature be monitored continuously during the procedure, that central venous pressure be measured intermittently during and after the procedure, and that absolute sterile technique be employed.

Other potential problems associated with exchange transfusion include the development of hypoglycemia, hypocalcemia, and respiratory and metabolic acidosis. Hypoglycemia is most commonly a rebound phenomenon due to increased insulin release in response to the rather large glucose load represented in ACD (acid-citrate-dextrose) exchange blood. When the procedure is concluded, the glucose (dextrose) is suddenly cut off, leaving the high levels of insulin unopposed to produce hypoglycemia, unless an infusion of 10 per cent glucose water is maintained and gradually tapered off after the exchange. Hypocalcemia should not be a problem if adequate amounts of 10 per cent calcium gluconate (½ cc. after every 50 cc. of blood exchanged) are given during the procedure. In premature babies with limited ventilatory reserves or the added problem of hyaline membrane disease, this may pose a real threat to life. CPD (citrate-phosphate-dextrose) blood is preferred here since it presents less of an acid load to the baby. Intermittent or continuous ventilatory support in these very small babies with respiratory distress is frequently required.

THE INFANT OF A DIABETIC MOTHER

The infant of a diabetic mother (IDM) has long been a prime example of the newborn at

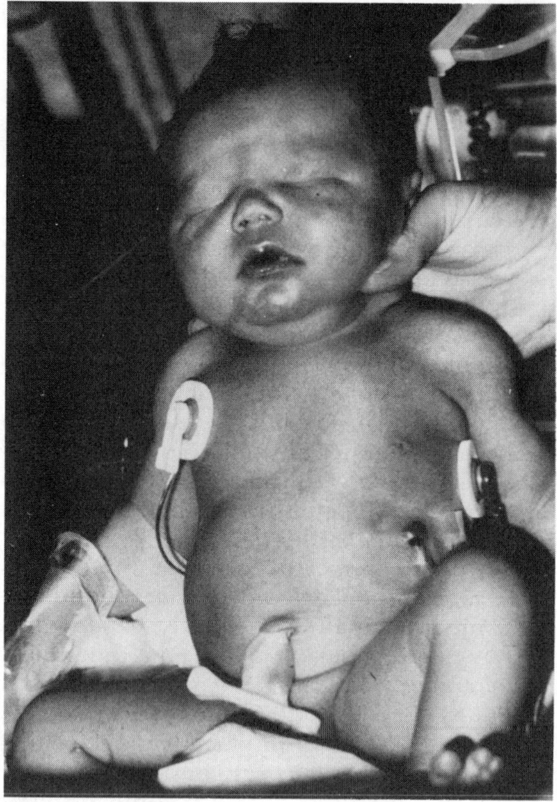

FIGURE 37-15. Infant of a diabetic mother.

risk. Indeed, the IDM is at great risk to die before birth (stillbirth) or in the immediate newborn period. Mortality is about equally divided between stillbirths and neonatal deaths, with the mortality rate dependent upon both the severity of the mother's disease and how well the mother and baby are managed during the perinatal period.

The severity of maternal disease is classified from A through F. Class A diabetics, also called "gestational diabetics" because they only test abnormal during or immediately after pregnancy, require no insulin to remain metabolically stable. In contrast, class B through F diabetics are all insulin dependent and fall into the various categories according to age of onset, duration of disease, and presence of vascular or renal complications. Perinatal mortality rate approaches 20 per cent in the latter classes, but may be reduced by more than half by hospitalizing mothers at 34 weeks of gestation, monitoring closely for signs of placental insufficiency, going to term whenever possible, and by affording the infants transitional and neonatal intensive care.

Morbidity also depends upon the severity of the mother's disease, as attested to by the fact that infants of gestational diabetics (IGDM) have a considerably lower incidence of neonatal problems associated with maternal diabetes than do those from class B through F mothers. This will be brought out as we discuss the individual problems of the IDM.

Clinically, the IDM is easily identified (Fig. 37-15). The baby is usually large-for-date, being above the ninetieth percentile for both weight and length at birth. The overall body size is large (macrosomia) as is the heart (cardiomegaly), liver (hepatomegaly), spleen (splenomegaly) and umbilical cord (part of splanchnomegaly). He is plethoric (ruddy in appearance) and full-faced (cushingoid facies). All IDM's look remarkably alike, except those born of mother's with advanced vascular or renal disease. Such babies tend to be SGA rather than LGA, and better exemplify the problems of that risk group (see above).

A closer look at the body make-up of an IDM reveals that the increased size is a result of increased fat tissue and glycogen stores in the organs, rather than increased tissue fluid or edema. In fact, the total body water of IDM's is reduced at birth and diminishes even further over the next day or two. This is due to their high urinary excretion rates (high urine output) in response to the freeing of intracellular water as glycogen stores are being broken down for energy purposes.

A number of the problems encountered in infants of diabetic mothers have been discussed above in conjunction with other high-risk newborn categories. Rather than reiterate points regarding anticipation, assessment, and supportive treatment for these problems, this discussion will be restricted to those pathophysiologic aspects of the problems that are unique to the IDM.

The *hypoglycemia* encountered in about one out of six IGDM's and four out of six IDM's is largely due to a state of functional hyperinsulinism (relatively high insulin-producing capacity) in the affected newborn. During pregnancy, maternal glucose crosses the placenta but insulin does not because of its large size. The fetus is thus required to adjust to the higher-than-normal sugar levels of the diabetic mother by producing increased amounts of insulin himself. The beta cells of his pancreatic islets that produce the insulin become hypertrophied (enlarged) to meet the increased demand. At the time of birth, he is suddenly cut off from the maternal glucose supply, although he does have considerable initial glycogen stores to fall back on. However, due to his relatively high insulin levels and large energy requirements, these stores are quickly depleted. The rate at which his blood glucose falls in the first hours after birth is directly proportional to how high the cord blood glucose was, and provides us with a measure of how severe the problem is likely to become.

Recent studies have also demonstrated an impaired epinephrine release in response to hypoglycemia in infants of diabetic mothers. Epinephrine is a substance largely produced in the medulla (inner portion) of the adrenal glands, and it acts to raise blood glucose levels by stimulating mobilization of glucose from glycogen in the liver, and by inhibiting further release of insulin from the pancreas. In IDM's, it is as if their regulatory mechanism for handling situations in which the blood sugar level gets low has not yet been learned, since the fetal glucose level was generally kept high by the mother.

As mentioned above in the section on *hyaline membrane disease*, the increased incidence of this disease in IDM's can be largely accounted for by the increased frequency of premature deliveries and/or cesarean sections. Whether there is an additional factor that increases the incidence of HMD in IDM's beyond this is still open to debate. The incidence of IRDS in IGDM's is approximately 1 in 20, and in IDM's 1 in 4.

Hyperbilirubinemia seen so frequently in infants of diabetic mothers is also directly related to gestational age at the time of birth. IDM's born between 32 to 34 weeks of gestation have a greater than 50 per cent incidence of hyperbilirubinemia, whereas those born after 37 weeks of gestation have a rate of about 15 per cent. Since many of these babies are also *polycythemic*, there is this additional load of bilirubin to be cleared from the natural process of red blood cell breakdown, as described in the previous section on postmaturity. In conjunction with their problems of low total body water, increased urinary excretion in the first day or two of life, and the osmotic diuresis associated with glycosuria (see above), this polycythemia in a baby who is already suffering from relative *dehydration* makes the IDM particularly vulnerable to *blood hyperviscosity* (thick blood that tends to sludge or circulate poorly) and subsequent *venous thrombosis* (clotting). Indeed, the frequently lethal complication of *renal vein thrombosis* is seen almost exclusively in infants of diabetic mothers. It should also be mentioned that the IDM seems to have an excess amount of extramedullary erythropoiesis (points of new red blood cell production outside the usual location in the bone marrow). These foci of generating blood cells are largely found in the liver and spleen (see discussion above on erythroblastosis), and may have an adverse effect on liver function and bilirubin clearance.

The *hypocalcemia* frequently seen in these babies (about 20 per cent in IGDM's and nearly 30 per cent in IDM's) probably can be totally accounted for by the associated high incidence of premature delivery and asphyxia at birth (see previous discussion on hypocalcemia). Tissue damage incurred during the frequently difficult delivery of these LGA babies adds to the phosphate load which is so difficult for the neonate to clear and accounts for some of the depression of serum calcium levels.

Birth injury as well as *asphyxia neonatorum* (incidence of 20 per cent in IGDM's and 35 per cent in IDM's; see previous discussion) is not at all uncommon in infants of diabetic mothers because of their large body size (macrosomia). Damage occurs most frequently to the head and neck and may take the form of cephalohematomas (subperiostial collection of blood over one of the skull bones), facial nerve paralysis due to difficult forceps delivery, fractured clavicles, and brachial plexus palsies (paralyses of the nerves coming from the cervical [neck] spinal cord and going to the arm). There are two main types of the latter injury, the Erb's paralysis and the Klumpke's paralysis.

The *Erb's paralysis* (most common) or upper arm palsy involves cervical nerve roots 5 and 6, and is the result of excessive traction (pulling) on the arm or shoulder (as in a difficult breech delivery) or excessive traction downward on the head to deliver the shoulder, thereby overstretching the neck and the nerve roots inside (as in a difficult cephalic presentation). This results in a drooping shoulder girdle on that side and an arm that hangs limply to the side with extended elbow and inwardly rotated wrist (palm faces outward in the "waiter's tip position"). If the roots themselves are avulsed (torn) close to the cord or if cervical nerve root 4 is also involved, there may be paralysis of the diaphragm on that side (*diaphragmatic hemiparalysis*) with subsequent respiratory distress. This possibility should always be checked in a baby found to have an Erb's palsy. Respirations are rapid and breath sounds weaker on that side. The upper abdominal wall and umbilicus may be shifted to that side on deep inspiration.

Treatment of Erb's palsy is supportive in all cases, and may include midpositioning of the joints, passive range of motion exercises without overstretching the paralyzed muscles, and pulmonary physiotherapy. On rare occasions involving diaphragmatic paralysis, ventilation may need to be supported or the diaphragm muscle surgically plicated (sewn over on itself to shorten or tighten it). A loose, floppy (lacking nervous innervation) diaphragm actually works against the baby's efforts to breathe, since it goes up (as intrathoracic pressure becomes negative) on inspiration rather than down as it should (paradoxical diaphragmatic movements).

The *Klumpke's paralysis* (extremely rare) or lower arm palsy involves the lower cervical nerve roots (eighth cervical root and first thoracic root), and is the result of obstetric maneuvers which cause excessive traction on the arm when it is already hyperabducted at the shoulder (moved away from the midline of the body). In contrast to the Erb's palsy, the elbow can be bent (flexed), but the hand grasp (grip) is lost. The wrist cannot be actively flexed but the fingertips can, leading to a "claw hand" deformity. It is not uncommon to have the cervical sympathetic nerve fibers also involved, since they are contained in the first thoracic root. This leads to the *Horner syndrome* (ptosis or droopy eye lid, miosis or contraction of the pupil of the eye, and enophthalmos or retraction of the eye into the orbit), and can often result in delayed pigmentation of the iris in the eye on that side.

There is also an increased incidence of serious *congenital anomalies* in infants of diabetic mothers. The overall incidence is close to 6 per cent of IDM's in contrast to the usual rate of about 2 per cent in all deliveries. SGA infants born of diabetic mothers with vascular complications seem to be at particular risk. The most common anomalies involved are *CNS malformations* such as anencephaly (lack of upper brain and skull), encephalocele (herniation of brain substance out of the skull along the midline), meningomyelocele, and hydrocephalus. The next most common group of anomalies seen in IDM's has been termed the *caudal regression syndrome.* These malformations include sacral agenesis (failure of formation of the sacral spine with lower limb weakness and/or deformities), absence of the femoral head with fixed hip joints, and shortening or deformities of the upper legs. Other malformations seen with increased frequency in infants of diabetic mothers include tracheoesophogeal fistula and congenital heart defects.

BIBLIOGRAPHY

General Texts

Behrman, R. E. (ed.): *Neonatology, Diseases of the Fetus and Infant,* C. V. Mosby, St. Louis, 1973.
Klaus, M. H. and Fanaroff, A. A.: *Care of the High-Risk Neonate,* W. B. Saunders, Philadelphia, 1973.
Schaffer, A. J. and Avery, M. E.: *Diseases of the Newborn,* ed. 3. W. B. Saunders, Philadelphia, 1971.
Young, D. G. and Weller, B. F.: *Baby Surgery, Nursing Management and Care.* University Park Press, Baltimore, 1971.

Topical References

Abramson, H. (ed.): *Resuscitation of the Newborn Infant,* ed. 3. C. V. Mosby, St. Louis, 1973.
Chapter 2: *Physiology and biochemistry* by James, L. S. (transition from fetal to extrauterine life).
Chapter 10: *The first sixty seconds of life* by Apgar, V. and James, L. S. (assessment at birth).
Chapter 21: *Surgical emergencies in respiratory difficulties of newborn inants* by Coryllos, E. (mechanical problems involving the airways and lungs).

Assali, N. (ed.): *Pathophysiology of Gestation, vol. 3: Fetal and Neonatal Disorders.* Academic Press, New York, 1972.
Part I: *Disorders of circulation.*
Part II: *Disorders of respiration.*

Avery, M. E. and Fletcher, B. D.: *The Lung and Its Disorders in the Newborn Infant,* ed. 3. W. B. Saunders, Philadelphia, 1974.
Part II: *Disorders of respiration in the newborn period* (mechanical problems involving the airways and lungs, malformations of the thorax and diaphragm, hyaline membrane disease, meconium aspiration, pulmonary air leak).

Cornblath, M.: *Disorders of Carbohydrate Metabolism in Infancy.* W. B. Saunders, Philadelphia, 1966.
Part II: *Problems of the newborn and neonate.*

Duffey, M., et al. (eds.): *Current Concepts in Clinical Nursing, vol. 3.* C. V. Mosby, St. Louis, 1971.
Chapter 8: *Nursing care of high-risk infants* by Harris, C. H. (Feeding and intravenous therapy, care of the baby with respiratory distress, psychologic and emotional problems in the intensive care nursery).

Lough, M.D., et al. (eds.): *Pediatric Respiratory Therapy.* Year Book Medical Publishers, Chicago, 1974.
Chapter 3: *Evaluation and care of the newborn infant* by Fanaroff, A. A. and Klaus, M. H. (resuscitation, transport, temperature control, oxygen theapy, treatment of hyaline membrane disease, assisted ventilation).
Chapter 6: *Mechanical ventilation* by Lough, M. D. (assisted ventilation equipment and techniques).

Oski, F. A. and Naiman, J. L.: *Hematologic Problems in the Newborn,* ed. 2. W. B. Saunders, Philadelphia, 1972.
Chapter 4: *Polycythemia in the neonatal period.*
Chapter 7: *Erythroblastosis fetalis* (Rh and ABO erythroblastosis, kernicterus, exchange transfusion).

Ross Laboratories Nursing Education Aids, No. 7: *Congenital Heart Abnormalities.* Columbus, Ohio, 1961.

Rowe, R. D. and Mehrizi, A.: *The Neonate with Congenital Heart Disease.* W. B. Saunders, Philadelphia, 1969.
Chapter 3: *Physical examination of the cardiovascular system of the newborn.*
Chapter 6: *The frequency of various cardiac malformations.*
Chapters 13, 21, 16, 20, 14, 17, 11, 25, 12, 29 and 9: (patent ductus, tricuspid atresia, pulmonary atresia, pulmonary stenosis, tetralogy of Fallot, total anomalous venous return, transposition, truncus arteriosis, VSD, ASD, and coarctation).

Stave, U. (ed.): *Physiology of the Perinatal Period, vol. 2.* Appleton-Century-Crofts, New York, 1970.
Part VII: *Hypoxia neonatorum.*
Chapter 35: *Metabolic Effects in Hypoxia Neonatorum,* by Stave, U. and Wolf, H. (asphyxia neonatorum).

Thaler, M. M.: *Perinatal bilirubin metabolism.* Schulman, I. (ed.): Advances in Pediatrics, vol 19. Year Book Medical Publishers, 1972, pp. 215–235. (physiologic jaundice of the premature and hyperbilirubinemia).

Winters, R. W. (ed.): *The Body Fluids in Pediatrics.* Little, Brown and Company, Boston, 1973.
Part II: *Disorders of the neonate.*
Chapter 9: *Acid-base changes in the perinatal period* by James, L. S. (fetal distress and asphyxia neonatorum).
Chapter 11: *Pathophysiology of birth asphyxia and resuscitation* by James, L. S. (asphyxia neonatorum and resuscitation).
Chapter 17: *Late metabolic acidosis of premature infants* by Kildeberg, P.

Selected Articles for Review

Behrman, R. E., et al.: *Treatment of the asphyxiated newborn infant.* J. Pediat. 74:981, 1969.

Choi, M.: *A comparison of maternal psychological reactions to premature and full size newborns.* Mater. Child Nurs. J. 2:1, 1973.

Daily, W. J. R., et al.: *Apnea in premature infants: Monitoring, incidence, heart rate changes, and an effect of environmental temperature.* Pediatrics 43:510, 1969.

Davis, L.: *Neonatal respiratory emergencies.* Nurs. Clin. North Am. 8:441, 1973.

Desmond, M., Rudolph, A. and Phitaksphraiwan, P.: *The transitional care nursery: A mechanism for preventive medicine in the newborn.* Ped. Clin. North Am. 16(3):651-669, 1966.

Dubowitz, L. M. S., et al.: *Clinical assessment of gestational age in the newborn infant.* J. Pediat. 77:1, 1970.

Edelmann, C. M., Jr. and Spitzer, A.: *The maturing kidney.* J. Pediat. 75:509, 1969.

Eng, G. D.: *Brachial plexus palsy in newborn infants.* Pediatrics 48:18, 1971.

Evans, J.: *Fundamentals of infant resuscitation.* Int. Anesthesiol. Clin. 11:141, 1973.

Fenner, A. et al.: *Periodic breathing in premature and neonatal babies: Incidence, breathing pattern, respiratory gas tensions, response to changes in the composition of ambient air.* Pediat. Res. 7:174, 1973.

Finnegan, L. and Machew, B.: *Care of the addicted infant.* Am. J. Nurs. 74:685, 1973.

Freeland, E.: *Long-term follow-up studies of prematurely born infants. I. Relationships of handicaps to nursery routines.* J. Pediat. 80:501, 1972.

Galloway, K.: *Early detection of congenital anomalies.* J. Obstet. Gynecol. Nurs. 2:37, 1973.

Gilien, N.: *Determinants of Birth Weight.* In Duffey, M., et al. (eds.): *Current Concepts in Clinical Nursing, vol. 3.* C. V. Mosby, St. Louis, 1971, pp. 169–177.

Gillen, J.: *Behavior of newborns with cardiac distress.* Am. J. Nurs. 73:254, 1973.

Gregory, G. A., et al.: *Treatment of idiopathic respiratory distress syndrome with continuous positive airway pressure.* N. Eng. J. Med. 284:1333, 1971.

Harris, C. H.: *Some ethical and legal consideration in neonatal intensive care.* Nurs. Clin. of North Am. 8:521, 1973.

Harris, C.: *Social problems surrounding the high-risk infant.* In Anderson, E., et al. (eds.): *Current Concepts in Clinical Nursing, vol. 4,* C. V. Mosby, 1973, pp. 100–110.

Hasselmeyer, E.: *Indices of fetal welfare.* In Bergersen B., et al. (eds): *Current Concepts in Clinical Nursing, vol. 2,* C. V. Mosby, St. Louis, 1973, pp. 298–317.

Jones, C., et al.: *Intravenous feeding of the newborn.* Nurs. Times 69:1364, 1973.

Katz, V.: *Auditory stimulation and developmental behavior of the premature infant.* Nurs. Res. 20:196, 1971.

Klaus, M. H. and Meyer, H. B. P.: *Oxygen therapy for the newborn.* Pediat. Clin. North Am. 13:731, 1966.

Kumpe, M., et al.: *Care of the infant with respiratory distress syndrome.* Nurs. Clin. North Am. 6:25, 1971.

Lees, M. H.: *Cyanosis in the newborn infant: Recognition and clinical evaluation.* J. Pediat. 77:484, 1970.

Lubchenco, L. O. and Bard, H.: *Incidence of hypoglycemia in newborn infants classified by birth weight and gestational age.* Pediatrics 47:831, 1971.

Lucey, J.: *Effects of light on the newly born infant.* J. Perinatal Med., Vols. I and III, pp. 147–150, 1973.

Lutz, L., et al.: *Temperature control in newborn babies.* Nurs. Clin. North Am. 6:15, 1971.

Maisels, M. J.: *Bilirubin—on understanding and influencing its metabolism in the newborn infant.* Pediat. Clin. North Am. 19:447, 1972.

Mast, F.: *Flight to life.* J. Obstet. Gynecol. Nurs. 3:15, 1974.

Meyers, R. E.: *Two patterns of perinatal brain damage and their conditions of occurrence.* Am. J. Obstet. Gynecol. 112:246, 1972.

Michaelis, R., et al.: *Activity states in premature and full term infants.* Dev. Psychobiol. 6:209, 1973.

Mingeot, R.: *The functional status of the newborn infant.* Am. J. Obstet. Gynecol. 115:1138, 1973.

Neal, M.: *Nursing care of the prematurely born neonate.* In Bergersen, B., et al. (eds.): *Current Concepts in Clinical Nursing, Vol. 2,* C. V. Mosby, St. Louis, 1969, pp. 332–339.

Neal, M. and Nauen, C.: *Ability of the premature infant to maintain his own body temperature.* Nurs. Res. 17:396, 1968.

Pildes, R. S.: *Infants of diabetic mothers.* N. Engl. J. Med. 289:902, 1973.

Reed, B.: *Management of the infant during labor, delivery and the immediate neonatal period.* Nurs. Clin. North Am. 6:3, 1971.

Reynolds, E.: *Neonatal intensive care, Parts I and II.* Nurs. Times 69:1220, 1972.

Roberts, J.: *Suctioning the newborn.* Am. J. Nurs. 73:63, 1973.

Slumek, M.: *Screening newborns for hearing loss.* Nurs. Outlook 19:115, 1971.

Robinson, R.: *The pre-term baby.* Brit. Med. J. 4:416, 1971.

Sinclair, J. C.: *Heat production and thermoregulation in the small-for-date infant.* Ped. Clin. North Am. 17:147, 1970.

Sinclair, J., et al.: *Supportive management of the sick neonate: Parenteral calories, water, electrolytes.* Pediat. Clin. North Am. 17:863, 1970.

Strickland, M.: *Fetal assessment techniques: A challenge to the nurse practitioner.* In Duffey, M., et al. (eds.): *Current Concepts in Clinical Nursing, Vol. 3,* C. V. Mosby, 1971, pp. 179–188.

Strickland, M.: *Environmental influences on the fetus.* In

Anderson, E., et al. (eds.): *Current Concepts in Clinical Nursing*, vol. 4, C. V. Mosby, St. Louis, 1973, pp. 216–229.

Tempesta, L.: *The importance of touch in the care of newborns.* J. Obstet. Gynecol. Nurs. 1:17, 1972.

Todd, R. M.: *The baby of the diabetic mother.* Nurs. Times 69:1322, 1973.

Tsang, R. C., et al.: *Possible pathogenetic factors in neonatal hypocalcemia of prematurity.* J. Pediat. 82:423, 1973.

Tsang, R. C. and Oh, W.: *Neonatal hypocalcemia in low birth weight infants.* Pediatrics 45:773, 1970.

Tucson Medical Center: *Policies, Procedures and Guidelines for Regular and Special Nurseries, 1974.* Copies at cost for printing may be obtained by request to: Tucson Medical Center, 5301 E. Grant Road, Tucson, Arizona, 85733.

White, M., et al.: *Recognition and management of hypoglycemia in the newborn infant.* Nurs. Clin. North Am. 6:67, 1971.

Zwerdling, M. A.: *Factors pertaining to prolonged pregnancy and its outcome.* Pediatrics 40:202, 1967.

Winters, R.: *Principles of Pediatric Fluid Therapy.* Abbott Laboratories, 1970.

Zelson, C.: *Infant of the addicted mother.* N. Engl. J. Med. 288:1393, 1973.

Zelson, C., Rubio, E. and Wasserman. E.: *Neonatal narcotic addiction.* Pediatrics 48:178, 1971.

38 *Care of the High-Risk Neonate*

DYANNE D. AFFONSO, R.N., M.N.
THOMAS R. HARRIS, M.D.

The theoretical bases for understanding certain categories of pathophysiologic processes unique to the newborn were discussed in the preceding chapter. The purpose of this chapter is to apply such knowledge to the nursing care of the high-risk neonate. Intensive neonatal nursing care involves a collaborative relationship among health professionals, especially between nurses and physicians. This chapter evolved from such a close working relationship, and is thus authored by both a nurse and a physician. It is hoped that this example will serve as a model of interdisciplinary collaboration in this field. The authors strongly believe that such collaboration is necessary for the delivery of optimal care to the high-risk neonate.

The high-risk neonate appears to have two main classifications of needs, upon which the content of this chapter is organized:

1. Immediate attention for protection from deleterious effects of the pathophysiologic processes which, if not treated, can be fatal to the infant. These are immediate or acute needs.
2. Supportive care which helps the infant to maintain optimum physiologic functioning to enhance his ability to cope effectively with the pathophysiologic processes. These are referred to as supportive needs or health care maintenance.

In the first part of this chapter, the role of the nurse in providing health care maintenance to the high-risk neonate is explored. Although the nurse plays an important role in meeting the neonate's acute needs, frequently such needs are most aptly met by medical intervention. During acute emergency situations the neonate is a recipient of a barrage of manipulations from various health professionals. Such attention is usually intense until the infant stabilizes. After the infant emerges from his distressed state, attention from various health professionals decreases in frequency and duration, except that from the nurse. The neonate's contacts with the nurse continue because his daily life activities are monitored and nurtured by the nurse.

The second part of this chapter focuses on nursing care to meet the neonate's unique needs which arise from the specific pathophysiologic processes presented in the previous chapter.

HEALTH CARE MAINTENANCE

There are general needs which the nurse must meet when caring for any neonate at risk. Such needs manifest after the neonate has survived the acute distress, regardless of etiology. These needs provide direction for the goals of intensive neonatal nursing care.

MAINTENANCE OF ADEQUATE VENTILATION

To support the infant to maintain adequate ventilation during his distressed state, the nurse should 1) ensure patency of the airway, 2) provide oxygen as necessary, and 3) position the infant in a manner that does not interfere with his breathing. Other nursing measures for the care of a neonate with respiratory problems will be discussed under the category of respiratory distress.

Suctioning to Ensure Patency of the Airway. Newborns may have difficulty getting rid of their secretions. The nurse assists the infant to keep his airway patent by suctioning either with manual or electrical devices. Electrical suctioning can result in trauma to the mucosal lining if excessive negative pressure is applied. The maximum recommended pressure is 80 cm. of water. Also, vigorous, continuous suction can leave the infant airless, as oxygen is aspirated along with the secretions. Suction can also be done manually, as with the rubber bulb syringe of the DeLee mucus trap. The DeLee mucus trap is most effective since the catheter can reach farther down into the throat to clear its contents. The head should be positioned downward and neck hyperextended during the procedure because this position raises the tongue from the posterior pharyngeal wall, thus aiding the removal of secretions.

Special soft suction catheters (#5, 8, or 10 French) with rounded tips should be used. There should be more than one hole (multihole) at the end of the catheter to reduce the likelihood of occlusion when suction is first applied. The rationale is that multiple holes offer a wider distribution of the suction pressure so that the mucosal lining is less likely to be drawn over all holes at once. A small container of sterile water should be used to lubricate the catheter as well as to clear its contents between suctionings. The infant should be in a supine position and its head held securely while the catheter is gently inserted into the nostril and passed into the throat. The infant will gag as it reaches the esophagus or choke if it enters the trachea and for this reason suctioning is best done prior to feedings. The actual suction should be applied after the tube is in place and slow rotating motions should be made as the catheter is withdrawn. Suction should never be just a routine procedure, but in response to a need to help the neonate rid secretions. Frequent and prolonged suctioning creates two major detrimental effects. First, mucus production increases due to mucosal irritation involved, and second, bradycardia may occur from resulting vagal stimulation.

Administration of Oxygen. A detailed discussion of this subject will be presented later in this chapter.

Infant Position. There is not enough appreciation of the significance positioning plays in an infant's ventilation. Breathing is a whole new "happening" for the neonate and anything which helps him to accomplish the task can only be viewed as an asset. Improper positioning can hinder the infant's ability to exchange air during respirations. Examples of positions which facilitate ventilation are:

1. The supine position allows free expansion of the thoracic cage. (The prone position inhibits chest expansion because the infant's body weight is a burden on the chest and abdomen.)
2. Slight elevation of the head and trunk (when not contraindicated for other reasons) will decrease pressure on the diaphragm from the abdominal organs.
3. Slight extension of the neck (when not contraindicated) allows opening of the trachea. This can be done by placing a diaper roll under the shoulders. Guard that the roll does not go under the infant's head causing flexion of the neck which narrows the tracheal opening.
4. Flexion and abduction of the arms en-

hances thoracic expansion. Guard that the arms do not rest on the abdomen or chest as this increases the weight for chest elevation with inspirations.

5. Do not constrict the abdominal area with diapers or other objects because the abdominal muscles aid in respirations.
6. Positional changes from side to side help to drain any fluids accumulated in the thoracic cavity. For the infant too weak to change its own position, positional changes should be done at a minimum of every two hours.

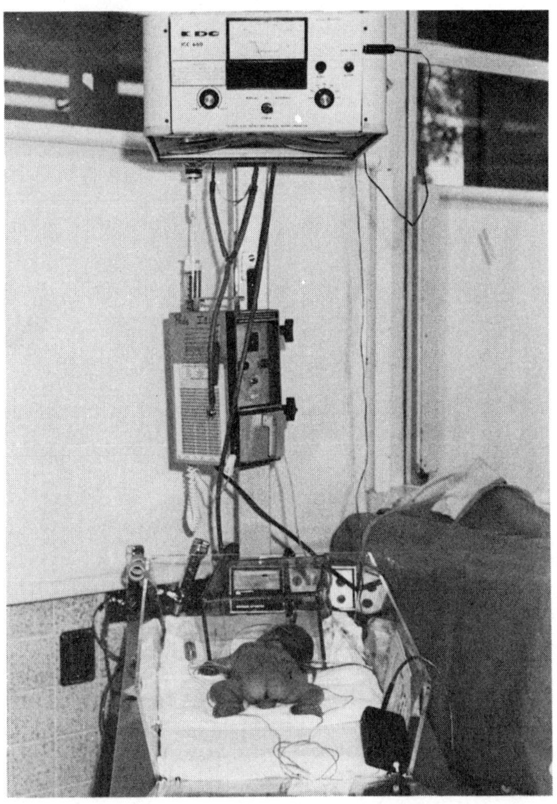

FIGURE 38-1. The open radiant-heat warmer permits easy accessibility to the infant for nursing care. Note the IVAC infusion pump beneath the heating element.

ENVIRONMENTAL PROVISION FOR BODY HEAT MAINTENANCE

Most neonates at risk will need support in maintaining body temperature. Currently, the best environmental heating devices are enclosed incubators or open radiant heat warmers (Figure 38-1). Maintenance of a safe thermal environment is among the most important aspects of nursing a sick neonate.

Temperature Regulation

The goal in providing thermal support to the neonate is to maintain an environmental temperature whereby the baby utilizes the *least* possible amount of energy to maintain stable body temperature. The environmental temperature range in which energy expenditure (measured by oxygen consumption) by the baby is minimal, is called the *thermal neutral zone,* or *range of thermal comfort.* The extent of this range depends upon the size and age of the baby; the younger and/or smaller the infant, the narrower the range. Table 38-1 provides an estimate of the thermal neutral zone for babies of various weights. The reader is referred to Klaus and Faranoff[1] for a more detailed listing of thermal neutral environmental temperatures.

The nurse must be alert to other factors which may influence incubator temperature and/or heat loss or gain in the baby. They

TABLE 38-1. Estimates of Thermal Neutral Zone for Babies of Various Weights

Weight	*Initial Environmental Temperature for Thermal Neutrality*
1000 grams (under 2 lb.)	37° C (98.6° F)
1000–1500 grams (2–3½ lb.)	35° C (95.0° F)
1500–2500 grams (3½–5½ lb.)	34° C (92.0° F)
2500–3500 grams (5½–7¾ lb.)	32° C (89.5° F)

include proximity to air conditioners, presence of direct sunlight on the baby, frequency of opened portholes, and the climate (temperature extremes and humidity) of the locale. For this reason, the temperature of both the infant and the incubator must be monitored frequently and systematically. The infant's axillary temperature should be taken and the incubator should have an internal thermometer and control dials for necessary adjustment.

When it is desired that an infant's temperature be elevated, it is recommended that the thermostat be increased two degrees above the infant's present temperature. Some incubators have an internal thermostat and skin thermistor for servo-control which automatically regulates the incubator temperature to maintain the infant's temperature at the prescribed level (thermostat setting). The thermistor (skin probe) is attached securely with tape to the skin of the trunk, rather than to an extremity (Fig. 38-2). The rationale for this is that trunk temperature is less susceptible to alterations in peripheral circulation and better reflects core temperature. Attaching the thermistor to the infant's abdominal side allows the baby more freedom of movement and the nurse more convenience in changing the infant's position. However, in open radiant heat warmers, the thermistor must always be on the upper surface of the baby, in direct line of sight with the heat source.

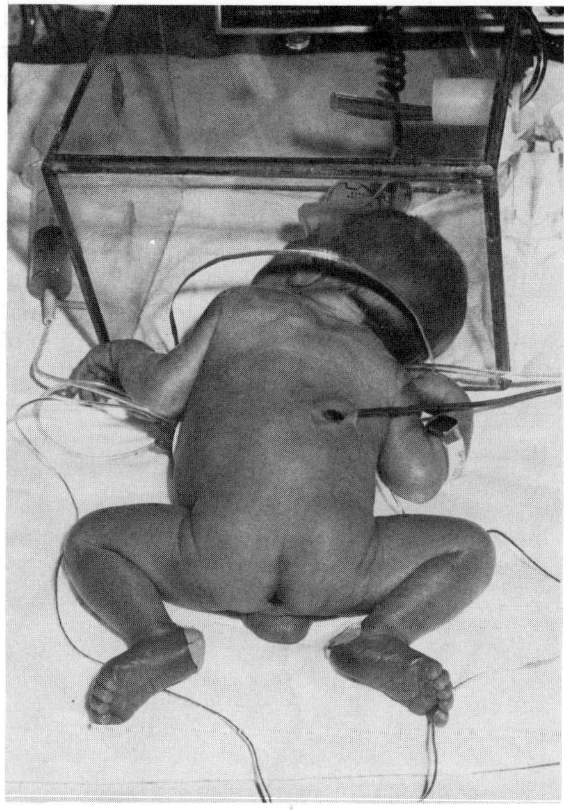

FIGURE 38-2. The thermistor is attached to the infant's trunk rather than to an extremity.

Some assessment factors the nurse should consider regarding temperature regulation are:

1. Check if infant's body or extremities are cool to touch. If so, consider an underheated incubator or heat loss due to radiation to a cold incubator wall.
2. Check activity level of infant. Hyperactivity, restlessness, or short sleep duration may indicate lack of thermal comfort.
3. Be aware of external causes for temperature elevation (above 99° F or 37.2° C) in the baby. Consider an overheated incubator, radiation heat increase from direct sunlight, or sign of impending illness.
4. Likewise, be alert to any sudden drop in infant's temperature as it may indicate a cool incubator or early sepsis.

When the incubator is used to maintain the baby's temperature at a prescribed level, the infant should be undressed and uncovered to allow direct body contact with the flow of warm air. When total support for body temperature is no longer deemed necessary, a weaning procedure is instituted. The infant should be slowly weaned rather than removed abruptly from the incubator. The first step is to dress the baby with a diaper, and then a shirt, and gradually lower the incubator temperature. Frequent monitoring of the infant's temperature to assess his response is necessary. The infant may be transferred to an open bassinette when the incubator temperature approximates room temperature and the infant is maintaining an axillary temperature between 97 to 98° F or 36.0 to 36.6° C.

Humidity Control

Humidification for the neonate is important for the following reasons:

1. Reduces heat loss.
2. Reduces insensible water losses through the skin and lungs.
3. Loosens secretions of the upper airway (especially important after extubation).

Currently, there are mixed views about the value of adding water to the incubator for increased humidity. A major concern is that any water pooling in an incubator reservoir provides an excellent environment for bacterial growth, especially Pseudomonas. Another concern is that any visual obstruction of the infant by fogging is undesirable as it interferes with continuous observations. As long as the room humidity in the nursery is maintained above 50 per cent and inflowing gases are humidified, the humidity within the incubator will be adequate without addition of water to the reservoir.

PROVIDING CALORIC, FLUID AND ELECTROLYTE REQUIREMENTS

The neonate at risk has greater nutritional and fluid requirements because of increased energy needed to cope with the stresses. Stress rapidly depletes available energy stores and increases cellular metabolic processes. This in turn increases oxygen consumption. Carbohydrate is the most important energy source used by the central nervous system (CNS). Therefore, lack of adequate blood sugar levels can create CNS disturbances. If the increased caloric requirements are not met, hypoglycemia (low blood sugar level) ensues. Infants under physiologic stress are prime candidates for hypoglycemia because of increased metabolic demands as well as reduced glycogen stores and reduced ability to convert glucose from fat and protein. Unfortunately, hypoglycemia is manifested by only subtle symptoms, or none at all. Observable signs in the neonate may be lethargy, hypotonia, refusal to eat, restlessness, jitteriness, peripheral cyanosis, or mottled skin color. Such signs should immediately clue the nurse that the infant may be sick and appropriate diagnostic work-up should be done. More details on hypoglycemia will be presented later in this chapter.

Another consideration is that high-risk neonates, because of their illness, frequently have increased caloric needs. They are unable to be fed orally during the acute phase of illness. Whenever oral feedings are withheld, increased calories must be supplemented by parenteral means to minimize tissue catabolism and to reverse a negative nitrogen balance.

The neonate in distress frequently has greater fluid requirements. Dehydration in premature infants ensues rapidly due to relatively large body surface area, mandatory water losses, as well as the restricted intake in volume during acute illness. Likewise electrolyte requirements may vary considerably because of the disease itself or from overzealous therapeutic medical interventions (iatrogenic diseases).

The specific calculated electrolyte needs for an individual infant can be determined by laboratory analysis, the degree of deviation from norm, and the infant's body weight.

Infants in stress are usually too weak to maintain adequate nutrition. Their sucking and swallowing reflexes may be absent, weakly present, or easily fatigued. These infants often require a modified, predigested formula which aids the reabsorption process.

Parenteral Therapy

Intravenous feedings are usually indicated for infants in respiratory distress, any acute trauma which restricts oral intake, after major surgery, serious infections, dehydration, or any time that difficulties are encountered with oral feeding. In the newborn, suitable peripheral veins for the site of infusion can be found on the scalp, back side of the hand, antecubital fossa of the arm, and the dorsum of the foot. Cutdowns are usually performed at the ankle. Nutrients can also be infused through umbilical arteries or vein catheters with special precautions taken. Important technical considerations during intravenous therapy include:

1. Ensuring asepsis of equipment used.
2. Ensuring that the IV equipment is cleared of air.
3. Securing needle or catheter at infusion site.
4. Controlling flow rate as prescribed.
5. Assessing that the equipment is functioning properly.

The neonate is vulnerable to rapid fluid-electrolyte imbalance from improper intravenous therapy because his body surface is large in proportion to his size and weight. One important nursing action is the use of infusion pumps or other equipment which can be precisely set to deliver the desired quantity of fluid (even very small amounts) to an infant. Infusion pumps are an asset because they provide accurate and constant flow rate (see Fig. 38-1). Another important nursing action for any infant on intravenous therapy is to monitor intake and output. All urinary output should be measured and tested for specific gravity. Specific gravity can provide an indication as to degree of hydration in the newborn (if sugar and protein are not being spilled in the urine). An elevated reading (above approximately 1.012) indicates a concentrated urine possibly reflecting inadequate fluid intake (or spillage of sugar or protein). A reduced reading (less than 1.004) may indicate overhydration. Finally, a most important nursing action is daily weight of the infant. Infants should not gain more than 1 to 1½ ounces per day. If more weight gain is observed, possible overhydration and/or heart failure must be considered.

Gavage or Tube Feeding

When an infant survives the critical phase of physiologic stress and larger feedings are no longer contraindicated, he will graduate to tube feedings called gavage. These infants are still too weak to obtain adequate nourishment by sucking and swallowing (nippling) alone. Therefore their nutritional requirements are gradually introduced via a tube inserted in the nostril or mouth, passing down the esophagus into the stomach. Gavage is definitely a nursing procedure. Nurses not only insert the tube and instill the formula, but also play a role in determining the amount and frequency of feedings by evaluating the infant's responses to the procedure.

It is imperative that nurses delivering neonatal intensive care be able to perform the gavage procedure skillfully and with knowledge as to its rationale. Therefore, a comprehensive discussion on the gavage procedure follows.

Preparation of Equipment. Assemble the following at the infant's bedside:

1. *Feeding tube.* The tube should be

selected according to the infant's size, a #5 to 8 French tube is usually adequate. The size refers to the diameter of the lumen which will influence the flow rate. The 15-inch length tube is the most frequently used.
2. *Reservoir to hold the formula.* A 10 to 30 cc. syringe is usually used. The syringe should be clear and calibrated to allow exact measurement of the amount.
3. *Stethoscope.* It is used to assess if the tube is inserted properly into the stomach and is regarded as the preferred tool for assessing tubing placement.
4. *Tape.* Used to mark the desired length the tube is to be inserted and to secure the tube.
5. *Sterile water.* A container of sterile water is used to lubricate the tube and clear its contents as necessary.
6. *Formula.* The formula should be at room temperature rather than cold.

Preparation of the Infant. The head and trunk should be slightly elevated to promote gravity flow of the formula into the stomach. The view of the chest and abdomen should be unobstructed to allow visible assessment for signs of distention or respiratory distress during the feeding. An active baby may need to have its arms gently restrained to prevent dislodgment of the tube by the infant's movements.

Determination of Route for Tube Insertion. Opinions vary as to which is the preferred route, the nose or mouth, and whether the tube should be reinserted for each feeding or left indwelling. Advocates for oral insertion state that nasal insertion creates problems by occluding the nasal passage (infant is an obligatory nose-breather). The tube can also irritate the mucosal lining which will increase mucus secretions in the nose. This can interfere with ventilation as well as predispose to otitis media (infection of the inner ear) by causing swelling at the opening of the eustachian tube leading to the inner ear. Oral insertion also has the additional benefit of preparing the baby for oral intake by activating his sucking, swallowing, gagging, and vagal reflexes. Advocates of nasal insertion are usually also advocates of the indwelling tube feeding since fixation is easier and the baby tends to readily adapt to the nasal tube over longer periods. If an indwelling tube is used it should be changed at least every 1 to 2 days and reinserted in the other nostril.

Each neonatal nurse should make a judgment regarding route for tube insertion based on the unique needs and responses of the individual baby. For general health care maintenance, use of the oral route is preferred.

Tube Measurement (Fig. 38-3).

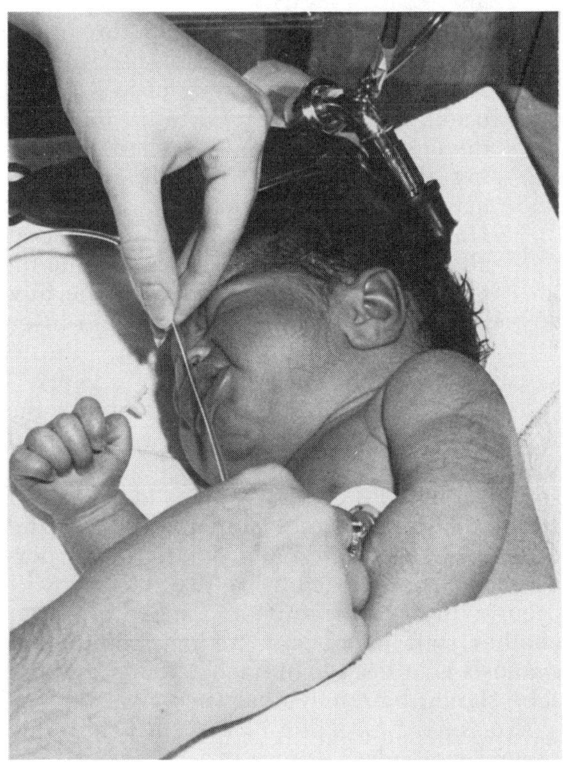

FIGURE 38-3. The nurse measuring the tube from the bridge of the nose to the xiphoid process for oral insertion.

1. *Oral route.* Measure from the bridge of the nose to the xiphoid process (lower end of the sternum).
2. *Nasal route.* Measure from the tip of the nose to the ear lobe, and then to the xiphoid process.

Tube Insertion.

1. *Oral route.* Lubricate the tip of the tube with water, insert into back of the throat, gradually easing it down until the desired mark is at the infant's lips. The swallowing reflex may be stimulated which lifts up the glottis, opens the upper end of the glottis, and makes passage of the tube easier with each swallow.
2. *Nasal route.* Aim the tube down and toward the midline of the nose and not along the bridge of the nose (straight back). It may be helpful to lift the tip of the nose, like a pug nose, when performing this procedure. A little resistance may be felt at the turn into the throat. Holding the tube straight, rather than allowing it to bend, helps ease it into the pharynx. Sometimes, stiffening the tube by chilling it in ice water will aid insertion.

Tube insertion often creates anxiety for the novice nurse, sometimes leading to a hurried insertion. However, the tube should be inserted slowly. Force has no place in gavage. If strong resistance is met, stop and redirect the tube, and gently try again. If resistance persists and there is concern that trauma will occur, withdraw the tube and seek help from another staff member. Choking, gasping, or cyanosis is indicative of tracheal entry and the tube should be removed at once.

Assessment for Tube Placement. There are several methods:

1. Attach the syringe to the tube and insert a couple of cc.'s of air through the tube while listening to the upper left abdomen with a stethoscope (Fig. 38-4). Hearing a swishing, bubbling, growling sound indicates that the tube is positioned correctly in the stomach. Remember to withdraw the instilled air.
2. Immerse the proximal (nearest, closest to you) end of the tube in a container of water and observe for bubbles. If bubbles appear in timing with the infant's respirations, the tube is in the trachea and must be removed at once. Sometimes a few bubbles appear, then the bubbles stop, indicating some air in the stomach. For this reason it is not regarded as a

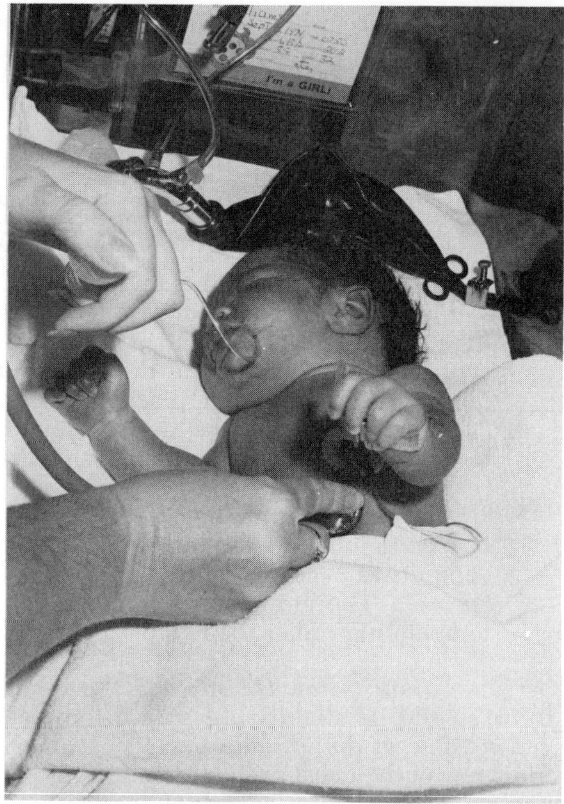

FIGURE 38-4. The nurse is listening for the sounds of air instilled to assess if the tube is correctly placed in the stomach.

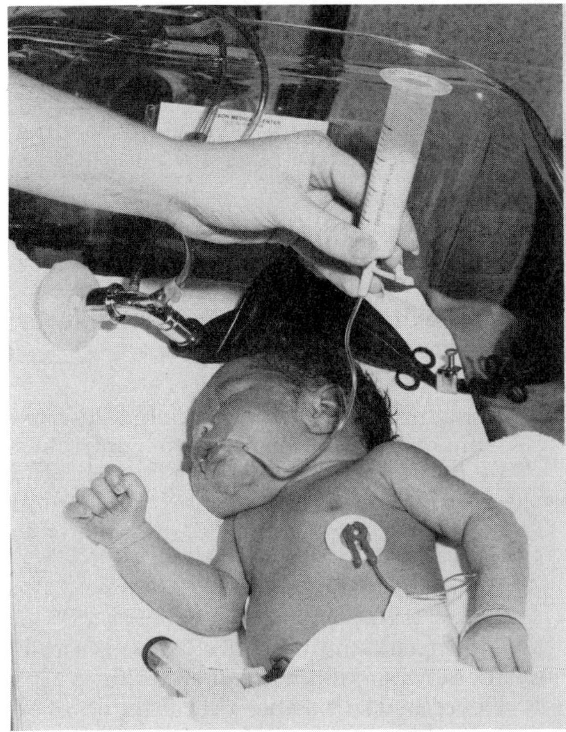

FIGURE 38-5. The nurse allows the formula to flow in by gravity and observes the infant's reactions during the feeding.

reliable assessment method.

3. Gently aspirate the tube and observe for return of gastric contents indicating proper placement in the stomach. Return these contents to the stomach before proceeding.

When the tube is assessed to be in place, tape it securely.

The Feeding. Before each gavage feeding, the amount of gastric contents should be evaluated. This is done by aspirating stomach contents into a syringe. If the amount is more than 1 to 3 cc. (depending on the size of the baby) the current feeding should be reduced by that amount. If excessive amounts are aspirated, this indicates lack of absorption of the previous feeding and it might be best to skip the feeding after consultation with the physician. Allow the formula to flow in by gravity (Fig. 38-5). Sometimes it is necessary to start the flow with a gentle push of the plunger, but once the flow starts, further forced injection should be avoided. Gravity flow usually approximates 5 cc. intake in a 5 to 10 minute period and the average time for gavage is usually 20 to 25 minutes (depending on the amount). Factors that affect the flow rate are size (diameter) of the tube, height the syringe is held over the stomach (usually approximately 6 inches), and the size and fullness of the stomach. Rapid flow is undesirable as it forcibly expands the stomach and may lead to bradycardia (slow heart rate) due to vagal stimulation. Excessive amounts of gavage feeding pose the danger of regurgitation due to abdominal distention and interference with peristalsis. Continue the feeding until the desired intake is achieved or the gravity flow ceases which is indicative of a stomach filled to capacity.

Termination of Feeding. Pinch the tube and withdraw quickly to prevent leakage of the tube contents which may be aspirated as the tube passes the pharynx. An indwelling tube should be cleansed with 2 to 3 cc. of water and clamped until the next feeding. The infant should be bubbled. The infant should then be positioned on the right side to facilitate emptying of the stomach.

Assessment and Recording of the Infant's Reaction to Gavage. This provides direction for the amount of the next feeding and the infant's readiness for oral intake. Significant factors to assess and record are:

1. Observe the abdomen for postprandial (after feeding) distention. Distention makes the infant more vulnerable to aspiration as well as to respiratory difficulties secondary to restriction of the diaphragm.
2. Observe the infant's activity level during the feeding. Restlessness and agitation indicate that the tolerance limit has been

reached and no more formula should be given. A lack of further gravitational flow supports this assumption.

3. Observe for any sucking on the tube which may indicate readiness for nippling.
4. Record the amount of gastric contents aspirated prior to feeding, amount of intake, amount of regurgitation, presence of any abdominal distention, activity during feeding, sucking motions, and so forth.

Oral Feeding

The change from gavage to breast or bottle feeding should be a gradual process. This allows the infant time to adjust to active sucking and swallowing, and will minimize fatigue during feeding. In general, oral feeding should not exceed 20 minutes. Ninety-five per cent of what the infant will ultimately receive is taken in the first 10 minutes; the remaining 10 minutes primarily fulfill sucking needs. Beyond 20 minutes of feeding the infant is likely to become fatigued.

A good way to begin the weaning process is to nipple every third or fourth feeding. This process allows meeting nutritional requirements without overextending the infant's energies. Frequency of nippling is increased as tolerated until all feedings are by bottle or breast. If the bottle is used, certain factors must be considered to aid the infant:

1. Use a soft nipple with an adequate opening (drips one drop per second when held upside down).
2. Help the infant, when necessary, to learn to open his mouth and begin sucking. This can be done by gentle pressure with the nipple on the chin or lips.
3. Do not rush the baby; let him proceed at his own pace. However, if the baby sucks rapidly the nurse must be prepared to remove the bottle if the milk flow is too fast.

The nurse also needs to assess the pattern of oral intake. Should the infant be reluctant to suck on two or more successive feedings, he may be communicating that he is not ready for such a venture. Also, a change in feeding pattern may be the first clue of illness such as sepsis.

PROTECTION FROM INFECTION

Infants in distress are more vulnerable to infection for numerous reasons:

1. Immobility due to the restricted environment and attached equipment contributes to pooling of secretions, mucus, and circulating fluids, providing a good medium for pathogenic organisms to grow.
2. Breakage of the body's first line of defense (skin) by catheters inserted for electrical monitoring, intravenous therapy, suctioning, and so forth.
3. Decreased resistance because of overextended energy requirements in face of stress and accompanying fatigue.
4. The incubator environment or the respiratory therapy equipment may be sources of bacterial infection (such as Pseudomonas) if inadequately cleaned or sterilized.

A sick neonate may not be able to cope with the additional stress of an infectious process. Nursing care to protect the infant from infection focuses on manipulation of three potential categories of sources of infection: people, places, and things. *People* can be excellent carriers of infection through their noses, mouths, hands, and so forth. Personnel caring for sick neonates should be periodically screened with cultures to detect any pathogens. Enough cannot be said about proper handwashing technique (see Chapter 31) in intensive neonatal nursing. Traffic through the nursery should be limited, especially personnel from other departments. It is desirable that one person from the laboratory or x-ray department be assigned to perform procedures in the nursery. In terms of *place,* infants should be adequately spaced from their companions. Although an incubator is considered an individual isolation unit, incubators should also be spaced because pathogens can easily be transmitted when the portholes are open during care tasks. *Things* should be individualized as much as possible, each infant having his own supplies and linens. Asepsis should be ensured in the use of any equipment which must be placed in an internal orifice. Detailed nursing actions will be presented in the discussion of perinatal infection.

PROMOTION OF REST

During a stressful experience, all available energy is directed toward coping with the stressors. This is a priority for survival, usually made at the expense of normal, routine bodily activities. For example, the role of proteins and carbohydrates in promoting physical growth must be delayed until after the infant's survival is ensured. In the battle for its life, the infant is easily fatigued and exhausted. Every effort must be made to conserve his available energy. This can be done by meeting his daily needs and arresting the disease or risk factor. For example, maintenance of respirations, body heat, and fluid and nutritional requirements conserves energy by supporting essential body functions. Medical therapy which minimizes the stress of disease frees the available energy for other functions besides coping with the physiologic stresses. It is essential that the nursing care plan incorporate measures to conserve energy, for example:

1. Organization of care to ensure minimal handling and protection of the infant from overstimulation.
2. Removal of all possible environmental input which can hinder rest and sleep, e.g., excessive noise, glaring lights, and excessive heat or cold, to allow replenishment of energy cells.
3. Proper positioning of the infant. Improper positioning, especially when the infant must support the weight of his own body parts, leads to fatigue.
4. Assess the infant's activity level. Lethargy may indicate sepsis.
5. Assess sleeping patterns. Lack of uninterrupted sleep may indicate a pathophysiologic disturbance, such as gastroenteritis.

STIMULATION FOR BEHAVIORAL DEVELOPMENT

The infant at risk is in jeopardy not only from the point of view of his physical well-being but also his emotional or mental health. Obviously, when the infant is acutely ill the overriding concern is for physical care which will ensure survival. This is rightly so, because at such a time the infant is hardly able to assimilate input from the environment. He must also be protected from environmental stimuli because they fatigue him and waste his valuable energy supplies. Frequently the baby is restrained to prevent accidental displacement of equipment used to sustain his life. Thus, the baby is denied kinesthetic stimulation which occurs from his own responses when normal activity puts his muscles and joints through a range of motion.

However, once the baby is improved, stimulation for behavioral development must be provided (Fig. 38-6). Too often the pattern of providing only physical care has been set. Even after the infant is well, nurses and doctors continue to focus only on such aspects of care as body temperature, amount of intake and output, and vital signs. The baby at risk continues to be deprived of routine stimulations given to his healthy counterparts. He is frequently not held, talked to, or even allowed eye-to-eye contact. Thus, he is denied opportunities to familiarize himself with the

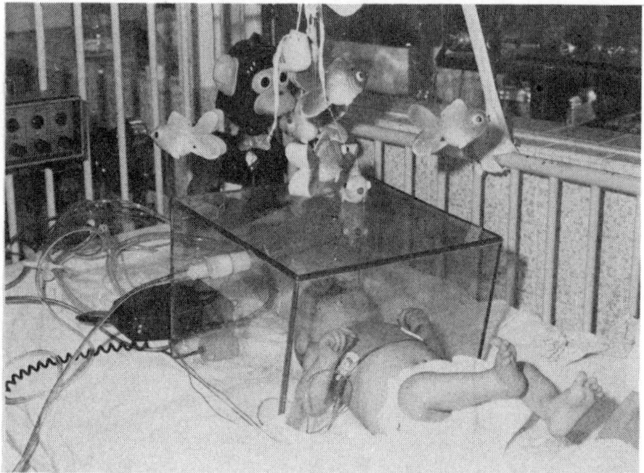

FIGURE 38-6. Nurses have provided a mobile for behavioral stimulation in spite of the baby's need for an oxygen hood.

human world. It would be sad indeed if our health care delivery system focused only on ensuring physical life without regard for behavioral and mental health. The nurse is in a unique position to promote behavioral development. Infant stimulation can be integrated into daily nursing tasks.

Regardless of where the infant is, isolette or basinette, once stimulation is no longer a danger to him, the nurse should provide it. Nurses should talk, touch, and be within the baby's visual field during routines such as feeding, diapering, and linen changes. Encourage eye-to-eye contact by bringing yourself to the baby and be sure there is an unobstructed view between the baby and you. This helps him to explore you and familiarize himself with the human world. Take a moment to cuddle, stroke, or pat an infant after feeding, weighing, and bathing. Allow the baby freedom of movement whenever possible so he can stimulate himself. He may need help in changing his position so that he can incorporate aspects of the environment into his view. The nurse must use her creativity in providing sensory stimulation from inanimate objects. Examples include the use of rocking or swinging devices in isolettes, colorful mobiles, and soothing musical sounds. Remember, the preferred stimulus is the human one, so nurses should make a conscious effort to provide such stimuli. No matter what the mode used, its effects are likely to be positive when the nurse genuinely values her or his role in promoting behavioral development in this beginning phase of life. One last note, always remember to share such actions with the parents. They need to value the significance of infant stimulation so that it can be continued at home. The hospital environment provides a unique setting for parents to stimulate their infants. There, under the guidance of nurses, they can receive help when needed and have their concerns about the baby answered or clarified. They can also receive praise for their efforts which becomes a reinforcement for continuation of behaviors for infant stimulation. Here is an example of a simple nursing action to involve parents. First, the environment is manipulated to allow mother and baby to have an unobstructed view of each other. The nurse helps position mother, explaining the value to the infant if he can see his mother's face, especially her eyes, and hear her voice. The nurse provides a chair for the mother and allows the mother and baby to explore each other in private, proceeding at their own pace.

CRISIS INTERVENTION FOR PARENTS

This is included as a supportive need for the neonate at risk, based on the premise that you cannot foster health or well-being in infants unless the parents are also physically and emotionally healthy. Having an infant at risk is stressful to parents and can lead to crisis. The nurse's role in helping parents emerge successfully through such a crisis is crucial. Parents need to see their infant and be allowed to ask questions about the infant's behaviors and the numerous pieces of equipment (Fig. 38-7). They also need help in expressing their feelings and concerns for the life of their baby or

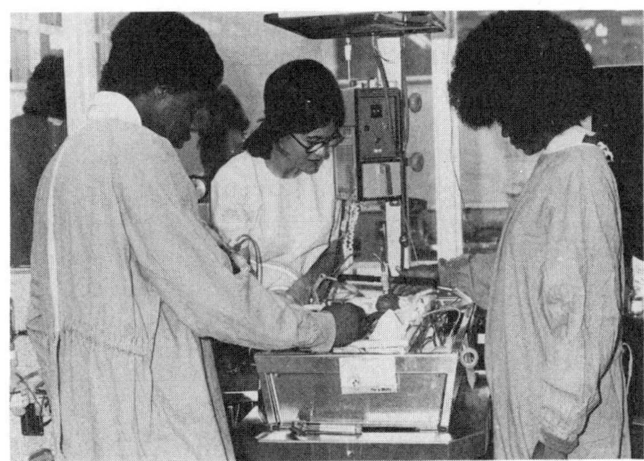

FIGURE 38-7. The nurse clarifies the infant's status to the parents. Note the mother and father's attempts to touch their critically ill baby.

possible effects should the baby survive. A thorough discussion of specific nursing actions for crisis intervention will be presented in Chapter 41, using the example of the birth of a premature infant. Such principles can be applied in working with all parents whose infants are at risk, regardless of causative factors.

NURSING CARE RELATIVE TO PATHOPHYSIOLOGIC PROCESSES

This section discusses nursing care relative to the risk categories presented in the preceding chapter. Specifically, the following aspects of the nursing process will be explored:

1. *Assessment.* What are the conditions, events, and recognizable signs which indicate that a pathophysiologic risk is present or can be anticipated?
2. *Special Needs or Goals.* What are the special needs of the neonate which must be met, thus becoming nursing goals? These are needs beyond the normal provision of care which arise as a result of physiologic stress.
3. *Intervention.* What actions will protect the infant from detrimental effects of the physiologic stress? Most of the actions to nurture and stimulate have already been discussed under Health Care Maintenance. However, actions unique to a pathologic condition are introduced as appropriate. The role of the nurse in supporting medical therapy is emphasized. The rationale for this is that medical therapy is mandatory to protect the infant from effects of the pathophysiologic processes. The physician may initiate the therapy, but its maintenance is the responsibility of the person continuously present, namely, the nurse.

In the care of a sick neonate, nurses are beginning to expand their roles by assuming responsibilities which allow them to become primary care agents in collaboration with the physician.

ASPHYXIA, RESPIRATORY DISTRESS, AND APNEA

The role of the nurse in the assessment process of the neonate who is asphyxiated, in respiratory distress, or apneic, is threefold:

1. Identification of infants who are vulnerable to such risks due to factors that occurred in the prenatal, intrapartal, or immediate postpartal periods. The nurse must be aware of events in a newborn's prenatal and perinatal history which will classify the baby as being at risk for difficulties involving respiratory functions. Examples of such factors are asphyxia at birth as demonstrated by a low Apgar score, prematurity, difficult labor and delivery, maternal bleeding, infants of diabetic mothers, and meconium staining of the amniotic fluid. Such awareness helps the nurse to anticipate which in-

fants will have respiratory difficulties.

2. Recognition of the manifestations of respiratory difficulties through close observation of infants who are identified as high risk. The nurse should be able to share observations that will be most helpful toward making a medical diagnosis.
3. The nurse should be able to grade the severity of the difficulties with respirations. Thus, assessment data should reflect time of onset, duration and frequency of clinical manifestations, as well as ability to correlate one symptom with another. When the nurse is able to apply knowledge of the pathophysiologic process of the disease, she will then be able to recognize the various symptoms which are interrelated. For example, the astute nurse will not merely tell the physician a baby is grunting, but will also share data on other observations such as presence or absence of retractions, nasal flaring, and so forth.

The nurse is able to make a significant contribution in the assessment of the neonate's condition primarily because of constant contact with the baby. Thus, onset of a clinical manifestation or sudden change in the infant's status may be identified initially by the nurse.

Asphyxia

Nursing Assessment

Knowledge to guide the nurse in recognition of asphyxia in the neonate has been presented in the preceding chapter. A review of the Apgar scoring system, which provides data on the degree of asphyxia which may be present, is recommended.

Nursing Intervention

The nurse has an important role in intervention because frequently the infant's life and future well-being are in jeopardy if no immediate action is taken. The nurse is right there with the neonate and while awaiting the physician's arrival can initiate measures that may prove life-saving or can turn the tide at a crucial point and avoid extensive or prolonged future therapy.

Resuscitation

All infants are exposed to some asphyxia during normal birth, from which the healthy neonate easily recovers. However, if asphyxia is greater than the norm inherent in the birth process, major measures of resuscitation need be taken. An outline of these measures and their rationale were described in the preceding chapter. This section deals primarily with the specifics of resuscitation.

Any infant who does not cry vigorously or initiate rhythmic breathing within seconds after birth will need immediate help. This implies that the nurse is appraising the infant immediately from the moment of birth, with special attention paid to the pattern of respirations (rhythm) and the ease or difficulty of making the first few breaths.

The Apgar scoring system helps to clue the nurse as to which infants will need minimal or extensive treatment. Infants with Apgar scores of 4 to 6 usually need some form of intervention such as brief pharyngeal suctioning, stimulation by flicking the soles of the feet, or brief administration of oxygen with a face mask. Most infants usually respond successfully to such treatment. Other infants may be severely depressed (Apgar score of 0 to 3) and may need extensive treatment such as tracheal suctioning, intubation, assisted ventilation and artificial lung expansion, and/or closed chest cardiac massage.

A priority need for any infant prior to initiation of breathing is a clear (patent) airway. This is usually provided by brief pharyngeal and nasal passage suctioning with a bulb

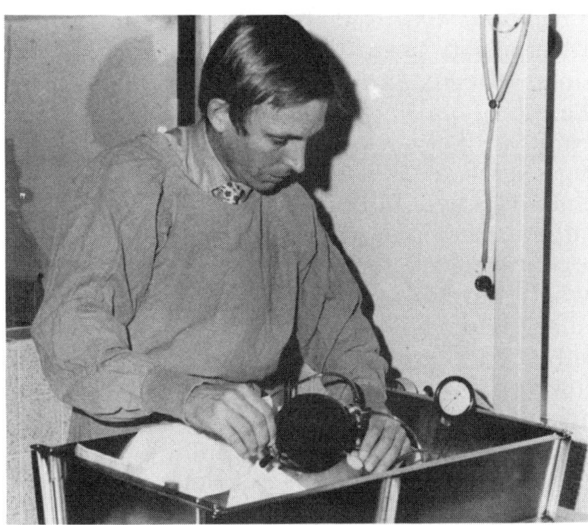

FIGURE 38-8. Physician checks the amount of pressure being delivered during assisted ventilation with an anesthesia bag and mask set-up capable of delivering IPPV and CPAP.

syringe. The next priority is for initiation of respiratory movements. If these are not spontaneous, or if there is no response to suctioning, the infant should be *bagged* or manually assisted in his ventilation.

Assisted ventilation for the depressed infant is usually performed with an Ambu-bag that has a safety pop-off valve set at 35 cm. H_2O pressure, or with an anesthesia bag connected to a monometer which indicates exact pressures generated (Fig. 38-8). If such equipment is not available, mouth-to-mouth or mouth-to-tube breathing is indicated.

The rationale for this bagging procedure is to forcefully expand the lungs setting off reflex responses that stimulate further spontaneous respiratory efforts, increase blood flow through the lungs, and provide initial gas exchange. The expected results of such actions are spontaneous gasping efforts and crying, improved heart rate, and increased muscle tone. If there is no response to one minute of bagging with a mask (no respiratory effort and the heart rate continues to fall) *intubation* should commence. This involves:

1. Visualization of the glottis with a laryngoscope.
2. Suctioning of any material obstructing the view of the glottis or entrance to the trachea.
3. Insertion of a curved endotracheal tube into the trachea (intubation).
4. Inflation of the lungs by means of intermittent and then continuous positive pressure application.

If the heart rate remains below 60 to 70 beats per minute in spite of assisted ventilation for more than 15 to 30 seconds, *external cardiac massage* should be started (Fig. 38-9). This is

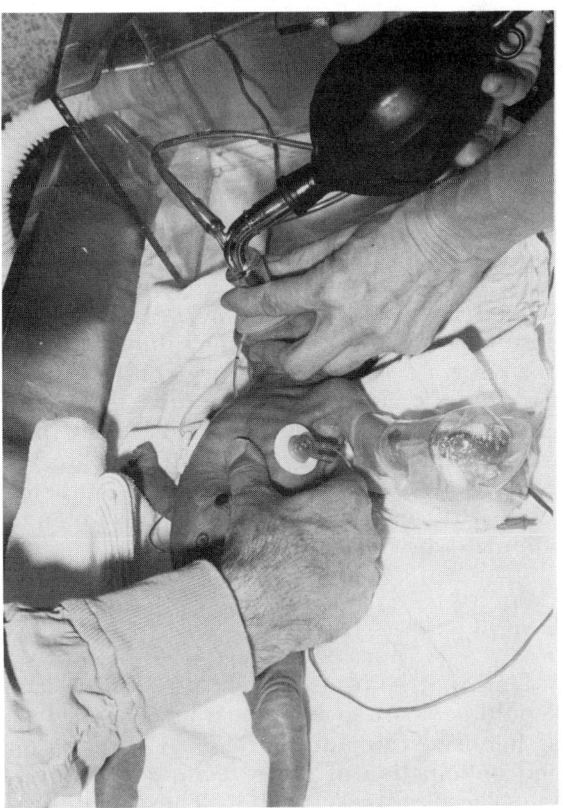

FIGURE 38-9. External cardiac massage being applied with the thumb, approximately two compressions per second. Assisted ventilation is simultaneously provided.

accomplished by compressing the heart at a rate of 100 to 120 times per minute (about 2 times per second). This procedure of manual compression of the heart maintains the circulation, forcing blood out to the lungs and body to maintain blood pressure and provide nutrients and oxygen to the tissues. Effective cardiac massage is indicated by palpable peripheral pulses (brachial or femoral arteries). It may be discontinued when the spontaneous heart rate has risen above 80 to 100 beats per minute. Administration of drugs such as sodium bicarbonate and epinephrine will be of little help during circulatory collapse since they will not be taken to their site of action. This is another reason why maintaining the circulation by external cardiac massage during resuscitation is so important.

If there is still no satisfactory response to assisted ventilation and external cardiac massage within 2 to 3 minutes, the nurse should anticipate immediate placement of an umbilical catheter for infusion of medications to correct acidosis and stimulate the heart. *Sodium bicarbonate* at half strength (0.5 mEq. per cc., or the standard 1 mEq. per cc. solution diluted half-and-half with sterile water) at a dose of 3 mEq. (or 6 cc. of the dilute solution) per kilogram body weight is given to correct the acidosis. *Epinephrine* at one tenth the usual strength (1/10,000 or 0.1 cc. of 1/1000 solution drawn up to 1 cc. with sterile water) at a total dose of ½ to 1 cc. through the catheter while cardiac massage is continued is given to stimulate the heart.

Complications

During the resuscitation procedure, care should be taken to avoid heat loss. Transfer to an intensive care nursery for close observation and anticipation of future complications follows successful resuscitation. These complications, the reasons for their development, and the basic modes of therapy to be anticipated by the nurse are presented here.

Hypoglycemia. Asphyxia represents a tremendous stress on the infant that rapidly depletes already limited energy supplies. Furthermore, oral intake and reabsorption of nutrients is likely to be severely curtailed following asphyxia. For these reasons, infusion of glucose is generally indicated. If an umbilical catheter has been placed, 10 per cent dextrose in water at a rate of 2 to 3 cc. per kg. body weight per hour (or 50 to 75 cc. per kg. per 24 hours) is the infusion solution of choice with calcium added as described below. Care must be taken to avoid fluid overloading of the child since cerebral edema may also develop after severe asphyxia.

Hypocalcemia. Because of the acidosis (low pH) that invariably accompanies asphyxia, calcium comes out of the bone to buffer (neutralize) the hydrogen ion (acid) and in part is lost through the urine. When the acidosis is then corrected with alkali (sodium bicarbonate), the little remaining calcium goes back into the bone leaving the level in the blood very low (hypocalcemia). Therefore, calcium should be added to the infusion solution at a dose of 200 to 400 mg. per 100 cc. of solution, or given by slow IV push by the physician if he chooses to put the bicarbonate into the solution. (Calcium salts and sodium bicarbonate do not mix in an IV solution since a precipitate of calcium bicarbonate forms.)

Seizures. Twitching or frank seizure may develop after asphyxia due to metabolic reasons (hypoglycemia, hypocalcemia), cerebral edema (brain swelling), or hypoxic damage to the brain cells themselves. These may also present as cyanotic or apneic episodes. If adequate treatment of the metabolic disturbances has been achieved and seizures persist, anticonvulsant therapy (e.g., phenobarbital) may be necessary.

Respiratory Distress

Nursing Assessment

There are several clinical appraisal tools

available which can help the nurse to recognize respiratory distress in the newborn. Examples of such tools are:

1. Silverman-Anderson Score[2] (Fig. 38-10)
   This involves a clinical appraisal of signs of respiratory retractions as identified below:
   a. Retraction of the upper chest as compared with abdominal respirations during inspiration.
   b. Retraction of lower intercostal muscles (lower chest).

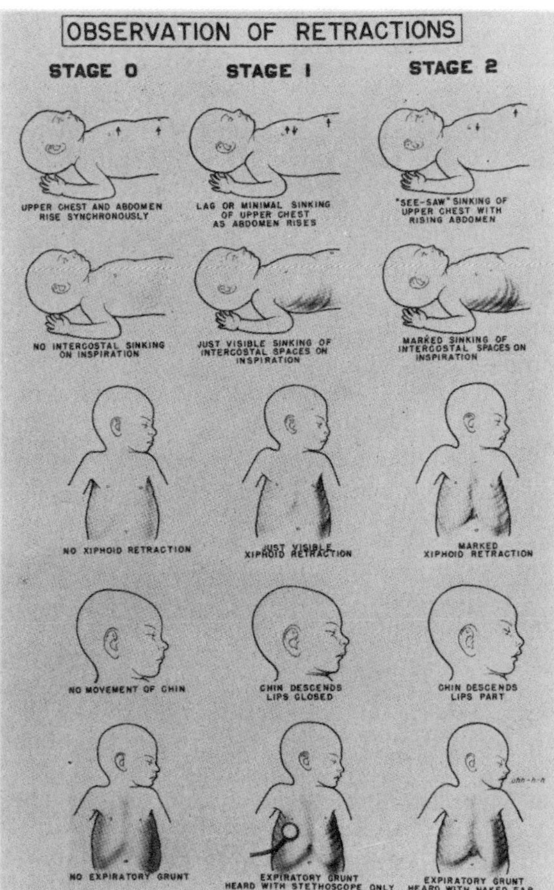

FIGURE 38-10. The Silverman-Anderson Score. (From Silverman, W. and Anderson, D. Pediatrics 17:1, 1956, with permission.)

   c. Retraction of the xiphoid.
   d. Movement of the nares with inspiration.
   e. Expiratory grunt.

   In this tool, the higher score (maximum of 10) indicates poor ventilation and severe distress.
2. The Miller Score[3] (Fig. 38-11)
   This tool classifies infants into three groups: normal, precautionary or those requiring close observation, and critically sick babies.
   a. *Normal*: infants who breathe 40/minute ± 15/minute from birth on.
   b. *Precautionary*: infants who start breathing at higher rates (greater than 60/min.) but show no significant increase over the first hour, and then begin decreasing their rate, slowly coming back to the normal range.
   c. *Critical*: infants whose respirations persist at a rate of 15+/min above the normal mean during the first 48 hours.

   Miller advocates that all neonates (especially preterm babies) have their respirations counted at least 2 to 3 times in the first hour after birth, at least every 2 hours within the next 48 hours, and then every 4 hours until stable.
3. Stanford Scoring Scale (Fig. 38-12)
   A simplified system developed at Stanford scores three different parameters repeatedly and allows a trend to be recognized:
   a. *Grunting*: score 0 for none, 1 for stethoscopically audible, 2 for obviously audible.
   b. *Flaring*: score 0 for none, 1 for minimal, 2 for marked.
   c. *Retracting:* score 0 for none, 1 for minimal, 2 for marked.

The nursing should also be alert to signs indicative of respiratory distress as listed in Table 38-2.

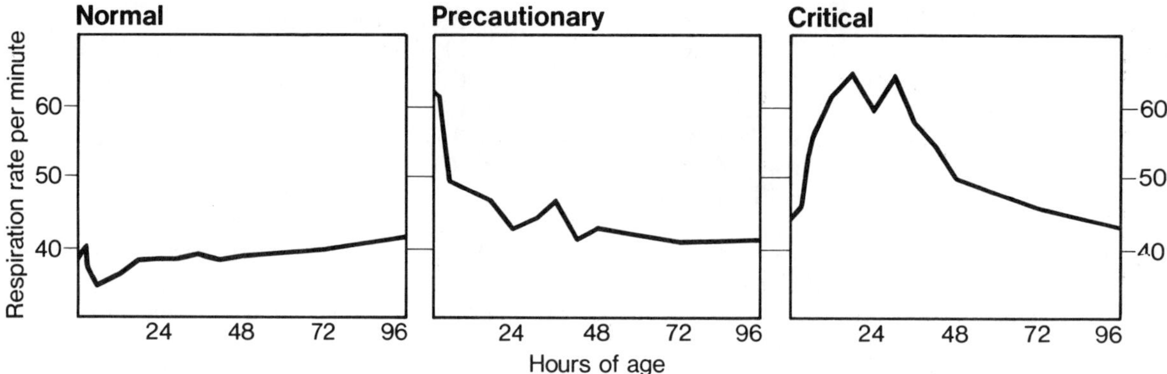

FIGURE 38-11. The Miller Score for evaluating rates of respiration. (From Miller, H. C.: *Respiratory disorders: Clinical evaluation of respiratory functions in newborn infants.* Pediatr. Clin. North Am. 2:17, 1957, with permission.)

TIME	RESPIRATORY STATUS		
	G	F	R
0810	0	1	1
0825	0	1	1
0840	0	1	0

GFR	SCORE		
	0	1	2
Grunting	None	Stethoscopically audible	Audible
Flaring	None	Minimal	Marked
Retracting	None	Minimal	Marked

FIGURE 38-12. The Stanford Scoring Scale.

Nursing Intervention

The special needs of the infant in respiratory distress are 1) assistance of ventilation, 2) assurance of adequate oxygenation, and 3) correction of the acid-base imbalance. In addition to these three extraordinary measures, the infant needs the following health care maintenance support to avoid any worsening of the respiratory distress: 4) assistance in maintaining body heat, 5) protection from infection, 6) provision of adequate caloric and fluid intake, and 7) protection from overstimulation.

Assisted ventilation

This section briefly describes the various means of assisting ventilation, the rationale for their use, and the problems the nurse may anticipate in the course of such therapy.

Assisted ventilation implies supporting or assisting the infant in doing what he normally does himself in the process of breathing. Basically this involves two functions, the *bellows function* or process of moving air in and out of the lungs, and the *antiatelectasis function* or process of keeping the alveoli (air sacs) partially expanded even at the end of expiration.

For the infant to adequately move air in and out of the lungs (*bellows function*) in sufficient quantity to bring in enough oxygen and blow off enough carbon dioxide, he needs 1) a functioning respiratory center to regulate the rate and depth of breathing, 2) intact nerves from the brain to the muscles of breathing to carry the messages of how often and how hard to contract or relax, 3) enough energy to supply the respiratory muscles with the strength they need to do the work of breathing, and 4) a free airway to allow passage of air in and out of the lungs. If 1) the respiratory center is depressed (as when large amounts of sedative drugs have crossed over to the baby while he was still in the mother), or 2) if the nerves running to the muscles of breathing are injured (as in the high type of Erb's palsy where overstretching of the brachial plexus nerves during delivery damages the phrenic nerve innervating the dia-

TABLE 38-2. Signs Indicative of Respiratory Distress in the Neonate

Clinical Data	*Rationale for Manifestation*
Tachypnea (respiratory rate greater than 60/minute)	Indicates stiffening of the lung or mild hypoxia, and represents an attempt by the baby to move more air with less effort and increase the amount of oxygen being brought into the lungs.
Expiratory grunting (audible sound made by exhaling against a partially closed glottis)	Indicates hypoxia and a tendency for the alveoli to collapse, and represents an attempt by the baby to keep open his alveoli with back pressure until the very end of expiration and allow more oxygen exchange.
Retractions or depression of the sternum and sucking in of the suprasternal notch (space above the sternum), intercostal spaces (between the ribs) and subcostal margin (below the ribs) on each inspiration.	Retractions are indicative of decreased lung compliance (stiffness or difficulty expanding the lungs) and represent an increased effort by the baby to overcome this. The increased negative pressure thus generated in the intrathoracic space (between lung and chest wall) sucks in the tissues between and around the ribs.
Flaring of the alae nari (nostrils) on inspiration.	Attempt to allow more air flow into the lungs by widening the external passageways.
Cyanosis (dusky blue color of the skin)	Indicates desaturation of the hemoglobin (reduced amount of bound oxygen) in the presence of still adequate circulation.
Pallor (pale, clammy skin)	Pallor reflects poor circulation to the periphery, usually in conjunction with severe hypoxia and circulatory collapse.
Apneic spells (cessation of breathing with change of color and dropping heart rate)	Indicates an immature or depressed respiratory center unable to maintain spontaneous rhythmic respirations without additional stimulation or support.
Bradycardia (heart beats less than 100 times per minute)	Associated with apneic episodes and hypoxia leading to reduced cardiac activity.
Hypothermia (reduced body temperature)	Low body temperature reflecting inability to produce body heat by metabolic processes requiring oxygen.
Hypotonia and hyporeflexia (reduced muscle tone and weak reflex responses)	Indicates a depressed central nervous system from drugs, trauma, hypoxia or exhaustion.

phragm), or 3) if the baby tires or runs out of energy to do the work of breathing (as in hyaline membrane disease where the work of breathing has increased due to stiffening of the lungs), or 4) if the airway is partially obstructed (as after aspiration of thick meconium), then the infant may very well require some form of assisted ventilation to tide him over until the basic problem is resolved.

The same is true of the *antiatelectasis function* or process of keeping the alveoli partially expanded even at the end of expiration. If the air sacs tend to collapse completely at the end of each breath (as in hyaline membrane disease where there is a lack of surfactant on the inner surface of the alveoli to reduce their surface tension and overcome their tendency to collapse), then the baby is forced to take the difficult "first breath" over and over again. This represents a tremendous amount of extra work. Also, there would be no reserve oxygen left in the lungs to tide him over between breaths. And since blood may continue to flow through those areas of the lung that are totally collapsed, it may return to the left side of the heart and then to the body without having picked up the needed amount of oxygen. Assisted ventilation in this situation involves some method of helping the baby hold the alveoli open even at the end of expiration. It may or may not be combined with some form of assisted bellows function, depending on whether the baby's respirations are depressed or if he is becoming tired.

Respiratory failure means the child is no longer able to keep up his blood oxygen level even when breathing 100 per cent O_2, or he is retaining carbon dioxide to the point that he is being anesthetized by the high CO_2 level. The blood gas limits that are widely accepted as defining respiratory failure are an arterial Po_2, (Pao_2) below 50 mm. Hg while breathing 100 per cent O_2, or a Pco_2 above 80 mm. Hg in spite of periodic bagging. It is at this point that some sort of assisted ventilation must be instituted or the baby will die. In babies weighing less than 1500 grams at birth, one need not wait until the child is in 100 per cent O_2, but rather start assisted ventilation when the Pao_2 drops below 50 mm. Hg while the baby is breathing 60 to 70 per cent oxygen. Prolonged or intractable apnea is also an indication to begin assisted ventilation.

The simplest form of assisted ventilation is performed by using a *bag and mask set-up* which forces air into the lungs when the bag is squeezed. An adaptor piece connects the bag to a tight-fitting face mask or directly to an endotracheal tube (going from nose or mouth to the trachea). The bag is either self-inflating or is flow-inflated. In the *self-inflating bag,* the bag springs back to its original shape after being squeezed and thereby sucks in surrounding air through an "in-only" entryway separate from the "out-only" passageway going to the baby. An example of this type of a set-up is the Hope resuscitator pictured in Figure 38-13. The advantages of the Hope bag include the fact that it may be used anywhere (requires no compressed gas source), and is fairly safe even in inexperienced hands, since it has an automatic pop-off valve to prevent excessive pressure buildup. The disadvantages of this type of set-up are that you cannot accurately regulate the oxygen concentration being delivered to the baby, nor can you apply CPAP (continuous positive airway pressure; see below). Also it is most difficult to get a "feel" for bagging with this type of self-inflating resuscitator.

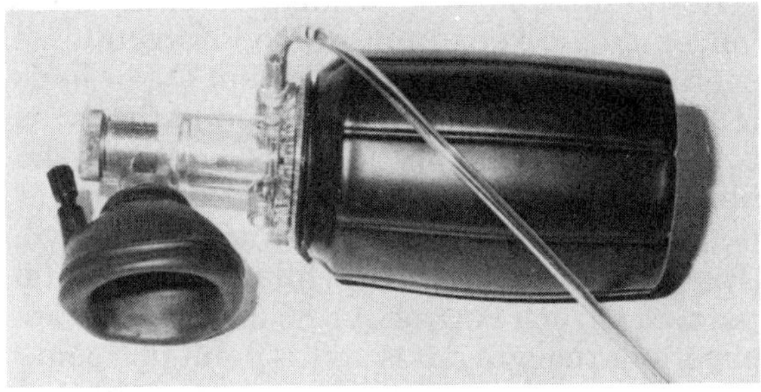

FIGURE 38-13. Hope infant resuscitator, an example of a self-inflating bag and mask set up. Oxygen enrichment of variable amount is brought in through the side port.

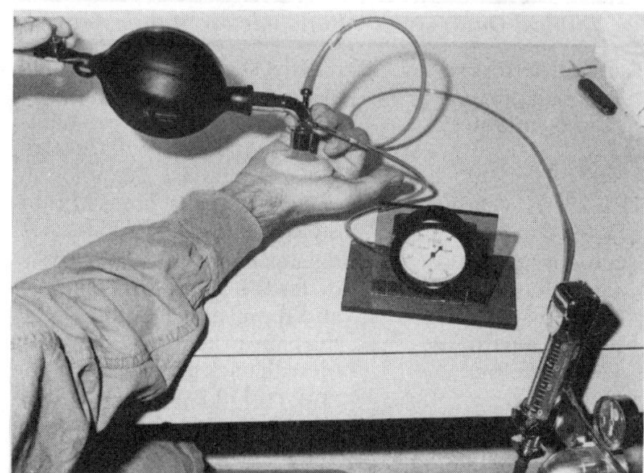

FIGURE 38-14. Modified flow-inflated anesthesia bag set-up which allows application of CPAP and IPPV while monitoring pressure within the system on the attached manometer.

Flow-inflated bag and mask set-ups require a source of compressed air and/or oxygen to fill them. The concentration of oxygen flowing into the bag can be regulated exactly by a blender or Y-tubing from air and oxygen sources, and there is no mixing of this with an undetermined amount of air drawn in through a separate entryway as in the Hope bag. By the simple addition of a side port at the metal elbow of the usual flow-inflated anesthesia bag set-up, and connecting this to a manometer, one can monitor the amount of pressure being delivered (Fig. 38-14). The open end of the rubber anesthesia bag is fitted with an adjustable screw clamp to regulate the amount of gas escaping from the system. If more gas flows into the bag from the top than is allowed to flow out through the end, pressure will build up in the system (assuming there is no leak at the face mask) and is transmitted by way of the mask to the baby's airway and alveoli. The baby continues to breathe spontaneously against this continuous positive airway pressure which helps to hold open his alveoli by maintaining a higher pressure on the inside than on the outside, even on end expiration when alveolar pressure normally drops to zero or atmospheric pressure. The CPAP pressure applied is registered on the manometer and regulated by adjusting the screw clamp. In cases where the infant is having difficulty ventilating (moving air, reflected by P_{CO_2}) as well as oxygenating (getting oxygen into the blood, reflected by P_{O_2}), one can also support ventilation by squeezing the bag smartly in timing with the baby's spontaneous inspiratory efforts. Thus, intermittent positive pressure ventilation (IPPV) can be administered as well as CPAP, making the system as versatile as it is simple and inexpensive. Such a bag and mask set-up is ideal for resuscitation in the delivery room or at the bedside of any infant at risk for apneic episodes. It may also be used to apply CPAP and/or IPPV in referral hospitals until the transport team arrives, as well as in transit, rather than struggling with a cumbersome and temperamental respirator.

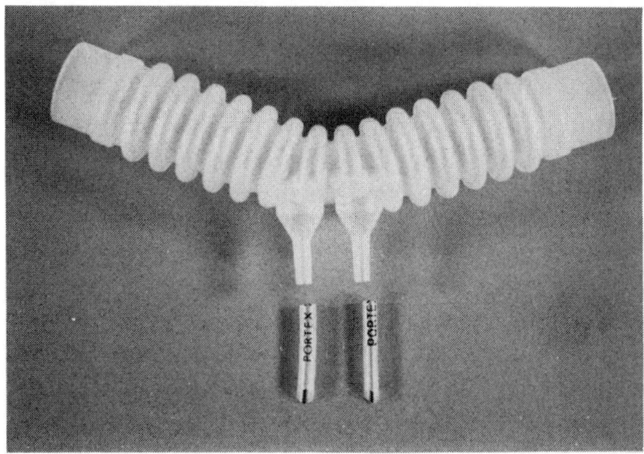

FIGURE 38-15. Central portion of nasal CPAP circuit showing soft rubber flex tube with holes cut for Bennett adaptors and nasal prongs cut from the end of standard Portex endotracheal tubes.

For prolonged assisted ventilation a more permanent CPAP arrangement or respirator for mechanical ventilation is used. Continuous positive airway pressure may be applied by way of an endotracheal tube, face mask, nasal prongs, or tightly-fitting head box. Each has its advantages and disadvantages. The *nasal prong system* is widely used because of its easy application, inexpensive components, ready access to the entire body including the

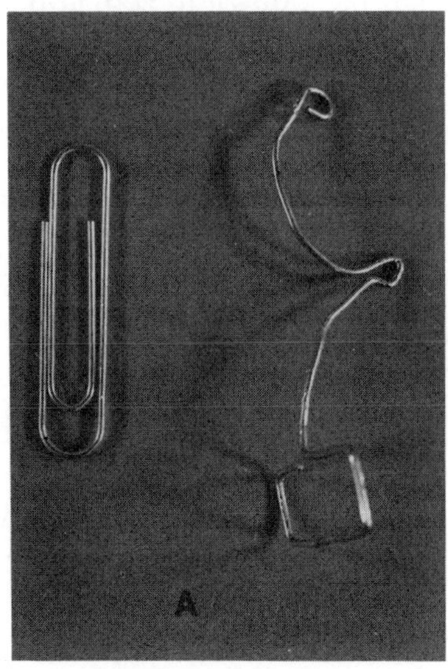

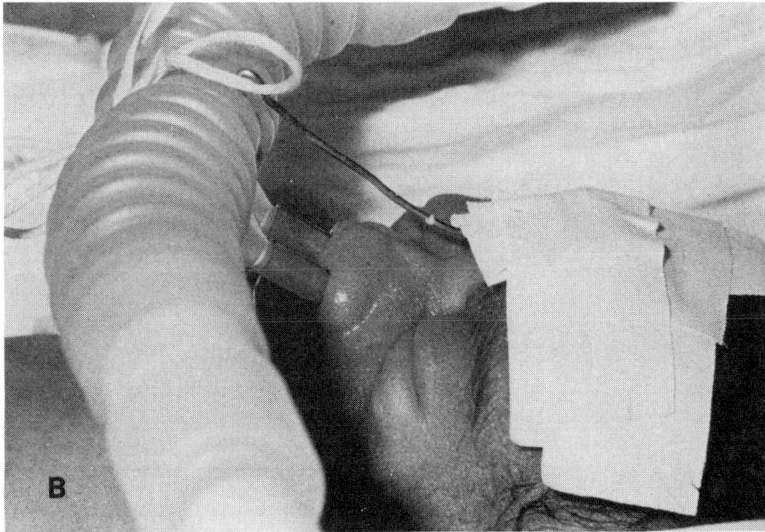

FIGURE 38-16. *A*, Head mount frame constructed from a large paper clip. *B*, Head mount taped to forehead and supporting flex tube and nasal prongs for nasal CPAP.

mouth, and the apparent safety of the method in terms of low incidence of pulmonary air leak (pneumothorax, pneumomediastinum, and so forth). The central components (Fig. 38-15) include a soft rubber flex tube, two Bennett tracheostomy adaptors, and two 1-inch cut-off tips of Portex ET-tubes: they may be resterilized and reused indefinitely. The head mount is constructed from a large paper clip and 1-inch adhesive tape (Fig. 38-16), and when the system is attached to the support arms of a Bourns infant cradle, it provides a secure yet flexible system in which the baby can be repositioned at will (Fig. 38-17). The effect upon oxygenation (Po_2) of applying CPAP to an infant with hyaline membrane disease is illustrated in Figure 38-18.

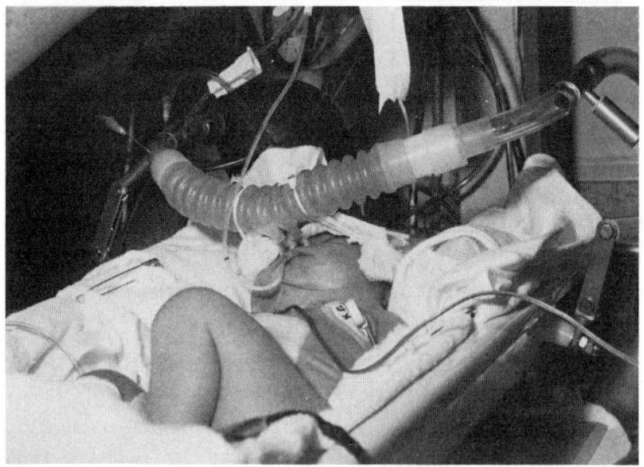

FIGURE 38-17. Baby on nasal CPAP in Bourns cradle that provides support for the circuit and allows easy repositioning.

The early *respirators* (Fig. 38-19) used to mechanically ventilate newborns provided only IPPV, and advanced gas into the lungs during the inspiratory cycle by generating pressure or flow in a preset pattern for a chosen length of time (time-cycled), or until a predetermined volume of gas had been delivered (volume-cycled), or until flow from the respirator had fallen below a certain critical point (flow-cycled). Improvements on the older models and the development of newer models now allow one to provide the baby with PEEP (positive end expiratory pressure) or background CPAP as well as IPPV to assist both the antiatelectatic function and bellows function of breathing. In respirators providing IPPV and PEEP, pressure in the closed system is not allowed to fall back down to zero at the end of expiration, holding alveoli open which

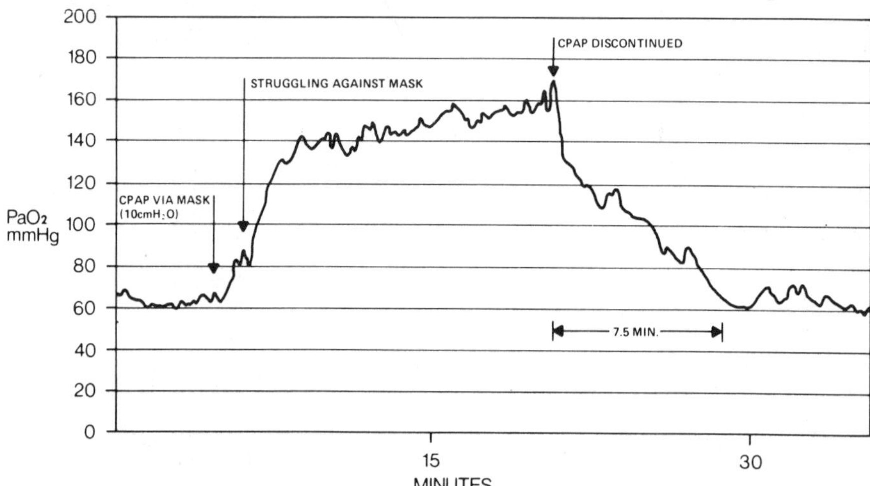

FIGURE 38-18. The effect on arterial Po_2 of applying CPAP via bag and mask for approximately 10 minutes to an infant with severe hyaline membrane disease weighing 1,815 grams. (From Harris, T. and Nugent, M.: *Continuous arterial oxygen tension monitoring in the newborn infant.* J. Pediatr. 82:934, 1973, with permission.)

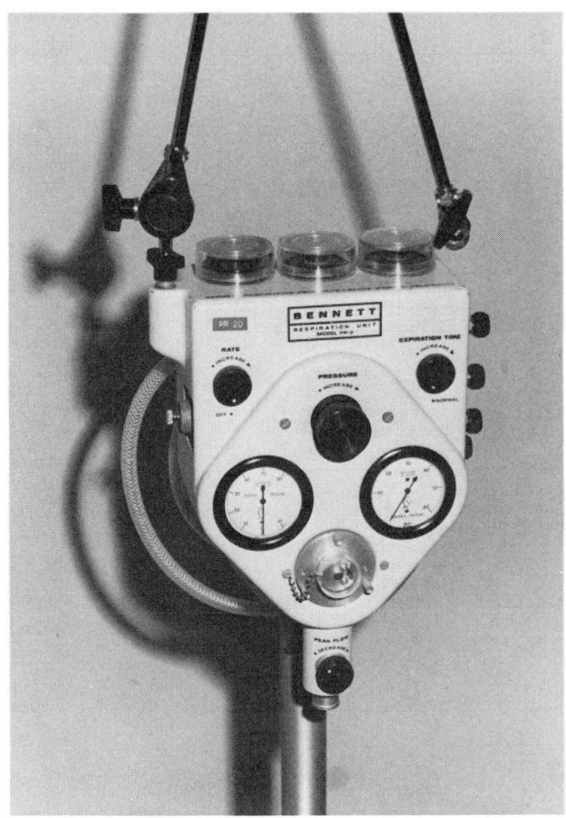

FIGURE 38-19. Bennett PR-2 flow-cycled positive pressure respirator for assisting ventilation by providing IPPV.

would otherwise collapse and thus improving oxygenation (Fig. 38-20). In those that use background CPAP and intermittently provide positive pressure inspiratory support (also known as intermittent mandatory ventilation, or IMV) at an adjustable rate, the same thing is accomplished as regards never allowing pressure in the airway and alveoli to drop to zero. Here, however, the baby always gets fresh gas if he breathes out of phase with the respirator, since the CPAP is maintained by a constant gas flow. As the infant improves and gets stronger, he is allowed to do more and more of the work of breathing himself as the IMV rate is turned down further and further. This provides a very smooth "weaning" of the baby

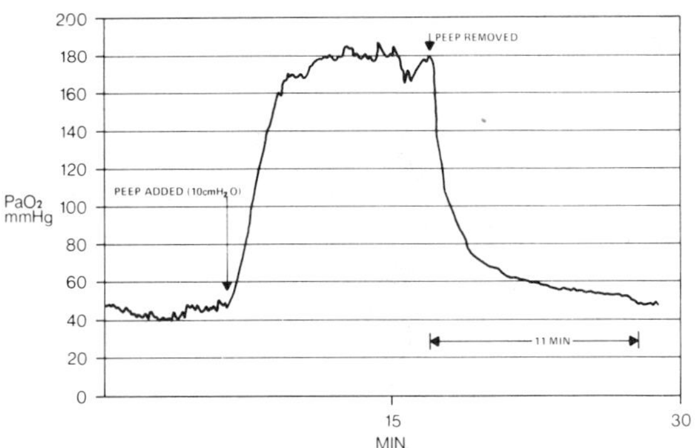

FIGURE 38-20. Effect on arterial P_{O_2} of adding PEEP to a respirator delivering IPPV to an infant with severe hyaline membrane disease weighing 1,300 grams. (From Harris, T. and Nugent, M.: *Continuous arterial oxygen tension monitoring in the newborn infant.* J. Pediatr. 82-934, 1973, with permission.)

TABLE 38-3. Complications of Assisted Ventilation of Newborns*

Complication	*Number of Babies*	*Incidence*	*Survival*
Pulmonary air leak (pneumothorax, pneumomediastinum, pneumopericardium, interstitial emphysema)	52	25%	50%
Chest tube perforating lung	2	1%	50%
Bronchopulmonary dysplasia (chronic respiratory lung disease)	15	7%	60%
Accidental extubation	10	5%	67%
Tracheal stenosis requiring trachiostomy	2	1%	50%
Nasal strictures	5	2.5%	100%
Blindness	3	1.1%	100%
Total number of babies in sample	206		63%

* Data reflects the experience of assisting ventilation in 206 newborns at Tucson Medical Center over a period of 34 months, August 1, 1961 to May 30, 1974.

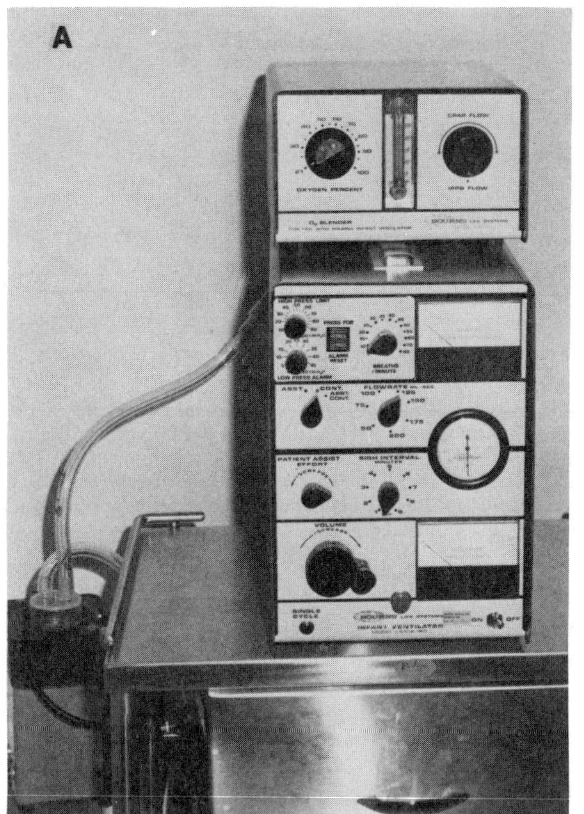

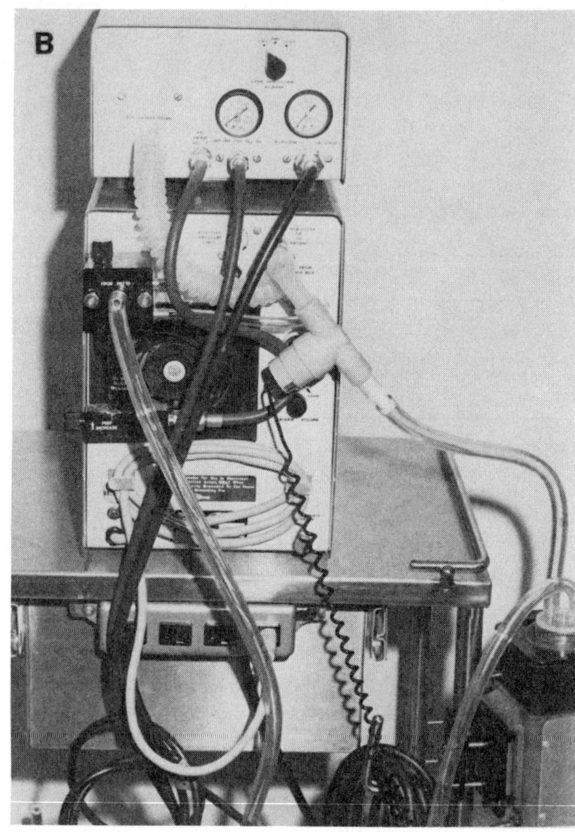

FIGURE 38-21. *A*, Front view of Bourns infant respirator. *B*, Back view of Bourns infant respirator showing retrofittings for PEEP assist and IMV (control IPPV and background CPAP) modes.

from the machine. The most versatile of the infant respirators is the retrofitted Bourns, shown in Figure 38-21, which allows one to use IPPV alone or with PEEP in both "assist" (the patient triggering the machine) and "control" mode, or CPAP alone or in conjunction with IMV.

Assisted ventilation of the newborn is a highly developed science (and art) and requires a team of experts including nurses, doctors, and respiratory therapists, as well as 24-hour back-up x-ray and laboratory support facilities. Some of the many nursing responsibilities involved in the care of an infant receiving assisted ventilation are discussed below. Complications encountered in a large series of babies receiving assisted ventilation, their incidence, and effects on ultimate survival are listed in Table 38-3.

The type of sophisticated respiratory care involved in assisting ventilation of newborns should not even be attempted in a small hospital. Rather, all efforts would be directed toward developing a referral system whereby mothers-at-risk or infants born with respiratory distress may be safely transferred to regional high-risk obstetric and neonatal intensive care centers for such care. Both mortality rates and cost can thus be kept to a minimum, while still providing access to superior perinatal care for every high-risk mother and infant in the region.

The Role of Nursing

What are some of the problems the nurse must anticipate when a neonate is on assisted ventilation therapy? The following is a brief outline of aspects to be integrated into the nursing care plan:

The Neonate on the Respirator

Problems	*Suggested Actions for Management*
1. Extubation (dislodging of the tube)—Recognized by: a. Baby struggling to breathe, out of phase with the respirator. b. Breath sounds heard out of phase with respirator.	Bag baby with 100% O_2 by mask after tube removed. Decompress stomach of air by aspirating NG tube. Anticipate setting up equipment for reintubation.
2. Blockages of ET (endotracheal) tube—Recognized by: a. Baby making gasping respirations out of phase with the respirator. b. Marked increase in respirator pressures. c. Reduced breath sounds.	Suction ET tube after instilling 0.5–3 cc. of normal saline, making sure that suction catheter goes beyond end of ET tube (length of tube should always be posted at bedside). Percussion, postural drainage, and suction are part of the routine in cases of prolonged intubation. Turning q1–2h prevents stasis and promotes drainage.
3. Trauma to trachea or nose—Recognized by: a. Blood-tinged tracheal aspirate. b. Inflammation around nares.	Secure ET tube firmly; prevent excessive movement of head. Apply antibiotic ointment to skin at entrance to nares. When suctioning, limit suction pressure to minus 80 cm. H_2O.
4. Pneumothorax (alveolar rupture allowing air to enter into the pleural space)—Recognized by: a. Decreased chest movement and breath sounds on affected side. b. Rapid onset of tachypnea, cyanosis, and eventual bradycardia. c. Sudden abdominal distention. d. Heart sounds heard on the right side if pneumothorax on the left.	Raise ambient oxygen concentration to 100%. Call for stat chest x-ray. Alert physician immediately and assist in the therapy which may include: a. Needle aspiration of the air in extreme emergencies. b. Chest tube placement with connection to one-way valve (Heimlich) or underwater seal.

5. Malfunctioning of equipment—Recognized by: a. Sounding of no-flow or pressure alarms. b. Sudden change to extremely high or low respirator pressures. c. Sudden deterioration of the baby (cyanosis, bradycardia).	Listen for machine alarms and look for sudden pressure changes. Check heart rate, respiration, other vital signs being monitored. Check settings of respirator every hour. Observe baby for signs of sudden change. Check all tube connections and assure they are snugly fitted. Be systematic in assessment of equipment; begin at the ET tube and follow back to the respirator and gas source. Check to be sure oxygen concentration is at desired level. Analyze the amount of oxygen the infant is receiving hourly.
6. Decubiti Formation—Recognized by: a. Inflammation of the skin. b. Actual breakdown of the skin.	Consider meticulous skin care; skin kept clean, dry, free of pressure. Turn baby q1–2h to alleviate pressure and promote circulation. Use ordered medications to areas vulnerable to decubiti or areas of skin already breaking down. Use of a water pillow or pressure-alternating mattress pad when feasible.

The Neonate Receiving Nasal CPAP

Problems	*Suggested Actions for Management*
1. Possible drying of mucous membranes which causes thick tenacious mucus to form that may block off the posterior pharynx or glottis obstructing breathing.	Maintain full humidification of gas flowing in CPAP circuit to decrease formation of thick mucus. Suction baby as ordered on a routine basis. Normal saline may be instilled periodically into the nostrils to loosen up secretions prior to suctioning.
2. Possible irritation to nares, oral cavity.	An ointment may be ordered for application around the outside of the nares. Oral hygiene (such as with lemon and glycerine swabs or glucose water) to prevent drying.
3. Possible near-drowning because of malfunction of equipment or too much condensation of humidity in tubing.	Keep checking the level of humidity in the circuit. Be sure there is no condensation in the tubes that may flow downward to the baby.

4. Aspiration of gavage feeding secondary to air distention of the stomach.	Aspirate stomach to remove air prior to gavage feeding. Tilt bed so that head is elevated during gavage feedings. Keep the gavage tube in place and connected to open syringe barrel suspended above the level of the abdomen. If regurgitation occurs, reflux will be up into the barrel rather than up into the pharynx where it could be aspirated into the lungs.
5. Pulmonary air leak such as pneumothorax.	Actions for these have been discussed in the preceding section.
6. Skin breakdown, decubiti.	Actions for these have been discussed in the preceding section.

Oxygen Administration

The distressed neonate may need enriched oxygen to breathe. Stressors increase the metabolic rate and, therefore, oxygen consumption. Furthermore, the high-risk neonate generally has low oxygen reserves which limit his ability to maintain adequate oxygenation. The primary purpose for giving enriched oxygen to breathe is to increase the amount of oxygen delivered to the tissues.

The word oxygen is almost synonymous with life or saving-life. However, as a drug, it has the potential for complications when used injudiciously. Therefore, the nurse must have knowledge as to the proper use of oxygen. What is the nurse's role in oxygen therapy? Major nursing goals relative to the use of oxygen in the neonate are:

1. Maintain the prescribed concentration of ambient (surrounding) oxygen needed by the neonate.
2. Alert the physician to changes in the neonate's clinical status which may indicate increased or decreased need for oxygen.
3. Appreciate that blood oxygen tension levels, when high, can also have toxic effects. Therefore, blood gas monitoring is necessary whenever high ambient oxygen concentrations are used.

Maintenance of the Prescribed Ambient Oxygen Concentration. The physician orders the prescribed oxygen concentration based on clinical findings and laboratory blood gas analyses. Prescribed oxygen levels should be ordered in exact concentrations (per cent or fraction of inspired oxygen [F_IO_2]) instead of liters per minute, since inflow of oxygen is only one of the many determinants of the oxygen concentration in an enclosed space. Therefore, the nurse should question any medical order for oxygen written in liters per minute.

There are two types of oxygen analyzers generally in use, the older *paramagnetic* type and the newer *polarographic* type.

The first (and previously most commonly used) type of instrument takes advantage of the *paramagnetic* properties of oxygen, namely its attraction *into* a magnetic field. Nearly all other gases such as nitrogen and helium which make up the air we breathe are diamagnetic, that is, they are repelled *out* of a magnetic field. By measuring force changes in a magnetic field when various samples of gas are brought into the field, one can tell how much oxygen is in the sample compared with the other gases. One is thus measuring the percentage of oxygen in the total gas sample, or the portion of the total which is oxygen. The gas sample is brought into the magnetic field or measuring chamber of the instrument by pumping or squeezing a bulb a number of times. This must be done before taking each new reading, and thus the instrument gives intermittent rather than continuous values.

The newer oxygen analyzers which do provide continuous read-out of ambient oxygen concentration operate on the *polarographic* principle. A voltage from a battery in the instrument is constantly applied to the cathode of the sensing electrode cartridge polarizing it and attracting oxygen. The oxygen diffuses through a membrane over the cathode and is electrochemically reduced at the cathode, giving up electrons which then migrate by way of an electrode paste to the anode in the same electrode cartridge. The current (flow of electrons) moving between the cathode and anode is equal to the amount of oxygen being reduced, which in turn is directly proportional to the oxygen concentration in the surrounding air. The amount of current thus reflects the concentration of oxygen, which is then displayed on the dial of the instrument. Problems with the battery losing strength, the electrode paste drying out, or the membrane changing its characteristics all require that this type of instrument be recalibrated at frequent intervals.

Alert the Physician to Changes in the Neonate's Clinical Status. It is obviously desirable to use the lowest concentration of oxygen possible to maintain pink skin color in the neonate (see discussion on cyanosis in the preceding chapter). The nurse should be able to assume responsibility for rapidly increasing the oxygen concentration when the neonate's condition warrants (as after aspiration or in cyanosis).

Appreciate the Toxic Effects when High Concentrations of Oxygen Are Used. High concentrations of oxygen can be detrimental to the newborn. Organs most vulnerable to deleterious effects are the eyes (retrolental fibroplasia) and the lungs (bronchopulmonary dysplasia). Damage to the eyes is due to high levels of dissolved oxygen in the arterial blood (increased PaO_2), while damage to the lungs is a direct effect from breathing high concentrations of oxygen.

Retrolental fibroplasia is a disease unique to the premature infant. Immature vessels in the retina are susceptible to vascular constriction when exposed to increased arterial oxygen tension during breathing of high O_2 concentrations. This vascular constriction causes hypoxia to the areas of the retina normally supplied by the constricted blood vessels. New vessels are formed (neovascularization) in response to the hypoxia but are susceptible to breakage and hemorrhage. The result is retrolental (behind the lens) fibroplasia (scar tissue formation) which later may constrict to produce retinal detachment and eventual blindness (Fig. 38-22).

When a newborn breathes high concentrations of oxygen for prolonged periods, the effects are toxic to the lungs and contribute to *bronchopulmonary dysplasia.* High oxygen exposure lowers surfactant production causing atelectasis (collapse of air spaces) as well as capillary proliferation, thickening of the alveolar basement membrane, and hypertrophy of bronchial mucous glands.[4]

The nurse helps to protect the newborn from detrimental effects of oxygen therapy by assuring safe administration of prescribed oxygen concentrations. This involves frequent measuring of the neonate's oxygen levels in the blood, and dictates that blood gas measuring capabilities be available on a 24-hour basis. The nurse should assure that blood gas mea-

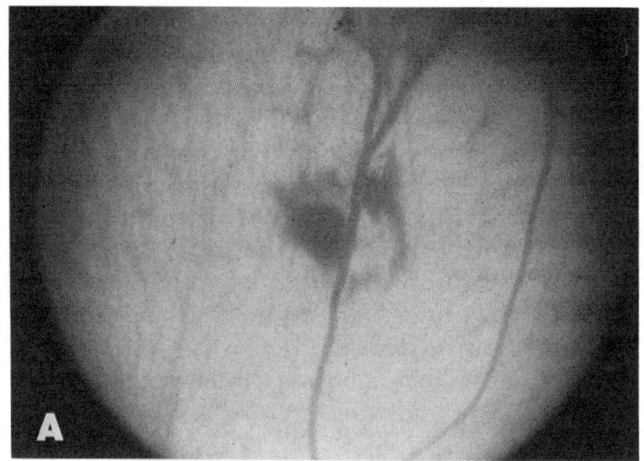

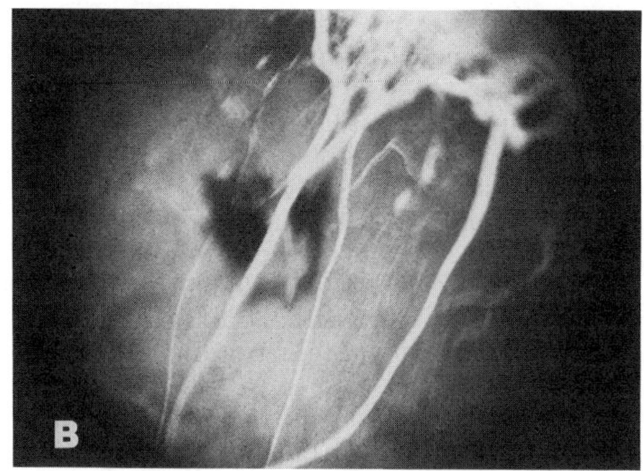

FIGURE 38-22. *A*, Retrolental fibroplasia in a 3-month-old infant. The darkened area in the center shows an intraretinal hemorrhage surrounding a large arteriole. Note the fan-shaped network of new vessels. *B*, Fundus photograph of area shown in figure *A*, taken while vessels were filled with fluorescent dye in order to clearly show the vasculature. (Photographs courtesy of Harold E. Cross, M.D., Ph.D., University of Arizona College of Medicine.)

surements are done whenever a neonate is on oxygen above 30 per cent, and that such results are available to serve as guidelines for the prescribed levels of oxygen to be given. If the nurse finds herself in a clinical setting without facilities for blood gas measurement, the following method is suggested as a way to provisionally estimate the O_2 concentration to be used:

> Lower the surrounding oxygen concentration 5 to 10 per cent at a time until a point is reached at which the infant just appears slightly cyanotic. Then increase the oxygen no more than 10 per cent so that the baby is held at a level that just maintains pink skin color.

To illustrate the above, a nurse would gradually lower the oxygen concentration by 10 per cent reductions and if the infant appears cyanotic at 30 per cent concentration, then a relatively safe level of oxygen therapy would be estimated to be 40 per cent.

Blood gas measurements are an integral part of an oxygen therapeutic plan because they allow oxygen concentrations delivered to meet the unique needs of the baby rather than by generalizations (Fig. 38-23). For example, it was once accepted that an oxygen concentration of 40 per cent or less was a safe therapeutic level. However, this generalization is no longer applicable for clinical use because infants in severe respiratory distress can die of hypoxia if restricted to 40 per cent O_2,

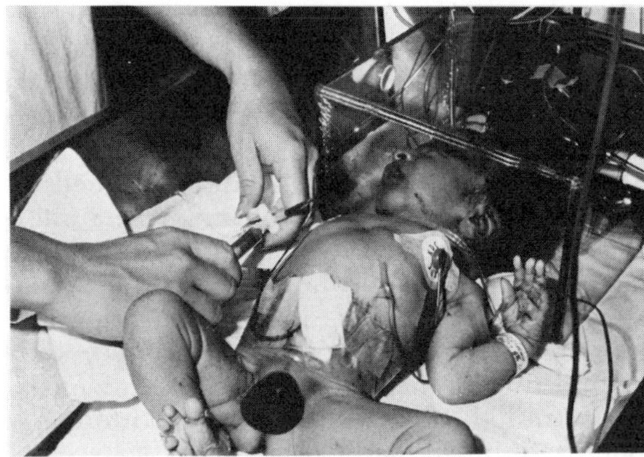

FIGURE 38-23. Blood being drawn for blood gas measurements. Such monitoring is an integral part of intensive neonatal care.

while small preterm infants may be damaged by oxygen concentrations of even less than 40 per cent.

The nurse also assures that every infant exposed to high oxygen concentrations has its fundi checked periodically during the therapy if possible, and most certainly before discharge from the nursery. During the administration of high oxygen concentrations, resulting arterial constriction of the retinal vessels may be detected by opthalmologic examination by experienced personnel.

The role of the nurse during oxygen therapy has undergone radical changes. At one time nurses were advised to gradually reduce or increase the amount of oxygen in accordance with their clinical observation of the neonate's appearance (primarily the presence or absence of cyanosis). However, rough estimates in the regulation of oxygen therapy no longer have a place in newborn care. This releases nurses from the overwhelming burden of trying to regulate oxygen to the newborn through data obtained primarily from clinical assessment, a task insurmountable even for physicians. Modern oxygen therapy dictates the need for frequent intermittent or continuous monitoring of the neonate's response. It is therefore advocated that should nurses ever find themselves in situations in which adequate monitoring devices are not available, they should use the method described previously, only until the baby can be transported to a better-equipped medical facility.

Correction of acid-base imbalance

Acidosis may be due to the retention of carbon dioxide secondary to depressed respirations or inadequate ventilation due to tiring of the baby, or it may be due to the collection of fixed acid as a result of poor oxygenation or poor circulation. That is to say, the acidosis seen in babies with respiratory distress may be of respiratory or metabolic origin, or a combination of both. In cases of respiratory acidosis (pH low, P_{CO_2} high), the only treatment is to assist ventilation to effectively blow off the CO_2. The nurse needs to know that the correction of respiratory acidosis involves a different mode of therapy from that for metabolic acidosis. Giving bicarbonate in this situation will only further increase the level of CO_2. In cases of combined respiratory and metabolic acidosis, it is necessary to both assist ventilation and administer alkali. Considerations for nursing care when acidosis is corrected with alkali therapy include:

1. Knowledge on preparation of the alkali solution (sodium bicarbonate is the preferred drug). For calculation of dosages, each milliliter of the usual 44.5 solution contains 1 mEq. of sodium bicarbonate. Always check the label on the vial for confirmation.
2. Dosages of sodium bicarbonate must be diluted because it is very hypertonic. A safe dilution is with equal amounts of distilled water.
3. The prescribed dosage is determined by the doctor according to blood gas measurements. However, in an emergency, when time precludes determination of blood gases a generally accepted dosage is 3 mEq. sodium bicarbonate per kilogram of body weight. The nurse can save precious time by having the dosage readily available. Thus, the nurse must know the infant's body weight in kilograms. If time allows, a slow rate of infusion such as 2 to 3 mEq./min. is recommended.

Health Care Maintenance During Respiratory Distress

A neonate in respiratory distress is particularly vulnerable to hypothermia because of limited oxygen to support the metabolic processes for heat production. If the baby is forced to produce heat from processes that do not require oxygen (anaerobic pathways), the result is a buildup of lactic acid or metabolic acidosis. Both the cold itself and metabolic acidosis are thought to cause pulmonary vasoconstriction (narrowing of the pulmonary arteries), thus further decreasing blood flow and oxygen uptake in the lungs which worsens the problem of tissue hypoxia. Some important nursing actions for these babies are:

1. During any procedure which requires that the baby be exposed (e.g., resuscitation, umbilical catheterizations), supply the infant with heat from an overhead radiant source (warmer or heat lamp).
2. Movement or transfer of infants should be carried out in a protected environment. One can provide either a) protection against heat loss or b) an artificial source of heat production en route.
   a. Means of preventing heat loss include the traditional method of wrapping the baby with warm blankets, or the newer technique of wrapping the baby in transparent, double-layered plastic bags in which the two layers are separated by large, self-contained air bubbles which provide insulation but still permit visualization of the baby.
   b. An artificial source of heat production is provided en route in battery-powered transport incubators that produce either convective (circulating warm air) or radiant (heat dome) sources of heat.
3. Remember that humidified, compressed gas (air or oxygen) in itself is cold, so that it becomes necessary to protect large surface areas of the baby from exposure to the gas flow. Furthermore, the greater the gas flow, the more heat loss due to this increased convection and evaporation. Nursing actions include:
   a. Limiting the exposed area to the head and face whenever possible,
   b. Increasing the warmer or incubator temperature to compensate for this increased heat loss, or
   c. Using oxygen therapy equipment which prewarms the inflowing gas.

Periodic Breathing and Apneic Episodes

The theoretical basis for periodic breathing and apneic episodes as well as the assessment for infants most vulnerable to apnea have been presented previously in Chapter 37. Apnea in the newborn is probably the most frequent emergency situation encountered by the nurse in the nursery. Therefore, it is essential that the nurse be able to implement actions immediately which will save the neonate's life. Specific nursing actions, in order of priority, are:

1. A bag and mask connected to O_2 and/or air, and suction catheter connected to wall suction should be in the infant's incubator for ready use.
2. If apnea alarm sounds or you observe infant not breathing, first attempt to reinitiate respiration with manual simulation.
3. Determine if vomitus is in mouth or if there is bradycardia (pulse less than 100/min.).
4. Suction if necessary.
5. If in Bradycardia, bag until heart rate is back up to previous resting level.
6. If prolonged bagging is necessary, insert #8 or larger feeding tube as soon as possible to act as vent for air that may enter stomach while bagging.
7. Check heart rate frequently. If patient remains bradycardiac, call physician immediately and continue bagging.
8. Record each apneic episode and details of any difficult resuscitation.
9. If there is no improvement:

a. Check patency of airway.
b. Suction again.
c. Check for leaks around the mask.
d. Check for adequate pressure and O_2 inflow into bag.
e. Check breath sounds while bagging to see if adequate ventilation is being provided.

10. If pulse drops below 60, maintain circulation by applying external cardiac massage.
11. Have all necessary further resuscitation equipment and medications available at the bedside. Call Respiratory Therapy for ventilator support.

PERINATAL INFECTIONS

Factors that make the fetus and neonate vulnerable to infections have been discussed in Chapters 30 and 34. This section provides guidelines for identifying infants suspected of infection.

Infection Acquired by the Transplacental Route. Maternal infections can be transmitted across the placenta to the infant. Examples of maternal infections and their effects on the fetus are found in Table 38-4. Suspect infants are all those whose mothers had a known infection during pregnancy or who manifest certain physical signs and symptoms as listed in Table 38-5.

Infection Acquired by the Ascending Route. This refers to entrance of pathogenic organisms into the uterine cavity through the cervix. Infection can occur directly into the amniotic sac or indirectly by spreading along the uterine wall through the maternal-fetal vascular system. The intact amniotic membranes can protect the fetus from ascending infection, although organisms can penetrate the sac causing amnionitis (infection of the amniotic fluid). Suspect infants are those with prolonged rupture of membranes (over 24 hours prior to delivery), foul smelling or discolored amniotic fluid, or maternal fever.

Difficult Labor and Delivery. Difficult, prolonged labor and delivery make the infant vulnerable to skin breakdown or mucosal abrasions from the trauma associated with obstetric manipulation. Also, the stress of a difficult delivery increases the hazard of aspiration. Fluid aspirated into the lungs can cause pneumonia, and infected fluid in the middle ear can create otitis media leading to meningitis. The breakdown of the skin allows entrance of pathogens and the damaged tissues provide a good medium for bacterial growth. Suspect infants are those with prolonged, difficult labor, indications of fetal distress (e.g., meconium-stained amniotic fluid, fetal bradycardia) or signs of neonatal respiratory distress.

Infections Acquired during Passage through the Birth Canal. During birth the infant may acquire pathogens harbored in the vaginal canal. Examples are gonococus, monilia, herpes, listeria, and beta hemolytic streptococcus. Suspect infants are those from mothers with signs of vaginal infection.

Infections Acquired in Newborns in Less Than Optimal Condition. A sick neonate is particularly vulnerable to infection due to his basic disease process and the manipulative procedures employed to save his life. In addition to lowered resistance and available energy to combat infection, manipulative measures carry a degree of hazards. For example:

1. Resuscitation can cause injury to the mucosal lining and expose the baby to "water bugs" (see below) from prolonged ventilatory assistance.
2. Catherization of umbilical vessels can bring with it introduction of organisms directly into the central circulation, rather than cause just localized infection at the site of peripheral vein infusion.
3. Babies who undergo surgery involving opening of the intestines are exposed to gram-negative organisms such as E. coli

TABLE 38-4. Effects of Maternal Infection on Fetus and Neonate*

	Effects on Fetus and Neonate	*Associated Factors*	*Prognosis of Infant*
Coxsackie virus	? congenital malformations in first trimester. Transplacental meningoencephalitis and/or myocarditis. Acquired infections.	Maternal infection mild.	Depends on the extent of the disease.
Cytomegalic inclusion body disease	Intrauterine death. Premature delivery. Severe generalized disease—jaundice, hemolytic anemia, thrombocytopenia, hepatosplenomegaly, central nervous system disease including cerebral calcification and chorioretinitis), microcephaly, and undergrowth.	Half the women in early childbearing years show no immunologic response to this virus. Mothers are asymptomatic.	Early death in majority of severely affected infants. Severe mental and motor retardation in some survivors.
Hepatitis (serum)	Abortion. Neonatal hepatitis.	Circumstantial evidence incriminates hepatitis virus.	
Herpes simplex	Mild infection with a few skin lesions; infant does not appear ill. Viremia, severe generalized disease, CNS involvement. ? congenital malformations.	Maternal herpetic vulvovaginitis usually present. Transplacental infection of fetus may occur.	Mild disease—recovery. Severe disease—usually fatal.
Influenza	Increased incidence of abortion and premature labor. Occasional association of congenital malformations, especially anencephaly and meningomyelocele.	Active immunization by an attenuated vaccine should not be given during pregnancy for fear of fetal damage.	
Listeriosis	Infants infected either through direct invasion or from birth contamination. Generalized disease, skin rash, meningitis, pneumonia, etc. Fetal involvement with scattered foci of necrosis (granulomatosis infantiseptica). Delayed infection of the newborn infant, usually listerial meningitis.	4% of pregnant women harbor *Listeria monocytogenes* in the cervix or vagina. Occasionally influenza-like symptoms in the mother. Amniotic fluid noted to be dirty brown.	Mortality and morbidity high, especially from CNS complications.
Malaria	Direct transmission of *P. falciparum* occurs rarely. Diminished growth with placental involvement.	Placental involvement 10 times more frequent than fetal involvement.	
Mumps	Abortion, premature birth or stillbirth not unusual. ? cause of endocardial fibroelastosis.		
Mycoplasma	Chronic reproductive failure. Interstitial pneumonia or generalized sepsis.	Mycoplasma isolated from genital and lower urinary tracts of women and men.	Abortion in early pregnancy. Neonatal death common, generally from respiratory involvement.

* From Klaus and Faranoff,[1] with permission.

TABLE 38-4. *Continued*

	Effects on Fetus and Neonate	*Associated Factors*	*Prognosis of Infant*
Poliomyelitis	Abortion. Rare congenital or acquired poliomyelitis. Growth retardation in chronic, severe, maternal, paralytic poliomyelitis.	Widespread use of immunization procedures has all but eliminated this disease as a pregnancy problem. Use of Sabin live virus vaccine during pregnancy is contraindicated. May safely administer Salk vaccine.	Fetal and neonatal loss — 33%.
Rubella	Abortion. Congenital malformations of heart, eye, ear, brain; dermatoglyphic abnormalities. Systemic involvement with or without malformation, anemia, thrombocytopenia with purpura, jaundice, hepatosplenomegaly, bone changes, myocarditis, encephalitis, pneumonia, etc.	Maternal infection usually mild, occasionally arthritis and/or encephalitis. Strict isolation for neonates with congenital rubella as long as virus is present in pharynx or urine.	Residua and sequelae for the neonate depend on time during pregnancy when mother acquires the disease, virulence of the virus, and extent of the infectious process. Incidence of malformation in the infant is 35% in first month, 25% in second month, and 16% in third month of gestation. After 4th month, abnormalities are uncommon.
Rubeola (measles)	Interruption of pregnancy. Congenital or neonatal measles, with or without bronchopneumonia (typical dermal lesions are in same stage as those in mother).	Measles vaccine should be given to all nonimmune women prior to but not during gestation.	Maternal rubeola at any time during pregnancy is responsible for increased perinatal death rate. Great majority of infants are normal.
Smallpox and vaccinia	Increased fetal wastage in all stages of pregnancy. Congenital malformations not more frequent, but congenital infections with skin lesions reported.	Primary vaccination and revaccination against smallpox must be deferred until after delivery because vaccinia often causes fatal widespread fetal visceral and cutaneous lesions.	
Syphilis	Major cause of mid-trimester abortion, fetal death in utero, or premature labor and delivery. Early congenital syphilis (septicemia, skin lesions, anemia, jaundice, periostitis). Late congenital syphilis.	If maternal infection occurs less than 1–2 years prior to gestation, fetus probably will be affected seriously. When onset of disease occurs in early pregnancy, congenital infection usually occurs. Transmission of infection is rare before the 5th month of gestation.	40–50% of infants affected in untreated mothers. 40% of above show clinical signs at birth.
Toxoplasmosis	High incidence of abortion. Premature delivery. Generalized disease — hepatosplenomegaly, jaundice, chorioretinitis, microphthalmia, convulsions. Later manifestations — hydrocephalus or microcephaly, mental retardation, cerebral calcifications.		Poor

TABLE 38-4. *Continued*

	Effects on Fetus and Neonate	*Associated Factors*	*Prognosis of Infant*
Tuberculosis	Small infants born to mothers with active disease. Congenital tuberculosis – rare. Acquired infection readily contracted.	Severe maternal disease and malnutrition. Essential to segregate mother with pulmonary tuberculosis from her infant to avoid neonatal infection.	Great majority of infants unaffected.
Varicella (chickenpox)	Premature delivery. Congenital varicella.	Low maternal immunity; most mothers have had the disease and developed immunity in childhood; therefore, congenital varicella is rare.	Mortality high.

and Klebsiella, whereas those requiring deep-vein hyperalimentation with hypertonic solutions are often exposed to Candida fungus.

Infection Acquired from Environmental Sources. People, equipment, and neighboring babies are possible carriers of pathogens. Moisture is an excellent medium for bacterial growth, and special consideration should be given to cleaning anything that comes in contact with water or moist gases. Specifically, the use of humidity with oxygen in an isolette or wet tubings should not be ignored as areas for possible bacterial growth. Epidemics of septicemia, meningitis, conjunctivitis, and pneumonia have been caused by organisms found in one or more of the following sources, which are specific examples of such objects or equipment:

- suction machines and reused suction catheters
- face masks and other resuscitation apparatus
- humidifiers for wall outlet gas
- sink faucets
- dirty soap dispensers and soap trays
- pans used for giving baths
- solutions used for irrigations (e.g., for the eyes)
- solutions used for cold sterilization (e.g., Zephiran)
- isolettes with water in the humidity reservoir.

Unfortunately, physical manifestations of infection in the newborn are subtle and vague so that they may go unnoticed in the early stages of the disease. When later identified, it may be already too late. The classic signs of infection in the adult, such as fever, may be absent in the newborn. Therefore, it is crucial that the nurse recognize early subtle signs that will arouse suspicion of possible infection in a newborn (see Table 38-5). The role of the nurse in casefinding infants at risk for infection is vividly expressed by Klaus and Fanaroff:

> . . . it is the nurse who usually alerts us (physicians) to the diagnosis by observing subtle changes in color, tone, activity or else in feeding the infant. Unless an excellent working relationship between the nurse and physician exists, early diagnosis is impossible.[5]

A good nursing rule is to suspect infection in any infant who is "not doing well," as reflected in daily patterns (feeding, sleeping, activity, elimination).

Role of the Nurse

When an infant is suspected of having an infectious disease, laboratory diagnosis helps to identify the etiologic agent and guides prescription of antimicrobial therapy. Some of

TABLE 38-5. Clinical Presentation of Infection*

"Not Doing Well"

Poor Temperature Control
- Fever
- Hypothermia

Central Nervous System
- Lethargy/irritability
- Jitteriness/hyporeflexia
- Tremors/seizures
- Coma
- Full fontanelle
- Abnormal eye movements
- Hypotonia/increased tone

Respiratory System
- Cyanosis
- Grunting
- Irregular respirations
- Tachypnea/apnea
- Retractions

Gastrointestinal Tract
- Poor feeding
- Vomiting (may be bile-stained)
- Diarrhea/decreased stools
- Edema/erythema abdominal wall
- Hepatomegaly

Skin
- Rashes/erythema
- Purpura
- Pustules/paronychia
- Omphalitis
- Sclerema

Hematopoietic System
- Jaundice
- Bleeding
- Purpura/ecchymosis
- Splenomegaly

Circulatory System
- Pallor/cyanosis/mottling
- Cold, clammy skin
- Tachycardia/arrhythmia
- Hypotension
- Edema

* From Klaus and Faranoff,[1] with permission.

TABLE 38-6. Rationale for Laboratory Investigations to Aid in Diagnosis of Infection in the Newborn

Laboratory Investigation	*Rationale*
Cultures and Sensitivities Of greatest importance are cultures from blood, spinal fluid, urine, skin, ear, stool, gastric aspirate, and umbilical cord area. Microscopic examination and gram-staining of these specimens may also be done.	By definition, a positive blood culture indicates septicemia. The spinal fluid must also be examined because some infants with septicemia have meningitis. Direct microscopic examination helps to identify the organisms.
Cervical smears (Papanicola) from mother	A Pap smear is usually done if infection is suspected.
Samples from the mother's blood, urine, and lochia may also be done.	Provides clues of pathogens acquired from mother via placenta or passage through the birth canal. Knowledge of the etiologic agent helps in initiating effective therapy.
Complete Blood Count (CBC) White blood cells, differential for polymorphonuclear leukocytes, hematocrit, hemoglobin, platelet count.	Provides valuable data indicating conditions which need therapy because they can complicate the infectious process placing the infant in further jeopardy. For example, anemia, clotting deficiencies, abnormal erythrocytes, etc.
Blood Chemistry pH, sugar, electrolytes such as calcium and potassium, bilirubin levels, coagulation factors.	Reveals valuable data indicating conditions which can be side effects of the infectious process or complicate it further. For example, hyperbilirubemia is associated with congenital viral infections and acidosis; hypoglycemia can augment the infectious process creating jeopardy to the infant's life.

TABLE 38-6. *Continued*

Laboratory Investigation	*Rationale*
Radiologic Studies X-ray of the chest, skull, and long bones of the extremities.	Reveals possible infiltration of the pathogen into the lungs as in pneumonia and into the long bones as with congenital syphilis and rubella. Cerebral calcifications may be seen with toxoplasmosis and cytomegalic inclusion disease (CID).
Serologic Studies VDRL, FTA, serum immunoglobulins, or specific antibodies.	Findings on VDRL and FTA can indicate syphilis. Findings on serum immunoglobulins, especially IgM levels on cord blood and serial blood samples, may indicate exposure to an intrauterine infection such as rubella. Such findings alone are not sufficient because they do not identify the etiologic agent but rather indicate exposure to infection. Presence of rising titers of specific antibodies may identify the exact organism or agent.

the laboratory procedures done and their rationales are found in Table 38-6. The nurse's role focuses on assurance that samples for laboratory analysis are free from contamination. For example, blood samples should be obtained only after the skin is cleansed prior to puncture, and a new, clean needle should be attached to the syringe before the blood is inserted into the culture container. Urine samples for culture must be obtained via cathetization or suprapubic aspiration. If a spinal tap procedure is to be performed, the nurse must ensure sterility of the equipment and field of work, in order to guarantee a reliable sample.

Isolation of the Infant

Infants suspected of having an infection should be physically separated from healthy infants to prevent transmission of the pathogens. Infants who have positive laboratory cultures should be isolated into an isolette or moved into another room. There are certain principles the nurse must value to ensure effective isolation techniques:

1. Isolation does not merely mean separation in distance, but should also incorporate separation of anything coming in contact or produced by the infant. For example, catheters, feedings, linens, clothing, as well as excretions such as stools and vomitus should be discarded into the infant's individual receptacle and disposed of properly.
2. Remember, although an isolette is an individual isolation unit, portholes left open can allow transmission of pathogens. When giving care to the infant in an isolette, hands should be washed up to the elbows and sleeves on a gown rolled up to the elbow to avoid contamination of the gown.
3. Use a gown when caring for infants with positive laboratory cultures. The rationale for the use of a gown is to prevent transmission of pathogens which can be acquired on the staff's clothing during close contact with the infant. Ideally, the nurse should use the gown during delivery of nursing care and dispose of it when the care is completed. If the gown must be reused (due to shortage of linens or other reasons), the nurse must carefully remove the gown to prevent contamination of the inside of the gown by contact with the gown's outside surfaces. Hands should be washed prior to untying the gown at the neck to keep this area clean. The gown should then be folded lengthwise with uncontaminated

surfaces to the inside. It should be hung by placing the shoulder seams over the hook.

4. Handwashing is especially important when caring for a baby in isolation. It should never be sacrificed, especially prior to or after giving care, or having come in contact with bodily excretions or drainage.

Antibiotic Therapy

At present, antibiotics are the primary therapy for infectious disease. With the use of antibiotics, consideration must be given to the uniqueness of the newborn in absorption, breakdown, distribution, and excretion of the drug as contrasted with adults (absorption, detoxification, and excretion may be delayed in the newborn). Antibiotics and other drugs commonly used in the newborn period are listed, with dosages and indications, in Table 38-7. The role of the nurse during such therapy is to:

1. Ensure adequate parenteral infusion in terms of flow rate, and correct drug and dosage. The intravenous therapy should be periodically checked for signs of infiltration at the site of the needle (Fig. 38-24).
2. Observe the infant for reactions to the drug.
3. Maintain proper recording of the antibiotic therapy in the patient's chart.

TABLE 38-7. Antibiotic Therapy Commonly Used in the Newborn

Penicillin	50,000 units/kg./24 hr. ÷ 2 doses
Kanamycin	15 mg./kg./24 h. ÷ 2 (IM)
Ampicillin	100 mg./kg./24 hr. ÷ 2
Gentamicin	5 mg./kg./24 hr. ÷ 2 (IM or IV)
Methacillin	100–150 mg./kg./24 hr. ÷ 3 then ÷ 4
Carbencillin	400 mg./kg./24 hr. ÷ 3 then ÷ 4

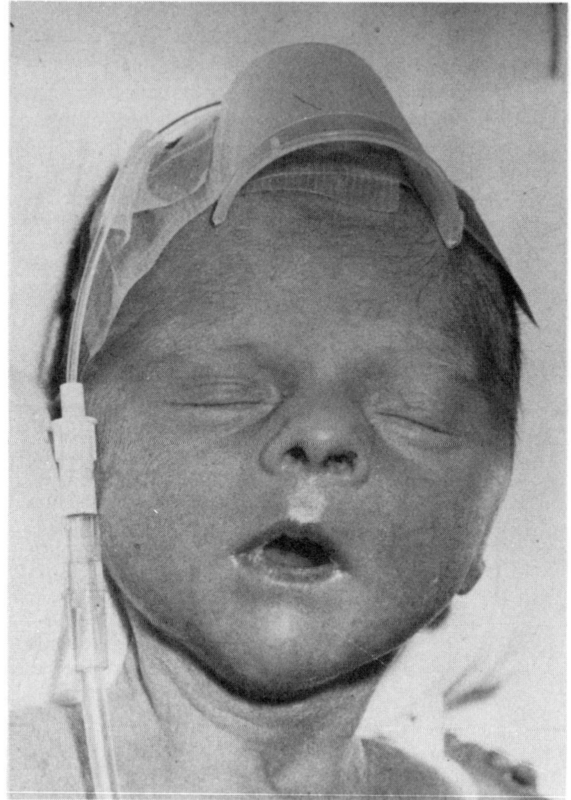

FIGURE 38-24. Infant receiving antibiotics intravenously. Note how the nurses have protected the IV site with the use of a medicine cup.

4. Monitor the infant's input and output during the intravenous therapy.

In addition to the above, the nurse must have knowledge about the following to protect the neonate from therapy that is not recommended:

1. Antibiotics should not be given prophylactically (meaning as a routine measure to prevent possible infection in the future). Therapy should be in response to the presence of a definite infection or suspect infants with histories as

described previously. One danger from "prophylactic antibiotics" lies in the neonate's different capacities to absorb, detoxify, and excrete drugs, exposing a number of infants unnecessarily to the possibility of drug toxicity. Another danger is that strains of bacteria resistant to the usual antibiotics will be selected out with the indiscriminate use of prophylactic antibiotics.

2. Certain antimicrobial or bacteriostatic drugs are not recommended for use in the newborn. Examples are erythromycin, streptomycin, tetracycline, sulfonamides, and bacitracin. Although such drugs are widely used in adults, the neonate's different absorption, detoxification, and excretion abilities can create toxicity to the liver and kidney. Also, the effectiveness of these drugs appears to have declined by a buildup of resistance to their action by pathogens most likely affecting the newborn. This is illustrated by streptomycin, which has declined in its effectiveness in the last decade, to be replaced by kanamycin (Kantrex). The latter drug, in turn, is now frequently replaced with gentamycin (Garamycin) because of the development of resistant organisms. The nurse must keep abreast of the latest information regarding drug resistance and new, promising drug replacements. With such knowledge, the nurse can be in a position to professionally assess the physician's order regarding the choice of drug for antibiotic therapy.
3. Antibiotic therapy in the newborn is usually given parenterally. This allows more rapid and effective assimilation of the drug.

Besides antibiotic therapy, blood transfusions are sometimes given to the infant with severe infection. The rationale for such therapy is that whole blood provides factors which enhance phagocytosis by the leukocytes as well as provides some specific antibodies. Depending upon the severity of the infection, anemia and/or shock can occur, and whole blood may be needed to correct such complications.

Supportive Therapy

In addition to eradicating the pathogenic agent, the septic infant must be supported in his needs for warmth, maintenance of ventilation, fluids and electrolytes, and be monitored for vital signs. Nursing actions relative to these needs were discussed earlier in this chapter.

Environmental Monitoring

This involves controlling the spread of infection in the nursery by ensuring techniques that prevent transmission of pathogens by people and things. In this regard, the nurse is probably the most significant person in the nursery. The nurse is in more close, continuous, and repeated contact with the infant than any other member of the health team. Thus, the nurse can be either the infant's protector or may unwittingly jeopardize his life by being a transmitter of pathogens. To assume the role of protector, the nurse must have knowledge of and value the following:

1. Proper handwashing technique is a cardinal rule for nursing care in the nursery. Under no circumstances should it be ignored—an inexcusable act reflecting lack of professionalism in the nurse. The significance of this simple act is expressed by Korones:

   > Failure to wash hands properly between handling of different infants is undoubtedly the principal mode of infection by any organism. Nothing is more fundamental to proper nursery hygiene than handwashing.[6]

Hands should be washed up to the elbows (sleeves rolled above elbows) when caring for an infant in an isolette.

2. Regarding dress attire, the use of caps, masks, and hairnets is no longer necessary and some institutions allow the use of a scrub gown over the regular uniform. The American Academy of Pediatrics recommends the use of a short-sleeved scrub gown. Whatever the nursery policy, the nurse should remember that the attire should allow proper handwashing up to the elbows. If the sleeves of a gown become wet, the gown is considered contaminated and should be changed.
3. Touching any part of one's face or head is considered contaminating the hands. Therefore, any personnel touching their hair, eyes, nose, ear, mouth, etc., should wash their hands before renewed contact with an infant.
4. When coming into intimate contact with an infected infant, such as during restraining an infant for a procedure or holding the infant close to one's body, the nurse should use a gown. This is important to protect other infants from possible contact with pathogens carried on the nurse's attire. Discard the gown after such contacts.
5. Regarding admission to the nursery, the nurse should have knowledge as to which people can enter or be excluded. The nurse should assess for factors described below:
   a. *Infants*: Infants should not be allowed in a regular nursery if they have diarrhea, herpes simplex, draining lesions, or were born to a mother with a communicable disease. Infants born of pregnancies complicated by prolonged ruptured membranes, or mothers with temperatures above 38° C should be bathed or isolated immediately before being allowed in the open nursery. Infants suspected of bacterial meningitis, septicemia, pneumonia, or other infections should be isolated by incubator or separate room from well infants.
   b. *Parents and Personnel*: Exclude anyone who has a febrile condition (fever), any draining lesions, or acute respiratory or gastrointestinal tract infections (diarrhea, productive coughs). Remember however, that parents of infected infants should not be separated from their infants only because of the disease. Undesirable effects from separation have been demonstrated in the developing parent-child relationship. The nurse's role is to teach parents the proper technique for handwashing and gowning while in contact with their infants. Teaching is always enhanced with a demonstration by the nurse. To keep total exposure of the infants to a minimum and reduce traffic through the nursery, it is recommended that the same auxiliary hospital personnel (e.g., x-ray technicians, phlebotomists) be regularly assigned to the nursery for doing diagnostic procedures.
6. Regarding infant care, such as bathing and cord care, it is recommended that the antiseptic soaps or solutions used be effective against gram-negative, as well as gram-positive organisms. Currently, there is controversy about the use of hexachlorophene in bathing infants. Cases of cerebral damage in extremely small prematures repeatedly exposed to hexachlorophene have been reported. There is also evidence that reduction of staphyloccocal colonization with the use of hexachlorophene has created an increase in gram-negative colonization of newborns in nurseries. Thus, an antiseptic solution effective against gram-negative organisms such as iodophor

(Betadine) should also be available for handwashing by the nursery personnel. Regarding protection of the infant from pathogens that can be acquired from equipment and fixtures, the following should be considered:

a. Cultures at regular intervals should be obtained from equipment or fixtures exposed to moisture because certain gram-negative organisms thrive in dark, damp areas and may cause clinically significant infection in a premature or debilitated infant. Such "water bug" infections may be caused by the following organisms: Pseudomonas, Aerobacteria, Achromobacter, Flavobacterium, Serratia, and Erwinia. Examples of areas to be cultured are the water traps of incubator humidifiers, soap containers, plumbing fixtures, and respiratory therapy equipment.
b. Equipment exposed to moisture should be changed every 8 to 24 hours to safeguard against bacterial growth. Examples are tubing for humidified gases, respirator circuits, and face masks.
c. Ensure proper cleansing and disposal of equipment. Examples:

TABLE 38-8. Principles of Management during a Major Nursery Epidemic*

1. Identify source.
2. Determine extent of outbreak (culture of contacts and nursery personnel).
3. Re-evaluate techniques (handwashing, antiseptic bathing and cord care, cleaning and sterilizing of equipment).
4. Notify local hospital infection committee and proper health authorities.
5. Follow up infants previously discharged from nursery (including cultures).
6. Continue surveillance after epidemic (culture infants, personnel, equipment, etc. May do cultures on admission and discharge).

COMMON EXAMPLES:

	E. coli	*Streptococcus*	*Staphylococcus*
Nursery	Close to new admissions. Reduce census. Culture fomites and equipment.	Do not close nursery. Culture all new admissions.	Close nursery if serious epidemic. May colonize all infants with low virulence Staphylococcus. Re-evaluate techniques.
Affected infants	Antibiotics and fluids.	Penicillin × 10 days	Methicillin/cloxacillin
Infant contacts	Culture stools. Antibiotics (neomycin** 50 mg./kg./day; colistin** 10 mg./kg./day	Culture cords. Oral penicillin (150,000 units/kg. in 3 divided doses) while in nursery + 48 hours after discharge. If positive culture, treat for 10 days.	Culture cords and noses. If severe epidemic, colonize infants with low virulence Staphylococcus.
Personnel	Stool culture.	Nose and throat culture. If positive culture, move from nursery.	Culture nose. Remove personnel with Staphylococcus aureus lesions but not nasal carriers.

The six principles outlined above apply in all cases.

* From Klaus and Fanaroff,[1] with permission.
** Give orally in four equally divided doses every six hours throughout nursery stay and for 48 hours after discharge.

1. Cribs and isolettes should be cleansed weekly or between infants.
2. Reusable equipment should be cleansed via autoclave or gas sterilizer; otherwise, such equipment should not be reused.
3. Ensure asepsis for any equipment or solution which will be inserted or administered internally.

d. Beware of multi-use containers of disinfectant. They are a potential source for bacterial growth, especially if cotton balls are stored in the solution. For example, stored solutions of Zephiran with cotton balls have been found repeatedly to contain Pseudomonas; benzalkonium chloride compounds (Zephiran) are in fact used by bacteriologists to enhance the growth of Pseudomonas in laboratory studies.

e. When caring for an infant suspected of infection, isolation precautions should also be extended to the cleansing and disposal of equipment that comes in contact with the infant. Dispose of supplies, linens, and waste into proper receptacles.

Finally, every nurse should be aware of the measures to be taken should an epidemic occur in the nursery. Table 38-8 summarizes necessary procedures during an epidemic.

CONGENITAL ABNORMALITIES

It is beyond the scope of this text to present a detailed discussion of all the various deviations that can occur in fetal growth due to developmental pathology (genetic or adverse intrauterine conditions). Chapter 18 discussed congenital malformations in fetal development and it may be helpful to the reader to review that content. The major congenital deviations that can manifest in a neonate are listed in Table 38-9. This section discusses the nursing role in caring for neonates with congenital anomalies, focusing on two principal areas. First, nursing care to neonates with anomalies of the gastrointestinal tract will be presented. The rationale for selection of this body system is that these defects usually present with symptoms identified initially by the nurse. Second, the nursing care to the neonate requiring surgery will be explored, primarily because surgical intervention is a primary mode of treatment for most congenital anomalies.

TABLE 38-9. Major Congenital and Chromosomal Anomalies Identifiable in the Neonate

Body System/Tissue	*Defect*	*Description*	*Clinical Signs/Manifestations*
Congenital Malformations			
Central Nervous System	Hydrocephalus	Accumulation of cerebrospinal fluid in the intracranial cavity due to obstruction in the flow and reabsorption of the fluid.	Enlarged head size which rapidly increases, appears prominent with accentuated veins. Anterior fontanel wider, feels tense, may be bulging. Sutures widely separated. High-pitched, shrill cry. Irritability, restlessness. Vomiting, convulsions. Setting sun sign of eyes.
	Spina bifida occulta	Incomplete closure of the spinal canal due to failure of fusion of spines and laminae. Commonly occurs in the lumbar sacral region.	Neurologic signs may or may not be present, depending upon the defect and its location. Spina bifida occulta usually is asymptomatic.

TABLE 38-9. *Continued*

Body System/Tissue	*Defect*	*Description*	*Clinical Signs/Manifestations*
	a. Meningocele	Protrusion of the spinal cord membranes (meninges) and cerebrospinal fluid through the spina bifida giving a saclike bulging appearance (cystic tumor).	Meningoceles may be asymptomatic unless they rupture or become ulcerated by irritation to the overlying skin.
	b. Myelomeningocele	Protrusion of nerves (spinal cord) in the cystic tumor, in addition to the meninges and spinal fluid.	Depends upon the nerve roots involved. Increased pressure in the cerebrospinal fluid can cause neurologic signs. Neuromuscular involvement may be reflected in paralysis, flaccidity, or spasticity in the lower extremities. Lack of bowel and bladder control may be evidenced by loose stools and frequent (dribbling) voidings. If the tumor ruptures or perforates, it easily leads to infection or meningitis.
Skeletal Muscle (there are two major defects unique to the neonate)	Talipes equinovarus (clubfoot)	Extension and inversion of the foot caused by unequal pull of the muscles due to intrauterine position or imbalance in muscular development.	Foot is inverted, heels drawn upward making it difficult to walk on the soles of the foot. If the foot can be passively moved in a corrective direction beyond the middle position, the defect is "positional" and needs no correction. If not, casting is usually required.
	Dislocation of hip	The head of the femur is displaced from the acetabellum resulting in instability of the ball socket joint.	Resistance to abduction and outward rotation of the thighs is met on the affected side or sides. If one persists in application of pressure in these directions, the head of the femur wili suddenly relocate itself into the acetabulum, making a palpable and sometimes audible click (Ortolani's click). Asymmetry in the gluteal and inguinal fold may also be seen on the affected side.
Genitourinary System	Exstrophy of the bladder	Failure of the abdominal wall to fuse with the anterior wall of the bladder creating a fissure which exposes the bladder mucosa and ureter openings. The defect involves the abdominal wall, anterior wall of the bladder, symphysis pubis, and urethra. It is usually associated with other congenital anomalies.	The bladder mucosa is exposed showing numerous red folds; area sensitive to the touch; located below the umbilical area. More common in males.

TABLE 38-9. *Continued*

Body System/Tissue	*Defect*	*Description*	*Clinical Signs/Manifestations*
	Hypospadias	Failure of the urethra to extend the length of the penis, with the meatal opening on the underside (ventral surface) of the glans penis.	Detected by observing site or urination.
Gastrointestinal Tract	Cleft lip and palate	Failure of the maxillary and palatal processes to fuse between the 5th–8th weeks of embryonic development. Results in fissure in the midline of the roof of the mouth (cleft palate) and/or fissure of the upper lip (cleft lip).	Cleft lip is common in males while cleft palate (with or without cleft lip) is more common in females. The lip involvement is obvious while the palate involvement may not be suspected until difficulties with feeding occur or the inside of the mouth is inspected.
	Esophageal atresia with or without tracheoesophageal fistula	Most common type involves the upper esophagus ending in a blind pouch while the lower portion connects to the trachea by a fistula.	There are 3 classic symptoms: 1. Excess accumulation of mucus in the mouth or bubbling of saliva from the mouth (excess drooling) 2. Continuous or episodic respiratory distress 3. Aspiration if feeding attempted.
	Intestinal stenosis or atresia	Obstruction to any portion of the small or large intestines.	Vomiting, abdominal distension and frequent stools that are pasty and pale if the obstruction is below the entrance of the bile duct in the duodenum.
	Imperforate anus	Lack of an anal opening. A membrane may exist where the anus should be.	Inspection or inability to pass a rectal thermometer or catheter.
	Omphalocele	Herniation of the abdominal contents through the umbilical cord. May or may not be covered by a thin membrane.	The larger herniated protrusions are clearly visible. More discrete herniation a short distance into the cord may be overlooked and carries the danger of damage to a loop of bowel when the cord is clamped.
Respiratory System	Descriptions and illustrations of the major obstructive and restrictive congenital defects of the airways and lungs may be found in Chapter 37.		
Circulatory System Defects known as Congenital Heart Disease	Descriptions and illustrations of the major congenital heart defects may be found in Chapter 37.		

TABLE 38-9. *Continued*

Body System/Tissue	*Defect*	*Description*	*Clinical Signs/Manifestations*
Chromosomal Deviations	*Autosomal Defects*		
Chromosomal defects may occur during the meiotic or mitotic phases of cellular division. Half of the defects involve the autosomes (first 22 pairs of chromosomes) and the other half involve the sex chromosomes (remaining pair of chromosomes)	Trisomy or translocation for #21. Known as Down's syndrome or mongolism	In this form of trisomy there are 3 chromosomes instead of 2 in pair #21, making a total of 47 instead of 46. It occurs because of the chromosome pair #21 fails to separate, called nondisjunction. This is more frequent in children born to mothers over 35 years of age. The extra #21 chromosome can be translocated to another chromosome. This would result in a normal total of 46 but clinical signs would manifest because of the presence of the extra chromosomal material.	Classical physical features are: Round, flat face Close set eyes Epicanthal folds Eyes slanting upward at the sides Speckling spots on the iris Small head with flat occiput Short, broad, pudgy neck Short, flat nose Small ears with folded upper helix Large, protruding tongue Broad hands; short, stubby fingers; transverse palmar creases Poor muscle tone; able to assume unusual postures Large toe abnormally separated from the others Increased incidence of cardiac malformation Signs of mental deficiency
	Trisomy 13	Nondisjunction in Group D chromosomes (#13–15)	Condition is rare with severe defects to the brain, nose, eyes (arhinencephaly, microphthalmia, anophthalmia. Defects in the face: cleft palate and/or lip Polydactyly Associated with congenital heart defects and severe mental retardation
	Trisomy 18	Nondisjunction in Group E chromosomes (#16–18). More prevalent in offspring of mother above 30 years old	Prognosis is poor for survival beyond a year Severe retardation and congenital heart defects Low birth weight for gestational age Low-set abnormal ears Flexion contractures of fingers Rocker-bottom feet Micrognathia Increase in genitourinary anomalies Spasticity in muscle tone Umbilical, inguinal, and diaphragmatic hernias are common Frequently noted to have one umbilical artery

TABLE 38-9. *Continued*

Body System/Tissue	*Defect*	*Description*	*Clinical Signs/Manifestations*
	Sex chromosome Defects		
	Turner's syndrome	A female who has lost an X chromosome resulting in a 45,XO karyotype	Usually infertile Few secondary sex characteristics Hypoplastic nipples Broad chest Underdeveloped ovaries Short in stature; webbed neck Normal in intelligence Manifest perceptual disturbances
	Klinefelter's syndrome	A male with an extra X chromosome resulting in a 47, XXY karyotype	Usually sterile Testicles atrophy

Gastrointestinal Tract Anomalies*

Abnormalities of the gastrointestinal tract occur less frequently than those of the central nervous system or cardiovascular systems. Gastrointestinal anomalies occur in about two out of every thousand births (Fig. 38-25).

There are many historical and clinical symptoms which aid in the early diagnosis of a gastrointestinal anomaly. A good history of the pregnancy is necessary to identify such problems as polyhydramnios. In polyhydramnios, there is an increase in the volume of amniotic fluid in excess of 2,000 cc. This condition often is the first evidence of a high alimentary tract obstruction and is rarely seen with obstructive lesions of the lower small or large intestine. Since amniotic fluid is normally swallowed by the fetus in utero and absorbed in the intestinal tract, amniotic fluid accumulation in the mother may denote inability of the fetus to swallow and absorb the fluid, hence a high obstruction. A maternal history of repeated miscarriages or the presence of anomalies in siblings may also aid in an early diagnosis.

* This content was prepared by Kathy Puls, R.N.; C.N.M., based on a paper presented in Tucson, Arizona, 1973.

Gastrointestinal anomalies in the newborn may be indicated by:

- regurgitation or vomiting
- excessive oral mucus
- abdominal distention
- paroxysmal bouts of crying
- poor feeding
- dehydration
- diarrhea
- constipation
- absence of stools
- respiratory distress

In most neonates with an obstruction, regurgitation or vomiting is present, sometimes on the first day of life. The characteristics of the emesis should be noted and charted: time of onset, quantity of the emesis, projectile or slow flow, presence of bile, flecked with blood, presence of fecal matter. Is the vomiting instigated by the introduction of food or medication, and what was the infant's physical condition following vomiting (color, respirations)?

An excessive mucous accumulation in the infant's mouth, so that he produces froth and bubbles around his mouth and nose, usually is

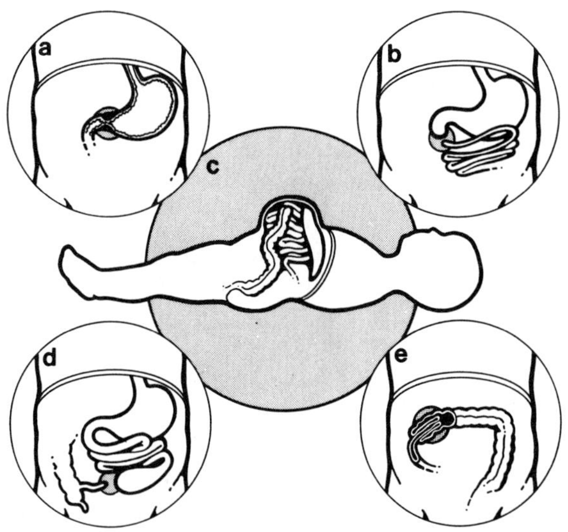

FIGURE 38-25. Gastrointestinal tract anomalies. *a,* Pyloric stenosis. *b,* Duodenal atresia. *c,* Omphalocele. *d,* Ileal atresia. *e,* Intussusception (rarely seen before 6 months of age).

an early symptom of esophageal obstruction, frequently an atresia, which may be associated with a fistula. Abdominal distention to some degree is usually associated with gastrointestinal anomalies. If the obstruction is high, the distention may be less marked and limited to the upper abdomen. Lower obstruction will produce distention that is more diffuse. Visible peristaltic waves may be detected and can be produced for diagnostic purposes by feeding small amounts of formula or water.

Absent or scanty stools even with digital examination are common with distention. Approximately 94 per cent of newborns pass about a cupful of dark meconium in the first 24 hours of life. Occasionally infants with incomplete or high obstruction may pass small amounts of light-colored, greyish, or gray-green meconium, which should not be confused with a normal meconium stool. In some cases of partial obstruction, chronic constipation with periods of diarrhea may be evident. Pain is evident by paroxysmal bouts of crying, facial grimaces, clinched fists, and kicking feet, all symptoms common in the neonate with an obstruction. Symptoms of respiratory distress such as grunting, episodes of cyanosis, apnea, and retractions due to pressure on the diaphragm from a distended abdomen may also be evident. Some later effects of partial obstruction are loss of weight or failure to gain weight, and fever due to dehydration.

Nursing Care

The nursing management of a baby who is vomiting large amounts of bile-stained material, has generalized abdominal distention, has grunting respirations, has had no stools since birth and is very irritable, would be to achieve the following objectives: make the baby as comfortable as possible and protect it from further complications. To achieve these objectives, stop feeding the infant and suction the baby's mouth and nasal pharynx. To prevent him from aspirating stomach contents, pass a tube into the stomach and leave connected to gravity drainage. The neonate's urine should be frequently checked for the presence of sugar, protein, and blood. The pH, the specific gravity, should be checked to monitor kidney function for onset of dehydration or hemorrhaging. The stools, as well as the gastric aspirate, should also be checked for the presence of blood. The infant needs good oral care with lemon and glycerine swabs or saline swabs at least every two hours to prevent breakdown of tongue, gums, and lips. The infant's position should be changed and bony prominences padded with sheepskin. A water bed, made from a large irrigating solution bag partially emptied will prevent pressure areas and flattening of the head if the infant must lie in one position (e.g., if he is on a respirator). Special attention must be paid to the skin in the perineal area, since it will break down easily if the infant has diarrhea. Keep the area clean and dry, exposing it to air or a warm lamp to help heal the area.

Frequently these infants are extremely irritable. Handling gently, and cuddling the baby when possible, frequently talking to the baby, and using a pacifier will help to keep the infant calm and quiet. As the infant becomes older, he will respond to sounds, lights, and brightly colored objects, as well as mobiles and radios.

The infant and parents need to spend time together, as they begin to build a parent-child relationship. The infant's parents should be given the opportunity to touch and hold the baby as much as possible. Many parents feel guilty that they did not bring a perfect child into the world. The nurse should allow them opportunities for ventilating these feelings. She may find it helpful to emphasize the potential for normalcy within the infant. The nurse may demonstrate caring, handling, and talking to the baby, thereby giving the parents opportunity to see the infant suck, follow voices and sounds with his eyes, grasp, and as he gets older, smile or perhaps begin to vocalize. Parents vary in their rate of acceptance of the infant; therefore, the nurse should not hurry them into this relationship with their child but she should be aware of clues concerning how they are doing and use every opportunity to support them in this relationship. Calling the infant by name is helpful in establishing the infant as an individual to whom the parents can relate.

Prior to surgery, the infant will probably have a venous cutdown or a hyperalimentation line inserted. These two types of catheters need to be constantly monitored for evidence of infiltration and infection. The line needs to be frequently checked for patency and precipitate, and should include a micropore filter to prevent precipitate and bacteria from entering the infant's blood stream. The insertion site should be inspected daily for signs of infection and dislodgment. The neonate's general wellbeing should be monitored closely for any signs of systemic infection.

Since surgery is the usual treatment for gastrointestinal obstruction or anomalies, the infant will need the same gentle meticulous care following his corrective procedure.

Surgery*

Most congenital abnormalities result in surgical corrections. Therefore, it is important to examine how the nurse cares for a baby before and after surgery.

Preoperative Care

The objective of preoperative care is to prepare the neonate for the best possible health status for optimal coping with the stressors of surgery. What are some general actions for implementation of quality preoperative care?

1. Assure that the neonate's temperature is normal and support him through use of a thermal neutral environmental device (isolette or warmer). Stressors can easily create thermoregulation problems. Transfer the neonate to surgery via a heating-type conveyance.
2. Assure adequate status in terms of hydration, electrolyte, and caloric needs. Parenteral therapy is usually instituted to: 1) assure adequate energy supply to tolerate the surgery, 2) provide a route for medications, 3) ensure hydration because the infant will be restricted in oral intake (NPO) at least 4 to 6 hours prior to elective surgery, and 4) to correct any fluid and electrolyte imbalance.
3. Monitor vital signs (temperature, pulse, respirations).
4. Suctioning should be readily available to ensure patent airway.

*An excellent source for details in this area is *Baby Surgery,* by D. Young and B. Weller. University Park Press, Baltimore, 1971.

5. Oxygen and resuscitation equipment should always be available.
6. Special attention in the form of hygiene to the proposed operative site. The area should be clean, protected from drying, irritation, and infection. The site may need to be shaved or washed with an antibacterial agent. The umbilical area should also be clean, dry, and crust-free.
7. Attention to skin care by adequate changes in position, massage to bony prominences, freedom from moisture (such as drainage, urine, feces).
8. The infant should be accompanied to surgery by relevant data: roentgenograms, proper identification, chart containing age, weight, diagnosis, laboratory reports, progress notes, doctor's orders and consultants' reports.

Other specific preoperative nursing actions are found in Table 38-10.

*Postoperative Care**

Surgery is now performed successfully on many more neonates mainly because of the following:

1. Infants are transferred earlier to neonatal intensive care centers and better stabilized before surgery.
2. There is better, less stressful anesthesia and in-surgery care of the infant.
3. Most importantly, there is improved postoperative care being extended to these infants in the neonatal intensive care nursery.

A large portion of this improved postoperative care being extended to the neonate is attributable to three major factors:

1. Better understanding of the pathophysiology of the postoperative period.
2. Improved monitoring capabilities to detect deviations early.
3. Setting the primary goal of postoperative care as maintenance of homeostasis and support of physiologic functions.

Monitoring of the neonate during the postoperative period is defined broadly as following the course of vital signs and key parameters to early detect deviations from the norm or trends toward abnormality. The goal is to detect problems before they become overwhelming and at a time when simple countermeasures can be instituted to reverse the trend (Fig. 38-26).

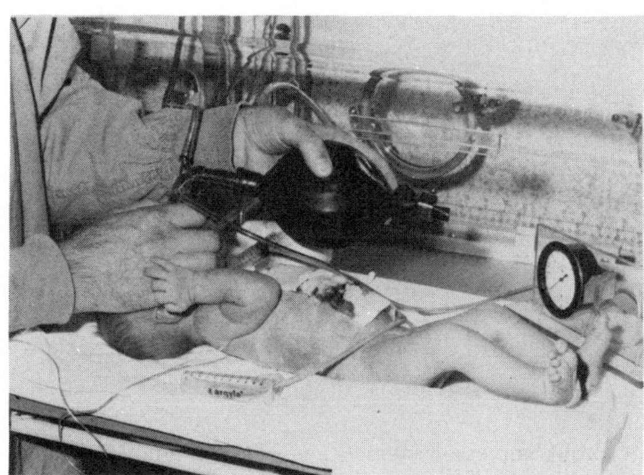

FIGURE 38-26. Intermittant bagging and application of CPAP to overcome postoperative atalectasis of the lung in a baby who underwent surgical repair of an omphalocele.

What are some of the major problems encountered in the postoperative period in the neonate? The following is a brief discussion of the major problems to anticipate as well as measures for monitoring and managing such problems.

Prolongation of Unconsciousness or Persistance of Coma. This may be caused by 1) anesthetic overdose, 2) extreme CO_2 retention with CO_2 narcosis, and 3) electrolyte or

*Adapted from a speech given by Thomas Harris, M.D. Pediatric grand rounds, Denver Children's Hospital, 1972.

TABLE 38-10. Special Nursing Actions beyond General Preoperative and Postoperative Care in Neonatal Surgery of Selected Body Systems

Body System/Condition	*Preoperative Care*	*Postoperative Care*
Gastrointestinal Tract Examples: Esophageal atresia Tracheoesophageal fistula Pyloric stenosis Duodenal atresia Intestinal obstruction	Insert nasogastric tube and aspirate to prevent secretions from entering the trachea and lungs. Leave NG tube open to allow drainage of gastric contents into container kept level with the infant. Lavage or emptying of the gastric contents via the NG tube may be ordered. Fluid and electrolyte replacement needed, especially if vomiting occurs. Position infant to prevent aspiration of vomitus or secretions.	NG tube remains for aspiration of secretions and gastric contents. Suctioning may be necessary as often as every 30 minutes in the first 24 hours. In the first 24 hours fluids may be limited because the normal response to surgery is fluid retention. Fluid therapy needs to incorporate assessment of electrolytes and volume lost through gastric aspirate, diarrhea, vomiting, etc. Daily weights, intake and output critical. Initial feeding directly into the stomach via gavage, usually beginning with dextrose water, then formula. Other feeding method may be by gastrostomy (opening into the stomach via the abdominal wall). The nurse should have knowledge of the special care of an artificial opening into the gastrointestinal tract (esophagostomy, gastrostomy, ileastomy, colostomy). Certain aspects to value in such nursing care are: a. Apply nonadherent dressings around it and secure with tape. b. Check position of catheter; protect it from slipping back internally. c. Use cream to protect area from excoriation and bacteria. d. Check area for any bleeding, report immediately. e. Catheter should be changed monthly.
Central Nervous System	Do the following for any infant having surgery for CNS involvement: a. Regular measurement of the occipitofrontal head circumference. b. Note fontanels (bulging, depressed?) c. Note position of extremities and abnormalities in movements. d. Note state of consciousness in infant (drowsy, irritable). e. Note vomiting and protect from aspiration. f. Protect from convulsions.	Continue head circumference measurements and assessment for neurologic functioning.
Myelocele/Meningomylocele	Note muscle activity of lower extremities, bowel/bladder control to determine neuromuscular involvement Get x-ray of spinal column Cover lesions with sterile saline gauze to prevent drying Gentle handling and positional changes to prevent irritation to lesions	If neuromuscular involvement, may need to perform passive range of motion to extremities

TABLE 38-10. *Continued*

Body System/Condition	*Preoperative Care*	*Postoperative Care*
Hydrocephalus	Ventriculograms or EMI scan done to determine level of obstruction and size of ventricles. Shave head. Be sure head and neck free of skin irritation or infection.	Ensure that drainage shunt is functioning properly. Continue head circumference measurements.
Respiratory System	Suctioning to aspirate pharyngeal secretions. Gastric contents aspirated as needed. Oral airway may be inserted. May need ventilation support, via mask-bag apparatus.	A tracheostomy may be performed. Important aspects for its care are: a. Ensure that tracheostomy tube will not be displaced; make sure tapes are secure to the neck. b. Position infant with head extended with a roll or pad under the head. c. Assessment for activity, respirations every 15 minutes. d. Normal saline (0.5 ml.) is introduced into the tracheal tube every half hour and then aspirated along with secretions. e. Maintain high humidity to prevent drying of the secretions leading to obstruction. f. Use oxygen as needed. g. Keep area clean, free from obstruction by clothing, linens. After thoracic surgery an intercostal drainage system is needed to allow fluid and air to escape from the pleural cavity and re-expansion of the lung. General factors to remember to ensure functioning of the drainage system are: a. Never lift bottle above level of patient or fluid and air may re-enter the pleural cavity. b. Be sure the system is an airtight seal; fluid in the underwater seal bottle should cover the drainage tube connected to the bottle. c. Clamp tubing if patient is to be moved or tubing changed, but unclamp immediately if patient becomes distressed. d. Record respiration and amount and type of chest drainage. After the drainage system is removed, postural drainage with percussion may be needed to encourage removal of bronchiole secretions. Frequent change in infant position also helps to re-expand the chest.

TABLE 38-10. *Continued*

Body System/Condition	*Preoperative Care*	*Postoperative Care*
Cardiovascular System Congenital Heart Diseases	These infants may be in respiratory distress, necessitating actions to ensure patent airway and ventilatory assistance as needed. Some infants require sedation to ensure rest and energy conservation. Position semi-upright to facilitate breathing.	Care of a tracheostomy or chest drainage may be indicated. Knowledge needed of medicinal therapy such as: a. Digitalis to strengthen cardiac output b. Diuretics to decrease fluid retention c. Antibiotics to prevent infection d. Alkali therapy should metabolic acidosis occur Intake and output, and conservation of energy are crucial
Cleft Lip and Palate (Discussed separately because of the unique preoperative needs relating to feeding.)	The major needs of these babies during the neonatal period are orthodontic treatment and maintenance of feeding. Orthodontic treatment may be necessary before surgery to align parts of the maxilla which form the alveolar arch; the bones are molded by gentle pressure from a prosthesis inserted into the mouth. The nurse should assure cleanliness of any orthodontic equipment. Feeding: the nursing goal is to prevent the infant from choking, possible aspiration and respiratory infections. One objective is to prevent hard sucking attempts because the baby cannot create suction. Use of a rubber-tipped syringe, a soft, large-hold nipple or a special cleft palate nipple helps to achieve this. Some babies are given feedings by spoon. Some factors to consider during the feeding are: a. Direct formula flow to the side of the mouth. b. Feed quantity and rate that the baby can tolerate without choking. c. Position semi-upright to facilitate swallowing and gravitational flow into stomach. d. Frequent bubbling as air may be swallowed during feeding. e. Keep suction equipment nearby in case of aspiration. f. Position on side after feeding to prevent aspiration should regurgitation occur. g. Cleanse mouth from food debris with water after feeding to prevent upper respiratory infection which can lead to otitis media. h. Feedings should be supplemented with vitamins and iron to prevent anemia.	Surgical repair for cleft lip usually is done at 2–3 months (6–8 weeks) and at 12–15 months for cleft palate. The rationale for this delay is the oral cavity is too small for adequate repair in the neonatal period. Postop nursing care: a. Oral and pharyngeal suction as needed. b. Protect suture area (on lip) by preventing drying with use of creams; restraining the infant to prevent contact on area; position on side, not abdomen, to avoid irritation to lip.

metabolic disturbances derived from surgery such as hyponatremia (low sodium), hypothermia or hypoxia (with acidosis or hypoglycemia). Thus, the newborn needs to have neuro-checks such as for pupillary response and response to pain. Also, blood gases should be closely monitored and intravenous sodium and glucose provided as needed.

Hypothermia and Hyperthermia. The sick neonate may be unable to mobilize his usual mechanisms for regulating body temperature, namely by peripheral vasoconstriction and metabolising fat and protein for heat. If hypoxia exists, the infant cannot increase his oxygen consumption which is needed for heat production. If the infant is dehydrated or hyperosmolalic, fever results which does not necessarily indicate infection. However, fever in the presence of normal osmolality is an indication of infection. The infant's rectal temperature is monitored and ideally a skin probe can be applied which is attached to a radiant-heat system (described earlier under Health Care Maintenance).

Airway Obstruction. Simple obstruction of nasal passages is a potentially lethal problem because the neonate is an obligatory nose-breather. Thus, it is undesirable to leave indwelling nasogastric tubes in the nose which obstruct half of the upper airway unless a nasal endotracheal tube is in place. The nurse must value the need for oral suctioning and prevention of aspiration. Tracheal swelling or subglottic edema can be a problem after short-term endotracheal intubation. Thus, such postoperative babies are usually placed in isolettes or oxygen hoods in which the air is humidified. Also, the tip of the endotracheal tube may be smeared in advance with cortisone to minimize any local reactions. Lower airway obstruction is more difficult to assess. Wheezing and prolonged retractions are important clinical signs. Wheezing is usually treated with a nebulized aerosol medication such as isoproteranol in a dilute strength.

Hypoventilation and Tendency toward Atelectasis. This usually follows such events as 1) excessive sedation, 2) hypothermia and apnea secondary to accompanying acidosis, 3) hyperthermia and increased incidence of periodic breathing or apnea, and 4) airway obstruction. The premature infant is especially vulnerable to atelectasis. Measures found to overcome atelectasis include:

1. Intermittent bag and mask ventilation or stimulating to cry.
2. Intermittent application of CPAP by mask.
3. Combination of intermittent bagging and CPAP.

Cardiovascular Insufficiency. A major concern in the postoperative period is cardiovascular insufficiency which can be reflected through peripheral vasoconstriction with poor tissue perfusion and resulting acidosis, systemic hypotension (low blood pressure), or actual heart failure and cardiac arrest. Currently, blood pressures can be monitored directly through an arterial catheter or indirectly by means of a photoelectric cell or utilizing the Doppler effect.

Water Retention with or without Salt Retention and Edema. The neonate handles an excessive water load very poorly. The reduced liver metabolism in the sick neonate with less than adequate protein intake and poor liver perfusion makes the infant vulnerable to hypoproteinemia and edema. There is also the problem of capillary damage and fluid leakage secondary to transient hypoxic damage. Thus, the following parameters should be monitored:

intake
urinary output
urine specific gravity
total serum solids (of which about 70 per cent is albumin)
hematocrit
electrolytes

occasionally serum osmolality and urinary electrolytes (dehydration can best be assessed by osmolality)

Electrolyte Imbalance. Hypokalemia, hyperkalemia, hypocalcemia, and hyperphosphatemia can occur for reasons discussed previously.

Hypoxia and Hyperoxia. The effects of too little or too much oxygen on brain, eyes, and lungs must be appreciated in postoperative care. Thus, the O_2 concentration the baby is breathing and the level in the blood must be monitored. This can be done intermittently or continuously, as mentioned previously.

Caloric or Dietary Imbalances. Provisions must be made to maintain adequate caloric intake. This may be done through some form of hyperalimentation therapy until oral feedings can ensure a balanced diet.

The above are examples of problems the nurse should anticipate when providing postoperative care to the neonate. In addition to supporting medical interventions to meet such problems, the nurse should value the following as an integral part of the care plan.

Provision for safety and comfort. Hygiene care helps to protect the baby from possible infection. The skin should be clean and dry. Oral hygiene at frequent intervals helps to stimulate salivation which is the best way to keep the mouth moist and clean. Use sterile equipment as needed.

Ensure anatomic position to prevent muscle tension, fatigue and interference with bodily functions such as respiration.

Change position at least every two hours to stimulate circulation, facilitate drainage of secretions and prevent decubiti.

Use gentle restraints to protect the infant from dislodging equipment by spontaneous movements.

Check to ensure patency of catheters and proper functioning of equipment. This implies a double monitoring process: the nurse monitors the equipment which is monitoring the infant's status.

Check all dressings for bleeding, drainage, or signs of infection.

Promote energy conservation by organizing care to allow the infant rest and sleep.

There may be unique needs regarding preoperative and postoperative neonatal care relative to surgery on selected bodily systems (see Table 38-10).

Inborn Errors of Metabolism

There are numerous inborn errors of metabolism, the discussion of which is beyond the scope of this book. The unique contribution of the nurse is to initially raise the question of a possible metabolic disturbance based on a number of astute observations. Table 38-11 lists a number of clinical clues which can alert the nurse to the possibility of an inborn metabolic error.

TABLE 38-11. Clinical Phenomena Suggestive of Inborn Errors of Metabolism*

In newborns:
Previously affected sibling or a positive family history
Unexplained seizures
Unusual physical appearance
Sexual ambiguity
Persisting jaundice
Edema
Vomiting and anorexia
Unexplained acidosis
In older infants and children:
Failure to thrive (failure to grow)
Mental retardation, seizures, spasticity, coma
Specific physical abnormalities—dislocated lens, renal tones, deafness, rickets, liver disease, cataracts, renal disease, thrombosis, hematuria, speech defects, osteoporosis

* From Barness, L. and Morrow, G.,[7] with permission.

Many inherited disorders are clinically asymptomatic during the newborn period but may be detected by metabolic screening procedures.[7] Early detection is imperative if brain damage is to be prevented and/or minimized in many of these disorders. However, many of these tests presently available for such early detection remain prohibitively expensive or impractical. The one test that has found almost universal acceptance today is that for the inborn error of protein metabolism called *phenylketonuria.* Phenylketonuria involves the buildup of phenylalanine in the blood due to genetically controlled lack of the enzyme system phenylalanine hydroxylase. Blood phenylalanine levels may not be elevated until after two or three days of milk feedings, so screening tests should be delayed until that time. Appropriate therapy involves a restricted dietary intake of phenylalanine. Therefore, the usual milk feedings must be substituted with a special formula (Lofenelac) which contains reduced amounts of phenylalanine. This formula is expensive, not very palatable, and requires that blood phenylalanine levels be monitored carefully by laboratory analysis. Recognition of this disorder is crucial in the newborn period because brain damage can occur as early as six months of life and dietary therapy is totally ineffective after two years of age.[8]

Special Modes for Nutritional Intake

Feeding (supplying nutrients) is best accomplished through the gastrointestinal tract, since generous quantities of all the different types of foodstuffs can be offered and the body can pick and choose what it needs while allowing that which it doesn't to pass through. For the newborn and especially the premature, special care must be taken regarding the particular formula and amount offered, since reabsorption is limited and the ability to discharge the waste is markedly reduced. Nevertheless, it still remains our goal to supply all of the baby's caloric and fluid needs by the natural oral route of feeding.

However, when dealing with high-risk neonates, it is often temporarily impossible to accomplish this goal. Oral feedings simply may not be tolerated, and persistent attempts may actually threaten the baby's life by leading to regurgitation and aspiration, or resulting in bowel perforation and peritonitis. In such situations we must seek alternative routes of providing nourishment until the baby's condition stabilizes and oral feedings may be reinstituted.

The three most commonly used alternative modes of feeding sick neonates are deep-vein parenteral hyperalimentation, peripheral hyperalimentation, and nasojejunal feeding. A brief description of the techniques, advantages, and disadvantages of these methods follows.

Deep-vein parenteral hyperalimentation involves infusing of a concentrated solution containing glucose, amino acids, electrolytes, and vitamins directly into the central circulation. A small catheter is placed under local or general anesthesia in the superior vena cava by way of the external or internal jugular vein in the neck or the axillary vein of the arm. The baby is taken to surgery for this procedure, and meticulous sterile technique is maintained. Other precautions to avoid infection, which is the primary complication of this form of therapy, include tunneling the catheter under the skin to come out some distance away from the incision over the vein, preparing all infusion solutions under a laminar flow hood, and inserting a Millipore filter in the line to remove particulate matter or micro-organisms. In spite of all precautions, however, bacterial and fungal septicemia is a frequent, life-threatening complication of deep-vein hyperalimentation. Other problems of this form of therapy include the risks of taking these sick infants to surgery, difficulty in placing the catheters in the appropriate location, perforation of vessels by the catheter, clots forming at the tip of the catheter, dehydration due to osmotic diuresis if the volume or concentration of the solution is increased too rapidly, withdrawal hypoglycemia if the infusion has to be suddenly discontinued, and hyperammonemia (high ammonia levels) and other serious metabolic disturbances if the solution infused overloads the baby's system and exceeds his ability to metabolize it. The great advantage of this form of parenteral nutrition is that relatively high caloric intake can be achieved by infusing rather small amounts of fluid.

Peripheral hyperalimentation, in contrast, involves infusing dilute solutions in large (even huge) amounts in order to provide comparable numbers of calories. Peripheral IV's are used instead of catheters, avoiding most of the infection and deep-vein complications of central hyperalimentation. However, there is the need to frequently restart the IV when it infiltrates, and the danger of local tissue damage (and even skin sloughing) if it does. As with central hyperalimentation, the same care must be taken to maintain metabolic equilibrium, with frequent laboratory checks assuring continued normal blood levels of electrolytes, urea nitrogen (BUN), pH, ammonia, and glucose. Likewise, urine must be frequently tested to rule out the possibility that glucose or protein is being lost in any significant quantity. Most important in peripheral hyperalimentation is the need to monitor body weight and intake and output; when fluid volumes as high as 200 to 250 cc. per kg. per 24 hours are being infused, the danger of fluid overload and/or heart failure is relatively great. This form of therapy obviously cannot be used in babies with poor kidney function or cardiovascular problems.

The most recently advocated mode of improving nutrition in the low-birth-weight infant unable to take adequate amounts of formula by mouth or gavage is that of *continuous nasojejunal infusions* through a thin tube passed through the nose and on down into the proximal jejunum. The #5 French feeding tube, long enough to extend from the base of the nose to the heel on an outstretched leg, is passed manually into the stomach in the usual fashion of gavage feedings, and then passed further by spontaneous peristaltic action to end in the jejunum. Thus, the stomach is bypassed, which avoids the problems of regurgitation and aspiration. On the other hand, life-threatening intestinal perforation by these tubes has been reported, as well as various stages of necrotizing enterocolitis and a radical change in the normal bacterial flora of the small intestine.

Nursing care in all three of these alternative modes of feeding involves avoidance of contamination of the catheter site or the infusion solution, as well as close observation and early detection of any of the above-mentioned complications.

BIRTH TRAUMA

The neonate is subjected to considerable pathologic risk in the process of being born. Trauma complicating labor and delivery can result in transitory and/or permanent injuries to muscles, nerves, bones, tissues, and the central nervous system. Although many birth injuries are not extremely hazardous to the infant's immediate survival, such injuries do create much anxiety for the parents. Therefore, the nursing role, in addition to assessment and supporting medical treatment, is to explain the phenomenon and its immediate and potential long-term effects on the infant to the parents. Such information-sharing will help parents to understand the true significance of the injury and alleviate unnecessary anxiety. The nurse must therefore have a clear understanding of the various types of birth injuries that can commonly occur in a neonate.

Trauma Involving Muscles and Peripheral Nerves

The facial nerve may become paralyzed temporarily when pressure is exerted upon it during delivery, especially by a forceps blade. The nurse can recognize such injury because the affected side of the face will be immobile,

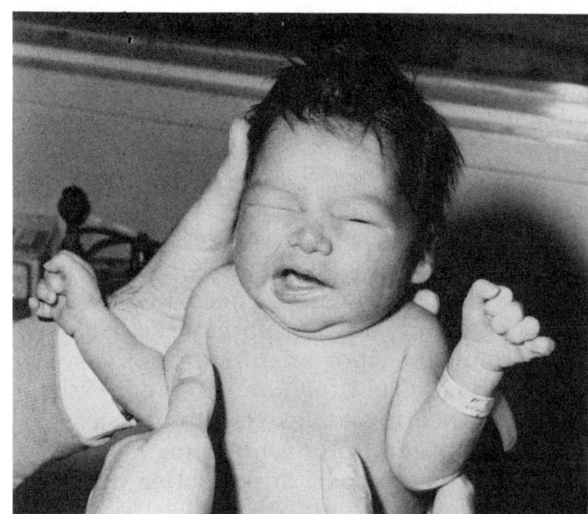

FIGURE 38-27. Facial nerve paralysis. Note the lopsided facial appearance. The mouth is drawn toward the unaffected side and the eye on the affected side is unable to close.

the baby's facial muscles will not move (in the forehead, cheeks, mouth area), especially when the baby cries. The face will appear lopsided because the mouth will be drawn toward the unaffected side, and the eye on the affected side may not be able to close (Fig. 38-27). Nursing care is directed to helping the infant with feeding because difficulty with sucking may occur. The use of a soft, small nipple or gavage feedings may be indicated. The nurse also protects the eye from contact with external objects and keeps the cornea moist with artificial tears (eye drops). The injury is usually transient, requiring no neurosurgical treatment.

Trauma can also occur to nerves in the brachial plexus creating partial or complete paralysis of certain muscles in the arm as well as the diaphragm. This problem was discussed in detail in Chapter 37. The treatment for brachial plexus palsy consists of proper positioning and passive exercises to prevent contractures of the paralyzed muscles. The nurse needs to help maintain the arm in an abducted, externally rotated position. The arm may be elevated at the shoulder and the elbow kept flexed at a right angle, as shown in Figure 38-28. The nurse needs to use her creativity to maintain the arm in such a position by making improvised slings or splints which can be pinned to the mattress or by simply pinning the infant's gown to the desired position on the mattress. The nurse must take special precautions while handling the arm. In the normal routine of dressing the infant, the nurse should remove clothing from the affected arm first, and redress the unaffected arm first so that the clothing can be easily slid off the involved arm. These aspects of treatment must be shared with the mother to ensure continuity of prescribed care in the home setting.

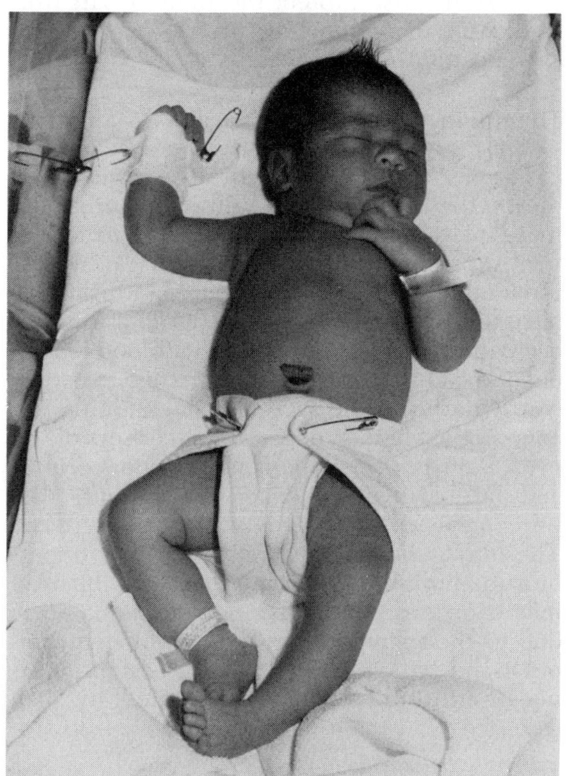

FIGURE 38-28. Proper position for treating brachial plexus palsy. The arm is elevated at the shoulder and the elbow is kept flexed at a right angle.

Trauma Involving Bony Structures

Delivery may result in breakage or fractures of bones most susceptible to injury, such as the clavicle and long bones of the extremities. Fractures are suspected if an infant has limited arm or leg movement, the Moro reflex is asymmetrical, or spasms are seen in related muscles. If such occurs, careful palpation of the area is indicated. One will feel bone crepitation, or a sand-grating sensation over the fracture. Healing is enhanced when the involved part is immobilized in the appropriate position. This can be done by wrapping the involved part with supportive material, or up against another limb or the body trunk. The nurse must also protect the injured part from stretching or undue pressure during carrying or repositioning of the baby.

Trauma Involving Soft Tissues

Tissues can be easily bruised or abrased during the birth process. Vulnerable areas are those of the presenting parts. For example, vertex presentation can result in caput succadaneum or cephalhematoma. Manifestations of tissue injuries are edema, discoloration, or ecchymoses due to extravasation (blood leaked out of the circulation) into the tissues, petechia (particularly on the face and neck), and subconjunctival hemorrhages at the corners of the eyes. Soft tissue trauma is usually not serious, and rarely involves special treatment. The bruising usually resolves within a few days. The nurse should note, however, that hyperbilirubenimia can occur in extensively bruised infants or those with large cephalohematomas due to the increased breakdown of hemaglobin in the extravasated blood. Careful monitoring of bilirubin levels is indicated in such cases.

Trauma Involving the Nervous System

One of the most serious forms of birth trauma is intracranial hemorrhage. Bleeding may occur in the subdural, subarachnoid, or intraventricular spaces of the brain. Infants vulnerable to intracranial hemorrhage are those whose deliveries involve the following:

1. Rapid, precipitous delivery which results in sudden changes in pressure, causing breakage of the blood vessels, particularly the bridging veins penetrating the dura mater and causing subdural hematomas.
2. Prolonged labor or difficult delivery resulting in sustained or extreme pressures and shearing forces resulting in tears of the falx cerebri or tentorium.
3. Hypoxia or anoxia during labor, delivery, or shortly after birth which results in cerebral vessel damage and periventricular and/or intraventricular hemorrhage.
4. Prematurity is associated with fragile blood vessels and a tendency toward bleeding as well as coagulation defects in the postnatal period.

The nurse should be able to recognize signs indicative of intracranial hemorrhage so it can be reported immediately and therapy implemented when possible. Clinical signs correlate to the degree of cerebral involvement and may appear at birth or later:

- cyanosis
- irregular respirations and apnea
- pale, cold, clammy skin
- decreased sucking or failure to suck, forceful vomiting
- eyes in staring position
- restlessness, irritability
- absence of or weak Moro response
- flaccidity followed by spasticity (diminished and then increased muscle tone)
- fontanels tense
- opisthotonic position
- seizures

A spinal tap may be done to determine the

presence of blood in the cerebral spinal fluid. The nurse should support management of the baby by minimal handling, promoting quiet rest, protecting the baby from self-injury during seizures, ensuring warmth and oxygen or resuscitation as needed. Intracranial hemorrhage in the newborn carries a high degree of mortality and morbidity. One must be extremely cautious of projecting successful outcome for the future when discussing the baby's problems with the parents.

METABOLIC DISTURBANCES

There are numerous metabolic disturbances that can occur in the neonate. This section highlights two specific conditions: hypoglycemia and hypocalcemia. These conditions as well as assessment and therapy factors were discussed in detail in Chapter 37 and the reader is encouraged to review that content. The focus here is to explore the nurse's role in the clinical management of these two conditions.

Hypoglycemia

In addition to an awareness of which neonates are most vulnerable to develop the condition, and the ability to identify early symptoms, the nurse must be capable of performing selected screening procedures for early detection and treatment of hypoglycemia in high-risk newborns.

1. Dextrostix screening procedure involves a color reaction brought about by bringing a drop of blood from a simple heelstick puncture onto a reagent stick and correlating the resulting color changes from comparable blood glucose levels. It is not considered an exact test for blood glucose levels. However, the test does allow the nurse to rapidly identify infants suspected of hypoglycemia and who need accurate laboratory assessment of blood glucose levels.
2. The nurse should ensure that blood sugar levels are properly monitored in the neonate with hypoglycemia. Such levels are usually monitored at intervals of 1 to 2 hours while receiving therapeutic doses of glucose to ascertain whether the condition is being corrected or whether the infant is receiving too much glucose (hyperglycemia).
3. The nurse must ensure that any termination of intravenous glucose therapy is done gradually, since an abrupt cessation of the glucose supply can lead to a rebound hypoglycemia (due to the interim elevated insulin secretion).
4. The infant at risk for hypoglycemia who can tolerate oral feedings should have early feedings instituted before symptoms appear. Such infants may be given glucose water as early as 1 to 2 hours after birth. If infants are unable to tolerate oral feedings, the nurse and physician will collaborate to support glucose intake via gavage or intravenous infusions.

Hypocalcemia

In addition to knowledge on recognizing and assessing infants at risk for hypocalcemia, the nurse needs to value some specific actions to be carried out during its treatment:

1. Anticipate the possible complication of bradycardia during IV administration of calcium by having cardiac monitoring capability set up prior to the infusion.
2. Infants receiving IV calcium are best monitored by an audio or visual pulse counting or EKG device. Continuous auscultation with a stethoscope is also acceptable.
3. Ensure that no infiltration of the solution occurs because of its damaging effects

(skin sloughing and later calcification formation).

4. Oral supplement is often given as soon as the baby's condition improves and the dangers of neonatal tetany have subsided.

THE DRUG-ADDICTED NEONATE

A baby born to a mother with a narcotic addiction may passively acquire the addiction. The drug crosses the placental barrier to enter the fetal circulation and the narcotic withdrawal syndrome can manifest because birth abruptly terminates the infant's narcotic supply. Between 50 to 90 per cent of infants born to narcotic mothers exhibit withdrawal. The degree of infant withdrawal is dependent upon the duration and type of maternal addiction and the mother's drug level immediately prior to delivery. The closer to delivery a mother takes heroin, the greater the delay in onset of withdrawal but the more severe the symptoms in the neonate.[9]

The nurse must be able to recognize manifestations of the withdrawal syndrome. This includes recognition of signs of addiction as well as the ability to predict which infants are likely to exhibit symptoms later.

Most addicted neonates appear healthy at birth. Thus, the nurse needs knowledge about the time of onset of narcotic withdrawal signs. For general approximations, it is safe to predict that almost all cases of neonatal narcotic addiction will manifest within 3 to 4 days and at least by a week or 10 days.[10] Symptomatology relates largely to irritability of the central nervous system and gastrointestinal disturbances. The signs of narcotic withdrawal in the neonate are:

Irritability, restlessness, sleeplessness, excessive crying
Tremors
Vomiting and poor feeding
High-pitched, shrill cry
Diarrhea
Hypertonicity and hyperactivity (muscle rigidity)
Respiratory distress
Fever, sweating
Sneezing, mucus, stuffy nose
Convulsions
Yawning, hiccups, salivation
Scratching face, other skin abrasions.

What are some of the ways the nurse can assess for signs suggestive of neonatal narcotic withdrawal? Four major symptoms indicate *central nervous system irritability.* They are identified below with suggested approaches for assessment:

1. *Hyperactivity.* Does not lie still when positioned in isolette; if not on stomach may crawl around; activity may shake bassinet or bang sides of isolette.
2. *Hypertonicity.* In the stepping response (reflex) the legs appear rigid and straight as though providing support to the body weight instead of legs sagging. In the traction response the body is rigid and the head at the level of the arms. Elevation of the infant by the heels while he is lying on a flat surface also reveals hypertonicity.
3. *Tremors.* Shaking, flapping movements noted in the extremities; elicitation of the Moro reflex reveals tremors of arms and legs; startling the infant produces tremors and a shrill, high-pitched cry.
4. *Irritability.* Lack of ability to have undisturbed sleep for any duration, especially after a feeding; difficult to comfort; low consolability factor.

The following is assessment for the major signs of *gastrointestinal disturbance* suggestive of narcotic withdrawal:

1. *Poor Feeding Ability.* Sucking and swallowing reflexes appear uncoordinated; inability to take average amount of for-

mula within a reasonable time; feeding ability comparable to that of a premature.
2. *Vomiting.* Regurgitates large portion of feeding; projectile vomiting.
3. *Diarrhea.* Frequent loose stools.
4. *Hunger.* Appears constantly hungry; noted to be sucking fists, hand, fingers, bed, clothing; exaggerated rooting reflex.

Other signs may give the impression that the baby has a cold (stuffy nose, sneezing, mucus) or is experiencing an infection (fever, sweating). Narcotic-addicted infants also tend to be lower in birth weight and have shorter gestations.

The maternal history may also present data suggestive of delivery of an addicted infant. Examples are minimal or no prenatal care due to lack of interest and awareness for the care of the self, a history of venereal disease, hepatitis, tetanus, or septicemia, as well as needle marks, scars, or thrombosed veins and bruises from nurturing the drug addiction.[11] The drug pattern appears to affect the menstrual cycle creating a history of amenorrhea, dysmenorrhea, or variations in cycle duration. The mother may arrive at the hospital in late first stages of labor because of decreased sensitivity to labor contractions. During the hospital course the mother may request medications frequently, needing higher dosages for medications to be effective; there may be an urgent desire for early hospital discharge because of need to nurture the drug habit; delivery is often from the breech presentation due to the fetus' low birth weight.

Suggested goals for the nursing care of the drug-addicted infant are:

1. Identify the neonate at risk for withdrawal and observe closely for symptomatology.
2. Support the neonate to emerge successfully from the syndrome via management of the symptoms. Support drug therapy when indicated.
3. Protect from pathophysiologic processes to which the addicted infant is vulnerable.
4. Promote maternal-infant acquaintance.

To achieve the above goals the nurse must assess for the neonatal withdrawal syndrome. The nurse should remember to collect urine for toxicologic studies before 24 hours of life because narcotic metabolites rapidly disappear. Suggested nursing actions to manage the withdrawal symptoms are described in Table 38-12. The nurse also has a responsibility to support any drug therapy used to control symptomatology. Numerous pharmacologic agents are used for treatment. Currently, the most common agents are phenobarbital, chloropromazine (Thorazine), diazepam (Valium), and paregoric. When such drugs are used, the nurse must be on the alert for side effects of depression from excessive sedation. Examples are respiratory distress, possible aspiration leading to pneumonia, lethargy, reduced sucking, and hypotonia. The nurse may need to help the infant maintain caloric and fluid balance by parenteral intake, help prevent aspiration by positioning or suctioning, and be prepared for resuscitation if severe respiratory distress occurs. One important note, infants who are jaundiced should not be given Valium because it contains a substance (caffeine sodium benzoate) which competes with the bilirubin-albumin binding capacity, predisposing the infant to hyperbilirubinemia.

Another important nursing responsibility is protection of the infant from pathophysiologic processes to which it is vulnerable. Such disturbances are related primarily to the infant's possible low birth weight and immaturity. The nursing care for these processes (hypoglycemia, hypocalcemia, hypothermia, anoxia, sepsis) has been discussed in this chapter.

The nurse must consciously implement actions to promote maternal-infant interaction. This is a critical goal because there may be a total lack of or only minimal initiative by the mother to establish contact with the baby. The reasons are numerous: the addicted mother usually has a negative self-concept and low self-esteem creating increased anxiety about her ability to care for the baby; the baby may make the mother feel guilty or may be seen as a punishment for the mother's lifestyle of drug dependency; the baby may be seen as a socioeconomic burden, or interfering with her financial ability to nurture her drug dependency. Such mothers may use the defense of projecting their guilt, anger, and frustrations upon others by being critical of the baby's management or even of the baby's normal behavior.

TABLE 38-12. Nursing Care of the Drug-Addicted Neonate*

Infant Behavior	*Nursing Observations*	*Nursing Intervention*
High-pitched cry	Note onset. Note length of time cry persists—is it continuous? Is it high-pitched and piercing as though infant were in pain? Observe infant for other causes of abnormal crying patterns (meningitis, intracranial bleeding, etc.) Is anterior fontanel full or bulging? Are cranial sutures widely separated? Is head circumference increased? Does infant stare without blinking and exhibit adder's tongue? Is cry aggravated or alleviated when infant is picked up?	Soothe infant by wrapping him tightly in blankets (swaddling), or holding him tightly and close to one's body, or both. Decrease feeding intervals and/or implement a demand-feeding schedule. Reduce environmental stimuli.
Inability to sleep	Note how long infant sleeps after feeding. Note general sleep and wake patterns. If drug therapy has been initiated, note changes in sleep patterns, ability to rest, and whetehr there is decreased activity which may indicate drug overdose.	Decrease environmental stimuli. Swaddle. Feed small amounts at frequent intervals.
Frantic sucking of fists	Note onset and amount of sucking. Observe for blisters on fingertips and knuckles. If blistering occurs, observe sites for signs of infection.	Use infant shirts with sewn-in sleeves for mits to prevent skin trauma. Keep skin area clean; use aseptic technique.
Yawning	Note onset and frequency.	None
Sneezing Nasal stuffiness	Observe onset and frequency. Note severity of nasal stuffiness and determine whether it hinders feeding. If mucus is excessive, consider possibility of other underlying problems such as esophageal fistula, and congenital syphillis.	Aspirate nasopharynx. Give frequent nose care. Allow more time for feeding with rest between sucking. Aspirate trachea if tracheal mucus is increased. Check rate and character of respirations frequently.
Poor feeding	Note sucking pattern—is infant uncoordinated in his attempt to suck? Observe for other possible causes of poor feeding (sepsis, hypoglycemia, immaturity, bowel obstruction, pyloric stenosis).	Feed small amounts at close intervals. Maintain fluid and caloric intake required for infant's weight.

* From Finnegan and Macnew,[9] with permission.

TABLE 38-12. *Continued*

Infant Behavior	*Nursing Observations*	*Nursing Intervention*
Regurgitation Vomiting Loose Stools	Note when regurgitation or vomiting occurs. Is there a precipitating factor (medication, handling, manipulation, position, etc.)? Observe for signs of dehydration: poor skin turgor sunken anterior fontanel sunken orbits around eyes marked weight loss. Note time, color, consistency, and quantity of vomitus and/or stool. When stools are loose, estimate amount of water loss with stools. Note whether vomiting is nonforceful or projectile. Observe for electrolyte balance.	Maintain IV at prescribed rate. Maintain infant in side-lying position to prevent aspiration of vomitus. Give skin care to prevent excoriation of neck folds, buttocks, and perineum.
Tachypnea mottling	Note onset of respiration over 60/min. If tachypnea worsens, note HR and report if more than 180/min. Note retractions, their severity (mild, moderate, severe) and location (subcostal, intercostal, sternal, suprasternal, supraclavicular). Note presence of nasal flaring. Note infant's color—is there pallor? Cyanosis? If cyanosis is present, note location (extremities, circumoral, generalized) and degree (mild, moderate, severe). Observe for other possible underlying pathophysiological causes (anemia, aspiration pneumonia, congenital heart disease, etc.) Is mottling precipitated by factors such as handling, hypothermia? Watch closely for apnea.	Maintain infant in semi-Fowler's position. Hyperextend head slightly to assure patient airway. Minimize handling and manipulation. Correlate RR, HR, retractions, and color with infant's progress, general condition, and blood gases. If infant is receiving O_2 and is premature, observe color closely, correlate with blood gases, and reduce O_2 if Po_2 exceeds 85–90. Maintain warmth since hypo- or hyperthermia increases O_2 consumption. Place infant on cardiac-apnea monitor. If apnea occurs, resuscitate.
Hyperactive Moro reflex	Is reflex moderately or markedly exaggerated? If drug therapy has been started, note a diminished or absent Moro reflex. Is there asymmetry of the reflex? Asymmetry may indicate underlying pathophysiology—Erb's palsy, fractured clavicle, intracranial hemorrhage.	
Hypertonicity	Note degree of increased muscle tone (mild, moderate, or severe) by: Attempting to straighten arms and legs and recording degree of resistance Picking up by hands and noting rigidity with degree of head lag (a withdrawing	Change infant's position often since prolonged or marked rigidity predisposes him to develop pressure areas. Use sheepskin to reduce pressure. Decrease environmental temperature if infant's temperature goes above 99° F.

TABLE 38-12. *Continued*

Infant Behavior	*Nursing Observations*	*Nursing Intervention*
	infant often exhibits trunk rigidity and holds his head on a plane with his body for a prolonged time). Raising infant by arms and letting him stand. (a withdrawing neonate exhibits marked leg rigidity and can support his body's weight for considerable periods.) Correlate mother's obstetrical history and delivery with infant's condition and observe baby for other pathophysiology—hypocalcemia, hypoglycemia, meningitis, asphyxia neonatorum, and intracranial hemorrhage. Observe for reddened areas over heels, occiput, sacrum and knees. Observe temperature frequently; increased activity may cause pyrexia.	
Tremors Convulsions	Note if tremors occur when infant is disturbed and/or undisturbed. Note location of tremors: upper extremities lower extremities generalized Note whether degree of tremor is mild, moderate, or severe. Observe skin over nose, elbows, fingers, toes, knees, heels for excoriation. Observe for face scratches. Observe for underlying pathology mentioned above under Hypertonicity. Check temperature often for pyrexia. Observe for seizures. If they occur, note onset, length, origin, body involvement, whether tonic, clonic, or both, eye deviation and infant's color.	Change position frequently to prevent excoriation. Give frequent skin care (cleansing, ointment, and exposure to air and/or heat lamp.) Use sheepskin. Observe excoriations for healing, worsening, infection. Decrease environmental temperature if infant exhibits pyrexia. If infant convulses, maintain patent airway and prevent self-trauma. If infant is apneic after seizure, begin resuscitation. Decrease environmental stimuli.

HYPERBILIRUBINEMIA

The steps in the process of clearing bilirubin (a toxic substance) from the blood which make the premature infant particularly vulnerable to developing elevated serum bilirubin levels (hyperbilirubinemia) have been described in detail in the preceding chapter, along with normal bilirubin values and the rationale for major modes of therapy. Table 38-13 was developed to guide the nurse in predicting which newborns will be vulnerable to hyperbilirubinemia or pathologic (in contrast to physiologic) jaundice. The basic pathophysiologic mechanisms involved are again stressed.

Assessment or diagnostic work-up for causes of hyperbilirubinemia includes clinical observation and laboratory testing. Clinical assessment includes the following observations:

1. Blanching the skin by applying pressure

TABLE 38-13. Nursing Guide for Predicting Neonates at Risk for Hyperbilirubinemia or Pathologic Jaundice

Contributing Factors	*Mechanisms*
Incompatibility of blood group factors between mother and infant. Infants at risk are those who are Rh positive with an Rh negative mother or infants with type A or B blood with an O type mother.	A sensitization process occurs involving an antigen-antibody reaction that leads to hemolysis of red blood cells (Rh or ABO erythroblastosis).
Family history of hemoglobin or red cell abnormalities such as G-6-PD deficiency, thalassemia, hereditary spherocytosis, etc.	Infants who have abnormalities of hemoglobin or the metabolic activities of their red blood cells show changes in the shape, contour, or life span of the cells and are vulnerable to increased hemolysis.
Polycythemia or increased quantity of red blood cells. Infants at risk are those who had delayed clamping of the cord, the larger of monovular twins in the feto-fetal transfusion syndrome, and babies receiving a maternal-fetal transfusion.	The amount of hemoglobin released during normal red blood cell destruction (turnover) is directly proportional to the total red blood cell volume. Remember, for every gram of hemoglobin released, approximately 35 mg. of bilirubin is formed.
Hemorrhage into extravascular spaces. Infants at risk are those with a history of traumatic or precipitous delivery, and/or findings of cephalohematomas, extensive ecchymosis, and petechiae.	Accumulated blood outside of the circulation (extravasated) is rapidly broken down and increases the amount of hemoglobin to be converted to bilirubin.
Reabsorption of bilirubin from the gastrointestinal tract (enterohepatic circulation). Infants at risk are those with bowel obstruction (possibly preceded by polyhydramnios), delayed passage of meconium, and intestinal bleeding or swallowed blood.	Obstruction or delayed emptying allows absorption of pigment (hemoglobin or bilirubin itself) from blood or meconium in the bowel, or the reabsorption of bilirubin already excreted by the liver in the form of bile.
Prematurity	See discussion in Chapter 37.
Hypoxemia. Infants at risk are those with asphyxia, hyaline membrane disease, and other respiratory or cardiac disorders.	Transport of bilirubin into and out of the liver as well as conjugation itself are energy-consuming processes requiring oxygen.
Hypoglycemia. Infants at risk are prematures, SGA, LGA, IDM, and those with delayed oral intake.	Bilirubin is conjugated with glucuronic acid which itself is formed from glycogen, the storage form of glucose.
Exposure to drugs. Infants at risk are those whose mothers received drugs such as aspirin or sulfonamides, and babies who receive Valium or heparin.	These drugs either compete with bilirubin for conjugation or for binding to the albumin.
Breast feeding	Breast milk jaundice is due to a substance in the milk (pregnanediol) which suppresses the conjugation process. Reduced fluid and caloric intake until the mother's milk comes may also be a factor.
Infection	Toxins released during the infection may cause hemolysis, or infection process may involve the liver, interfering with secretion of bile.

and quickly releasing to assess the underlying yellow discoloration, especially on the tip of the nose or over the sternum. This is especially helpful in the child who is plethoric (has accentuated redness of the skin due to increased blood hematocrit).

2. Noting distribution of the jaundice. Is it limited to the head and upper chest, or does it extend over the entire body? Pathologic levels of bilirubin are not reached until jaundice has spread to the lower trunk and extremities.
3. Relating appearance of jaundice to time after birth. Any jaundice that appears within the first 24 to 36 hours of life is considered early onset jaundice (icterus praecox) and is pathologic and not physiologic. It generally represents some type of hemolysis caused by a blood group or type incompatibility.

Laboratory assessment may include any of the following tests:

1. Blood typing and grouping of mother and infant to rule out Rh and ABO incompatibilities.
2. The Coombs' test (antihuman globulin test) to determine the presence of antibodies on the baby's red cells (direct Coombs' test) or in the mother's or baby's serum (indirect Coombs' test).
3. Reticulocyte count to rule out rapid production of young red cells indicating hemolysis.
4. Hematocrit to rule out polycythemia.
5. Examination of the peripheral blood smear to rule out structural abnormalities of the red cells which one sees in hemolytic diseases due to incompatibilities or inherited metabolic or hemoglobin defects affecting the red cells.
6. Blood, urine (by suprapubic aspiration), or spinal fluid cultures to rule out sepsis and meningitis.

Assessment always includes a thorough review of the maternal pregnancy and delivery history as regards possible infection or receipt of medications.

The nurse's role in the *therapy* of jaundice or hyperbilirubinemia is crucial, as the avoidance of complications is largely up to her. *Early feeding* techniques have been described previously. Supplemental feedings of 5 per cent glucose water (10 per cent glucose given by mouth will quickly lead to diarrhea) between feedings, or postprandial formula if the mother is breast feeding is an important adjunct (helpful addition) form of therapy.

The procedure for *phototherapy* is not complex. The infant is placed under a canopy of fluorescent lights and as much of his skin as possible is exposed to the light. Cool white or blue lamps with a high percentage of light with wave lengths between 400 to 500 mm. are the most effective for the photo-oxidation process. Blue lights alone are the most effective, but loss of the ability to clinically assess the baby's skin color for cyanosis makes their exclusive use inadvisable.

When phototherapy is instituted, the nurse must incorporate the following into the care plan of the infant:

1. Protect the retina from damage due to the high-intensity light by shielding the infant's eyes. They must be protected from corneal abrasion. These things can be accomplished by first placing a soft oval eye patch over each eye. Tape the eye patches to the head with nonallergic tape, or secure them with an overlying "bili mask" (Fig. 38-29). Both eyes must be completely covered by the patches; if any portion of the eyes is visible, turn off the lights and reapply the patches. Remove the eye patches with each feeding so the baby can a) receive visual stimulation, and b) have each eye examined for signs of infection or irritation.
2. Monitor the infant's skin and core temperature frequently at the beginning of

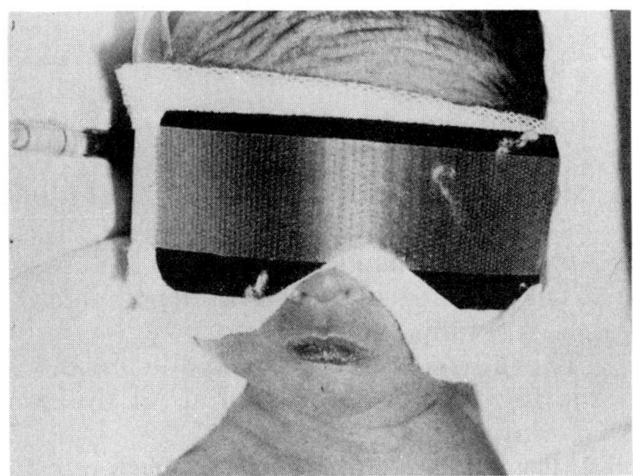

FIGURE 38-29. The "bili mask" to protect the infant's eyes during phototherapy.

phototherapy until his temperature is stable within the thermal neutral zone. Hypothermia and hyperthermia are common complications of phototherapy. Remember, hypothermia leads to acidosis, hyperthermia may lead to apneic episodes in the premature, and both result in increased oxygen consumption.

3. Provide extra fluid intake, as insensible water losses and stool water losses are increased under phototherapy.
4. The nurse must closely assess the infant's daily patterns to detect any notable changes in such things as food ingestion, bowel and urination patterns, sleep and waking rhythms, and so forth.

The nurse's role in assisting with an *exchange transfusion* involves the following actions:

1. Determine that the donor blood is the correct type and group, and that the unit's identification matches that of the patient. Confirm this by checking with a doctor or another nurse.
   a. In cases of Rh erythroblastosis, O Rh negative blood or group-specific (same blood group as baby) Rh negative blood should be used.
   b. In cases of ABO erythroblastosis, *only* O group Rh type-specific (same Rh type as baby) blood should be used.
   c. In cases of nonhemolytic hyperbilirubinemia requiring an exchange transfusion, type- and group-specific blood should be used whenever possible. O Rh negative blood (universal donor) is also acceptable.

   It is extremely important in premature or sick infants that the blood be as fresh as possible (within a day or two) since older blood tends to have high levels of acid and potassium which are poorly tolerated by the premature or sick neonate.
2. The blood should be warmed close to body temperature before use. This can be done in a pail of warm water or a special blood warming device. Guard against overheating the blood because this destroys blood cells.
3. Prepare the necessry equipment. With the exception of special instruments sometimes needed for placement of the umbilical catheter, equipment for an exchange now comes as a disposable set and includes syringes, 4-way stopcock, catheters, 10 per cent calcium gluconate, collection bag, ruler for venous pressure measurements, and sterile drapes and gloves. The nurse makes available the antiseptic solution, swabs, and so forth, and circulates to bring any other needed equipment during the procedure.
4. Prepare the infant. The last scheduled feeding prior to an exchange should have been withheld. Stomach contents are now aspirated to prevent possible regurgitation and aspiration during the procedure. A source of radiant heat or a warming mattress is set up to assure temperature maintenance throughout the exchange. A telethermometer skin or rectal probe is taped in place to con-

tinuously monitor the baby's temperature. Skin leads for EKG or heart rate monitoring are also secured in place so that uninterrupted cardiac monitoring is provided during the entire procedure. Equipment for emergency suctioning and resuscitation is made immediately available, first having been checked to assure that it is functioning properly.

5. Once the umbilical catheter is in place and blood samples for pre-exchange laboratory tests (bilirubin, hematocrit) have been taken, the baby is usually "primed" with albumin to enhance the removal of larger amounts of bilirubin in the process of exchange. The dosage is approximately 1 gram of albumin (25 per cent salt-poor human albumin) per kilogram body weight of the infant, and is given over a 10 to 15 minute period. To keep the catheter open until the actual exchange commences (preferably 30 minutes after the albumin), one attaches a heparin lock (heparinized-saline flush solution on a 3-way stopcock hooked up to the catheter and periodically flushed through in small increments) or an intravenous solution of 10 per cent dextrose in water is hung for a constant infusion.
6. The unit of fresh blood, after having been checked for identification (see #1 above), is attached to the standard blood filter set and then to a warming coil which is placed in the blood warmer or pail of warm water (approximately 37° C or 98.6° F; see #2 above). The person to perform the exchange attaches the 4-way stopcock and syringe, clears the line of air, and proceeds under strict sterile technique.
7. During the exchange transfusion, besides circulating to provide additional equipment and materials, the nurse keeps an exact log or record of all that proceeds in the course of the exchange:
   a. Exact times.
   b. Vital signs q15 minutes or more frequently.
   c. Amount "blood in" and "total blood in" to that point.
   d. Amount "blood out" and "total blood out" to that point.
   e. Mediations given.
   f. Pertinent observations as to infant's reactions, and so forth.

   The nurse is also responsible for monitoring the sterile technique of the procedure.
8. After the procedure the infant should be closely monitored for potential aftereffects of the exchange transfusion. The nurse should be particularly alert for signs of hypoglycemia, hypocalcemia, acidosis, and sepsis.

PREMATURITY, SGA INFANTS AND LGA INFANTS

Chapter 37 discussed infants in these categories, the problems for which they are at high risk, their physiologic handicaps, their behavioral manifestations, and the therapeutic plan for management of the diseases and conditions to which they are vulnerable.

What are the major nursing goals in the care of the premature, the SGA infant, and LGA infant? The following are of particular value:

1. Protect the infant from pathophysiologic processes to which he is vulnerable.
2. Nurture the infant by maintenance of his daily life activities (see Health Care Maintenance above).
3. Stimulate the infant toward a higher degree of wellness in terms of physical growth and behavioral development.

Nursing actions to achieve the above goals encompass an integration of content previously presented throughout this chapter. The following is a brief summation.

Nursing Actions Which Protect

Respiratory Distress. The nurse monitors the infant closely for clinical signs indicative of difficulty in maintaining ventilation and shares significant observations with the physician so that early therapy can be instituted. The nurse should anticipate that the infant may require ventilatory and metabolic resuscitation. Resuscitation equipment, drugs, suction apparatus, and oxygen should be readily available. Since the SGA infant is prone to aspiration of amniotic fluid leading to pneumonia and possible pneumothorax and/or pulmonary hemorrhage, the nurse should be alerted to the symptoms of these complications which include increased respiratory rate, retractions, gasping, sudden change in color, absent or reduced breath sounds on one or both sides of the chest, and a shift of cardiac sounds. The nurse should assist in taking chest roentgenograms, as well as anticipate a chest-tube insertion and/or umbilical vessel catheterization. (Nursing actions for these procedures were described earlier in this chapter.) The nurse should also anticipate that the premature infant is most vulnerable to apnea and will need close observation and monitoring.

Hypocalcemia. Be alert to signs of hypocalcemia (twitching, trĕmors, irritability) in the premature infant and SGA infant, especially when previously treated with bicarbonate for metabolic acidosis secondary to neonatal asphyxia.

Hyperbilirubinemia. The immature infant should especially be watched for signs of jaundice and be monitored for bilirubin levels. He is in jeopardy due to both increased bilirubin production and decreased bilirubin clearance.

Hypoglycemia. This is commonly found in the prematures, infants of diabetic mothers, and SGA babies. The nurse can anticipate that hypoglycemia is most likely to occur in the first 12 hours of life, but also as late as 48 hours. Therefore the nurse should be sure that the blood sugars are monitored, and that these babies do not have undue delay in initiation of feeding. Dextrostix measurements can easily be done by the nurse every hour in the initial period after birth or as specifically ordered. The nurse should be prepared to institute parenteral glucose therapy via peripheral IV or central (umbilical) catheter.

Thermoregulation. The nurse should ensure that incubator thermal settings maintain a desired infant skin temperature between 35.8 and 36.5° C. Skin temperatures should be monitored appropriately to protect the baby from hypothermia and hyperthermia. Hyperthermia can cause apnea in the premature infant.

Infection. Intensive neonatal nursing care involves constant awareness of environmental factors that pose risk of infection. The nurse must be aware that some SGA babies have failed to grow in utero because of congenital infection and will require immediate treatment and possible isolation.

Polycythemia. SGA, LGA, and postmature infants are most vulnerable to elevated red blood cell volume. The nurse should be alerted to its symptoms which include tachypnea, tachycardia, peripheral cyanosis, and possible convulsions. In extreme cases, the nurse may need to prepare for an abbreviated exchange transfusion using fresh-frozen plasma rather than whole blood. The nurse should ensure that the baby's hematocrit is monitored.

Congenital Malformations. The incidence of congenital malformations (anomalies) is particularly high in SGA and IDM infants. Thus, screening procedures and observations should be done carefully in such infants to detect any hidden anomalies.

Nursing Actions Which Nurture

Feeding. The nurse's greatest contribution in the area of health maintenance involves feeding. Maintenance of caloric and fluid intake is an essential life activity. Feeding SGA and premature infants is a particular challenge

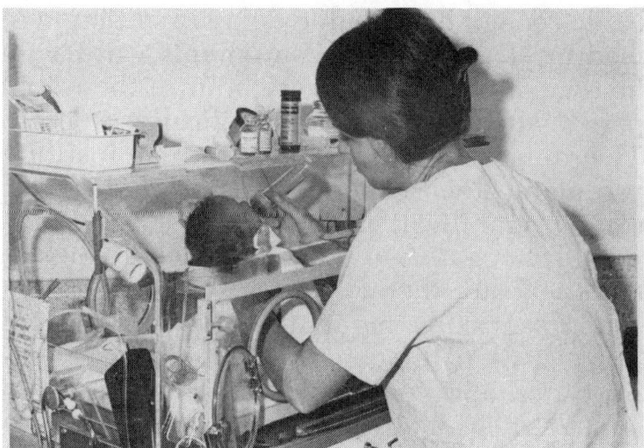

FIGURE 38-30. Feeding the small infant is a nursing challenge.

(Fig. 38-30). Some important aspects of feeding the small infant are considered below:

1. Decision to initiate feeding is based upon successful extrauterine adaptation. Infants should have normal breathing pattern, good color, tone, cry, and normal skin temperature before feeding is instituted.
2. When extrauterine adaptation is compromised, intravenous therapy should be used to maintain caloric and fluid balance.
3. If the gag reflex is absent or weak, and sucking and swallowing are poor, the baby should be fed by gavage.
4. In infants who are prone to have increased fluid contents in their stomachs at birth, such as those born via cesarean section or with polyhydramnios, gastic contents may need to be aspirated by lavage prior to feeding.
5. Small frequent feedings may be indicated because of the limited gastric capacity.
6. Do not delay feeding unnecessarily since premature and SGA infants are particularly vulnerable to hypoglycemia which is accentuated by prolonged fasting.
7. Appreciate that feeding may initially be a stressful activity to the immature infant. Watch for any periodic breathing or apnea that may occur approximately 15 minutes after feeding. The infant is also vulnerable to regurgitation and aspiration because large amounts of air may be swallowed during feeding.
8. Protect the infant from overfeeding. Abdominal distention, vomiting, and "spitting up" may indicate too much volume for the gastric capacity. "Spitting-up" should not be taken lightly, and the amount of each feeding should be reduced until it no longer occurs.
9. Coordinate feeding attempts with the unique "suck pattern" in the immature infant. It is characterized by short sucking bursts preceded or followed by swallows, as contrasted to prolong sucking bursts with multiple swallows simultaneously with the sucking as seen in the full-term sucking pattern. The nurse needs to frequently stop the flow of milk to coordinate with the baby's attempts to swallow. This immature sucking pattern is viewed as a compensatory, protective mechanism to prevent overloading of the limited capacity of the esophagus and stomach. The reader is referred to two excellent articles by Gryboski describing these mechanisms in detail.[12,13]
10. Frequent bubbling and positioning to allow gravity flow of any regurgitation is a must.
11. Formulas should be adequate in calories, electrolytes, iron, and vitamins to meet specific nutritional requirements of premature and SGA infants.

Monitor Intake, Output, and Growth Indices. The small, immature baby should be assessed as to adequate voiding, stools, and any drainage products. Such infants may have numerous tubes from which fluid and electrolytes can be lost. Monitoring the infant's growth is done by frequently measuring weight, length, and head circumference. Weights should be taken in grams and any changes noted from the weight taken previously. These findings are charted regularly on standard growth charts, and serve as baseline norms for future reference.

Conservation of Energy. Promote rest and sleep by minimal handling and organize care so baby is not disturbed unnecessarily. Supporting the infant's normal physiologic functions such as respirations and temperature regulation will contribute to energy conservation and thus enable him to better cope with other stressors.

Positioning. The nurse needs to value the importance of changing the infant's position regularly (every two hours is generally accepted). This has numerous benefits such as stimulating circulation, preventing stasis of accumulated secretions, and minimizing irritation to the skin. The nurse also needs to value proper anatomical position and positions which facilitate respirations.

Safety and Comfort. The infant needs to be kept physically clean through bathing and oral hygiene. He needs to be protected from self-injury due to his own random movements, and from injury by equipment. Be sure portholes are kept closed, as the small infant may work his way out through the opening.

Nursing Actions Which Stimulate

Possibly the most "fun" and rewarding aspect of neonatal intensive care is when the nurse uses imagination and creativity in helping the sick baby gain input which will help him grow and develop. After the infant is no longer acutely distressed, the nurse should meet his kinesthetic needs which help to increase his sensory input and release muscle tension. The creative nurse will devise means to rock, sway, and tactilely stimulate the baby. The nurse also needs to value the fact that although the baby is small and possibly immature, his sensory abilities to hear, smell, and touch are nevertheless active. Thus, the nurse should exercise such capacities by providing sensory input (touch, sounds, sights) to encourage the development of the neonate's interaction potential. A higher level of wellness is not possible unless the infant is allowed interaction with his parents. Parents are the vital link in helping the infant achieve maximum health capacity within the unique habitat of the family. Thus, intensive neonatal nursing care should make every attempt to promote parent-child interaction. This is done by keeping the parents informed, allowing them to express their feelings, encouraging their contact with the baby, and allowing their participation in the care of the infant.

The nurse must also be cognizant of the fact that birth of an infant who is sick from pathophysiologic processes creates a tremendous financial burden on the family. The results of a cost analysis study of the expense to the family of babies who survived various mortality risk diseases are illustrated in Figure 38-31. It is essential that the nurse help mobilize other resources to work with the family so that a financial problem-solving plan can be instituted. Social workers, and public health or visiting nurses provide invaluable services to the sick newborn's family. Neonatal intensive care nursing demands a great deal of expertise, skill, and knowledge. The nurse who can implement a plan that protects, nurtures, and stimulates the sick baby and his family receives unending rewards.

TRANSPORT OF THE ILL NEONATE*

In order to give optimal care to the critically ill neonate, very specialized equipment and

---

*Kathy Puls, R.N., C.N.M., contributed to the preparation of this section.

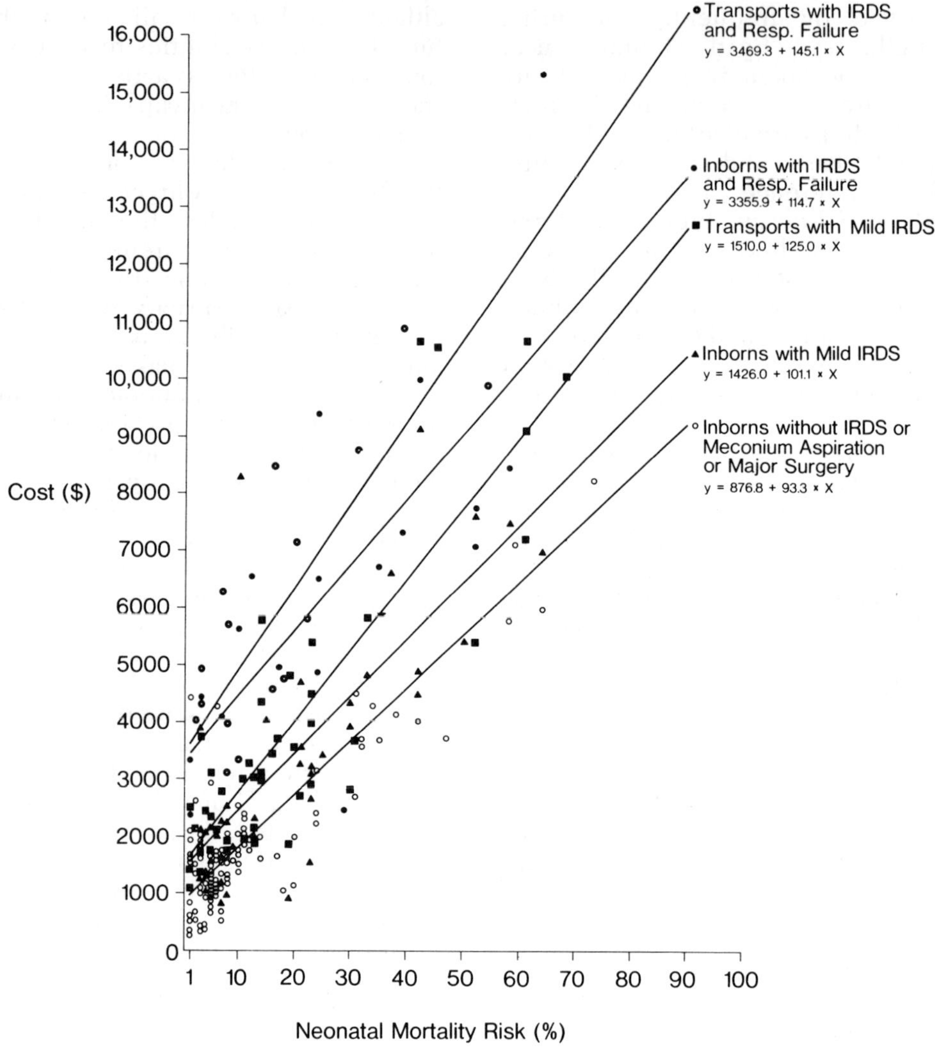

FIGURE 38-31. Graph showing estimation of cost to patient according to mortality risk percentage for certain groups of inborn or transported babies admitted to Tucson Medical Center, November 1, 1971 to May 30, 1973.

trained personnel are required. Because of the expense of such equipment, and the limited number of qualified (and willing) personnel to provide the needed specialized services, it has become necessary to regionalize perinatal care and establish centralized newborn intensive care centers.

Although it is desirable for an infant to be cared for in the hospital closest to his family, it becomes more important for everyone concerned that he be transferred to the regional newborn intensive care center if he is assessed to require care beyond the capabilities of the hospital of birth. Table 38-14 lists specific

TABLE 38-14. Criteria For Transport of the Neonate*

Babies to be Transported	*When to Transport*
All prematures weighing less than 4½ lb. (2,000 g.)	Immediately
Babies weighing less than 5 lb. showing any signs of respiratory distress	Within two hours
Babies over 5 lb. in severe respiratory distress	Immediately
Infants who will probably require an exchange transfusion:	
a. Rh sensitized babies with cord hemoglobins less than 14 g.% and positive Coombs' test	Immediately
b. ABO incompatability with bilirubin greater than 10 mg.% by 24 hours or 15 mg.% by 32 hours	Within a few hours
c. Any baby with bilirubin greater than 18 mg.%	Immediately
Any baby who requires greater than 40% oxygen to stay pink	Within an hour
Any baby severely asphyxiated at birth (Apgar less than 3) and requiring greater than 5 minutes to establish adequate spontaneous respirations	Immediately
Babies having cyanotic, apneic, or bradycardic spells	Within a few hours
Babies with seizures	Within a few hours
Infants thought to be septic or possibly having meningitis	Immediately
Babies with possible surgical problems:	
a. Prolonged abdominal distension	Within 12 hours
b. Babies who have not urinated within 24 hours or stooled within 48 hours	Within 12 hours
Newborns with major congenital malformations: congenital hydrocephalus, encephalocele, meningomyelocele; choanal esophageal, intestinal or anal atresia; diaphragmatic hernia; cyanotic heart disease, etc.	Within a few hours or immediately

* Developed by T. Harris, M.D., medical director of the Southern Arizona State Newborn Transport and Intensive Care Program.

indications for the transport of newborns and the time when the referral should be initiated.

Full therapeutic support capabilities for the ill neonate must be provided in transport. This dictates that a fully trained and equipped team come from the regional newborn care center to pick up the baby, and not that the baby be placed hurriedly in a local ambulance to be transported unprotected to the center. There are a number of general needs of the infant that must be fulfilled during transport; they include:

1. Thermal control.
2. Vital signs monitored (pulse, respirations, temperature, blood pressure).
3. Oxygen requirements.
4. Ventilation needs.
5. Caloric and fluid needs.
6. Medication needs.
7. Protection from infection.

To meet these needs, specific types of equipment are required. First and foremost is a compact, portable incubator with its own power supply and the capability of using alternate power sources such as may be provided by the airplane or ambulance batteries or the wall outlets of the referral hospital. The incubator must be able to carry portable tanks of oxygen and compressed air and to blend them to meet the infant's specific oxygen needs. It must also provide space to carry the appropriate battery-powered monitoring equipment, and allow visual display of the parameters monitored. Such a transport incubator is shown in Figure 38-32.

Self-inflating as well as flow-inflated bag and mask set-ups must be available to ventilate or administer continuous positive pressure to the baby as necessary. Supplies for starting both perepheral IV's and placing umbilical vessel catheters are needed, along with the appropriate intravenous infusion fluids. Medications such as sodium bicarbonate, calcium gluconate, epinephrine, heparin, antibi-

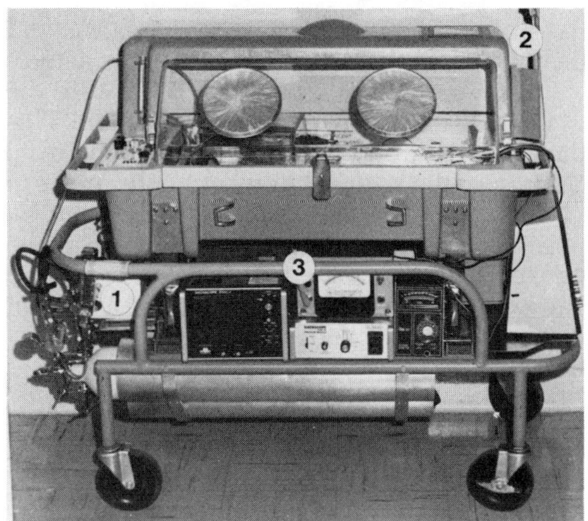

FIGURE 38-32. Modified newborn transport isolette to provide 1) "Dial-in" gas mixtures for head hood or assisted ventilation equipment. Compressed air and oxygen are pre-set mixed by a blender. 2) Constant IV infusion by way of battery-powered roller pump. 3) Monitoring capabilities for heart rate, temperature, direct or indirect blood pressure, F_1O_2 (ambient oxygen concentration) and PaO_2 (arterial oxygen tension). Scope display of EKG and pulse or blood pressure waveform. Modification design by Dr. T. Harris for Tucson Medical Center.

otics, Nalline or Narcan, salt-poor albumin, phenobarbital, Lasix, and Digoxin must be included. Equipment for intubation and insertion of chest tubes must also be available. Frequently, one or two large "tool chests" are necessary to contain all the required equipment and supplies.

After receiving notification from the medical director of the transport program that an ill neonate with specific problems needs to be transported, the nurse, accompanied perhaps by another nurse, house officer, or neonatal fellow, departs from the regional center by helicopter, ambulance, or airplane to the referring hospital. The transport nurse has been specially prepared to perform physical assessment of the infant, order and utilize specific laboratory and x-ray data, and determine a plan of management for stabilizing the infant and handling all emergencies that may arise in transit. She has been trained to administer fluids and medications, provide respiratory support and perform necessary procedures such as umbilical vessel catheterization, intubation and chest-tube insertion. The nurse is also skilled in interviewing parents and is able to provide psychologic support relative to parental concerns which arise from the infant's illness and impending separation. After examining the baby, carrying out the necessary emergency procedures, and talking with the parents, the transport nurse calls the neonatologist at the regional center to discuss her plan of management, and to describe the seriousness of the infant's condition so that appropriate preparations at the regional center for receipt of the new admission can be undertaken.

When the infant has been stabilized, and only then, the return trip begins. The transport nurse must continue her treatment regimen and make modifications as the infant's condition continues to change according to her repeated assessments. These modifications may include increasing the ambient oxygen concentration, applying continuous positive airway pressure by face mask as the airplane increases altitude, or administering sodium bicarbonate via an umbilical catheter to correct suspected acidosis secondary to poor perfusion or continued cyanosis. Assisted ventilation in the form of IPPV to lend support to the infant's own inadequate or irregular respiratory efforts may also be required. If ventilation by way of a face mask proves ineffective, it may be necessary to intubate the baby and apply assisted ventilation directly through the endotracheal tube. During the entire trip, the nurse must frequently monitor the infant's vital signs, including heart rate, respiratory rate, blood pressure, and temperature, and record her observations and treatments on a flow sheet. Good hand-care technique is necessary to prevent infection, and may include the use of an antiseptic foam or other prepackaged cleaning agent prior to each handling of the infant.

Upon arrival at the regional center, the infant is weighed and placed under a radiant-heat warmer attached to the various monitoring devices, cultured (internal and external sites) to rule out present colonization or infection, and the necessary diagnostic tests begun. The transport nurse reports her observations and treatment to the neonatologist and staff nurses, turning over the infant's further care to them. She then replaces the supplies she used from the transport equipment and cleans the incubator in preparation for the next run.

During the infant's hospitalization, the parents are encouraged to visit and participate in the infant's care as much as possible. This participation may include holding, feeding, and bathing the infant, and giving such treatments as percussion and postural drainage, especially if such procedures are to be continued after discharge from the hospital. If an infant is unable to suck, the parents are taught to gavage feed the infant.

The transport nurse should also communicate with the nurses of the referral hospital who were initially involved in the baby's care. They are always anxious to know of the baby's progress, and this is an excellent opportunity to suggest to them how future care of such infants may be improved.

Follow-up care of these infants is important for the parents, the ongoing medical management of the infants themselves, and the future management of babies with similar conditions. The parents of the infants may have unanswered questions or untold concerns, and may require counselling or social service support as well as instruction on how to provide better care for the babies' ongoing medical problems. The babies themselves may need the benefit of further specialized diagnostic tests, or the primary physician in the referring city may need advice as to how best to handle ongoing or anticipated medical problems. Data on growth and development, as well as on pulmonary and neurologic functions are most important for assessing the quality of the patients being saved, and helping to critically evaluate the efficacy of various treatment regimens. It is also most rewarding for the medical and nursing personnel to see the fruits of their labor, especially a healthy and normal child some months or years later being "shown off" by grateful parents.

REFERENCES

1. Klaus, M. and Faranoff, A.. *Care of the High-Risk Neonate.* W. B. Saunders, Philadelphia, 1973, p. 68.
2. Anderson, W. and Andersen, D.: *A controlled clinical trial of effects of water mist on obstructive respiratory signs, death rate and necropsy findings among premature infants.* Pediatrics 17:1, 1956.
3. Miller, H. C. and Conklin, E.: *Clinical evaluation of respiratory insufficiency in newborn infants.* Pediatrics, 16:427, 1955.
4. Northway, W., Rosan, R. and Porter, D.: *Pulmonary disease following respirator therapy.* N. Engl. J. Med. 276:357, 1967.
5. Klaus and Faranoff: op. cit., p. 212.
6. Korones, S.: *High-Risk Newborn Infants, The Basis for Intensive Nursing Care.* C. V. Mosby, St. Louis, 1972, p. 210.
7. Barness, L. and Morrow, G.: *Clinical Clues to Diagnosis of Metabolic Disorders.* Clin. Pediatr. 9:605, 1970.
8. Blake, F., Wright, F. and Waechter, E.: *Nursing Care of Children,* ed. 8. J. B. Lippincott, Philadelphia, 1970.
9. Finnegan, L. and Macnew, B.: *Care of the Addicted Infant.* Am. J. Nurs. 74:685, 1974.
10. *Narcotic Addiction in the Newborn.* Programmed Instruction, Johnson & Johnson Meducation, 1972.
11. Finnegan and Macnew: op. cit.
12. Gryboski, J.: *The swallowing mechanism of the neonate. I. Esophageal and gastric motility.* Pediatrics 35:445, 1965.
13. Ibid.: *Suck and swallow in the premature infant.* Pediatrics 43:96, 1969.

BIBLIOGRAPHY

General Texts

Behrman, R. E. (ed.): *Neonatology Diseases of the Fetus and Infant,* C. V. Mosby, St. Louis, 1973.

Klaus, M. H. and Fanaroff, A. A.: *Care of the High-Risk Neonate*, W. B. Saunders, Philadelphia, 1973.

Schaffer, A. J. and Avery, M. E.: *Diseases of the Newborn*, ed. 3. W. B. Saunders, Philadelphia, 1971.

Young, D. G. and Weller, B. F.: *Baby Surgery, Nursing Management and Care.* University Park Press, Baltimore, 1971.

Topical References

Abramson, H. (ed.): *Resuscitation of the Newborn Infant*, ed. 3. C. V. Mosby, St. Louis, 1973.
Chapter 2: *Physiology and biochemistry* by James, L. S. (transition from fetal to extrauterine life).
Chapter 10: *The first sixty seconds of life* by Apgar, V. and James, L. S. (assessment at birth).
Chapter 21: *Surgical emergencies in respiratory difficulties of newborn inants* by Coryllos, E. (mechanical problems involving the airways and lungs).

Assali, N. (ed.): *Pathophysiology of Gestation, vol. 3: Fetal and Neonatal Disorders.* Academic Press, New York, 1972.
Part I: *Disorders of circulation.*
Part II: *Disorders of respiration.*

Avery, M. E. and Fletcher, B. D.: *The Lung and Its Disorders in the Newborn Infant*, ed. 3. W. B. Saunders, Philadelphia, 1974.
Part II: *Disorders of respiration in the newborn period* (mechanical problems involving the airways and lungs, malformations of the thorax and diaphragm, hyaline membrane disease, meconium aspiration, pulmonary air leak).

Cornblath, M.: *Disorders of Carbohydrate Metabolism in Infancy*. W. B. Saunders, Philadelphia, 1966.
Part II: *Problems of the newborn and neonate.*

Duffey, M., et al. (eds.): *Current Concepts in Clinical Nursing, vol. 3*. C. V. Mosby, St. Louis, 1971.
Chapter 8: *Nursing care of high-risk infants* by Harris, C. H. (feeding and intravenous therapy, care of the baby with respiratory distress, psychologic and emotional problems in the intensive care nursery).

Lough, M.D., et al. (eds.): *Pediatric Respiratory Therapy.* Year Book Medical Publishers, Chicago, 1974.
Chapter 3: *Evaluation and care of the newborn infant* by Fanaroff, A. A. and Klaus, M. H. (resuscitation, transport, temperature control, oxygen therapy, treatment of hyaline membrane disease, assisted ventilation).
Chapter 6: *Mechanical ventilation* by Lough, M. D. (assisted ventilation equipment and techniques).

Oski, F. A. and Naiman, J. L.: *Hematologic Problems in the Newborn*, ed. 2. W. B. Saunders, Philadelphia, 1972.
Chapter 4: *Polycythemia in the neonatal period.*
Chapter 7: *Erythroblastosis fetalis* (Rh and ABO erythroblastosis, kernicterus, exchange transfusion).

Ross Laboratories Nursing Education Aids, No. 7: *Congenital Heart Abnormalities.* Columbus, Ohio, 1961.

Rowe, R. D. and Mehrizi, A.: *The Neonate with Congenital Heart Disease.* W. B. Saunders, Philadelphia, 1969.
Chapter 3: *Physical examination of the cardiovascular system of the newborn.*
Chapter 6: *The frequency of various cardiac malformations.*
Chapters 13, 21, 16, 20, 14, 17, 11, 25, 12, 29 and 9: (patent ductus, tricuspid atresia, pulmonary atresia, pulmonary stenosis, tetralogy of Fallot, total anomalous venous return, transposition, truncus arteriosis, VSD, ASD, and coarctation).

Stave, U. (ed.): *Physiology of the Perinatal Period, vol. 2.* Appleton-Century-Crofts, New York, 1970.
Part VII: *Hypoxia neonatorum.*
Chapter 35: *Metabolic Effects in Hypoxia Neonatorum*, by Stave, U. and Wolf, H. (asphyxia neonatorum).

Thaler, M. M.: *Perinatal bilirubin metabolism.* Schulman, I. (ed.): Advances in Pediatrics, vol 19. Year Book Medical Publishers, 1972, pp. 215–235. (physiologic jaundice of the premature and hyperbilirubinemia).

Winters, R. W. (ed.): *The Body Fluids in Pediatrics.* Little, Brown and Company, Boston, 1973.
Part II: *Disorders of the neonate.*
Chapter 9: *Acid-base changes in the perinatal period* by James, L. S. (fetal distress and asphyxia neonatorum).
Chapter 11: *Pathophysiology of birth asphyxia and resuscitation* by James, L. S. (asphyxia neonatorum and resuscitation).
Chapter 17: *Late metabolic acidosis of premature infants* by Kildeberg, P.

Selected Articles for Review

Behrman, R. E., et al.: *Treatment of the asphyxiated newborn infant.* J. Pediat. 74:981, 1969.

Choi, M.: *A comparison of maternal psychological reactions to premature and full size newborns.* Mater. Child Nurs. J. 2:1, 1973.

Daily, W. J. R., et al.: *Apnea in premature infants: Monitoring, incidence, heart rate changes, and an effect of environmental temperature.* Pediatrics 43:510, 1969.

Davis, L.: *Neonatal respiratory emergencies.* Nurs. Clin. North Am. 8:441, 1973.

Desmond, M., Rudolph, A. and Phitaksphraiwan, P.: *The transitional care nursery: A mechanism for preventive medicine in the newborn.* Ped. Clin. North Am. 16(3):651-669, 1966.

Dubowitz, L. M. S., et al.: *Clinical assessment of gestational age in the newborn infant.* J. Pediat. 77:1, 1970.

Edelmann, C. M., Jr. and Spitzer, A.: *The maturing kidney.* J. Pediat. 75:509, 1969.

Eng, G. D.: *Brachial plexus palsy in newborn infants.* Pediatrics 48:18, 1971.

Evans, J.: *Fundamentals of infant resuscitation.* Int. Anesthesiol. Clin. 11:141, 1973.

Fenner, A. et al.: *Periodic breathing in premature and neonatal babies: Incidence, breathing pattern, re-*

spiratory gas tensions, response to changes in the composition of ambient air. Pediat. Res. 7:174, 1973.

Finnegan, L. and Machew, B.: *Care of the addicted infant.* Am. J. Nurs. 74:685, 1973.

Freeland, E.: *Long-term follow-up studies of prematurely born infants. I. Relationships of handicaps to nursery routines.* J. Pediat. 80:501, 1972.

Galloway, K.: *Early detection of congenital anomalies.* J. Obstet. Gynecol. Nurs. 2:37, 1973.

Gilien, N.: *Determinants of Birth Weight.* In Duffey, M., et al. (eds.): *Current Concepts in Clinical Nursing, vol. 3.* C. V. Mosby, St. Louis, 1971, pp. 169–177.

Gillen, J.: *Behavior of newborns with cardiac distress.* Am. J. Nurs. 73:254, 1973.

Gregory, G. A., et al.: *Treatment of idiopathic respiratory distress syndrome with continuous positive airway pressure.* N. Eng. J. Med. 284:1333, 1971.

Harris, C. H.: *Some ethical and legal consideration in neonatal intensive care.* Nurs. Clin. of North Am. 8:521, 1973.

Harris, C.: *Social problems surrounding the high-risk infant.* In Anderson, E., et al. (eds.): *Current Concepts in Clinical Nursing, vol. 4,* C. V. Mosby, 1973, pp. 100–110.

Hasselmeyer, E.: *Indices of fetal welfare.* In Bergersen B., et al. (eds.): *Current Concepts in Clinical Nursing, vol. 2,* C. V. Mosby, St. Louis, 1973, pp. 298–317.

Jones, C., et al.: *Intravenous feeding of the newborn.* Nurs. Times 69:1364, 1973.

Katz, V.: *Auditory stimulation and developmental behavior of the premature infant.* Nurs. Res. 20:196, 1971.

Klaus, M. H. and Meyer, H. B. P.: *Oxygen therapy for the newborn.* Pediat. Clin. North Am. 13:731, 1966.

Kumpe, M., et al.: *Care of the infant with respiratory distress syndrome.* Nurs. Clin. North Am. 6:25, 1971.

Lees, M. H.: *Cyanosis in the newborn infant: Recognition and clinical evaluation.* J. Pediat. 77:484, 1970.

Lubchenco, L. O. and Bard, H.: *Incidence of hypoglycemia in newborn infants classified by birth weight and gestational age.* Pediatrics 47:831, 1971.

Lucey, J.: *Effects of light on the newly born infant.* J. Perinatal Med., Vols. I and III, pp. 147–150, 1973.

Lutz, L., et al.: *Temperature control in newborn babies.* Nurs. Clin. North Am. 6:15, 1971.

Maisels, M. J.: *Bilirubin—on understanding and influencing its metabolism in the newborn infant.* Pediat. Clin. North Am. 19:447, 1972.

Mast, F.: *Flight to life.* J. Obstet. Gynecol. Nurs. 3:15, 1974.

Meyers, R. E.: *Two patterns of perinatal brain damage and their conditions of occurrence.* Am. J. Obstet. Gynecol. 112:246, 1972.

Michaelis, R., et al.: *Activity states in premature and full term infants.* Dev. Psychobiol. 6:209, 1973.

Mingeot, R.: *The functional status of the newborn infant.* Am. J. Obstet. Gynecol. 115:1138, 1973.

Neal, M.: *Nursing care of the prematurely born neonate.* In Bergersen, B., et al. (eds.): *Current Concepts in Clinical Nursing, Vol. 2,* C. V. Mosby, St. Louis, 1969, pp. 332–339.

Neal, M. and Nauen, C.: *Ability of the premature infant to maintain his own body temperature.* Nurs. Res. 17:396, 1968.

Pildes, R. S.: *Infants of diabetic mothers.* N. Engl. J. Med. 289:902, 1973.

Reed, B.: *Management of the infant during labor, delivery and the immediate neonatal period.* Nurs. Clin. North Am. 6:3, 1971.

Reynolds, E.: *Neonatal intensive care, Parts I and II.* Nurs. Times 69:1220, 1972.

Roberts, J.: *Suctioning the newborn.* Am. J. Nurs. 73:63, 1973.

Slumek, M.: *Screening newborns for hearing loss.* Nurs. Outlook 19:115, 1971.

Robinson, R.: *The pre-term baby.* Brit. Med. J. 4:416, 1971.

Sinclair, J. C.: *Heat production and thermoregulation in the small-for-date infant.* Ped. Clin. North Am. 17:147, 1970.

Sinclair, J., et al.: *Supportive management of the sick neonate: Parenteral calories, water, electrolytes.* Pediat. Clin. North Am. 17:863, 1970.

Strickland, M.: *Fetal assessment techniques: A challenge to the nurse practitioner.* In Duffey, M., et al. (eds.): *Current Concepts in Clinical Nursing, Vol. 3,* C. V. Mosby, 1971, pp. 179–188.

Strickland, M.: *Environmental influences on the fetus.* In Anderson, E., et al. (eds.): *Current Concepts in Clinical Nursing,* vol. 4, C. V. Mosby, St. Louis, 1973, pp. 216–229.

Tempesta, L.: *The importance of touch in the care of newborns.* J. Obstet. Gynecol. Nurs. 1:17, 1972.

Todd, R. M.: *The baby of the diabetic mother.* Nurs. Times 69:1322, 1973.

Tsang, R. C., et al.: *Possible pathogenetic factors in neonatal hypocalcemia of prematurity.* J. Pediat. 82:423, 1973.

Tsang, R. C. and Oh, W.: *Neonatal hypocalcemia in low birth weight infants.* Pediatrics 45:773, 1970.

Tucson Medical Center: *Policies, Procedures and Guidelines for Regular and Special Nurseries, 1974.* Copies at cost for printing may be obtained by request to: Tucson Medical Center, 5301 E. Grant Road, Tucson, Arizona, 85733.

White, M., et al.: *Recognition and management of hypoglycemia in the newborn infant.* Nurs. Clin. North Am. 6:67, 1971.

Zwerdling, M. A.: *Factors pertaining to prolonged pregnancy and its outcome.* Pediatrics 40:202, 1967.

Winters, R.: *Principles of Pediatric Fluid Therapy.* Abbott Laboratories, 1970.

Zelson, C.: *Infant of the addicted mother.* N. Engl. J. Med. 288:1393, 1973.

Zelson, C., Rubio, E. and Wasserman, E.: *Neonatal narcotic addiction.* Pediatrics 48:178, 1971.

UNIT 10

CRISES DURING CHILDBEARING

39 *Adolescence*

ANN L. CLARK, R.N., M.A.

In spite of the fact that females today have more latitude in the control over their reproductive systems, pregnancy and motherhood in the adolescent population is on the increase, particularly among the 15 and under age group. In a recent U.S. Maternal and Child Health Service Report,[1] from one fifth to one third or more of maternity patients in representative local maternity projects supported by Maternal Child Health Services are teenagers. This is of great concern to medical and social agencies since adolescent pregnancies are associated with many high-risk factors. Two statistically significant findings are a higher rate of premature births and an increased rate of toxemia whenever consistent comprehensive prenatal care is not available or not utilized by the young woman (Table 39-1).

Aside from these biologic dangers, the lives of pregnant teenagers are disrupted, and their prospect for completing their education and becoming contributing members to the society are reduced. They face motherhood prematurely, often before their own nurturing has been completed. Pregnancy for the adolescent in our society is not often a maturing experience, especially for the very young. It imposes multiple stresses for the individual, as we shall see.

It is not known how many adolescent girls become pregnant each year, but we do know that over 200,000 school-age girls deliver babies each year and that their numbers are

TABLE 39.1. Complications in Teenage Pregnancies*

Investigators	*Nonwhite, %*	*Toxemia During Antepartum Period, %*	*Prematurity, %*	*Perinatal Loss, %*
Aznar and Bennett	90	9.8	18.7	5.0
Marchetti and Menaker	99	19.7	14.8	3.8
Morrison	95	21.0	16.0	3.8
Poliakoff	72	17.7	17.4	5.9
Sarrell and Klerman	97.5	5.0	10.8	0.8
Dickens et al.	95	5.0	12.0	1.0

* From Dickens, H., et al.: *One hundred pregnant adolescents, treatment approaches in a university hospital*. Am. J. Pub. Health 63:796, 1973, with permission.

increasing by about 3,000 annually.[2] Profiles of women and girls who now seek abortions are almost direct parallels of the women who previously released their children for adoption.[3] About 15 per cent of school-age girls are placing their babies for adoption, while close to 85 per cent are attempting to mother the child. Indeed, it is the very young, who frequently lack the experience and resources to rear a child alone, who are least likely to release the child for adoption; and it is in this age group in which pregnancy out-of-wedlock is increasing. Thus a substantial number of our young population is beginning family life at a very young age.[4]

GROWTH AND DEVELOPMENT

The adolescent girl has a very definite need to achieve her own developmental goals first, and this development is vital to her performance as a mother. Indeed, the very young adolescent is totally unready to mother her child. Moreover, the extent to which an individual can be successful in achieving her own developmental goals ultimately enhances her potential as a mother.[5]

ADOLESCENT MATURITY—A CRISIS

Adolescence is in itself a crisis period. It is, in fact, the crisis period that must precede maturity. Resolution of this period will bring about changes in the personality structure, but the resolution is never a smooth one. Because the adolescent is a "new person" in a sense, his ego is inexperienced in dealing with the numerous different tasks with which he is faced.[6]

The adolescent must deal with two normative crises—the crisis of independence and the crisis of self-discovery. The crisis first comes into view sometime after puberty, usually between 15 and 18 years of age.[7] In dealing with the crisis of independence the young person must emancipate himself from home and from dependence on his parents. In dealing with the crisis of self-discovery, he must search for self-identity which has previously lain unseen. He must discover the self that is a psychologic, and in a certain sense, a biologic entity which underlies the varying uses of the "ego" self. Self is the human organism seen through its own eyes.

The last step in the development of self is self-cognition. The self-concept of most persons is determined by the internalization of the behavior of others toward them. Thus, those accorded high esteem by others should reflect a higher self than those poorly regarded.[8] This is a vulnerable developmental stage of life and has great relevance for the subject under consideration, i.e., pregnancy and particularly out-of-wedlock pregnancy.

The development of the self-concept is dynamic. It arises from the complex of the person's interpersonal relationships and according to Sullivan[9] is determined by the way one organizes his experience to avoid or diminish anxiety.

Maturation is a threefold process. Each phase of the process—physical maturity, emotional maturity, and intellectual maturity—unfolds, to a degree, independently, but at the same time each process is inescapably interwoven with each of the other processes. The significance of each developmental phase is understood only as one views the total person. The major tasks facing an adolescent are:

1. To integrate growth in physical, social, and psychologic spheres.
2. To accept, develop, refine, and master a new identity.
3. To lay the groundwork for long-term mutual interpersonal relationships.
4. To develop patterns of work behavior that are consistent and reasonable for adult occupations and careers.[10]

PHYSICAL MATURATION

The spurt of physical growth during adolescence is nothing short of phenomenal. After a prepubertal period when the rate of growth is fairly even, there is a remarkable increase in the velocity of growth.

The changes in glandular secretions bring about changes in height, weight, body contour, and voice. Even though these may be desirable attributes, they may nonetheless prove to be embarrassing to young persons. Their bodies seem strange to them; they have, in fact, lost their old familiar bodies.

One of the major developmental tasks the adolescent girl must solve is to become acquainted with and integrate the bodily changes which take place. They tend to deny bodily changes until all others have noticed them, but finally these physical changes will necessitate a reorganization of the body image. Not all young people are pleased with what they see when they gaze in a mirror. Jersild's[11] study showed that of 83 girls interviewed, 38 were disturbed over their physical characteristics. Concern for physical appearance seems to have direct correlation with personal esteem.[12] These physical changes are superimposed on a vast number of experiences that have molded the young person's perception of her physical self and have impressed her with the importance of her physique and physical power.[13]

The young girl of today matures physically earlier than did the previous generation. She looks older and at times her sophistication leads one to expect greater maturity than she is capable of having at this stage. She has opportunities for boy-girl relationships which her mother was never allowed. This may well be reflected in the statistics stated earlier.

After menarche, a girl is potentially capable of becoming a mother and yet hardly acquainted with her new body or accustomed to her new clothes. Her counterpart, a boy, often so young that it seems incongruous to picture him as a father, is nevertheless her potential mate.

PREGNANCY

All adolescents who become pregnant are high medical risks. The younger the girl, the greater the risk to her and to her infant, for the additional nutrient demands of pregnancy may compromise her growth potential and that of her fetus. Unfortunately, many adolescent girls who become pregnant are from deprived socioeconomic backgrounds, where health facilities both quantitatively and qualitatively leave much to be desired. The girl may not seek early and consistent prenatal care because of society's response to her unwed condition. Indeed, even today it is not possible in some clinics for a girl to obtain an examination to determine if she is pregnant or to receive prenatal care unless parental consent is obtained.[14] This means that some girls go without prenatal care until very late in the pregnancy, jeopardizing their health and that of their unborn children.

The pregnant adolescent presents different management problems during all phases of her obstetric care.[15] Anemia and toxemia are common problems. Some authorities believe this reflects the nutritional status of teenagers rather than their chronological age. The very young adolescent may have cephalopelvic disproportion necessitating cesarean section. There are more births of infants who are premature or of low birth weight, resulting in increased hazards of neurologic handicaps.

Throughout the nation there are now prenatal adolescent clinics developing which combine education and medical and social service care. This results in much improved care for the expectant and new mother and her infant.[16–19] Family planning is made available to these young people during the early puerperium and encouragement and support are available to them as they assume the mothering role. Peer group interaction is encouraged.

PSYCHOSOCIAL MATURATION

The psychologic events of adolescence in our society are not necessarily counterparts of the physical changes of puberty, but a cultural invention—not a deliberate one, but a product of an increasing delay in the assumption of adult responsibilities.[20] In the early part of this century, young people, physiologically ready for sexual experiences, married and mated early. The culture sanctioned this behavior and there were adequate situational supports to assist the young couple to establish a home and a family. Readiness to assume a responsible position in life and to support a family today takes many more years to achieve. In the meantime, young people have all the usual sexual drives. Psychiatrists who work with adolescents have an opportunity to study the varied ways these drives are manifested. They see both extremes—asceticism with its exaggerated denial of sexuality, and teenagers who for one reason or another "engage in sexual experimentation in the manner of a child in a candy store."[21] Through sexual conquest or prowess they may be seeking acceptance from peers of the same or opposite sex. They may be looking for a way to express rebellion and defiance, or they may have found a way in which they can fulfill the negative prophecy of an angry parent. None of this is focused on getting pregnant, bearing, and rearing a child, although there may be unconscious wishes in that direction also.

One of the major developmental tasks and problems an adolescent girl must resolve in order to become an adult is to make choices which determine what kind of a feminine person she is going to be. For many girls today, there are a great many more conflicting pressures than there were for the girls of former generations. A girl may not have a clear understanding about what is appropriate, for example, how to evolve some standards of sexual behavior when conflicting pressures seem to be voiced with an equal degree of authority.[22]

As an aid in maturation, and with the loss of some of the ties to the parent, the adolescent turns to contemporaries for support, sometimes almost desperately. Social pressures and sexual anxieties are hidden by being "like everyone else" and a great deal of support is derived from peers. These factors are particularly important in adolescent pregnancies. Sometimes social workers are impressed by how little concern the young adolescent shows for the baby and how much she is concerned, comparatively, about the disruption of her peer relationships.[23]

Developmental tasks of this period of life, according to Erikson[24] are:

Crisis of Adolescence—Establishment of one's own identity
Crisis of Young Adulthood—Development of intimacy in relationships
Crisis of Adulthood—Generativity.

The adolescent who becomes pregnant finds herself struggling to solve the developmental crisis of growth, that of establishing one's own *identity*, while she is facing still another developmental crisis, that of *generativity* (an adult developmental task of creating and nurturing life). She may very likely be straddling still another developmental task which comes between these two, that of the crisis of *intimacy*. She has a lot of work to do, and needs a number of environmental supports to resolve these crises.

EMOTIONAL IMPACT OF PREGNANCY ON THE ADOLESCENT

Pregnancy for any woman is always accompanied by considerable emotional changes—some somatopsychic, others psychogenic. The former are produced by the hormonal and metabolic changes of pregnancy. These bring about mood swings, introversion, and passivity.[25] The psychogenically induced changes are frequently linked to the sexual aspects of pregnancy, i.e., pregnancy as an outcome of sexual relations. As pregnancy develops, a woman tends to ignore this factor and to focus her attention on the developing fetus and the motherhood aspects. She daydreams about the baby and turns her attention inward to "self." Any conflict which a woman may have in her sex life is likely to be stimulated by the fact that she is pregnant. The vicissitudes of her own previous sexual development are likely to be mirrored in her attitude toward pregnancy.[26]

The married adolescent, who may not as yet have developed a stable sense of self, or have worked out a meaningful sex relationship with her husband, and who finds herself pregnant with all the attendant psychogenic and somatopsychic changes may be in for a very difficult time indeed. If the marriage was necessitated by a premarital pregnancy, there may also be anxiety and guilt. Furthermore, the struggle for independence may be deterred by the need to turn to one or both sets of parents for financial aid. If a baby is born to an individual so young that motherhood is overlaid on the needs and wishes of the adolescence, there may be intense conflict between the wish to grow up and the wish to hold on to the security of childhood dependence and freedom from responsibility.[27] Consequently, a firm base on which motherliness can develop will be missing. Some girls literally turn their infants over to their mothers to rear, continuing to assume the role of daughter in the home, and the role of sibling to their own children.

The security which comes to an expectant mother through the understanding and support of a mature husband may also not be available to the girl married to an adolescent husband. Thus, the developmental task of adolescent maturity and the developmental task of mothering may both suffer, each compounding the other.

EMOTIONAL IMPACT OF PREGNANCY ON THE UNMARRIED ADOLESCENT

There is an acute emotional crisis brought on by an out-of-wedlock pregnancy and the attendant feelings of guilt and of being "trapped." Many unwed teenage expectant mothers find that their struggle to free themselves from dependency on their families is served a painful blow, for now the only way out of the dilemma is submission to the parents. It must be remembered also that the etiology of the problem is often a disturbed parent-child relationship with feelings of lack of love and security. Being unloved, internalized as being unloveable, may very well have already had an effect on the value system of the adolescent. The sexual relationship that resulted in the pregnancy represents a synthetic substitute for love.[28] If the sexual partner now rejects or refuses to acknowledge his paternity and abandons the expectant mother, her feeling of worthlessness is reinforced. Many unwed teenagers have related to the author their serious consideration of suicide as a way out of a crisis where "no one cares anyway." Although they did not carry out the act, the fact that they considered it gives some indication of the degree of distress.

Since the unwed mother is also subjected to the same hormonal and metabolic changes as any pregnant woman, it is very difficult to know the basis for any given emotional upset that the girl may experience. That she does have emotional upsets is evidenced by her acting out of anxiety through hostility, rebellion, and anger, and by her frequent psychosomatic complaints. She may be terrified of labor and during the experience may be so anxious that she nears the panic stage.

If the decision is made to relinquish the baby, the adolescent mother is now faced with coping with separation anxiety, grief, and bereavement—crises she is poorly prepared to resolve. One of the expressions of grief may be projection of hostility onto others. It may also include expression of sorrow and, frequently, verbalization of guilt. These behaviors are readily observable in a home for unwed mothers. She may, of course, keep her child. This may come about by choice, or be necessitated by the lack of adoption demands for certain cultural groups. The support and care of the child may necessitate further dependence on the parents, thereby continually blocking emotional maturity.

The total experience of unwed pregnancy and the reactions of society to the girl and her situation will be potent forces on this adolescent's self-concept. Although the pregnancy may be a purposive acting out of inner drives and the best solution the person could find to her emotional dilemma, it is nevertheless responsible for even more psychologic problems in her life.

Successful motherhood is a positive outcome of a new maturational crisis presented by pregnancy.[29] The maturational crisis of adolescence must be faced and resolved first, however, before one can confidently expect the young person to resolve the maturational crisis of parenthood.

INTELLECTUAL MATURATION

School-age girls who become pregnant are concerns for every school system in the United States. Unfortunately, they are still too often seen as problems to be solved by banishment rather than as long-range concerns to be dealt with openly. A number of young people, therefore, are left without sufficient education and marketable skills, so that they end up becoming social risks. Pregnancy is a major cause of school dropouts among girls in the United States. Many of these girls do not return to school following their deliveries. This leads to limited employment opportunities, unemployment, and increased dependence on welfare.

There is a way to counter this trend, and fortunately more and more interdisciplinary teams of teachers, social workers, nurses, and physicians are involved in bringing about a change. In 1968 the Children's Bureau sponsored the creation of Cyesis Programs Consortium. Through research, demonstration, and grants, communities are given assistance in providing comprehensive programs for school-age parents. At present, more than 150 communities offer these programs.[30] Some programs also offer services to the mothers of the pregnant adolescents and to the adolescent fathers.

Many comprehensive programs have goals that encompass intellectual maturation in addition to their goals for physical care. One program states its goals as:

> To offer a pregnant young woman opportunity and encouragement to develop her inner strengths, examine her alternatives, make the best choice to meet her needs and those of her family; to help her to mature; and to foster her feelings of hope for the future.
>
> To assure mother and child the best obstetrical care and knowledge obtainable during pregnancy and to motivate young families to continue to pursue medical care.
>
> To offer a young mother opportunity to continue her public school education; to encourage her to approach education as a means of self-realization; and to aid her and her family in developing future educational or vocational plans.[31]

Through such programs, young expectant and new mothers are offered an opportunity to continue their education, modified if necessary in keeping with their condition of pregnancy. In some programs she remains in her own school, in others she attends a special school, and in still others special classes are offered in a center where medical and social care are also provided. She may continue in these special schools for a time after her delivery, with infant care in a nursery provided for her child during class hours.

The program gears prenatal education to the level of the student. Peer group instruction has been found to more nearly meet the needs of the adolescent, promoting the teaching-learning process and reducing the tension level of individual members.

The programs also facilitate the learning of parenting skills. It is important that the teaching of childrearing skills be made relevant to the practices of various ethnic and racial groups, for the learning of childrearing skills encompasses attitudes, values, and beliefs. However, certain practices, such as a balanced diet and the need of infants early environmental enrichment, transcend cultural differences.[32]

WHO BECOMES AN UNWED MOTHER?

Who are the girls who become unwed mothers? This question is asked first to put it to rest. Stereotyping individuals by race, culture, socioeconomic stratum, and so forth will not be useful to the discussion of unwed mothers. To begin with, we have no accurate statistics on the number of such pregnancies. It is probably much larger than the number mentioned in the beginning of this chapter. Some cultures and socioeconomic groups must turn to public facilities to resolve, at least in part, the problems of pregnancy out of wedlock. The more affluent members of our society are often able to do so without assistance. Birth certificates are likely inaccurate. The life style of some segments of our society does not include medical assistance at the time of birth and the recording of the newborn individuals. Suffice it to say, pregnancy out of wedlock is to be found in every social and cultural group. It has occurred down through the ages but is more evident today in the more open society in which we live.

WHY ARE THERE UNWED MOTHERS?

Since out-of-wedlock pregnancies so frequently signal the beginning of a cycle of new unstable families that often end in divorce, or failure of continuing formal education and dependency on the state's welfare system, it seems appropriate to ask why. In asking the question and exploring all possible answers to it, nurses should be better prepared to understand the client and to assist her, her infant, and others significant to her in dealing with the crisis.

In working with pregnant adolescents, one finds, as with adult women, that

being pregnant,
having a baby, and
nurturing an infant

can often all be very separate events. Sometimes none of the events are desired; sometimes only one is desired. These facts help in understanding the behavior that leads to

pregnancy
submission to an abortion
producing a baby
relinquishing the baby
keeping and nurturing the baby
keeping the baby, but turning its caretaking over to others.

According to Notman,[33] pregnancy in an unwed girl is usually an unrealistic attempt at some solution of her *conflict*. The causes are complex. Some very few are genuine accidents. Most are determined by the concurrence of several causal factors: the conscious and unconscious *meaning of the pregnancy* to both parents, but particularly the girl; her *state of mind and emotions at the time pregnancy occurs*; her *life situation*, and her *mode of expression of wishes and defensive patterns*. A girl is more likely to expose herself to pregnancy if she has a character pattern of living out unconscious wishes in an *impulsive* manner, and if she has a tendency to *overlook realities when under pressure* either from inner feelings or outer circumstances.

The above paragraph contains a number of

key words which are helpful in

understanding the girl
understanding the environment in which she became pregnant.

These words are included below in question form:

1. What behaviors does the girl display that give clues that there is a *conflict*? (See Chapter 8 on Frustration and Conflict.)
2. What are the goals that bring about the *conflict*?
3. What does the pregnancy and/or baby *mean* to the girl?
4. What were her *state of mind* and *emotions* just prior to the sexual relationship which resulted in the pregnancy?
5. What were her *state of mind* and *emotions* when she learned she was pregnant?
6. What is her *life situation*?
7. Over a period of time, what mode does she use to *express wishes*? What *defensive patterns* does she utilize?
8. Does she act *impulsively*?
9. Faced with a *pressure*, is she *reality* oriented?

The girl may have a wish for a baby. This wish may be of considerable importance to her even though she may be too young or too immature to really care for the infant. Sometimes this infant is seen as something that belongs "just to me." This may occur when the girl has suffered loss of significant figures in her life. Most significant is the loss of her mother, especially if there has been no adequate and consistent mothering available. Other losses, such as father's desertion or death of a beloved and supportive grandmother, may be contributing factors. Many young women have never had a stable relationship with a supportive figure, having lived in numerous foster homes or institutions.

Even if the mother was present, the young person still may have experienced a deprived childhood if the mother was too busy or too unconcerned to nurture the child. In this sense the girl is attempting to recreate a closeness which she may long for and idealize because she has never had an adequate one. On the other hand, the wish for a baby may result from a feeling of emptiness and chronic inner depression. The girl may fantasize that the baby will fill the void, in that she will be loved by the baby.

In other cases, neither pregnancy nor motherhood may be desired. It may be that the girl is seeking a relationship which will overcome the feelings of solitude and depression by sampling the "forbidden pleasures" of sex. The pregnancy and the infant are unplanned and undesired outcomes of her attempt to fill a void. When the girl's environment has lacked tenderness, she may turn to any mate whom she feels she can trust to give her the tenderness without considering the sequelae of pregnancy and a baby. She may simply feel the strong need to get close to someone, to feel contact, while the specific sexual nature of the closeness may be secondary.

The girl's fantasies regarding the pregnancy often involve some aspect of her relationship with her mother. Strict physical punishment in early childhood may have produced a rebellious individual. This rebelliousness is expressed in terms of acting out behavior, sexually and socially. Thus she retaliates by physical means. In some instances it is a desperate means of finally enlisting the mother's assistance or of finally getting some attention. The mother may have failed to serve as an adequate feminine image with which the girl can identify, thus growth and development of the self-concept as a feminine figure is underdeveloped.

Sexual curiosity, brought about by erotic allurement of our mass media and our "fun society" may result in an undesired pregnancy. Coupled with this, there would need to be an unrealistic expectation that "pregnancy couldn't happen to me," so no precautions against conception are taken. Peer pressure coupled with a weak ego, even in the face of lack of pleasure in the sexual relationship, may be strong enough to provide an experience in which pregnancy may occur.

A young girl who is not succeeding in school may well be a prime candidate to become an unwed mother. The pregnancy represents a way of escaping from an unsatisfactory educational experience.

Family patterns, too, seem to have implications. When the mother, and/or older sisters have born babies out of wedlock, the girl may come to expect that she has little control over what happens and acknowledge the inevitable by following in their path.

There is a disproportionate number of young women with physical defects who become unwed mothers. It is felt this represents a need to bear a child and to keep it as evidence of her wholeness, desirability, and femininity.

In a recent study by Perez-Reyes,[34] three different behavior patterns were discerned in pregnant girls in *early* adolescence:

1. The very young, inexperienced, passive girl who "submits" to intercourse under pressure of an older and casual male partner.
2. The adolescent who has started forming heterosexual relations and as part of the sexual experience between her and her boyfriend, reaches intercourse before she becomes fully aware of the possible consequence.
3. The adolescent with a history of emotional problems starting from early adolescence, increased marked conflict between her and her parents, who practices intercourse as part of a pathological pattern of behavior to fulfill unsatisfied emotional needs.

There are many other reasons for pregnancy out of wedlock. Early relationships with the male parent, pressure of the male partner to prove his virility, and rape are some of these.

The conflict that the pregnancy is supposed to resolve often leaves the young person in a vulnerable position. The pregnancy generally constitutes a crisis, for which situational support is needed. Moreover, more conflicts ensue because of the pregnancy and birth. There are many role conflicts to be found in being a daughter, a mother, and a student. Peer relationships may well change. The pregnant adolescent finds herself estranged from friends. The adolescent task of self-identity no longer has the advantage of peer input and feedback. Conflict is incumbent in the need to mature as an adolescent individual first, while at the same time being pressured to mature beyond one's years as a mother.

The pregnant adolescent may present a picture of bewilderment. Fright, anxiety, rebelliousness, insecurity, and self-destruction may constitute some of her feelings and behaviors. She may also feel guilty and feel great concern over her parents' response to her problem. She may hunger for attention and present interesting ways of attention-getting. Sometimes the mother's attention to her and to her problems is most gratifying—one suspects the overall motive may have been just that.

THE UNWED FATHER

In the past, little was known about the unwed father, since there were no valid followup studies about him. He was generally viewed as someone who had "taken advantage" of the girl and then refused to stand by her in her crisis. However, social workers, nurses, and others knew of many instances when he had been a supportive person. Frequently the pregnant girl refused to divulge his name or even to inform him of his impending paternity. If he was informed, he sometimes refused to acknowledge his paternity. To complicate matters, families of young people often stepped in with legal council. This often broke up an otherwise supportive relationship between the two. The law in many states could punish the putative father on the grounds of rape or of assaulting a minor. Therefore, many girls did not reveal the name of the father because of fear of repercussions.

Only recently has counseling been made available to the unwed father. There is also now some research which begins to clarify the relationship between the unwed mother and her mate. Although there are many variations to this relationship, often it is a relatively enduring one the couple has after knowing each other for some time, and the male often remains in the picture offering support in varying ways to the expectant mother. Some of these relationships lead to marriage, often after the infant's birth. Girls have stated they wanted it that way in order to "see how he treats the baby and me," or "that way they can't say he was forced to marry me." Other girls paradoxically state, "I like him, but I wouldn't want to marry him or have him raise my child."

It is important that we learn as much as we can about the unwed father, for as Pannor[35] has pointed out:

> Helping unwed parents to reshape their lives and to act responsibly will make them better people, strengthen the generation that is to follow, and the one after that—an important goal for the helping professions.

The unwed father, like his mate, tends to be surprised when the relationship results in a pregnancy. He often knows about contraceptives but uses them sporadically or not at all, stating that to do otherwise would debase the relationship.

Often he is as frightened as the expectant mother when he learns he is about to become a father. It is not unusual for him to drop out of school because of his girl friend's pregnancy. He may feel a deep sense of responsibility for this young woman and the child. Some young men have gone as far as to commit suicide in their despair.

Today many agencies that offer a comprehensive program for adolescent parents include the father in this program. Since he, too, is struggling with the developmental tasks of adolescence, and particularly with his developing sexuality, he often admits to unsatisfactory sexual relationships leaving him depressed, guilty, and anxious, and would take advantage of counseling if it were available to him. He needs to understand how and why he became a father and the serious implications to the mother, the child, and himself. He needs to know the legal implications of his actions and his legal rights. He needs help to understand his sexual feelings and beliefs. He needs to have an appropriate part in decisions related to his paternity. Accepting responsibility for his actions and making decisions related to resolution are maturing experiences for him.

All unwed fathers are not as pictured above. Some are only slightly known to the unwed mother. He may have been a necessary part of her impregnation, but having served his purpose, she may not wish to identify him. Some men refuse to admit their paternity and reject the expectant mother, adding to her feeling of worthlessness.

Some men who father a child are unlikely prospects for marriage. This may bring added shame to the girl's family, which may be what she had in mind when she chose him as her sexual mate. Knowledge about the man who fathers the child and about the relationship between the girl and her mate can be of assistance in helping to better understand the unwed mother as well.

THE NURSING ROLE

THE NURSE AND THE PATIENT

Pregnancy out of wedlock is seldom a welcomed state. Even though moral standards seem to have changed (society seems more tolerant), attitudes toward the pregnancy are negative. The negative aspects may run the gamut from "inconvenient" to "disastrous," depending upon the girl's circumstances. Some nurses, due to the transmission of values by their own culture, have many strong feelings about the unwed mother. All nurses have some feelings about the appropriateness of the pregnancy. These feelings vary and each nurse responds in a different manner, depending on who it is that is pregnant and how the patient responds to the pregnancy.

The important point to be made here is that it is essential for the nurse to recognize these feelings and try to understand what causes them. Some patients for whom the nurse plans and administers nursing care will come from her own socioeconomic class. Many will come from a culture about which she understands little. Unless the nurse is fully aware of what her feelings are, she may do one of two things, neither of which will be helpful. She may 1) overidentify with the girl, or 2) begin to stereotype individuals. When she does either of these two things, she fails to develop a professional nursing identity with the pregnant adolescent and she limits her efficacy as a therapeutic person.

ASSESSMENT*

Assumptions made about how a specific unmarried mother feels or how she perceives her pregnancy are of little use to a nurse. All patients do *not* feel guilty, although many do. All patients do *not* have a negative attitude toward the pregnancy, although many do. Some women want to remain anonymous, others are not concerned. A few patients seem to easily relinquish their babies, others find it difficult or impossible to do so. The nurse needs to *assess* how stressful each part of the situation is, how the patient is coping with the stress, what factors in her environment hinder her coping, and what factors in her environment support her coping. On this basis she can then plan nursing care which will protect and nurture the individual.

Culture

With the exception of some more primitive cultures, out-of-wedlock pregnancy is recognized and some pronouncements are made about it. Even within a given culture, it is important to recognize that cultures have strata. Within that culture, certain members will be upwardly mobile, while others will be downwardly mobile. All of this will have impact on the expectant mother and her need for care. Cultural pronouncements will provide the nurse with some general ideas about the impact that the experience will have on a specific patient. One must then validate this implied impact with the individual who is one's patient.

In the Black and Puerto Rican cultures, marriage is considered desirable and most persons do marry. However, consensual unions are an acceptable alternative. Relationships with more than one man at a time are considered pernicious. Thus, if a sexual relationship is established prior to marriage, it should ideally be a meaningful one and often it is indeed a stable one.[36]

Culture defines what stigma, if any, is attached to being an unwed mother. A girl may have been born out of wedlock, but when she becomes pregnant her own mother generally expresses disappointment. This is often less of a moral sanction than a concern over the problems and hardships her daughter will face. If a girl from one socioeconomic level does not feel guilt in the same way as a person from another level, it may only indicate that guilt is accepted more stoically.

---

* Adapted, in part, from Nursing History, Young Women's Maternity Clinic, developed by Eleanor W. Smith under U.S. Public Health Services Contract No. N1H 72-4216 granted to Department of Family Health Care Nursing, School of Nursing, University of California, San Francisco.

Some cultures strongly disapprove of placing a child for adoption. High value is placed on children by both Puerto Ricans and Blacks. Perhaps this in itself is an important factor in making out-of-wedlock pregnancies more acceptable to them.[37]

Part of the nurse's assessment process should therefore include:

1. Culture
2. Socioeconomic strata of society
3. Responses of significant members of the girl's family to the pregnancy.

Relationship with Significant Others

It is important that the nurse have an awareness of who is significant to the young unwed mother and what her relationship is with them. The family constellation and the girl's place in the family will help the nurse to plan care, using whatever situational supports the girl has or that can be mobilized in her behalf. They can become a balancing factor in helping to resolve the crisis in which the girl finds herself. The nurse should therefore assess:

1. Is her mother and/or father living and does she reside with one or both of them?
2. If one parent is not living or resides in some other place, at what age did the break occur?
3. If she resides with someone else, who is this person(s) and how long has she resided with them?
4. Number and ages of siblings. Her place in the family constellation.
5. With whom does she have the most meaningful relationship and why?
6. Does she have close relatives living nearby and, if so, how often does she see them?
7. What changes would she like to make in her present living arrangements?

In relation to the girl's mother:

1. How does she get along with her mother? During childhood? In adolescence? Now?
2. Her mother's response to her pregnancy? (If she has not been informed, are there plans to do so?)
3. What has the mother told her daughter about her own pregnancy, labor, and delivery?
4. If she plans to keep her child, will she and her mother agree about how to raise a child?

In relation to the baby's father:

1. His age, education, work.
2. How long has their relationship existed? Is it continuing now?
3. How do they get along with each other?
4. What was his response upon learning of the pregnancy? (If he has not been informed, are there plans to do so?)
5. How is he helpful/not helpful to the girl?
6. Since the pregnancy occurred, have changes occurred in his education, job, or future goals?
7. What kind of help does he need? (Education, vocational training, work, learning about childbearing and childrearing.)

Sex and Sex Education

Adolescents are individuals striving to understand their sexuality and to evolve some standards of sexual behavior. An increasing number of young women, some very young indeed, are becoming sexually active, sometimes with a variety of sexual partners. This fact appears to be associated with an increased incidence of cervical cancer. Moreoever, the life style of many young persons leads to vaginal infections including venereal diseases, to the development of condylomas, and to hepatitis. A knowledge of the girl's manner of relating sexually, her use of contraceptives, and her knowledge of sex generally will be a necessary part of assessment. This information is needed during the pregnancy for counseling purposes and after the pregnancy is terminated:

1. How old was she when she first had sexual relations?
2. How does she feel about them? (Enjoys it, doesn't like it, is indifferent to it.)
3. What did her parents tell her about sex and where else did she learn about sex?
4. How frequently does she have sexual relations?
5. What does the present relationship with the baby's father mean to her and how (if at all) would she like it to be different?
6. Has she used any method of preventing pregnancy? If so, what, and what is her opinion of the method(s) used?
7. Has she regularly used any method of preventing pregnancy that failed to work for her?
8. How does the baby's father feel about birth control for her? What kind of birth control does he prefer? Would he be willing to take responsibility for birth control, e.g., use a condom as a temporary form of contraception until an I.U.D. can be placed or a pill cycle completed?
9. Does her mother want her to use birth control?
10. When does she want her next baby and what does she wish to do to prevent pregnancy until she is ready?
11. What else would she like to learn about sex? About birth control?

Self-Concept

We have explored earlier in this chapter the adolescent developmental task of self-discovery. The concept of self may have been a causative factor in the girl having become pregnant. It will most surely enter into the experience of pregnancy. The adolescent is often ashamed of and uncomfortable with her pregnant body. The bulging abdomen is proof of her sexual activity and is embarrassing to her. Assessment of her self-concept should include:

1. Is there anything about herself she would like different or changed? (Appearance, behavior, getting along with others, etc.)
2. How does she view her pregnant body?
3. Other concerns.

There should also be an accurate assessment throughout pregnancy of:

1. Grooming
2. Posture
3. Dress
4. Behavior.

Anxiety and Coping Behaviors

Anxiety is experienced when there is a threat to a biologic need or a threat to the security of self. Although it is simple to say that pregnancy out of wedlock would be both a biologic threat and a threat to the self system, it is unwise to use one's own standards to judge how another will experience or respond to a stress. Age, past experiences, and physical states may bring about differences in the way one views a threat. Anxiety is identifiable (see Chapter 9 on the Concept of Anxiety). The nurse needs to recognize the stresses her patient is experiencing and observe the manner in which she is coping with them. Moreover, preparation for the many events of pregnancy, labor, birth, and childrearing can be anticipated and prepared for. Preparation for an event can reduce the threat, and thus anxiety may be avoided or lessened. When anxiety is observed, it is important to also recognize the level of anxiety in order to intervene appropriately. Assessment for stress and anxiety should include:

1. Was the pregnancy planned?
2. Why does she think she got pregnant?
3. What were her feelings when she first realized she was pregnant?
4. What did she do to try to start her missed period?
5. How does she consider resolving the pregnancy? (Abortion, marriage, adoption, suicide, etc.)
6. Whom did she first tell about her pregnancy and what was their response? What were her feelings about their response?
7. How will the pregnancy change her life?
8. Does she or has she felt nervous, upset, anxious?
9. What does she do to help herself when she gets upset? (Cry, talk, clean house, walk, yell, throw things, withdraw, think things out, etc.)
10. Does she feel she has someone with whom she can talk out her feelings and problem?
11. Does she feel her relationship with others has changed recently? (Have they indicated she is hostile, sarcastic, belittling, noncommunicative? Does she feel that they are behaving in any of these ways?)

Observe also for:

1. Changes in voice (quality, rate, tone).
2. Flood of talk, repetitive talking, stuttering.
3. Activity (trembling, tapping, doodling, pacing, etc.).
4. Selective inattention to some aspects of the problem.
5. Disassociating, or excluding from awareness, certain topics.
6. Distortion of reality.

Collect data on:

1. Insomnia
2. Psychosomatic responses (diarrhea, nausea, etc.)
3. Palpitation.

Expectant Parent Education And Care

Nursing care plans for the adolescent mother include transmission of information related to the physiologic and psychologic changes of pregnancy, hygiene of pregnancy, and preparation for labor, delivery, and for the care of the child. To be effective, this education must be modified to meet the adolescent's needs and is preferably taught with her peers. As with any educational preparation, it should be based on what knowledge she already brings to the sessions and geared to her felt needs, but supplemented by the knowledge the nurse anticipates she will also find useful in the future. Assessment should include:

1. What she feels she needs or wants to know about having a baby, being a good mother, building a sound marriage relationship, doing what she wants with her life, and being the kind of person she wants to be.
2. Her concerns about her health, her pregnancy, her baby, her relationships with the baby's father, and her relationships with her family.

Some more specific assessment would include:

1. Does she know anyone who has had a good experience during pregnancy, labor, and delivery (the details) or someone who has had a bad experience?
2. What does she anticipate labor will be like for her?
3. Has anything happened to her in the

past, or is happening presently, that worries her about her pregnancy? About her baby?

4. What is her usual health? How does she feel different (if at all) now that she is pregnant?
5. Has she ever been hospitalized? What was the experience like? (Good or bad.) Did she prefer to share a room with others or to be alone? Did she feel things were done to her that she did not understand?
6. What does she think will help her when she is in labor? Who would she like to have with her while she is in labor? (Is this wish realistic?)
7. Does she regularly take any medications? Any "street" drugs?
8. Has she ever seen a newborn?
9. Has she had any experience in caring for small babies?
10. What will she do when the baby cries?
11. How does she plan to feed the baby? How did she arrive at that decision?
12. Who will help her to care for herself and the infant when she leaves the hospital?
13. What are her fantasies (daydreams) about her baby?
14. What preparation has she made for the baby? Is a name chosen?
15. What are her feelings when the fetus moves (hurt, disturbed, pleased, etc.)?
16. Does the fetus move too much, too little?
17. If she returns to school or to work, who will care for the baby? Is that arrangement satisfactory to her?

The Future

The nurse will need specific data related to the girl's plans and goals for the future. This data will be useful and is built on the present:

1. Her school and the last grade completed.
2. Her feeling about school. What she does well and what subjects give her the most difficulty.
3. What work experience she has had.
4. Her hobbies. How she spends an average day.
5. Her plans to continue in school or to receive vocational training.
6. The kind of work she would like to do (expects to do). Is this realistic or more of a fantasy?
7. The kind of work she really expects to be able to do (reality-based).
8. Her responsibilities outside of school and/or work.
9. What changes she thinks this pregnancy will make in her educational and vocational plans.

PLANS FOR NURSING ACTION

Crisis theory will prove most useful to nurses in assisting the adolescent unwed mother to work through the disequilibrium she will likely experience. By using crisis theory, it can be anticipated that better problem solving and an increased potential for self-realization and maturity will ensue. The nurse can and undoubtedly will enter into any one of the balancing factors in helping to restore equilibrium and to negate the possibility of future crisis, i.e.,

Establishing a realistic perception of the event
Finding adequate environmental support
Finding useful coping mechanism
Helping with anticipatory planning.

The assessment process itself will facilitate three things:

1. It will indicate to the nurse that the tension, anxiety, depression, and degree of inability to function makes the diagnosis of crisis appropriate.

2. The assessment will give the nurse a clear picture of what factors can be relied upon to help the girl to establish equilibrium and what factors are missing.
3. The assessment process in itself becomes part of the technique in the crisis intervention, for the process will bring feelings out in the open and can be used to help the girl to gain intellectual understanding.

In the young unwed mother, disequilibrium due to lack of adequate coping mechanisms may occur time and time again. Anticipating some of these periods is helpful:

Discovery of the pregnancy.
Response of significant others to the girl.
Crisis of education.
Decision to carry the pregnancy to term or to have an abortion.
Labor and birth.
Decisions related to keeping the child and rearing it or to place it in a foster home or to place it for adoption.
Planning for the future.

Hopefully, the nurse will have other professionals in a team with whom she can work. However, except for medical assistance, she may be the one to assume major responsibility in assisting the girl to resolve the crisis. The remainder of this chapter discusses the role of the nurse in applying crisis theory during the periods listed above.

APPLICATION OF CRISIS THEORY

Discovery of the Pregnancy

The interview will be the method of choice in which nurse and patient can examine the fear, if indeed there is a fear, realistically. Obviously, either the girl is pregnant or she is not, and a diagnosis needs to be made. The nurse is in a position to collect significant data to establish the possibility, remembering that some very young people may still believe they can become pregnant even though sexual relations have not occurred. If the girl has engaged in sexual relations, it is possible in some "walk in" clinics for the nurse to collect a urine specimen and make the diagnosis. Even if the girl is not pregnant, but admits to being sexually active, the nurse needs to help her with anticipatory planning and to grasp the reality of the situation, i.e., that unless she is using conception control she could become pregnant. If the nurse cannot make the diagnosis of pregnancy, she should refer the girl to a physician. The nurse would then explore who, if anyone, could accompany her to the medical office. She should explain to the girl what the physician will include in his examination and how the diagnosis of pregnancy will be made.

Denial may be the girl's method of coping with any stressful events. Even in the face of obvious abdominal and breast enlargement and fetal movements, the girl may deny she knew she was pregnant. Indeed, she may deny having ever had sexual relations and that therefore the whole possibility of pregnancy is unacceptable. These are often not falsehoods, but a real attempt to use an actual psychotic mechanism to distort the reality which is perceived.[38] Through a trusting relationship, she can be helped to accept the reality. In sharing the reality, the nurse can assist the girl to begin to look at the alternatives at her disposal in dealing with the real fact that a baby is growing within her.

Response of Significant Others

Once the diagnosis of pregnancy is made, it is very likely that other persons significant to the young woman will need to be informed. Parents, siblings, or the sexual partner can be potent forces in supporting the young woman. On the other hand, they may reject her, punish her, or abandon her. Realistically, it must be recognized that when the diagnosis is shared with family members the crisis expands to become a family crisis. Assessment of who can be relied upon to offer situational support is crucial. The young person may be very sure that her parents will not assist her in any way only to find that, after the response to the shock has been resolved, they show concern for her in a manner she has not experienced before. In a preliminary study conducted by Smith,[39] it appears that close mother-daughter relationships can occur during the period and are therapeutic in that they help the daughter to assume the role of mother to her own child, while at the same time they prepare the grandmother to finally relinquish the mothering role to her daughter. This closeness is of a very supportive nature in many instances. It is suggested by this study that, in appropriate instances, nurses can encourage the healthy aspects of this relationship by increasing the involvement of the mother with her adolescent daughter. By so doing, role identity of each can be facilitated.

It may be that the relationship of the mother and daughter is already fraught with pathology and neither is able or willing to be supportive. Older sisters, peers, or the sexual partner may offer the needed environmental support. Nurses, social workers, and others in the helping professions act first to assist the girl to find adequate support and, failing that, to become the situational support.

Bringing feelings out into the open, gaining understanding of the feelings, as well as the feeling of others, and learning new useful coping mechanisms to deal with the response of others to the pregnancy are techniques used by the nurse to intervene in the crisis.

Crisis of Education

If the girl is still in school, she must realistically face the consequences to her education. The nurse, knowing the alternatives, if any, open to the young woman, can help her to share her problem with the school authorities and work out ways to continue her education. The comprehensive service programs discussed previously include a provision for continued education during and after the pregnancy. Such programs are becoming more widespread. The nurse should encourage the girl to continue her education or seek vocational training. She shares with the girl the reality of the future, for whether the girl keeps the infant or gives it up for adoption, if she lacks formal education, she will be ill-prepared to support herself and her family and will more than likely be headed for a life on welfare.

Anticipatory planning must also include knowledge of self-care during pregnancy and knowledge of how to create a stable family unit in which a child can be nurtured and can grow. The literature is full of examples of the peer group method of meeting the informational and psychologic needs of a pregnant adolescent.[40] The climate of these groups is not easy to establish. The nurse should work to permit freedom to expose lack of knowledge and to seek answers. At the same time she must set some limits on behavior so that the topic in focus can be adequately explored before moving on to a new topic. Misconceptions about reproduction are frequent among adolescents. The birth process is usually seen as frightening and carries the possibility of mutilation and death. The realities of labor and birth must become a part of any expectant parent education program.

Visual aids are helpful, but should be used with care for the adolescent has a keen sense of the dramatic. Films may well feed her fantasies. Some nurses who conduct classes for adolescent expectant mothers feel that slides have a wider application than films. Whatever an instructor's preferences, flexibility is the key. Some groups will wish to view a film on birth. This can be successful with careful preparation. Prior knowledge of the physiology of birth, physical preparation for labor, and an explanation of the anxiety-producing scenes in the film are prerequisites. Individual preferences, even in a group, should be respected. There should be a full discussion of the film following its use. The kinds of questions asked often give the nurse insight into the felt anxiety. She can use this opportunity for learning, i.e., name the concept (anxiety) and help the group to relate their feelings to the threat they have just experienced.

Tours, role playing, and other creative methods of keeping interest, and enhancing understanding of the human body and of the needs of an infant, help the girl to prepare emotionally, physically, and pragmatically for motherhood.[41]

Besides meeting the needs for information and providing anticipatory guidance, a group discussion can help build self-esteem. Self-confidence and a sense of importance are nourished when a girl receives feedback that what she has to say is considered important by the group leader. The goal of the group can become one of utilizing the many ego strengths of each girl. Thus, the peer group method of learning may well fulfill some of the techniques of crisis intervention in that it can offer environmental support, help to discover useful coping mechanisms, help to establish realistic perceptions of events, facilitate the expression of feelings, and offer opportunity for anticipatory planning.

Decisions Related to the Pregnancy

The decision must be made whether to carry the pregnancy to term or to seek an abortion. However, these alternatives may not be available to all girls. Religious, medical, moral, and social pressures have to be considered. The girl's family will likely bring pressure to bear. The parents, for example, may not be willing and/or able to support the girl and her baby. There may not be infant care available so that the young woman can pursue her education or vocation. These are realities that must be explored and worked through.

Usually the decision related to continuing with the pregnancy or seeking an abortion must be made within a short period of time due to the increased danger of an abortion after the twelfth week of gestation. Too frequently the girl has dealt with the problem, adapting to a nonsolution by not sharing her knowledge of the pregnancy with others until few alternatives are possible.

All of the techniques for resolving a crisis situation can be brought to bear as the girl and her family work to solve the problem. Feelings need to be brought out into the open. The nurse can help by sharing her knowledge of community facilities and helping the girl achieve a realistic perception of the alternatives that are possible in resolving the crisis. Her concern for the girl may satisfy the girl's longing for a caring person. The girl's self-esteem may be enhanced simply because she is seen as someone who is not abandoned but is worthy of assistance. Whatever way the problem is resolved, the young person(s) involved will gain greater maturity if they have a part in the final decision. Once the decision is made, persons in the helping professions should respect the decision, even though it may not seem to be the "right" decision as they have defined it.

Labor and Birth

Once the decision is made to carry the infant to term, the nurse can become the key helping person in providing continuity, flexibility, and support so that the girl can emerge from the crisis of delivery with an increased potential for self-realization and maturity.[42]

The actual hospitalization and the physiologic changes that accompany labor may be unusual threats to an adolescent. She frequently maintains an objective anxiety in the early phases of labor. Manifestation of the stress experienced will be revealed by symptoms of dizziness, numbness, vomiting, and perspiration.

The adolescent, who is often quite modest, is distressed by the exposure which is necessitated by perineal preparation, vaginal examinations, and the delivery itself. Fears of soiling and uncontrollable loss of amniotic fluid increase her feeling of inadequacy. Actions are frequently provocative, demonstrated by rolling of the head, swearing, screams of "I can't! Wait! Don't do that now." The regression is obvious. She seems to have a need to create a stir and by demanding retaliatory actions from the nurse or physician she attempts to justify her feelings of anger and frustration.[43]

Labor and delivery are frequently short for the adolescent. With adequate prenatal preparation and with a supportive relationship with the nurse and the physician, it is quite possible for the young mother to successfully meet the challenge of giving birth and looking back on this adult task with pride. If she can emerge from this experience with a feeling of dignity and self-worth, she can better progress to motherhood. Her own needs must be met first. Solicitous nursing care she received during labor will help the more mature adolescent to ultimately achieve a readiness to nurture a child.

The adolescent mother is often put in a bind when she has to make a choice of *one* person who will be with her during labor and/or delivery, as is true in many hospitals. She may want the baby's father but fears that her mother will be angry if she's not chosen, and she's going to need her mother's help desperately in the future. On the other hand, she may very much want her mother, who has been through this herself and will "understand," but her boy friend expects to be the one who will support her and she doesn't want to anger him either. Often the nurse can help her to express her real wish and perhaps help her to find ways to meet her own needs. Again, close involvement with the grandmother and with the young father can be helpful in resolving this situation.

Decisions Related to the Child

Decisions about the baby can only be made when the baby is realistically acknowledged. A decision to keep the infant and nurture it must be made with full knowledge of the implications. Even if the inevitable decision is that the baby must be relinquished for adoption, it is the opinion of many authorities that the pregnancy and baby must not be denied as realities. The mother, except in extraordinary instances, needs to see her infant so she can remember with real pride that she has given birth to a normal healthy child. This is no small matter, and although it may increase the distress over separation from the child, she does need to have an opportunity to view the child and to be reassured about its reality.

If the decision is made to keep the child, the adolescent girl will need support while she develops mothering skills. She will wish assistance in learning to care for her child, but at the same time she will be very fearful that you, the nurse, will find out how very insecure she feels and how little she really does know. The telephone is often used as a literal lifeline to keep in touch with persons whom she believes understand her. These people are most often her peers. It would be erroneous to interpret this behavior as a lack of concern for her child.

The nurse who gains the adolescent's trust has an excellent opportunity to be a role model for the girl. Teaching parenting skills in a nonthreatening manner reduces feelings of inadequacy and builds feelings of maternal competency. As learning occurs, the nurse, by giving honest praise, strengthens the adolescent mother's self system.

Osofsky[44] states that adolescents do show strength in that they can display warmth and physical interaction with their infants. However, they show low verbal interaction. Since stimulation, both tactile and verbal are important to early infant development, the nurse needs to find tactful ways of transmitting this information and encouraging these young mothers to enrich their infants' environment.

There are imposing obstacles for a very young person to keep her child and mother it. Inability to support one's self and the child must be considered. The child's care will, in most instances, absorb her totally, leaving little time and a reduced number of outlets for the satisfaction of the girl's own needs.[45]

The very young (under 15 years old) adolescent is most frequently unready to care for her infant totally, mainly due to the overlay of her own developmental tasks. She can be helped to learn nurturing skills; however, the final responsibility for her child will have to be assumed by a more mature adult.

Finding surrogate mothering for her child can be accomplished without destroying the very young mother's pride in herself and her developing self-concept. She can be supported in her efforts to find good mothering for her child even though she cannot provide it herself while she is completing her own developmental processes. She can take pride in bearing a fine child, in her child's healthy growth and development even though she herself is not giving the greater part of the mothering care. She is providing some mothering for her child and thus is a good mother. She is growing and maturing herself in order that she may later provide what her child needs. The nurse who has assessed the family dynamics as well as the developmental level of her patient may be a key figure in helping the family either in building up the mothering role for the adolescent mother or in helping her to provide surrogate mothering for her infant. She thus may help the young person to fill her own needs and her child's needs with pride in these accomplishments. The grandmother is often the one who will provide the surrogate care. Again, an early involvement with the grandmother during the pregnancy can often lead to this kind of supportive and strengthening relationship between grandmother, mother, and grandchild, and the reinforcement of the young mother's developing feeling of self-worth and maturity.[46]

If the mother relinquishes her child for adoption, she can be expected to go through a grieving process related to the loss. It will be the nurse's responsibility to see that persons significant to her understand how they can support her during this grieving process. Parents and others will likely feel that they will be helping the girl "forget" by discouraging any discussion of the events of the previous months. The nurse must anticipate this possibility and intervene appropriately.

It would be naive, however, to expect that all girls who relinquish their babies for adoption care deeply about their children. Many do, but some do not. Assessment is of utmost importance here. The young woman who appears to easily relinquish her child should be very carefully assessed. She may be repressing her feelings as a coping mechanism. It can be expected that the feelings of loss and grief are always present and need to be dealt with to prevent them from reappearing later in life.

The girl's coping with the loss may take the form of hostility and breaks in interpersonal relationships with others, in restlessness, or in somatic distress. These are clues the nurse can use to formulate a nursing diagnosis and to mobilize someone in the girl's environment who can be supportive of her as she works through the grieving process.

The Future

The nurse will have already assessed the young person's ambitions and plans for the future in terms of her academic goals, life's work, and plans for her child. The nurse is now faced with the responsibility to help the girl look at these goals and plans realistically, perceiving not only the present but the future. Developing a sense of the future is an important feature of adolescent growth. An experience of out-of-wedlock pregnancy can leave a person with feelings of guilt, shame, failure, and hopelessness.

Sometimes the nursing assessment will elicit real sadness—helplessness and hopelessness, e.g., "I wanted to be a teacher . . . I always wanted that . . . but now . . . I'll probably be nothing." The nurse can then make a beginning of helping her to think positively and explore some of the resources that are available to her.

Sometimes the exploration elicits an unrealistic fantasy or a real desire that is unlikely to be achieved. The nurse can help her to look at the reality of her dreams. For example, if she says she plans to be an airline stewardess, the nurse can help her to answer the question, "What kind of hours does a stewardess work?" and then recognize that the responsibility of a baby would not permit a mother to be away from home for such long periods. The nurse could then explore what she might do. She might be able to work at an airline ticket counter and take some flights on holidays.

Feelings of hopelessness can lead to "dead end" relationships with repeated pregnancies. Family planning for the sexually active girl must be discussed and the issues related to the use of contraceptives must be explored. The nurse can be an effective model by 1) communicating to the girl that she is capable of making appropriate decisions and judgements about herself, and 2) providing the support and information basic to her making mature and reality-based decisions.[47] Peer group sessions give adolescents a chance to express their social and emotional problems in relation to family planning.

Followup is an extremely important aspect of contraceptive care for the young person. The nurse should be available for questions, discussions, and so forth until the young woman is thoroughly comfortable with her choice. If this is not possible, she should provide the patient with specific resources easily and quickly available to her. Many young women, no matter how well prepared for the minor complications or discomforts of the various methods of birth control, often panic and cease using the method. An easily and quickly available source of information which they trust may be crucial to continuance of contraception.

Reports of Coordinated Community Services[48] now indicate that many practical and realistic opportunities are offered to adolescent girls for continuing their education and vocational preparation, and with effective support from the team they can look forward to a more hopeful future for themselves and their children. Where no such services are available, the professional nurse has a responsibility to spearhead the development of such services.

Regarding general education, much of the information adolescent unwed mothers need should ideally be a part of every school curriculum. Health, sexuality, and reproduction can, and to an increasing extent are, being included in family life education courses. This education of all young people of both sexes would lessen the need to teach such basic facts under the stress of pregnancy. The total educational process should also include, for *all* young people, parenting skills. Young people should be learning the art of mothering and fathering at the same time that they are preparing for a vocational future. One is as important as the other. Nurses could well be the persons in the community to bring this to the attention of parents, teachers, and other members of the health profession.

REFERENCES

1. *Promoting the Health of Mothers and Children*. Report for Fiscal Year 1972 of the Maternal and Child Health Service, Health Services and Mental Health Administration, U. S. Department of Health, Education and Welfare, 1972, p. 59.

2. Howard, M.: *Pregnant school-age girls*. J. Sch. Health. 41:361, 1971.
3. Giovannini, D. H.: *Data indicates changing profile of unwed mothers*. Wisconsin's Health. 20:4, 1972.
4. Howard, op. cit.
5. Nelson, S. A.: *School-age parents*. Child. Today 2:31, 1973.
6. Sklansky, M. A. and Lichter, S. O.: *Some observations of the character of the adolescent ego*. Soc. Serv. Rev. 31:271, 1957.
7. Nixon, R.: *An approach to the dynamics of growth—Adolescence*. Psychiatry 24:18, 1961.
8. Mead, G. H.: *Mind, Self, and Society*. University Press, Chicago, 1934, pp. 144–149.
9. Sullivan, H. S.: *The Inter-Personal Theory of Psychiatry*. W. W. Norton, New York, 1953, p. 164.
10. Lamers, W. J.: *After office hours, understanding the teenager*. Obstet. Gynecol. 33:131, 1969.
11. Jersild, A. J.: *The Psychology of Adolescence*, ed. 2. Macmillan, New York, 1963, p. 63.
12. Ibid., p. 4.
13. Ibid, p. 68.
14. Howard, op. cit., p. 362.
15. Jorgensen, V.: *Clinical report on Pennsylvania hospitals' adolescent obstetric clinic*. Am. J. Obstet. Gynecol. 112:816, 1972.
16. Smith, E. W., et al.: *Adolescent maternity services: a team approach*. Children 18:208, 1971.
17. Howard, op. cit., p. 362.
18. Jorgensen, op. cit., p. 816.
19. Nelson, op. cit.
20. Stone, L. J. and Church, J.: *Childhood & Adolescence: A Psychology of the Growing Person*. Random House, New York, 1957, pp. 271–272.
21. Lamers, op. cit., p. 131.
22. Notman, M. T.: *Emotional impact of pregnancy on the unwed adolescent*. In Jeffries, J. E. (ed.): *The Adolescent Unwed Mother, Ross Roundtable on Maternal & Child Nursing*. Ross Laboratories, Columbus, 1965, p. 23.
23. Ibid.
24. Erikson, E. H.: *Childhood and Society*. W. W. Norton, New York, 1950.
25. Caplan, G.: *Concepts of Mental Health and Consultation*. U. S. Department of Health, Education and Welfare, Children's Bureau, 1959, p. 46.
26. Ibid., p. 4.
27. McFarland, M. and Reinhart, J.: *The development of motherliness*. Children 6:48, 1959.
28. Eisenberg, M. S.: *Out of wedlock pregnancy aspects of the mother-child separation crisis*. Casework Papapers, 1956, Family Service Association of America.
29. Bibring, G. L., et al.: *A study of psychological process in pregnancy and the earliest mother-child relationship*. Psychoanal. Study Child 26:9, 1961.
30. Lesser, A. J.: *Progress in maternal and child health*. Child. Today 2:12, 1972.
31. Smith, E. W., et al., op. cit., p. 209.
32. Nelson, op. cit., p. 33.
33. Notman, op. cit., p. 26.
34. Perez-Reyes, M. G. and Falk, R.: *Follow up after therapeutic abortion in early adolescence*. Arch. Gen. Psychiatry 28:120, 1973.
35. Pannor, R.: *The forgotten man*. Nurs. Outlook 18:36, 1970.
36. Cahill, I.: *Facts and Fallacies Concerning Pregnancy Out of Wedlock*. In Jeffries, J. E. (ed.): *The Adolescent Unwed Mother, Ross Roundtable on Maternal & Child Nursing*. Ross Laboratories, Columbia, 1965, p. 14.
37. Ibid., p. 15.
38. Notman, op. cit., p. 28.
39. Smith, E. W.: *Transition to the Role of Grandmother as Studied with Mothers of Pregnant Adolescents. A.N.A. Clinical Sessions*. Appleton-Century-Crofts, New York, 1970, p. 146.
40. Barnard, J. E.: *Peer group instruction for primigravid adolescents*. Nurs. Outlook 18:42, 1970.
41. Middleman, R. R.: *Unmarried pregnant teenagers*. Children 17:108, 1970.
42. David, L. and Grace, H.: *Anticipatory counseling of unwed pregnant adolescents*. Nurs. Clin. North Am. 6:581, 1971, p. 590.
43. Walker, E. G.: *Supporting the Unwed Adolescent through Labor*. In Jeffries, J. E. (ed.): *The Adolescent Mother, Ross Roundtable on Maternal & Child Nursing*. Ross Laboratories, Columbus, 1965, p. 61.
44. Osofsky, H. and Osofsky, J. D.: *Adolescents as mothers*. Am. J. Orthopsychiat. 40:825, 1970.
45. Eisenberg, M. S.: *Adolescence and Out of Wedlock Pregnancy*. Paper presented at Rutgers University, at N. J. Council on Maternal & Child Health, N. J. League for Nursing, 1965, p. 5.
46. Smith, E. W.: Personal communication.
47. Davis and Grace, op. cit., p. 589.
48. Smith, E. W.: Personal communication.

BIBLIOGRAPHY

Barnard, J. E.: *Peer group instruction for primigravid adolescents*. Nurs. Outlook 18:42, 1970.

Beckner, F. J.: *How do you respond to an unwed mother?* R.N. 33:46, 1970.

Bernstein, R.: *Helping Unmarried Mothers*. Association Press, New York, 1971.

Ibid.: *The maternal role in the treatment of unmarried mothers*. Social Work 8:58, 1963.

Bowlby, J.: *Attachment and Loss, vol. 1*. Basic Books, New York, 1969.

Claman, A. D., Williams, B. J. and Wogan, L.: *Reaction of*

unmarried girls to pregnancy. Canad. Med. Assoc. J. 101:328, 1969.

Clark, A.: *Maturational crisis and the unwed adolescent mother*. Nurs. Science 2:112, 1964.

Ibid.: *The crisis of adolescent unwed motherhood*. Am. J. Nurs. 67:1965, 1967.

Clark, M., et al.: *Sequels of unwanted pregnancy*. Lancet 2:501, 1968.

Cobliner, W. G., Schulman, H. and Romney, S. L.: *The termination of adolescent out-of-wedlock pregnancies and the prospects for their primary prevention*. Am. J. Obstet. Gynecol. 115:432, 1973.

Cochin, J. (ed.): *Drug abuse and contraception. Fifth International Congress on Pharmacology*. S. Karger, New York, 1973.

Curtis, F. L. S.: *Observation of unwed pregnant adolescents*. Am. J. Nurs. 74:100, 1974.

Daniels, A.: *Reaching unwed, adolescent mothers*. Am. J. Nurs. 69:332, 1969.

Davis, L. and Grace, H.: *Anticipatory counseling of unwed pregnant adolescents*. Nurs. Clin. North Am. 6:581, 1971.

De Lissovoy, V.: *Child care by adolescent parents*. Child. Today 2:22, 1973.

Dempsey, J. J.: *Analysis of Programs for Pregnant Adolescents*. Research to Improve Health Services for Mothers and Children, U. S. Department of Health, Education and Welfare, Rockville, Maryland, 1973.

Dempsey, M. O.: *The development of body image in the adolescent*. Nurs. Clin. North Am. 7:609, 1972.

Does anybody care? Am. J. Nurs. 73:1562, 1973.

Dwyer, J. F.: *Teenage pregnancy*. Am. J. Obstet. Gynecol. 118:373, 1974.

Friedman, H.: *The mother-daughter relationship: its potential in treatment of young unwed mothers*. Social Casework 47:502, 1966.

Furstenberg, F. F., Jr., et al.: *How can family planning programs delay repeat teenage pregnancies?* Fam. Plan. Perspect. 4:54, 1972.

Gabrielson, I. W., et al.: *Adolescent attitudes toward abortion: effects on contraceptive practice*. Am. J. Pub. Health 61:730, 1971.

Howard, M.: *Comprehensive service programs for school-age pregnant girls*. Children 15:193, 1968.

Iungerish, Z.: *High school for unwed mothers*. Am. J. Nurs. 67:92, 1967.

Jekel, J. F., et al.: *Factors associated with rapid subsequent pregnancies among school-age mothers*. Am. J. Pub. Health 63:769, 1973.

Jorgensen, V.: *One-year contraceptive follow-up of adolescent patients*. Amer. J. Obstet. Gynecol. 115:484, 1973.

Kaminetsky, H. A., et al.: *The effect of nutrition in teen-age gravidas on pregnancy and the status of the neonate*. Am. J. Obstet. Gynecol. 115:639, 1973.

Kane, F. and Lachenbruch, P.A.: *Adolescent pregnancy: a study of aborters and non-aborters*. Amer. J. Orthopsychiat. 43:796, 1973.

Klaus, M. et al.: *Human maternal behavior in the first contact with her young*. Pediatrics 46:187, 1970.

La Barre, M.: *Emotional crisis of school-age girls during pregnancy and early motherhood*. J. Child Psychiat. 11:537, 1972.

Lipper, I., et al.: *Abortion and the pregnant teenager*. Can. Med. Assoc. J. 109:852, 1973.

Marinoff, S. C.: *Contraceptives in adolescents*. Pediatr. Clin. North Am. 19:811, 1972.

Martin, C. D.: *Psychological problems of abortion for the unwed teenage girl*. Genet. Psychol. Monogr. 88:23, 1973.

McKay, M. J. and Richardson, H.: *Personality differences between one-time and recidivist unwed mothers*. J. Genet. Psychol. 122:207, 1973.

McMaster, A.: *Effective care of school age mother hampered by 'syndrome of failures'*. Hosp. Top. 49:71, 1971.

Mcmurray, G. L.: *Continuing education of teenage parents*. Nurs. Outlook 17:66, 1969.

Menken, J.: *The health and social consequences of teenage childbearing*. Fam. Plan. Perspect. 4:45, 1972.

National Council on Illegitimacy: *Illegitimacy: Changing Services for Changing Times*. National Council on Illegitimacy, New York, 1970.

Oppel, W. C. and Royston, A. B.: *Teen-age births: some social, psychological and physical sequelae*. Am. J. Pub. Health 61:551, 1971.

Osofsky, H. J.: *Pressures on pregnant unwed teenagers*. Briefs 34:103, 1970.

Ibid.: *The Pregnant Teen-ager: A Medical, Educational and Social Analysis*. Charles C Thomas, Springfield, Ill., 1968.

Osofsky, H. J. and Osofsky, J. D.: *Adolescents as mothers (results of a program for low-income pregnant teenagers with some emphasis upon infant's development)*. Am. J. Orthopsychiat. 40:825, 1970.

Pannor, R.: *The forgotten man*. Nurs. Outlook 18:36, 1970.

Pannor, R., Massarik, F., and Evans B. W.: *The Unmarried Father*. Springer, New York, 1969.

Perez-Reyes, M. G. and Falk, R.: *Follow up after therapeutic abortion in early adolescence*. Arch. Gen. Psychiatry 28:120, 1973.

Pierce, R.: *Single and Pregnant*. Beacon Press, 1970.

Pion, R. J., Wabrek, A. J. and Wilson, W. B.: *Innovative methods in prevention of need for abortion*. Clin. Obstet. Gynecol. 12:4, 1971.

Prevention of Pregnancy in Adolescents. New York Family Planning Resources Center, 1970.

Rosenberg, M.: *Society and Adolescent Self Image*. University Press, Princeton, N. J., 1965.

Sarrel, P. M., et al.: *The young unwed mother: the role of the obstetrician in the comprehensive care program*. Obstet. Gynecol. 32:741, 1968.

Sauber, M. and Corrigan, E.: *The Six-Year Experience of Unwed Mothers as Parents*. Research Dept., Community Council of Greater New York, 1970.

Smith, E. W.: *Transition to the role of grandmother as studied in mothers of pregnant adolescents*. In *A.N.A. Clinical Sessions, American Nurses' Association, 1970, Miami*. Appleton-Century-Crofts, New York, 1970.

Wallerstein, J. and Bar-din, M.: *Seesaw response of a young unmarried couple to therapeutic abortion*. Arch. Gen. Psychiatry 27:251, 1972.

40 Abortion

ANN L. CLARK, R.N., M.A.

Abortion is defined as termination of a pregnancy before the fetus has attained viability. Viability is generally considered possible after 28 weeks of gestation. A *spontaneous* abortion is one which occurs naturally, it is not induced by artificial means. An *induced* abortion is one which is brought on intentionally by drugs or mechanical means. The term *miscarriage* is often used by the lay public when speaking of spontaneous abortions to avoid connotations of illegality often associated with the word abortion.

SPONTANEOUS ABORTION

A large number of early pregnancies are lost through spontaneous abortions. Most of these occur in the first trimester of pregnancy (82 per cent) with a smaller number (18 per cent) occurring in the second trimester.[1] It is difficult to ascertain the proportion of pregnancies that end in spontaneous abortion. Many clinicians believe that the incidence is underreported in the first eight weeks of gestation. The woman herself may be unaware of being pregnant. When her menstrual period does finally occur, she is aware it is delayed and that the flow is somewhat heavier than normal, but she may not report it to the physician because she does not see it as significant. Figures on spontaneous abortions range from 10 to 15 per cent of all pregnancies to as high as 30 per cent.[2]

Whenever a woman loses a pregnancy, whether the pregnancy was originally welcomed or not, she wants to know the cause. In either case the termination of the pregnancy is significant to her. It may, in a number of instances, have impact from a psychologic point of view or it may have importance to the family's goal-directed plans related to family size.

Premature expulsion of the products of conception can occur for a number of reasons; however, for as many as 50 per cent of all lost pregnancies, a cause cannot be found.

ETIOLOGY

The causes of spontaneous abortion, when known, can be placed into three categories:

1. Abnormalities occurring in the ovum
2. Abnormalities of the female generative tract
3. Maternal host factors.

Abnormalities Occurring in the Ovum

All ova and all spermatozoa are not perfect specimens. If one of these imperfect cells takes part in conception and begins to grow, the defective germ plasma will produce a defective product of conception. The imperfection may be in the genes or in the chromosomes. Sometimes the zygote does not develop at all and the product is termed a blighted or a dropsical ovum. In other cases the zygote develops into a fetus with multiple imperfections incompatible with life. When the fetus dies, the uterus treats it as a foreign body, eventually initiating contractions which result in expulsion of part or of all of the products of conception. Sometimes the placenta is left in utero with subsequent vaginal bleeding.

There may also be imperfections in the implantation of the products of conception due to a faulty intrauterine environment. The most frequent lesion in spontaneous abortion is hemorrhage into the decidua basalis, followed by necrotic changes in the tissues adjacent to the bleeding. This in turn sets up an inflammatory reaction. Because of the hemorrhage and necrosis the ovum becomes detached. If the implantation is not such that intrauterine life can be sustained, the fetus dies and is expelled.

The placenta may also be defective, so that fetal life cannot continue. Sometimes large infarcts prevent adequate functioning of sufficient placental tissue to sustain fetal life. This interference with fetal circulation will bring about death of the fetus and expulsion.

Abnormalities of the Female Generative Tract

The anatomic development of the uterus has implications for conception, implantation, and successful term birth. Uterine anomalies, such as infantile uterus, double uterus, or adnexal inflammation, may be causes for an abortion. Tumors of the uterus, endocervicitis, and submucosal tumors in the lower uterine segment also may make retaining a pregnancy impossible. Retrodisplacement of the uterus may cause the incarceration of the uterine fundus as it enlarges, resulting in an abortion.

The midpregnancy abortion is sometimes due to an incompetent cervix. In such cases, the cervix painlessly dilates, the membranes rupture, and the pregnancy is expelled. The condition lends itself to repeated loss of pregnancies and is a frequent cause of habitual abortions.

Maternal Host Factors

Maternal infections are high on the list of causes of abortions. Any severe acute infection resulting in bacterial invasion to the fetus and the production of toxins in the mother may bring about abortion.

Endocrine imbalance and endocrine dyscrasias may be responsible for an abortion. Inadequate production of progesterone and estrogen, which are responsible for the maintenance of the decidual bed, may be responsible for the death of the embryo in early pregnancy. In later pregnancy, failure of the placenta to take over the steroidal functions of the corpus luteum and produce sufficient chorionic gonadotrophic hormones will cause loss of the products of conception.

Inadequate thyroid function has an impact on a woman's ability to nourish and carry a fetus to term. In a study by Jones and Delfs,[3] it was found that 63.5 per cent of women in their study had inadequate thyroid function and that in 35 per cent of the women, it was the sole factor found to be responsible for reproductive failure.

Maternal nutrition and fetal development are profoundly interrelated. Caloric intake in sufficient quantity and quality is essential to fetal growth. Deficiencies in vitamins A, B-complex, D, and E have been implicated in fetal malformations and in abortions. Defects in folate metabolism can affect the growing maternal/fetal tissue and can also be implicated in abortions.

Other diseases affecting intrauterine growth include: essential hypertensive vascular diseases; chronic nephritis; ABO incompatibility; and in the second trimester, syphilis. Rh incompatibility may bring about fetal death late in pregnancy, but is generally not considered a factor in abortion. Accidents, psychic trauma and surgery, may in rare cases be responsible for an abortion, but generally they are not so implicated.

TERMINOLOGY AND THERAPY

For greater clarity, spontaneous abortions are frequently subdivided to indicate their clinical nature.

A *threatened abortion* is one in which there is vaginal bleeding accompanied by pelvic cramping and backache. The free bleeding may be followed by expulsion of part or all of the products of conception. In other instances, the bleeding may be slight and persist for days or even weeks. However, all vaginal bleeding during early pregnancy is not due to a threatened loss of the pregnancy. Some women "spot" or have frank vaginal bleeding due to polyps, ruptured paraplacental blood vessels, erosions of the cervix, and other less defined causes. The pelvic cramping and backache, present in a threatened abortion, are usually absent. This fact is helpful in making a differentiation.

There is no reliable evidence that therapy of any kind really changes the course of the threatened abortion.[4] Most physicians do restrict the patient's activities and may prescribe a mild sedative. The patient is usually advised against coitus. In a number of instances bleeding ceases and pregnancy continues to term. In other instances bleeding continues, pelvic cramping increases and the condition is now termed an *imminent abortion*. The membranes then rupture, the cervix dilates, and all of the products of conception are lost or part of the placenta continues to adhere to the uterine lining. The latter case is termed an *incomplete abortion*. In such instances uterine bleeding may or may not be profuse. It can become massive to the point of profound shock due to the opening in the venous sinuses beneath the placenta. Treatment consists of supportive therapy (infusions, transfusions, etc.) and dilatation and curettage to remove the remaining tissue.

A *missed abortion* is one in which the fetus dies, but is not expelled. It can remain in utero with little or no untoward effects for two or more months. In such instances uterine growth ceases and breast changes brought about by pregnancy diminish. However, amenorrhea continues. Most missed abortions terminate spontaneously. If they do not, intravenous oxytocin may be used to stimulate uterine contractions or a hypertonic dextrose or saline solution may be injected into the uterine cavity to bring about expulsion of the dead fetus and other products of conception.

Habitual abortion is the loss of three or more consecutive pregnancies. This is a much more serious problem. The etiologic factors are often manifold, consisting of a combination of the conditions discussed earlier in this chapter. When the diagnosis is an incompetent cervix, surgery has been used to aid many of these patients in carrying their pregnancies to term. The weak cervix is reinforced by a kind of purse-string suture placed between 14 and 18 weeks of pregnancy. In successful cases, the suture may be removed by 38 or 39 weeks of pregnancy so that labor can progress normally. In other techniques, the suture is left in place and a cesarean section is performed near term.

Other therapy depends on clinical investigation of the etiology. Thyroid dysfunction is treated, as is inadequate secretion of progesterone. Nutritional deficiencies are corrected. Congenital malformations related to uterine growth are treated by surgery.

With therapy, many women (70 to 80 per cent) can carry a subsequent pregnancy to term and deliver a normal infant.

PSYCHOLOGIC IMPLICATIONS

There are a number of studies which indicate that there are identifiable personality characteristics that distinguish women who habitually abort from other women. Grimm[5] administered the Wechsler-Bellevue, Rorschach, and TAT (Thematic Apperception Test) to 61 habitual abortion patients who had no discernible organic basis for the abortions. She found that as a group they demonstrated an impairment in their ability to plan and anticipate, had poorer emotional control, more emphasis on conformity and compliance with the conventional, greater tension about hostile affect, stronger feelings of dependency, and greater proneness to guilt feelings. Psychologic testing carried out by Simon and coworkers[6] indicates that women who spontaneously abort have conflicts about sexual identity and sadomasochism. They suggest that pregnancy and the abortion may be seen as a primary way of acting out unconscious sadomasochistic conflicts. The abortion may be an alternative way of dealing with and acting out impulses and conflicts about the feminine biologic role. Emotionally-conditioned autonomic imbalance may produce uterine irritability leading to decidual hemorrhage and spontaneous abortion.

THE ROLE OF NURSING

Spontaneous abortion may constitute a crisis for the woman and her family. Vaginal bleeding is always anxiety-producing for any woman. The loss of a pregnancy may be regarded by a woman as a threat to her feminine biologic functioning as well as a threat to her life. Repeated losses of pregnancies are threatening to the life goals of families who wish to produce and to raise children.

The nurse caring for a patient who is threatening to abort or who has aborted needs to assess her physiologic functioning:

- Monitor vital signs
- Observe amount and type of vaginal bleeding
- Collect data related to area of pain, intensity, onset
- Take a nutritional history (after the crisis has subsided)
- Study the diagnostic clinical investigation (hematology, blood chemistry, pregnanediol assays, etc.).

She also needs to assess psychologic functioning:

- Happiness or sadness about loss of the pregnancy
- The coping behaviors manifested
- Anxiety exhibited
- Expressions of self blame, guilt
- Grief responses
- Depression.

The role of the nurse is to support both the physiologic and the psychologic functioning. The medical team is responsible for relating the clinical findings to the patient and her husband. The nurse should listen to what is told to the patient. Shock and depression may well result if the woman is told she was probably carrying an abnormal pregnancy. She needs time to mourn the loss of a desired pregnancy and an opportunity to verbalize her feelings. It is too early to have her focus on a future pregnancy with the hoped for happier outcome. The nurse can help set up lines of communication between the patient and others significant to her.

INDUCED ABORTION

THE ISSUES

Abortion by voluntary means is at once a moral, medical, legal, sociologic, philosophic, demographic, and psychologic problem not amenable to one-dimensional thinking.[7] There are no clear statistics on the number of induced abortions that have occurred in the United States. Prior to the Supreme Court's decision in 1973 which legalized induced abortions, it was believed that there were anywhere from 200,000 to 1.5 million illegal abortions performed every year.[8] Moreover, these illegal abortions were the largest single cause of maternal death in the United States.

By the middle of the twentieth century, many people, for many reasons, had developed strong and different feelings about induced abortion. They ranged all the way from "legalized abortion is a wicked price to pay for sexual emancipation of women, and abhorrent to the fundamental humanist tenets of society which are rooted in the Commandments,"[9] to a rejection of any morality which by giving *absolute* rights to the fetus, inescapably denies all rights to the woman, to her family and ultimately to society itself (here overpopulation was seen as a threat to civilization). The feminist view held that a woman had *absolute* right over her uterus, whether to fill it or to empty it. These intense and strongly diverse feelings grew into public controversy all over the nation. In 1968 the American Nurses' Association House of Delegates adopted a "Statement to Study State Legislation on Abortion." That statement reads:

> During the past biennium, there has been marked activity by individuals and lay and professional groups to change the existing abortion laws in the states.
>
> The changes recommended have followed the general provisions of the 1959 Model Penal Code of the American Law Institute, which provides for legal termination of pregnancy to preserve the life and health of the mother when either would be seriously jeopardized by continuance of pregnancy; when there is substantial risk of fetal anomalies; and when pregnancy results from rape or incest. The Penal Code also specifies that therapeutic abortions for the above reasons should be performed only by licensed physicians in accredited hospitals, after consultation with medical colleagues.
>
> The concern of the American Nurses' Association about this social health issue stems from the belief that the health and welfare of women and their families are seriously imperiled by the loose application of the present abortion laws and/or the disregard of them. It does not imply that nurses should make the decisions or perform abortions.
>
> The American Nurses' Association, the professional organization of registered nurses, concerned with the health and welfare of individuals and families, supports the movement to examine and modify existing abortion laws where they have proven to be inadequate to meet the needs of society in reducing the number of illegal abortions.
>
> Because nurses have a real and enduring interest in the well-being of people, the ANA endorses efforts to promote discussion and understanding of the moral, ethical and professional issues involved in making changes in the existing abortion laws.

THE LAW

From 1967 to 1973, 18 states passed new abortion laws which permitted voluntary interruption of pregnancy and other states were beginning discussion on the revision of their abortion laws.

Suddenly the controversy *seemed* to be over. The United States Supreme Court decision of January 22, 1973, in a 7 to 2 vote, eliminated all legal restrictions to abortions during the first three months of pregnancy except that the abortion must be performed by a licensed physician. It left to the individual states what restrictions should be placed after that period. Even then, any restrictions had to be "reasonably related to maternal health (including mental health)." The summation of the decision follows:[10]

Summation of the Majority Opinion
of the United States Supreme Court
in the Case of *Roe v. Wade*
by Justice Harry A. Blackmun
January 22, 1973 (No. 70-18)

To summarize and to repeat:

1. A state criminal abortion statute of the current Texas type that excepts from criminality only a *life saving* procedure on behalf of the mother, without regard to pregnancy stage and without recognition of the other interests involved, is violative of the Due Process Clause of the Fourteenth Amendment.

(a) For the stage prior to approximately the end of the first trimester, the abortion decision and its effectuation must be left to the medical judgment of the pregnant woman's attending physician.

(b) For the stage subsequent to approximately the end of the first trimester, the State in promoting its interest in the health of the mother, may, if it chooses, regulate the abortion procedure in ways that are reasonably related to maternal health.

(c) For the stage subsequent to viability the State, in promoting its interest in the potentiality of human life, may, if it chooses, regulate, and even proscribe, abortion except where it is necessary, in appropriate medical judgment, for the preservation of the life or health of the mother.

2. The State may define the term "physician," as it has been employed in the preceding numbered paragraphs of this Part XI of this opinion, to mean only a physician currently licensed by the State, and may proscribe any abortion by a person who is not a physician as so defined.

In *Doe v. Bolton, post,* procedural requirements contained in one of the modern abortion statutes are considered. That opinion and this one, of course, are to be read together.

This holding, we feel, is consistent with the relative weights of the respective interests involved, with the lessons and example of medical and legal history, with the lenity of the common law, and with the demands of the profound problems of the present day. The decision leaves the State free to place increasing restrictions on abortion as the period of pregnancy lengthens, so long as those restrictions are tailored to the recognized state interests. The decision vindicates the right of the physician to administer medical treatment according to his professional judgment up to the points where important State interests provide compelling justifications for intervention. Up to those points the abortion decision in all its aspects is inherently, and primarily, a medical decision, and basic responsibility for it must rest with the physician. If an individual practitioner abuses the privilege of exercising proper medical judgment, the usual remedies, judicial and intra-professional, are available.

Although many people were ecstatic with the passage of the law, others tended to agree with Callahan,[11] who states:

It may be counted a social and technological advance that abortion is becoming legally possible and medically safe as a method of procreation control *where other methods have failed*. But it is, at best, an advance to be looked upon with ambivalence. A single and faint cheer only is in order. Any method which requires the taking of human life, even though that life be far more potential than actual, falls short of the human aspiration, in mankind's better moments, of dignifying and protecting life. The time for loud cheering will come when, through a still more refined technological development, a method of birth control is discovered which does not require that we make a choice between the life of a conceptus and those other human values and goods we count important. It is possible to settle for and become comfortable with bad choices. It is better to seek good ones.

As the abortion laws took effect, it soon became apparent that the letter of the law was not being met. Many hospital quotas were quickly filled. Women who were less than eight weeks pregnant and could have their pregnancies terminated by a simple procedure often had to wait another six weeks when a more complicated and more dangerous procedure would be necessary. The cost of an abortion, as high as $600 to $700 made the law useless for many women. Although the law permitted abortions to be performed, obviously any hospital could and did pass their own policies related to it and physicians and nurses made individual decisions as to whether they would be involved with the procedure.[12] Walter,[13] speaking about physicians' attitudes, explained it this way:

> One of the largest deterrents to a liberalized abortion policy, in spite of the public clamor, is the health profession itself. Abortion is foreign to the attitudes fostered in physicians during their medical training; the gynecologist, the one to do the abortion, has a basic psychologic conflict. A whole generation of professional health workers refuses to let the myth die out that abortion will irreparably harm a woman and somehow place a stigma upon her. Physicians remain adamant. The male physician won't let the woman decide—reminiscent of the moralistic attitude about pain relief in childbirth before Queen Victoria demanded it for herself. The pregnant woman symbolizes proof of male potency, and if the male loosens his rule over women and grants them the right to dispose of that proof when they want to, the men then feel terribly threatened lest women can, at will, rob them of their potency and masculinity. This flaunting of traditional subservience may be one of more powerful and less conscious determinants of our irrational opposition to granting women the right to decide matters in this crucial area of their lives. It may also function in the frequent professional insistence upon sterilization as a "package deal" with abortion. In this way the male physician can maintain control.

Views among physicians were often not so much liberalized as they were polarized. Each hospital whose policies permitted abortions to be performed had several physicians willing to do the operation. Other physicians often looked on these physicians with disdain. Thus, conservatism of institutions and physicians became a barrier to obtaining the free benefits of the new abortion law.

Nurses, too, found that a voluntary abortion threatened their basic values. It was particularly difficult for nurses whose life goals have been to care for women who were producing life to suddenly find patients in these same beds exhibiting behaviors strange to them in the face of giving up life. Nurses were made anxious when they lacked skills to support these women. Moreover, ambivalent feelings regarding conflicting goals and religious beliefs and the increased volume of patients left nurses with feelings of fatigue and irritability. They felt angry when they were left alone to care for women patients and dispose of the products of conception, some of whom showed signs of life. Their ego was threatened when colleagues or family made derogatory remarks about the type of nursing they were engaged in.

Since the days when the laws were changed, certain conditions have improved or are being focused on for improvement. These include:

Opportunity of health personnel, physicians, nurses, and others to discuss their concerns and feelings about abortion and to receive psychologic counseling when indicated.

- Improved understanding of the stressors experienced by the abortion patient and better ways of intervening to support her.
- Improved insurance coverage for abortion patients.
- Improved knowledge related to the importance of seeking early care, about the methods used and the advantages and side effects.
- Family life, sex, and reproduction education introduced into the school curriculum.
- Conception planning integrated into abortion services.
- Preabortion and postabortion counseling.
- Streamlined abortion services consistent with good health care.

In many states the controversy over making abortion services available to minors without parental consent is still going on.

There are still many persons and groups, some of them physicians and nurses, who are actively working to repeal the liberalized abortion law and to place increased restrictions on its use. At the same time, research is going on to improve conception control so that abortion can be used only as a "back up" emergency procedure.

FACTORS WHICH INFLUENCE THE WOMAN'S DECISION

What are the factors which enter into the decision-making process of a woman regarding the termination of a pregnancy? According to Steinhoff,[14] there are four areas of psychologic relevance to be explored:

- The woman's relationship with the man involved in the pregnancy.
- The context of the decision-making after conception occurred.
- The woman's extramaternal aspirations.
- The woman's self-concept regarding her sexual activity.

Relevant decision-making and behavior of pregnant women can be located at three points in time: 1) Were they doing anything to prevent conception if they did not want a child? 2) What did they decide to do after becoming pregnant? 3) What will they do to prevent another pregnancy?

Preliminary analysis of data in one study[15] suggests that preconception decision-making is quite *irrational*. It appears much of the failure to use a proper contraceptive control method is due to the denial process in which the woman avoids seeking a stable contraception method because she cannot admit to herself that she is going to be sexually active. This situation is exacerbated when she derives little personal pleasure from sex and uses the lack of contraception as an excuse to avoid it. At the same time, she is likely to succumb to pressures and to continue to engage in sexual activities, unprepared to prevent pregnancy.

On the other hand, the decision to abort the pregnancy is based on the *objective* factors and is related to the woman's capacity to take care of the child. Her extramaternal aspirations and her relationship with the male, figure heavily in the decision to have the child or to have an abortion.

In a study by Abernathy,[16] there seems to be a predisposition to risk an unwanted pregnancy by ineffective use of contraceptions when the girl, married or single, has a history of "role redefinition in the family of origin." The principle components of role redefinition are:

- The daughter taking over some elements of her mother's role as wife or housekeeper.
- The daughter's alienation from the mother.
- Intimacy between the father and daughter which excludes the mother.

In addition to some combination of the above circumstances being present during adolescence, these girls and women relate that they feel they have received inadequate support from female friends and relatives and that their most important relationships have been with men. Moreover, they relate that they dislike sex and sexual relations.

Comparatively few women seek abortion on strictly medical grounds. Women say they seek legal abortions for very familiar reasons:

Reluctance to interrupt career plans.
Lack of money.
Fear of losing personal freedom.
Uncertainty about their relationship with the man involved.
Unmarried.
Have had enough children.
Need more time between children.

Abortions are used as methods of birth control by women from all religions, ethnic groups, and ages. They are students, housewives, clerical workers. They are married and they are single. However, most, if not all women seeking abortions have become pregnant at a time when they are experiencing crisis in their lives. There may be problems with the sexual mate, marital problems, problems with parents or career, economic crisis, or loss of significant others. It is said few pregnancies occur by accident. Miscalculations, missed pills, omitted spermicidal foam, and forgotten or improperly used diaphragms and condoms may be unconscious efforts to prove fertility or femininity by a pregnancy.

Some legislators and community leaders have, of course, expressed concern about changes in the law. They see it as a threat to morality and fear that ultimately abortions will be used as a major source of birth control. These are difficult questions to answer and more time is necessary before research can give us the answer. Nearly everyone agrees that abortion is a wasteful human experience and should only be used as a "back up." However, it seems from some of the studies reported earlier, there will always be women for whom availability of family planning information and technology will not be enough. For them, psychologic interference with contraception use must be recognized and treated.[17]

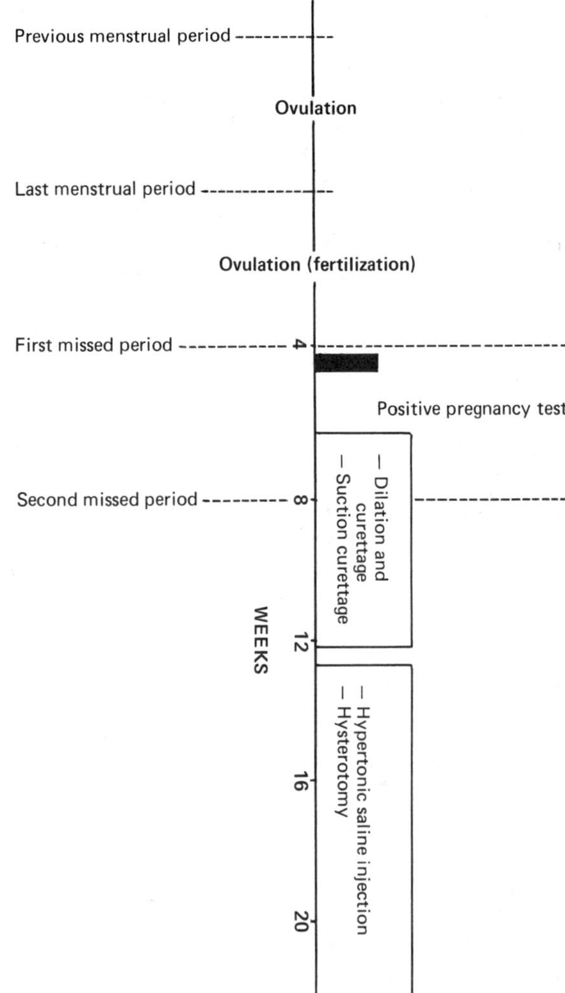

FIGURE 40-1. Usual methods for terminating human pregnancy and their application as a function of gestational duration. Shaded region represents "neglected area" of professional involvement. (From Pion et al.,[18] with permission.)

METHODS

If an abortion is going to be performed, it should be done as early in pregnancy as possible. Pregnancies that have reached or exceeded 12 weeks of gestation increase the danger to the individual. Hospitalization, with its costs, is prolonged and the patient experiences many stressors during the procedure, including the contractions of labor.

There are a number of methods used to induce abortion. Considerable research is underway to perfect existing techniques and to develop new ones. All induced abortions must be preceded by certain safeguards. A complete medical and psychosocial history is taken. Laboratory studies include, as a minimum, a CBC, Rh factor, blood typing, typing and cross-matching for RhoGAM, urinalysis, and cervical culture for gonorrhea.

Preabortion counseling is essential, although not carried out in all clinics or private physicians' offices as yet. Some state laws specify that the procedure must be performed in a hospital, others permit abortions to be performed on an out-patient basis.

The periods of pregnancy when certain methods of interruption of pregnancy are utilized are shown in Figure 40-1.

First Trimester

Menstrual Extraction. This method of forced endometrial shedding can be accomplished by a suction method immediately following a missed menstrual period, even prior to a possible diagnosis of pregnancy being made.[18] The technique is described below under Vacuum Aspiration.

Morning After Pill. This is the administration of a relatively high dose of a synthetic estrogen during the first three days after possible conception. The medication causes endometrial shedding. Unfortunately, this method is accompanied by nausea and vomiting for many patients.

Vacuum Aspiration. Pregnancies of less than 10 weeks of gestation may be terminated by aspiration using a cannula and suction. Cervical dilatation is first required prior to the suction. This dilatation may be accomplished by one of two methods: a laminaria tent (the dried stem of a sea tangle, fashioned in the form of a cone which swells, slowly dilating the cervix overnight) or by the introduction of progressively larger sounds until the cannula can be introduced. In very early pregnancies the cannula is 4 to 5 mm. The suction is by a closed-system 60 cc. syringe. Later in pregnancy, it is necessary to use a 6 to 10 mm. cannula and a small vacuum pump to remove the products of conception.

The patient is placed in lithotomy position, the vulva is cleansed with an antiseptic solution, and a speculum is used to expose the cervix. The cervix is fixed with a tenaculum. A paracervical block may be performed using 1 per cent lidocaine (Xylocaine) or one of the related anesthetic agents. (Some physicians do not feel the paracervical block is needed.) A preabortion oral analgesic may be given one hour prior to the procedure and "vocal anesthesia," i.e., the presence of a counsel to provide emotional and physical support to the patient, is provided. The procedure usually takes less than five minutes. Following the suction, completeness of the evacuation may be checked by exploring the uterine cavity with a small curette.

The patient may experience mild cramping and some discomfort during the procedure. Following the procedure, she should have no pain and only minimal vaginal bleeding. The patient is usually discharged within one hour of the procedure with an appointment to return in two weeks for a postabortion visit.

Prostaglandin. Research is being conducted on the use of prostaglandin, an effective abortifacient drug which mimics the action of the oxytocic hormone and causes contractions of the smooth muscles of the uterus. It is applied by means of vaginal instillation into the cul de sac or administered intravenously. The dosage depends on the compound used. The time needed to dilate the cervix and bring about expulsion of the products of conception varies with the length of the pregnancy. Eight to 31 hours are reported, with a mean average of 24 hours.

There are some side effects from the drug's use. Sometimes the placenta is retained and it is necessary to complete the abortion by means of curettage. Other side effects are vomiting, diarrhea, chills, and tissue reaction at the site of injection.

Dilatation and Curettage. This procedure must be performed before 12 weeks of pregnancy. It may be accomplished under local or general anesthesia and consists of dilation of the cervix with sounds until a curette, a small spoon-like instrument, can be introduced to remove the embryonic material. The procedure takes about 15 minutes and may be accompanied by some uterine cramping. After recovery from the anesthesia and a short period of rest, the patient may be discharged with written instructions for self-care and an appointment to return for a postabortion examination.

Second Trimester

Saline Induction. This procedure carries with it the greatest danger. It is reserved for second trimester abortions and is usually not performed until 16 weeks of gestation when the uterus is high enough in the abdominal cavity and amniotic fluid is sufficient to perform a safe amniocentesis.

The patient is hospitalized for the procedure. The bladder is emptied, the abdomen shaved and an enema is given to lessen the pressure and discomfort experienced at the time the fetus is expelled. The abdomen is prepared and the site of injection is anesthesized with 1 per cent lidocaine. The needle (18 spinal) with stylet is introduced through the abdominal wall and through the uterine wall to the amniotic cavity. A small amount of amniotic fluid is withdrawn and tested with nitrozine paper to be sure the amniotic sac has been penetrated. Then, up to 250 ml. of amniotic fluid are withdrawn. A test dose of 10 ml. of hypertonic saline is injected. Severe side effects such as dryness of the mouth, flushing, tinnitus, tachycardia, or severe headache may occur. If all goes well following the test dose, 30 to 40 grams of NaCl, diluted in 200 to 240 ml. of fluid are infused into the amniotic sac. The quantity may be injected in a relatively short period of time or it may be given by drip method. The patient experiences little pain during the procedure, but some cramping and a feeling of fullness are experienced once the injection is completed. These usually disappear within an hour. The patient may now be permitted to ambulate and to have food as she wishes. Fetal death usually occurs within one hour of the injection.

Some clinics begin an infusion of an oxytocin about six hours after the amniocentesis to speed labor; other physicians believe this is unnecessary since labor ultimately begins within 24 hours.

The cervix usually dilates to 4 cm. before the abortion occurs. This may take some hours; the average is 22. It is accompanied by uterine contractions and pain. An analgesic may be administered every 3 to 4 hours,[19] and the patient encouraged to relax and use controlled breathing during the contractions. She must use the same bearing down efforts with contractions to expel the fetus as she would with a full-term delivery.

The placenta may be retained at the time the fetus is expelled but is usually expelled spontaneously within one to two hours. If not, a curettage may be required to remove it. As with any delivery, postabortion hemorrhage must be guarded against.

Saline induction is not without serious complications. It is for this reason that researchers are trying to find other drugs that will be less toxic. Alcohol has been injected.[20] Alcohol seems to cause hemolysis of the erythrocytes in the cord vessel, causing fetal death. Urea has also been used experimentally for induction of midtrimester abortion.[21] Urea is a potent osmotic diuretic which causes fetal death. And, as discussed previously, prostoglandin, used as a first trimester abortifacient, is also used in the second trimester. When introduced into the amniotic sac, it causes contractions of the uterus and expulsion of the fetus and placenta.

Hysterotomy. A hysterotomy, an incision into the uterus, may be chosen as a method of voluntary interruption of pregnancy if there are contraindications against using other methods. It is also the method of choice if the patient wishes to be permanently sterilized by a tubal ligation. The usual preoperative and postoperative care is planned for the patient as well as special care as indicated due to the stress attendant with having a voluntary interruption of pregnancy.

It is anticipated that methods for interrupting pregnancies will continue to change. Some women's motivation for birth limitation becomes activated only after they have missed a menstrual period. Self-administration of some abortifacient, such as prostoglandin, by vaginal route in the form of a tampon is a future possibility. Marketing of prostoglandins in the United States is not permitted. They have, however, been used with promising results experimentally.

TABLE 40-1. Psychologic Evaluation in 250 Cases*

Category†	*Per cent*
Predominant Mood	
Very unhappy	4.2
Moderately unhappy	10.5
Neutral	20.7
Moderately happy	20.0
Very happy	44.6
Physical Emotionality	
Much crying	8.2
Moderate crying	7.6
Neutral	15.8
Moderate smiling	19.0
Much smiling	49.4
Feelings about Abortion	
Negative—much guilt	8.2
Moderate guilt	15.6
Neutral	13.4
Moderate relief	14.8
Positive—much relief	48.0
Attitudes toward Self	
Negative—angry	1.5
Moderate anger	7.2
Neutral	12.6
Moderate happiness	17.6
Positive—happy	61.1

* From Osofsky,[22] with permission.
† Ratings from negative = 1, to positive = 5

PSYCHOLOGIC IMPACT

Studies are beginning to accrue which indicate that for most women, markedly negative responses are rare. In a study by Osofsky and colleagues,[22] it was shown that 64 per cent of the women were moderately or very happy following the procedure, 10.5 per cent displayed a moderate amount of sadness, and 4.2 per cent felt very sad. Further statistics are listed in Tables 40-1 and 40-2. In summarizing this psychologic data, these investigators state:

> Few women have felt strong guilt, unhappiness or self anger; relatively few have been objectively distressed. Although many have physically feared the procedure and although a considerable number would have liked to bear the child if possible, given the existent social and/or economic circumstances, the predominant moods have been relief and happiness. Physical relief has also been apparent to the staff.[23]

Burnell and colleagues[24] conducted postabortion group therapy and reported that most women expressed a sense of relief once the procedure was performed. They reported a reduction of emotional tension, insomnia ceased, depression and somatic complaints faded. Five per cent still had guilt feelings and residual ambivalence and doubt about the decision. In discussing the guilt feelings and depression, they tended to see it as a part of their deserved punishment. This subgroup, for

TABLE 40-2. Decision-Making Regarding Abortion*

	Per cent
Difficulty of Decision	
Not difficult	52.5
Mildly difficult	19.5
Considerably difficult	28.0
Reasons for Difficulty of Decision	
Desire for the child	32.6
Psychologic discomfort	20.1
Physical discomfort	3.3
Reasons for Abortion	
Single	43.9
Financial	32.2
Wanted child but could not have it	13.4
Wanted to finish school	10.9
No positive feelings for the father	9.2
Medical reasons	8.8
Too many children	6.7
Does not want child	5.9
Too many children close in age	3.3
Parental advice	3.3
Husband not father of child	2.1
Unwilling intercourse	0.8

* From Osofsky,[22] with permission.

the most part, consisted of

Women with long-standing marital conflicts.
Teenagers with severe identity problems.
Older women with long histories of social and psychologic maladjustments.

For these women, the unwanted pregnancy and the abortion represented one of many crises in their lives. Burnell feels that, for these women, the pregnancy and the abortion led to an intense emotional crisis that reactivated underlying conflicts about femininity, motherhood, self-esteem, self-control, and acceptance or rejection. He believes that they now need psychotherapy.

It is well to look at the differences among individuals and their life situations to predict what sequelae, if any, will follow an induced abortion. A woman with a complex family relationship who thinks she is pregnant and is extremely ambivalent about her desires to be a mother is vulnerable. She becomes more vulnerable if there are conflicting pressures from her family and from her sexual partner. This woman's response to an abortion may be expected to be quite different from a mature woman who, due to contraceptive failure is quite sure she must interrupt this pregnancy. The presence or absence of personal or religious scruples will also affect the psychologic impact. If there are no conflicts the woman can be expected to complete the experience without psychologic trauma. She will still appreciate and benefit from some nursing support with her coping.[25]

The reader is advised to review the literature as more studies are reported. We will soon have a more accurate report of the impact of induced abortion as an increasing number of women elect to terminate their pregnancies in this manner.

NURSES AND NURSING

An acute identity crisis occurred for many nurses, as mentioned earlier, when laws legalizing abortions were passed. Unfortunately, few persons foresaw this development and it was necessary to deal with the problem at the same time clinical departments were already overloaded with patients, and when administrative routines were being established and adequate staff was being assembled.

Nursing has long been aware that the attitude of the nurse influences the kind of care she is able to administer and the patient's response to that care. Nurses do have attitudes about abortions. Many nurses have sufficient awareness and insight into their attitudes that they are able to offer supportive care to abortion patients. Any nurse who contemplates an assignment to an obstetric-gynecologic ward which cares for abortion patients or to a special ward for abortion patients should make a personal assessment in order to arrive at an understanding of her own feelings. To do this, she needs to understand how her early education and the attitude of her parents, church, and culture have molded her conscience about abortions. Next, she needs to consider abortion from her present rational position. It is possible that the nurse will then realize she has some conflicting attitudes about induced abortions and about women who undergo such procedures. In-service education can be most helpful to the nurse in ascertaining the problems the abortion patient faces prior to making her decision. It can also be helpful in recognizing the coping behavior the patient exhibits during the procedure. If the nurse can separate professional responsibility from her personal attitudes, even when they are ambivalent, she can meet the patient's needs. Some nurses, however, should ask not to be assigned to care for abortion patients, for no one should be asked to modify their moral and ethical beliefs. Their feelings, as well as patient's needs, should be respected. The nurses who care for abortion patients should have professional counseling accessible to them should they wish to verbalize their problems and feelings.

Schorr, in an editorial in the *American Journal of Nursing*, speaks eloquently on the issue of nursing the abortion patient:

> Issues of Conscience
>
> A nurse called us recently to say she had accompanied a patient who was admitted to a small private New York hospital for an abortion.
>
> "I was appalled and ashamed," she said, "to see how some of the nurses treated those kids, many of them only 14 or 15 years old, from all over the country. It was like Bedlam. They were herded like cattle, given no counseling, no support at a time of such crisis in their young lives."
>
> It's difficult—sometimes impossible—to submerge one's view of another's behavior. Yet there is no place in the nursing care of any patient for punitive action based upon personal moral judgments.
>
> The abortion patient is particularly vulnerable to attitudinal assaults. She has made a difficult decision, and often she has made it alone. She needs support, she needs skilled counseling, she needs help in considering her sexual future realistically and in learning how to avoid pregnancy until she can accept motherhood. She needs the shelter of a separate service where her grief and her guilt can be minimized, not an obstetric unit on which hostility toward her will be almost inevitable. She needs thoughtful care . . . and she needs to be in a setting planned with administrative wisdom. . . .
>
> There are many nurses who see an abortion as an unconscionable act, and certainly they should never be placed in the position of having to nurse patients who have chosen to have their pregnancy terminated. Just as a patient's freedom to choose must be respected, so must a nurse's. But it is also that nurse's responsibility to protect both the patient's freedom and her own by refusing to work in a situation which she finds morally offensive.
>
> It would be easier in nursing, or in journalism, or in life not to struggle with ethical issues. But the search for moral values is part of what makes one human. Respecting the rights of others in their search also makes one humane.[26]

PREABORTION COUNSELING

It is generally agreed that preabortion counseling, either on an individual basis or in groups, helps the patient to gain insight into her feelings about the pregnancy and the abortion, to better cope with the abortion procedure, and to complete the experience with a minimum of painful emotional aftereffects. The following are suggested by Gedan[27] as factors supporting the need for preabortion emotional counseling.

1. An abortion is a significant event in the patient's life. It will leave its mark on her as any important event would. The meaning a prospective abortion has to the patient and the way that she handles her reaction to that prospect will determine what effect the procedure will have upon her.
2. Patients seeking abortion are often experiencing some crisis in their life; a woman may be having marital problems, a teen-age girl may be having trouble with her family or a young single woman may be having difficulty working out satisfactory relationships with men. These are the problems that may have led the patient to seek an abortion and are the appropriate topics for emotional counseling. If the patient's feelings about these problems are repressed, they may then reappear as an "emotional reaction to abortion."
3. Because abortion is only now becoming a common and respectable procedure in many states, patients still have fears and misconceptions about the abortion process. Ventilating their feelings about their fears and clarifying what will happen to them is an important part of preoperative care.
4. The fact that unconscious motivations very often result in pregnancies which are attributed by the patient to missed pills, accidents, miscalculations, slip-ups and the like should come as no surprise. Exploring these motivations with the patient in some depth helps her realize needs that probably influenced her to become pregnant. This experience is a beginning in meeting her needs in a more appropriate fashion. It will (hopefully) contribute to her general well being and help to avoid a second abortion trip.
5. Even without any extraneous emotional complications, most patients have feelings about being pregnant and about terminating their pregnancy. Counseling aimed at handling these normal emotional reactions can relieve postoperative guilt, anxiety and depression.

These beliefs about the importance of preabortion counseling are so universally accepted that nurses should take the lead, if necessary, in seeing that such opportunities are provided for their patients. Moreover, counseling sessions can in themselves be further used as assessment tools for the planning of appropriate nursing care for the preabortion, abortion, and postabortion patient.

The abortion counseling usually encompasses three major aspects:

1. Emotional feelings related to the experience of pregnancy and the anticipated experience of the interruption of pregnancy.
2. Preoperative orientation to the procedure.
3. Anticipatory guidance in relation to the future in learning how to avoid pregnancy until motherhood can be accepted.

Group discussion is needed as a problem solving-activity where open expressions of thoughts, feelings, doubts, and fears can be expressed. Relief of tension comes about through verbalization. Having an opportunity to express feelings and explore what precipitated the feelings is therapeutic. Moreover, it increases one's sense of personal worth to have an interested, supportive audience. Verbalization helps to clarify one's thoughts and to find better ways to solve problems. Sharing feelings with others and becoming cognizant of the fact that others feel the same way reduces the feeling of being alone, different, or even of having reprehensible feelings about one's self. When concerns and fears are expressed, the group leader (nurse) has an opportunity to help the group members examine them realistically.

It is the practice of some agencies to offer individual preabortion counseling for some patients. For example, 1) adolescent patients, 2) patients who evidence ambivalence about going ahead with the abortion, 3) patients who state they are being forced to submit to an abortion, and 4) patients who had already had one or more abortions.

Again, crisis theory will be useful in assessment, counseling, and planning other aspects of nursing care.

Perception of the Event

In order to intervene in the crisis of abortion, health personnel need to collect data relating to the woman's fantasies of invulnerability, unrealistic expectations, rationalization for yielding to impulses, and defense mechanisms of denial, if any. These factors are unrealistic perceptions of events that have led to having a pregnancy which is undesired and which the woman wishes to have terminated by an abortion.

Verbalizing feelings about the pregnancy and about the way she feels she must resolve the problem are essential elements in helping the woman to eliminate the need to repeat the experience in the future. Accepting the responsibility for the pregnancy and for having the abortion must ultimately be faced by the individual and worked through. Perceiving the reality of the event is one of the steps in the resolution of the crisis.

The nursing assessment of the patient and her problems should include:

1. Where and at what age did the woman receive information about sexual relationships, pregnancy, and family planning?
2. What is the woman's pattern of relating sexually (the age it began, her sexual partner[s])?
3. Her knowledge and her use of birth control methods?
4. The duration of the pregnancy and at what point she decided on having the abortion? (If pregnancy is advanced, denial may be a coping mechanism.)
5. Her reaction to the pregnancy and to the abortion? (This will include what she *thinks* about abortions and people who have abortions [her conscience] and what she *feels* about having an abortion [the reality of the decision].)

Situational Support

The nurse needs to assess who is available to the woman to support her during this stressful event, for situational support will be needed. The woman will benefit if this person is already known to her. If there is someone available, but not being utilized, the nurse should encourage the woman to make contact. It may be necessary for the nurse to personally intervene in manipulating the environment so someone is available to the woman.

Women who are having abortions at the same time often will reach out and be supportive to each other. Patients often ask to be placed with another individual and not to be left alone during the abortion. This is particularly true with saline inductions. The patient's preference should be sought. Maternity wards are generally not appropriate places for abortion patients. They cause undue stress for both new mothers and abortion patients. Administrative planning must take this into consideration.

From the assessment data the nurse may well find that she must become the major supportive figure for the woman. *Guilt* is one feeling often expressed to the nurse. The woman may have decided that an abortion is the only rational way out of her predicament, but at the same time she may believe that in doing so she is a "shameful person." The nurse encourages her to talk about herself as a person and to act out her feelings (tears, shouting, any kind of behavior is appropriate). This helps her to reduce the tension precipitated by the feelings of guilt. At this point she can be guided to talk about her needs, particularly needs that were involved in and affected by the decision to have an abortion. This will permit her guilt to become more bearable.[28]

Some information relative to the development of the fetus may also be useful to the woman and should be shared, if she shows interest in this aspect. Many women have unrealistic beliefs about the developing fetus and even in the earlier weeks of gestation believe the development to be quite advanced. This knowledge for some women reduces their guilt.

Ambivalence about having an abortion or having the baby may also be a factor which needs exploration. The woman may feel a sense of pride in her feminine capacity and yearn for the baby. She may have developed quite a fantasy life with the developing fetus. On the other hand she knows rationally that she cannot have a baby at this time. She needs encouragement to express these feelings. The nurse can anticipate that the woman will experience grief and sadness following the abortion, and can help the woman to begin the grieving process.

Denial of feelings about being pregnant may be expressed. This is a defense mechanism and requires energy, needed for other aspects of living, to maintain it. Persons who use denial in coping may find that it fails to work for them at some point. This leaves them particularly vulnerable candidates for overwhelming anxiety, leading to panic and the danger of a psychic breakdown. The nurse needs to confront the woman with her denial and help her to validate and verbalize how denial is affecting her. Anger, disappointment, and/or sadness may be expressed when the woman can give up denial and discuss her feelings.[29] She can be encouraged to use nurses during the procedure by telling them of her fear, her sadness, and in openly expressing her feelings through crying, and other behaviors.

The individual facing an abortion procedure needs information relating to the technique to be used. Most women fear the hospital, its routines, and the abortion procedure. Knowing what to expect and whom they can depend on is good anticipatory guidance. On the other hand some women have very unrealistic ideas of how simple the procedure will be and then experience great anxiety when faced with the reality. For example, patients facing saline induction may not be aware of the method of saline instillation, the time involved to bring about the abortion, or that they will experience labor. The patient needs specific knowledge of the hospital, the examination, the technique, and the recovery period. Since the patient's anxiety levels may be so high as to inhibit learning, some of this information should be made available in printed form, particularly the postabortion care. Anticipatory planning for the experience may well keep a stressful experience from becoming a crisis.[30,31]

As a method of pain control, the patient having a saline induction will benefit from learning techniques of relaxation and controlled breathing.[32,33] Nurses need to teach the technique and then act as coach in helping the woman to utilize the method.

During the abortion procedure the nurse acts in a situational role by:

- Monitoring vital signs
- Monitoring intake and output
- Encouraging fluid intake
- Protecting the patient from infection
- Reducing physical discomfort by reinforcing relaxation techniques, giving sacral support, and providing medication as needed
- Reducing psychologic discomfort by providing an opportunity to express feelings, and providing an explanation of progress.

Following the abortion procedure the nurse supports the patient by:

- Teaching her self-care (diet, hygiene, breast care, awareness of danger signs, awareness of bleeding, facts about menstruation and resumption of sexual intercourse)
- Teaching her conception control based on her level of comprehension
- Providing sex education as indicated
- Making appropriate referral.

Coping

Some types of coping activities reduce or short circuit stress reactions by modifying stress-induced threat appraisals, and others presumably provide an opportunity for anticipatory coping, that is, for working out, prior to impending crisis the harms and threats to be faced. Patients in hospital treatment rooms and wards for saline induction vary greatly in their coping ability. The nurse assesses this behavior and supports that which has growth potential. At the same time she helps other patients to use coping behaviors that will reduce the stress and will help by reducing the fears and the physical and psychologic pain. The following ongoing assessment will help the nurse to observe the patient's level of coping and to indicate to the nurse when intervention is appropriate.

- Ability to express feelings and verbalize reactions. These feelings should be accompanied by congruent behaviors.
- Ability to verbalize needs regarding pain, fear, loneliness, etc.
- Ability to seek information and accept information and reassurance.
- Ability to focus on information and utilize information, including self-help technique.
- Ability to accept involvement with others in the health facilities.

The patient facing and experiencing voluntary interruption of pregnancy exposes a great deal about herself as a person and some of the most intimate details of her life. The nurse who exhibits attitudes of warmth, acceptance, objectivity, and compassion creates an atmosphere in which the woman can face and resolve this stressful experience and return to a state of equilibrium better prepared to face future crises in life which we all must expect. The nurse's attitude and her knowledge can make the difference.

REFERENCES

1. Panjabi, J. and Krishna, U.: *Problem of recurrent abortion.* The Clinician 37:105, 1973.
2. Roth, D.: *The stale egg concept in spontaneous abortion.* Obstet. Gynecol. 19:411, 1962.
3. Jones, G. E. S. and Delfs, E.: *Endocrine patterns in term pregnancies following abortion.* J.A.M.A. 146:1212, 1951.
4. Eastman, N. J. and Hellman, L. M.: *Williams' Obstetrics*, ed. 13. Appleton-Century-Crofts, New York, 1966, p. 515.
5. Grimm, E. R.: *Psychological investigation of habitual abortion.* Psychosom. Med. 24:369, 1962.
6. Simon, N. W., et al.: *Psychological factors related to spontaneous and therapeutic abortion.* Am. J. Obstet. Gynecol. 104:799, 1969.
7. Callahan, D.: *Abortion: Law, Choice and Morality.* Macmillan, New York, 1970.
8. Schulder, D. and Kennedy, F.: *Abortion Rap.* McGraw-Hill, New York, 1971, p. 9.
9. Noonan, J. T.: *The Morality of Abortion.* Harvard Press, Boston, 1970.
10. Lader, L.: *Abortion II.* Beacon Press, Boston, 1973.
11. Callahan, op. cit., p. 506.
12. Hall, R. E.: *Abortion: Physicians and hospital attitudes.* Am. J. Pub. Health 61:517, 1971.
13. Walter, G.: *Psychologic and emotional consequences of elective abortion.* Obstet. Gynec. 36:483, 1970.
14. Steinhoff, P.: *Pregnancy decisions: locating the psychological factors.* Pacific Health 4:11, 1971.
15. Ibid., p. 12.
16. Abernathy, V.: *The abortion constellation.* Arch. Gen. Psychiatry 29:346, 1973.
17. Ibid., p. 350.
18. Pion, R. J., Wabrek, A. J. and Wilson, W. B., Jr.: *Innovative methods in prevention of the need for abortion.* Clin. Obstet. Gynecol. 11:1313, 1971.

19. Cronenwett, L. R. and Choyce, J. M.: *Saline abortion.* Am. J. Nurs. 71:1754, 1971.
20. Gomel, V. and Carpenter, C. W.: *Induction of mid-trimester abortion with intrauterine alcohol.* Obstet. Gynec. 41:455, 1973.
21. Weinberg, P. C. and Shepard, M. K.: *Intraamniotic urea for induction of mid-trimester abortion.* Obstet. Gynec. 41:451, 1973.
22. Osofsky, J. D., et al.: *Psychologic effects of legal abortion* In Schaefer, G. (ed.): *Legal Abortions in New York State.* Clin. Obstet. Gynecology 14:215, 1971.
23. Ibid., p. 231.
24. Burnell, G. M., Dworsky, W. A. and Harrington, R. L.: *Post-abortion group therapy.* Am. J. Psychiat. 129:134, 1972.
25. Harting, D. and Hunter, H.: *Abortion technique and services: a review and critique.* Am. J. Pub. Health 61:2085, 1971.
26. *Editorial.* Am. J. Nurs. 72:61, 1972.
27. Gedan, S.: *Pre-abortion Emotional Counseling. A.N.A. Clinical Sessions, 1972.* Appleton-Century-Crofts, New York, 1972, p. 219.
28. Smith, E. D., Veolitze, M. and Merkatz, R.: *Social aspects of abortion counseling for patients undergoing elective abortion.* Clin. Obstet. Gynecol. 14:204, 1971.
29. Gedan, op. cit., p. 221.
30. Keller, C. and Copeland, P.: *Counseling the abortion patient is more than talk.* Am. J. Nurs. 72:102, 1972.
31. Clancy, B.: *The nurse and the abortion patient.* Nurs. Clin. North Am. 8:469, 1973.
32. Whitley, N.: *Second trimester abortion: a program of counseling and teaching.* J. Gynecol. Obstet. Nurs. 2:15, 1973.
33. Velvosky, I., et al.: *Painless Childbirth through Psychoprophylaxis.* Foreign Language Publishing House, Moscow, 1960, p. 26.

BIBLIOGRAPHY

Planned Parenthood of New York City: *Abortion: A Woman's Guide.* Abelard-Schuman, New York, 1973.

Abortion: the lonely problem. R.N. 33:34, 1970.

Addelson, F.: *Induced abortion: source of guilt or growth?* Am. J. Orthopsychiat. 43:815, 1973.

Ballard, C. A. and Quilligan, E. J.: *Midtrimester abortion with intra-amniotic saline and intravenous oxytocin.* Obstet. Gynecol. 41:447, 1973.

Bernstein, N. R. and Tinkhma, C. B.: *Group therapy following abortion.* J. Nerv. Ment. Dis. 152:303, 1971.

Bowlby, J.: *Attachment and Loss, vol. 1.* Basic Books, New York, 1969.

Bracken, M., et al.: *Abortion counseling: an experimental study of three techniques.* Am. J. Obstet. Gynecol. 117:10, 1973.

Branson, H.: *Nurses talk about abortion.* Am. J. Nurs. 72:107, 1972.

Burnell, G. M., Dworsky, W. A. and Harrington, R. L.: *Post-abortion group therapy.* Am. J. Psychiatry 129:220, 1972.

Burnett, L. S., Colston, W. and King, T. M.: *Technique of pregnancy termination.* Obstet. Gynec. Surv. Part I (Dec.) 1973, Part II (Jan.) 1974, pp. 6–42.

Cahill, I. D.: *Conflicts in values: staff attitudes toward therapeutic abortion.* In Duffey, M., et al. (eds.): *Current Concepts in Clinical Nursing, vol. III.* Mosby, St. Louis, 1971.

California Committee on Therapeutic Abortion: *Abortion and the Unwanted Child.* Springer, 1970.

Callahan, D.: *Abortion: Law, Choice and Morality.* Macmillan, 1970.

Clancy, B.: *The nurse and the abortion patient.* Nurs. Clin. North Am. 8:469, 1973.

Clark, M., et al.: *Sequels of unwanted pregnancy.* Lancet 2:501, 1968.

Cobliner, W. G., Schulman, H. and Romney, S. L.: *The termination of adolescent out-of-wedlock pregnancies and the prospects for their primary prevention.* Am. J. Obstet. Gynecol. 115:432, 1973.

Connell, E. B.: *Abortion: patterns, technics, and results.* Fertil. Steril. 24:78, 1973.

Cronenwett, L. and Choyce, J. M.: *Saline abortion.* Am. J. Nurs. 71:1754, 1971.

David, H. P.: *Abortion in psychological perspective.* Am. J. Orthopsychiat. 42:61, 1972.

Gabrielson, I. W., et al.: *Adolescent attitudes toward abortion: effects on contraceptive practice.* Am. J. Pub. Health 61:730, 1971.

Gedan, S.: *Pre-abortion emotional counseling. A.N.A. Clinical Sessions, 1972.* Appleton-Century-Crofts, New York, 1972.

Goldman, A.: *Learning abortion care.* Nurs. Outlook 19:351, 1971.

Gomel, V. and Carpenter, C. W.: *Induction of mid-trimester abortion with intrauterine alcohol.* Obstet. Gynecol. 41:455, 1973.

Hall, R. E.: *Abortion: physician and hospital attitudes.* Am. J. Pub. Health 61:517, 1971.

Harper, M. W., et al.: *Abortion: do attitudes of nursing personnel affect the patient's perception of care?* Nurs. Res. 21:327, 1972.

Harting, D. and Hunter, H. J.: *Abortion techniques and services: a review and critique.* Am. J. Pub. Health 61:2085, 1971.

Hausknecht, R. W.: *Free standing abortion clinics: a new phenomenon.* N. Y. Acad. Med. 49:985, 1973.

Hausknecht, R. U.: *The termination of pregnancy in adolescent women.* Pediatr. Clin. North Am. 19:803, 1972.

Heckman, M. K.: *What if it were I?* Am. J. Nurs. 66:768, 1966.

Howells, J. G.: *Termination of pregnancy.* In Howells, J. G. (ed.): *Modern Perspectives in Psycho-obstetrics.* Brunner-Mazel, New York, 1972.

Kane, F. and Lachenbruch, P. A.: *Adolescent pregnancy: a study of aborters and non-aborters.* Am. J. Orthopsychiat. 43:796, 1973.

Kane, R. J., Jr., et al.: *Motivational factors in abortion patients.* Am. J. Psychiatry 130:290, 1973.

Keller, C. and Copeland, P.: *Counseling the abortion patient is more than talk.* Am. J. Nurs. 72:102, 1972.

Lipper, I., et al.: *Abortion and the pregnant teenager.* Can. Med. Assoc. J. 109:852, 1973.

Malo-Juvera, D.: *Preparing students for abortion care.* Nurs. Outlook 19:347, 1971.

Martin, C. D.: *Psychological problems of abortion for the unwed teenage girl.* Genet. Psychol. Monogr. 88:23, 1973.

Meikle, S., et al.: *Therapeutic abortion: a prospective study.* Am. J. Obstet. Gynecol. 115:339, 1973.

Neubardt, S. and Schulman, H.: *Techniques of Abortion.* Little, Brown, and Company, Boston, 1972.

Newman, S. H. (ed.): *Abortion, Obtained and Denied Research Approaches.* Population Council, New York, 1971.

Perez-Reyes, M. G. and Falk, R.: *Follow up after therapeutic abortion in early adolescence.* Arch. Gen. Psychiatry 28:120, 1973.

Personal experience at a legal abortion center. Am. J. Nurs. 72:110, 1972.

Saltman, J.: *Abortion Today.* Charles C Thomas, Springfield, Ill., 1973.

Sarvis, B., and Rodman, H.: *The Abortion Controversy.* Columbia University Press, New York, 1973.

Vorherr, H.: *Contraception after aborton and post partum.* Am. J. Obstet. Gynecol. 117:1002, 1973.

Wallerstein, J., Bar-din, M.: *Seesaw response of a young unmarried couple to therapeutic abortion.* Arch. Gen. Psychiatry 27:251, 1972.

What nurses think about abortions. R.N. 33:40, 1970.

Wilson, R. R.: *Problem Pregnancy and Abortion Counseling.* Family Life Publications, Saluda, N. C., 1973.

Zahourek, R.: *Therapeutic abortion and cultural shock.* Nurs. Forum 10:9, 1971.

41 *Prematurity*

ANN L. CLARK, R.N., M.A.

Delivery prior to term can be a crisis situation to the parents. This chapter discusses parental problems related to the birth of a premature infant, but not the care of the infant. The preterm infant, with his physiologic handicaps, has been discussed previously in Chapters 37 and 38, since his care is similar to that of many other high-risk infants.

PREMATURITY AS A CRISIS

Very few women expect to deliver prior to term. Even though a woman may have experienced bleeding or other medical problems early in pregnancy, she hopes, and indeed expects, to deliver a fully developed infant. Labor which occurs prematurely is usually totally unexpected and is a stressful experience for the whole family. The psychologic preparation for labor and delivery has not been completed. Plans for caring for other siblings and for preparing the home for a new child are incomplete. The events that surround the labor, birth, and infant's care cause much disorganization. The fantasy of the "dream child," which now is not to be, brings about a sense of loss. Premature labor and the birth of a premature infant almost always constitute a crisis for the woman and her family.

ETIOLOGY

Frequently, the cause of a premature labor is not known. Even when the event can be explained medically, the mother usually searches for something that she may have done or may not have done to bring about this state of affair.

Studies appear to indicate that life experiences for many women who fail to carry to term seem to have been more stressful than for women who reach their estimated dates of confinement. A study by Gunter[1] implies that the physical, psychosomatic, and neuropsychiatric characteristics, and the social or life situation of the mother are related to and may in part determine the outcome of the pregnancy in terms of birth weight of the infant. These women were described as immature, dependent individuals. Many of these women gave social histories of neglect and desertion by their mothers. They saw themselves as being inadequate as a female, as rejecting heterosexual relationships, and as associating sex with guilt. They felt that they are less able to adapt to stressful life situations and less able to solve their own problems. It has been suggested that in internalizing their feelings they have expressed them somatically by giving birth prematurely.

Although other studies appear to support this hypothesis, the reader is cautioned to keep an open mind on the subject until more conclusive studies are completed on a wider social and ethnic population.

Blau and colleagues'[2] study of women who

delivered prematurely indicates that these women had more negative attitudes toward pregnancy, greater emotional immaturity, more body narcissism, and less resolution of familia (oedipal) problems. Downs[3] conducted a study indicating that maternal stress in primigravidas was a factor in the production of neonatal pathology. Prematurity and other neonatal pathology rates were higher for women who had experienced stress during the first trimester of pregnancy according to her findings.

LABOR AND DELIVERY

The recognition and acceptance that labor has indeed begun is often delayed for many women who go into labor prematurely. When it is accepted, it is experienced as an emotional shock for which the woman is unprepared. The journey to the hospital is of an emergency nature. The admission and the care in labor foster an atmosphere of danger. The fetal heart rate is checked frequently. The expectant parents' spoken and unspoken fears are answered in a guarded, noncommittal manner. The mother is told she will be given no analgesia or anesthesia in order to protect the infant's delicate structure. It is obvious that in no way is this a normal event and that the outcome is fraught with danger.

When the infant is delivered, it is quickly cared for by a number of individuals and then wisked away. The mother may not have heard the cry and immediately fears for its life. She may have only been given a fleeting glance of her child, enough to impress her with its small size, cyanotic color, and unattractive features, or she may not see the infant at all.

The distraught husband, after the stressful trip to the hospital or home from his place of employment, may be frantically trying to mobilize care for the other children. At the same time he is concerned for his anxious wife and his new baby which he perceives, possibly realistically, as being in grave danger.

PARENTAL RESPONSE TO THE BIRTH

The mother's stay in the hospital is a particularly trying time for her. Her anxiety is heightened due to concern for her baby and concern for self. How is it that she failed in this first task of mothering, that of carrying her child to term?

The atmosphere may still be filled with the perception of dangers. Is the child physically whole? When the parents visit the nursery they are frightened by the size and features of the infant. The mother may view the infant as a reminder of her failure. If she is an individual with a deprived social history, the baby is one more reflected appraisal of her self concept.

The equipment in the nursery, necessary to sustain life activities, may well leave the parents with great concern about their ability to assume responsibility for this child.

The environment for both parents is devoid of the usual rewards and recognitions accorded parents of a normal healthy child. No congratulatory notes or cards arrive, and few, if any, flowers. Visitors and callers speak with caution and with sympathy. The mother is not encouraged to feel proud, happy, and to get a good rest. She cannot share the baby with others for she experiences no feelings of success. Indeed, she feels lost and lonely.

The mother may roam aimlessly about the maternity department, expecting any minute to hear that her child has had a turn for the worst or has died. She responds somatically with sleepless nights and a loss of appetite. She may experience spells of weeping and of depression.

The staff may experience the mother's anxiety empathically and reduce their contact with her. They may feel unsure about their role. There may be no prompt and open discussion with the mother as to the cause or prognosis and the mother is kept in a state of suspense.

What information is imparted to her may be couched in guarded tones.

Sometimes the staff discusses the condition of the baby in an inconsistent manner with each of the parents. The father may be informed but cautioned "not to worry" his wife. This causes a breakdown in communication between the couple at a very important point during the crisis.

The father may experience guilt as to his own involvement in the infant's premature birth. He may well see it as a reflection on his masculinity. He is deprived of the usual pride in boasting of the child's size and features, and foregoes the usual cigar distribution and other cultural prerogatives.

REACTING AND COPING

Kaplan and Mason[4] state that the mother has four psychologic tasks to accomplish in coping with the birth of a premature infant:

1. Prepare for possible loss of the child whose life is in jeopardy. This "anticipatory grief"[5] involves a withdrawal from the relationship already established with the child so that the mother still hopes the baby will survive but simultaneously prepares for its death.
2. Face and acknowledge maternal failure to deliver a full term baby.
3. As the baby improves, she must now respond with hope and anticipation in this change. The baby's improvement symbolizes to the mother the possibility of retrieving, from what has been a total disappointment, a good measure of her hopes during the pregnancy. She now must resume the process of relating to the baby which had previously been interrupted.
4. Come to understand how a premature baby differs from a normal baby in terms of its special needs and growth patterns. This is in preparation of the imminent job of caring for the infant. In order to provide the extra amount of care and protection, the mother must see the baby as a premature with special needs and characteristics. But, it is equally as important for her to see that these needs are temporary and will yield in time to more normal patterns.

MATERNAL ATTACHMENT

It must be anticipated that maternal attachment may be more difficult to establish when the infant is premature. The many life-saving support systems may separate the mother from her infant for an extended period. The three sensory modalities involved in attachment need careful consideration so that modifications of hospital procedures and routines can be made for these mothers.[6] These modalities are:

Touch
Eye-to-eye contact
Caretaking.

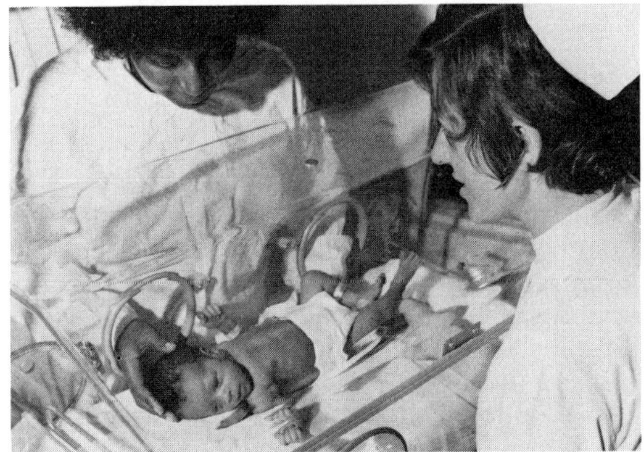

FIGURE 41-1. The mother of a premature infant begins the acquaintance process. (Courtesy of Louise Warrick. Photograph by Wometco Photo Services.)

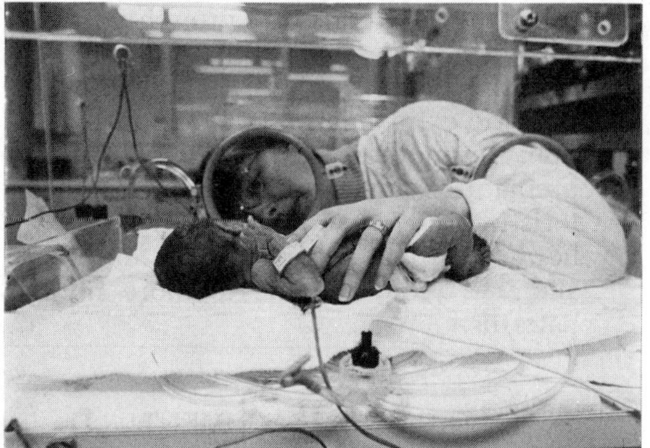

FIGURE 41-2. The mother in the en face position. (From Klaus, M., *Human maternal behavior in the first contact with her young*. Pediatrics 46:187, 1970, with permission.)

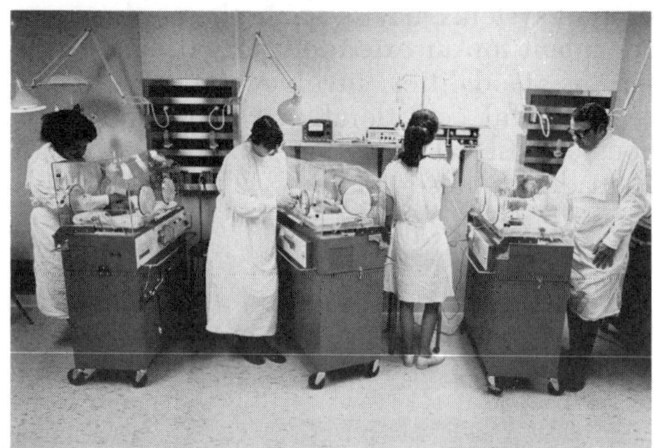

FIGURE 41-3. Parents of premature infants learning to care for their children. (Courtesy of Marshall Klaus.)

Figure 41-1 shows the premature's mother using touch to become acquainted with her infant. Each mother moves at her own rate, depending upon her perception of what is appropriate. Appropriateness depends upon how she perceives her child, i.e., how delicate his condition is, and how she interprets his response to her touching. Figure 41-2 shows the eye-to-eye contact in the en face position. Note that the mother tilts her face in line with the infant's so that the eye contact is direct. Figure 41-3 shows mothers carrying out their first mothering responsibility, that of giving physical care to their tiny infants. It may take some women a considerable time before they can reach this stage.

The mothers of many premature infants experience severe deprivation in one or several of these necessary components of interaction due to hospital policies, the condition of the infant, or the necessity to transfer the infant to another facility for the intensive care he needs. It is hypothesized that mothers who cannot establish the necessary attachment bonds to their infant during the critical attachment period (considered to be the first 10 to 14 days of life) due to enforced separation may, in turn, ultimately deprive their infants of adequate stimulation when they become largely responsible for their care. [7] Not only are attachment and commitment to the infant at stake, but the

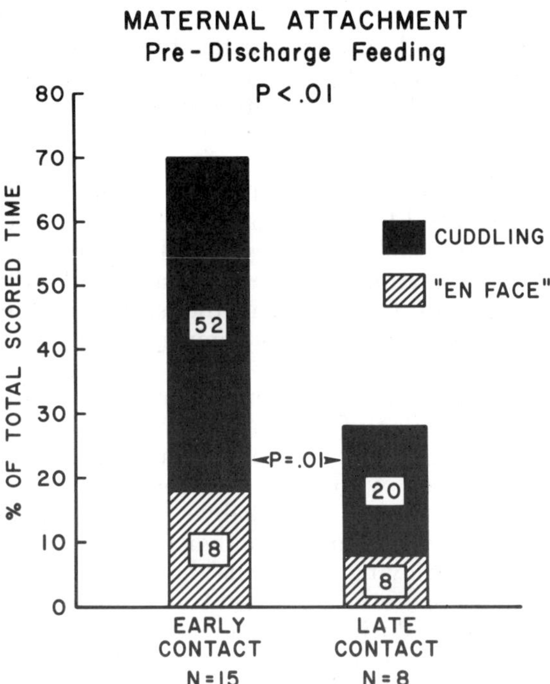

FIGURE 41-4. Percentage of en face and cuddling time in early and late contact mothers of premature infants. (From Klaus, M. and Kennell, J.: *Mothers separated from their newborn infants*. Pediatr. Clin. North Am. 17:1015, 1970, with permission.)

mother who is unable to care for her helpless infant cannot develop confidence in her ability to do so. Confidence is an important component of motherliness.

Decreased maternal attachment may ultimately be reflected in altered maternal behavior.[8] Figure 41-4 shows the difference in the amount of cuddling time and en face position between mothers who had opportunity to have early contact with their premature infants and those who did not. A large number of premature infants are later returned to the hospital with failure to thrive. Studies have shown that 15 to 30 per cent of these infants have no organic disease. Moreover, a significant number of children who are battered by their parents are prematurely born.[9] It is suggested that where maternal-infant separation is prolonged and grief advances unduly, close ties of affection may never be established securely.[10]

Fortunately, an increasing number of modern high-risk nurseries are permitting mothers and fathers into the nursery. The parents simply have to scrub their hands and wear a gown over their clothes. They can touch their infant and begin the acquaintance process.[11] The acquaintance process proceeds through three steps which answer the questions:

What are you really like?
What do you think of me?
What do I really think of you?

As Kennedy points out,[12] the developing maternal-infant relationship may be easily influenced in a negative direction by the acquisition of invalid or insufficient information from or about the infant, or by the mother's faulty or negative assessment of the baby's attitude toward her. Nurses can help the mother in her assessment process, but the mother must have access to her infant and must have assistance in collecting data about the baby.

Before the infant goes home, the mother who is permitted to meet some of her infant's physical needs has developed some confidence in her ability to care for the infant.

BALANCING FACTORS

There are various patterns with which families respond to the birth of a premature infant. Some of the patterns are more healthy in a psychologic sense than are others.

Healthy Patterns	Patterns Which Require Intervention
	Perception of the Event
Is willing to acknowledge reality of the danger.	Anxiety low or denied displaced or suppressed.
Is openly worred about the infant's chance of survival, about possible abnormality.	Naive or flippant attitude about infant's size and its health problems.
Judgment about the event is based on reality assessment.	Unrealistic explanation of cause of prematurity either in relation to self or others.
Reassurance by authority figures must be based on facts.	Accepts reassurance by authority figures, does not question rationality.
Realistic explanation of the cause of the prematurity.	Handles guilt and anxiety by blaming others.
Is aggressively active in her effort to learn about the baby and its progress.	Fails to come to grips with fears over the baby by not seeking information.
Keeps in touch with the hospital staff and makes frequent visits to the infant.	Infrequent visits to hospital, less verbal in seeking information about the infant.

Situational Support	
There is a mutual support system between the parents with division of responsibility.	Parents unable to express fear and grief with each other (often conscious agreement between parents).
There are qualities of warmth displayed between members of the immediate and extended family.	Use of denial or avoidance on part of the parents reduces opportunity for family or friends to offer support.
Family actively seeks help with the tasks related to dealing with negative feelings coping with the anticipated grief.	Reluctant to enlist or to use help. Apparent conflicts between husband and wife. Relatives may be hypercritical.
Agency help with cognitive grasp of the situation, accepts and encourages verbalization of feeling, encourages parental acceptance.	Agency has regulations which delay and limit parent-infant contact. Agency does not offer added environmental support.
Coping Behavior	
Anxiety level moderately high, openly evident, and acknowledged.	Little or no verbal expression of negative feelings, guilt, depression, anxiety.
Expresses feelings in words and nonverbally (e.g., crying) with resultant lessening of tension.	Thinks of escape from the hospital, sleeps to escape.
Maternal attachment shown through touch, focus on infant's emotional levels, learns to care for infant.	Maternal attachment shows passivity, with low activity in relation to attachment.
Objects to separation from the infant.	Rising tensions precipitate aggressive outbursts, blaming and other behavior not related to problem solving.
Plans for infant's homecoming. Seeks information and skill in caring for the infant.	Awaits news of the baby. Leaves outcome up to "fate". Little conscious planning for child care in the future.

NURSING ROLE

The nurse, with knowledge of the favorable and the less favorable manners in which individuals cope with the crisis of a premature birth, can apply her knowledge of the concept of crisis to help families redirect their efforts along more productive lines.

Her assessment must include some information related to the early life experience of the mother of the infant. Knowledge related to a deprived childhood will help the nurse understand the mother better and alert her to maternal performance that may lack depth and warmth. Positive feedback with the mother's ongoing personality development can be planned so that a nonspecific maturing effect can take place.

Assessment of the families' balancing factors as detailed previously will indicate to the nurse where she may "load" the balancing factors so that the family is assisted in resolving the crisis and improving their problem-solving methods for future crisis. Much is at stake in resolving this crisis, namely: a mother's mental health, a mother-infant relationship which will support the development of a healthy personality, and family stability.

It is important that the physician-nurse team keep each other apprised as to the information given to the parents and the parents' response to the events. Until the mother can visit the nursery, the nurse, as well as other members of the health team, should help her arrive at a realistic perception of the event.

The mother should be encouraged to express her feelings about herself, her labor, the premature birth, and the crisis in general. The fears and the loss need to be openly shared by the two parents. If the nurse observes a reluctance on the part of parents to share their common concerns, she should intervene. She can indicate that not discussing mutual concerns in order to "protect" another who is equally upset denies both individuals needed support. Crying should be expected and not be discouraged.

If anxiety is denied, the nurse will need a period of time to develop a trusting relationship with the individual and then to help the person express their fears for the infant's chance for survival, its normality, and their ability to care for the infant.

If the infant is gravely ill, the nurse may expect the parents to display anger at being deprived or abandoned. Feelings of purposelessness and shame may be experienced and verbalized or acted out.

It will be useful to explore with the parents what they think a premature infant is like and how it can be expected to develop. It is altogether possible that they may have had close contact with persons who are parents of prematures. Their own feelings, positive or negative, may be influenced by prior contacts.

If the mother saw the infant at the time of birth, she should be asked to describe what she saw and her feelings about the infant. More detachment should be expected if the mother does not describe the child with human features. Prior to the visit to the premature unit, the mother should be given a verbal orientation as to what she will see. The baby, if normal, should be described as "small, but quite normal in every way", for it is important at this point for the mother to know she has produced a normal child. The equipment should be described and its use related to her child. She can also be informed regarding when it can be discontinued and what this signifies about her child's progress.

When the mother visits the child, the nurse takes her cues from the mother, at the same time allowing her free access to her child, in keeping with its physiologic handicaps. The mother may be unready or unwilling to become involved with the infant for fear she may ultimately have to give the child up. Her tolerance level during the first week or so may only permit her to look at the baby. Until the mother can focus on the infant, the nurse focuses on the mother. As soon as possible, a porthole of the incubator should be opened and the mother encouraged to touch and to explore the child. The nurse can help the mother by pointing out certain features of the child and how perfectly it responds. She can be helped to note the infant's behavior and to gather cues as to his response. A communication system can be set up and the mother asked to try to determine what the baby likes and then send a message to him by verbal or nonverbal means.

Besides the support of the health team, the nurse should be aware of the quality of support that other individuals significant to the parents are offering. If there seems to be a paucity of support, the nurse should enquire as to who could be available, and encourage the parents to seek such assistance. Family, friends, clergy, and community agencies should be used to the fullest extent.

When the mother leaves the hospital she may well experience an acute sense of deprivation and a reinforcement of her failure. The health team must now put into action a plan to facilitate as close a contact between the parents and the child as possible, taking into consideration the mother's responsibilities to her other children and to transportation problems. The parents should be encouraged to visit as often as possible and to involve themselves in the infant's care. The mother's claiming progress should be carefully noted. The maternal visiting pattern is a crude but simple technique for predicting maternal performance.[13] Infrequent, uninvolved visiting may indicate that maternal claiming is not progressing normally. Concern for possible aberrant maternal acceptance should be noted. It would be well for high-risk nurseries to keep a log of all calls and visits to the infant. Notation of the mother's response to the infant should be recorded—whether she touches, feeds, or communicates with the infant in other ways. The length of the visit and the questions asked should also be noted. These are all important assessment data to identify the mother at risk. Maternal competence and attachment should be criteria for discharge from a premature unit.[14]

When the mother does visit, she should be afforded some privacy with her infant. "Love making" requires being alone and is an important element in the maternal attachment process.

Telephone calls should be encouraged. When the parents call they should be able to speak directly to those who are responsible for the infant's care. If the nursery makes plans to call the parents, the time should be preplanned so that anxiety is not experienced by the parents with each call.

There should continue to be some time set aside at intervals during which the parents can talk about themselves; their problems, their emotional feelings, and their somatic responses to the events related to being the parents of a premature infant. Verbalization reduces tension and helps individuals gain a new perspective of the problems facing them. Moreover, this kind of interest on the part of the nurse denotes respect for the parents and may be an important element in the process of regaining an acceptable view of self.

THE MOTHER AND THE NURSE

The mother may well experience some feelings of jealousy toward the nurse who cares for her infant. The nurse should keep this possibility clearly in mind and make certain she does not behave in a possessive manner. As the mother views the competent nurse caring for *her* child she may have mixed emotions of gratitude and resentment. The mother may be suspicious and resistive in fear of competition with the nurse for her child.[15] This response probably has little to do with the present situation but is a flash-back for the mother to prior life experiences with other persons.

Sometimes the nurse is a target of parental aggression or hostility. In such instances the nurse needs to see the behavior for what it is, a person's method of "holding on." The hostility is directed at "self," but finds expression interpersonally. It is not meant for the nurse personally. The nurse can assist the individual by responding to the assault in a therapeutic manner, not in a social one. Once the emotion is spent, the nurse can help the mother explore what precipitated the behavior and to express the feeling in a more acceptable manner.

The nurse can do much to help the mother feel it is indeed her child. When she discusses the child, she uses the term, "your son" or "your daughter." When the mother begins to care for the infant, she gives her tasks at which she can succeed and makes every effort not to let her fail at any task. The nurse, in her awareness of competition strivings that may arise due to the mother's dependence on others, avoids criticism at all costs.[15] The mother needs to renew her self-concept and the nurse can find many opportunities for input. "You did a great job," and "what a perfect little baby you have" can go a long way in meeting this need.

The nurse can assist the mother in feeling close to the infant as her own child by suggesting some small remembrance be left with the infant (a ribbon, a safe toy, etc.). The nurse herself should not furnish clothing or gifts for the infant; this will only foster unnecessary feelings of competition.

Some nurses have devised ingenious communication methods between the infant and its mother. A simple note pinned to the crib can assist—such as, "Gee, I'm happy. My mommie is coming to give me my next bath. Dave."

Parents who live such distance from the unit that they are unable to visit could be assisted in feeling a greater closeness by notes sent by the staff and signed by the infant.

HOSPITAL TO HOME

As indicated earlier, plans for sending the infant home are based on:

infant weight and progress
maternal competence
maternal attachment

Plans for homecoming should be initiated as soon as the infant's progress indicates that he will survive. Whenever possible, referral to the community health nurse should be made. This nurse in the community can then begin to coordinate plans with the hospital staff to continue the needed support. Assessment should be shared.

The nurse in the community helps the mother to talk about herself, her feelings of frustration, conflict, and fatigue. She can help the parents to think of ways the infant can take its place in the life of the family.

Siblings will need preparation for the arrival of their new brother or sister and the nurse should enquire into the preparation of them. Prior to homecoming, parents can be encouraged to take a picture of the infant for the children.[17] The children should discuss the feelings of competitiveness and jealousy they may well feel and be encouraged to talk to their parents when these feelings occur.

The mother will need to be helped to keep a realistic perception of the infant so that it is not overprotected. She may need continued support to develop competence so that she can find the time to enjoy and love the baby freed of the focus on food intake and weight gain.

REFERENCES

1. Gunter, L.: *Psychopathology and stress in the life experience of mothers of premature infants.* Am. J. Obstet. Gynecol. 86:333, 1963.
2. Blau, A., el al.: *The psychogenic etiology of premature births: a preliminary report.* Psychosom. Med. 25:201, 1963.
3. Downs, F.: *Maternal stress in primigravidas as a factor in the production of neonatal pathology.* Nursing Science 2:348, 1964.
4. Kaplan, D. M. and Mason, E. A.: *Maternal reactions to premature birth viewed as an acute emotional disorder.* Am. J. Orthopsychiatry 30:539, 1960.
5. Douglas, J. W. B.: *Factors associated with prematurity: results of a national survey.* J. Obstet. Gynaecol. Brit. Emp. 57:143, 1950.
6. Barnett, C., et al.: *Neonatal separation: the maternal side of interactional deprivation.* Pediatrics 45:197, 1970.
7. Rubenstein, J.: *Maternal attentiveness and subsequent exploratory behavior in the infant.* Child Develop. 38:1089, 1967.
8. Kennell, J. H. and Klaus, M. H.: *Care of the mother of the high-risk infant.* Clin. Obstet. Gynecol. 14:926, 1971.
9. Helfer, R. and Kempe, C., (eds.): *The Battered Child.* University of Chicago Press, Chicago, 1968.
10. Kennell and Klaus, op. cit., p. 936.
11. Newcomb, I.: *The Acquaintance Process.* Holt, Rinehart and Winston, New York, 1961.
12. Kennedy, J. C.: *The high risk maternal–infant acquaintance process.* Nurs. Clin. North Am. 8:549, 1973.

13. Fanaroff, A. A., Kennell, J. and Klaus, M.: *Follow-up on low birth weight infants–the predictable value of maternal visiting patterns.* Pediatrics 49:287, 1972.
14. Ibid., p. 289.
15. Prugh, D. G.: *Emotional problems of the premature infant's parents.* Nurs. Outlook 1:461, 1953.
16. Ibid., p. 462.
17. Warrick, L. H.: *Family centered care in the premature nursery.* Am. J. Nurs. 71:2134, 1971.

BIBLIOGRAPHY

Balu, A., et al.: *The psychogenic etiology of premature births.* Psychosom. Med. 25:201, 1963.

Bowlby, J.: *Attachment and Loss, vol. 1.* Basic Books, New York, 1969.

Callon, H. F.: *The premature infant's nurse.* Am. J. Nurs. 63:103, 1963.

Caplan, G.: *Patterns of parental response to the crisis of premature birth.* Psychiatry 23:365, 1960.

Cohen, R. L.: *Pregnancy stress and maternal perception of infant endowment.* J. Ment. Subnormality 12:18, 1966.

Downs, F.: *Maternal stress in primigravidas as a factor in the production of neonatal pathology.* Nurs. Science 2:348, 1964.

Eggli, O. W.: *Follow up care of the premature baby.* Am. J. Nurs. 58:231, 1958.

Fanaroff, A. A., Kendall, J. and Klaus, M.: *Follow-up of low birth weight infants.* Pediatrics 49:287, 1972.

Gunter, L.: *Psychopathology and stress in the life experience of mothers of premature infants.* Am. J. Obstet. Gynecol. 86:333, 1963.

Kaplan, D. and Mason, E.: *Maternal reactions to premature birth viewed as an acute emotional disorder.* Am. J. Orthopsychiat. 30:539, 1960.

Klaus, M. and Kennell, J.: *Mothers separated from their newborn infants.* Pediatr. Clin. North Am. 17:1015, 1970.

Klaus, M., et al.: *Human maternal behavior in the first contact with her young.* Pediatrics 46:187, 1970.

Mason, E.: *A method of predicting crisis outcome for mothers of premature babies.* Public Health Rep. 78:1031, 1963.

Moore, M. L.: *The Newborn and the Nurse.* W. B. Saunders, Philadelphia, 1972.

Owens, C.: *Parents' response to premature birth.* Am. J. Nurs. 60:1113, 1960.

Rubin, R., Rosenblatt, C. and Balow, B.: *Psychological and educational sequelae of prematurity.* Pediatrics 52:352, 1973.

42 *Death*

ANN L. CLARK, R.N., M.A.

Both childbearing families and health personnel working with expectant and new families experience grief when the anticipated joyous event of birth turns into a loss. Young parents often have few, if any, coping mechanisms to help them with the loss. Nurses and physicians, too, need new insight into their feelings, so that they can mourn the loss, but also allow themselves to assist the parents in their grief.

Since there are more deaths in the first few days of life than at any other time during childhood, and since most of these deaths and nearly all stillbirths occur in the hospital, certain policies and procedures have been developed to assist the grieving parents. We shall explore some of these in this chapter.

THE NURSE'S RESPONSE

When a death occurs on a maternity unit, it is an unexpected event and calls for an entirely different set of interpersonal skills[1] than one generally uses on such a unit. In every instance the nurse will be called upon to support the parents who are experiencing grief. It is therefore necessary for the nurse to have a clear understanding of the process of grief both as it affects her and as it is affecting her patient. Unless she recognizes how she handles her own feelings, she may not allow herself to give of "self" to others. Indeed, she may impede the mourning process of her patient.

The nurse must take into consideration her own personality and defenses against death. She needs insight not only into her feelings, but recognition of her own limitations.[2] Perhaps some questions and possible responses will help the reader to think more deeply about her feelings and defenses.

1. What are your feelings about the death of a fetus or a neonate?
   Do you feel sad? Are you frightened? Do you feel angry? Is it "God's will"? Do you feel helpless? Are you feeling a little guilty? Are you made anxious by the question? What else do you feel?

2. What would you say to an expectant mother whose fetus is dead?
   Would you avoid her? Talk about something else? Refer her to the physician? Encourage her to keep hoping and praying? What else would you do?
3. What do you feel is a proper way to respond to the loss of a fetus or a baby?
   Is it all right to cry? All right for the woman to cry but not the man? All right for the man to cry, or should he remain the strong member of the family? Should parents be left alone to grieve in privacy?

4. How do you feel about people who scream, swear, throw things, and blame others during their grief?
   Is that inappropriate behavior? Is it okay if it doesn't disturb others? Is it okay period?
5. Could you inform parents their infant had just died?
   Do you think that is not a nurse's responsibility? Would you want to be any place else but with the parents? Would you cry too? If you did cry, would that be "unprofessional" behavior?
6. Should the mother or parents ask to see the stillborn child? Is that inappropriate behavior?
   Would you agree to such a request or try to talk them out of it? Would you ask someone else to carry out the request? Do you think it would be too upsetting for a parent to see the body?

These are only a few of the questions that may help the reader to consider how the crisis of fetal or neonatal death might affect her or others.

When a nurse assumes closeness and emotional involvement with the expanding family, her commitment, in case of a death, may leave her with tangled emotions. Maternal and infant nursing is committed to protect and to nurture. When a fetus or neonate dies, the nurse may have a feeling of failure. This feeling of failure will make her feel guilty, perhaps helpless, angry, and undoubtedly anxious. She is vulnerable at this point and experiences internal conflicts. She must be careful not to work out her own problems (not deliberatively but as a defense) at the expense of her patient.[3]

The nurse most closely involved with the mother and infant, will need time to grieve, just as her patient will. She will also need environmental support, particularly an opportunity to talk about her feelings of failure, about the lost baby, the parents' feelings and responses to the loss. She needs others to temporarily assume her work load. In her feelings of sadness that she shares with the parents, there is no harm in her showing sympathy and expressing grief in the early mourning stage.[4]

The nurse can be seen to pass through the cardinal phases of mourning which according to Seltz and Warrick [5] could be expressed as:

Not me!
Why me?
If me—
Can I?
I can, I must!

The nurse who assesses where both she and her patient are in the grief process, grows personally and professionally through the experience of grief.

The nurse needs to be prepared for the tears and the outbursts that may well be her patient's response to the loss. Caught off guard, she may avoid or abandon the patient.[6] Often the mother's culture or her religious beliefs may dictate expressions of loss quite different from those with which the nurse is familiar. [7] When another's method of grieving does not "match," avoidance and even rejection are possible. The nurse needs to use objectivity in studying another person's mourning behavior. Adequate assessment can reduce the subjectivity.

THE AGENCY'S RESPONSE

The policies and procedures of an agency related to management at the time of fetal or neonatal death, if they are to be truly therapeutic, should be scientifically supportable. Kennell and colleagues[8] suspect that they are most often based on the convenience of the institution or of the staff. They are more likely to be a mixture of traditions, common assumptions, and staff's personal reaction. There is very little research to support the decisions made in relation to the parents, their grieving responses, and the care of the infant's body. The decisions are often made unilaterally, without consulting the parents as to their preferences. One might pose the following questions:

1. Should a mother see and touch her critically ill infant who may die?
   Does she mourn longer if she does touch? Is she more upset at the death? Does she regret or feel grateful for the experience?
2. After a stillbirth, what about the mother?
   Should she remain on the maternity unit, be transferred to a single room, transferred to another unit of the hospital? Should she be sent home?
3. Who should tell the mother of her infant's death?
   Should the father be told and he should tell his wife? Should it be the pediatrician? The obstetrician? The nurse? The health professional having the closest emotional ties with the mother?
4. If the fetus is unexpectantly born dead, should the mother be told immediately?
   Should she be given a tranquilizer and told later? Should she be kept under tranquilizers?

PARENTAL RESPONSES TO LOSS

THE MOTHER

Every mother and father mourns for their dead child. The absence of grief is not a healthy sign but rather a cause for concern. Even if the infant is nonviable at birth and lives only a few minutes, mourning takes place.[9] This is an indication that attachment begins well before birth. Even without the maternal nurturing experience, a mother is capable of deep love for the baby while it is still a "dream child."

The stages of mourning discussed in Chapter 10 will be the same for the parents of a dead neonate. The initial stage of shock and disbelief can be expected. If the death comes without prior warning, the first stage, accompanied by denial may be lengthy.[10] If the mother is under heavy sedation during the labor, remembers little or nothing of the delivery, and does not see the dead baby, she may awaken from the experience feeling nothing except she has had a very bad dream. With no mental picture of the infant, she may beg to see the child's body.[11] During the acute mourning stage, weeping and occasionally hysterics can be expected. If the woman's culture and/or the persons in the institution support this behavior, "grief work" can begin. However, loud crying is generally not culturally accepted in most of America. She may be silenced by tranquilizers and/or referred for psychiatric consultation, either of which may increase her anxiety and her feelings of guilt. Indeed, the stronger the mourning reaction is in the early period of grief, the more favorable the outcome can be expected to be.[12] The use of tranquilizers to subdue the woman's grief is no doubt more for the staff who, by controlling and legitimizing her behavior, feel more comfortable themselves.[13]

Feelings of guilt very often accompany the grieving process and they are extremely painful for the mother of a dead neonate. She reviews what she has done, what she has not done, and even what she has thought of doing. The mother may blame sexual activity, moving, climbing, nutritional intake, and hundreds of other activities for the loss. Her fantasies regarding the power of any negative feelings may be particularly stressful to the woman. One or both parents or their families may imply that genetic, social, or psychologic "weakness" was responsible for the loss. All of this can be ego destructive to the mother.

The grieving mother may behave in a hostile manner, become enraged, and verbally blame the staff for the infant's death. Expressed anger is part of the mourning process. It is part of the acceptance of the reality and finality of the event. However, blaming, unless the blame is indeed valid, impinges on acceptance and impedes the resolution of the grief process.

The intensity and duration of the grieving appear to relate to the duration of the woman's pregnancy and the concomitant evolution of her maternal identity.[14] A good mother does not harm her baby and the thwarted mother is now faced with insulating herself from the overwhelming feelings of shame and guilt. Her failure, her sense of maternal identity, and her self-esteem are at stake.[15]

Handling the death of an expected baby requires some strange and unique cognitive powers. The reader will recall that during the resolution of the earliest tasks of pregnancy, the mother asks:[16]

Who me?
Now?

That task must have been completed if grieving for the dead fetus ensues. Now the woman must reverse the process and ask:

Not now? Oh no!
Why me?

The mourning that occurs is an elaborate process. The mother's ego is regained bit by bit. The final resolution will come when, according to McLenahan,[17] the mother is freed from the bondage of the baby who is gone and makes adjustments in her life without the anticipated baby, forms other relationships, and finds other interests. This may take anywhere from three months to a year, with an average of six months. The important point to keep in mind is that mourning and grief should not be suppressed and cannot be compressed.[18]

The mother will exhibit any number of the cardinal features of mourning:

somatic distress
intense subjective distress
preoccupation with the image of the infant (real or imagined)
feelings of guilt for possible negligence or minor omissions
breakdown in normal patterns of conduct, including hostility toward others.

According to a study by Kennell and colleagues,[19] a higher degree of mourning can be expected of women in four circumstances:

pleasure at being pregnant
prior loss of a baby
touching the baby before its death
lack of communication with the husband about the loss.

In their study, all mothers experienced sadness and preoccupation with thoughts of the dead baby and even after the grieving was past, there were waves of sadness. All but two of the mothers experienced insomnia and disturbance with the usual patterns of their daily life. All but three experienced unusual irritability and all but four experienced loss of appetite.

Certain women are particularly vulnerable when they experience the loss of an expected baby. The physical health of the individual will make a difference, for ill health leaves the woman more defenseless. Further, the number and the nature of previous losses and the way they were resolved is important. Loss tends to be cumulative in its effect.[20] A recent loss tends to revive an earlier loss, particularly if it has been left unresolved.[21]

If the loss is expected, some grief work may occur before the actual death. In any case, the supportive factors will enter into the resolution of the crisis. Relatives and friends, religious faith and cultural values, beliefs and practices are all potential sources of support. According to Engle,[22] "the clearest evidence of successful healing is the ability to remember comfortably and realistically both pleasure and disappointment of the lost relationship."

Some women develop pathologic responses to the loss. Any of the following *may* indicate such a response:[23]

- Displays increased activity and intensified focus on external affairs.
- Does not weep.
- Expresses no feelings of pain or loneliness.
- Displays marked hostility, often toward those caring for the deceased.
- Verbalizes exaggerated degrees of guilt.
- Projects "wooden" or formal manner.
- Carries on activities detrimental to own safety, social or economic existence.
- Demonstrates agitated depression.

THE FATHER

A culturalization of male behavior begins very early in life. "Boys don't cry, but girls can." "Men are strong and do not show emotions." These concepts cause real problems when a man faces the loss of a child—problems for himself and often problems for his wife. The fact is, men, like all human creatures, grieve over such losses. Whether a man will mourn overtly and resolve his grief will depend on his self-concept as a man. Some men deny grief and plunge into their work, even taking on extra work. When they experience the feelings that accompany grief, they are perplexed. Distortion of pre-existing husband-wife relationships may follow.[24] The husband may feel that any discussion of the loss with his wife will further distress her. Sometimes he tries to bring his wife out of her depression. On the other hand, the wife may be moving ahead with her "grief work" while the husband is still maintaining denial with an "everything will be all right" attitude. In his inability to cope with the situation he may feel impatient and, lacking support, will withdraw from the event. Perhaps that is what the man who takes on extra work is doing. There is always the possibility that he will feel and even display anger toward his wife for failing to give him the anticipated child. It is important that synchrony of grieving between the husband and wife occurs, lack of synchrony leads to dissonance. The parents need to talk to each other about their sadness. Some couples find physical closeness and sexual relations most comforting and meaningful during these times.

THE CHILDREN

Regardless of their age, children in a family that loses an expected baby will be affected by the loss in some way. The age of the child, his concept of death, his parents' response to the loss, and their attitude about sharing the loss with the children will be the key issues.

In our culture we are now, according to Fromm,[25] in an "era which simply denies death. It even seems to be a matter of bad taste to mention it. Death is passed off as a morbid topic to be ignored if at all possible." Yet we all develop some personal concept of life and of death—much of it from our parents.

Explaining death to children is not a simple task, but when an expected sibling fails to materialize it is important that there be a free communication flow between the parent and the child. The infant's death and the sadness that the parents feel should not be withheld from the child. The child will be well aware that something has happened and that his parents are upset. If it is not discussed, the secretness teaches the child that certain subjects are taboo, in this case the discussion of death. If it is so awful to talk about it, then it must be fearful indeed. This leaves the child to fantasize and the fantasies may be more terrifying than the true story told by loving parents. The death can be converted into a positive life experience for the child through the sharing of feelings. The sadness which the parents feel can be shared with the child, teaching him that loss is appropriately grieved. The child also learns how much parents can care. Open communication can protect the child from feeling that somehow he was responsible for the death of the baby.

What and how does a parent tell a child about death? Much depends on the age of the child and on the parents' religious concepts. Even then, it is no simple matter to clearly convey the concept to a child. The parents will be burdened with their own personal grief and may themselves be struggling with a question for which there is no answer. The resolution of "why" their neonate did not live must be based on some faith.

For all children it is important to use the correct terms, e.g., "died," "dead," "buried." Children think in concrete terms and they can deal with these explanations.[26] The baby did *not* go into a long sleep. To believe this is to make the child fearful of going to sleep himself.

Preschool children do not conceive of the finality of an event. They can easily believe that a person can be gone and then can return again. We teach children that this is a causal world, that things just don't happen, but that they are caused.[27] We don't always get the message across that *they* are not the cause. In this instance, the child needs to be reassured that no one, including he himself, caused the baby to die. The preschool child can usually accept death as a matter of fact and without emotions. In Gartley's study,[28] preschool children who had been taught that heaven was to be their final destiny were still sometimes unclear whether they could return to earth after they had died. Their expressed concern about dying and going to heaven was that they "couldn't play up there." Perhaps the parents best approach to this age child is to report the event, share their sorrow with the child, and give him every assurance that he is loved.

Children 5 to 10 years of age perceive a loss differently. They begin to personify death and to believe that it can happen and that it is final. It is at this age that the child begins to believe in boogie men and scary all-powerful ghosts. They can easily believe that some dreadful person carried the baby off.[29] These children may feel fearful of the implication of death and fear for their own safety. The child needs to be assured that he is loved and that he is safe. Holding the child closely while the story is related will convey that message. If it is the parents' belief that the soul goes to heaven, this can be shared with the preteen child. In any event, an open parent-child communication system is necessary in which questions can be posed and fears expressed.

The adolescent sees death as a personal loss, something which has occurred and which is irrevocable.[30] They should be given an adult explanation of the loss and encouraged to discuss the event with their parents. Depending upon their emotional involvement with the anticipated sibling they may have "grief work" to do, and they may experience guilt.

It is important that we all develop a healthy understanding of death. It's unhealthy to pretend we will live forever and it is just as unhealthy to be morbidly preoccupied with death. It would appear that frank, honest, simple explanations are more advisable than trying to conceal death from children.[31] Healthy grieving should not be suppressed. The way in which parents handle the subject of death with their children says much about how they are permitting themselves to grieve.

In the review of the literature, there is to be found a paucity of answers to how to explain death to a child but a lot of statements of what not to say.

Honesty is the best approach. If the parents believe that there is a spiritual body which leaves the physical body at death and that God makes the determination when that shall occur, there is no reason to fear telling this to the child. It can be done in a manner that will not convey to the child that God is a vengeful being who might "swoop down and carry him off next." The same rationale can be applied in explaining to the child that the infant was too weak, too ill, or not completely developed and therefore God made a place for his soul in heaven. This need not make the child more fearful for his own life when he becomes ill sometime in the future.

NURSING ASSESSMENT

The *behavior dynamics* of the grieving individual will form the basis for nursing assessment. Most often the loss of a fetus or neonate is an unexpected event. The suddenness of the event leaves the nurse with little or no time to plan and in a position where the collection of some useful data is, for the time being, inappropriate.

The grieving parents' response to the loss, both as individuals and as a couple, will help the nurse to assess what nursing action is appropriate.

Are the mother and father open in expressing their grief and sadness, both verbally and nonverbally?

What is the extent of their weeping, anger, guilt, hostility?

Are they experiencing insomnia, loss of appetite, irritability, somatic distress, or changes in patterns of conduct with others?

Bibring[32] states that parents who hide their feelings and avoid talking about the traumatic event continue to exhibit symptoms of grief longer than those who communicate their grief freely.

The nurse will want to know if there is synchrony between the parents in the grieving process. There are nursing implications if one parent is denying the loss or is refusing to communicate with the other. This may be a serious problem. Culberg's[33] study indicates that a severe breakdown in husband-wife communication may have contributed to more than one third of the mothers in his study developing severe psychiatric problems within one to two years of the tragic event.

The nurse will want to know what the parents have been told about the cause of death and if they personally have other explanations for the event. Through interview the nurse would want to ascertain what guilt feelings the mother may be experiencing and how she feels about herself as a feminine person. She will want to learn what impact the loss has on the father's concept of self.

The nurse will want to know if the parents have seen the dead infant and if they have requested to see the infant. If the infant was born alive, she will want to know if the mother has seen, touched, or cared for the infant.

The religious beliefs of the parents, particularly in relation to life and death, will be necessary data. The nurse will wish to know if the family has seen, has asked to see, or wishes to see a member of the clergy. The cultural beliefs and practices of the family will be useful data for the nurse to obtain.

Other useful data which must await a closer nurse-patient relationship are:

Feelings about becoming pregnant, being a mother.

Other major losses in life and particularly the loss of a child. How she has responded to these losses. If she has ever had a friend who has lost a baby.

The nurse will want to enquire who are the significant people in the couple's lives who can now be depended upon to support them in their grief. There may be no one, which has significant implications for nursing.

Finally, the nurse will need data about the other children in the family: their ages, what they have been told about the coming baby, and how the parents plan to inform them of the infant's death.

NURSING INTERVENTION

The nursing acts planned and carried out in the interest of parents of stillborn infants and parents of neonates who die are essentially directed toward promoting a resolution of the grief process. The nurse cannot give to the grieving parents the child they so desperately want. She can assist them through acts of protection, nurturing, and stimulation, to face the grief, to mourn, and ultimately to accept the reality in a healthy manner. Acceptance of the loss in a healthy manner is of extreme importance. Beyond the grievous loss is a reassessment on the part of both parents of the concept of self. To give birth to an infant who is too ill or too incompletely developed to survive is a threat to one's ego.

This discussion first explores some universal acts of nursing that are applicable to the loss of a neonate and then focuses on some specific incidents that need special intervention. Protecting, nurturing, and stimulating will be found in nursing actions that

promote the resolution of the grief process
offer ego support to protect and enhance the self system.

The nurse faced with a family who has just sustained the loss of an infant may well feel there is little she can do. However, "with our present concept of maternity care focused upon the woman's acceptance of her maternal identity and maternal role, it is impossible to ignore or view lightly the meaning of the infant's death to the mother" according to Seltz and Warrick.[34] Every nurse can carry out acts of nursing care that conserve energy. This is an important first step, for grieving takes energy. Offering comfort measures to the woman is one way of demonstrating "caring." The extra attention of a cup of tea, a back rub, assembling bath equipment and accompanying her to the shower, and so forth are not only physically comforting but convey the reassuring message that she is worthy of such added attention. Dependency in the early puerperium is to be expected; it should not only be permitted but encouraged. Studies indicate that women do not want to be left alone during their grief, but it is not easy to stay with a weeping and grieving individual. What does the nurse do? What is appropriate and helpful to say? Staying with the woman shows that the nurse feels compassion for her. Listening to her, encouraging her to talk about her disappointment, her fears, her concerns, are all helpful. By simply remaining, she demonstrates her feelings of worthiness for the individual. Some women may want to cry, others to be silent, to gesticulate, to talk. The nurse offers the mother an opportunity to do what she has to and accepts her unique manner of expressing her loss. If the form of grieving is upsetting to other patients, the nurse finds a place where the woman can have privacy.[35] Kennell and Klaus[36] believe that tranquilizers divert the grief work and should not be given except to facilitate sleep at night.

Most women are further distressed by having to share a room with another mother whose baby is brought to her,[37] so that a private room or a room with another woman who does not have a baby should be made available. It is generally agreed that to remove the woman from the maternity unit is a denial of reality.[38] It is probably true that the maternity nurse can best plan for the total care of this patient, but, the patient's desires should be taken into consideration. It is very important, no matter where the patient is placed, that all members of the staff who have contact with the patient know what has happened and verbally acknowledge that the woman is experiencing a difficult task. Patients understandingly become very angry when they are asked if they "had a boy or a girl" or are told to "get ready, babies will be brought out soon." The woman may choose anyone, the cleaning lady, the volunteer, or others, to relate her loss. All women in a study by Yates[39] expressed an overwhelming need to talk about the experience. She may need to repeat the story over and over again. It is not necessary for the nurse, or indeed for others who come in contact with the woman, to have all the scientific, logical, or spiritual answers to the "why?" What the woman needs is a caring attitude in which she is free to explore her own feelings about the "why." Verbal acknowledgment of others as to the pain she must be experiencing and the difficult task she is facing will be of great assistance. In permitting the woman to explore her own version of the cause for the death, erroneous and guilt-laden material may be verbalized. She may state that she is being punished for past wrongdoings.[40] The woman may not have really heard or understood the physician's discussion with her. The nurse can fill a useful role in clarifying and reiterating what has been communicated. However, the nurse's most useful role will be in the supportive relationship she builds with the mother, not in explaining the "why." The patient can look to the physician for the etiology, to the clergy for a religious interpretation; the nurse supplements those functions, but she has a unique contribution due to her knowledge and the opportunity to have close contact with the mother and with the family.

Once the loss has occurred, special consideration should be given to the patient. Visiting hours should be relaxed so that supportive family and friends can visit. If the woman wishes, the clergy should be notified. It is the nurse's responsibility to remember to check the mother's data sheet for her religious preference and ask the mother if clergy should be summoned.

The woman's concept of self will be interrelated with details of the baby. The nurse who perceives of the baby as an accepted, special human being will be helping to preserve the woman's feminine identity.[41] When the baby can be described as "perfect," "beautiful," "brown hair like yours," the mother will feel less shame over the outcome and an increased sense of dignity and personal worth.[42]

The nurse may be faced with an angry patient (or family). The nurse recalls it is a part of the grieving process and accepts it as such. The anger moves the grieving process forward,[43] thus nursing efforts must not be withdrawn. This may be a difficult experience for the nurse but she cannot respond to it in a social frame of reference. Once the anger has been spent, the nurse can help the individual to understand its cause.

Talking with the grieving parents about the pattern that mourning can be expected to take, including the waves of sadness that may persist for a time and the length of the experience, may be very useful. This sharing of the universality of feelings and behaviors may well reduce the alarm a person may experience.

It is inappropriate to suggest that the mother replace the lost baby with another pregnancy. No future child can take the place of this one. Many women become angry when the focus is diverted. However, the couple will at some point want to know if they can produce a normal child sometime in the future. Deutsch[44] tells us that having a baby soon after the death of a neonate is "not characteristic of real grief but corresponds to the effect of the nonfulfillment of a wish fantasy." In a study by Wolff,[45] 50 per cent of the women planned never to become pregnant again and four women (2 per cent) had permanent sterilization procedures performed. One could speculate that these women did so out of fear of being hurt again. It might have been a method of self-punishment. If the family does state that they do not wish to have more children, the nurse needs to assess if they have adequate conception control information and should fill any needs.

It is also inadvisable to suggest that the mother remember that she is blessed with other children. She needs to work through this present loss, she cannot focus on other aspects of her life at this time. When the woman does inquire about her chances of having another *normal* child, the nurse must not give in to her desire to reassure the mother. Although it may be true that the overwhelming chances of having a normal child are in her favor, to go further than this is to give false optimism, for no one can assure her, or for that matter anyone, that the next pregnancy will result in a normal live child.

Some special attention should be centered on returning home. Some writers suggest that the mother should return to her home as soon as she is physically able to do so. An assessment of the home environment should precede the final decision. The woman can expect tearful encounters with family and friends. Some of them will know and may be very supportive, others will know and find themselves unable to discuss the tragedy, and others will not know of the loss and may make painful enquiries. The nursing data collection will help the nurse to give the woman anticipatory guidance. She can help her to think through how she will tell others. There will need to be decisions made about the disposition of the assembled layette. Having someone "wisk it away" is a form of denial. The woman may not be able to deal with storing or disposing of the baby's equipment at first; when she does do so, it will take its place in the "grief work" to be accomplished. A referral to the community health nurse may be an appropriate nursing decision. The mother should be warned not to rush back to work, not to try to "pull herself together." The sad feelings and the disappointment need to be shared, the painful feeling will then slowly lessen until the finality is accepted and becomes a part of life. Positive accomplishment leaves the individual with more coping ability to face future crises in life.

If the infant is born alive, it is important that during the infant's terminal illness both parents be given the *same* report about the infant's progress. It should be given to both parents at the same time if possible. "Shading" the report to one member of the family leads to breakdowns in communication, something that must be guarded against at all costs.

Should the mother of a critically ill neonate have contact with her infant? Should she touch it, care for it? Is it psychologically safe? Will there be pathologic grieving following such contact? Studies by Kennell and colleagues[46] indicate that unless the woman has had a history of hospitalization for a psychiatric disease, the mother is not unduly upset. The mourning response may likely be of a higher degree when the mother does touch her child but no pathologic grieving results. Indeed, it is said that the stronger the early mourning reaction is, the more promising the outcome.[47] The mother should not be denied the right to share life with her child, even for such a brief period. The staff who do deny the mother, feeling that it would be "too cruel" are more than likely protecting themselves by the use of denial and rationalization as defenses.

When the infant dies, the nurse caring for the infant should make herself available to the mother. The time spent with her can be used to answer her questions and clarify the event. This nurse more than anyone can assure the mother that she, the mother, has done all that is humanly possible to give her baby the best chance to survive and to let her know that she has not neglected her baby.[48] A repeat visit to the mother the following day may be most therapeutic.

Some parents ask to view the body of the stillborn child and this, too, should not be denied them. It is most important to the self-esteem of the parents to view the body of their well-formed infant. Even when there are malformations or incomplete development, the parents' fantasies may be more destructive than the reality. Prior to bringing the dead infant to the parents, the nurse explores with them their experience in viewing a dead body. The nurse explains what they will witness—a white, cold, stiff body and something of the appearance of the baby as well. She will also warn them that the experience will be painful, but that if they wish to see the baby, it will be useful to the grief process. They can then make the decision about viewing the body on a personal basis. With this kind of prior preparation, hysterical responses are rarely encountered. When the infant is brought to the parents it should be clean, wrapped in a colorful blanket and handled with care, indicating that it is valued. The parents should have privacy but the nurse should remain with them as appropriate.

It is most important that parents be encouraged to share their grief and to talk with each other about their feelings after such an experience. Men, especially in the American culture, may need help and permission to express their grief. He needs to know that grieving is a universal experience and that its expressions are valid, vital, and appropriate. Kennell and colleagues'[49] study indicates that high mourning was associated with a failure of communications between husband and wife or when there was no husband or mother with whom to share the grief. Physical symptoms of grief are alarming to the parents, they may fear they are "losing their minds." They may complain of strange visceral sensations, such as "whirling around," "pressure in the head," "heartaches," and "stomach pains," accompanied by sighing and restlessness.[50] Some feel immobilized, unable to even care for themselves at all.

The concerns for the couple must not end when the mother is discharged from the hospital. At the 4 to 6 week checkup and again at 3 to 4 months postpartum a member of the health team (it could well be the nurse) should see the couple together, enquire of their health and learn how well they have worked through their grief. The autopsy findings, complete by the second contact, should be shared with the parents.[51] These sessions have two purposes. They show the concern felt for two individuals who have faced a painful experience. This in itself is ego-supportive. It also gives the physician or the nurse an opportunity to assess for any distortions in the resolution of the grief and to make appropriate referrals, if necessary.

FETAL DEATH: SPECIAL IMPLICATIONS

The fetal heart may suddenly stop during pregnancy, usually without warning, and often for no explainable reason. Indeed, an etiology cannot be found for over half of the fetal deaths, even after an autopsy.[52] The expectant mother may first notice the lack of fetal movements and report it to the physician. These are extremely anxious days until the physician can make a final determination as to the condition of the fetus. Once the determination is made that the fetus has succumbed, both expectant parents should be told, if at all possible, at the same time. They need to have mutual understanding of the problem and to be encouraged to talk together about the problem and their feelings. In 75 per cent of women, labor spontaneously ensues within two weeks of fetal death.[53] This is a difficult two weeks. The nurse should make herself available to the parents and encourage them to verbalize their feelings. Listening, allowing the tears, and tolerating the anger helps the expectant mother to feel she is not alone in her grief. It is a difficult experience to carry a dead baby even for two weeks, but it may be four or five weeks before induction of labor can safely be started. Even then, the induction, as discussed in Chapter 40, is not without dangers.

The nurse should make herself available to the expectant mother for extra visits and for telephone calls during the wait. The nurse can call the woman between visits, signifying that even in the face of failure the expectant mother has worth and value. The expectant mother may greatly need this kind of communication for it is likely family and friends may find it difficult to discuss or even permit the expectant mother to discuss her tragedy.

The labor and delivery of a woman who is carrying a dead fetus is a particularly stressful experience for both the woman and her husband. The woman must now face a physically painful experience, no doubt made more painful due to the cumulative stress. She is not only fearful of the pain of labor, but of the final confirmation of the death. No matter how sure she is that the fetus is dead, she does not want to give up hope.[54] At the same time she wants some sign that those who care for her during labor know of her "special" situation and she studies each one who comes into her room for such confirmation. Under *no* circumstances should a member of the staff use the stethoscope or Doppler to "check once more."

The expectant father, like his wife, may undergo a painful experience during his wife's labor. He may feel guilty for subjecting his wife to such stress, frustrated that he cannot help her, and ashamed of his "lack of masculinity." He needs an opportunity to talk with a caring individual also.

Whatever induction method is chosen by the physician, the woman will need a clarification of the procedure and the support of a caring nurse during her labor. She will not want to be left alone. It is possible that the woman may use the labor to accomplish further "grief work." The nurse may expect behavior such as denial, anger, bargaining, and depression. The nurse can create an atmosphere in which it is safe to express feelings and to verbalize fears for there is no "real" purpose in this labor. The nurse may well feel she doesn't know what to say to this patient, and verbalizing this to a patient would be entirely appropriate.

> I don't know what to say. There are no right words when we lose a baby—but we all feel your loss.[55]

Once the delivery is accomplished and the baby is pronounced dead, the "grief work" can continue. Prolonged shock and disbelief must now give way to acceptance. When denial is continually used, the nurse will gently confront the patient with the reality of the baby's death. This will be difficult, but it is important.[56] The mother will at some point seek information about her baby. Some women will want to be involved in naming the baby, consenting to the autopsy, making funeral arrangement, etc. The decisions each individual makes will be right for them. The words the nurse uses and the actions she takes will depend on the needs and problems of each individual. Assessment will make the response relevant for that individual.

MEDICAL MANAGEMENT

If labor does not begin spontaneously after the death of the fetus, it is induced by the fourth or fifth week.[57] Weekly fibrinogen determinations are carried out after the fetal death occurs, for decreased fibrinogen content in the maternal blood may result from the retention of a dead fetus.[58] The release of thromboplastin into the maternal circulation from degenerating fetal tissues results in defibrinogenation by promoting maternal intravascular clotting.[59]

Labor may be induced by a dilute infusion of an oxytocic or by the intrauterine injection of a hypertonic saline solution (20 per cent) or a hypertonic glucose solution (50 per cent). These have been discussed previously in Chapter 40. Induction of labor is not without danger to the woman and research continues in order to discover a safer way to successfully terminate these pregnancies.

REFERENCES

1. Engel, G. L.: *Grief and grieving.* Am. J. Nurs. 64:93, 1964.
2. McLenahan, I. G.: *Helping the mother who has no baby to take home.* Am. J. Nurs. 62:70, 1962.
3. Bruce, S.: *Reactions of nurses and mothers to stillbirths.* Nurs. Outlook 10:88, 1962.
4. Zahourek, R. and Jensen, J. S.: *Grieving and loss of the newborn.* Am. J. Nurs. 73:836, 1973.
5. Seitz, P. and Warrick, L.: *Perinatal death: the grieving mother.* Am. J. Nurs. 74:2028, 1974.

6. Zahourek, loc. cit.
7. McLenahan, loc. cit.
8. Kennell, J. H., Slyter, H. and Klaus, M. H.: *The mourning response of parents to the death of a newborn infant.* N. Engl. J. Med. 283:344, 1970.
9. Ibid.
10. Zahourek, loc. cit.
11. Ibid.
12. Klaus, M. and Farnaroff, A.: *Care of the High Risk Neonate*. W. B. Saunders, Philadelphia, 1973, p. 117.
13. Zahourek, op. cit.
14. Seitz and Warrick, op. cit.
15. Ibid.
16. Rubin, R.: *Cognitive style in pregnancy*. Am. J. Nurs. 70:502, 1970.
17. McLenahan, op. cit.
18. Kennell, J. H. and Klaus, M. H.: *Care of the mother of the high risk infant.* Clin. Obstet. Gynecol. 14:926, 1971.
19. Kennell, H. H. Slyter, H. and Klaus, M. H.: *The mourning response of parents to the death of a newborn infant.* Child and Family 9:221, 1970.
20. Engel, op. cit.
21. Ibid.
22. Ibid.
23. Zahourek, op. cit., p. 837.
24. Kennell, op. cit.
25. Fromm, E.: *Man for Himself.* Fawcett, Greenwich, Conn., 1965, p. 72
26. Gartley, W. and Bernasconi, M.: *The concept of death in children.* J. Genet. Psychol. 110:71, 1967.
27. Layman, W. A.: *Grief and grieving.* In Clark, A., et al. (eds.): *Parent-Child Relationships: Role of the Nurse.* Rutgers University, New Brunswick, N. J., 1968, p. 13.
28. Gartley, loc. cit.
29. Lyman, loc. cit.
30. Ibid.
31. Gartley, loc. cit.
32. Bibring, G. L.: *The death of an infant: A psychiatric study.* N. Engl. J. Med. 283:370, 1970.
33. Culberg, J.: *Mental reactions of women to perinatal death.* In Morris, N. (ed.): *Psychosomatic Medicine in Obstetrics and Gynecology.* Karger, New York, 1972.
34. Seltz and Warrick, loc. cit.
35. McLenahan, op. cit., p. 71.
36. Kennell and Klaus, op. cit.
37. Ibid.
38. Kennell, Slyter and Klaus, op. cit.
39. Yates, S. A.: *Stillbirth—What staff can do.* Am. J. Nurs. 72:1592, 1972.
40. Johnson, J. M.: *Stillbirth—A personal experience*. Am. J. Nurs. 72:1595, 1972.
41. Seitz and Warrick, loc. cit.
42. Ibid.
43. Klaus, M.: Unpublished paper presented at First Week of Neonatal Life Conference. Oshkosh, Wisconsin, November, 1973.
44. Deutsch, H.: *Psychology of Women, vol. 2.* Grune and Stratton, New York, 1945.
45. Wolff, J. R., Nielson, P. E. and Schiller, P.: *The emotional reaction to a stillbirth.* Am. J. Obstet. Gynecol. 108:73, 1970.
46. Kennell, Slyter and Klaus, op. cit.
47. Ibid.
48. Queenan, J. T.: *Communication: emotional guidance for perinatal problems.* Contemporary OB/GYN 2:33, 1973.
49. Kennell, Slyter and Klaus, op. cit.
50. Bergman, A. B., Pomeroy, M. A. and Beckwith, J. B.: *The psychiatric toll of the sudden infant death syndrome.* G.P. 40:99, 1969.
51. Kennell and Klaus, op. cit.
52. Danforth, D.: *Textbook of Obstetrics and Gynecology.* Hoeber, New York, 1971, p. 306.
53. Ibid., p. 307.
54. Yates, op. cit.
55. Seitz and Warrick, loc. cit.
56. Zahourek, op. cit.
57. Queenan, loc. cit.
58. Danforth, op. cit., p. 307.
59. Ibid.

BIBLIOGRAPHY

Bowlby, J.: *Attachment and Loss, vol. 1.* Basic Books, New York, 1969.

Downs, F.: *Maternal stress in primigravidas as a factor in the production of neonatal pathology.* Nurs. Science 2:348, 1964.

Hardgrove, C. and Warrick, L.: *Perinatal death: how shall we tell the children?* Am. J. Nurs. 74:448, 1974.

Johnson, J. M.: *Stillbirth—a personal experience*. Am. J. Nurs. 72:1595, 1972.

Kennedy, J. F.: *Implications of Grief and Mourning for Mothers of Defective Infants.* Unpublished doctoral dissertation, Smith College, School of Social Work, Northampton, Mass., 1969.

Kubler-Ross, E.: *On Death and Dying.* Macmillan, New York, 1969.

Wolf, A. W.: *Helping Your Child to Understand Death.* Child Study Assoc. Publication, New York, 1958.

Yates, S. A.: *Stillbirth–what a staff can do.* Am. J. Nurs 72:1592, 1972.

43 *Abnormality*

ANN L. CLARK, R.N., M.A.

All expectant parents dream of and have a deep desire to produce a normal healthy infant. Consider how frequently the question "Do you want a boy or a girl?" is answered "It doesn't matter, as long as it is healthy." However, it often does matter. The expectant parents often would prefer one sex over the other, but not in their wildest dreams would they prefer a child of either sex to be a damaged child. Overwhelmingly, infants are born normal and whole. However, an alarming percentage of babies enter this world with abnormalities (statistics range from 24.4 per 1,000 to 40 per 1,000 births).[1,2] Some mothers fear such a catastrophe during their pregnancies, but they do not frequently share this fear. Mothers who are considered high risk are well aware that the risk is to both their expected child and to themselves. Some women have such a low concept of themselves that they fear that anything they produce, including a child, is likely to be defective.

ABNORMALITY AS A CRISIS

The American culture places high value on perfection, beauty, and superior intelligence. Persons receive praise if they possess these qualities and persons who have physical defects, particularly if these defects are visible, are likely to be devalued. These values are instilled very early in childhood. We cruelly "poke fun" at the ugly, fat, and "stupid" classmate. Since beauty, perfection, and intelligence are so highly valued, parents who produce a child who is less than perfect may experience shame and embarrassment. They may feel that the child is a visible manifestation of their own biologic inadequacies.

Many cultures have believed, and some cultures still believe, that the birth of a congenitally damaged child is retribution for some sin. This thought may be lurking in the mind of a parent whose child is atypical. The birth of an abnormal child represents a threat to the parents' sense of adequacy and is a blow to their self-esteem. The defect in the child may be viewed as tantamount to a defect in one's self.[3]

The new mother's ego status is particularly vulnerable. During pregnancy the psychologic tasks require an increase in narcissism as the expectant mother turns her attention and her concern onto herself and the fetus she carries within her body. When an abnormal infant arrives, the mother experiences a deep narcissistic wound.[4]

The unmet expectations of both parents are responsible for the high anxiety experienced. The birth of an imperfect child therefore represents a crisis for two reasons:

1. The parents are deprived of the "dream child" which they desire.

2. The parents must cope with public appraisal of their ability to produce a "whole" child.

RESPONSE TO THE EVENT

There are many common themes in the response to the birth of a less than normal child. Although culture, personality, and experience with previous pregnancies and with other children may produce variations in the theme, the knowledge that one's child is not normal will be experienced as a tragic loss. Whether the damage is seen or unseen, severe or minor, it can overwhelm the parents. For most parents the more the infant deviates from normalcy, the more powerful the impact, but some parents react with great distress even to minor physical defects. The concept of loss explains the response of the parents, but there are differences in the theme of this loss—the loss of a much desired, idealized child. Self-image, self-concept, and the concept of the family are involved in the grieving that follows. The grieving takes the form of a painful *mental process* which has two parts:

1. Disorganization and disequilibrium
2. Coping and reorganizing.

The stages of the process follow, although it should be remembered that there is much overlapping from one stage to another.

STAGE I. Disorganization and Disequilibrium

Reaction	*Response (behavior/feelings)*
a. Shock	Feelings of numbness. Mute crying. Hysteria.
b. Denial/disbelief	Wish to flee. Denial that they could have produced a baby like that. May commit baby to an institution. Make rounds to other physicians searching for one who supports their denial. Withdraw by refusal to talk about the event, pull curtains about bed. Long periods of sleep. Psychosomatic complaints.
c. Sadness/anger	Blame themselves, the hospital staff. Ask "why me?" Anger at everyone, feel this anger is intolerable. Hate, resentment, and frustration are felt. Keeps distance from infant.

STAGE II. Coping and Reorganizing

Reaction Stage	*Response (behavior/feelings)*
a. Acceptance	Searches for a cause. Struggles to look for normal aspects of the child, relates child to themselves. Greater mastery of feelings. Waves of depression experienced. Anxiety is reduced. Fearful of the future and how they will manage.
b. Adaptation	Search for clues of acceptance of self and of child (husband, siblings, family and friends). Movement toward attachment to the child. Mobilizes health care facilities to correct or ameliorate the defect.

The process follows a pattern of 1) grief for self, 2) grief for the loss of the perfect child, and finally 3) attachment to a child with an imperfection. The attachment may follow a pathologic route or total rejection may occur. Moreover, parents may cope with the situation by excesses in work, drink, food, sleep, and so forth.

All members of the immediate family and the extended family will in some way be influenced by the birth of an atypical child.

The husband and wife mutual support system is of utmost importance in the resolution of the crisis. Open communication will assist both parents. It is important that the couple move through the grief process in a synchronous manner. If the husband withdraws in his own grief, his wife's anxiety may become acute.[5] Just as the mother needs understanding and support in coping with her grief, so does the husband. His anger and anxiety may be high as he reviews the events and reflects on his own manhood. Assisting him in coping will also help him in providing the love for his wife which she badly needs. Not only are two lives affected, but the marriage may also be at stake.

The siblings of the atypical child need some explanation of their brother or sister who is different from them, and it is the parents' responsibility to furnish this information. This will not be an easy task for the parents. The probing questions the children may ask can be a source of more pain. Having an atypical child in the family may divert some of the attention the older children have come to expect from their parents. On the other hand, loving and nurturing such a child can be of benefit to both the children and the parents.[6] No family would wish to plan for such an event, but should it occur, the problem-solving methods learned to cope with the event may strengthen the family.

Members of the extended family may offer the necessary support to the grieving parents. On the other hand, a complete breakdown in relationships may occur. In their anger and resentment the parents may withdraw, severing relationships which could have been counted on to help resolve the crisis.[7] Some members of the extended family may feel pity for the parents and great anxiety in approaching them, not knowing how to express their feelings. Other members of the family may feel that the stigma of a damaged child in the family may be reflected on themselves, or fear for a similar outcome in their own lives.

MOTHER-INFANT RELATIONSHIP

The initial mother-infant relationship will be influenced by the mother's resolution of her grief. Her responses to the child are useful clues in assessing that process. She may refuse to see the child at first. When she does see the child there will be staring, particularly at the defect. There is usually not an attempt to make eye-to-eye contact. Indeed, eye contact may be low for a considerable period. Many mothers cannot touch the defect and will not permit the infant's random movements to touch the defect. Their early tolerance of the infant may be low. They may only permit the child to remain in the room if the nurse remains. The initial difficulty in touching and caring for the child with a defect and the feelings of shock, anxiety, grief, and guilt will result in an inability of the mother to develop a relationship.[8] The mother-infant relationship will be influenced by whether she can ultimately see the defect as a realistic problem. Excessive concerns, in the face of reality, indicate that the child is not seen as one with a defect but as a defective child.[9] If she continues to view the child as proof of her own inadequacies and visible evidence of her own imperfection, there can never be relaxed pride in her mothering ability. If, because of the defect, the infant is unable to respond to the mother in a normal manner, the developing maternal attachment will be handicapped.[10] Benedek[11] has observed that a healthy, thriving infant leads to maternal self-confidence. An unhealthy, frustrated infant leads to mothering that is unsuccessful and frustrating.

Some mothers ultimately lavish unusual time and care on the child with a defect. It is almost as though such care will magically cause the defect to be erased. This overprotection will lead to problems in personality development for the child as well as family problems between the mother and her husband or between the mother and her other children. In spite of this overconcern, McGregor[12] has shown that, if there are other children in the family, the child with a defect is never the favorite child.

IMPACT OF THE BIRTH ON THE STAFF

When an atypical infant is born it may constitute a crisis for the maternity unit and the staff on that unit. It immediately poses a problem of when to tell, who to tell, how much to tell, and what and how to tell.

Most studies indicate that how the parents are told and when they are told are powerful forces in the grief process. Both parents should be informed (together if at all possible) as soon as a definite diagnosis is made. Even when a defect is suspected, and the parents make inquiry, they have a right to the information about their child, and the truth must be shared, as far as it is known.[13] There should be no "shading" of what is told to each parent. Both should know of the extent of the problem and the prognosis. If the diagnosis is definite, the telling should be carried out with conviction, thus reducing the possibility that denial will take the form of "shopping around" for another opinion.

There should be privacy provided for the parents at the time of the telling and great warmth displayed toward the parents in their grief. The parents should see the child as soon as the mother and the child are in satisfactory condition. Exposure to the reality of the problem is important and usually less disturbing than the parents' fantasies.[14]

The person who has had the longest and closest relationship with the parents should inform the parents. That person might be the obstetrician, nurse-midwife, or maternal nurse practitioner. Following the early disclosure, the person assuming major responsibility for the infant, usually the pediatrician or the pediatric surgeon, keeps the parents informed of the prognosis. It is preferable that one person assume this major role, but all members of the team must be kept informed and reinforce each other. The nurse, because of psychologic and physical closeness to the parents, particularly the mother, has a unique role to play.

The anxiety the parents will experience will reduce their ability to hear or even to accept fully the implications of the defect. Therefore, all aspects of the problem must be gone over with the parents more than once.

The staff, too, may have feelings of guilt. Relating to the parents may be difficult. The nurse who retreats from the parents, leaving them alone in their grief, only adds to their burden of feelings of worthlessness and inadequacy which they already feel. Feelings of anxiety, helplessness, and anger on the part of the nurse may make her so uncomfortable that she may respond to the parents in ways that seem to imply "detachment," lack of interest.[15] The nurse needs to guard against this.

In an attempt to spare the parents, the nurse may give false reassurance. The staff may feel so uncomfortable in caring for the child and in communicating with the parents that they may prematurely transfer the infant to another unit of the hospital, thus removing any evidence of their "failure."[16] In other instances, parents have been counseled to promptly institutionalize their infant without receiving help to study all the alternatives. Again, this behavior may be a method of reducing the stress which the staff finds unbearable.[17] The mother should have access to her child for as long as possible in order for affectional bonds to form. The ultimate relationship between the mother and infant may depend on this early contact.

If the infant remains in the newborn nursery, the staff may "hide" the infant in some room off the nursery or mark the crib "not to be shown." These responses easily communicate to the parents that their child is not acceptable and that they have done something (parented this child) of which they should be ashamed. This behavior increases the difficulty of the parents in working through their feelings of grief and guilt.[18]

NURSING ASSESSMENT

There are many similarities in the data needed to plan the appropriate nursing care for any family facing a crisis of childbearing.

There are also differences. The parents of a child with a defect, unlike the parents of a dead neonate, face not only the loss of their "dream child" but the care of "another" child. Very often the decisions to be made about the other child are emergency in nature and need to be made even before the grief process has been resolved.

As has been indicated earlier, both parents experience loss when their child is born with a defect. It is important to ascertain something about their relationship with each other and the solidarity of their marriage. The grieving each experiences needs to be mutually shared. The nurse will wish to know if they have discussed their loss with each other and if they have shared it with significant others in their lives. The responses of others, and the parents' feelings about those responses are important clues to the amount of support which the parents have available to them. If the mother does not have a supportive relationship with a partner, this needs to be known also.

The degree of energy the mother has at the time she receives this psychologic blow will have implications for nursing care. The woman who has cumulative stressful experiences during pregnancy and labor will have depleted emotional and physiologic reserves and will need appropriate care based on that assessment.

The interview and careful observations of verbal and nonverbal responses to the loss will inform the nurse where the patient is in relation to the process of grief. Using the stages of the process as related earlier in this chapter, the nurse can ascertain the mother's readiness for receiving and caring for her child.

The place of the baby in the family needs to be known. The total responsibilities of the mother not only for other children, but for other adults, will have an impact on the energy she can commit to this special child. The nurse will also want to know what information about the infant she has shared or plans to share with her other children.

Social, cultural, and economic factors affecting the lives of the parents are important aspects of the assessment process.

The mother's maturity and her maturing process will influence how she will resolve this crisis in her life. Her ability to meet stress and her tolerance for frustration will be observed. Her experience with others who have congenital defects will affect her feelings about her child and may reactivate unconscious feelings. The nurse will want to know what, specifically, the parents have heard or have read about the condition which affects their child. It is important to know what the defect means to the parents in a personal sense. They cannot be expected to see the child and what the defect means to the child until they achieve mastery over their own feelings.[19] Assessment begins that process.

NURSING ACTIONS

Basically, nursing actions will focus on two goals:

1. To help the parents resolve the grief process.
2. To facilitate parent-infant relationships.

The appropriate nursing action will depend upon the nurse being able to "tune in" to the parents in relation to where they are in the grieving process. Until the parents have grieved for and given up the dream child, they cannot be expected to care for or care about the child they now have in its place.

RESOLVING GRIEF

There is considerable psychic work to be accomplished before the "dream child" can be released. This work is accompanied by painful feelings and intense longings. The parents should be encouraged to react fully to their feelings. This is the first step in giving up the feelings.[20] The parents need many opportunities to talk about their disappointment, their feelings about self, their sense of failure, and their feelings of frustration and helplessness. Even as the parents struggle with final acceptance and adaptation, opportunity should be provided for them to talk about themselves and their feelings. Concern can appropriately be expressed for the parents' difficult life experience and they can be praised for their accomplishments.

Anger is to be expected. The nurse must recognize that the anger is a part of the grief process. The parents have a right to feel anger at what has occurred to them. When anger is expressed to the nurse, it is not meant personally. The nurse does not abandon the parents at this time but stays close by. This is an excellent opportunity to collect data about the parents' relationship with each other and their manner of coping.

The nurse must help the parents to deal with the realities of the situation; false reassurance usually is used by the nurse to reduce her own tensions. The parents are only confused by reports which give varying prognoses. They are also confused and left to feel helpless when the nurse uses professional and technical language which they cannot comprehend.

Dependency is to be expected during this early period of the puerperium. Persons who have been narcissistically wounded are even more dependent and display regressive behavior.[21] The nurse's care for them helps to heal the lacerations of the ego. The nurse who permits dependence and who provides special care and physical rest will be ego-supportive as well as facilitating physiologic recuperation. An atmosphere of warmth and acceptance of the parents will be the best means whereby the nurse can communicate with them. The parents need to know that their feelings and responses are not unnatural. This, too, helps the parents to regain their self-esteem.

The nurse should be prepared to repeat the information given the parents as often as is necessary. Due to the anxiety, their ability to hear and to comprehend the event will be reduced.

FACILITATING AN ATTACHMENT PROCESS

The nurse uses her assessment of the mother to find an appropriate time to help the mother to begin to relate to the child she now has. The nurse should expect that each mother-infant contact will reactivate the mother's feelings of disappointment and sorrow. The nurse should be sensitive to times when the care of the infant represents too great a task and should permit the mother to withdraw from the infant without being labeled a "rejecting mother." If she senses the mother needs a period of privacy away from the infant, she responds to that need with warmth and understanding.

The parents will be acutely aware of manner in which the nurse handles their child. They will be very conscious of her acceptance of the infant through handling and expression of warmth and meticulous care. They will be sensitive to any expression of withdrawal from the infant. Indeed, the nurse can become an excellent role model for the parents.

The nurse first helps the mother to touch and to hold her child. These contacts reduce the feeling of separation and reduce the fantasies about the abnormality. The nurse helps the mother to see the normal aspects of the child and to relate them to herself and to the family. She helps her to study the child in order to recognize the unique individual she has. She helps the mother to care for her infant; first to feed the child and later to learn to give whatever special care the infant may require. She recognizes the difficulty the mother is experiencing and praises her successes. She anticipates problems the mother may have and helps her to surmount them. She manipulates the environment so that the mother may experience successes. These experiences not only facilitate the mother-infant adaptation, but help the mother to regain her sense of self-esteem.

Most infants with a congenital defect will need long-term care. The nurse helps the parents to find community facilities that will help them to obtain the best possible care for their infant. Advocacy services, community health nursing referrals, and temporary relief of household pressures through the use of Home Health Aids are some of the ways the nurse can help the parents of an atypical child.

REFERENCES

1. Khalili, A., et al.: *An approach to the estimation of the true number of congenital malformations.* Pediatrics 46:712, 1970.
2. Hay, S. and Mackeprang, M.: *Estimation of true number of congenital malformations.* Pediatrics 47:1094, 1971.
3. Waechter, E. H.: *The birth of an exceptional child.* Nurs. Forum 9:202, 1970.
4. Ibid.
5. Ibid.
6. Golden, D. A. and Davis, J. G.: *Counseling parents after the birth of an infant with Down's syndrome.* Child. Today 3:7, 1974.
7. Waechter, op. cit.
8. Mercer, R.: *Mothers' responses to their infants with defects.* Nurs. Research 23:133, 1974.
9. Banks, M. J.: *The Reactions of a Family to a Malformed Infant. A.N.A. Clinical Sessions, 1966.* Appleton-Century-Crofts, New York, 1966, p. 69.
10. Rubin, R.: *Basic maternal behavior.* Nurs. Outlook 9:683, 1961.
11. Benedek, T.: *Organization of the reproductive drive.* Int. J. Psychoanal. 41:11, 1960.
12. MacGregor, F. M. C. et al.: *Facial Deformities and Plastic Surgery: A Psychosocial Study.* Charles C Thomas, Springfield, Ill., 1953.
13. National Association for Mental Health Working Party: *The birth of an abnormal child: telling the parents.* Lancet 2:1075, 1971.
14. Kennell, J. H. and Klaus, M. H.: *Care of the mother of the high-risk infant.* Clin. Obstet. Gynecol. 14:926, 1971.
15. Waechter, op. cit.
16. Kennell and Klaus, op. cit.
17. Golden and Davis, op. cit.
18. Waechter, loc. cit.
19. Ibid.
20. Ibid.
21. Ibid.

BIBLIOGRAPHY

Bowlby, J.: *Attachment and Loss, vol. 1.* Basic Books, New York, 1969.

Byers, M. L.: *Grief work of a mother of a child born with defects.* In *A.N.A. Regional Clinical Conferences, A.N.A. 1965, vol. 3.* American Nurses' Association, New York, 1965.

Cohen, R. L.: *Pregnancy stress and maternal perception of infant endowment.* J. Ment. Subnormality 12:18, 1966.

Cummings, S. T., et al.: *Effects of the child's deficiency on the mother: a study of mothers of mentally retarded, chronically ill, and neurotic children.* Am. J. Orthopsychiatry 36:595, 1966.

Downs, F.: *Maternal stress in primigravidas as a factor in the production of neonatal pathology.* Nurs. Science 2:348, 1964.

Fackler, E.: *The crisis of institutionalizing a retarded child.* Am. J. Nurs. 68:1508, 1968.

Forrer, G. R.: *The mother of a defective child.* Psychonal. Q. 28:59, 1959.

Jordan, T.: *The family aspects of physical disability in children.* Child and Family 4:78, 1965.

Kennedy, J. F.: *Implications of Grief and Mourning for Mothers of Defective Infants.* Unpublished doctoral dissertation, Smith College, Sch. of Social Work, Northampton, Mass., 1969.

Klaus, M. and Kennell, J.: *Mothers separated from their newborn infants.* Pediatr. Clin. North Am. 17:1015, 1970.

Klaus, M., et al.: *Human maternal behavior in the first contact with her young.* Pediatrics 46:187, 1970.

Mandelbaum, A. and Wheeler, M. E.: *Meaning of a defective child to parents.* Social Casework 41:360, 1960.

Rose, J. A.: *The prevention of mothering breakdown associated with physical abnormalities of the infant.* In Caplan, G. (ed.): *Prevention of Mental Disorders in Children.* Basic Books, New York, 1961.

Solnit, A. and Stark, M.: *Mourning and the birth of a defective child.* Psycholanal. Study Child 16:523, 1961.

Tisza, V. B. and Gumpertz, E.: *The parents' reaction to the birth and early care of children with cleft palate.* Pediatrics 30:86, 1962.

Warkany, J.: *Birth defects through the ages.* In Fishbein, M. (ed.): *Birth Defects.* J. B. Lippincott, Philadelphia, 1963, pp. 18-24.

Winick, M.: *Birth defects.* Child and Family 6:12, 1967.

UNIT 11

CURRENT ISSUES

44 Legal, Moral, and Ethical Considerations

ANN L. CLARK, R.N., M.A.
DYANNE D. AFFONSO, R.N., M.N.

During this century many changes have occurred that relate to mothers, infants, families and society. The changes present definite issues to be resolved without any easy answers to be found. Society has, until recently, passively accepted these changes. Now individuals and groups of individuals are raising their voices to question if these changes are necessary or are even beneficial. Hospitals, health personnel, and the whole health care system are being challenged.

At the same time, advances in medical science have brought about conditions which promote issues never before faced. Questions related to who shall produce, who shall survive, and the importance of the quality of life now confront health professionals as well as persons in theology, law, and economics. It is now possible for life-saving equipment to keep alive infants who a very short time ago could not have been conceived, would not have been born alive, or would have died within a short time of their birth. Many of these infants begin life congenitally damaged, but live to become a burden to themselves, their parents, and society. At the same time, society's genetic pool is having added to it an increasing number of disorders which will affect future generations.

There are questions related to moral differences between an act of commission and an act of omission in preserving the life of an individual. Questions arise about the rights of the *fetus*, the rights of a *defective neonate*, the rights of *parents*, and the rights of *society*. Who should decide what is the best course of action? The family? The medical staff? The courts? Who?

The authors believe that nurses, who are unquestionably involved in all of these issues, should be carrying on a dialogue within their own profession and with their professional colleagues. In raising the following issues, we do not propose to give the answers. We are presenting some of the aspects of the issues to assist with the discussion. The nine issues presented are pertinent to maternal and infant nursing, but they are not all of the issues. Indeed, more formidable issues are just over the horizon. Since nursing cannot avoid being involved, we dare not refuse to try to resolve the dilemmas facing individuals and society.

IS THERE CULTURAL WARPING OF THE CHILDBIRTH EXPERIENCE IN AMERICA?

There are medical writers who believe that the birth experience is no longer a normal physiologic process but that it has been distorted into a pathologic event in American hospitals.[1] In this process, they contend, the family has been separated so they are unable to support each other during childbearing;

labor and birth have been distorted and the fetus and neonate have been compromised,[2] and unnecessary neurologic damage has occurred.[3,4] It is true that the infant mortality rate in the United States ranks below those for 14 other developed countries. Moreover, being born alive is not our only goal; to be well born is equally important.

A number of interventions are implicated as being responsible for distorting labor and birth. Among them are

- elective induction of labor
- medications given during labor, and anesthesia administered during delivery
- chemical stimulation of labor
- routine forcep extraction
- conduct of labor
- position for delivery
- routine episiotomy
- separation of family members during the childbearing experience.

These issues are briefly reviewed below.

Elective induction of labor has certainly changed the birth scene. It is now possible for many women to be delivered on a selected day. Outside of America, this is viewed as idiosyncratic. It is only countenanced by physicians abroad if there is a clear medical indication for its use. It does carry some possible hazards, such as prematurity, prolonged latent stage of labor, fetal distress due to anoxia, intrapartal infection, prolapsed cord, premature separation of the placenta, lacerations, uterine rupture, and postpartal hemorrhage.[5] The issue could also include the legal consequences of a practice resulting from the mother's uninformed consent, for it is questionable if she is ever fully informed of the risk involved. The other part of the issue relates to the convenience of women being admitted to the hospital and then labor being induced. Patients who live long distances from the hospital or who have experienced rapid precipitant labors are spared this anxiety. Physicians feel they can better practice obstetrics when they can plan to spend time with the woman in labor or with their prenatal patients without unexpected interruptions.

Neonatal respiratory distress is one of the most obvious hazards from sedation given to the woman in labor to counteract the pain of uterine contractions. The respiratory center of the infant is highly vulnerable to sedatives and anesthetic drugs. Many infants are born with delayed or sluggish respiration following the administration of drugs, particularly if they are administered near the time of birth.[6] The added burden on the new born of having to detoxify intrauterine acquired obstetric medication as he adjusts to extrauterine life is the subject of much scientific literature.[7-9] Even the recovered infant may still be jeopardized, with irreversible brain damage occurring. Besides the long-term effects, the neonate's ability to suckle may be adversely affected for several days. This could lead to dehydration as well as to a delayed or distorted mother-infant relationship.

Not only is the outcome of the infant involved but also that of the mother who is experiencing the stresses of labor. Perhaps the place of birth is also involved in the outcomes. When the woman labored at home, she had the emotional support of concerned individuals as her companions. In the hospital setting, individualized support from nurses and from the woman's mate does make a considerable difference in the woman's need for obstetric medication. Physical and emotional preparation for the experience of labor also reduces the need for medication and tends to shorten the labor process.[10] Many American physicians still rely heavily on narcotics to allay the pain of labor and much research continues to discover an effective medication which has a minimal effect on the fetus. Only a small percentage of women are prepared to cope with the discomforts of labor and birth through classes on preparation for parenthood. There are still many American hospitals which deny women the companionship and support of their mates during labor, yet do not substitute adequate staff support for the women. They state that the overworked staff will find the addition of a husband one more patient to care for. They voice concern over legal implications and over the transmission of infections to the labor and delivery areas of the hospital.

The conduct of labor in our American hospitals is also seen as an issue. Labor is not only induced, but normal labors may be stimulated by oxytocic agents. Women are confined to bed during labor, the perineal area is shaved, food and fluids are denied, and delivery is performed with the woman in lithotomy position with her legs elevated and widely separated. Forceps are routinely used to deliver many infants and a routine episiotomy is performed.

Ambulation during labor is frequently discouraged in American hospitals, partly because early labor facilities are not available and partly because of concern for safety. The administration of drugs for pain control makes ambulation unsafe. Unless her membranes have ruptured, there are advantages for a laboring woman being up and about during early labor. Ambulation encourages a more rapid engagement of the fetal presenting part. It distracts the woman from the discomforts of her uterine contractions and facilitates better maternal circulation.

The practice of withholding fluids and light food from women in labor began with the use of general anesthesia for delivery. Although general anesthesia is not frequently used today, light food and fluids are still generally withheld and intravenous feeding is substituted. It is true that the effects of withholding food and fluids on the mother and fetus have not been sufficiently investigated, but the substitution of an intravenous set in the labor room has surely detracted from the naturalness of the scene.[11]

The lithotomy position for birth is preferred by nearly every American physician, and for good reason—it is more convenient for him. On the other hand, it is said not to serve the woman's purpose in delivering her child spontaneously or even in her assisting with the birth. It inhibits the mother's voluntary efforts to expel her infant. She can be much more effective in a semi-sitting position, with her feet resting on the bed or delivery table. Morever, the lithotomy position tends to adversely affect the maternal circulatory system and pulmonary ventilation, and this in turn affects the fetus.[12]

There are times when fetal distress, prolonged labor, malpositions of the presenting part, and other conditions dictate the use of forceps to facilitate the safe delivery of the fetus. However, forceps are used in up to 65 per cent of all deliveries in some American hospitals, whereas in other countries they are rarely used in more than 5 per cent of births. Butler[13] states that there is no scientific support for the *routine* application of forceps during delivery. Forceps can reduce the length of labor by from 30 minutes to one hour or more, but they can also lead to damage to the infant's facial nerves or to the brachial plexus, or to intracranial hemorrhage.[14]

There is little agreement between the factions which say that a routine episiotomy reduces the incidence of relaxation of the pelvic floor musculature and reduces neurologic impairment to the fetus and those who believe that it is unnecessary. The latter group state that an intact perineum, strengthened by postpartal exercises is more apt to result in better sexual satisfaction for both the male and the female. [15] There is also a middle-of-the-road group who believe that some women need an episiotomy to avoid severe perineal laceration, but that other women could deliver without the surgical incision if they were placed in a semi-sitting position and if the perineum were allowed to be slowly stretched.

Finally, cultural warping is said to occur because the family is separated and do not have access to each other even in time of crisis.

As has been stated earlier, husbands are not always permitted to be with their wives during labor and even fewer husbands are permitted to be present during the delivery. Following delivery, the infant is quickly transported to the nursery after only a fleeting contact with its mother. The father views his child through a glass partition. In a majority of American hospitals the infant is kept in a central nursery and brought to the mother at specified hours for feedings. The logic for these procedures relates to keeping the infant warm and reducing infection to the mother and infant. However, such policies do not always meet the needs of the individual. Set hours for infant feedings do not necessarily meet his hunger needs. Maternal responses to nurturing the infant are interfered with when the mother cannot have free access to her infant. The father is frustrated in his desire to have contact with his child.

The common American practice of prohibiting the toddler and other children from visiting the mother during her hospital stay is said to be a hardship for all concerned. The policy is generally set to avoid having infection brought into a maternity unit. Experience in other countries and in several hospitals in the United States suggests that when children are allowed to visit a short explanation as to the importance of not bringing communicable diseases into the hospital seems to be effective in controlling infection (Fig. 44-1).

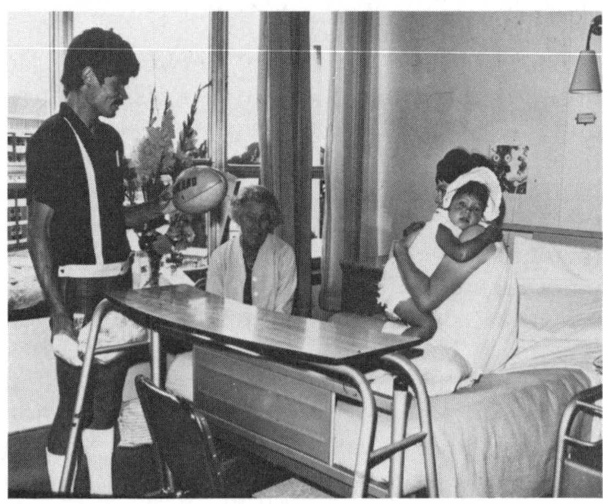

FIGURE 44-1. A new mother is visited by her family in a New Zealand hospital. (From Haire, D.: *The Cultural Warping of Childbirth*. International Childbirth Education Association, 1972, with permission.)

Perhaps the issue of caring for mothers and infants separately rather than as a unit continues because traditionally in America one group of nurses assumes care for mothers while another group cares for the infants in a central nursery. This distorts the mother-infant relationship.

All of the above issues are of great importance to families experiencing childbirth and to the health professions who provide needed care.

WHAT ARE THE COMPONENTS IN THE DECISION-MAKING PROCESS CONCERNING THE RIGHT TO LIFE AND ITS QUALITY?

Gone are the days when recipients of health care were complacent, allowing events to occur without any questions and remaining uninvolved in decisions which would influence their health status. We are in an era of consumer advocacy; the "rights" of the individual regarding the delivery of health care are highlighted. There is a community spirit toward an individual's rights: "bill of rights" for the hospitalized, "right to life" of the fetus, "right to die" of the terminally ill, and the "right to medical care" regardless of ethnic, religious, or socioeconomic differences. The upsurge of community action for the individual's "rights" is bringing to the surface many moral, ethical, and social dilemmas. Within the childbearing experience, the issues are heavily focused on forces involved in decision making concerning the "right to life and its quality."

Who should make decisions on whether to treat or to withhold treatment of sick newborn infants?

There is a movement that says that parents should be given the right to decide for their babies whether medical treatment should be given or withheld. The issue arises from "informed consent," the patient's right to know all the facts concerning his health situation so he can make a decision about his health care after weighing all the alternatives. Shaw comments there is a dilemma of "informed consent" when the patient is a minor because in such situations "a parental decision rejecting recommended treatment is subject to review when physicians or society disagree with the decision"[16] Some of the issues in the "informed consent" dilemma are:

1. At times "informed consent" is not complete or is biased. For example, parents may be told all the choices for treatment, but not given the option for refusing treatment. Another example is that the information given by the physician may be based upon what the physician has already decided should be done.[17]
2. To allow participation in decision making, informed consent must break away from old, traditional ways of presenting information. Instead of only information on cost, length of hospitalization and possible risks, parents need to know not only the proposed treatments but also the consequences of treatment or the consequences of refusing to consent.
3. What is the impact on the medical staff when parental decisions differ from their own? Shaw describes the issue:

    The lingering death of a newborn infant whose parents have denied consent for surgery can have a disastrous effect on hospital personnel as illustrated last year by the well publicized Johns Hopkins Hospital case, which raised a national storm of controversy. The baby's lingering death (15 days) severely demoralized the nursing and house staffs. In addition, it prolonged the agony for the parents, who called daily to find out if the baby was still alive.

    Once the parents have made a decision, should members of the medical staff support them in their decision regardless of their own feelings? (This support may be important to assuage recurrent feelings of guilt for months or even years after the parents' decision.)[18]

At present, the painful decision concerning the giving or withholding of health care rests primarily on the physicians, with some advancements in parental rights to decide. Also emerging are legal actions whereby courts have reversed decisions made by parents and physicians. In such legal actions, the courts claim to be protecting the infant's life by law because determination of the value of the infant's life is seen as beyond the scope of medical practice.

What about the quality of life?

A new concern for the quality of life is emerging. Whereas at one time the focus was to implement life-saving measures at all cost, now the issue is consideration of whether such efforts are in the best interest of the infant and the society as a whole. It is no longer possible to be preoccupied only with individual problems. Consideration must be given to the consequences on society in terms of factors such as financial burdens, pollution of the genetic pool, and psychosocial stressors on family life with the presence of a handicapped child. The issue is: When is the right time to abandon interventions and allow the infant the right to die? There are those who claim it is no longer enough merely to help a baby survive but consideration must be given to the baby's potential to achieve meaningful "humanhood" (a state in human existence characterized by such features as the ability to interact with others, to love and be loved, and to feel self-awareness).[19] Thus, some physicians elect to make no attempts to preserve life when the consequences are an inability to attain humanhood. There are others who feel that allowing a baby to die is wrong, a criminal act, and against the principles of the Hippocratic oath.[20] The issue is not a lack of concern for life but rather a concern for its quality. Quality of life penetrates beyond physical health into the realm of psychosocial development. We have knowledge demonstrating that normal, healthy children exposed to parental and social deprivation experience disastrous effects to their behavioral development. A child with physical defects is more vulnerable to restricted social and parental interactions because of the defects.[21] Lasagna vividly describes the issue:

> We may as a society scorn the civilizations that slaughtered their infants, but our proposed treatment of the retarded is in some ways more cruel.[22]

What are the rights of the fetus, the parents, and society?

Currently, there is another issue focusing on when a human being is considered a person and what are its rights to life. One precipitating factor for this issue is the Supreme Court's ruling which legalized abortion. The dilemma involves several factors:

1. There is the issue of whether a fetus is a person. In 1973, the U. S. Supreme Court ruled that the newborn, whether in the zygote, blastocyst, embryo, or fetus stage, is not a "person" entitled to the constitutional protections of due process and equal protection of the laws.[23] There is currently a proposal to amend the U. S. Constitution to include the following:

   > Neither the United States nor any State shall deprive any human being, from the moment of conception, of life without due process of law; nor deny to any human being from the moment of conception, within its jurisdiction, the equal protection of the laws. *

   Obviously the proposed amendment is a direct opposition to legalized abortion but it will bring to the surface many presently unknown issues on the rights of the fetus. For example, one such issue will be what are the legal rights of an infant whose human existence was jeopardized because of alterations in its intrauterine environment from factors such as smoking, drugs, or maternal accidents. Possibly this issue is not too far in the future as exemplified in a change in court viewpoints whereby claims are granted to children who were victims of prenatal injuries.[24]
2. There is the issue of whose property the fetus is. Currently, court decisions have allowed that a woman has the sole right to determine the fate of the fetus (abortion or carried to term). Such legal decisions have nearly eliminated any decision-making participation on the part of the male. The two opposing forces are those who claim the fetus is a creation of two individuals and thus the property of both; while others claim that requiring a mate's consent would create problems, e.g., if he were not available, or if he and the

* Proposed Amendment to the U.S. Constitution, introduced in the House by Representative Lawrence Hogan (R-Md.) (H.J. Res. 261) and in the Senate by Senator Jessie Helms (R-N.C.) (S.J. Rec. 130).

woman disagree. This issue of the right to "co-decide" the fate of the fetus[25] will need to be resolved or it may create strain on a marriage, leading to family disintegration.

3. There is also the issue regarding the use of live, aborted fetuses for research. Once again, the issue is whether the aborted fetus should be viewed as a person or merely as a by-product of the human body (as if it were a removed organ). The National Institutes of Health has banned Federal funding of research which uses live, aborted fetuses[26] after public outcry that such fetuses, by the fact that they are viable, have a right to death unmutilated by research manipulations. The medical profession, on the other hand, is proclaiming that restrictions on live fetal research will impede progress in perinatal medicine.

The issues concerning the right to life and its quality are not for the future but are confronting the present society. Unfortunately, questions are emerging more rapidly than solutions.

IS THE HOSPITAL THE MOST CONDUCIVE ENVIRONMENT FOR CHILDBIRTH?

Chapter 2 described the many advantages and disadvantages that resulted from the move of the birth from the home to the hospital. There are groups of people who believe that the advantages do not outweight the disadvantages. Home deliveries are occurring in increasing numbers among the counterculture groups. Although these births constitute only a small percentage of the nation's total, home delivery is an important issue. The reasons why people wish to have their babies born outside of the hospital setting should be important to providers of health care. Many feel that the naturalness of the home setting, the participation of the mate and others in the birth process, and the feeling that the hospital is cold and dehumanizing make home delivery more desirable. The soaring costs of hospital care coupled with the desire to extend the natural life style has prompted a number of young people to opt for home delivery. Groups who favor home deliveries can be found in large metropolitan cities, in less populated areas, and in rural settings.[27-29]

When a couple decides to have their baby at home, it is exceedingly difficult in most areas of America to find a physician who will care for the mother and deliver her at home. Some young people accept prenatal care in a hospital clinic but choose to deliver at home. The fear that pressure would be put on them to deliver in a hospital by refusing to provide continued medical care keeps them from sharing their plans with clinic staff.

The Santa Cruz Birth Center, not unlike other groups, has developed a clinic of their own. They have also published a *Birth Book*, complete with prenatal care, equipment needed for a home delivery, technique of labor and delivery, and care of the neonate, including the technique of resuscitation. It also includes many informative photographs of the delivery phase. This birth center is staffed, for the most part, with members of the group who provide prenatal care and act as the birth attendants. Most are not trained in any of the health professions. Frediani, writing a historical prospective of childbirth in *Birth Book,** perhaps gives the clearest account of why their culture is choosing home delivery.

> But where has all this innovation of modern medicine brought us today? We, as women, are still forced to endure some of the most outrageous insults possible. We are still expected to labor and bear our children in hospitals which are centers of disease and

* Frediani, J.: In Lang, R.: *Birth Book.* Genesis Press, Ben Lomond, Calif., 1972.

infection. Once we have entered them and entrusted our lives and the control we have over them to the authority of doctors, we are insulted with one indignity upon another. Thus a woman in the midst of labor is first required to juggle the bureaucratic red tape of the institution. Then we are given an enema, an experience that can be more painful when combined with uterine contractions. We must then have all our beautiful pubic hair shaved off in the name of sanitation. At least one third of our body is considered "sterile field" and beyond the boundary of our own touch.

We are handled by strangers and separated from our mate, barring us from one of the most intimate experiences we will ever share. Then we are administered all kinds of drugs, very often against our will, and must spend our energy on the delivery table turning away from persistent offerings of gas. Our movements and choice of position are restricted, and we are most often forced to deliver strapped down to the modern, cold, hard delivery table which instinctively feels too high from the floor. And then after a delivery including numerous potent drugs, perhaps the use of forceps and a compulsory episiotomy, our child is taken from us to be observed by strangers in a nursery full of screaming babies. At this point, if the mother is undrugged, she is overwhelmed by maternal feelings. She wants to examine, touch and hold this baby she has waited so long to see. Instead the baby is detached from the sounds, smells, tastes and closeness that are her/his birthright. The father often gets his first look through a pane of glass. Where is there room for love? How can mother, father, and child share the true bond of these moments so vital to their mutual growth?

This is modern obstetrics, 1972. In light of this type of treatment, we women are now taking the responsibility of childbirth out of the hospital, into our own hands. It is only with the changing consciousness of our times, that once again recognizes man as a being of the spirit who lives in a material world, that we are able to recover the joy and beauty of childbirth. Modern science has removed the medieval horrors of childbirth. The difficult labor no longer need end in tragedy. But in the technological advance, the uncomplicated labor has been neglected. Today, we are attempting to bring childbirth back to nature wherever possible. Women are learning how to listen once more to their long buried instinctive selves. Our children are once again being born at home in an atmosphere of love and beauty. We have taken the joyous task of bearing our young back into our own hands! And our mates are by our sides in fullfledged support. We have not neglected the advances of scientific knowledge, but we have realized that through a new understanding we must now bring birth and motherhood back to its rightful place. Childbirth is a natural process; we need only to relearn to work in harmony with nature.

Is home delivery a symptom of a failure in our society as some have said? Does our health care system lack people who care? Cannot this issue be resolved by health care professionals working with consumers of our services? Cannot maternity centers be both safe and at the same time meet the needs of all who use the facilities?

IS CIRCUMCISION A MEDICAL NECESSITY OR A MEDICAL RITUAL?

Circumcision is not a new procedure. It is known that the Egyptians practiced it 5,000 years ago, as a form of sacrifice. It was performed at the age of 13 on Egyptian youths. It has been practiced by the Hebrews, as an initiation into Judaism, for more than 20 centuries. In America, circumcision has become a nearly routine procedure within the past three decades. Circumcision is said to be done primarily to facilitate cleansing of the penis and to prevent accumulation of smegma under the foreskin. It is also necessitated by phimosis (a narrowing of the foreskin so it cannot be retracted over the glans penis). It has also been said that the uncircumcised penis (and the accumulation of smegma under the foreskin) was responsible for cancer of the penis, prostrate, and cervix.[30] This discussion would not be complete without looking at the other side of the procedure, the complications and disadvantages. The procedure itself, although usually free from complications, has resulted in excessive bleeding and in infection. Since the prepuce acts as a shield to the glans penis, danger of injury may be increased with circumcision. It is also claimed that the glans may lose some tactile sensitivity when constantly exposed to air.[31]

Today routine circumcision is being questioned as necessary or even as desirable. Faber[32] has refuted most of the advantages, stating that cleansing of the penis can be readily done by retraction and daily cleansing. He further states that phimosis in uncircumcised males is rare after age 2 or 3. Finally, it has not been possible in animal research to induce cancer with smegma, thus the case for circumcision as a means of avoiding cervical or penile cancer is not proven. It would seem that multiple sexual partners, venereal disease, and general lack of hygiene are more to be implicated.

Many young parents are questioning the need for circumcision of their male child and some are refusing to permit this procedure. What is clearly needed is a re-evaluation of circumcision as a routine procedure, based on research.

WHAT ARE THE ISSUES REGARDING CONTROL OF FERTILITY TO EASE THE POPULATION EXPLOSION?

The decade of the seventies heralded an increased awareness for the need to conserve the world's available resources. Community action programs infiltrated everyday life styles by advocating the need to avoid pollution of natural resources, reduction of wastage such as through recycling campaigns, and control of human reproduction. The latter was viewed as very important because possibly the greatest force to create a burden on the world's resources is the human one. Each human being contributes significantly in decreasing the food supply, increasing consumption of energy resources, and adding to pollution merely by the everyday efforts for survival.

The interest for the control of fertility increased further when psychosocial research revealed that many pregnancies were unwanted but individuals did not have sufficient knowledge or resources whereby they could control their fertility. There is also evidence that lack of family planning can be a health hazard. One study indicated that frequent pregnancies and increased family size posed risks not only to mother and fetus but the entire family. Such risks were increased mortality rate; higher prematurity rate; greater likelihood of child abuse; increased incidence of infectious disease; poor growth, both height and weight, among preschool and school children; and lower intelligence quotient scores among children.[33] It is hypothesized that important advantages of a smaller, planned family are better marital relationships and better parent-child relationships.[34]

Worldwide interest in the control of human reproduction was exemplified in the formation of such organizations as the International Planned Parenthood Federation. In the United States, the need for fertility control became more than an interest when the President, in 1969, "called for a 'national goal' to provide family planning services to all who want but cannot afford them and for 'essential' continued research to find additional . . . birth control methods of all types."[35]

In spite of the surge of interest, the first systematic worldwide survey on the practices of fertility control revealed that needs for fam-

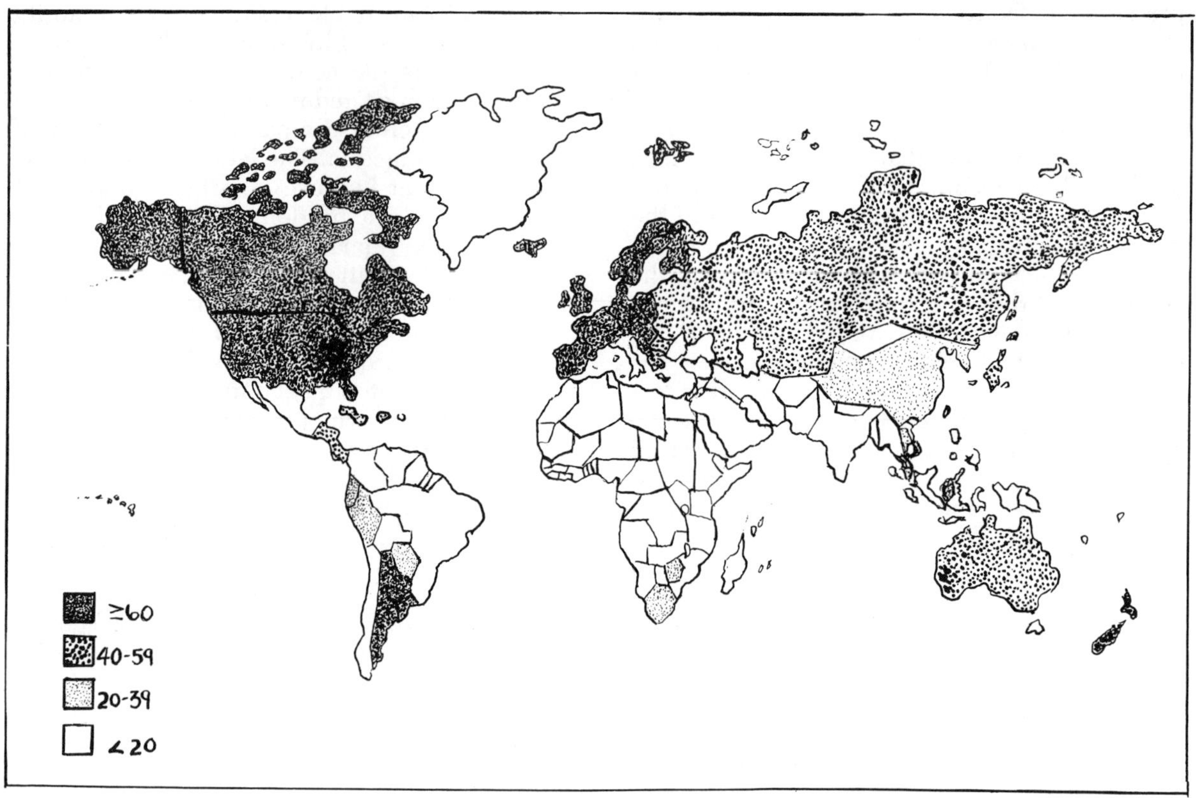

FIGURE 44-2. Per cent of women at risk of unwanted pregnancy who were practicing contraception, 1971. (From Family Planning Perspective 5:233, 1973, with permission.)

ily planning were essentially unmet[36] (Fig. 44-2). The results are summarized below:

1. Seven in 10 of an estimated 500 million women at risk from having an unwanted pregnancy were using no contraceptive at all. This is equivalent to an estimated 70 per cent who were not using contraceptives.
2. Of the 30 per cent who used some contraceptive method, only one in seven used the most effective methods such as the pill, IUD, or sterilization. Others used less effective, traditional methods such as the condom, rhythm, spermicidals, douche, or withdrawal. More than 55 million women terminated their pregnancies by induced abortion, legal or illegal. Essentially this meant four abortions for every 10 babies delivered.
3. In developed, industrialized countries, 60 per cent of couples at risk used contraceptives. In less developed countries other than China, 12 per cent used contraceptives. In China, which accounts for nearly one fourth of the world's population, 35 per cent were using contraceptives.

Table 44-1 presents a summary of the worldwide picture on contraceptive practices.

In the United States, statistics also reveal incomplete success in controlling fertility, in spite of the fact that the rate for contraceptive use is among the highest in the world and birth rate has declined.[37] The Commission on Population Growth and the American Future has regarded the incidence of unwanted pregnancy as reaching "epidemic proportion".[38] Studies also describe that unintended pregnancies frequently result from contraceptive failure.[39,40]

What are some of the issues confronting efforts to control human population and curtail population growth?

> While the present types of contraceptives are being significantly improved, no radical new departures in birth control technology are currently in sight. This leads to two conclusions. One is that family planning for years to come will have to rely on technology which is too expensive, too complicated, too dependent on the medical profession, and too hard to distribute to be easily applied in low-income countries; the second is that continued attention to fundamental research on human reproduction must be assured and concentration only on contraceptive technology would be a mistake.[41]

The first conclusion focuses on the issues on education, cost factors, safety, and availability of contraceptive methods. Let us examine these factors. The worldwide survey of 1971 revealed that "knowledge about contraceptives were at low levels, especially among rural couples and young people".[42] There has been a surge of audiovisual materials produced to fill the knowledge gap. The issue is not the amount of materials produced but whether the message is readily accessible and comprehensible. Too often in the United States, contraceptive information is written only in English, using technical terms, and found only in select locales such as a physician's office or other medical facility. Sometimes materials can be obtained by mail request, but even then, the addresses are usually to be found in selective (professional-type) magazines. Many times the request must be accompanied by money. One current response to making contraceptive information more available is known as Tel-Med. It allows the individual to receive 3 to 5 minute taped-

TABLE 44-1. Estimated number and per cent distribution of women at risk of unwanted pregnancy and number and per cent practicing contraception, by method used; for 208 countries, by development status (numbers in millions).*

			Contraceptors		*Method used, and per cent distribution of contraceptors*					
	At risk				*Pill/IUD*		*Sterilization*		*Other and unknown*	
Countries, by development status	*No.*	*%*	*No.*	*% of all at risk*	*No.*	*%*	*No.*	*%*	*No.*	*%*
All countries (N = 208)	496	100	153	31	48	31	24	16	81	53
Developed (N = 44)	141	28	85	60	22	26	4	5	59	69
Less developed (N = 164)	355	72	68	19	26	38	20	29	22	32
China	112	23	39	35	13	33	13	33	13	33
Less developed other than China	243	49	29	12	13	45	7	24	9	31

Note: Per cents may not add to 100 because of rounding.

*From Robbins, J.: *Unmet needs in family planning: a world survey.* Family Planning Perspectives, 5:234, 1973, with permission.

recorded messages by a physician on family planning through toll-free telephone networks.[43] Tel-Med achieved a certain degree of success and received wide publicity through newspapers, radio, and television. It has the advantage of making basic contraceptive information as available as a telephone. However, because Tel-Med is primarily an information-giving program, the individual who is uncertain and confused about family planning is not able to implement fertility control measures. Such a person still needs a resource person to whom feelings can be expressed and by whom questions can be answered. This leads into another issue. Who should this resource person be? Should this resource person be found only in acute-health-care settings such as the hospital, or in out-patient health care clinics? Take a minute and reflect on the environment and function of these health care settings. Frequently, clinics are understaffed for their large caseloads. More often than not, the environment is limited in space so that a worker cannot sit down and listen to a person without being interrupted. One response to this issue has been the increased interest in over-the-counter contraceptives and the role of their distributor—the pharmacist. The pharmacist is becoming appreciated as a very important community educational resource, perhaps because he or she is the most readily accessible member of all health professionals.[44] The attitudes of the pharmacist toward contraception and the practices employed regarding the sale and display of nonprescription contraceptives can contribute or hinder the possibility of the neighborhood drug store becoming a resource setting for contraceptive information. There should be exploration of other disciplines and their possible contribution toward community action to enhance contraceptive knowledge. Examples are teachers conveying information through sex education in schools and businessmen supporting campaigns for advertising information through radio, television, magazines, and newspapers.

Another issue confronting fertility control is the cost factor. Whether the individual or the government pays, the financial burden must be assumed not only for the method per se, but also for training and research programs. The 1971 worldwide survey revealed that of the $3 billion spent worldwide for fertility control, $1.9 billion came from individuals who paid for their own services. A principal obstacle to the success of family planning was the unwillingness or inability of governments to allocate sufficient resources to the programs.[45] Thus, we can conclude that the majority of people in the world must finance their own family planning. The cost for contraceptives varies with the method. The over-the-counter drug store type measures are probably the least expensive, with procedures involving hospitalization being most expensive, while prescription type measures are intermediate. The prescription type measures carry the additional financial burden of the cost for a visit to the physician. Hospitalization appears to be a major factor in elevating costs for elective medical contraceptive procedures; thus vasectomy costs less than any female sterilization procedure because it requires virtually no hospitalization.[46] The issue is clearly how to make fertility control less expensive to the consumer.

In addition to making fertility control more readily available and financially feasible for a larger majority of the world's population, there is another important issue. Presently, contraceptive methods are not without risks. The current concern is that many contraceptive measures which were believed to be safe when first introduced, now are revealed as being medically hazardous. For example,

1. There is a possible association between the use of intrauterine devices and acute, first episode pelvic inflammatory disease.[47]
2. The pill, which is regarded as the single most influential factor for contraceptive success,[48] has been linked to increased

incidences of thrombosis and hemorrhagic cardiovascular disorders. The risks of myocardial infarction and stroke are increased when the use of oral contraceptive is in combination with other risk factors such as smoking, hypertension, high serum cholesterol, diabetes, obesity, and other medical disorders.[48-51] Oral contraceptives have also been known to create dermatologic side effects such as acne, darkening of the skin, and hirsutism. Such effects are usually minimized by carefully selecting an appropriate combination of estrogen and progesterone.

3. Vasectomy was once viewed as virtually risk- and discomfort-free. However, current research reveals such complications as recanalization and granulomas, sometimes manifesting many years later but clearly indicating their incidence after an average vasectomy.[52] Also, there is evidence that men have more discomforts after the procedure than reported by physicians. Most discomforts were considered mild but involved specific complaints such as heavy oozing, tenderness, and swelling. Sometimes complaints persisted one month or more after the procedure.

The major issue relating to fertility control concerns the attitudes and values of the society toward contraception. Attitudes will be either a major obstacle to or a major force for contraceptive success worldwide. Currently there are two differing attitudes. One exerts social pressure to establish the "ideal" and "expected" family size in America for childbearing couples, the ideal reflecting an acceptable family size limit of 2 to 4 children.[53] Community action programs campaign to make contraceptives readily available to the younger population who are more vulnerable to unwanted pregnancies. It is advocated that contraceptive services be available in college and school settings, and even be accessible to teenagers. The opposing force reflects the traditional, less rigid attitudes toward sex and control of its consequences. These attitudes of society are still very much alive as reflected in the fact that nearly half of the states have statutes which prohibit or restrict contraceptive information and practices.[54] The issue becomes even more complex regarding contraceptives for minors. The Commission on Population Growth and the American Future states:

> The major difficulty is balancing "religious and ethical reasons" for requiring parental consent for the contraceptive services with "the facts of life . . . that sexual involvement by minors is widespread and increasing." To deal with both issues, the report recommended "that states should formulate statutes establishing [contraceptive information and service] programs with due regards to the interests of parents, the sensitive nature of the problems involved in teenage sexual activity and the long range social objectives of promoting healthy and sexually responsible citizens.[55]

Currently, the American Bar Association is advocating abolishment of statutes which restrict access to contraceptive information and practices.

The issues on fertility control will not be resolved quickly. Time is a necessity for the change of attitudes, especially when related to human sexual functioning and activities. One major challenge facing health professionals concerns how to better motivate individuals to control fertility and to control it prior to conception.

ARE THERE CONSEQUENCES FROM THE NEW VEGETARIAN DIETS FOR MOTHERS AND INFANTS?

The importance of nutrition during pregnancy and during infancy has been discussed in detail in Chapter 17. There is a new vogue in eating patterns among an increasingly large number of people in America, many of them young people of childbearing age. The following is a review of the more prevalent dietary cultists:

Vegetarian: one who lives wholly or principally upon vegetable foods.
Lacto-ovo-vegetarian: one who lives on vegetable foods, milk, milk products and eggs.
Fruitarian: one who restricts the variety of plant foods he eats to fruits and nuts with or without the addition of grains and legunes.
Theosophist: one who believes in a system claiming a knowledge of nature more profound than that obtained from empirical sources, thus only "natural" foods.
Macrobiotic: one whose food intake is intended to prolong life. A complicated series of graduated diets with food selection based on acidity and alkalinity is used.
Omophagist: one who eats of raw flesh.

In our country, there are many vegetarian groups, e.g., the Trappist monks of the Catholic Church, members of the Seventh Day Adventist Church, adherents of Mazdaism, an ancient Persian philosophy, and followers of Jainism, a religious sect closely resembling Buddhism.

Probably the largest group is composed of individuals with multiple vague reasons for adherence to a vegetarian diet. Their beliefs are supposedly based largely on nonviolence. Within this group are the ranks of a subculture or counterculture which state an aversion to established American food practices and substitute ill-defined dietary patterns of vague origin. Many of the youth culture combine several of the diets and add their own beliefs to decide their food intake.

Vegetarian diets usually find their most serious deficiency in the lack of protein. Iron is also low and if milk is excluded from the diet calcium becomes another problem. Pregnant women, nursing mothers, and infants need all of these components. Pregnant and lactating women and their infants appear to be particularly vulnerable to the inadequacies of the Zen macrobiotic diet.[56] The infants are of low birth weight and gain little or no weight during breast feeding. The pregnant women lose body fat and muscle and often suffer from severe anemia and all of the signs of hypoproteinemia. Erhard states that

> anyone who tries to help these people professionally has to understand each cult in the context of its own terms and must appreciate the influences that govern food-selection if he hopes to effect changes for the better, where such are necessary. Reinforcement of the positive aspects of the dietary practice helps to change the more negative aspects in the vegetarian's belief system. We have found that in making such attempts at education we have been tolerant and even overlook the abuse that many of these people wish to impose upon themselves.[57]

Bancroft [58] working with the counterculture in the Haight-Ashbury Free Clinic states that most of the counterculture see nurses as having some knowledge about nutrition, therefore their advice is regarded as fairly reliable. However, they reserve the right to disagree and expect to be treated with respect if they reject some of the advice.

Group pressure within the commune influences the expectant mother's nutrition. Some communes make an added effort to see that her diet is adequate, even though they reject the added foods otherwise. Other communes put pressure on the expectant mother to adhere to the prescribed beliefs and reject the advice of medical teams to increase the intake of animal proteins.

The reader is referred to Chapter 17 where information related to vegeterian diets is included.

Good nutrition for the next generation clearly is an issue.

WHAT ARE THE ISSUES RELATING TO MAN'S ABILITY TO MANIPULATE HIS GENETIC CONSEQUENCES?

We are in a period of historical development in which advancements in the science of genetics have placed man on the threshold of being able to consciously control and engineer the composition of future human population.[59] Genetic engineering, the processes by which man can manipulate genetic consequences, is described as having two goals: the improvement of the individual (euphenics), and the improvement of society or the population as a whole (eugenics).[60] Genetic engineering is creating a new moral and ethical dilemma because euphenic and eugenic efforts frequently produce consequences which are in conflict with each other. For example, attempts to improve the individual might create a negative impact on the population's future genetic health.

The dilemma arising from genetic engineering is presented here as an issue because attempts to manipulate genetic consequences must occur within the childbearing phase of the life cycle (involving individuals with reproductive organs and some capacity to procreate a new human product). It is not feasible to describe in detail the factors relating to ethical considerations in human heredity. Rather, some of the issues society must face are briefly discussed below.

As we become more effective in euphenic treatment for genetic diseases (such as diabetes and hemophilia), we allow more individuals to live to adult life. Are we not jeopardizing mankind's future "genetic pool" as these individuals reproduce and pass their defective genes to the next generation, whereas previously they did not live to reproduce? What eugenic consequences are the price for euphenic success? The financial burden on society for the care of a single genetically defective individual who cannot be self-sustaining is great. The issue is that as society allows itself to be surrounded by an increased population of individuals with genetic risks, it is increasing a genetic load of detrimental genes with which it must deal. The burden is not only financial but in terms of social and psychologic effects on the family and productivity of the society. Also, can we afford polluting the "genetic pool" for the future?

Technology has brought an era in which various laboratory analyses (culture of skin cells, amniocentesis) allow identification of chromosomal disorders. It is speculated that multiple testing to identify heterozygous genetic disorders will be made as simple and as cheap as those existing for homozygous defects.[61] Heterozygous genetic disorders involve individuals who are normal but carry a recessive gene capable of producing disorders when combined with a similar recessive gene. Heterozygous carriers constitute 1 per cent of the population, creating a risk toward genetic misfortune as great or greater in frequency than those for homozygous disorders.[63] It is speculated that tests for heterozygous conditions will be conducted in maternity hospitals for each baby, similar to routine testing for blood typing, and results recorded in a computer system for determining how to handle those with genetic risks.[63] Herein lies the issue: What measures will be appropriate when heterozygous carriers are identified? The questions facing society and the individual who knows he is a carrier, or his parents, are best summarized below:

1. Advances in genetic technology appear to be the stimulus which is creating a crisis in current human values. Therefore, what are these advancements which the nurse should be aware of in order to get involved in attempts to avoid detrimental effects from genetic engineering?
   a. Before the year 2000, human reproductive cells will be able to be kept in a frozen state in "laboratory banks" for

future use.[64] Genetic strains identified as superior can thus be preserved and used to produce a more genetically healthy individual and future generation.

b. We will see the day when there will be genetic surgery by which geneticists will locate and transform defective genes; this is speculated to be done in very young embryos, before cells begin to multiple, or in the reproductive cells.[65] This will allow active manipulation to ensure a genetically healthy product of pregnancy.

c. The practice of "prenatal adoption" will emerge in which a healthy embryo will be implanted into a foster mother's womb allowing the full experience of parenthood from development of the fetus to a labor-delivery event terminating in a desired product.[66] It is believed this will engender maternal and paternal feelings because the childbearing experience is almost totally complete except for the initial conception phases.

d. Currently the practice of artificial insemination is responsible for an estimated 10,000 babies a year in the United States[67] in a population who would otherwise be deprived of a childbearing experience.

e. It will one day be possible to choose the sex of a child.[68] Studies indicate there is a preference for sons rather than daughters.[69]

2. What will be the process of selection as to which reproductive cells will be banked and who is entitled to their use?
3. What will be the rights of the individual in the decision-making process relating to genetic outcome? For example, will a couple be able to say yes or no regarding the termination of a genetically malformed pregnancy? What will be the rights of the couple in terms of producing children when they are found to be carriers for heterozygous genetic disorders? Will parents be able to decide to have genetically superior children by use of genetic technology instead of letting nature take its course?
4. What will be the responsibility of society in decision making relating to genetic outcome? Will society, through legal statutes, be able to exert control to protect the genetic pool by limiting procreation of individuals with genetic risks? It is speculated that eugenics will be related simply to the measures for population control; through genetic testing those not at risk in genotype will be permitted to procreate.[70] This presents the problem of who determines a "good" genotype, as almost everyone carries some defective genes, averaging about eight.[71]

The nursing profession cannot be oblivious to events in genetic engineering because "processes that influence our genetic future have begun; several have been under way for some time."[72]

WHERE ARE WE IN RELATION TO UTILIZING THE CHILDBEARING EXPERIENCE FOR PREDICTING AND CHANGING THE COURSE OF EVENTS LEADING TO CHILD ABUSE?

Parental abuse of children is not new as evidenced by a historical review demonstrating that parents are a powerful control over the life or death of their child. Parents once were the sole determinants as to whether their child would be fed and clothed, abandoned, sold as a slave, sent to work at an early age, or disciplined through beatings. However, time brought a growing awareness that many children were physically injured by parental actions. This awareness was heightened in the forties when many roentgenologic studies revealed unexplained multiple fractures of bones in conjunction with subdural hematomas in young children.[73] Currently, abuse of children is viewed as a medical and social problem of such magnitude that community action is mandatory to protect the children. The problem of child abuse is expressed aptly by Kempe and Helfer:

> The problems of child abuse and neglect require a multidisciplinary approach in any attempt at solution. Failure to assist these children and their families result in multiple social, physical and emotional ills of all those involved. Unless interrupted in some way, the cycle of child abuse and neglect is endless. With few exceptions, children who survive this form of rearing develop into parents who rear their children as they were reared.[74]

The phenomenon of child abuse is complex, involving many interrelated forces which are beyond the scope of this chapter for discussion. The focus here is to explore the issues relative to child abuse which are associated with the childbearing experience. Childbearing exerts an important influence on whether a parent will develop the potential toward child abuse. This occurs primarily because of the factors involved in the development of parent-child relationships. This section is an exploration of events during pregnancy and the early postpartal period which can make a parent(s) vulnerable toward an abusive pattern.

Kempe and Helfer[75] have identified major criteria which lead parents toward an abusive pattern:

> In order for a child to be physically injured by his parents or guardian several pieces of a complex puzzle must come together in a very special way. To date, we can identify at least three major criteria.
>
> First, a parent (or parents) must have the *potential to abuse*. This potential is acquired over the years and is made up of at least four factors:
>
> 1. The way the parents themselves were reared, i.e., did they receive the "mothering imprint?"
> 2. Have they become very isolated individuals who cannot trust or use others?
> 3. Do they have a spouse that is so passive he or she cannot *give*?
> 4. Do they have very unrealistic expectations from their child (or children)?
>
> Second, there must be a *child*. As obvious as that might sound we point it out because this is not just *any* child, but a very special child. One who is seen differently by his parents; one who fails to respond in the expected manner; or possibly one who really is different (retarded, too smart, hyperactive, or has a birth defect). Most families, in which there are several children, can readily point out which child would have "gotten it" if the parents had the potential to abuse. Often the perfectly normal child is "seen" as bad, willful, stubborn, demanding, spoiled or slow.
>
> Finally, there must be some form of *crisis*, or a series of crises, that sets the abusive act into motion. These can be minor or major crises—a washing machine breaking down, a lost job, a husband being drafted, no heat, no food, a mother-in-law's visit and the like. It would seem most unlikely for the crisis to be *the* cause for the abuse, as some would like to believe; rather it is the precipitating factor. The simplistic lay view that child abuse is caused by parents who "don't know their strength" while disciplining their child has been shown to be false.
>
> It is this combination of events that, when they occur in the right order and at the right point in time, lead to physical abuse.

Utilizing the above framework on the abusive pattern, the following outline was developed to help identify possible issues confronting the nursing profession in working to break the tendency toward parental abuse of children.

Abusive Pattern	*Influencing Factors during Childbearing*	*Issues*
I. The Parent		
A. The way parents themselves were reared, i.e., did they receive "mothering imprint?"	Unsatisfying family relationships existed during childbearing, leading to fears that such unpleasant relationships will continue in the present family unit. Dependency on one's own parents is so great that there is an inability to problem solve without seeking the parents. Because there was no open communication with one's own parents, but rather fear and guilt, these feelings may arise frequently during attempts to communicate with others.	What are we doing to help prospective parents express their feelings about how they were reared and/or concerns about how they will rear their child after the pregnancy? When parents share feelings of guilt, anger, fear, or whatever else, do we criticize or make a judgment about what has been said, or are we able to accept what we hear and show some understanding and compassion? Do the behaviors of health professionals help to make communication attempts satisfying or do we also reinforce feelings of fear and guilt by our behavior? [This is an important point because frequently the only sense of worth and self-esteem the person has is related to a relationship in which there were constant attempts to please the parents. Thus when they feel they are not pleasing the health professionals, the impact is a blow to the ego.]
B. Have they become very isolated individuals who cannot trust or use others?	The individual's personality is such that she is not able to seek help openly from others during and after the pregnancy. Pregnancy occurs in a new community, or away from family and friends. The living environment does not offer freedom of space, accessibility to neighbors, health care facilities, or outlets for recreation.	Does our health care system help to minimize feelings of loneliness or isolation when individuals come to receive prenatal, intrapartal, and postpartal care? Or does the mode for delivery of health care generate such feelings, thus intensifying the existing loneliness? Where are we in relation to initiating community action programs to offer health care and

Abusive Pattern	*Influencing Factors during Childbearing*	*Issues*
		opportunities to interact with others for the childbearing family who are in locales where human population is concentrated, and there is a sense of nonexistence of the individual?
C. Do they have a spouse that is so passive he or she cannot give?	The marital pattern prior to and during pregnancy is such that there is no open communication by which a husband or wife can freely express how they feel or what they want from the other. Attempts to seek help from the spouse lead to disappointment and anger.	How much longer will society expect young adults to enter the childbearing age without some knowledge on the realities of marriage and family living? Are we providing service by which adults can seek help to improve their adult relationships or do we expect individuals to be able to solve their problems on their own?
D. Do they have unrealistic expectations from their child (children)?	A couple may have no knowledge about the normal appearance and behavioral patterns of a newborn infant. The perception of the baby may be distorted by mass media or by experiences shared by family or friends.	What are we doing to better educate adults of childbearing age to the expected behavioral patterns of the neonate? Are we helping parents to recognize the clues that the neonate can give reflecting his needs? Are we helping parents to learn to respond appropriately to the newborn's behavioral clues so there will be increased satisfactions in the early interactions between parent and infant? Does our health care system value reinforcement and praise for efforts in "parenting" or are we constantly critical toward efforts by parents to meet the needs of their child?
II. The child		
The abused child is frequently perceived as or is different, and does not respond in	Frequently the newborn does not coincide with the parents' expectations, dreams, fantasies, in terms of:	Are we incorporating in maternity nursing care assessment for parental expectations of their baby-to-be?

Abusive Pattern	*Influencing Factors during Childbearing*	*Issues*
the expected manner as perceived by the parents.	a. Sex b. Activity pattern c. Physical appearance d. Feeding patterns e. Sleep patterns f. Bowel/bladder functions	When a baby is born who is different from what was desired or expected, do we allow parents the right to a grieving process which is a normal manifestation? Or do we force them to interact with the baby and make critical judgments when parents react differently from the expectations of the health professionals.
III. Crisis Usually a crisis event, minor or major, is the precipitating factor for child abuse, but not the cause for the abuse.	Pregnancy is a time of increased physical and emotional stress as discussed throughout this book.	Where are we in relation to implementing crisis intervention to the family unit during their childbearing experience? What progress have we made in identifying families at risk during childbearing; risk not only to physical health but also emotional-mental health?

WHAT ARE THE OBSTACLES TO OPTIMAL DELIVERY OF HEALTH CARE DURING CHILDBEARING?

The United States is regarded as one of the most economically and scientifically advanced nations. However, the health status of its people is not the most desirable as evidenced by higher morbidity and mortality rates in comparison with other countries. Although the United States has some of the finest health care resources, its health care services "have developed unevenly resulting in a mixture of technical virtuosity and inadequacies in the delivery of minimum essential care."[76] What are some of the issues confronting Americans in their efforts to improve health care during childbearing?

One issue concerns the accessibility of health care as a right to all, whereby the "national goal is to assure the highest level of health attainable for every person." [77] There are many obstacles to converting the right to health care into an actuality in which services are readily available to the people. One obstacle is cost factors. Health care services are so expensive that there is some truth to the cliche that "only the very rich or the very poor can afford health care."[78] Therefore, there is a current movement toward some kind of national health care program to help individuals cope financially with the system, and to avert the "danger of inflated health costs that do not produce increased services or increased availability and access to improved services."[79]

Other obstacles emerge from the health care delivery system itself. The present system seems to have various disadvantages:

While manpower, facilities, and services are lacking in some areas, as observed earlier, they are in excess in others. There is also functional as well as geographical maldistribution, causing most notably the nearly nationwide inadequacy in primary care while medical specialties often exceed requirements. The market mechanism works imperfectly in meeting needs for health care; there is a distortion in incentives and pricing, and functions are poorly organized and often inefficient. Nor has there been an adequate effort at overall planning . . .

The very programs intended to help people meet rising costs have contributed unintentionally to further increases in cost. For example, the most prevalent kind of health insurance coverage is hospital care, whereas ambulatory-care benefits still are scantily insured; this has contributed to the overuse of expensive hospital facilities at the same time that it has discouraged the development of badly needed ambulatory-care services. Likewise, reimbursing providers of care by tolerating the pass-through of costs has reduced or eliminated incentives for economy.[80]

Another issue relates to the belief that the current health care system is really a nonsystem that "now defies standardization and the sensible application of resources in a national network of information and management."[81] A contributing factor is "incomplete and irregular medical records and the absence of a system of continuing audit serves to buttress the traditional educational system that relies on memory oriented pedagogy. . . ."[83]

There is also the issue concerning how to "turn on" individuals to health care during their childbearing experiences. Unfortunately, we are still plagued by attitudes which foster the belief that the prime period when health care is needed is during hospitalization for the birth of the baby. The value of preventive health has not fully impressed the public. Thus, prenatal care is not a reality for a large portion of the childbearing population. The health care system contributes to the problem because of its emphasis on hospital facilities as described previously. Also, the time has come when the people delivering health care must no longer ignore the impact of their own personal behavior on the individuals they serve. Too often the pregnant woman may be "turned off" to prenatal care because of the verbal and/or nonverbal behaviors of nurses, doctors, and others. One major obstacle is that people are not receiving enough positive feedback for their efforts in seeking prenatal health care. We must change current practices in which the individual is made to feel judged, criticized, or treated as if he has no rights or knowledge about his health care status. One approach to change this is implementation of the "patients' bill of rights."[83] Every person in the health care system has a responsibility to work toward making individuals feel more satisfaction and pleasure when they seek health care.

REFERENCES

1. Haire, D.: *The Cultural Warping of Childbirth.* International Childbirth Education Association, Hillside, New Jersey, 1972.
2. Richards, M. and Bernal, J.: *Effects of obstetric medication on mother-infant interaction and infant development.* International Congress of Psychosomatic Medicine in Obstetrics and Gynecology, London, April, 1971.
3. Gordon, H.: *Fetal bradycardia after paracervical block.* N. Engl. J. Med. 297:910, 1968.
4. Ploman, L. and Persson, B.: *On the transfer of barbiturates in the human fetus and their accumulation in some of its vital organs.* J. Obstet. Gynaecol. Brit. Emp. 64:706, 1957.
5. Hellman, L. and Pritchard, J.: *William's Obstetrics,* ed. 14. Appleton Century-Crofts, New York, 1971, p. 434.
6. Ibid.
7. Windle, W.: *Brain damage by asphyxia at birth.* Sci. Am. 77:83, 1969.
8. Brazelton, T. B.: *Effect of maternal behavior on the neonate and his behavior.* J. Pediatr. 58:513, 1961.
9. Adamson, K. and Joelsson, I.: *The effects of pharmacological agents upon the fetus and newborn.* Am. J. Obstet. Gynecol. 96:437, 1966.

10. Enkin, M., et al.: *An adequately controlled study of the effectiveness of P.P.N. Training.* Third International Congress of Psychosomatic Medicine in Obstetrics and Gynecology, London, April, 1971.
11. Haire, op. cit., p. 18.
12. Blanfield, A.: *The optimum position for childbirth.* Med. J. Australia 2:666, 1965.
13. Butler, N.: *A national long term study of perinatal hazards.* Sixth World Congress, Federation of International Gynecologists and Obstetricians, 1970.
14. Hubinont, P., et al.: *Effects of vacuum extractor and obstetrical forceps on the fetus and newborn–a comparison.* Fifth World Congress on Gynaecology & Obstetrics, Sydney, Australia, 1967.
15. Haire, op. cit., p. 24.
16. Shaw, A.: *Dilemmas of "informed consent" in children.* N. Engl. J. Med. 289:885, 1973.
17. Wilson, R.: *Decision-Making. Moral, Legal and Institutional Implications.* In *Report of the Sixty-Fifth Ross Conference on Pediatric Research: Ethical Dilemmas in Current Obstetric and Newborn Care.* Ross Laboratories, Columbus, Ohio, 1973.
18. Shaw, op. cit., p. 886.
19. Fletcher, J.: *Indicators of Humanhood: a Tentative Profile of Man.* In *The Hastings Center Report Vol. 2, No. 5.* Hastings-on-Hudson, New York. Institute of Society, Ethics and Life Sciences, Nov. 1972, pp. 1-4.
20. *The Hardest Choice.* Time, March 25, 1974, p. 84.
21. Duff, R. and Campbell, M.: *Moral and ethical dilemmas in the special-care nursery.* N. Engl. J. Med. 289:892, 1973.
22. Lasagna, L.: *Life, Death and the Doctor.* Alfred A. Knopf, New York, 1968, p. 185.
23. Dilpel, H.: *The fetus as a person: Possible legal consequences of the Hogan-Helm Amendment.* Fam. Plann. Perspect. 6:6, 1974.
24. Bernard, W.: *Injury During Pregnancy May Pose Double Damage.* In *Tucson Daily Citizen,* Dec. 5, 1973.
25. Etzioni, A.: *The Fetus: whose property?* Commonweal. 98:493, 1973.
26. *NIH bans research on live fetuses.* Science News, 103:253, 1973.
27. *Home delivery–advance or retreat?* Briefs 37:104, 1973.
28. Lang, R.: *Birth Book.* Genesis Press, Ben Lomond, California, 1972.
29. Converse, T. A., Buker, R. S. and Lee, R. V.: *Hutterite midwifery.* Am. J. Obstet. Gynecol. 116:719, 1973.
30. Faber, M. M.: *Circumcision revisited.* Birth and Family 1:19, 1974.
31. Ibid., p. 20.
32. Ibid., p. 21.
33. Siegel, E. and Morris, N.: *Family Planning: Its Health Rationale.* Am. J. Obstet. Gynecol. 118:995, 1974.
34. Lieberman, E.: *Reserving a womb: Case for the small family.* Am. J. Pub. Health 60:87, 1970.
35. *Editorial.* Fam. Plann. Perspect. 5: (cover page), 1973.
36. Robbins, J.: *Unmet needs in family planning: A world survey.* Fam. Plann. Perspect. 5:232, 1973.
37. Harkavy, O. and Maier, J.: *Research in contraception and reproduction: A status report, 1973.* Fam. Plann. Perspect. 5:213, 1973.
38. Commission on population growth and the American future: *Population and the American Future.* U. S. Government Printing Office, Washington, D.C. 1972, p. 97.
39. Ryder, N.: *Contraceptive failure in the United States.* Fam. Plann. Perspect. 5:133, 1973.
40. Jaffe, F.: *Commentary: Some policy and program implications of contraceptive failure in the United States.* Fam. Plann. Perspect. 5:144, 1973.
41. Bell, D.: *Summary, Third Bellagio Conference on Population, May 10-12, 1973.* Rockefeller Foundation, New York, 1973.
42. Robbins, op. cit., p. 234.
43. Millstone, D.: *Resources in review.* Family Plann. Digest 3:11, 1974.
44. Roffman, D., Speckman, C. and Gruz, N.: *Maryland pharmacists ready for family planning initiative.* Fam. Plann. Perspect. 5:243, 1973.
45. Robbins, op. cit., p. 235.
46. *Four factors affect cost of sterilization.* Fam. Plann. Digest 3:4, 1974.
47. *IUD use linked to pelvic infection.* Fam. Plann. Digest 3:1, 1974.
48. Jaffe, op. cit.
49. *Smoking and high blood pressure increase stroke risk among oral contraceptive users.* Fam. Plann. Digest 3:6, 1974.
50. *Stroke risk higher among pill users.* Family Plann. Digest 2:12, 1973.
51. Radford, D. and Oliver, M.: *Oral contraceptives and myocardial infarction.* Br. Med. J. 3:428, 1973.
52. *Men report more complications than MDs; recanalization sometimes found to occur.* Family Plann. Digest 3:14, 1974.
53. Griffith, J.: *Social pressure on family size intentions.* Fam. Plann. Perspect. 5:237, 1973.
54. *Lawyers favor end to restrictive laws.* Family Plann. Digest, 3:7, 1974.
55. Ibid., p. 8.
56. Erhard, D.: *The new vegetarian–vegetarianism and its medical consequences.* Nutrition Today 8:4, 1973.
57. Ibid., p. 12.
58. Bancroft, A. V.: *Pregnancy and the counter culture.* Nurs. Clin. North Am. 8:67, 1973.
59. Nagle, J.: *The dilemma of genetic engineering.* Mental Health Digest 5:42, 1973.
60. Ibid.
61. Glass, B.: *Human Heredity and Ethical Problems.* In Katz, J. (ed.): *Experimentation with Human Beings.* Russell Sage Foundation, New York, p. 452.
62. Ibid., p. 452.

63. Ibid.
64. Ibid., p. 454.
65. Ibid., p. 455.
66. Ibid., p. 452.
67. Nagle, op. cit., p. 43.
68. *Choice of child's sex soon a possibility?* Family Plann. Digest, 3:14, 1974.
69. *Most couples prefer boy as a first child.* Family Plann. Digest 3:14, 1974.
70. Glass, op. cit., p. 456.
71. Ibid.
72. Nagle, op. cit., p. 42.
73. Gil, D.: *Violence against Children.* Harvard University Press, Cambridge, Massachusetts, 1970, p. 2.
74. Kempe, H. and Helfer, R.: *Helping the Battered Child and His Family.* J. B. Lippincott, Philadelphia, 1972, p. 294.
75. Ibid., pp. xvi and xv.
76. *Toward National Health Care.* Research and Policy Committee of the Committee for Economic Development, Current Report, June, 1973, p. 32.
77. Ibid., p. 36
78. Ibid., p. 46
79. Ibid., p. 36.
80. Ibid., pp. 37 and 40.
81. Weed, L.: *Medical Records, Medical Education, and Patient Care.* Press of Case Western Reserve University. 1971, (inside cover).
82. Ibid.
83. Quinn, N. and Somers, A.: *The patient's bill of rights.* Nurs. Outlook 22:240, 1974.

BIBLIOGRAPHY

Bloch, H.: *Dilemma of "battered child" and "battered children."* State J. Med. 73:799, 1973.

Converse, T. A., Buker, R. S. and Lee, R. V.: *Hutterite midwifery.* Am. J. Obstet. Gynecol. 116:719, 1973.

Edey, H.: *Psychological aspects of vasectomy.* Medical Counterpoint 4:19, 1972.

Eiduson, B. T., Cohen, J. and Alexander, J.: *Alternatives in childrearing in the 1970's.* Am. J. Orthopsychiat. 43:720, 1973.

Erhard, D.: *The new vegetarians–the Zen macrobiolic movement and other cults based on vegetarianism.* Nutrition Today 9:20, 1974.

Fontana, V.: *The Maltreated Child.* Charles C Thomas, Springfield, Ill., 1964.

Gil, D.: *Violence against Children.* Harvard University Press, Cambridge, Mass., 1970.

Glass, B.: *Human heredity and ethical problems.* In Katz, J. (ed.): *Experimentation with Human Beings.* Russell Sage Foundation, New York, 1972.

Harkavy, O. and Maier, J.: *Research in contraception and reproduction: a status report, 1973.* Fam. Plann. Perspect. 5: 213, 1973.

Harris, C. H.: *Some ethical and legal considerations in neonatal intensive care.* Nurs. Clin. North Am. 8: 521, 1973.

Helfer, R. and Kempe, C. (eds.): *The Battered Child.* University of Chicago Press, Chicago, 1968.

Home delivery—advance or retreat? Briefs 37:104, 1973.

Johnston, C. M. and Deisher, R. W.: *Communal child rearing.* Pediatrics 52:319, 1973.

Kempe, H. and Helfer, R.: *Helping the Battered Child and His Family.* J. B. Lippincott, Philadelphia, 1972.

Lang, R.: Birth Book, Genesis Press, Ben Lomond, Calif., 1972.

Lederberg, J.: *Experimental genetics and human evolution.* In Katz, J. (ed.): *Experimentation with Human Beings.* Russell Sage Foundation, New York, 1972.

Lieberman, J.: *Reserving a womb: case for the small family.* Am. J. Pub. Health 60:87, 1970.

Liley, A.: *The foetus as a personality.* Mental Health Digest 5: 2, 1973.

Love of children, a myth. Clin. Pediatr. 7:703, 1968.

McDonald, H.: *Implanting human values into genetic control.* Science and Public Affairs 30:21, 1974.

Nagle, J.: *The dilemma of genetic engineering.* Mental Health Digest 5:42, 1973.

Nitowsky, H. M.: *Prenatal diagnosis of genetic abnormality.* Am. J. Nurs. 71:1551, 1971.

Robbins, J.: *Unmet needs in family planning: a world survey.* Fam. Plann. Perspect. 5:232, 1973.

Siegel, E. and Morris, N.: *Family planning: its health rationale.* Am. J. Obstet. Gynecol. 118:995, 1974.

Stone, F. A.: *Psychological aspects of early mother-infant relationships.* Brit. Med. J. 4:224, 1971.

Zeller, W.: *The new morality—re-evaluated: a psychiatrist's point of view.* Am. J. Obstet. Gynecol. 119:24, 1974.

APPENDICES

1. Glossary
2. Maternal-Newborn Nursing Assessment Forms
3. Family Planning Nursing Assessment Forms
4. United Nations Declaration of the Rights of the Child

GLOSSARY

abortion (ah-bor′shun). Termination of pregnancy prior to viability of the fetus (28 weeks of gestation). **spontaneous a.,** one that has not been induced by artificial means. **induced a.,** one that is intentionally brought on by drugs or mechanical means.

abruptio placentae (ah-brup′she-o plah-cen′ta). Premature separation of a normally situated placenta.

accoucheur (ah-koosh-er′). One skilled in midwifery; an obstetrician.

acinus (as′i-nus). The smallest division of a gland; a group of cells surrounding a saccular or tubular cavity.

adnexa (ad-nex′ah). Appendages; adjunct parts.

afterbirth (af′ter-berth). The placenta and membranes.

afterpains (af′ter-pānz). Painful uterine contractions following delivery.

airway. (1) The passage through which air passes from outside the body to the pulmonary alveoli; (2) a curved, semi-rigid tube which, when inserted into the mouth, permits the passage of air from the lips to the glottis.

albumin (al-bu′min). Any simple protein soluble in water and dilute salt solutions, and coagulable by heat. **serum a.,** a specific protein normally present in human blood.

albuminuria (al′bu-mi-nu′re-ah). The presence of albumin in the urine (proteinurea).

aldosterone (al-dos′ter-on). An electrolyte-regulating hormone of the adrenal cortex.

alveolus (al-ve′o-lus). An air sac in the lung.

ambient (am′be-ant). Completely surrounding, encompassing. Environment.

amenorrhea (a-men-o-re′ah). Absence of menstruation.

amino acid (am″in-o as′id). One of the basic compounds of which protein is composed.

amnesia (am-ne′se-ah). Lack or loss of memory.

amniocentesis (am′ne-o-sen-te′sis). Procedure whereby amniotic fluid is removed from the uterine cavity by insertion of a needle through the abdominal and uterine walls and through the amniotic sac.

amnion (am′ne-on). The inner of the two fetal membranes forming the sac that encloses the fetus within the uterus.

amniotic (am-ne-ot′ik). Pertaining to the amnion. **a. fluid,** liquid contained in the amniotic sac. **a. sac,** the sac that incloses the fetus in utero. Loosely, the sac formed by the amnion and chorion.

amniotomy (am-ne-ot′o-me). Artificial rupture of the amniotic sac.

analgesia (an-al-je′ze-ah). A medication which relieves pain.

analogue (an′ah-log). A part or organ similar to another. In chemistry, a compound which is structurally similar to another but differs in that one molecule or radical has been replaced by one of the same valence. In logic, one thing is inferred to be similar to another in certain respects.

androgen (an'dro-jen). Internal endocrine secretions manufactured mainly by the testes when stimulated by the pituitary gland.

anemia (ah-ne'me-ah). A condition in which the blood is deficient in red blood corpuscles, hemoglobin, or both.

anencephalus (an-en-sef'ah-lus). A congenital deformity characterized by absence of most of the brain and spinal cord, the cranium being open throughout its whole extent and the vertebral canal converted into a grove.

anesthesia (an-es-the'ze-ah). Loss of feeling or sensation, with or without loss of consciousness.

anesthesiologist. A physician specially trained in the science of anesthesia and the use of medicinal gases.

anesthetist. Anyone administering an anesthetic agent.

anomalous, anomaly (ah-nom-ah-lus). Irregular; marked by deviation from the natural order.

anoxia (an-ok'se-ah). Literally, absence of oxygen. See Hypoxia.

anteflexion (an-te-flek'shun). State of being bent forward.

antenatal (an-te-na'tal). Occurring (to a fetus) before birth; less accurately, occurring (to a pregnant woman) before delivery.

anterior (an-te're-or). In front of.

anteroposterior (an"ter-o-pos-te're-or). Front to back.

anteversion (an-te-ver'zhun). A state of being turned forward.

anthropoid (an'thro-poid). Ape-like.

antibiotic (an'ti-bi-ot-ik). Any variety of substances both natural and synthetic which inhibits growth of or destroys microorganisms.

antibody (an'te-bod-e). Any substance in the blood serum or other fluid of the body which exerts a specific restrictive or destructive action on bacteria, cells, or other noxa, or neutralizes their toxins.

antipyretic (an"te-pi-ret'ik). Relieving fever; cooling.

antiseptic (an-te-sep'tik). An agent that will prevent the growth or arrest the development of microorganisms.

antitoxin (an-te-tok'sin). A substance specifically antagonistic to some particular toxin.

anuria (ah-nu're-ah). Complete failure of the kidneys to secrete urine.

anus (a'nus). Distal end and outlet of rectum.

aorta (a-or'ta). Main artery of the body, originating at the left ventricle of the heart and terminating by bifurcating into the two common iliac arteries.

aortography. X-ray delineation of aorta after injection of a contrast medium into it.

areola (a-re'o-la). Darkened ring around a part. Pigmented ring about the nipple of the breast. **secondary a.**, a ring which, during pregnancy, surrounds the areola papillaris.

asepsis (a-sep'sis). Absence of septic matter, or freedom from infection.

aseptic technique. Sum total of procedures designed to prevent the introduction of pathogenic organisms into a patient; less commonly, similar procedures to prevent transfer of such organisms from a patient to some other person, or from one part of the body to another.

asphyxia (as-fik'se-ah). A condition in which there is a deficiency of oxygen in the blood and an increase in carbon dioxide in the blood and tissues.

asphyxia neonatorum (as-fik'se-ah ne'o-na-tor'um). Delayed onset of breathing at the time of birth.

atelectasis (at'e-lak'tah-sis). Collapse of air sac in the lungs.

atonic (a-ton'ik). Characterized by lack of normal tone or tension.

atrophic (a-trof'ik). Characterized by shrinkage and degeneration of vital components, resulting in partial or total loss of function.

attitude (at'e-tūd). Posture of the fetus, especially flexion or extension of its spine.

auscultation (aws-kul-ta'shun). Listening.

autogenous (aw-toj'e-nus). Self-generated;

originated within the body. **a. vaccine,** a vaccine for use in a specific patient, prepared from bacteria secured from that patient.

bacteria (bak-te′re-ah). Microorganisms of the plant class Schizomycetes, many kinds of which produce disease in man.

bag-of-waters. The membranes which enclose the liquor amnii and the fetus.

ballottement (bal-ot-mon′). The bobbing motion produced by striking a solid body floating in a liquid.

Bandl's ring. Abnormal circular constriction of uterus which occasionally develops during labor and interferes with delivery.

Bartholin's (bar′to-linz) **glands.** The vulvovaginal glands.

basal metabolism (ba′sal me-tab′o-lism). The minimal amount of energy or number of calories required to support the basic metabolic processes of an individual at rest.

basal temperature. The lowest sustained temperature maintained by a normal individual in the course of a typical 24 hour period; for practical purposes, the body temperature, determined orally or rectally, present on awakening after a normal night's sleep.

bear down. To increase the intra-abdominal pressure for the purpose of expelling the contents of the bladder, rectum, or vagina.

bifurcate (bi-fur′kat), **bifurcated, bifurcation.** Forking into two nearly equal divisions; Y-shaped.

bilirubin (bil′i-roo′bin). Pigment produced by the breakdown of hemoglobin in cell elements and in the red blood cells.

bimanual (bi-man′u-al). With both hands; performed by both hands, especially pelvic examination with the fingers of one hand in the vagina and the other hand on the abdomen.

biopsy. Removal and microscopic examination of a small piece of tissue.

bipolar. Having or concerned with two poles.

birth. The act or process of being born. **b. canal,** the channel through the bony pelvis through which the baby passes during delivery.

blastoderm (blas′to-derm). The germinal membrane of the ovum.

blastodermic vesicle (blas-to-der′mik ves′ik-l). Blastocyst; the stage in development of a fertilized ovum in which the morula acquires a fluid-filled internal cavity.

Braxton Hicks contractions (braks′ton hiks). Light, irregular, painless contractions of the uterus during pregnancy.

breech (brēch). The buttocks. **b. presentation,** the condition in which the buttocks of the fetus lie directly above or in the birth canal.

bregma (breg′ma). Region of the anterior fontanel.

bulge (bulj). To swell or jut out; bend outward.

bullous. Characterized by large blebs or blisters.

bronchopulmonary dysplasia (brong′ko-pul′mo-ner′e dis-pla′ze-uh). An abnormality of development of the lungs and bronchi.

caput (ka′put). Any head or head-like structure. **c. succedaneum** (suk-se-da′ne-um). A swelling formed on the presenting part of the fetal head during labor.

cardiotocography (kar′de-o-to-cog′ra-fe). Method of continuous monitoring and recording of the fetal heart rate.

caul (kawl). Detached portion of the fetal membranes occasionally found covering the fetal head after the head has delivered.

cephalhematoma (sef″al-he-ma-to′ma). An accumulation of blood under the periostium of any of the cranial bones; especially one, induced by the trauma of birth, developing in a newborn.

cephalic (se-fal′ik). Pertaining to the head, or directed toward the head of the body.

cerebral edema (ser′e-bral e-de′ma). Swelling of the brain, especially of the cerebral hemispheres.

cerclage (sair-klahge′). The operative procedure of encircling the cervix with a ligature to prevent its premature dilatation; often called Barter or Shirodkar procedure.

cervix (ser′viks). Any neck-like part; the neck;

c. uteri, the lower end of the uterus.

cesarean section (se-za're-an). The operation consisting of cutting through the abdominal and uterine walls, and delivering one or more fetuses of viable size.

Chadwick's sign. Violet color of the vaginal mucous membrane during pregnancy.

choanal atresia (ko-a'-nal a-tre'ze-ah). Congenital obstruction of the posterior cavity of the nares.

chloasma (klo-az'ma). A cutaneous discoloration occurring in yellowish-brown patches and spots; the skin color change forming the "mask of pregnancy".

chorioepithelioma (ko"re-o-ep-i-the-le-o'ma). A cancerous tumor derived from placental tissue.

chorion (ko're-on). The outer of the two membranes forming the sac that encloses the fetus in the uterus.

chorionic gonadotrophin (ko-re-on'ik go-nad'o-trof'in). A hormone, with properties similar to those of leuteinizing hormone, that is secreted by the placenta during gestation. It is found in substantial amounts in human urine during pregnancy.

chorionic villi (ko-re-on'ik vil'e). Terminal fern- or frond-like microscopic subdivisions of chorionic (placental) tissue, each containing a single loop of a capillary of an umbilical artery-vein system. They project into the maternal uterine blood lakes or sinuses, or adhere to the decidua (anchoring villi).

chromatin (kro'ma-tin). Minute particles seen in the nuclei of stained cells. Just before cell division, chromatin condenses into clumps (chromosomes). It is the specific substance which transmits characteristics to new cells (inheritance).

chromosome (kro'mo-sōm). One of several microscopic rod-shaped bodies within the nucleus of a dividing cell.

cilia (sil'e-ah). (1) Eyelashes. (2) Minute hair-like processes.

circumcision (ser-kum-sizh'un). The removal of the end of the prepuce or foreskin of the penis.

cleft lip. Congenital fissure of the lip.

cleft palate (pal'it). Congenital deformity caused by the failure of the bones of the roof of the mouth to fuse in the midline.

clitoris (kli'tor-is, klit'or-is). A female organ homologous with the penis of the male.

coagulation time (ko-ag-u-la'shun). The amount of time required for blood to coagulate.

coitus (ko'i-tus). Sexual connection or intercourse; coition, copulation.

colostrum (ko-los'trum). Colorless, sticky secretion of the breasts during pregnancy and before lactation.

complete tear. Perineal tear which divides the anal sphincter completely; third degree tear.

conception (kon-sep'shun). The fecundation of the ovum.

congenital (kon-jen'i-tal). Existing at or before birth.

conjugate (kon'ju-gāt). An anteroposterior diameter of the bony pelvis. **external c.,** distance from the symphysis pubis to the depression below the spine of the last lumbar vertebra. **diagonal c.,** distance from the bottom of the symphysis pubis to the promontory of the sacrum. **obstetric c.,** the shortest distance from the symphysis pubis to the promontory of the sacrum. **true c.,** from the top of the symphysis pubis to the promontory of the sacrum. **c. vera,** true c.

conjugation (kon'ju-ga'shun). The act of joining or coupling.

contraception (kon-tra-sep'shun). The prevention of conception.

contractions, uterine. Shortening of the muscular fibers of the uterus during labor.

copulation (kop-u-la'shun). Sexual intercourse.

coronal suture (kor'o-nal su'ture). The suture between the frontal and parietal bones.

corpus (kor'pus). 1. The body. 2. The main part of any organ. 3. Any mass of specialized tissue. **c. luteum** (lu'te-um), a solid, yellow structure which develops following the rupture of, and replaces, a graafian follicle.

cortisone (kor'ti-sōn). A carbohydrate-regulating hormone from the adrenal cortex.

cotyledon (kot-e-le'don). Rounded segment or subdivision of the uterine surface of the placenta.

Couvelaire uterus (koo-vel-air' u'ter-us). Uterus with blood forced within the uterine walls between the muscle fibers. May occur in premature separation of the placenta.

Credé prophylaxis (kreh-da' pro-fi-lak'sis). Instillation of 1 per cent silver nitrate solution into the conjunctival sacs of a newborn for the purpose of preventing gonorrheal ophthalmia.

Credé's method. Method of expressing the placenta by firmly squeezing the fundus.

crown. The top of the head. **crowning,** stage in delivery when the fetal head presents at the vulva.

cul-de-sac of Douglas (kul'de-sahk). The lowermost posterior portion of the peritoneal cavity, lying between the rectum and uterus in proximity to the posterior vaginal fornix.

cyanosis (si-an-o'sis). Blueness of the skin due to insufficient oxygenation of the blood.

cystocele (sis'to-sēl). Hernial protrusion of the urinary bladder into the vagina.

decidua (de-sid'u-ah). The endometrium during pregnancy. **d. basalis** (ba-sa'lis), that part of the decidua which unites with the chorion to form the placenta. **d. reflexa** (re-fleks'ah) or **d. capsularis,** the part of the decidua which lies between the conceptus and the uterine cavity. **d. vera** (ve'ra), the true decidua; the portion of the decidua which lines the uterus except at the site of attachment of the placenta.

defibrination (de-fi'bri-na'shun). Removal of fibrin from the blood or lymph.

deliver, delivery. Expulsion or extraction of a baby from the mother's body. Loosely, expulsion or extraction of an organ or mass through a normal or abnormal body opening.

deoxyribonucleic acid (de-oks'e-ri-bo-nu-kle'ic). See DNA.

diastasia (di-as'ta-sis). 1. Separation of the epiphysis of a bond. 2. The last part of cardiac diastole. 3. Lateral separation of the rectus muscles of the abdomen.

digital (dij'it-al). Pertaining to the fingers.

dilatation (dil-a-ta'shun). The condition of being dilated or stretched beyond the normal or usual dimensions.

disproportion (dis-pro-por'shun). Lack of normal relationship, especially as to size; the condition when the fetal head is larger than the bony birth canal.

diuresis (di-u-re'sis). Increased secretion of urine.

dizygotic (di-zi-got'ik). Derived from two fertilized cells.

DNA. Deoxyribonucleic acid, one of the fundamental components of chromatin.

Döderlein's bacillus (ded'er-līnz). The normal, nonpathogenic bacillus of the vagina.

Doppler ultrasound sensor. A device used to monitor the fetal heartbeat.

dry labor. One in which the liquor amnii escapes prior to labor.

ductus arteriosus (duk'tus ar-te-re-o'sus). A fetal blood vessel extending from the pulmonary artery to the aorta.

ductus venosus (duk'tus ve-no'sus). Continuation of umbilical vein which passes directly to the vena cava.

Duncan's mechanism. Delivery of the placenta with the maternal surface outermost.

dysmenorrhea (dis-men-o-re'ah). Painful and difficult menstruation.

dyspareunia (dis-pa-ru'ne-ah). Painful coitus.

dyspnea (disp-ne'ah). Difficult or labored breathing.

dystocia (dis-to'se-ah). Cessation or interference with the normal process of labor.

ecchymosis (ek'i-mo'sis). Escape of blood into the tissues producing superficial blotchy areas of superficial discoloration (bruise).

Echo ultrasound. A diagnostic technique to assess fetal growth, fetal-maternal relationships, and maternal structures.

eclampsia (e-klamp'se-ah). Toxemia of pregnancy accompanied by high blood pressure, albuminuria, oliguria, tonic and clonic convulsions, and coma. May occur before, during, or after childbirth.

ectoderm (ek'to-derm). The epiblast or outer layer of the primitive (two-layered) embryo; from it develop the epidermis and the neural tube.

ectopic pregnancy (ek-top'ik). Implantation of the ovum outside of the cavity of the uterus.

edema (e-de'ma). Excessive accumulation of fluid in tissues.

effleurage (ef-lu-rahzh'). Gentle stroking of the abdomen, used during labor in the Lamaze method of childbirth.

embolus (em'bo-lus). Any material which is carried by the blood from one part of the body to another and obstructs a blood vessel.

embryo (em'bre-o). The fetus in its earlier stages of development, especially before the end of the third month.

endometritis (en'do-me-tri'tis). Inflammation of the endometrium.

endometrium (en-do-me'tre-um). The mucous membrane that lines the cavity of the uterus.

en face (ohn fass). Face-to-face, with eye-to-eye contact.

engagement. Passage of the largest diameter of the presenting part of the fetus into the pelvic brim.

engorgement. Hyperemia; local congestion; excessive fullness of an organ or passage.

entoderm (en'to-derm). The hypoblast; the inner layer of the blastoderm.

epigastric (ep-e-gas'trik). Pertaining to the upper middle portion of the abdomen, over or in front of the stomach.

episiotomy (e-piz-e-ot'o-me). Surgical incision of the perineum toward the end of second stage of labor to facilitate delivery and avoid laceration.

ethnocentrism (eth'no-sen'triz-im). The belief in the inherent superiority of one's own group and culture accompanied by a feeling of contempt for other groups and cultures.

Erb's paralysis. Paralysis of certain muscles of the arm and shoulder due to injury to the fifth and sixth cervical nerves. In obstetrics, usually produced by excessive lateral flexion of the neck of the baby during delivery.

erectile tissue (e-rec'tile). Tissue containing specialized blood vessels, which, when engorged with blood, cause the tissue to stand up or away from the surrounding nonerectile tissue.

erythema (er-i-the'ma). Redness, usually due to capillary dilatation.

erythroblastosis fetalis (e-rith-ro-blas-to'sis fee-tay'lis). A hemolytic anemia of the fetus and newborn occurring when the blood of the fetus contains an antigen lacking in the mother's blood, stimulating maternal antibody formation against the infant's erythrocytes.

estrogen (es'tro-jen). Female sex hormone manufactured in the ovaries. Production is intensified during ovulation, pregnancy, and menstruation.

etiologic (e"te-o-log'ik). Pertaining to the cause of disease.

expression. Squeezing or expelling by pressure.

expulsion (ex-pul'shun). Driving or forcing out; tending to expel.

extension (ex-ten'shun). 1. The straightening of a flexed part. 2. Going beyond a previous limit.

external rotation. Movement or turning of a body situated or occurring on the outside; performed outside the body. The spontaneous turning of the head after its delivery.

extraction, breech. The process or act of pulling or drawing out the fetus when the buttocks present.

extraperitoneal (ex"tra-per-it-o-ne'al). Situated or occurring outside the peritoneal cavity.

extrauterine pregnancy (ex'tra-u'-ter-in). Ectopic pregnancy; development of the ovum outside of the cavity of the uterus.

fallopian tube (fal-lo'pe-an). An oviduct.

fertilization (fer'til-iz-a'shun). The combining of basic male and female elements within an ovum, normally followed by the development of a fetus.

fetal (fe′tal). Pertaining to a fetus.
fetus (fe′tus). Undelivered baby, especially after the third month of gestation.
fibrinogen (fi-brin′o-jen). A normal blood constituent necessary for the formation of clots.
fibroid (fi′broid). A tumor made up of connective and muscular tissue. Commonly used to refer to myoma, liomyofibroma, and leiomyofibroma of the uterus.
fimbriated (fim′bre-a-ted). Fringed.
flaccid (flak′sid). Characterized by complete relaxation or lack of tone.
flexion (flek′shun). The act of bending; a bent state.
follicular (fol-lik′u-lar). Of or pertaining to a follicle, cyst, or sac.
fontanel, fontanelle (fon-tan-el′). Relatively wide unossified area along a cranial suture of a fetus or baby.
foramen ovale (for-a′men o-va′le). Opening between the atrial auricles of the fetal heart. It normally closes shortly after birth, but occasionally remains open or "persistent."
forceps (for′seps), **obstetric.** Forceps for grasping and making traction on the fetus to aid delivery.
fornix (for′niks). Substance forming an arch or vault. Also the space beneath an arch. The blind inner termination of the vagina, divided by the cervix into anterior, posterior, and lateral fornices.
fourchette (foor-shet′). The fold of mucous membrane at the posterior junction of the labia minora.
frenulum (fren′u-lum). Any part that serves as a curb or check, or limits the movements of an organ or part.
frontal bone. The bone of the forehead.
fundus uteri (fun′dus). The portion of the uterus distal to the point at which the oviducts traverse the uterine wall; loosely, the upper (away from the cervix) part of the body of the uterus.
funic souffle (fu′nik soof′fl). A hissing sound synchronous with the fetal heart sounds, heard over the umbilical cord.
funis (fu′nis). A cord; but chiefly the umbilical cord.
gavage (gah-vahzh′). Feeding through a tube directly into the stomach.
genetic load. The accumulated deleterious mutant genes in a population, including those maintained by mutation and selection.
gestation (jes-ta′shun). 1. Pregnancy. 2. Length of time a pregnancy is carried.
glycosuria (gli-ko-su′re-ah). The presence of glucose in the urine.
gonad (go′nad, gon′ad). A sex gland (ovary, testicle).
gonadotrophic (go-nad-o-trof′ik). Affecting or stimulating the gonads or sex glands.
Goodell's law. When the cervix is as hard as one's nose, pregnancy does not exist; when it is as soft as one's lips, pregnancy is probable.
graafian follicle (graaf′e-an). Ovarian cyst or sac containing an ovum.
gravid (grav′id). Pregnant; with child; containing a fetus.
gravida (grav′id-ah). A pregnant woman.
Hegar's sign. Softening of the lower segment of the uterus, suggesting pregnancy.
hemoconcentration (he′mo-kon′sen-tra′shun). Increase in the proportion of formed elements in the blood.
hemorrhage (hem′or-ij). A copious escape of blood. **postpartal h.,** loss of more than 500 cc. of blood over a short period of time after delivery.
heterozygous (het′er-o-zi-gus). Having different alleles in the two members of a pair of genes.
hiatus hernia, hiatal hernia. Herniation of a portion of the stomach through the esophageal foramen of the diaphragm.
HMD. Hyaline membrane disease.
homozygous (ho′mo-zi-gus). Having identical alleles in both members of a pair of genes.
hormone (hor′mōn). A chemical substance originating in a gland or organ which is conveyed through the blood to another part of the body where it exercises influence.

hyaline membrane disease. An often fatal disease of newborns. They exhibit the respiratory distress syndrome. Microscopic examination of the lungs reveals that extensive areas of the air sacs and passages are lined with a layer of homogeneous foreign material, source unknown, which apparently prevents the passage of oxygen from the air to the blood. Much more common in premature babies than full-term babies, and in babies delivered by cesarean section.

hydatidiform mole (hi-dah-tid'i-form mōl). A mass formed by the degeneration and swelling of the chorionic villi, resulting in multiple cysts that reasemble a bunch of grapes.

hydramnion, hydramnios. Excessive amount of amniotic fluid; also termed polyhydramnion, polyhydramnios.

hydrocephalus (hi-dro-sef'al-us). Excessive amount of cerebrospinal fluid in the brain cavities, surrounding the brain, or both.

hydrops fetalis (hi'drops). Massive edema (anasarca) of a fetus or newborn, usually due to Rh incompatibility (erythroblastosis).

hymen (hi'men). Membranous fold which partly closes vaginal orifice.

hyperbilirubinemia (hi-per-bil'i-roo'bine'me-ah). Excess bilibubin in the blood.

hypertonicity (hi'per-to-nis'i-te). State or quality of being hypertonic. Increased tonicity or tension.

hypocalcemia (hi'po-kal-se'me-ah). Diminished calcium in the blood.

hypofibrinogenemia (hi'po-fi-brin'o-je'meuh). Deficiency of fibrinogin in the blood.

hyperreflexia (hi'per-re-flek'se-ah). Exaggeration of reflexes.

hypoglycemia (hi'po-gli-se-me-ah). Abnormally low level of sugar (glucose) in the blood.

hypoplasia (hi'po-pla'ze-ah). Incomplete development of an organ or tissue.

hypoxemia (hi-poks-e'me-ah). Low oxygen tension in arterial blood.

hypoxia (hi-poks'e-ah). Insufficient available oxygen to the body tissues.

icterus neonatorum (ik'ter-us ne-o-na-to'rum). Jaundice in a newborn, usually physiologic jaundice as opposed to that of sepsis, erythroblastosis, etc.

iliac (il'e-ak). Pertaining to the ilium.

ilium (il'i-um). Flat upper part of innominate bone.

imperforate anus (im-per'fo-rāt a'-nus). Congenital anomaly in which there is no anal opening.

impetigo contagiosa (im-pet-e'go con-ta-je-o'sa). A contagious skin disease, caused by staphylococci, and characterized by vesicles which become pustular, rupture, then form a scab or crust.

implantation (im-plan-ta'shun). The insertion, penetration or grafting of one object in or on another.

impregnation (im-preg-na'shun). Fertilization of an ovum.

incision (in-sizh'un). A cut or wound or the act of cutting, specifically a surgical cut into, in contradistinction to cutting off (amputation) or cutting out (excision).

induction of labor. Labor brought on by artificial means.

inertia, uterine (in-er'she-ah). Sluggishness of the uterine contractions.

innominate bone (in-om'i-nāt). One of the two hip bones.

intercristal (in-ter-kris'tal). Between two crests. **i. diameter,** in pelvimetry, the greatest distance between the iliac crests.

internal rotation. One element of the mechanism of labor, characterized by rotation, within the birth canal, of the presenting part of the fetus.

interspinous (in-ter-spi'nus). Between two spinous processes. **i. diameter,** in pelvimetry, the distance between the iliac or ischial spines, usually the latter.

interstitial (in-ter-stish'al). Pertaining to or situated in the interstices or interspaces of a tissue.

intracranial hemorrhage (in-tra-kra'ne-al). A hemorrhage occurring within the skull.

intrapartal (in'tra-par'tal). Occurring during birth or delivery; broadly, during labor.

inversion (in-ver'zhun). A turning inward, inside out, or upside down.

inverted nipple. Congenital or acquired deformity of the nipple which prevents the projection of the bulk of the nipple from the surface of the breast.

involution (in-vo-lu'shun). The return of the pelvic organs to the nonpregnant state after the termination of pregnancy.

IRDS. Idiopathic respiratory distress syndrome.

ischemia (is-ke'me-ah). Local diminution in the blood supply due to obstruction in the supply or to nasoconstriction.

ischium (is'ke-um). The lower hind part of the innominate bone.

Isolette. Trade name for a self-contained incubator permitting isolation and manipulation of an infant.

jaundice (jawn'dis). Yellowness of the skin, eyes, and secretions, due to the presence of bile pigments in the blood.

joy. A positive emotion of fulfillment.

Kegal exercise. An exercise to strengthen the perineal muscles.

kernicterus (ker-nik'ter-us). A condition in the neonate marked by severe neural symptoms, associated with high levels of bilirubin in the blood.

ketosis (ke'to-sis). The accumulation of large quantities of ketone bodies in the body tissues and fluids.

kinesthesia (kin'es-the'ze-ah). Positioning and movement of various parts of the body. Receiving stimuli within the body due to stimulation of muscles, points and ligaments.

labia majora (la'be-ah ma-jo'ra). Skin-covered fat pads forming the two lateral halves of the vulva.

labia minora (la'be-ah mi-no'ra). The two folds of delicate skin between the labia majora which form the boundaries of the vestibule.

labor. The physiologic process by which the fetus and the associated placenta and membranes are expelled from the body.

laceration (las-er-a'shun). A wound produced by cutting or tearing.

lactation (lak-ta'shun). 1. The secretion of milk. 2. The period of the secretion of milk.

lambdoid, lambdoidal suture (lam'doid). A cranial suture between the occipital and parietal bones.

lactogenic (lack'to-jen'ick). Stimulating the production of milk.

laminaria tent (lam'i-nar'e-ah). A cone made of dried seaweed which swells when in contact with moisture. Used to dilate the cervix in induced abortion.

lanugo (la-nu'go). The fine hair on the body of the fetus and newborn.

lightening (li'ten-ing). The sensation produced by the descent of the presenting part into the pelvic cavity prior to labor.

linea nigra (lin'e-ah ni'gra). Narrow line of pigmentation which sometimes develops in the midline of the skin of the anterior abdominal wall during pregnancy.

liquor amnii (li'kwor am'ne-i). Amniotic fluid; fluid surrounding the embryo or fetus in utero.

lobule (lob'ule). Any small lobe.

lochia (lo'ke-ah). The vaginal (uterine) discharge present for several weeks after delivery.

lunar (lu'nar). Pertaining to the moon. **l. month,** 28 days (4 weeks).

luteotropic hormone (LTH) (lu-te-o-tro'pic). One of the gonadotropic hormones produced by the anterior pituitary gland. LTH stimulates the full development of the corpus luteum initiated by luteinizing hormone.

macerate (mas'er-āt). To cause to waste away; to soften by steeping in a liquid.

malformation (mal-for-ma'shun). Defective or abnormal formation; deformity.

malpresentation. A faulty, abnormal, or untoward fetal presentation.

mammary (mam'a-re). Pertaining to the breast.

mammary glands. The mammae; the milk-secreting organs.

mask of pregnancy. Brown pigmentation of the face seen in pregnancy; chloasma.

mastitis (mas-ti'tis). Inflammation or infection of the breast.

mechanism of labor. The series of passive movements undergone by the fetus in passing through the birth canal.

meconium (me-ko'ne-um). The fecal matter discharged by the newborn. It is a dark green substance, consisting of mucus, bile, and epithelial shreds.

membrane (mem'brān). A thin layer of tissue which covers a surface or divides a space or organ.

menstrual cycle (men'stru-al). (1) Periodic series of changes in female reproductive organs in preparation for pregnancy. If pregnancy does not occur, menstuation results. (2) The interval between the onset of successive menstrual periods.

mesoderm (mes'o-derm). The middle of the three layers of the primitive embryo.

metritis (me-tri'tis). Inflammation of the uterus.

micrognathia (mi'kro-nath'e-uh). Abnormal smallness of the lower jaw.

micropore filter. Filter used in intravenous sets to prevent bacteria from entering the system.

midwife. A woman who delivers parturient women.

monitrice. An individual specifically trained to support women in labor using a psychoprophylactic method.

monozygotic (mon-o-zi-got'ik). Derived from one fertilized cell.

monstrosity (mon-stros'it-e). 1. Great congenital deformity. 2. An anomaly of formation; fetal monstrosity.

mons veneris (monz' ven'er-is). A rounded prominence at the symphysis pubis of a woman.

Montgomery's glands. Sebaceous glands of the mammary areola, also called areolar glands.

morbidity (mor-bid'it-e). 1. The condition of being diseased or morbid. 2. The sick rate, or proportion of disease to health in a community. 3. Significant elevation in body temperature. **puerperal m.,** oral temperature of 100.4°F, (38°C.) or higher on any two of the second to tenth days postpartum (temperatures to be taken every 4 hours).

Moro reflex (mor'o). Flexion of an infant's thighs and knees, fanning and then clenching of fingers, with arms thrown outward and then brought together as though embracing something.

mortality rate. Number of deaths expressed in relation to a standard number of persons, usually expressed in percentage or in the number of deaths per 1000 or 10,000 patients or persons. **fetal m. r.,** strictly, the mortality rate among fetuses (unborn babies). Loosely, mortality rate of fetuses and newborns, now usually referred to as **perinatal m. r.** Many reports include babies up to one month of age. **maternal m. r.,** mortality rate among pregnant women and (variously) within 3 to 12 months after delivery, usually reported in relation to total live births. **neonatal m.r.,** mortality rate among newborns up to one month of age.

morula (mor'u-la). The solid mass of cells formed by the division and redivisions of the fertilized ovum.

multipara (mul-tip'a-ra). A woman who has borne two or more children; loosely, any pregnant woman who has had a child.

Nägele's rule. Method of estimating the expected date of confinement (EDC). Count back 3 months from the first day of the last menstrual period and add 7 days.

narcosis (nar-ko'sis). A state of profound unconsciousness produced by a drug.

natal (na'tal). Pertaining to birth.

navel (na'vel). The umbilicus.

neonate. A baby less than four weeks of age.

neonatologist (ne-o-na-tol'o-jist). A pediatrician specially trained in the care of the neonate.

nidation (ni-da'shun). Implantation of fertilized ovum in the endometrium.

nullipara (nul-ip'a-ra). A woman who has never borne a child.

obstetrician (ob-ste-trish'an). One who practices obstetrics.

obstetrics (ob-stet'riks). The art and science of caring for pregnant women.

occiput (ok'si-put). The back part of the head.

oligohydramnios (ol'e-go-hi-dram'ne-os). Scantiness of the liquor amnii.

ophthalmia neonatorum (of-thal-me-uh ne'o-na-to'rum). Purulent conjunctivitis of the newborn; gonorrheal conjunctivitis.

orifice (or'i-fis). Normal opening.

os innominatum (os in-nom-e-na'tum). Innominate bone: one of the two lateral bones of the adult pelvic girdle. It is composed of three bones—ilium, ischium, pubis—which are indistinguishably fused.

os uteri. Mouth of the uterus: the external uterine cervical opening.

oxytocic (oks-e-to'sik). Agent which stimulates uterine contractions. Given to speed the process of childbirth.

$PaCO_2$. Partial pressure of carbon dioxide in arterial blood.

palpation (pal-pa'shun). Digital examination or exploration by the hand.

PaO_2. Partial pressure of oxygen in arterial blood.

Papanicolaou smear. A specially fixed and stained microscopic slide, using scrapings from the cervix or fluid aspirated from the vagina. The P. smear is extremely valuable in the early detection of cancer. Often called a Pap smear or test.

papilla (pap-il'lah). The nipple of the breast; any nipple-like projection.

para (par'ah). Used as a combining form to indicate a woman who has produced viable offspring. Used as a prefix to indicate number of pregnancies that have resulted in viable offsprings as para o (none), para 1 (one), etc.

parietal (par-i'e-tal). Pertaining to, or forming, the wall of a cavity. **p. bone,** one of the pair of bones comprising the top and sides of the middle portion of the skull.

paroxismal (par-oks-iz'mal). A sudden attack, re-appearance or increase in the intensity of symptoms.

parturient (par-tu're-ent). 1. Giving birth. 2. A woman in labor.

parturition (par-tu-reh'shun). The act or process of giving birth to a child.

pelvic. Pertaining to the pelvis. **p. brim,** the plane of the upper boundary of the true pelvis, bounded by the promontory of the sacrum, the linea terminalis and the symphysis pubes. **p. cavity,** the space within the true pelvis. **p. floor,** the soft tissues closing the pelvic outlet. **p. outlet,** the lower end of the true pelvis, bounded by the pubic arch, the tuberosities of the ischia, and the coccyx.

pelvis. 1. Any basin-like cavity or structure. 2. The skeletal structure to which the spinal column and the lower extremities are attached. In the adult the pelvis is composed of four bones (two innominate, sacrum, the coccyx). Each innominate bone is composed of three bones (ischium, ilium, and pubis) which are firmly fused. 3. The space within the pelvis. **false p.,** that portion of the pelvis above the linea terminalis and symphysis pubis. **true p.,** the portion of the pelvis below the linea terminalis.

perinatal mortality. Death of a fetus or infant weighing 1000 gm. or over which occurs between 28 weeks of gestation (period of viability) and 4 weeks of age (neonatal period).

perineal body (per-e-ne'al). Pertaining to the perineum.

perineorrhaphy (per"i-ne-or'a-fi). Suture of the perineum, especially after restoring normal anatomic relationship.

perineum (per-e-ne'um). Loosely, the floor of the pelvis. In obstetrics, the tissues between the lower end of the vagina and the anal canal and lower rectum.

petechia (pe-tek'e-ah). Small punctate red

flecks in the skin that do not blanch when pressed.

phenylketonuria (fen-il-ke′to-nu′re-ah). A rare metabolic abnormality of infants characterized by the excretion of phenylketones in the urine and resulting in severe mental retardation. Abbreviated PKU.

phimosis (fi-mo′sis). The condition in which the foreskin of the penis cannot be retracted over the glans because the preputial orifice is too small.

phlebitis (fle-bi′tis). Inflammation of a vein.

phlegmasia alba dolens (fleg-ma′ze-ah al′ba do′lens). Thrombophlebitis or phlebothrombosis resulting in blanching, pain, and swelling of the thigh and lower leg. Milk leg.

phototherapy (fo′to-ther′ah-pe). Treatment of disease by light rays. Used in the neonate to aid in bilirubin clearance.

pica (pi′ka). Craving for unnatural articles of food. Ingestion of non-nutrative substances.

placenta (pla-sen′ta). A spongy structure that grows on the wall of the uterus during pregnancy, and through which the fetus is nourished; also called afterbirth. **circumvallata p.**, one encircled with a raised white nodular ring, the attached membranes being doubled back over the edge. **p. previa**, one located in the lower uterine segment, encroaching upon or covering the cervix of the uterus.

polar body. A portion of a maturing ovum which is extruded from it and discarded.

polarity (po-lar′i-te). The status of the fetus in regard to which end (head or breech) of the long axis is at the pelvic inlet.

polycythemia (pol′e-si-the′me-ah). Abnormal increase in the erythrocyte count or in hemoglobin concentration.

polyhydramnios (pol′e-hi-dram′ne-os). Excess in the amount of the liquor amnii.

position. The relation of the direction of the presenting part to the maternal pelvis.

posterior (pos-te′re-or). Behind or back of.

postpartal (post-par′tal). Occurring after delivery or childbirth.

postprandial (post-pran′de-al). After a meal.

Poupart's ligament (poo-pars′). A fibrous band running from the anterior superior spine of the ilium to the spine of the pubis.

precipitate (pre-sip′i-tāt). Hasty, rapid.

preeclampsia (pre-ek-lamp′se-ah). Toxemia of pregnancy characterized by edema, albuminuria, and hypertension. Threatened eclampsia.

prematurity (pre′ma-tur-it-e). State of being born before the usual or expected time. Less than 37 weeks of gestation.

prenatal (pre-na′tal). Existing or occurring before birth.

presentation (prez-en-ta′shun). The part of the fetus which enters the pelvis first.

presumptive (pre-sump′tive). Based on probable evidence.

primigravida. A woman during her first pregnancy.

primipara (pri-mip′ah-ra). A woman who has given birth or is giving birth to her first child.

prodromal labor. A variable period at the beginning of labor, during which there is only slight change in the cervix.

progesterone (pro-jes′te-rōn). A steroid with progestational activity. Isolated from human ovaries, adrenal cortex, and placenta.

prolactin (pro-lak′tin). One of the gonadotropic hormones of the anterior pituitary, promotes the growth of breast tissue and is responsible for lactation.

prolapsed cord. The presence of the umbilical cord beside or ahead of the presenting part.

pronucleus (pro-nu′kle-us). 1. The half-nucleus of the mature ovum. 2. The nuclear portion of the spermatozoon after fertilization of the ovum.

prostaglandin (pros-ta-glan′din). Active biologic substance which affects the cardiovascular system and smooth muscles. Stimulates the uterus to contract.

prothrombin (pro-throm′bin). A glycoprotein present in the plasma that is converted into thrombin during the second stage of clotting.

proteinuria (pro′te-in-u′re-ah). Presence of protein (albumen) in the urine.

pruritus (pru-ri′tus). Intense itching.

ptyalism (ti′ah-lizm). Excessive secretion of saliva.

puerperal sepsis (pu-er′per-al sep′sis). Sepsis (infection) during the puerperium, originating in the pelvic organs.

puerperium (pu-er-pe′re-um). The period from delivery to completion of involution.

pyloric stenosis (pi-lor′ic sten-o′sis). Stenosis or narrowing of the orifice of the pylorus (distal end of the stomach).

pylorospasm (pi-lo′ro-spazm). Spasm of the pylorus or of the pyloric portion of the stomach.

quickening (quick′en-ing). The first perceptible movement of the fetus.

radioimmunoassay. A test for pregnancy based upon the antigen-antibody reaction and measured by sensitive radioisotope technique.

rectocele (rek′to-sel). Hernial protrusion of a part of the rectum, particularly through the rectovaginal septum.

rectovaginal fistula (rek-to-vaj′in-al). An opening between the rectum and vagina.

regurgitation (re-gur-ji-ta′shun). The casting up of undigested food; vomiting.

respiratory distress syndrome (RDS). A poorly defined disease of newborns, characterized by cyanosis, abnormal respiratory pattern, grunting respiration, and retraction of the chest wall during inspiration.

restitution (res-ti-tu′shun). The rotation of the presenting part of the fetus outside of the vagina.

retrolental fibroplasia (ret-ro-len′tal fi-bro-pla′si-ah). An oxygen-induced retinopathy of premature infants.

Rh factor. A potentially antigenic blood factor.

Ritgen's maneuver. Method of control of fetal head during delivery by pressure through the mother's postanal tissue against fetal forehead and chin.

RNA. Ribonucleic acid, one of the fundamental components of chromatin.

sagittal (saj′it-al) **suture.** The suture between the parietal bones.

scan. Study of a large area, in a systematic fashion.

Scanzoni's maneuver. Forceps rotation of the occiput to an anterior position from a posterior position.

scapula (skap′u-la). The shoulder blade.

Schultze's mechanism. Delivery of the placenta with the fetal surface outermost.

sebaceous (se-ba′shus). Pertaining to sebum (natural skin oil).

secundines (se-kun′dinz). The afterbirth; the placenta and membranes.

SGA. Small for gestational age. Weighs less than 2500 gm.

Skene's glands (skenz). Two glands opening just within the meatus of the female urethra, regarded as homologues of the seminal vesicles.

smegma (smeg′ma). A thick, cheesy, ill-smelling secretion found under the prepuce and around the labia minora.

somatization (so-ma-ti-za′shun). Using a bodily organ to symbolically express a problem.

somnolence (som′no-lens). Sleepiness; also unnatural drowsiness.

spasticity (spas-tis′it-e). The state or quality of being spastic; marked hypertonus of muscles.

spermatozoon (sper-mah-to-zo′on). The male generative cell, consisting of a head or nucleus and a flagellum or tail.

spina bifida (spi′na bif′i-da). Congenital defect of failure of closure of the spinal canal, usually posteriorly.

sterilization. 1. The process of rendering free of living bacteria. 2. Any operation or procedure intended to destroy the ability to procreate.

stilbestrol (stil-bes′trol). Diethylstilbestrol. An estrogenic compound.

stillbirth. The birth of a dead fetus.

striae gravidarum (strī′ē gra-vi-da′rum). Fine pinkish-white or gray lines seen in parts of the body where skin has been streched. Often found on abdomens and breasts of women who have been pregnant.

stridor (stri′dor). Harsh, high-pitched sound during respiration.

subinvolution (sub′in-vo-lu′shun). Incomplete involution; failure of a part to return to its normal size and condition after enlargement from functional activity, as subinvolution of the uterus.

suboccipital-bregmatic (sub-ok-sip′it-al breg-mat′ik). Situated between the lower part of the occiput and the bregma.

sulcus (sul′kus). A groove or furrow.

supine hypotension syndrone. Symptoms of bradycardia and lowered blood pressure when in a supine position late in pregnancy. Due to compression of the inferior vena cava by the gravid uterus.

surfactant (ser-fak′tant). A substance formed in the lungs that helps to keep the small air sacs expanded by virtue of its ability to reduce surface tension.

suture (su′ture). 1. Junction of cranial bones. 2. Material used as thread in surgical sewing. 3. The act of surgical sewing.

symphysis pubis (sim′fi-sis pu′bus). The junction of the pubic bones.

tachypnea (tak′ip-ne′ah). Rapid respiration.

teratogen (ter′ah-to-jen). An agent causing damage in the developing embryo.

tetanic contraction (te-tan′ik). One during which the muscle remains tense for some time.

tetany (tet′an-e). A state characterized by excessive muscular tonicity, usually due to hypocalcemia or hyperventilation. **uterine t.,** prolonged uterine contraction.

thermal neutral zone. Environmental temperature wherein the individual can utilize the least possible amount of energy to maintain a stable body temperature.

thermoregulation (ther′mo-reg′u-la′shun). Heat regulation. Balance between heat loss and heat production.

thrombophlebitis (throm′bo-fle-bi′tis). Thrombosis combined with inflammation of a vein or veins.

tine test. Initial screening test for past or present infection by the tubercle bacilli.

thrush. Mycotic stomatitis; fungus infection of the mouth or throat caused by a yeast or mold and characterized by multiple adherent white lumps of what looks like curdled milk or cottage cheese. If scraped off, a bleeding surface is left.

tonic. Characterized by prolonged excessive muscular contraction.

toxemia (toks-e′me-ah) **of pregnancy.** A specific complication of pregnancy characterized by a sustained rise in blood pressure and often by edema and albuminuria (preeclampsia) and occasionally by convulsions (eclampsia).

trophoblast (trof′o-blast). Layer or layers of cells forming the outer or maternal surface covering of the blastodermic vesicle, and, later, of the chorionic villi.

umbilical cord (um-bil′ik-al). The attachment connecting the fetus to the placenta.

umbilical hernia. Protrusion of the bowel or omentum at the navel.

umbilicus (um-bil-i′kus). The navel; the point at which the umbilical vessels enter and leave the body of the fetus and newborn. After the cord drops off, the umbilicus is the depressed scar formed by the obliterated umbilical vessels and the area of fusion of the cuff of skin which formed the original base of the umbilical cord.

uterine bruit (u′ter-in broot). Uterine sounds caused by the maternal circulation in the uterine blood vessels.

uterine sinuses (u′ter-in si′nus-es). Venous canals in the wall of the uterus.

uterine souffle (soof′fl). A sound made by the blood in the arteries of the gravid uterus; it is synchronous with the maternal heart beat.

uterus (u′ter-us). The womb; a hollow muscular organ, in which the embryo and fetus develop. **u. bicornis,** congenital malformation of the uterus characterized by division of the body and fundus into two parts, caused by failure of complete fusion of the müllerian ducts.

vagina (va-ji′na). Canal from the vulva to the cervix uteri.

vascularity (vas-ku-lar′it-e). The condition of being vascular: the condition of having large numbers of blood vessels.

vasospasm (vas′o-spazm). Vasoconstriction.

vernix caseosa (ver′nix ka-se-o′sa). Sebaceous material found in varying quantity on the skin of a fetus.

version (ver′zhun). The act of turning; especially the manual turning of the fetus. **cephalic v.** (sef-al′ik), version which causes the fetal head to present. **podalic v.** (pod-al′ik), version which causes the feet to present.

vertex (ver′teks). The summit or top; the crown of the head.

vesicovaginal fistula (ves″ik-o-vaj′in-al). An opening from the bladder into the vagina.

vestibule (ves′ti-bule). The space below the clitoris and between the labia minora.

viability (vi-ab-il′it-e). Ability to live; state of development theoretically compatible with extrauterine survival.

viable (vi′a-bl). Capable of living; said of a fetus that has reached a stage of development such that it can live outside of the uterus (28 weeks of gestation).

vulva (vul′va). The external female genitalia or pudenda.

vulvovaginal glands. Bartholin's glands; the pair of mucus-secreting glands which lie in the posterior portion of the labia majora and empty into the vestibule.

Wharton's jelly (whar′tunz). The jelly-like material forming the bulk of the umbilical cord.

X-chromosome. Sex-determining chromosome found in all ova and in half of all sperm.

Y-chromosome. Sex determining chromosome found in half of all sperm.

zona pellucida (zo′na pel-lu′sid-ah). The transparent layer surrounding a discharged ovum.

Maternal-Newborn Nursing Assessment Forms

The assessment forms that follow were developed by the Family Concerns Committee* and finalized and implemented by the nursing staff of Hennepin County General Hospital, Minneapolis, Minnesota. They represent an example of cumulative data collection developed in the interest of promoting improved nursing care through communication.

The Antepartal Nursing Assessment is transmitted to the staff who plan intrapartal care. Significant data is assessed and recorded on the Intrapartum Nursing Assessment. These records are then sent to the Maternity Unit where the Postpartum Nursing Assessment is added and to the Newborn Intensive Care Unit where the Newborn Assessment is added.

Should the infant or the mother be readmitted, all nursing records are available on the chart with the physician's records.

---

* Committee was made up of Connie Benson, Pediatric Supervisor; Julie Boran, Newborn Intensive Care Supervisor; Elizabeth Colloton, Obstetric-Pediatric Coordinator; Karla Leaf, former Newborn Intensive Care Unit Supervisor; and Donna Peterson, Obstetric Supervisor.

HENNEPIN COUNTY GENERAL HOSPITAL

Subjective (sx)
Objective (obj)
Interpretation (int)

Plan
Treatment (rx)

Pt. Name
Pt. No.
Address
Phone No.

DATE	NARRATIVE
	AP NURSING ASSESSMENT --- DATA BASE
I	OBJECTIVE DATA:
	1. APPEARANCE
	2. FEELING TONE --- AFFECT
II	SUBJECTIVE DATA:
	1. HOW PATIENT DESCRIBES SUPPORT SYSTEM
	(relationship with father of baby, parents, close friends)
	2. CULTURAL, RELIGIOUS BACKGROUND
	3. SELF CONCEPT --- HOW PATIENT FEELS ABOUT HERSELF
	4. CONCERNS OF PATIENT AT THIS TIME
	5. PARENTING RECEIVED AS A CHILD.

HENNEPIN COUNTY GENERAL HOSPITAL

NARRATIVE NOTES

DATE	NARRATIVE
	6. WHAT IS PATIENT'S REACTION TO BEING PREGNANT?
	7. DESCRIBE ANY OUTSIDE STRESS DETERRING FOCUS ON PREGNANCY.
	8. SOCIAL SERVICE, COMMUNITY AGENCIES INVOLVED.
	9. PROBLEM SOLVING:
	A. Present, future goals (educational, occupational, birth control).
	B. Plans for baby --- Financial arrangement
	C. Plans for other children at home
	10. ABILITY TO COMPREHEND:

HENNEPIN COUNTY GENERAL HOSPITAL

NARRATIVE NOTES

DATE	NARRATIVE
III	IMPRESSION:
IV	PLAN:
A:	
P:	

HENNEPIN COUNTY GENERAL HOSPITAL

MATERNITY NURSING DATA BASE

Pt. Name
Pt. No.

Infant's Hosp. No.

DATE	INTRAPARTUM NURSING ASSESSMENT
	INVOLVEMENT OF SIGNIFICANT OTHERS:
	PREPARATION FOR LABOR AND DELIVERY:
	REACTIONS TO LABOR AND DELIVERY:
	Mother:
	Nurse:
	PARENTAL RESPONSE AND INFANT CONTACT:
	Immediate response to baby:
	Mother:
	Significant others:
	First physical contact with baby:
	Length of time after delivery:
	INITIAL PLAN FOR HOSPITALIZATION PERIOD:

HENNEPIN COUNTY GENERAL HOSPITAL

MATERNITY NURSING DATA BASE

POSTPARTUM NURSING ASSESSMENT

Pt. Name
Pt. No.

Infant's Hosp. No.

DATE:	MOTHER-INFANT RELATIONSHIP:
	Verbalized thoughts and feeling about baby:
	Interaction between mother and baby:
	Preparation for baby:
	CURRENT CONCERNS OF MOTHER:
	SUPPORT SYSTEM:
	Structure of family unit; persons available for child care, etc.
	Other children: How many? Ages?
	Resources (persons and/or agencies) mother feels free to use:
	MOTHER'S PLANS FOR THE FUTURE:

HENNEPIN COUNTY GENERAL HOSPITAL

Subjective (sx)
Objective (obj)
Interpretation (int)

Plan
Treatment (rx)

Pt. Name
Pt. No.
Address
Phone No.

DATE	NARRATIVE
	NEWBORN INTENSIVE CARE UNIT NURSING ASSESSMENT --- DATA BASE
S & O	Pertinent social information
	Perception and reaction to present situation
	Affects of baby's illness on family relationship
	Supportive persons available
	Present and future plans of mother and baby
	Progression of maternal identity
	Financial situation in relation to ill child
	Living arrangements
	Use of community facilities
	Mood, feelings, affect

*Family Planning Nursing Assessment Forms**

PART I: PHYSICAL ASSESSMENT

I. Data Base
  A. Subjective
    1. Purpose of visit
    2. Initial History
      a. Family history of relevant illness
        (1) congenital anomalies
        (2) multiple pregnancies
        (3) cardio-vascular disease
        (4) diabetes
        (5) tuberculosis
        (6) epilepsy
        (7) mental-emotional-psych
      b. Past Medical History
        (1) venereal disease
        (2) gyn. diseases
        (3) varicose veins
        (4) thrombophlebitis
        (5) convulsions
        (6) diabetes
        (7) heart disease
        (8) nephritis
        (9) hepatitis
        (10) allergies
          (a) meds.
          (b) other
        (11) emotional illness
        (12) other
      c. Menstrual History
      d. Obstetrical History
      e. Contraceptive History
      f. Sexual adjustment
      g. Immunizations

---

* Family Planning Nursing Assessment developed by: La Vohn Josten and Family Planning Staff. Grant Number: 05H 000054 awarded by PHS, DHEW Family, Planning Project #717, to Minneapolis Health Department, Minneapolis, Mn. Assessment contents are in no way the responsibility of the awarding agency.

3. Interval History
   a. Medical treatment since last visit?
   b. Evaluation of current method:

BCP
L.M.P. ________
Wt. gain ________
Edema ________
Spotting ________
Discharge ________
Pain ________
Dysmenorrhea ________
Varices ________
Mood ________
N & V ________
Headache ________
Dizziness ________
Visual problems ________
Chills, fever ________
Urin. Tract Symptoms ________
Other ________

IUD
L.M.P. ________
Pain ________
Bleeding ________
Discharge ________
Chills, fever ________
Urin. Tract
Symptoms ________
IUD in place? ________
Other ________

Foam, Condoms, Diaphragms
L.M.P. ________
Skin irritation ________
Discharge ________
Pain ________
Chills, fever ________
Urin. Tract Symptoms ________

B. Objective
1. Initial physical examination by physician.
2. Initial and Interval Evaluation
   a. Weight ________ Height ________
   b. B.P. ________
   c. Edema ________
   d. Varices ________
3. Laboratory values relevant to health
   a. Pap, G.C. culture, lab diagnosis of vag. discharge
   b. Serology, Hct.
   c. Urinalysis
   d. Sickle cell evaluation
4. Yearly laboratory evaluation
   a. Hct.
   b. Urinalysis
   c. GC culture
   d. Serology
   e. Pap Smear
5. Physical appearance
   a. Posture
   b. Facial expression
   c. Mannerisms
   d. Cleanliness

II. Impressions: Problems, Needs and Strengths (based on assessment)
  A. Purpose of visit
  B. Refer to interval evaluation
III. Plan
  A. Current
  B. Long-Term

PART II: PSYCHO-SOCIAL-COGNITIVE

I. Data Base:

Pertinent Psycho-Social-Cognitive information about the patient as it relates to her ability to reach her family planning goal.

Psych: Emotional functions
Social: Associations, relationships, cooperative, interactions
Cognitive: Come to know, awareness, judgments, perceptions

A. Subjective (personal symptoms, patient's comments, complaints)
  1. Family relationships (support system and nonsupportive relationships)
    a. Sexual partner: marital relationship, plans for marriage, marital adjustment and/or relationship, joint family planning goal, attitude toward family planning, attitude toward accidental pregnancy, sexual adjustment.
    b. Parents: relationship with mother and father especially important if young and/or unwed, family's knowledge of use of birth control.
    c. Children: coping ability with current children, reason why does or does not want more children.
    d. Social service agencies: mental health or marital counseling.
    e. Other supportive or nonsupportive relationships affecting family planning or adjustment, or self concept, friends, communal living, nurse.
  2. Emotional Status
    a. Self-image (description of feelings about self), ability to identify problems, concept of femininity.
    b. Concept of self in relation to total situation (overwhelmed, competent, coping, ability to ask for and receive help).
    c. Concerns of the patient, i.e., side effects, effectiveness, guilt, embarrassment, sexual adjustment, V.D., cancer.
    d. Stability of life situation, i.e., stress, frequent moves, promiscuous behavior, stable employment.
    e. Level of emotional maturity, i.e., completion of adolescent tasks, adult responsibilities.
  3. Cognitive
    a. Present knowledge of health condition, methods, health perception, misunderstandings and misinformation.
    b. Present goals.
    c. Ability to make decisions.

d. Comprehension—teaching learning ability.
e. Conviction and follow-up ability.

B. Objective (tests, measurements, specific findings, physical findings, facts aside from feelings)
1. Family income and economic practices
   a. Source of income, employment, agencies, other
   b. Use of income, regular expenses, indebtedness, other budgeting practices
   c. Plans for handling financial impact of unwanted pregnancy.
2. Education, vocational training, job potential of wage earner.
3. Living arrangements, who does she live with, adequacy of physical facilities for number of occupants.
4. Cultural background.
5. Religious background.
6. Use of community facilities, health, education, social care, clinics, schools, welfare organizations, churches, recreation.

II. Impressions: Nursing diagnosis, i.e., problems, needs, and strengths.
Inadequacies or conditions that may disrupt or interfere with the family planning goal and maintenance of health. Strengths and conditions that support family planning goal and aid in correcting health problems.

III. Plan:
Working diagnosis (contract) and treatment plan. Specific plans or activities which worker and patient agree to carry out.
A. Current
B. Long Term

PART III: ANTICIPATORY GUIDANCE—PREVENTIVE

(To be used as guideline for joint planning with patient. It is unlikely that a patient will be interested in discussing all of these topics.)

Pt. Name: ______________________________

(Date/Initial)	Checklist for Specific Methods				(Date/Initial)
HEALTH SUPERVISION					
Interpretation of Clinic	*BCP*				
Immunizations: DT, Polio, Mantoux	A. Effectiveness	____	____	____	____
	B. Mode of action	____	____	____	____
Medications	C. Specific instructions	____	____	____	____
Medical exam with pelvic & breast exam	BCP instruction sheet	____	____	____	____
	D. Normal side effects	____	____	____	____
Lab work & follow-up	vaginal bleeding	____	____	____	____
PHN referral	missed period	____	____	____	____
Routine Health maintenance	E. Danger signs	____	____	____	____
Medical care for other family members	AMA pamphlet	____	____	____	____
VD & lab follow-up					
Self Breast exam					

ANATOMY & PHYSIOLOGY
Conception-fert., & impregnation
Hygiene:
- rest, relax sleep
- discharge, vaginitis
- douches, sprays
- cotton panties

NUTRITION
Weight
Hct.
BCP; vitamins
IUD; iron
Preconceptual nutrition

RELATIONSHIPS
Meeting each other's needs
- Dependency
- Sexual

Stresses
- Financial
- Significant others
- Energy
- Living arrangements

FAMILY PLANNING
Goal
- Patient's
- Partner's

Methods
Motivation
Influencing factors: physical, social, psychological
Reasons: spacing children

PAMPHLETS
"VD"
"Vaginitis"
"Self-breast Exam"
"AMA Guide" for BCP
"C.H.C."

FOAM
A. Effectiveness
B. Mode of action
C. Specific instructions
   Foam instruction sheet
D. Side effects
   (i.e., rash, etc.)

CONDOMS
A. Effectiveness
B. Specific instructions
C. Relationship to V.D.

STERILIZATION
A. Vasectomy
B. Tubal ligation
   (pamphlet available)

IUD
A. Effectiveness
B. Mode of action
C. Specific instructions
   IUD instruction sheet
   Checking for string
D. Normal side effects
E. Danger signs
F. IUD consent form

DIAPHRAGM
A. Effectiveness
B. Mode of action
C. Specific instructions
   Diaphragm instruction sheet

RHYTHM
A. Effectiveness
B. Specific instructions

United Nations Declaration of the Rights of the Child

PREAMBLE

Whereas the peoples of the United Nations have, in the Charter, reaffirmed their faith in fundamental human rights, and in the dignity and worth of the human person, and have determined to promote social progress and better standards of life in larger freedom,

Whereas the United Nations has, in the Universal Declaration of Human Rights, proclaimed that everyone is entitled to all the rights and freedoms set forth therein, without distinction of any kind, such as race, color, sex, language, religion, political or other opinion, national or social origin, property, birth or other status,

Whereas the child, by reason of his physical and mental immaturity, needs special safeguards and care, including appropriate legal protection, before as well as after birth,

Whereas the need for such special safeguards has been stated in the Geneva Declaration of the Rights of the Child of 1924, and recognized in the Universal Declaration of Human Rights and in the statutes of specialized agencies and international organizations concerned with the welfare of children,

Whereas mankind owes to the child the best it has to give

NOW THEREFORE

THE GENERAL ASSEMBLY

PROCLAIMS

This Declaration of the Rights of the Child to the end that he may have a happy childhood and enjoy for his own good and for the good of society the rights and freedoms herein set forth, and calls upon parents, upon men and women as individuals and upon voluntary organizations, local authorities and national governments to recognize these rights and strive for their observance by legislative and other measures progressively taken in accordance with the following principles:

PRINCIPLE 1

The child shall enjoy all the rights set forth in this Declaration. All children, without any exception whatsoever, shall be entitled to these rights, without distinction or discrimination on account of race, color, sex, language, religion, political or other opinion, national or social origin, property, birth or other status, whether of himself or of his family.

PRINCIPLE 2

The child shall enjoy special protection, and shall be given opportunities and facilities, by law and by other means, to enable him to develop physically, mentally, morally, spiritually and socially in a healthy and normal manner and in conditions of freedom and dignity. In the enactment of laws for this purpose the best interests of the child shall be the paramount consideration.

PRINCIPLE 3

The child shall be entitled from his birth to a name and a nationality.

PRINCIPLE 4

The child shall enjoy the benefits of social security. He shall be entitled to grow and develop in health; to this end special care and protection shall be provided both to him and to his mother, including adequate pre-natal and post-natal care. The child shall have the right to adequate nutrition, housing, recreation and medical services.

PRINCIPLE 5

The child who is physically, mentally or socially handicapped shall be given the special treatment, education and care required by his particular condition.

PRINCIPLE 6

The child, for the full and harmonious development of his personality, needs love and understanding. He shall, wherever possible, grow up in the care and under the responsibility of his parents, and in any case in an atmosphere of affection and of moral and material security; a child of tender years shall not, save in exceptional circumstances, be separated from his mother. Society and the public authorities shall have the duty to extend particular care to children without a family and to those without adequate means of support. Payment of state and other assistance toward the maintenance of children of large families is desirable.

PRINCIPLE 7

The child is entitled to receive education, which shall be free and compulsory, at least in the elementary stages. He shall be given an education which will promote his general culture, and enable him on a basis of equal opportunity to develop his abilities, his individual judgment, and his sense of moral and social responsibility, and to become a useful member of society.

The best interests of the child shall be the guiding principle of those responsible for his education and guidance; that responsibility lies in the first place with his parents.

The child shall have full opportunity for play and recreation, which shall be directed to the same purposes as education; society and the public authorities shall endeavor to promote the enjoyment of this right.

PRINCIPLE 8

The child shall in all circumstances be among the first to receive protection and relief.

PRINCIPLE 9

The child shall be protected against all forms of neglect, cruelty and exploitation. He shall not be the subject of traffic, in any form.

The child shall not be admitted to employment before an appropriate minimum age; he shall in no case be caused or permitted to engage in any occupation or employment which would prejudice his health or education, or interfere with his physical, mental or moral development.

PRINCIPLE 10

The child shall be protected from practices which may foster racial, religious and any other form of discrimination. He shall be brought up in a spirit of understanding, tolerance, friendship among peoples, peace and universal brotherhood and in full consciousness that his energy and talents should be devoted to the service of his fellow men.

Index